Cardiopulmonary Bypass

Christina T. Mora
EDITOR

Robert A. Guyton   Donald C. Finlayson†   Richard L. Rigatti
ASSOCIATE EDITORS

Cardiopulmonary Bypass

Principles and Techniques of Extracorporeal Circulation

With 219 Figures

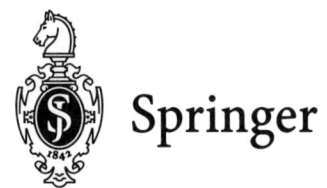

EDITOR
Christina T. Mora, M.D.
Department of Anesthesiology
Emory University School of Medicine
Atlanta, GA 30322
USA

ASSOCIATE EDITORS
Robert A. Guyton, M.D.
Division of Cardiothoracic Surgery
Emory University School of Medicine
Atlanta, GA 30322
USA

Richard L. Rigatti, B.S., C.T., C.C.T.
Perfusion Services
Emory University Hospitals
Atlanta, GA 30322
USA

Donald C. Finlayson, M.D., F.R.C.P.(C.)
†Deceased

Library of Congress Cataloging-in-Publication Data
Cardiopulmonary bypass : principles and techniques of extracorporeal
  circulation / [edited by] Christina T. Mora . . . [et al.].
    p.   cm.
  Includes bibliographical references and index.
  ISBN 0-387-94242-4. — ISBN 3-540-94242-4
  1. Cardiopulmonary bypass.   2. Blood—Circulation, Artificial.
  I. Mora, Christina T.
  [DNLM: 1. Cardiopulmonary Bypass.   2. Heart, Mechancial.   WG 168
C26622 1995]
RD598.C3546   1995
617.4'12059—dc20   94-29083

Printed on acid-free paper.

© 1995 Springer-Verlag New York Inc.
All rights reserved. This work may not be translated or copied in whole or in part without the written permission of the publisher (Springer-Verlag New York, Inc., 175 Fifth Avenue, New York, NY 10010, USA), except for brief excerpts in connection with reviews or scholarly analysis. Use in connection with any form of information storage and retrieval, electronic adaptation, computer software, or by similar or dissimilar methodology now known or hereafter developed is forbidden.
The use of general descriptive names, trade names, trademarks, etc., in this publication, even if the former are not especially identified, is not to be taken as a sign that such names, as understood by the Trade Marks and Merchandise Marks Act, may accordingly be used freely by anyone.
While the advice and information in this book are believed to be true and accurate at the date of going to press, neither the authors nor the editors nor the publisher can accept any legal responsibility for any errors or omissions that may be made. The publisher makes no warranty, express or implied, with respect to the material contained herein.

Production managed by Laura Carlson; manufacturing supervised by Rhea Talbert.
Typeset by Bytheway Typesetting Services, Inc., Norwich, NY.
Printed and bound by Maple-Vail, York, PA.
Printed in the United States of America.

9 8 7 6 5 4 3 2

ISBN 0-387-94242-4 Springer-Verlag New York Berlin Heidelberg
ISBN 3-540-94242-4 Springer-Verlag Berlin Heidelberg New York

This work is dedicated to:

My parents, Elizabeth and Jorge,
for their faith;
My husband, Dennis Mangano,
for his love and patience;
and to our son, Thomas Jorge,
for his gift of grace.

Foreword

Medical technology is so deeply indebted to so many scientific creditors that a late-coming analyst cannot easily trace the movements of intellectual capital that bankrolled a successful clinical enterprise. Cardiopulmonary bypass is one of the triumphs of medical technology, both in terms of volume (approaching one million procedures a year worldwide) and cost-effectiveness. If John Gibbon stands out as the tenacious broker who transformed a laboratory curiosity into a tool that surgeons would buy and use, contributions from many others — engineers, physiologists, and internists of all kinds — can also be recognized in the many facets of cardiopulmonary bypass. As its acceptance and use continue to expand, further investments of technology and clinical wisdom are still needed.

The Emory authors of this textbook have benefited from a long-standing local tradition of investigative work, clinical audit, and postgraduate education. Thirty years ago, in the pioneer days of cardiopulmonary bypass, attention was, of necessity, focused on devices and components, and on the degree of physiologic damage that could be tolerated to see the patient through a dangerous procedure. Nowadays, the emphasis is on the patient — or, more precisely, on the clinical impact of any procedure, material, component, or monitoring system that over the years has found its place in the care of cardiac patients.

The mechanics of cardiopulmonary bypass reflect the convergence of the efforts of several device manufacturers on a limited number of blood-contracting materials and gas-exchange and pumping systems, as well as much closer attention to quality control and cost containment. The procedure of cardiopulmonary bypass is reasonably well standardized. Physiology remains the frontier. New technology allows us to question accepted procedures, as exemplified by the advent of continuous-flow centrifugal pumps, warm retrograde cardioplegia, and normothermic body perfusion techniques. Yet innovation must be placed in the perspective of well-documented earlier experience, with proper attention to second-order effects on all organ systems. The physiologic consequences of cardiopulmonary bypass are much more extensive than was once thought, even though the morbidity of the procedure has been considerably reduced.

A better appreciation of the potential and the limits of cardiopulmonary bypass has allowed its recent application to special patient populations other than candidates for cardiac surgery. Its use as a mechanical or metabolic aid, after many false starts, now appears firmly established, even though the volume of cases in which its use is indicated is still quite small.

All of these issues are addressed in this text, which places innovation in the context of well-established knowledge. As a long-term observer of medical science and technology as applied to cardiopulmonary bypass, I congratulate Dr. Mora and her coauthors. I am confident that this textbook will enhance the proficiency of those who study it and will thereby contribute to continuing improvement in the quality of patient care in cardiac surgery.

Pierre M. Galletti, Ph.D., M.D.

Preface

Although the basic concept of extracorporeal circulation is almost 200 years old, the technique of cardiopulmonary bypass (CPB) has been used routinely in surgical procedures for only about 40 years. During the latter part of this century, however, the heart-lung machine has enabled the rapid growth of heart surgery, so that, by 1995, over 500,000 cardiac operations using CPB will have been performed in the United States alone.

The last decade has also witnessed an increase in the use of extracorporeal technology in the non-cardiac surgery patient. Cardiologists have brought the bypass circuit to the angioplasty suite; circulatory arrest is being used to facilitate intracranial surgery; and clinical trials to assess an intravenous oxygenator are underway. Although fatalities directly attributable to modern CPB techniques are remarkably few, extracorporeal support of cardiorespiratory function is still associated with multiple pathophysiologic processes and attendant morbidity. But with continued research and acquired knowledge, the adverse events that often accompany these life-saving techniques can be eliminated. With that goal in mind, *Cardiopulmonary Bypass* has been designed to provide a compendium of the current knowledge regarding the clinical practice, pathophysiology, and future direction of extracorporeal circulation.

The text is presented in seven parts. Part I, authored by a pioneer in the field of extracorporeal technology, recounts the history of the development of CPB. Part II outlines the physiology and pathophysiology of CPB. These chapters discuss both hemostasis and myocardial protection during bypass, and detail the effects of perfusion on the central nervous, respiratory, renal, hepatic, and immune systems and endocrine axis. Parts III and IV focus on the mechanics and conduct of bypass. These chapters describe the components of the heart-lung machine (oxygenators, pumps, heat exchange devices, etc.) and the procedural aspects of perfusion (cannulation, initiation and maintenance of bypass, discontinuation of bypass support, and management of perturbations). CPB in specific patient populations is explored in Parts V and VI. The use of extracorporeal circuits and oxygenators is increasing in non-cardiac surgery (intracranial, thoracic, liver transplantation, and high-risk angioplasty patients) and outside the operating room (ventricular assist devices in bridge-to-transplant patients or patients recovering from myocardial failure; extracorporeal membrane oxygenation in the pediatric and adult patient). Because the conduct of CPB in pediatric, obstetric, and thoracic surgery patients requires special expertise, the care of these patients during perfusion is considered in detail in Part V. Topics of current interest are found in Part VII and include normothermic bypass (Chapter 34) and blood conservation (Chapter 31) during cardiac surgery.

The book is intended to serve as a comprehensive text on the subject of CPB for surgeons, perfusionists, and anesthesiologists. This somewhat difficult task is accomplished by presenting both basic concepts and detailed knowledge on a given subject in language intended for all readers. A specific chapter may be of greater interest to one group, but every chapter contains essential information. For example, a grasp of basic pharmacokinetic principles (Chapter 4) is necessary to the perfusionist who requires a fundamental understanding of drug disposition during bypass, but who may be less likely to study the effect of bypass on a certain antibiotic. Similarly, the surgeon and anesthesiologist should understand the basic principles of extracorporeal oxygenation (Chapter 10) and heat exchange (Chapter 14), but may not need to know the specific thermal constants of the materials used in heat exchange devices. Several chapters, however—such as Chapter 17, on the discontinuation of bypass support, and Chapter 18, on the management of perturbations—will be vital to all readers. These chapters emphasize the importance of communication among the surgeon, perfusionist, and anesthesiologist during these critical events.

I would like to thank those who provided valuable assistance in the preparation of this text. I have been privileged to work with members of the Emory University School of Medicine, Department of Anesthesiology and the Division of Cardiothoracic Surgery; many of these colleagues gave generously of their time and support. Pierre Galletti, author of *Heart Lung Bypass* (1962), which served as the inspiration for this work, provided both direction and moral support during the course of this project. J. Devn Cornish kindly allowed me to recruit his expert help in editing many of the chapters on the technical aspects of perfusion, and the text benefited greatly from his contribution.

The day-to-day progress on this text was ensured by my secretary, Louise Evans, and I feel fortunate to have worked with this dedicated and tenacious individual. Helen Fontseré, editor for the Emory Department of Anesthesiology, polished each chapter and provided invaluable help in citing references, obtaining letters of permission, and addressing the myriad of tasks required to make a manuscript publisher-ready. Mary Lopez and Michele Mitchell offered encouragement and administrative support. Members of the Emory Department of Medical Illustration created many of the illustrations and photographs; Patsy Bryan, Nancy Mathews, Benjamin King, Jack Kearse, and Chuck Bogle never grumbled when I requested "one more" revision.

I am grateful to the publishers at Springer-Verlag for their enthusiasm and commitment to this book. Esther Gumpert, Laura Gillan, Andrea Seils, and the production staff contributed their seasoned expertise and ensured an orderly and timely production process.

Finally, I thankfully acknowledge the support of my husband, Dennis Mangano, who weathered the first year of our marriage in San Francisco while I completed this text in Atlanta.

Christina Mora Mangano, M.D.

Contents

Foreword vii
Pierre M. Galletti

Preface ix
Christina T. Mora

Contributors xv

Part I. The History of Cardiopulmonary Bypass

1. Cardiopulmonary Bypass: The Historical Foundation,
   the Future Promise 3
   Pierre M. Galletti and Christina T. Mora

Part II. Physiology of Cardiopulmonary Bypass

2. The Myocardium: Physiology and Protection During Cardiac Surgery
   and Cardiopulmonary Bypass 21
   Robert A. Guyton

3. Hypothermia, Cardiac Surgery, and Cardiopulmonary Bypass 40
   Willis H. Williams, Hakob G. Davtyan, and Milada Drazanova

4. Pharmacokinetics and Pharmacodynamics During Cardiac Surgery and
   Cardiopulmonary Bypass 55
   Richard I. Hall, Brian L. Thomas, and Carl C. Hug, Jr.

5. Hemostasis and Cardiopulmonary Bypass 88
   Markku T. Salmenperä, Jerrold H. Levy, and Laurence A. Harker

6. The Central Nervous System: Responses to Cardiopulmonary Bypass 114
   Christina T. Mora and John M. Murkin

7. The Respiratory, Renal, and Hepatic Systems: Effects of Cardiac
   Surgery and Cardiopulmonary Bypass 147
   James G. Ramsay

8. The Immunologic System: Perturbations Following Cardiopulmonary
   Bypass and the Problem of Infection in the Cardiac Surgery Patient 169
   *Bradley L. Bufkin, John P. Gott, Christina T. Mora,
   and Jerrold H. Levy*

9. The Endocrine System: Effects of Cardiopulmonary Bypass 180
   Carolyn F. Bannister and Donald C. Finlayson

Part III. Mechanics and Components of the Heart-Lung Machine

10. Oxygenators for Extracorporeal Circulation 199
    Philip D. Beckley, David W. Holt, and Richard D. Tallman, Jr.

11. Mechanical Pumps for Extracorporeal Circulation 220
    Christopher R. Trocchio and James O. Sketel

12. Conduits and Filters for Extracorporeal Circulation 229
    Kathy K. Spitzer and Charles T. Walker

13. Assembling and Monitoring the Extracorporeal Circuit 238
    Richard B. Davis, Jeffrey N. Kauffman, Terry L. Cobbs, and Sharon L. Mick

14. Heat Exchange in Extracorporeal Systems 247
    Richard L. Rigatti and Roger Stewart

Part IV. Conduct of Cardiopulmonary Bypass for Cardiac Surgery

15. Aortoatriocaval Cannulation for Cardiopulmonary Bypass 257
    Mark W. Connolly

16. Initiation and Maintenance of Cardiopulmonary Bypass 264
    James R. Zaidan

17. Discontinuation of Cardiopulmonary Bypass 281
    Luis G. Michelsen and Jack S. Shanewise

18. Safety and Management of Perturbations During
    Cardiopulmonary Bypass 298
    Scott M. Sadel

Part V(a). Cardiopulmonary Bypass in Special Patient Populations
Complete Cardiopulmonary Bypass

19. Pediatric Cardiopulmonary Bypass 311
    James M. Bailey and William L. Daly

20. Thoracic Aortic Surgery and Cardiopulmonary Bypass 329
    Tomas D. Martin

21. Intracranial Surgery with Cardiopulmonary Bypass 340
    Brian L. Thomas

22. Emergency Coronary Artery Bypass and Cardiopulmonary Bypass 347
    Joseph M. Craver

23. Chest Trauma and Emergency Cardiopulmonary Bypass 353
    Panagiotis N. Symbas

24. Pregnancy and Cardiopulmonary Bypass 359
    Christina T. Mora

Part V(b). Cardiopulmonary Bypass in Special Patient Populations
Partial Cardiopulmonary Bypass

25. Cardiopulmonary Bypass–Supported Angioplasty 379
    Steven K. Macheers

26. Closed Chest Bypass for Liver Transplantation 389
    Linda E. McLean, Scott M. Kreger, and Christina T. Mora

Part VI. Mechanical Assist of the Failing Heart and Lung

27. Ventricular Assist Devices 399
    Bradley L. Bufkin and Robert A. Guyton

28. Intraaortic Balloon Pump Counterpulsation 413
    John P. Gott

29. Extracorporeal Membrane Oxygenation for Severe Cardiorespiratory
    Failure 433
    J. Devn Cornish

30. The Intravascular Oxygenator, IVOX®: Augmentation of
    Blood-Gas Transfer 450
    Robert K. Wenger and JD Mortensen

Part VII. Special Considerations in Cardiopulmonary Bypass

31. Blood Conservation in Cardiac Surgery 461
    James G. Cormack, Robert W. Bolen, and Dirk A. Maisel

32. Religious Objections to Blood Transfusion 473
    Robert B. Lee and Tomas D. Martin

33. Medical-Legal Aspects of Cardiopulmonary Bypass 481
    Tomas D. Martin and Charles R. Hatcher, Jr.

34. Warm-Blood Cardioplegia and Normothermic Cardiopulmonary
    Bypass 484
    Robert A. Guyton

Index 493

Contributors

JAMES M. BAILEY, M.D., Ph.D., Assistant Professor of Anesthesiology and Pediatrics, Department of Anesthesiology, Emory University School of Medicine, Atlanta, GA 30322, USA

CAROLYN F. BANNISTER, M.D., Assistant Professor of Anesthesiology, Department of Anesthesiology, Emory University School of Medicine, Atlanta, GA 30322, USA

PHILIP D. BECKLEY, Ph.D., Assistant Professor of Circulation Technology, Director, Circulation Technology Division, School of Allied Medical Professions, College of Medicine, The Ohio State University, Columbus, OH 43210, USA

ROBERT W. BOLEN, B.S., C.C.P., Chief Perfusionist, Emory University Hospitals, Atlanta, GA 30322; Clinical Instructor of Circulation Technology, School of Allied Medical Professions, The Ohio State University, Columbus, OH 43210, USA

BRADLEY L. BUFKIN, M.D., Resident, Department of Surgery, Division of Cardiothoracic Surgery, Emory University School of Medicine, Atlanta, GA 30322, USA

TERRY L. COBBS, B.S., C.C.P., Perfusionist, Emory University Hospitals, Atlanta, GA 30322, USA

MARK W. CONNOLLY, M.D., Assistant Professor of Surgery (Cardiothoracic), Department of Surgery, Division of Cardiothoracic Surgery, Emory University School of Medicine, Atlanta, GA 30322, USA

JAMES G. CORMACK, M.D., Assistant Professor of Anaesthesia, Department of Anaesthesia, University of Alberta, Edmonton, Alberta T6G 2B7, Canada

J. DEVN CORNISH, M.D., Associate Professor of Pediatrics, Director, Division of Neonatology, Department of Pediatrics, Emory University School of Medicine, Atlanta, GA 30322, USA

JOSEPH M. CRAVER, M.D., Professor of Surgery (Cardiothoracic), Department of Surgery, Division of Cardiothoracic Surgery, Emory University School of Medicine, Atlanta, GA 30322, USA

WILLIAM L. DALY, B.S., C.C.P., Chief Perfusionist, Egleston Children's Hospital, Perfusion Services, Emory University Hospitals, Atlanta, GA 30322; Clinical Instructor of Circulation Technology, School of Allied Medical Professions, The Ohio State University, Columbus, OH 43210, USA

RICHARD B. DAVIS, Ph.D., Assistant Professor of Circulation Technology, Circulation Technology Division, School of Allied Medical Professions, College of Medicine, The Ohio State University, Columbus, OH 43210, USA

HAKOB G. DAVTYAN, M.D., Resident, Department of Surgery, Division of Cardiothoracic Surgery, Emory University School of Medicine, Atlanta, GA 30322, USA

MILADA DRAZANOVA, M.D., Clinical Research Assistant, Department of Surgery, Division of Cardiothoracic Surgery, Emory University School of Medicine, Atlanta, GA 30322, USA

DONALD C. FINLAYSON, M.D., F.R.C.P.(C.), Deceased

PIERRE M. GALLETTI, Ph.D., M.D., University Professor and Professor of Medical Science, Division of Biology and Medicine, Brown University, Providence, RI 02912, USA

JOHN P. GOTT, M.D., Assistant Professor of Surgery (Cardiothoracic), Department of Surgery, Division of Cardiothoracic Surgery, Emory University School of Medicine, Atlanta, GA 30322, USA

ROBERT A. GUYTON, M.D., Professor of Surgery (Cardiothoracic), Chief, Division of Cardiothoracic Surgery, Department of Surgery, Emory University School of Medicine, Atlanta, GA 30322, USA

RICHARD I. HALL, M.D., Associate Professor of Anaesthesiology and Pharmacology, Assistant Professor of Surgery, Department of Anaesthesiology, Dalhousie University; Director, Surgical Intensive Care Unit, Department of Anaesthesiology, Victoria General Hospital, Halifax, Nova Scotia B3H 2Y9, Canada

LAURENCE A. HARKER, M.D., Blomeyer Professor of Medicine, Director, Division of Hematology/Oncology, Department of Medicine, Emory University School of Medicine, Atlanta, GA 30322, USA

CHARLES R. HATCHER, Jr., M.D., Vice President for Health Affairs and Director, Woodruff Health Sciences Center, Emory University, Atlanta, GA 30322, USA

DAVID W. HOLT, B.S., C.C.T., Clinical Instructor of Circulation Technology, Circulation Technology Division, School of Allied Medical Professions, College of Medicine, The Ohio State University, Columbus, OH 43210, USA

CARL C. HUG, Jr., M.D., Ph.D., Professor of Anesthesiology and Pharmacology, Deputy Chairman for Research, Department of Anesthesiology, Emory University School of Medicine; Director, Cardiothoracic Anesthesia, The Emory Clinic, Atlanta, GA 30322, USA

Contributors

JEFFREY N. KAUFFMAN, B.C., C.C.P., C.C.T., Chief Perfusionist, Crawford Long Hospital of Emory University Hospitals, Atlanta, GA 30322; Clinical Instructor of Circulation Technology, School of Allied Medical Professions, The Ohio State University, Columbus, OH 43210, USA

SCOTT M. KREGER, M.D., Assistant Professor of Anesthesiology, Department of Anesthesiology, Emory University School of Medicine, Atlanta, GA 30322, USA

ROBERT B. LEE, M.D., Assistant Professor of Surgery (Cardiothoracic), Department of Surgery, Division of Cardiothoracic Surgery, Emory University School of Medicine, Atlanta, GA 30322, USA

JERROLD H. LEVY, M.D., Associate Professor of Anesthesiology, Department of Anesthesiology, Emory University School of Medicine, Atlanta, GA 30322, USA

STEVEN K. MACHEERS, M.D., Resident, Department of Surgery, Division of Cardiothoracic Surgery, Emory University School of Medicine, Atlanta, GA 30322, USA

DIRK A. MAISEL, B.S., C.C.P., Perfusionist, Emory University Hospitals, Atlanta, GA 30322, USA

TOMAS D. MARTIN, M.D., Associate Professor of Surgery, Department of Surgery, University of Florida, College of Medicine; Chief, Adult Cardiovascular Surgery, University of Florida Health Science Center, Gainesville, FL 32610, USA

LINDA E. MCLEAN, B.S., C.C.T., C.C.P., Perfusionist, Emory University Hospitals, Atlanta, GA 30322, USA

LUIS G. MICHELSEN, M.D., Assistant Professor of Anesthesiology, Department of Anesthesiology, Emory University School of Medicine, Atlanta, GA 30322, USA

SHARON L. MICK, B.S., C.C.P., Perfusionist, Emory University Hospitals, Atlanta, GA 30322, USA

CHRISTINA T. MORA, M.D., Assistant Professor of Anesthesiology, Department of Anesthesiology, Emory University School of Medicine, Atlanta, GA 30322, USA

JD MORTENSEN, M.D., President, Oxygenator Technology Development, Inc., Salt Lake City, UT 84116, USA

JOHN M. MURKIN, M.D., Professor of Anaesthesia, Department of Anaesthesia, University of Western Ontario, London, Ontario N66 3S5, Canada

JAMES G. RAMSAY, M.D., Associate Professor of Anesthesiology, Director, Critical Care Medicine, Department of Anesthesiology, Emory University School of Medicine, Atlanta, GA 30322, USA

RICHARD L. RIGATTI, B.S., C.T., C.C.T., Director, Perfusion Services, Emory University Hospitals, Atlanta, GA 30322; Clinical Instructor of Circulation Technology, School of Allied Medical Professions, The Ohio State University, Columbus, OH 43210, USA

SCOTT M. SADEL, M.D., Assistant Professor of Anesthesiology, Department of Anesthesiology, Emory University School of Medicine, Atlanta, GA 30322, USA

MARKKU T. SALMENPERÄ, M.D., Associate Professor of Anesthesia, Department of Anesthesia, Helsinki University, FIN-00290 Helsinki, Finland

JACK S. SHANEWISE, M.D., Assistant Professor of Anesthesiology, Department of Anesthesiology, Emory University School of Medicine, Atlanta, GA 30322, USA

JAMES O. SKETEL, B.S., C.C.P., Perfusionist, Emory University Hospitals, Atlanta, GA 30322, USA

KATHY K. SPITZER, B.S., C.C.P., C.C.T., Perfusionist, Emory University Hospitals, Atlanta, GA 30322, USA

ROGER STEWART, B.S.M.E., P.E., Cardiopulmonary Products, Cobe Laboratories, Arvada, CO 80004, USA

PANAGIOTIS N. SYMBAS, M.D., Professor of Surgery (Cardiothoracic), Department of Surgery, Division of Cardiothoracic Surgery, Emory University School of Medicine, Atlanta, GA 30322, USA

RICHARD D. TALLMAN, Jr., Ph.D., Associate Professor of Circulation Technology, Circulation Technology Division, School of Allied Medical Professions, College of Medicine, The Ohio State University, Columbus, OH 43210, USA

BRIAN L. THOMAS, M.D., Assistant Professor of Anesthesiology, Department of Anesthesiology, Emory University School of Medicine, Atlanta, GA 30322, USA

CHRISTOPHER R. TROCCHIO, B.S., C.C.P., Perfusion Education Coordinator, Emory University Hospitals, Atlanta, GA 30322; Clinical Instructor of Circulation Technology, School of Allied Medical Professions, The Ohio State University, Columbus, OH 43210, USA

CHARLES T. WALKER, C.C.P., Chief Perfusionist, Veterans Administration Medical Center; Perfusionist, Emory University Hospitals, Atlanta, GA 30322, USA

ROBERT K. WENGER, M.D., Resident, Department of Surgery, Division of Cardiothoracic Surgery, Emory University School of Medicine, Atlanta, GA 30322, USA

WILLIS H. WILLIAMS, M.D., Professor of Surgery (Cardiothoracic), Department of Surgery, Division of Cardiothoracic Surgery, Emory University School of Medicine, Atlanta, GA 30322, USA

JAMES R. ZAIDAN, M.D., Professor of Anesthesiology, Deputy Chairman for Education, Department of Anesthesiology, Emory University School of Medicine; Chief of Anesthesia, Emory University Hospital, Atlanta, GA 30322, USA

Part I
The History of Cardiopulmonary Bypass

1
Cardiopulmonary Bypass: The Historical Foundation, the Future Promise

Pierre M. Galletti and Christina T. Mora

Cardiopulmonary bypass (CPB) is used so routinely in hospitals around the world that most of the participants—surgeons, anesthesiologists, perfusionists, operating room nurses and, above all, patients—forget that this landmark in clinical technology is not even 40 years old. In fact, many of the pioneers are still active in the field. Yet, so much has been done to transform a once-hazardous procedure into standard medical practice—through basic science, quality control, and good manufacturing—that one hardly remembers the days (not so long ago) when "pump-oxygenators," as they were graphically called, were assembled just outside the operating room by tinkerers with a dream. The purpose of this chapter is to recall the inventiveness displayed by a small coterie of gifted investigators to whom we owe the mechanical and physiologic foundations of open-heart surgery, and to reflect on the new demands that continuing clinical advances will undoubtedly make on this technology.

The Origins of CPB

CPB hinges on twin postulates: that blood circulation can be sustained by mechanical pumps while the heart is arrested, and that venous blood can be artificially arterialized in an extracorporeal gas exchange device while blood flow is excluded from the lungs. Each of these mechanisms was established separately through animal experimentation over the course of slightly more than 100 years. In the 1950s, surgically oriented investigators combined the advances made by physiologists, pharmacologists, and engineers and turned them into the basic tool of cardiac surgery: the heart-lung machine.

The origins of CPB go back to the nineteenth century. Around 1813, when the anatomic course and mechanics of the cardiocirculatory system finally had been delineated, Le Gallois[1] suggested that artificial perfusion of a body part, separated from the heart, might preserve its function. To demonstrate that artificial circulation of venous blood could re-establish irritability in a dying mammalian muscle, Brown-Sequard in 1858 used the severed arms of beheaded criminals to show that reflex nervous activity could be maintained if perfusion was initiated promptly with oxygenated blood.[2] The Ludwig school of physiologists extended the concept of functional survival to *isolated*, perfused organs,[3] and Starling[4] applied this idea to the mammalian heart to elucidate cardiac autoregulation. The feasibility of *total* body perfusion after removal of the heart was established by Brukhonenko[5] in the 1920s, but this work remained largely ignored in the Western world.

The biochemistry of respiration—the exchange of oxygen and carbon dioxide as blood passes through the pulmonary and systemic capillaries—was not fully understood until the second half of the nineteenth century. The first system for extrapulmonary blood oxygenation was constructed by von Frey and Gruber[6] in 1885. In their device, arterialization occurred as blood was spread as a thin film over the surface of a slowly rotating cylinder in an oxygen atmosphere. While this early oxygenator operated within narrow margins (threatened as it was by the streaming, foaming, and clotting of blood), it showed the feasibility of blood arterialization as a continuous process, and it is widely acknowledged as the precedent that justified further efforts.

The Advent of the Heart-Lung Machine

The development of CPB was dependent on the emergence of a number of new and, at the time, revolutionary discoveries and techniques: the feasibility of temporary interruption of the venous return to the heart; the discovery of the A, B, and O blood groups; and the effectiveness of positive pressure ventilation. Most critically, the identification of a reliable, nontoxic anticoagulant, heparin,[7] and a safe antagonist, protamine,[8] made extracorporeal circulation possible. In 1934, DeBakey[9] reported on the value of the roller pump, a reliable mechanism for displacing large volumes of blood along a flexible piece of tubing. Long before DeBakey's report, the roller pump, or *die Beck'sche Mühle* (as it was called in German), had been used for person-to-person transfusion. Meanwhile, the pioneers of hypothermia, Bigelow,[10] Boerema,[11] Lewis,[12] and Swan,[13] demonstrated the feasibility of temporarily lowering the body temperature to decrease tissue metabolism and, consequently, perfusion needs during surgery. Table 1.1 summarizes the technical and scientific innovations that propelled the development of extracorporeal circulation.

The idea of coupling extracorporeal circulation and oxygenation to permit unhurried surgical interventions in adult patients originated with Gibbon.[14] Inspired by the tragic death of a gravid woman with a pulmonary embolism, he was the first to establish the feasibility of artificially supported circulation during temporary occlusion of the pulmonary artery. Over a period of 20 years (interrupted by World War II), Gibbon refined the technology of CPB. He was the first to succeed in using total extracorporeal circulation to facilitate cardiac surgery (Figure 1.1A and B). On May 20, 1953, he successfully closed an atrial septal defect in a young woman, Celia Bavolek[15] (Figure 1.1C and D).

Gibbon's initial laboratory models of blood oxygenators relied on rotating cylinders to spread blood in a thin film, in the tradition of von Frey and Gruber. The clinical model, built with technical support from IBM, and soon adopted by Kirklin's group at the Mayo Clinic,[16,17] was a *stationary film oxygenator* (Figures 1.2 and 1.3). This was a bulky device in which venous blood was evenly smeared over vertical wire mesh screens in an oxygen-enriched atmosphere. After undergoing gas exchange, the blood accumulated in an arterial reservoir, from which it could be pumped into a systemic artery. The primary problem with this design (besides its cumbersome dimensions) was blood streaming, which caused a constantly diminishing blood-gas exchange area. Dennis,[18] and later Kay and Cross,[19] tried to improve the system by replacing the Gibbon-Mayo-IBM (1958) stationary film support with rotating screens or rotating disks that were partially immersed in a blood pool (Figure 1.4). However, because blood conservation dictated a tight fit between the disks and the horizontal glass cylinder surrounding them, unacceptable foaming and hemolysis occurred at high spinning velocities. After a few years of use, these devices, as well as the rotating cylinder oxygenators pioneered by Crafoord and Senning,[20] were abandoned.

Physiologists first attempted to add oxygen and remove carbon dioxide from venous blood by bubbling pure oxygen through a stationary blood pool. *Bubble oxygenators* efficiently add oxygen to venous blood. Indeed, the smaller the bubbles, the larger the blood-oxygen exchange area developed by a steady stream of gas.[21] However, carbon dioxide removal is more difficult to control. Since the fractional concentration of carbon dioxide in the gas vented from a bubble oxygenator cannot exceed the partial pressure of carbon dioxide in arterialized blood, the carbon dioxide transfer rate is a direct function of the volume inflow rate of oxygen; therefore, the oxygen flow rate must exceed the oxygen uptake severalfold, as is the case for respiration in the normal lung (Chapter 10).

Four major advances propelled bubble oxygenators ahead of film oxygenators in the pioneer decade of cardiac surgery. The first was the identification of silicone-based defoaming compounds.[22,23] These compounds were significantly more effective in coalescing the blood foam than were previously used chemicals. The second was the quantitative process analysis by Clark and Gollan[21,23] which showed that, since small bubbles favor oxygen transfer because of their large overall exchange surface, and large bubbles are needed for carbon dioxide removal because of their large carrier gas content, an optimum size could be found in between, or alternatively, a mix of small and large bubbles should be used to balance oxygen and carbon dioxide exchange. The third important advance was the recognition that, when venous blood is spread on top of the foam in the gas exchange column of an oxygenator, gas transfer is mediated by spreading a continuously renewed blood film that cascades down the foam surface. Although often confused with bubble oxygenation, this mechanism is closer to the mode of operation of the stationary film oxygenator than to the upward bubbling process in a chimney. Carbon dioxide is effectively removed because of the large size of the gas cells in the foam, and the process is apparently gentler to blood elements than bubble oxygenation.[24] The fourth and critical advance was made simultaneously by Gott et al[25] and by Rygg and Kyvsgaard[26,27] in the late 1950s (Figures 1.5 and 1.6). These investigators replaced the cumbersome assembly of glass, steel, and ceramic components of the early bubble oxygenators with inexpensive plastic parts. This paved the way for the industrial manufacturing of disposable bubble oxygenators in which all functions needed for CPB, except pumping (ie, foaming, defoaming, filtration, oxygenation of blood, and removal of carbon dioxide) could

TABLE 1.1. Scientific discoveries and techniques that permitted the development of total extracorporeal circulation.

Successful temporary interruption of venous return to the heart
Discovery of A, B, O blood groups
Identification of reliable anticoagulant (heparin)[7]
Identification of anticoagulant antagonist (protamine)[8]
Implementation of roller pump[9]
Discovery of correlation between body temperature and metabolic rate[10-13]

FIGURE 1.1. Dr. John Gibbon, Jr., (A) prior to the first successful application of total extracorporeal circulation for cardiac surgery in humans, and (B) with his wife, Mary, several years later. (C) Celia Bavolek's admission papers to The Jefferson Hospital and her family's consent for Dr. John Gibbon, Jr., to perform open-heart surgery. (D) Celia Bavolek pictured with President Lyndon Johnson several years later as the spokeswoman for the Heart Fund. (Photos courtesy of the Mütter Museum of the College of Physicians of Philadelphia.)

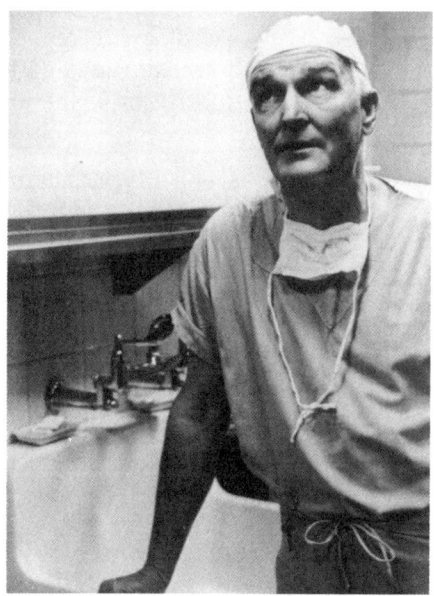
A

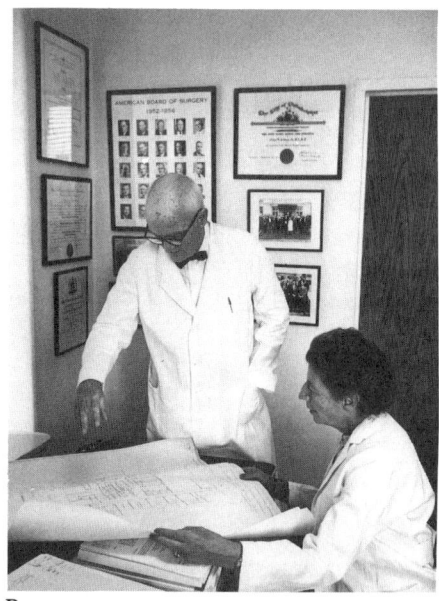
B

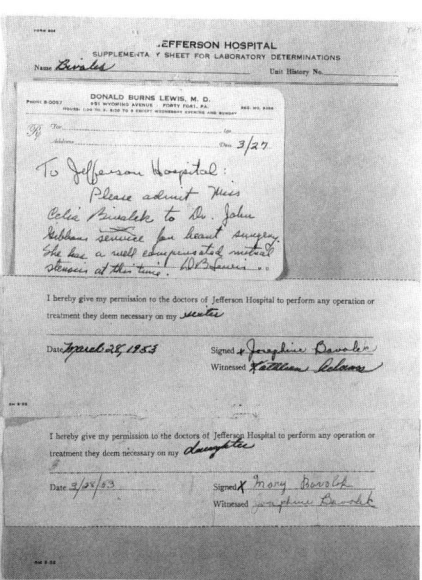
C

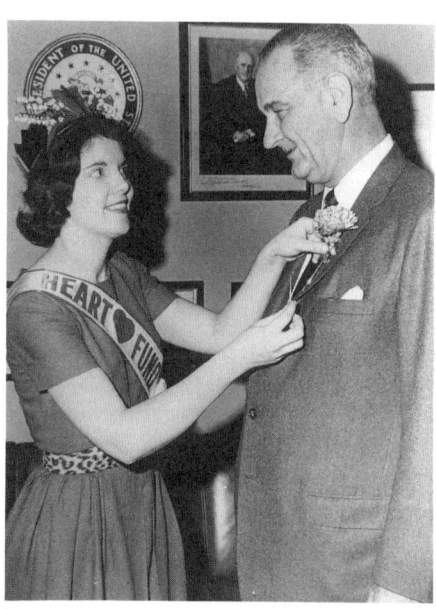
D

now be integrated. As a result, stationary film and disk oxygenators, which required careful cleaning, assembly, and sterilization, eventually disappeared, and disposable oxygenators came to dominate the field of CPB from 1960 to the early 1980s.

In the same time period, *roller pumps* replaced all other mechanisms as the blood propulsion device for the clinical heart-lung machine. This type of positive displacement pump, in which a roller progresses along a loop of flexible tubing so as to squeeze blood out of it, is such an old design that it is essentially impossible to decide whom to credit for its first application to extracorporeal blood handling. The higher flow capacity necessary for total extracorporeal circulatory support without unacceptable blood damage was made possible by the adaption of the early-design roller pumps to include large-bore flexible tubing; long, circular pumping chambers in over-dimensioned housings; and a fast, controllable rate of revolution of the rotor assembly (Chapter 11). Overall, it was the simplicity and sturdiness of the mechanical design, the long-term reliability, and the ability to use a hand crank in case of power failure that established the roller pump as the premier blood-pumping system in the operating room.

Clinical CPB

While Gibbon and colleagues proved that a pump oxygenator could be used for cardiac interventions, a number of pathology, thereby shortening the time needed for surgical repair (an important consideration when the duration of extracorporeal support had to be kept to a minimum).

Deep Hypothermia

Deep hypothermia (sometimes referred to as *surface hypothermia* because the patient was immersed in ice-cold water prior to cardiac surgery) served to lower body temperature and metabolism, and allowed a period of circulatory arrest (Figure 1.9). For a while it appeared to compete with CPB, and it was used for hundreds of cardiac operations throughout the 1950s.[30] Surface hypothermia did not require advanced technology and was relatively safe. However, this technique was cumbersome, time-consuming, and relatively inefficient, since external cooling was slow to reach the vital organs, and the surgeon had little time to proceed with complex repair procedures under cardiac standstill. However, the apparent desirability

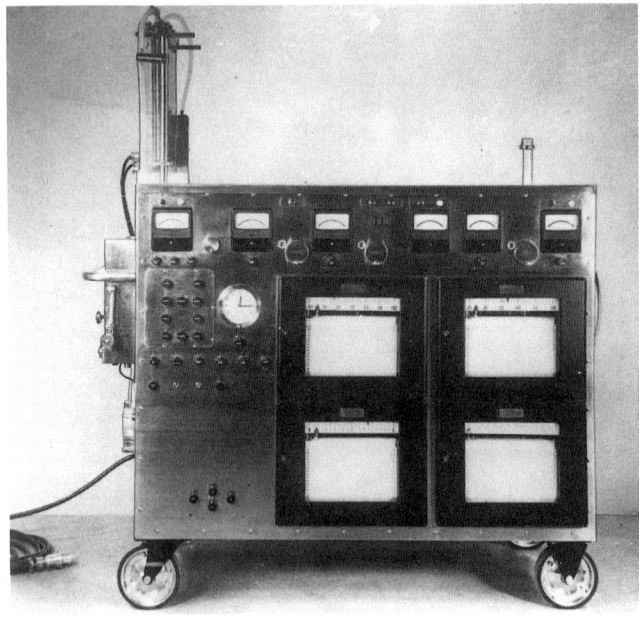

FIGURE 1.2. Gibbon's original battery-type stationary screen oxygenator. Venous blood entered from the top into a distributing chamber under the roof of the oxygenator casing and was spread over wire mesh screens through narrow slits in the floor of the distributing chamber. At the end of its descent in an oxygen atmosphere, arterialized blood collected in a reservoir at the bottom of the oxygenator casing. (Photo courtesy of Dr. Frederick B. Wagner and The Jefferson Medical College of Thomas Jefferson University.)

other important observations and advances were responsible for the progress of open-heart surgery (Table 1.2).

Cross-Circulation

In 1954, Lillehei[28] dared to pair a healthy adult donor with a blood-compatible child to repair a cardiac malformation. The procedure, dubbed *cross-circulation*, linked the two circulatory systems and provided CPB in the child through the heart and lungs of the adult donor (Figures 1.7 and 1.8). Over a period of 16 months, 47 patients were operated on, 28 survived, and none of the donors showed permanent harm. The clinical value of CPB had been demonstrated, and a major impetus was given to the development of appropriate machinery.

Cardiac Catheterization

Cardiac catheterization was another development critical to the advance of cardiac surgery. First performed by Forssmann[29] in 1927 and then by Cournand, Dickinson, and Richards in 1954, cardiac catheterization allowed the precise anatomic diagnosis of congenital or acquired cardiac lesions and also was an important advance in the nascent days of cardiac surgery. Cardiac catheterization oriented the surgeon to the exact nature of the cardiac

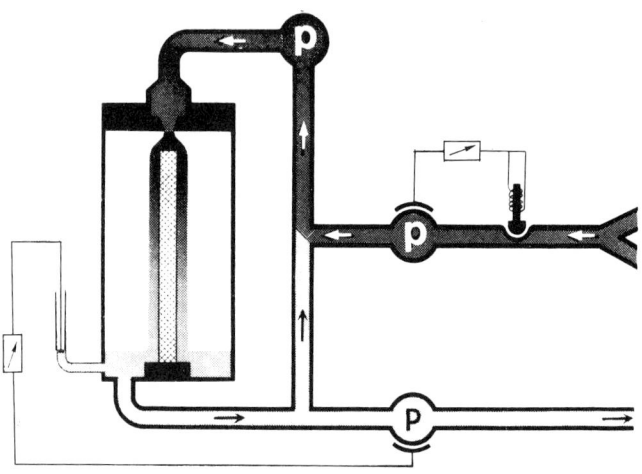

FIGURE 1.3. Diagram of Gibbon's original oxygenator. This design established one essential feature of an oxygenator, the necessity of maintaining a constant volume of blood in the extracorporeal circuit and, thereby, a constant thickness of the blood film, independent of fluctuations in blood flow to or from the perfused organism. The venous line included a segment of soft resilent tubing provided with a diameter-sensing device based on the principle of the differential transformer. If the venous pump generated too much suction, fluttering of the soft rubber tube actuated an electrical circuit that slowed the pump before actual caval collapse occurred. The recirculation pump (top P) was set at a constant flow rate which was always higher than that of the venous and arterial pumps. Consequently, there was always an upward flow of blood in the recirculating line (vertical connection between arterial and venous line). The rate of arterial pumping was automatically controlled by a level-sensing device in the collecting chamber, which tended to maintain a constant volume of blood in the extracorporeal circuit (electrical circuit acting on pump P on lower right side). (By permission of P. M. Galletti, *Heart-Lung Bypass*, Grune & Stratton, Philadelphia, 1962.)

Disc Reservoir-Oxygenator

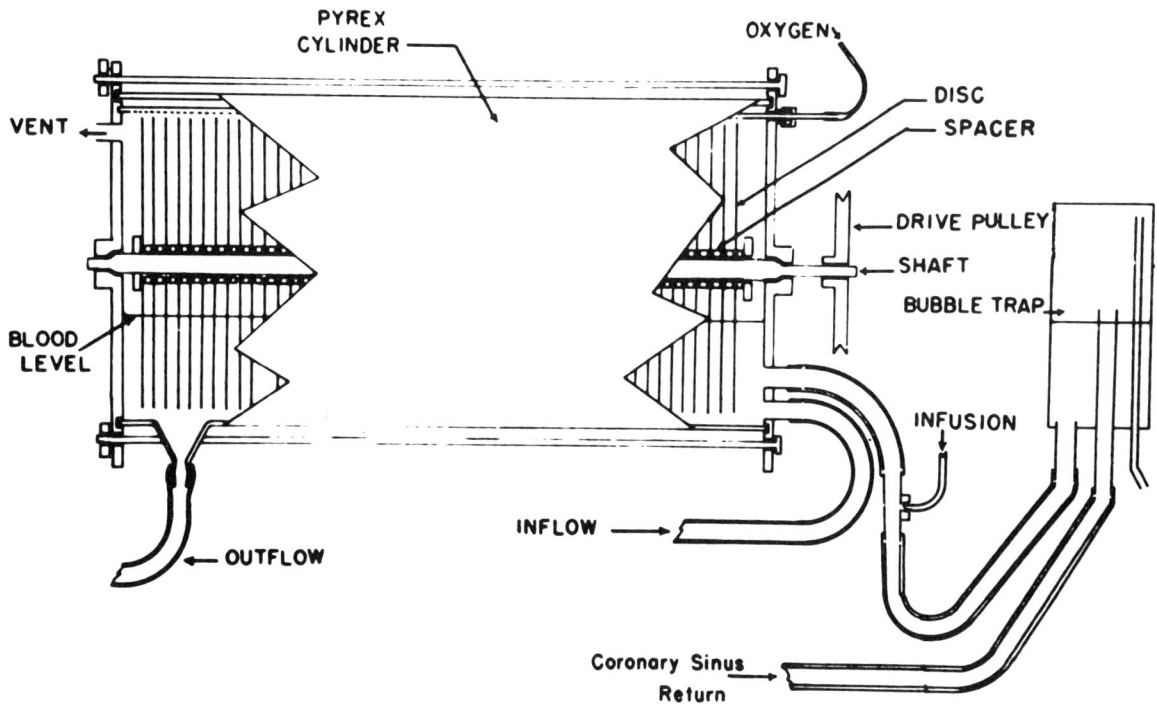

FIGURE 1.4. Diagram of the Kay-Cross disc oxygenator. This oxygenator consisted of 59 Teflon®-coated stainless steel (or entirely Teflon®) discs that were mounted 5 mm apart and enclosed in a cylinder of silicone-coated pyrex glass. With this arrangement, 0.84 m² of disk area was exposed to oxygen, and the maximum amount of oxygen that could be introduced into the blood was 207 mL/min. During actual perfusion at 2000 mL/min blood flow, the apparatus introduced 136 mL/min of oxygen into the blood. (From Cross et al,[19] by permission of Williams & Wilkins.)

of hypothermia led inventors to add heat exchangers to extracorporeal blood circuits in order to achieve *core hypothermia* — preferential cooling of those organs and tissues which receive the largest share of arterial blood flow.[31-34] Core hypothermia combines the advantages of mechanical cardiopulmonary support with those of reduced oxygen needs. The first blood-heat exchangers were sturdy, reusable devices built on the industrial model of automobile radiators. Following the trend toward disposable devices, heat exchangers have now become simple, mass-produced accessories that are commonly incorporated in the design of blood-gas exchangers.

Induced Myocardial Arrest

The ability to induce *myocardial* or *cardiac arrest* was also a major factor in the success of cardiac surgery in the early years. Surgeons recognized that cardiac surgery could be greatly facilitated by a quiet, flaccid heart. In 1953, Wesolowski and colleagues[35] demonstrated that myocardial anoxia, following interruption of the coronary circulation, resulted in myocardial arrest. Similarly, other investigators[36,37] noted that the infusion of potassium salts into the aortic root would provide an electromechanical arrest of the heart. Finally, investigators determined that myocardial hypothermia, induced by perfusion with cold blood or by surface irrigation with cold saline, would cause cardiac arrest.[38,39] Neither drug-induced nor hypothermic cardiac arrest, however, reduces myocardial metabolism to zero. Therefore, there is a time limit beyond which cellular damage will occur. Much has been learned since the 1950s about myocardial protection and intermittent coronary perfusion, and today surgery addresses more complex problems than were initially attempted. In spite of the recent resurgence of normothermic coronary perfusion, hypothermic cardiac arrest remains an important tool for cardiac surgery.

Myocardial Defibrillation

The heart recovering from induced cardiac arrest may go into ventricular fibrillation. Thus, techniques to defibrillate the heart and restore a normal rhythm were necessary for the growth of cardiac surgery. Kouwenhoven[40] in 1933 demonstrated that a fibrillating heart in a dog could be converted to sinus rhythm by an electric countershock. Wiggers[41] described the physiologic determinants of that transition, and in 1947 Beck[42] performed the first success-

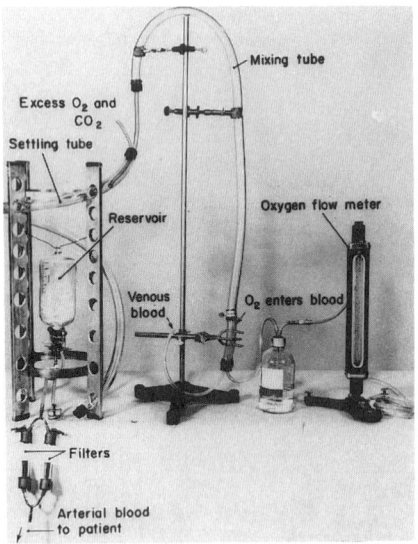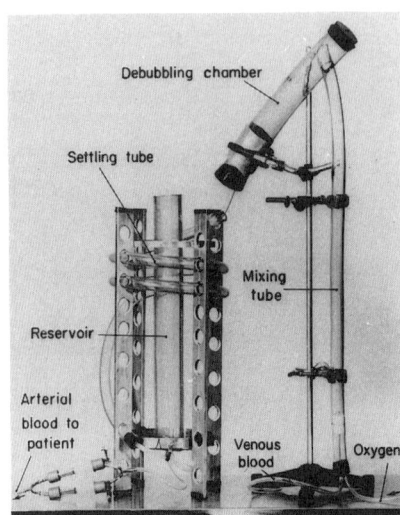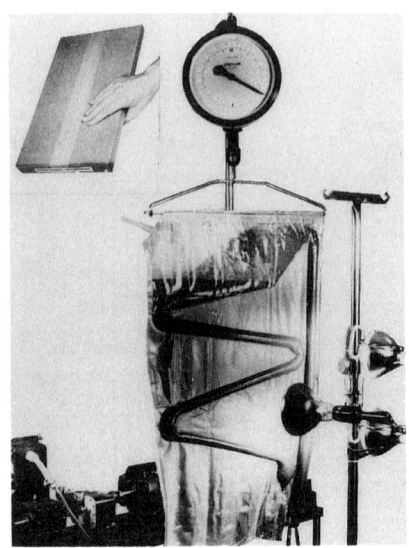

FIGURE 1.5. Evolution of the simple disposable DeWall-Lillehei bubble oxygenator for open heart surgery. *Left*: First 1955 model, successful in infants and small children. *Middle*: Late 1955, helix-reservoir model suitable for adults. *Right*: 1956, commercially manufactured model shipped sterile in a package (*inset*) ready to hang up and use. (Photo courtesy of C. Walton Lillehei.)

ful human defibrillation. Using an experimental hypothermic heart model, Bigelow et al[43] showed that after myocardial defibrillation, a cardiac rhythm can be reestablished with a primitive pacemaker. In 1957, Weirich, Gott, Paneth, and Lillehei[44,45] placed electrodes directly on the ventricle for the treatment of iatrogenic heart block in a cardiac surgery patient and restored adequate circulation. In 1966, Nachlass demonstrated the superiority of DC (direct current) over AC (alternating current) defibrillation.

Hemodilution

In the early days of CPB, when the highest achievable perfusion flow was often much below the resting cardiac output, *hemodilution* was believed to diminish unacceptably the oxygen-carrying capacity of the blood, and was therefore to be avoided. As the blood-gas transfer and the blood-flow capacity of pump oxygenators increased, so did the volume of blood required to prime the extracorporeal circuit. Eventually, blood banks could no longer supply all the blood requested for the growing number of cardiac procedures. Circuit blood dilution with saline, and the use of physiologic salt solutions, plasma expanders, or plasma became unavoidable. To the surprise of many surgeons, patients perfused with diluted blood suffered no harm; indeed, many seemed to have an improved postoperative course compared to patients who were not hemodiluted.[46] Improvement in tissue capillary perfusion was also noticed. Hemodilution was combined with hypothermia in order to attenuate the increase in blood viscosity at lower temperatures. Ultimately, hemodilution progressed from an unavoidable side effect of CPB to a deliberate, desirable feature of patient management.

The Ascent of Membrane Oxygenation

After World War II, the growing availability of commercially produced thin plastic films stimulated interest in the development of artificial membranes permeable to respiratory gases. The early observation that dark venous blood turned red while flowing through a long cellophane tube during hemodialysis suggested that blood-gas exchange occurs in synthetic systems.[47] Investigators hypothesized that the transition from a liquid-to-liquid exchanger of respiratory gases (on the model of a fish gill) to a flow-through, gas-to-liquid exchanger (as in an avian lung) was possible if a highly permeable membrane material could be identified that would separate blood from gas. The quest to find such a membrane material was excruciatingly slow. In desperation, disheartened surgeons tried to use excised animal lungs as gas exchange devices in extracorporeal circuits (*heterologous lung oxygenation*).[48-50] However, the fragility of animal lungs and the risk of transmitted infection made this technique clinically precarious, and it was abandoned once mechanical oxygenators became available.

The two major problems or challenges in membrane oxygenation are: (1) synthetic membranes as thin as the pulmonary alveolar wall cannot be fabricated; and (2) artificial blood distribution systems cannot match the fluid dynamic efficiency of the pulmonary circulation, in which a single feed vessel (the pulmonary artery) branches over

1. History and Future of CPB

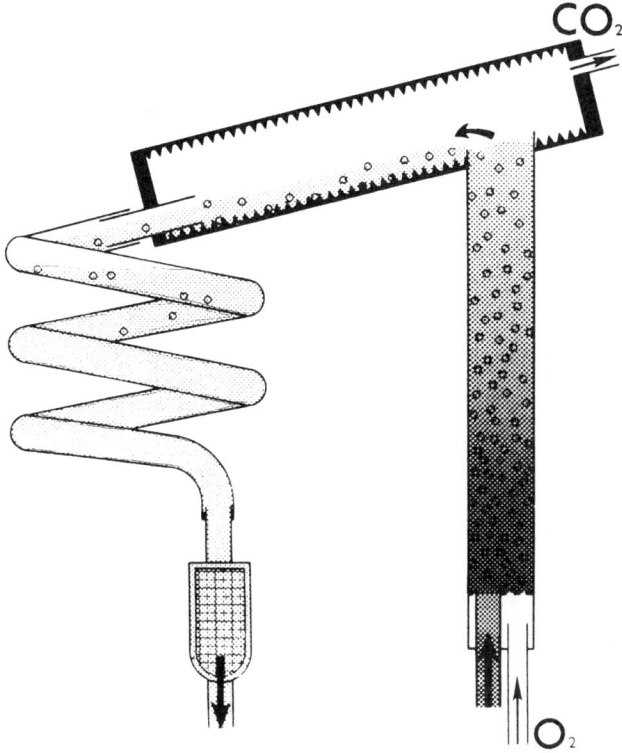

FIGURE 1.6. Diagram of the DeWall-Lillehei oxygenator. Venous blood (dark shading) and oxygen were injected simultaneously at the bottom of the oxygenating column. Oxygen bubbles ascended in the blood resulting in progressive arterialization. Antifoam-coated surfaces (black, vertical rhombs) in the debubbling chamber served to eliminate the excess oxygen and carbon dioxide which escaped into the atmosphere. The arterial blood accumulated in a settling chamber and passed through a filter (cross-hatching) before entering the arterial infusion line. (By permission of P. M. Galletti, *Heart-Lung Bypass*, Grune & Stratton, Philadelphia, 1962.)

a short distance into millions of tiny gas exchange capillaries the size of an erythrocyte, with a minimal loss of driving pressure. The first challenge has been addressed by the continuous improvement of microporous materials. The second awaits a technological breakthrough in the fabrication of thin-walled, branched tubes with several orders of arborization that mimic natural capillary beds.

TABLE 1.2. Observations and techniques facilitating the progress of open-heart surgery.

Cross-circulation (Lillehei[28])
Cardiac catheterization (Forssmann[29])
Deep hypothermia (Bigelow[10])
Myocardial arrest (Wesolowski,[34] Melrose[35])
Myocardial defibrillation (Beck[41])
External pacemaker (Lillehei[44])
Hemodilution (Zuhdi[45])

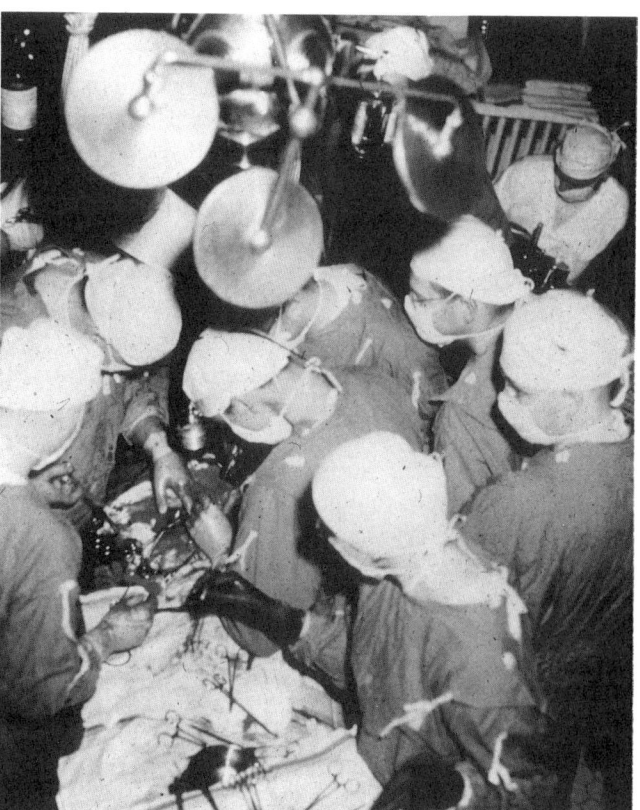

FIGURE 1.7. This photograph was taken at the University of Minnesota Medical Center on March 26, 1954, during the first successful open-heart procedure employing human cross-circulation for extracorporeal support. A ventricular septal defect was closed in a 12-month-old infant who was supported for 19 minutes of complete bypass by the father's heart and lungs. (The father-donor is seen in the far right of the photograph.) Dr. Lillehei is in the center of the photo and to the right of the scrub nurse, and Dr. R. L. Varco is opposite him. Also present are Dr. H. E. Warden (behind Dr. Lillehei) and Dr. M. Cohen, two residents who helped develop the technique in the dog laboratory. Dr. J. B. Aust (an assistant resident) and Dr. V. L. Gott (the surgical intern) are to the right and behind Dr. Varco, respectively. Dr. Norman Shumway, an assistant resident at the time, watched from behind Dr. Varco. The success of Dr. Lillehei's group served as a major impetus to the development of appropriate machinery for extracorporeal circulation. (Photo courtesy of C. Walton Lillehei.)

Membrane Materials

Membrane oxygenator development was initially predicated on the availability of materials for other uses, primarily from the packaging and capacitor industries. Besides the cellulosic membranes used for dialysis, the only hydrophobic polymers that could be cast in wide rolls of filmlike membranes devoid of pinholes were polyethylene and polytetrafluoroethylene (Teflon®). In the first systematic study of the permeability of polymer films in 1952, Karlson[51] concluded that an exchange area between

5 and 15 m² would be needed to meet the oxygen needs of a perfused patient. Undeterred by such calculations, Kolff and Baltzer[52] built a workable polyethylene coil oxygenator for experimental purposes. Clowes et al[53] recorded the first clinical use of a multilayered, ethyl-cellulose flat sheet, sandwich-type membrane lung. Shortly thereafter, Clowes and Neville[54] shifted to the less brittle and somewhat more permeable Teflon® membranes. The stacked oxygenator assembly of that era utilized two overlaid sheets of membrane material sealed around the edges to form an envelope through which the blood flowed (Figures 1.10 and 1.11). These blood envelopes alternated with porous spacers or meshes to provide a path for oxygen flow.

It took a while for investigators with medical backgrounds to appreciate that in an artificial membrane lung, carbon dioxide rather than oxygen transfer could be the limiting factor. This is because solid hydrophobic polymers have a low permeability to carbon dioxide, compared to the alveolar membrane.[55-57] This was indeed the major consideration which led to the progressive adoption of silicone elastomers as the choice transmembrane exchange material in the early days of membrane lungs.[58-60]

Blood Film Thickness

With the availability of more permeable membrane materials and the increased engineering sophistication in oxygenator design, the thickness of the blood film, rather than the permeability of the membrane, became the major obstacle to oxygen transport. Since under laminar flow conditions, a stationary boundary layer of blood forms adjacent to the membrane sheets and acts as a diffusion barrier, different systems were designed to promote mixing within the bloodstream; they included: (1) stretching the membrane between the peaks of external multiple point supports[61,62]; (2) embossing the blood-exposed side of the membranes with protruding cones[63]; (3) inserting mix-promoting screens in the blood envelopes[64]; and (4) compressing the entire sandwich assembly of blood and gas envelopes through pressurized bladders ("pneumatic shims").[65,66]

Early Bubble Versus Early Membrane Oxygenators

Even early membrane oxygenators had certain critical advantages over bubble oxygenators. Membrane oxygenators caused less damage to blood components, especially during long perfusions,[67] and required a relatively small and invariant priming volume. However, there were a number of problems that limited the clinical usefulness of membrane oxygenators. For example, three independent circuits had to be provided in the device for blood, gas, and temperature-control fluid. Venous, coronary, and ar-

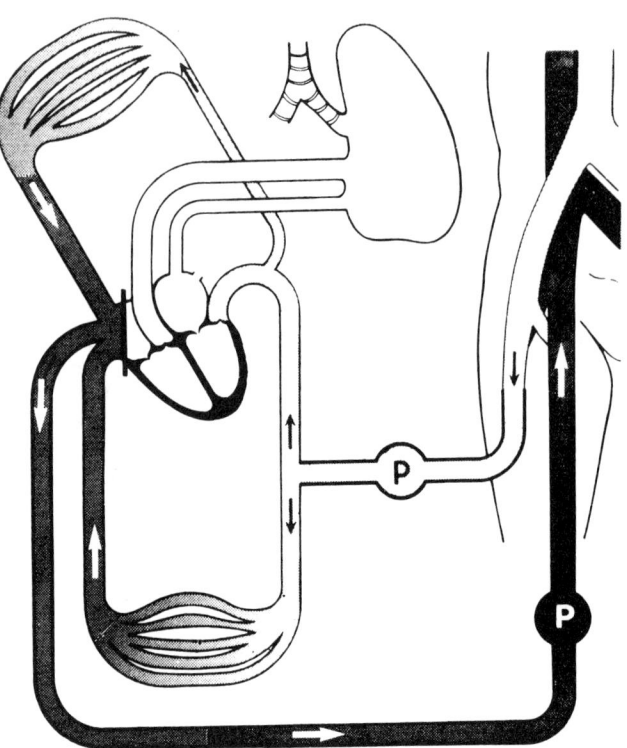

FIGURE 1.8. Diagram of cross-circulation. Blood from the arterial system of the donor was pumped into the arterial system of the receiver. Meanwhile, the blood accumulating in the venous system of the receive was prevented from entering the right heart cavities, and directed towards the venous system of the donor. Thereafter, the heart and lungs of the receiver were excluded from the circulation. Since the donor must carry, simultaneously, his own circulation and that of the donor, the organisms were different in size. An adult would usually act as a donor for a child. (By permission of P. M. Galletti, *Heart-Lung Bypass*, Grune & Stratton, Philadelphia, 1962.)

terial reservoirs could not be built in, since the oxygenator casing had to be rigid and often pressurized. On occasion, the gas space would be flooded through a membrane pinhole, or one of the parallel blood compartments would fail because of thrombotic obstruction of its feeding manifold. Most significantly, the rapid expansion of cardiac surgery in the period from 1965 to 1972 called for preassembled, sterile, disposable devices. At that time, membrane oxygenators could not be made as inexpensively, and as user friendly, as the bubble oxygenators.

Technology of Membrane Lungs

Industrial production of membrane oxygenators hinged on three major advances in material science and device technology: the development of gas-permeable hollow fibers and microporous membranes, and the appreciation

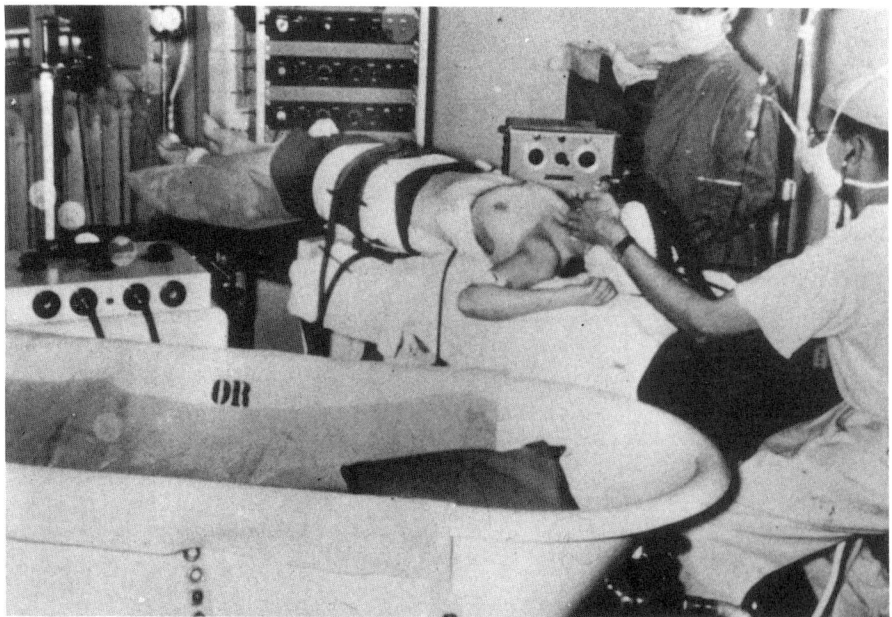

FIGURE 1.9. Photograph of anesthetized child being prepared for the induction of profound hypothermia through immersion in an ice-water bath. Rewarming was accomplished with the use of diathermy coils which, as seen in this photo, were well padded and wrapped around the pelvis. (Photo courtesy of Henry J. C. Swan.)

of secondary flows. These were the innovations that led to the membrane oxygenators of today (Chapter 10).

Gas-Permeable Hollow Fibers

By the early 1970s, 2- to 5-m^2 gas exchange units, containing as many as 50,000 silicone copolymer fibers in parallel,[68] were shown to have a gas transfer capacity approaching that of bubble oxygenators. However, blood distribution was a problem, and white platelet plugs formed where a single feed tube was separated into thousands of small, parallel capillaries. Over the next decade, better blood inflow and outflow manifolds were designed, and better materials and techniques for potting the fiber bundles and cutting the face sheet were identified. In 1983, Terumo (to be followed by Bentley) introduced the first commercial hollow-fiber oxygenator (Figure 1.12). However, the exchange area required for adult perfusion with the early gas-permeable hollow-fiber oxygenators was still large (on the order of 4 m^2), and carbon dioxide elimination remained a problem.

Microporous Membranes

During the 1960s, McCaughan and colleagues[69] proposed using porous hydrophobic polymer films to separate blood from gas in an exchange device relying on the surface tension properties of hydrophobic materials to prevent foaming. Further, the microporous materials of that period could not avert oozing when pressure was applied on the blood side of the membrane. Furthermore, it was believed that exchange devices made of microporous materials would include a direct interface between gas and blood and therefore would offer no advantage over bubble oxygenation in terms of blood handling. However, by the 1970s, an oxygenator appeared with an ultrathin silicone elastomer lining for blood passageways, which were insinuated into a thick, spongy composite of graphite and Teflon® particles through which the gas circulated. This device was found to be an efficient blood-gas exchanger with hematologic characteristics that compared favorably with those of nonporous membrane oxygenators.[70] Under normal operating pressures, blood did not penetrate the voids in the porous hydrophobic wall. Microporous membrane oxygenation was indeed possible.

The development of microfibrillar polytetrafluoroethylene (ePTFE or microporous Teflon®) in sheet form permitted the manufacturing of the first commercial microporous membrane oxygenator. With ePTFE membrane lungs, oxygen transfer capacity was as high as, or higher than, that with the most permeable solid membranes, and carbon dioxide removal was no longer a limiting factor.[71] Clinical experience verified the usefulness of the design.[72]

Secondary Flows

To further improve the gas transfer efficiency of membrane oxygenators, several methods were developed to improve mixing (secondary flows) in the bloodstream. All methods to induce the formation of secondary blood flows (ie, localized streaming patterns) within the main bulk flow rely on mechanical forces in association with well-defined geometric configurations. Secondary flows can typically increase oxygen transfer by a factor of two over the transfer under laminar flow conditions. Therefore, the membrane exchange area required for a standard

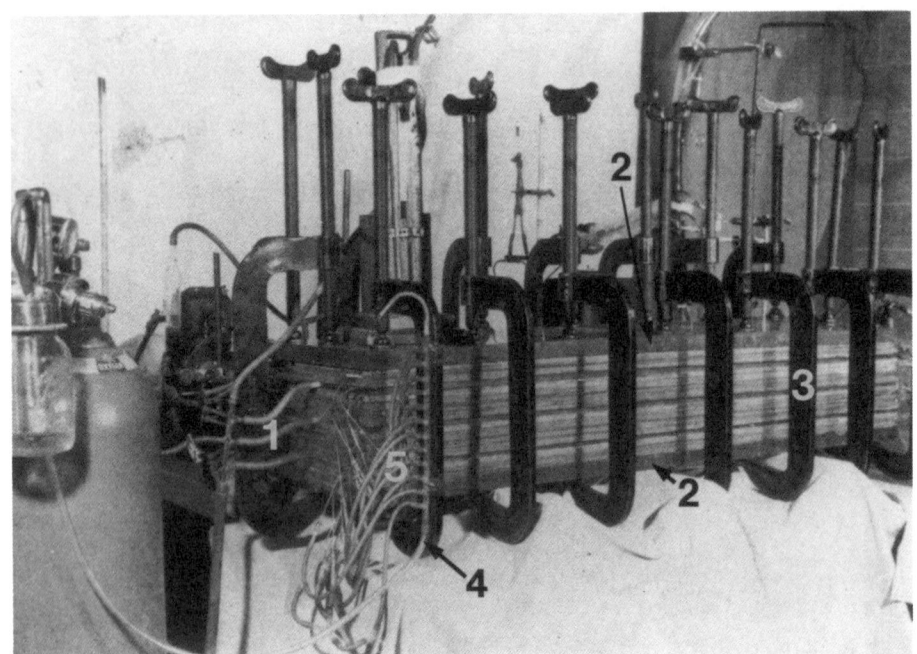

FIGURE 1.10. A 12-unit membrane oxygenator in operation as seen from the end into which venous blood was pumped. Venous blood was pumped (sigmamotor pump) into the three tubes (1) seen in the middle of the background. The stacked oxygenating units were sandwiched between heavy sheets of plastic (2), and the whole apparatus was clamped together with large C-clamps (3). Through the distributing manifold (4), oxygen entered each oxygenating unit through a flexible rubber tube (5) and flowed down the longitudinal space between the gaskets and the grooves. With the 12-unit system depicted here, it was possible to pump 300 mL/min of blood with an arterial-venous (A-V) difference of 16 volumes percent or 1200 mL with an A-V difference of 4 volumes percent. (From Clowes et al,[53] by permission of *J Thor Surg*.)

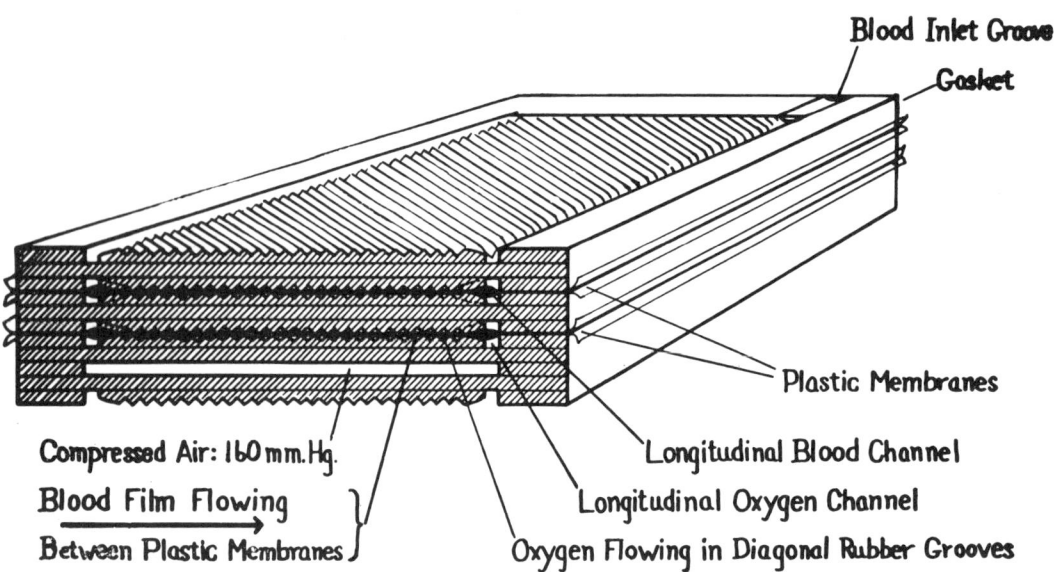

FIGURE 1.11. Cross-sectional diagram of the multiple-unit membrane oxygenator showing the course of blood and oxygen flow. Ethylcellulose (1 mm thick) and polyethylene (0.8 mm thick) plastic membranes permitted the introduction of approximately 8.6 and 5.0 mL of oxygen per square meter of surface area, respectively, into blood flowing at 100 mL/min. If the blood flow was reduced by 50%, the A-V difference did not double. The inventors of this oxygenator hypothesized that the reduced pumping pressure associated with lower flows would fail to open all the channels between the grooves, thus increasing blood shunting and decreasing oxygen uptake. (From Clowes et al,[53] by permission of *J Thor Surg*.)

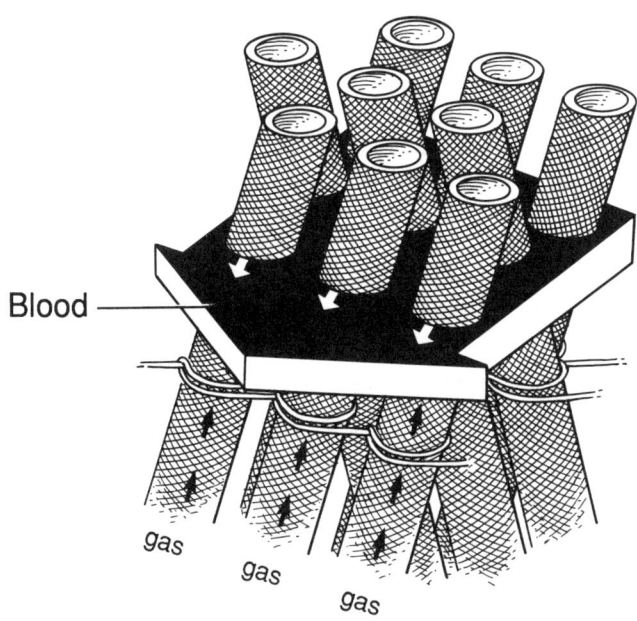

FIGURE 1.12. Representation of gas-permeable extraluminal flow (ELF) oxygenator fibers.

perfusion can be cut in half. By design or otherwise, secondary flows are a feature of all modern membrane oxygenators and have allowed a significant reduction in the size and cost of manufacturing membrane oxygenators.

Extraluminal Flow (ELF) Designs (Blood Outside, Hollow-Fiber Oxygenators)

Empirically, rather than analytically, the benefits of secondary flows were introduced in "blood outside" or "extraluminal flow" (ELF) oxygenators. In these devices, oxygen, rather than blood, flows through the lumen of the capillary tubes, while blood circulates outside of the hollow fibers through the chamber that houses the fiber bundle (Figure 1.13) (Chapter 10). Because the viscosity of oxygen is a thousand times lower than that of blood, gas flow through the narrow lumen of the hollow fibers does not require any excessive head of pressure (which could force gas to bubble through the pores of the material). Blood courses through a geometrically wider path than the sum total of the fibers' cross-sectional areas, and consequently the resistance to blood flow is reduced compared to the "blood inside" or intraluminal designs. The blood-gas exchange area is now the *outer* surface of the hollow fibers, which is larger than the inner surface of the same fibers. Clever juxtaposition or weaving of individual fiber bundles has been used to generate mixing in the bloodstream and (most likely) complex secondary flows, as individual streams are forced in curved or serpentine patterns.[73] Laboratory and clinical experience has shown that the membrane area required for a given level of gas exchange is reduced by 30% to 50% in "blood outside" hollow-fiber designs compared to "blood inside" models. Because ELF oxygenators are more efficient and are less costly to manufacture, they likely will replace "blood inside" devices.

From Artisanal to Industrial Production

In the early days of CPB, there were almost as many models of oxygenators as there were cardiac surgery teams. Custom-made gas exchange devices were assembled, sterilized, and then dismantled for each perfusion. However, with the development of disposable, transparent, soft-wall plastic bubble oxygenators in the 1960s, industrial production became limited to a few models. In response to the explosive growth of coronary bypass surgery in the 1970s, high-blood-flow, high-gas-transfer, hard-shell bubble oxygenators were manufactured, and a few models dominated the market for over a decade. However, as membrane oxygenators became clinically accepted, industrial production of bubble oxygenators declined in devel-

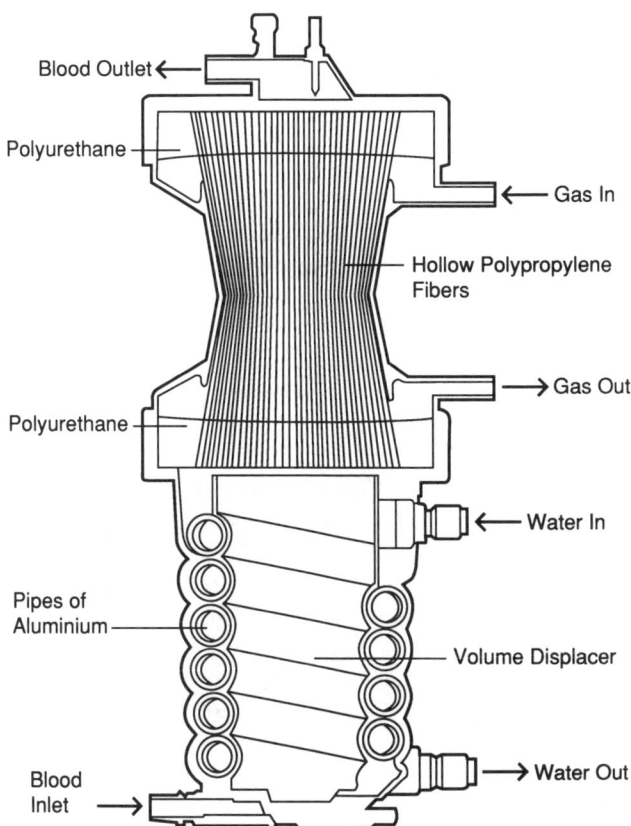

FIGURE 1.13. Diagram of the Bentley CM 40 hollow-fiber membrane oxygenator. The Terumo Capiox and Bentley BOS CM 40/50 were the first two membrane oxygenators to make use of hollow polypropylene fibers.

oped countries. Today, bubble oxygenators are no longer fabricated in the United States. In all of North America, Europe, and Japan, only 10 companies manufacture membrane oxygenators, each offering one or, at the most, two types. (The number of models is somewhat higher, since some types come in different sizes.) The majority of these oxygenators are capillary hollow-fiber exchangers, and the most recent ones use an ELF design. The membrane material is almost universally microporous polypropylene. A progressive convergence to fewer designs and fewer construction materials is typical of a mature device industry, paralleled, for instance, in the field of prosthetic cardiac valves. The high cost of entering a competitive market of sophisticated, disposable devices makes it unlikely that fundamentally new oxygenator designs will emerge in the coming years, except for specialized models, such as those for infant and pediatric perfusions, or intravenous oxygenation and chronic respiratory assistance.

Blood-Material Interactions

Hemolysis and defibrination were major problems in early perfusions. The pump and suction equipment, the large surfaces of foreign materials, and the fast flow and high shear conditions characteristic of early extracorporeal circuits had significant adverse effects on blood. Progressive improvement in bypass circuits has greatly attenuated the problems associated with blood handling. Today the damage observed in platelets and leukocytes is more subtle (Chapters 5 and 8). It is now known that most materials activate the coagulation as well as the complement cascade, and that there are interactions between these two mechanisms. Cardiopulmonary bypass activates some humoral amplification systems of the acute inflammatory reaction (involving both the chemical and the alternative complement pathway)[74,75] and initiates a systemic inflammatory reaction affecting multiple organs.[76] The resulting impairment of the immune system[77] includes neutrophil degranulation,[78] release of lysosomal enzymes,[79,80] changes in oxidative potential,[81] and diminished phagocytosis[82] and chemotactic activity.[83] (A more detailed discussion of the effect of CPB on the immune response is included in Chapter 8). Induction of interleukin-1 production generated by circulating monocytes[84] correlates directly with the postoperative increase in body temperature. The mechanisms involved have not been fully elucidated, and the clinical observations are not entirely concordant with in vitro studies or with animal studies,[85] but the role of blood-material interactions is now better understood.[86]

Heparin is still used as an anticoagulant in practically all clinical perfusions. However, heparin-bonded circuits may eventually obviate the need for systemic anticoagulation. Perhaps the most compelling demonstration of the feasibility of modifying material surfaces to minimize thrombus formation is provided by the early clinical experience with the intravenous oxygenator (IVOX). These devices,[87] which consist of a 1-m^2 bundle of hollow fibers that is introduced into the vena cava, have remained thrombus-free for up to a week, even in the absence of anticoagulation (Chapter 30). Until there is a major breakthrough in the formulation of circuit surfaces exposed to blood, the key to reducing the undesirable interactions of blood with the CPB circuit is to minimize the contact area in the bypass circuit.

Human-Machine Interactions

Perfusionists were trained to operate the heart-lung machine 30 years ago, and they are still needed today, since little progress has been made towards automation of the machine. Some of the uncertainties associated with the early equipment (eg, the amount of blood sequestered in the foam phase of the gas exchange device, the excessive content of a flexible venous or arterial reservoir) have been resolved. Some devices feature an electronic level control that precludes inadvertent emptying of the arterial reservoir by slowing down the arterial perfusion pump. Ultrasonic reflection analyzers or imagers have been used to identify the presence of gas bubbles or platelet aggregates in the arterial stream. The absence of stable, reliable, and inexpensive sensors for respiratory blood gases, pH, and hemoglobin content—parameters that are needed to assess the metabolic aspects of the procedure—has retarded the growth of automation in CPB. The interaction of these data with blood temperature (which, in turn, only indirectly reflects organ temperature) has discouraged the acceptance of software that could control the independent variables of blood flow, gas flow, and rate of cooling or rewarming. There is never a steady state during CPB. Indeed, surgical imperatives, as well as the desire to shorten the procedure as much as possible, have thus far precluded the development of automated controls.

Similarly, a method or device to provide on-line, automated control of anticoagulation and its later reversal is not available. Bolus doses of heparin are administered according to the clock or by some punctual measurements, and the dose of protamine is largely determined by a general formula that is only indirectly related to the individual patient. With serious perfusion difficulties limited to 1% to 3% of cases (and life-threatening ones to perhaps a fifth of that), it will be difficult to justify the cost of unproven automation. The empirical management of anticoagulation may also yield to the large-scale use of extracorporeal circuits coated with heparin and other bioactive substances, provided such materials can be fabricated at an acceptable cost. In the interval, most cardiac surgery teams continue to rely on the integration of every available element of information by an experienced *human mind.* Effective communication among all professionals on the team remains the best assurance of safety for the patient.

The Outlook for the Next Century

Is there a need for a new generation of pump oxygenators? Noseé has pointed out that, compared to improvements in the blood-gas exchange devices, the perfusion apparatus itself has remained virtually the same as it was 30 years ago. The pump console has, if anything, become larger and more complex than ever. As a result, the heart-lung machine occupies a large space in the operating room and requires a skilled perfusionist. The anesthesiologist, who has a major responsibility for the patient, has no designated space near the heart-lung machine and must relinquish direct control of the patient during the bypass period. Communication is a safeguard, but redesign and miniaturization of the bypass system, so that it would fit on the surgical instruments table or could be incorporated in the anesthesia equipment, would bring a revolution in CPB technology and cardiac surgery. The recent introduction of *centrifugal pumps* may be the harbinger for such a change (Chapter 11). Disposable and relatively inexpensive nonpulsatile rotary pumps are commonly used in circulatory assist procedures. Some surgical teams have already found them effective and affordable for routine CPB. These pumps demand little space and are easy to use. They are likely to become a significant factor with the expansion of infant surgery, the advent of fetal surgery under CPB, and the adoption of perfusion procedures by interventional cardiologists for high-risk coronary angioplasty procedures (Chapter 25).

Surface treatment of blood-gas exchange membranes is another likely area of change. It is known empirically that the gas transfer performance of microporous membrane oxygenators is limited by plasma leakage. Water vapor condensation on the gas side of the exchanger,[69] the inadvertent injection of surface-active agents into the bloodstream,[88] and, most significantly, the effect of high transmembrane pressures[89] can cause seepage through the voids of microporous polypropylene. Coating with a continuous polymer layer or glow discharge (physical plasma) treatment of the surface exposed to blood may answer this problem.

There are other reasons to consider polymer surface modification of the CPB circuit. Heparin coating of the extracorporeal circuit surfaces, originally introduced to prevent surface thrombosis and diminish the need for circulating heparin, also inhibits complement activation.[90,91] This is thought to reduce the release of leukocyte inflammation mediators.[92] Covalent bonding of heparin to the oxygenator surface has proven clinically effective and beneficial[93] and may, in coming years, have a more generalized application.

In medical biotechnology, there is a standard progression from what is initially *possible* to what becomes *promising*. In some cases, what is possible and promising is later recognized as *prudent* and is eventually *proven* to be safe and effective. The feedback loops of technology assessment will continue to guide the evaluation of CPB equipment and procedures.

Conclusion

At the American College of Surgeons Annual Meeting in 1939, John Gibbon presented for discussion his observation of the feasibility of total CPB for 20 minutes in cats. Leo Eloesser saw the human application of that technology as a Jules Verne science fiction story, whereas the more pragmatic Clarence Crafoord mused about its potential in the Trendelenburg operation for the removal of massive pulmonary emboli (the only relevant surgical indication at the time). By 1955, 2 years after the first successful open-heart operation by Gibbon, there were only five survivors, worldwide, who had undergone CPB for surgical correction of congenital heart malformations.

In the late 1950s, industrial pioneers introduced simple, transparent (but still "handmade") disposable bubble oxygenators to replace the more sophisticated and error-prone film devices. This left the open-heart team free to concentrate on the unsolved physiologic and surgical problems of that time, which, in retrospect, clearly overshadowed the imperfections of the oxygenator circuit. Ten years later, CPB became less hazardous, and there was a shift to reliable, quality-controlled, mass-produced gas exchange devices using the bubble principle. Similarly, the early membrane lungs were merely an engineering feat, although they established the blood-sparing value of this type of gas exchange system and brought attention to the problem of carbon dioxide elimination in CPB. Once Gerbode[94] brought membrane oxygenation to the clinical setting, new problems of device-patient interface had to be resolved through a dynamic adjustment among device fabrication, operational characteristics, and pathophysiologic observations in the operating room. The performance specifications for CPB equipment were progressively codified, starting a movement toward simplification of equipment which has led to the mass-produced hollow-fiber devices currently in use.

The application of CPB to cardiac surgery has proceeded historically in three phases. First it was used for the repair of congenital defects, the incidence of which, at that time, was inflated by the accumulated survival of patients for whom there had been no effective treatment. When Starr[95] paved the way for the surgical replacement of valve defects, a new burst of growth took place, enhanced again by the existence of a patient pool with valvular disease dating back many years. Then came the explosive growth of aortocoronary bypass surgery, leading to the third and biggest hump in the growth curve of operations under total body perfusion. During none of these phases was the next step quantitatively anticipated.

This observation should give us pause when we consider our ability to predict the future. The time course in the application of artificial organs to clinical problems is such that initially the focus is on the device itself. Once the device has proven effective, interest shifts to the clinical problems associated with the patient-machine interface. Eventually new problems arise from extending life or organ function beyond the natural history of the disease. Because of CPB, time is no longer a major factor in cardiac surgery. This should open the door to more complex and lengthy surgery some time in the future. However, we live in a timid and at times nearly paralyzed environment, beset by all sorts of regulations and threats of litigation. It is almost unimaginable that the adventurous saga of technology-based open-heart surgery could be replicated in the 1990s. A quantum leap forward will likely await an imaginative and largely unpredictable set of discoveries. Then, keen minds will foster their application to clinical problems. In the meantime, quality control in all aspects of patient management remains the key to confidence building and the spur to innovation.

References

1. LeGallois JJC; Nancrede NC, Nancrede JC, trans. *Experiments on the Principle of Life*. Philadelphia: M Thomas; 1813.
2. Brown-Sequard E. Recherches experimentales sur les propriétés physiologiques et les usage du sang rouge et du sang noir et leurs principaux éléments gazeus, l'oxygène et l'acide carbonique. *J Physiol de l'Homme (Paris)* 1858;1:95–122, 353–367, 729–735.
3. Ludwig C, Schmidt A. Das Verhalten der Gase, welche mit dem Blut durch den reizbaren Saugetiermuskel strömen. *Leipzig Berichte* 1868;20:12–72.
4. Starling EH. The Linacre lecture on the law of the heart. London: Longman Green Publishers; 1915.
5. Brukhonenko S. Circulation artificielle du sang dans l'organisme entier d'un chien avec coeur exclu. *J Physiol Path Gen* 1929;27:257–272.
6. von Frey M, Gruber M. Untersuchungen über den Stoffwechsel isolierter Organe. Ein Respirations-Apparat für isolierte Organe. *Virchow's Arch Physiol* 1885;9:519–532.
7. McLean J. The thromoboplastic action of cephalin. *Am J Physiol* 1916;41:250–257.
8. Chargraff E, Olson KB. Studies on the chemistry of blood coagulation. VI. Studies on the action of heparin and other anticoagulants. The influence of protamine on the anticoagulant effect in vivo. *J Biol Chem* 1937;122:153–167.
9. DeBakey ME. A simple continuous flow blood transfusion instrument. *New Orleans Med Surg J* 1934;87:386–389.
10. Bigelow WG, Lindsay WK, Greenwood WF. Hypothermia: its possible role in cardiac surgery: an investigation of factors governing survival in dogs at low body temperature. *Ann Surg* 1950;132:849–866.
11. Boerema I, Wildschut A, Broekhuysen L, et al. Experimental researches into hypothermia as an aid in the surgery of the heart. *Arch Chir Neerl* 1951;3:25–34.
12. Lewis FJ, Benvenuto R, Demetrakopoulos N. A new pump oxygenator employing polyethylene membranes. *Q Bull Northwest Univ Med School* 1958;32:262–267.
13. Swan HJC. Factors in the control of the circulation which may be modified during total body perfusion. *IXE Trans Med Electronics* 1959;6:32–33.
14. Gibbons JH Jr. Artificial maintenance of circulation during experimental occlusion of pulmonary artery. *Arch Surg* 1937;34:1105–1131.
15. Gibbon JH Jr, Dobell AR, Voigt GB, et al. The closure of interventricular septal defects on dogs during open cardiotomy with the maintenance of the cardio-respiratory functions by a pump oxygenator. *J Thorac Surg* 1954;28:235–240.
16. Kirklin JW, Theye RA, Patrick RT. The stationary vertical screen oxygenator. In: Allen JG, ed. *Extracorporeal Circulation*. Springfield, Ill: Charles C Thomas Publisher; 1958:57–66.
17. Kirklin JW, Dushane JW, Wood EH, et al. Intracardiac surgery with the aid of a mechanical pump-oxygenator system (Gibbon-type). Report of eight cases. *Proc Mayo Clin* 1955;30:201–206.
18. Dennis C. Certain methods for artificial support of the circulation during intracardiac surgery. *Surg Clin North Am* 1956;36:423–436.
19. Cross ES, Berne RM, Hirose Y, et al. Evaluation of a rotating disc type reservoir-oxygenator. *Proc Soc Exp Biol Med* 1956;93:210–215.
20. Crafoord C. Operationen am offenen Herzen mit Herz-Lungen-Maschine (Stockholmer Modell). *Langenbeck Arch Klin Chir* 1958;289:257–266.
21. Clark LC Jr. Blood gas exchange devices. *IRE Trans Med Electronics* 1959;6:18–21.
22. Thomas JA. Physiologie du coeur-poumon à membrane pulmonaire artificielle. *CR Acad Sci Paris* 1959;248:291–294.
23. Clark LC Jr, Gollan F, Gupta VB. The oxygenation of blood by gas dispersion. *Science* 1950;111:85–87.
24. Salisbury PF. Blood pump gas exchange system ("artificial heart-lung machine") of large flow capacity. *J Appl Physiol* 1956;9:487–491.
25. Gott VL, DeWall RA, Lillehei CW, et al. A self-contained disposable oxygenator of plastic sheet for intracardiac surgery. *Thorax* 1957;12:1–9.
26. Rygg IH, Kyvsgaard E. A disposable polyethylene oxygenator system applied in a heart-lung machine. *Acta Chir Scand* 1956;112:433–437.
27. Rygg IH, Kyvsgaard E. Further development of the heart-lung machine with Rygg-Kyvsgaard plastic bag oxygenator. *Minerva Chir* 1958;13:1402–1404.
28. Lillehei CW. Controlled cross circulation for direct-vision intracardiac surgery; correction of ventricular septal defects, atrioventricularis communis and tetralogy of Fallot. *Post Grad Med* 1955;17:388–396.

29. Forssmann W. Über Kontrastdarstellung der Hohlen des lebenden rechten Herzens und der Lungenschlagader. *Mün Med Wochenschr* 1932;78:789–792.
30. Swan HJC, Paton B. The combined use of hypothermia and extracorporeal circulation in cardiac surgery. *J Cardiovasc Surg* 1960;1:169–175.
31. Senning A. Extracorporeal circulation combined with hypothermia. *Acta Chir Scand* 1954;107:516–524.
32. Sealy WC, Brown IW Jr, Merrit D, et al. Hypothermia, low flow extracorporeal circulation and controlled cardiac arrest for open heart surgery. *Surg Gynecol Obstet* 1957;104:441–451.
33. Gollan F. Physiology of deep hypothermia by total body perfusion. *Ann NY Acad Sci* 1959;80:301–314.
34. Dubost C, Blondeau P. The association of the artificial heart-lung with deep hypothermia in open heart surgery. *J Cardiovasc Surg* 1960;1:85–93.
35. Wesolowski SA, Fisher JH, Welch CS. Recovery of the dog's heart after varying periods of acute ischemia. *Surg Forum* 1953;3:270–277.
36. Melrose DG, Dreyer B, Baker JBE. Elective cardiac arrest: preliminary communication. *Lancet* 1955;2:21–22.
37. Effler DB, Sones FM, Kolff WJ, et al. Elective cardiac arrest in open-heart surgery. Report of three cases. *Cleveland Clin Quart* 1956;23:105–114.
38. Shumway NE. A classification of elective cardiac arrest for open heart surgery. *Dis Chest* 1959;36:315–318.
39. Bjork VO, Fors B. Induced cardiac arrest. *J Thorac Cardiovasc Surg* 1961;41:387–394.
40. Kouwenhoven WB, Hooker DR, Lotz EL. Electric shock effects of frequency. *Electrical Eng* 1936;384–386.
41. Wiggers CJ. *Physiology in Health and Disease*. Philadelphia: Lea and Febiger; 1949.
42. Beck CS, Pritchard WH, Fell HS. Ventricular fibrillation of long duration abolished by electric shock. *JAMA* 1947;135:985–986.
43. Bigelow WG, Lindsay WK, Greenwood WF. Hypothermia: its possible role in cardiac surgery: an investigation of factors governing survival in dogs at low body temperature. *Ann Surg* 1950;132:849–866.
44. Paneth M, Weirich W, Lillehei WC, et al. Physiologic studies upon prolonged cardiopulmonary bypass with the pump oxygenator with particular reference to (1) acid-base balance, (2) syphon caval drainage. *J Thorac Surg* 1957;34:570–579.
45. Lillehei CW, Gott VL, Hodges PC, et al. Transistor pacemaker for treatment of complete atrioventricular dissociation. *JAMA* 1960;172:2006–2010.
46. Zuhdi N, McCollough B, Greer A, et al. The use of citrated banked blood for open-heart surgery. *Anesthesiology* 1960;21:496–501.
47. Kolff WJ, Berk HTJ. Artificial kidney: dialyzer with great area. *Acta Med Scand* 1944;117:121–134.
48. Jacobj C. Ein Beitrag zur Technik der kunstlichen Durchblutung überlebender Organe. *Arch Exp Path (Leipzig)* 1895;31:330–348.
49. Brukhonenko S. Appareil pour la circulation artificielle du sang des animaux à sang chaud. *J Physiol Path Gen* 1929;27:12–18.
50. Fleisch A. Ein automatisch regulierender Durchblutungsapparat mit fortlaufender Registrierung der Durchbkutungsgeschwindigkeit. In: Abderhalden E, ed. *Handbuch der biologischen Arbeitsmethoden*. 1935; Section V Part 8, Number 3, pp. 1007–1026.
51. Karlson KE. *The Problem of Construction of a Pump Oxygenator to Replace the Heart and Lungs for Brief Periods*. Minneapolis: University of Minnesota, 1952. Thesis.
52. Kolff WJ, Balzer R. The artificial coil lung. *Trans Am Soc Artif Int Organs* 1955;1:39–42.
53. Clowes GHA Jr, Hopkins AL, Neville WE. An artificial lung dependent upon diffusion of oxygen and carbon dioxide through plastic membranes. *J Thorac Surg* 1956;32:630–637.
54. Clowes GHA Jr, Neville WE. Further development of a blood oxygenator dependent upon the diffusion of gases through plastic membranes. *Trans Am Soc Artif Int Organs* 1957;3:52–58.
55. Melrose DG, Bramson ML, Gerbode F, et al. The membrane oxygenator. Some aspects of oxygen and carbon dioxide transport across polyethylene film. *Lancet* 1958;1:1050–1051.
56. Pierce EC II. Diffusion of oxygen and carbon dioxide through teflon membranes. *Arch Surg* 1958;77:938–943.
57. Galletti PM, Snider M, Silbert-Aiden D. Gas permeability of plastic membranes for artificial lungs. *Med Res Eng* 1966;5(2):20–23.
58. Kolobow T, Bowman R. Construction and evaluation of an alveolar membrane artificial heart-lung. *Trans Am Soc Artif Int Organs* 1963;9:238–243.
59. Bramson ML, Osborn JJ, Main FB, et al. A new disposable membrane oxygenator with integral heat exchange. *J Thorac Cardiovasc Surg* 1965;50:391–400.
60. Butruille Y, Chevallet J, Granger A, et al. Rhone-Poulenc oxygenator and associated pumping system. In: Zapol WM, Qvist J, eds. *Artificial Lungs for Acute Respiratory Failure*. New York: Academic Press-Hemisphere Publishing Corp; 1976:223–233.
61. Galletti PM, Hopf MA, Pierce EC II. A membrane lung-kidney. *Trans Am Soc Artif Int Organs* 1962;8:47–52.
62. Landé AJ, Parker B, Subramanian V, et al. Methods for increasing the efficiency of a new dialyzer-membrane oxygenator. *Trans Am Soc Artif Int Organs* 1968;14:227–230.
63. Pierce EC II, Mathewson WF Jr. Design and fabrication of blood oxygenator for circulatory assist devices. *Proc Artif Heart Prog Conf*. Washington, DC: US Dept of Health, Education, and Welfare; 1969:405.
64. Kolobow T, Zapol W, Pierce JE, et al. Partial extracorporeal gas exchange in alert newborn lambs with a membrane artificial lung via an a-v shunt for periods up to 96 hours. *Trans Am Soc Artif Int Organs* 1968;14:328–334.
65. Trudell LA, Friedman LI, Kakvan M, et al. Evaluation of a disposable membrane oxygenator. *Trans Am Soc Artif Int Organs* 1972;18:538–545.
66. Richardson PD, Galletti PM. Correlation of effects of blood flow rate, viscosity and design features on artificial lung performance. In: Dawids SG, Engell HC, eds. *Physiological and Clinical Aspects of Oxygenator Design, 29*. Luxembourg: Elsevier/North-Holland Biomedical Press; 1976.
67. Brinsfield DE, Hope MA, Geering RB, et al. Hematological changes in long term perfusion. *J Appl Physiol* 1962;17:531–534.

68. Friedman LI, Richardson PD, Galletti PM. *Blood Oxygenator Testing and Evaluation. Part II. Procedures and Results.* Bethesda, MD: Medical Devices Application Program, National Heart and Lung Institute; 1973. Report NIH-69-2047-2.
69. McCaughan JS Jr, Weeder R, Blakemore WS, et al. Evaluation of new non-wettable macroporous membranes with high permeability coefficients for possible use in a membrane oxygenator. *J Thorac Cardiovasc Surg* 1960;40:574–581.
70. Dantowitz P, Borsanyi AS, Deibert MD, et al. A blood oxygenator with preformed membrane-lined capillary channels. *Trans Am Soc Artif Int Organs* 1969;15:138–143.
71. Snider MT, Richardson PD, Friedman LI, et al. Studies of carbon dioxide transfer rate in artificial lungs. *J Appl Physiol* 1974;36:233–239.
72. Karlson KE, Murphy WRC, Kakvan M, et al. Total cardiopulmonary bypass with a new microporous Teflon membrane oxygenator. *Surgery* 1974;76:935–945.
73. Tanishita K, Nakano K, Richardson PD, et al. Augmentation of gas transfer with pulsatile flow in the coiled tube membrane oxygenator design. *Trans Am Soc Artif Int Organs* 1980;26:561–566.
74. Chenoweth DE, Cooper SW, Hugh TE, et al. Complement activation during CPB: evidence of generation of C3a and C5a anaphylatoxins. *N Engl J Med* 1981;304:497–506.
75. Kirklin JK, Westaby SW, Blackstone EH, et al. Complement and the damaging effects of cardiopulmonary bypass. *J Thorac Cardiovasc Surg* 1983;86:845–857.
76. Westaby SW. Organ dysfunction of cardiopulmonary bypass. A systemic inflammation reaction initiated by the extracorporeal circuit. *Intensive Care Med* 1987;13:89–95.
77. van Oeveren W, Wildevuur CRH, Kazatchkine MD. Biocompatibility of extracorporeal circuits in heart surgery. *Trans Sci* 1990;11:5–33.
78. Wachfogel YT, Kurick U, Greenplate J, et al. Human neutrophil degranulation during extracorporeal circulation. *Blood* 1987;69:324–330.
79. Gallin JR. Neutrophil specific granules: a fuse that ignites the inflammatory response. *Clin Res* 1984;32:320–328.
80. Antonsen S, Brandslund J, Clemensen S, et al. Neutrophil lysosomal enzyme release and complement activated during cardiopulmonary bypass. *Scand J Thorac Cardiovasc Surg* 1987;21:47–52.
81. Burrows FA, Steele RW, Marmer DJ, et al. Influence of operations with cardiopulmonary bypass on polymorphonuclear leukocyte function in infants. *J Thorac Cardiovasc Surg* 1987;93:253–260.
82. Lundstrom M, Olsson P, Unger P, et al. Effect of extracorporeal circulation on hematopoiesis and phagocytosis. *J Cardiovasc Surg* 1963;4:664–668.
83. Mayer JE Jr, McCullough J, Weiblen BJ, et al. Effects of cardiopulmonary bypass on neutrophil chemotaxis. *Surg Forum* 1976;27:285–287.
84. Haeffner-Cavaillon N, Roussellier N, Ponzio O, et al. Induction of interleukin-1 production in patients undergoing cardiopulmonary bypass. *J Thorac Cardiovasc Surg* 1988;22:51–53.
85. Rocatello D, Formica M, Cavalli G, et al. Changes in neutrophil oxidative potential in patients undergoing cardiopulmonary bypass with polypropylene hollow fiber oxygenators. *Artif Organs* 1990;14:69–72.
86. Plötz FB, van Oeveren W, Hultquist KA, et al. A heparin-coated circuit reduces complement activation and the release of leucocyte inflammatory mediators during extracorporeal circulation in a rabbit. *Artif Organs* 1992;16:366–370.
87. Bagley B, Bagley A, Henrie J, et al. Quantitative gas transfer into and out of circulating venous blood by means of an intravenacaval oxygenator. *Trans Am Soc Artif Int Organs* 1991;37:M413–415.
88. Gille JP. Personal communication, 1985.
89. Tamari Y, Tortolani AJ, Maquine M, et al. The effects of high pressure on microporous membrane oxygenator failure. *Artif Organs* 1991;15:15–22.
90. Nilsson L, Storm KE, Thelin S, et al. Heparin coated equipment reduces complement activation during cardiopulmonary bypass in the pig. *Artif Organs* 1990;14:46–48.
91. Videm V, Nilsson L, Venge P, et al. Reduced granulocyte activation with a heparin-coated device in an in vitro model of cardiopulmonary bypass. *Artif Organs* 1991;15:90–95.
92. Plötz FB, van Oeveren W, Hultquist KA, et al. A heparin-coated circuit reduces complement activation and the release of leucocyte inflammatory mediators during extracorporeal circulation in a rabbit. *Artif Organs* 1992;16:366–370.
93. von Saegesser LK, Weiss B, Garcia E, et al. Reduction and elimination of systemic heparinization during cardiopulmonary bypass. *J Thorac Cardiovasc Surg* 1992;103:790–799.
94. Gerbode F, Osborn JJ, Bramson ML. Experiments in the development of a membrane heart-lung machine. *Am J Surg* 1967;114:16–23.
95. Starr A, Edwards ML. Mitral replacement. A clinical experience with the ball valve prosthesis. *Ann Surg* 1961;154:726–746.

Part II
Physiology of Cardiopulmonary Bypass

2
The Myocardium: Physiology and Protection During Cardiac Surgery and Cardiopulmonary Bypass

Robert A. Guyton

Introduction

With the advent of endotracheal intubation and positive pressure ventilation in the 1940s, operative access to intrathoracic structures became possible. But the interior of the heart remained forbidden territory to the surgeon. Cardiopulmonary bypass (CPB) helped overcome this barrier, by temporarily substituting for the functions of the heart and lungs. But simple evacuation of blood from the perfused, beating heart did not provide suitable conditions for most cardiac surgery: aortic valve operations required that natural perfusion of the heart be stopped; precise coronary anastomoses could not be constructed upon the beating heart; and repair of complex congenital defects required a motionless, bloodless field. A breakthrough came when innovative surgeons developed systems for slowing or stopping the heart, facilitating exploration of its previously unknown interior.[1,2]

Goals of Myocardial Protection

The goal of myocardial protection techniques is to facilitate the operative repair of cardiac pathology by providing optimal operative conditions to the surgeon without damage to myocardial function.

Optimal operative conditions vary according to specific cardiac pathology and surgical requirements. For example, very difficult distal coronary anastomoses are best performed in a motionless, dry, bloodless operative field; mitral valve repair requires that left ventricular tone be maintained, so that the subvalvar apparatus may be appropriately adjusted; and repair of tetralogy of Fallot, via a right atrial incision, is facilitated by a flaccid, easily retracted heart.

Preservation of myocardial function presents different problems under various clinical conditions. Critical coronary stenoses may lead to acute myocardial ischemia upon induction of anesthesia, or initiation of CPB. The hypertrophied heart of aortic stenosis is especially vulnerable to ischemic damage, myocardial edema, and reperfusion injury. The failing myocardium that characterizes cardiogenic shock after infarction presents an opportunity to restore subcellular structure and integrity, not merely to preserve the preoperative status quo.

The clinical conduct of a cardiac operation is a compromise between ideal operative conditions and ideal myocardial preservation. The "optimal compromise" is unique for each clinical problem. The choice of a system of myocardial protection demands that the surgeon, anesthesiologist, and perfusionist understand both the clinical problem and a variety of myocardial protection techniques. This chapter will present a summary of basic concepts in myocardial protection, describe multiple clinical approaches to myocardial protection, and outline protection strategies appropriate for specific cardiac pathology.

Basic Concepts in Myocardial Protection

A useful analogy in understanding myocardial protection is to compare the heart to a swimmer who is asked to swim underwater through a long pipe from one lake to another. We can assume that before he undertook this effort, the swimmer would evaluate the length of the pipe and his own endurance and that he would demand some *margin of safety*. A conservative swimmer might insist that the pipe be no more than half as long as he is able to swim, while a very bold swimmer might not be concerned even if the pipe were almost as long as his longest effort. The bold swimmer is more likely to attempt the passage, but the conservative swimmer is less likely to drown. In myocardial protection, the heart must undertake a similar period of energy expenditure, without the ordinary means of energy supply. For each operation, the surgeon seeks an *adequate margin of safety*, such that the system of myocardial protection allows more time for the performance of the operative procedure than will be required. Just as a strong, well-rested swimmer can undertake a long passage through an underwater tunnel, a strong, metabolically prepared heart with a very simple system of myocardial protection can be subjected to a longer period of cardiac arrest. A weaker heart or a more complex operative procedure requires more sophisticated and individualized systems of myocardial protection, to give the patient an adequate margin of safety. This leads us to our first basic concept of myocardial protection. Just as the swimmer should not be asked to compete in a 500-meter race just prior to swimming through the underwater pipe, the heart should be well rested and well nourished prior to the interval of cardiac arrest.

Concept No. 1

Myocardial protection begins with preparation of the heart prior to arrest. Pre-CPB strategies to enhance myocardial protection are outlined in Table 2.1.

Metabolic Preparation

An unfortunate, but common, scenario includes a patient who is at the end of the operative schedule (his operation is difficult), whose operation is delayed (emergencies from the cardiac catheterization laboratory), and who becomes angry (too much delay). The patient, nutritionally deprived for over 14 hours, arrives in the operating room agitated, tachycardiac, hypoglycemic, and hypovolemic. This scenario can and should be prevented. Glucose loading prior to surgery increases glycogen stores and improves the heart's ability to tolerate ischemic arrest.[3,4] If the operation is scheduled for the afternoon, there is considerable advantage to giving IV glucose during the morning. Glucose, insulin, and potassium loading may provide further benefit, but, at the very least, some consideration should be given to IV glucose therapy preoperatively.

Hemodynamic Preparation

Induction of anesthesia, particularly in a hypovolemic patient with marginal cardiac function, is hazardous. Some studies have shown that myocardial damage begins in as many as 18% of patients *prior to the initiation of CPB*.[5] A smooth anesthetic induction, without tachycardia or hypotension, is especially important in patients with hypertrophied hearts and in patients with coronary artery disease.[2]

Cardiopulmonary bypass is particularly threatening to patients with coronary artery disease,[1] since *hypotension* often occurs when it is initiated. A mean blood pressure less than 60 mm Hg may lead to subendocardial ischemia, even in normal hearts,[6] and in hearts with coronary stenoses this harmful effect is exacerbated.[7-9] CPB also results in *hemodilution*, which has been shown to cause a coronary steal from vulnerable subendocardium in the presence of collateralized myocardium.[10,11] *Hypothermia* may eliminate the ability of the heart to autoregulate local blood flow, and it also leads to hypoperfusion of vulnerable areas.[12,13] *Ventricular fibrillation*, which often occurs as the heart is manipulated or cooled, can lead to subendocardial ischemia, particularly in hypertrophied hearts and those with coronary stenoses.[14-18] *Ventricular distention* may also accompany the initiation of CPB, resulting in decreased blood flow to the inner layers of the heart. An abnormally elevated preload is particularly threatening to the myocardium during ventricular fibrillation and during intervals of arterial hypotension. Ventricular distention is less threatening during the cardioplegic arrest interval, but it should be assiduously avoided prior to cardioplegic arrest.[19,20]

Ideally, CPB should be instituted *with coronary perfusion pressure maintained at prebypass levels*, as systemic cooling is accomplished. If hypotension does occur, α-adrenergic agonists (phenylephrine, norepinephrine) should be given to restore systemic blood pressure and coronary perfusion pressure. Unfortunately, these drugs have their own deleterious effects, with decreased blood flow to the subendocardium of collateralized regions.[8]

If ventricular distention occurs with the initiation of CPB, when the surgeon is not yet ready to arrest the heart, the heart should be vented.[2] The left ventricle can be vented either by active venting (placement of a suction catheter within the left atrium, left ventricle, or pulmonary artery) or by passive venting (placement of a catheter without suction or simply cutting a hole in the left atrium or pulmonary artery) (Figures 2.1 and 2.2). After cardioplegic arrest has been accomplished, venting may be

TABLE 2.1. Techniques and interventions to prepare the myocardium for induced arrest.

Metabolic preparation	Hydration
	Glucose loading
Hemodynamic preparation	Treat tachycardia with β-blockade
	Maintain coronary perfusion
	Phenylephrine
	Norephinephrine
Pharmacologic preparation	β-Blockers
	Propranolol
	Esmolol
	Lidoflazine
	CA^{2+} channel blockers
	Nifedipine
	Diltiazem
	Verapamil

achieved by active or passive venting of the aorta. The danger of active venting (suction) is that air is often introduced into the intracardiac chambers, and careful de-airing maneuvers must be carried out prior to ventricular ejection.[21,22]

Importantly, the prearrest CPB interval is a period during which myocardial cell integrity may be either greatly *compromised* or *enhanced*. If blood pressure is maintained, the heart can be rested and metabolically restored, but if hypotension occurs, the metabolic state of the heart begins to deteriorate. *In the presence of hypotension, the prearrest CPB interval should be kept short.* Cardioplegic arrest is much better for the heart than a prolonged interval of hypotension while cooling on the pump.

Pharmacologic Preparation

Early in the evolution of cardiac surgery, it was recognized that hypertrophied hearts are particularly vulnerable to ischemic contracture (a "stone heart"),[23] which could be prevented by administration of propranolol, a β-blocker. The reasons for the effectiveness of this intervention were incompletely understood, but it was one of the first important pharmacologic interventions to prepare the heart prior to ischemic arrest. β-Blockade decreases the metabolic rate of the heart, allowing nutritional replenishment of the myocardium prior to the arrest inter-

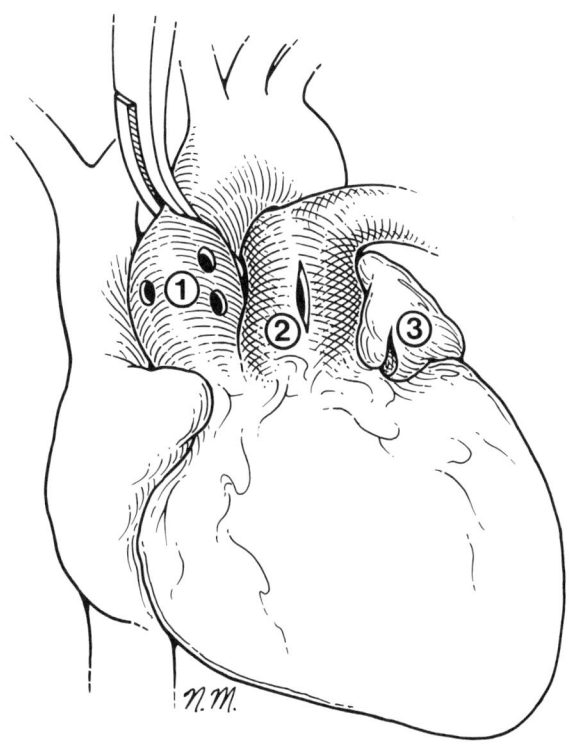

FIGURE 2.2. Three techniques for passive venting are depicted: (1) Passive venting may be accomplished by punching holes for proximal anastomoses into the aorta soon after placement of the aortic crossclamp. This allows passive venting of the aorta and left ventricle. (2) An incision may be made into the pulmonary artery to allow blood to passively flow from the pulmonary artery during the procedure. (3) An incision may be made in the tip of the left atrial appendage to allow blood to flow passively from the left atrium during the procedure. Techniques 2 and 3 may be used both before and after the crossclamp interval.

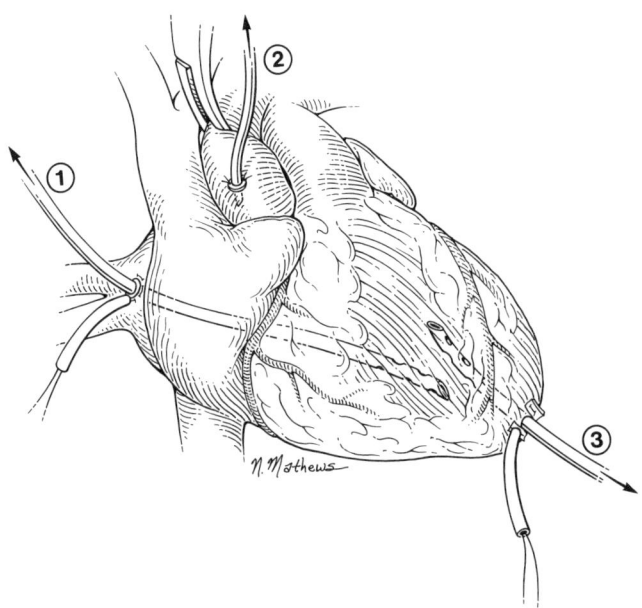

FIGURE 2.1. Three techniques for active venting are depicted: (1) A suction catheter is placed via the right superior pulmonary veins across the mitral valve into the left ventricle. (2) The cardioplegia catheter in the ascending aorta is placed on suction to vent the aorta and left ventricle. (3) A suction catheter is placed via the left ventricular apex into the left ventricle.

val.[24,25] Moreover, the metabolic rate prior to arrest seems to determine, in part, the metabolic rate during arrest.[26] Therefore, the heart not only enters the arrest interval in a stronger state, but the rate of nutritional depletion during the arrest interval is also decreased. β-Blockade with either propranolol or new, more specific β-blockers (esmolol) remains a very useful adjunct to virtually all techniques of myocardial protection. β-Blockade can be initiated after the patient has been placed on CPB, eliminating the threat of hemodynamic compromise. The author routinely uses propranolol, 5 mg IV, with the initiation of CPB in every patient with hypertrophied heart. Another instance in which β-blockade is particularly useful is in a patient who is metabolically hyperactive at the time of initiation of CPB. Isoproterenol pretreatment has been shown to be detrimental to myocardial recovery. The patient in cardiogenic shock, with tachycardia and massive sympathetic stimulation, may be similarly threatened.[27]

β-Blockade, upon initiation of CPB, decreases the metabolic rate of the heart acutely and allows replenishment of myocardial metabolic stores just prior to the arrest interval. β-Blockade should be considered in all patients with heart rates above 90 beats per minute at the initiation of CPB.

A number of other drugs have been tested as adjuncts to cardioplegic and myocardial protection techniques. Particularly notable among these drugs are lidoflazine and calcium channel blockers, such as nifedipine, diltiazem, and verapamil.[28-33] These drugs extend the heart's tolerance of ischemia and seem to increase the margin of safety with most myocardial protection techniques. Corticosteroids may be beneficial in preventing damage during ischemic arrest, but this benefit has been difficult to demonstrate.[1] Membrane stabilization with lidocaine or procaine seems to be useful, particularly in preventing postoperative arrhythmias.[34] Table 2.1 lists drugs that may improve myocardial preservation when given prior to cardioplegic arrest.

Concept No. 2

Metabolic requirements should be reduced during the arrest interval. Methods of decreasing myocardial metabolism during CPB are listed in Table 2.2.

Once the heart has been made as strong as possible prior to ischemic arrest, the second consideration is the reduction of the metabolic expenditure during the actual arrest interval. In the case of our swimmer, this means that the tunnel through which he must swim should be as short as possible. In the case of the heart, it means that a speedy surgeon, by keeping the arrest interval short, can reduce the total metabolic need during the arrest interval. Speed, however, is not always consistent with the execution of a precise cardiac operation. A meticulously executed operation is at least as important for the patient's long-term survival as a speedy operation. For this reason, the reduction of the *rate* of metabolism during the arrest interval has been a particularly effective method of reducing metabolic requirements during arrest. The two techniques most widely employed for this purpose are myocardial hypothermia and chemical (usually hyperkalemic) cardiac arrest.

Hypothermia

Hypothermia has been prominently employed in myocardial protection techniques since the beginning of heart surgery.[35] For every 10°C of temperature reduction in biologic systems, the metabolic rate of chemical processes is reduced by approximately a factor of two. Cardiac cooling may be accomplished with systemic cooling, iced saline irrigation, ice slush placed around the heart, cooling pads placed around the heart, or perfusion hypothermia (infusing cold blood or cardioplegic solutions directly into the coronary arteries or veins). All of these techniques are effective; however, the most efficient method of cooling the heart is perfusion hypothermia. Studies have shown that very cold solutions (as cold as 2°C) may be infused into the heart without damage to the myocardium. Considerable controversy exists, however, on the optimal level of myocardial cooling. With crystalloid solutions, myocardial temperatures as cold as 4°C have been achieved with nearly complete subsequent recovery. The optimal myocardial temperature for hypothermic blood solutions is probably a little higher (15° to 20°C). One disadvantage of perfusion hypothermia is that the heart is cooled in a heterogeneous manner, as the perfusate is heterogeneously delivered to the heart following the paths of least resistance. For example, if the right coronary artery is occluded, the right coronary region is poorly perfused, poorly cooled, and therefore not well protected.[36] Heterogeneous cardioplegic infusion leads to regionally variable myocardial recovery.[37] Addition of a topical hypothermic technique, such as local irrigation of the pericardium, ice slush, or cooling pads, greatly improves the homogeneity of myocardial cooling and is an important component of hypothermic techniques of myocardial protection.[38-40]

Systemic cooling can also be utilized to enhance myocardial cooling; it is particularly important in preventing the rewarming of the myocardium which occurs after the initial infusion of cold perfusate. Because of this rewarming, additional doses of cold solution are usually infused into the myocardium every 10 to 20 minutes. As a system of hypothermic myocardial protection is being developed, it is useful to monitor intramyocardial temperature with a temperature probe, using perfusion hypothermia and local cooling to maintain the myocardial temperature at 10° to 15°C. This is critically important if hypothermia alone is the primary method of myocardial protection.

There are problems with hypothermia which are incompletely understood. Metabolic processes in the myocar-

TABLE 2.2. Methods of decreasing myocardial metabolism during CPB.

Myocardial hypothermia	Cold solution infused into coronary arteries
	Antegrade
	Retrograde
	Local hypothermia
	Ice slush
	Local irrigation
	Cooling pads
	Systemic hypothermia
Cardioplegic arrest	Hyperkalemic solutions $[K^+] = 20\text{–}30$ mEq/L

dium are generally in balance at 37°C. As the heart is cooled, different chemical reactions undergo varying decreases in reaction rates. In particular, the rate of high-energy reactions, such as the ATP-requiring sodium-potassium pump, may be reduced four to six times for every 10°C reduction, in contrast to a decrease in the general metabolic rate of only two times per 10°C temperature decrease. Thus, as the heart is cooled, there is a gross disruption of myocardial homeostasis. Supplying oxygen and nutrients to a heart at 28°C will *not* result in the maintenance of all normal cellular functions of the myocardium, since the necessary chemical reactions are grossly out of balance. A hypothermic heart is a heart with a greatly reduced metabolic rate, but *one should never consider a hypothermic heart to be a metabolically intact heart.*[41]

Cardioplegic Arrest

One of the most effective ways of reducing metabolism is cardioplegic arrest. Oxygen consumption of the chemically arrested heart is approximately one fifth that of the empty, beating heart at 37°C. Indeed, as can be seen in Figure 2.3, oxygen consumption of the asystolic heart at 37°C is less than that of either the empty, beating heart or the fibrillating heart at 22°C.[42] A variety of solutions have been used for chemical arrest of the heart, but hyperkalemic solutions are the most widely used. The optimal potassium concentration for hyperkalemic arrest appears to be between 20 and 30 mEq/L. Higher concentrations of potassium may be damaging to the heart, particularly to the endothelium of the coronary vasculature.[43] Lower levels of potassium have been used to maintain cardioplegic arrest.[44] Subclinical electrical activity may resume in the heart with these lower levels of potassium, leading to increased oxygen consumption not apparent to the surgeon.[45]

Concept No. 3

A favorable metabolic milieu during arrest helps provide a margin of safety with reduced metabolism.

First, Do No Harm

Although metabolism may be profoundly reduced (and profoundly altered) during ischemic arrest, metabolism does continue, and it is important to provide a favorable metabolic milieu during this time interval. This has been accomplished, in general, by infusion of a cardioplegic solution into the coronary arteries. Requirements of cardioplegic solutions are summarized in Table 2.3. This solution is altered, not only to induce chemical cardiac arrest, but also to prevent damage to the heart during the arrest interval. It should also prevent interstitial and intracellular edema, prevent the loss of metabolites from the cell, maintain an appropriate acid-base balance, and, above all, *cause no further damage to myocardial cells.* Unfortunately, a number of solutions that have been used for clinical myocardial protection are cytotoxic.[46] This is particularly true of solutions that are dissimilar from interstitial fluid. These solutions may be successful in experimental situations, where carefully measured dosages may be uniformly delivered to the myocardium. In clinical situations, however, heterogeneous delivery of cardioplegia (because of coronary stenoses and hypertrophied myocardium) leads to underdosage of some regions of the myocardium and gross overdosage of other regions. The cardioplegic solution must, therefore, be protective and nondamaging both in low doses and in high doses: the effect must *not* be dose dependent.

A second important consideration in coronary operations is the effect of noncoronary collateral flow.[47] Even with the aorta crossclamped, some blood flow returns (in varying degrees) to the coronary vasculature, washing out cardioplegic solutions. If the basic cardioplegic solution

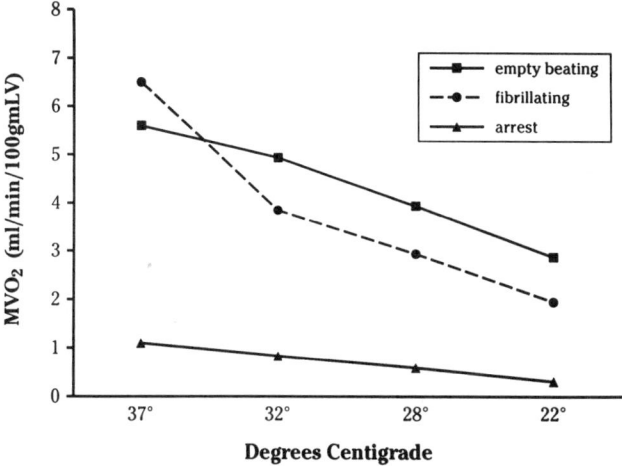

FIGURE 2.3. Oxygen consumption of the empty beating heart, the fibrillating heart, and the potassium-arrested heart at four different myocardial temperatures. Note that the potassium-arrested heart has the lowest oxygen consumption at any temperature. The empty beating heart has a higher oxygen consumption than does the fibrillating heart at a temperature below 32°C.[42]

TABLE 2.3. Requirements of cardioplegic solutions.

Induce myocardial arrest
Maintain favorable metabolic milieu
    Prevent interstitial and intracellular edema
    Prevent loss of cellular metabolites
    Maintain appropriate acid-base balance
    Provide metabolic substrate (oxygen and glucose)
Noncytotoxic

differs greatly from either blood or interstitial fluid, then the heart is exposed to wide fluctuations in the biochemical environment of the myocytes, as cardioplegic solution is infused, washed out, reinfused, washed out, reinfused, and washed out again. These considerations—the need for a noncytotoxic solution, the heterogeneity of cardioplegic infusion, and noncoronary collateral flow—mean that the basic cardioplegic solution should mimic either blood or interstitial fluid, with small amounts of other components added. Crystalloid cardioplegic solutions containing low sodium concentrations (<80 mEq/L) or very high dextrose concentrations (>400 mg%) should be avoided. Such solutions may be very successful in experimental situations (in which normal hearts may be protected in vivo under precise conditions), in experimental isolated heart situations, and in clinical transplant situations (where the heart is isolated). But in most clinical situations, where pathology varies from heart to heart, solutions that are greatly different from either interstitial fluid or blood may be hazardous.

The appropriate calcium concentration of cardioplegic solutions has been extensively studied, since intracellular and intramitochondrial calcium is prominent in ischemic damage. The appropriate level of calcium appears to be low, but some calcium should be present.[38-50]

Removal of Acid

Cardiac arrest usually leads to anaerobic metabolism with production of hydrogen ion (H^+) and lactic acid.[51] As the pH of the myocardium falls, metabolic reactions necessary for preservation of cellular integrity are shut down. Extremes of acidosis are usually associated with poor recovery after cardioplegic arrest. Therefore, most cardioplegic solutions contain some means of removing acid from the heart.

The most common buffer system used in crystalloid solutions is bicarbonate (HCO_3^-). For proper adjustment of pH in a cardioplegic solution with a bicarbonate buffer, some carbon dioxide (CO_2) must be equilibrated with the bicarbonate. Carbon dioxide is generated by aerobic metabolism and is also generated as hydrogen ions combine with the bicarbonate ion. Some investigators believe the crystalloid solution should be equilibrated with carbon dioxide–containing gases in order to prevent delivery of an excessively high-pH solution to the myocardium.[52-54]

Other buffer systems that have been advocated are Tham (tris(hydroxymethyl)aminomethane) and histidine, which have the advantage of improved transport across cellular membranes. In intact cells, there can be a considerable gradient between intracellular and extracellular pH, and there may be some advantage to buffer systems that can cross the cell membrane.[55,56]

Nutrient and Oxygen Supply During Cardioplegic Arrest

In some circumstances (for example, in preservation of the heart for transplantation), the heart can be arrested and myocardial metabolism can be almost completely shut down. In most clinical circumstances, however, clinical cardioplegia is heterogeneous (particularly with washout of cardioplegic solution related to noncoronary collateral flow), and some regions of the heart remain either fairly warm or incompletely arrested during some portion of the cardioplegic arrest interval. The heart does utilize oxygen during cardioplegic arrest, indicating continuation of metabolism, and lactate is produced, indicating that anaerobic metabolism also occurs. Therefore, as metabolism continues, the necessary substrates should be supplied. Oxygenation of both crystalloid and blood solutions has been shown to improve myocardial protection, particularly during longer intervals of cardioplegic arrest.[57-62] Most cardioplegic solutions, both crystalloid and blood, also contain glucose to provide substrate for metabolism.[63-65]

Blood Cardioplegia

Blood-based cardioplegic solutions have potential advantages, since blood provides trace elements, proteins, and enzymes that may not be found in analogs of interstitial fluid.[56,66] Blood provides a very effective protein buffering system for removal of acid, and it contains natural nutrients for the heart as well as large quantities of oxygen. The advantages of a blood cardioplegic solution are particularly important if a warm cardioplegic arrest circumstance is encountered. As noted above, some regions of the heart may be warm and metabolically active even when hypothermia is employed. In these circumstances, perfusion with blood is most likely superior to that with a crystalloid-based solution. If a warm cardioplegic arrest is utilized for myocardial protection, a blood-based solution should be used, since it offers an excellent means of providing oxygen, nutrients, buffers, and trace elements to the heart. However, if one relies upon profound myocardial hypothermia for myocardial protection, then a blood-based solution has certain disadvantages. Oxygen becomes tightly bound to hemoglobin at low temperatures so that the oxygen-binding capacity of hemoglobin becomes a disadvantage, rather than an advantage, at low temperatures.[67] Also, blood-based solutions present some difficulty in precise visualization of distal coronary anastomoses.

Blood cardioplegia appears to have a clear advantage over that with crystalloid solutions in the resuscitation of damaged myocardium. If the heart is exposed to an ischemic insult prior to the cardioplegic arrest interval, the use of blood cardioplegia, particularly warm blood cardioplegia, can resuscitate the myocardium during the arrest interval, leading to better recovery of myocardial function and structure.[68-70]

Concept No. 4

Reperfusion modification after an ischemic insult can minimize structural and functional damage to the myocardium.

After an ischemic insult, reperfusion of the heart with an unmodified blood solution may lead to explosive cell swelling, rapid and irreversible accumulation of intracellular calcium, ischemic contracture, and extensive cellular necrosis. Modification of the reperfusion conditions can reduce the subsequent loss of myocyte function and structure.[68-74]

Several factors have been shown to be important in reperfusion modification:

1. Metabolic requirements during reperfusion should be reduced by chemical cardioplegic arrest during the first 10 minutes of reperfusion.[75] Metabolic requirements should be further minimized by maintaining the heart in an empty, beating state for an additional 20 to 30 minutes before it is required to begin working.[76,77]
2. Abundant oxygen and substrate should be supplied for metabolic replenishment and aerobic metabolism.[78,79] Glutamate has been shown to be particularly important as a substrate for metabolism after an ischemic insult.[80,81] Aspartate may also be beneficial, although the evidence is less convincing.[82,83]
3. Relative hypocalcemia seems to prevent the rapid influx of calcium into myocytes in the first 5 to 10 minutes of reperfusion. After this interval, the metabolic integrity of cellular membranes is restored, and it is not so important to maintain low calcium levels. In particular, *hyper*calcemia in the first few minutes of reperfusion should be avoided.
4. An acidotic reperfusate seems to be inferior to an alkalotic reperfusate. This may be related to the ability of an alkalotic reperfusate to more rapidly restore intracellular pH to normal levels.
5. Oxygen-derived free radicals may be important in early reperfusion.[84] Xanthine oxidase inhibitors may reduce free-radical formation.[85] If the conditions of reperfusion are acidotic, the superoxide free radical is likely to be present and superoxide dismutase may be an important free-radical scavenger. In most clinical situations, an alkalotic reperfusate is used and the hydroxyl free radical predominates. In this situation, superoxide dismutase is less effective, and hydroxyl free radical scavengers, such as mannitol, are more effective.[86,87]
6. Leukocyte depletion may decrease damage consequent to reperfusion of ischemic myocardium by minimizing the acute local inflammatory response that occurs with reperfusion of ischemically damaged muscle. Table 2.4 summarizes methods and interventions that may be employed in the reperfusion period to reduce myocyte damage.

A number of concepts of reperfusion modification, mentioned above, have been tested in animal models. The benefits of reperfusion modification, at least under controlled experimental conditions, are demonstrable in both acute and chronic situations. The degree of benefit realized by reperfusion modification is variable, depending upon the animal model utilized. In pigs, very little collateral flow to infarcted regions exists, and minimal benefit from reperfusion modification can be realized after 60 to 90 minutes of ischemia. In dogs, natural epicardial collaterals exist, and considerable benefit can be realized from reperfusion modification after 2 hours of total coronary occlusion.[68,70] Some benefit may be realized as long as 6 hours after coronary occlusion in a canine model.[69] In humans, surgical reperfusion has resulted in improvement of regional ejection fraction with reperfusion 6 to 8 hours after infarction. This benefit seems to occur in those regions made ischemic by subtotal coronary occlusion or those regions receiving some collateral flow into the infarcted region. Without this limited inflow into the infarcted region, only minimal benefit was realized from late (>6 hours) surgical reperfusion.[88]

Clinical Systems for Myocardial Protection

Four very different systems for myocardial protection have been shown to be effective in clinical situations. Each of these systems utilizes the basic concepts discussed above, but the focus of each system is different. The first system, hypothermia with fibrillatory arrest, relies almost entirely upon hypothermia to decrease metabolic requirements. The second system, oxygenated cold crystalloid cardioplegia, relies heavily upon hypothermia and cardioplegic arrest to reduce metabolic requirements, with minimal emphasis upon metabolic supply. The third system,

TABLE 2.4. Methods of reducing myocyte damage during reperfusion.

1. Maintain or reinstitute cardioplegic arrest (first 10 minutes)
2. Provide oxygen and substrates (glutamate) for aerobic metabolism
3. Maintain relative hypocalcemia (first 5 to 10 minutes)
4. Avoid acidotic reperfusate
5. Consider oxygen free-radical scavenging (superoxide dismutase) and hydroxyl free-radical scavenging (mannitol)
6. Consider leukocyte removal from reperfusate

cold blood cardioplegia, relies less heavily upon hypothermia, but places more emphasis upon metabolic supply. The final system, continuous warm blood cardioplegia, utilizes cardioplegic arrest and decreased metabolic needs, does not utilize hypothermia at all, and focuses upon continuous metabolic supply. Each of these techniques has specific advantages and disadvantages in different clinical situations.

Hypothermia with Fibrillatory Arrest

Simple cooling of the heart, without chemical cardioplegia, was one of the early systems of myocardial protection, and still may be useful in certain clinical situations. Some surgeons use this technique as their primary system of myocardial protection.[89-91] If this technique is used, *attention to detail is crucial*. First, adequate myocardial cooling is essential. Since the heart continues to be perfused when this system of myocardial protection is used, myocardial cooling necessarily means systemic cooling. Ordinarily, systemic cooling is employed to 20° to 25°C. The heart is allowed to fibrillate as the body is cooled.

Second, active venting is always employed in order to prevent myocardial distention. This technique cannot be used if aortic regurgitation prevents adequate decompression of the left ventricle. Active venting is usually accomplished by a vent placed into the left ventricle via the right superior pulmonary vein. Such active venting poses a threat to the patient if negative intracavitary pressure occurs and air is introduced into the left atrium or left ventricle. This air is difficult to remove at the end of the operation. For this reason, several practitioners of this technique monitor the pressure within the left ventricle and maintain a positive intracavitary pressure of at least 5 mm Hg.

A third critical feature of this technique is that coronary perfusion must be maintained. Perfusion pressure is generally maintained at 80 mm Hg by systemic infusion of α-adrenergic agents. This provides enough oxygen and nutrients to the fibrillating, hypothermic myocardium to prevent myocardial damage. With these conditions—systemic hypothermia at 20° to 25°C, careful decompression of the heart with active venting, and maintenance of perfusion pressure at 80 mm Hg—excellent clinical results have been obtained. If one fails to cool or vent adequately, *or* fails to maintain perfusion pressures, described above, equivalent results should not be expected. Table 2.5 summarizes the clinical features of hypothermia with fibrillatory arrest for myocardial protection.

Oxygenated Cold Crystalloid Cardioplegia

Oxygenated crystalloid cardioplegia is a very effective and simple technique of myocardial protection.[61,88,92,93] A number of different solutions have been proposed for

TABLE 2.5. Clinical features of myocardial protection with hypothermia and fibrillatory arrest.

Systemic cooling (20°–25°C)
Active venting (intracavitary pressure at least 5 mm Hg)
Adequate coronary perfusion pressure (80 mm Hg)

crystalloid cardioplegia. As discussed above, the basic solution for cold crystalloid cardioplegia should be an analog of interstitial fluid. The compositions of two common crystalloid solutions are given in Table 2.6. The St. Thomas solution has been extensively used and is commercially available.[94] The solution described in the second column of the table is readily available by making small additions to commercially available interstitial fluid analogs.[61] The use of commercially available base solutions greatly reduces the risk of a catastrophic error in pharmacologic preparation of cardioplegic solutions. Because some commercially available solutions have a variable pH, bicarbonate or Tham should be added just prior to cardioplegic infusion. The potassium level of crystalloid cardioplegia should be 20 to 25 mEq/L, and the solution should be oxygenated. Our practice is to oxygenate the solution with 100% oxygen, but others advocate a gas mixture containing a small amount of carbon dioxide to provide a more reliable pH.[52,53,59] The final cardioplegic solution should be cooled to 2° to 4°C by circulation through a coil immersed in an ice bath. Infusion of 1 L of this cold solution (an initial infusion volume of approximately 15 mL/kg) leads to myocardial temperatures (in a normal-sized heart) of less than 15°C. Larger volumes may be necessary for larger hearts. Moderate systemic hypothermia (25° to 28°C) helps in myocardial cooling and prevents rewarming. Local irrigation of the pericardium with a very cold solution (again using an interstitial fluid analog) greatly enhances the homogeneity of myocardial cooling. In coronary bypass operations, the cardioplegic solution should be infused into each vein graft as it is completed. For longer crossclamp intervals, reinfusion of the solution into the aorta every 15 to 20 minutes is appropriate. Monitoring of myocardial temperature and maintaining the temperature below 15°C increase the margin of safety with this technique. Infusion of a dose of cardioplegia just prior to removal of the crossclamp (or infusion of cardioplegic solution into the aortic root with the crossclamp partially removed) assures that the heart will be metabolically quiescent for the first few minutes of reperfusion.

The infusion pressure appropriate for crystalloid cardioplegia varies with the clinical situation. In patients with very severe coronary disease, the infusion pressure should be increased to 100 to 150 mm Hg. In patients without coronary disease, an infusion pressure of 70 mm Hg is more appropriate.[95] Infusion pressures as high as 150 mm Hg

TABLE 2.6. Crystalloid cardioplegic composition.[a]

	St. Thomas solution[92]	Solution made by modification of balanced electrolyte solution[59]
Sodium	120	160
Chloride	160	98
Potassium	16	30
Calcium	1.2	0
Magnesium	16	3
Bicarbonate	10	20
Glucose	0	150 mg%

[a]Concentration in mmol/L except as noted.

have been tolerated without excessive myocardial edema or subsequent myocardial damage.[96]

Retrograde infusion of crystalloid cardioplegic solution via the coronary sinus is possible and particularly useful during valve operations or during reoperative coronary bypass surgery (Figure 2.4).[97-100] In the case of valve operations, use of coronary sinus retrograde infusion allows the valve procedure to be accomplished without interruption for subsequent cardioplegic infusion. In the case of coronary reoperations, retrograde infusion of cardioplegic solutions via the coronary sinus helps to flush out possible debris in the distal coronary arteries. This debris may embolize to the distal coronary circulation as a result of manipulation of old bypass grafts.

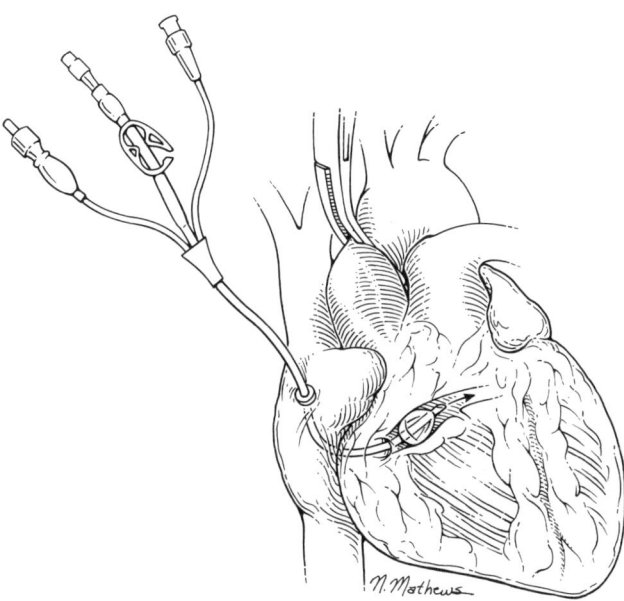

FIGURE 2.4. Placement of a retrograde coronary sinus catheter. The catheter is placed, through a small incision, into the right atrium and then into the coronary sinus. Inflation of a balloon occludes the coronary sinus, so that infusion of cardioplegic solution through a central channel leads to pressurized infusion of cardioplegic solution into the coronary sinus.

Cold Blood Cardioplegia

Cold blood cardioplegia has been a very successful cardioplegic technique[56,66] in which an infusion circuit (Figure 2.5) mixes blood from the pump oxygenator with a crystalloid solution to achieve a blood-crystalloid mixture with a hematocrit of 16 to 20, a potassium level of 20 to 25, a low calcium level, and an alkaline pH. Substrate enhancement (glucose, glutamate, aspartate, etc) is also possible. Table 2.7 gives an example of the cold blood cardioplegic solution popularized by Buckberg and colleagues.[56]

Several practitioners of blood cardioplegia advocate the use of a warm infusion at the beginning of the crossclamp interval.[101] This warm infusion is designed to replenish a metabolically depleted myocardium prior to the hypothermic arrest interval. Ordinarily, warm blood cardioplegic solution is infused for 5 minutes with a pressure of 50 mm Hg. Subsequently, the temperature of the cardioplegic infusate is reduced to 5° to 8°C by circulating it through a coil immersed in ice water or iced saline. The optimal temperature for blood cardioplegia (and the optimal temperature for the myocardium protected by blood cardioplegia) is probably slightly higher than the optimal temperature for crystalloid techniques.[102] The heart is cooled to 15° to 18°C. Prior to removal of the aortic crossclamp, warm blood cardioplegic solution is infused, restoring the metabolic state of the heart prior to unmodified blood reperfusion. This infusion is continued for 3 to 5 minutes, and it is particularly important because, as explained earlier, the cold heart is metabolically out of balance. When the crossclamp is removed, chemical cardioplegic arrest gradually dissipates and the heart begins to contract.

The technique of cold blood cardioplegia described requires a cardioplegic infusion circuit. Because a crystalloid solution is mixed with blood from the pump reservoir as it is infused into the patient, this technique usually allows only a single pass through the cooling coil prior to infusion into the patient. Therefore, cardioplegia temperatures are not as low as those usually achieved with crystalloid infusions. Also, since both a warm infusion and a cold infusion are desirable, a separate heat exchanger is

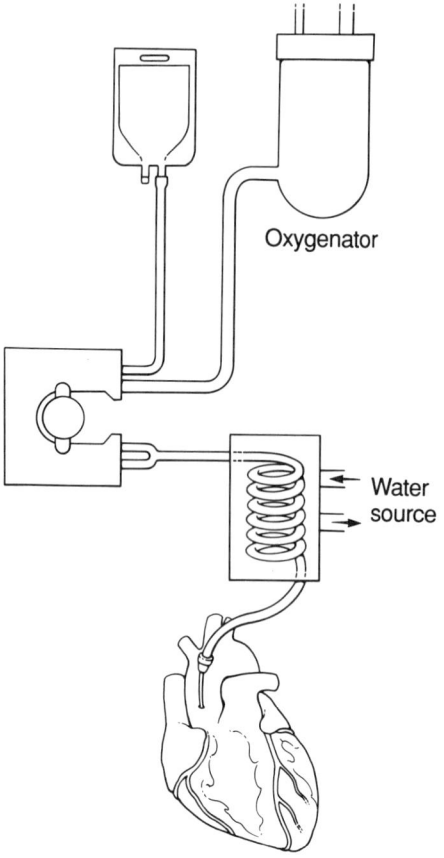

FIGURE 2.5. Schematic diagram of a blood cardioplegia circuit. Blood is taken from the oxygenator and mixed with cardioplegic solution from an intravenous fluid bag. The special roller pump uses calibrated tubing to mix the solutions in a predetermined manner (usually 4:1 blood-to-crystalloid mix). The solution is then passed through a coil and a heat exchanger to adjust the temperature of the solution prior to delivery into the ascending or the coronary sinus.

TABLE 2.7. Cold blood cardioplegic solution (Buckberg).[56]

Crystalloid component	
Glucose	16.2 g/L
Potassium	50 mEq/L
Tham	78 mmol/L
Magnesium	0
Citrate phosphate dextrose (CPD)	65 mL
Aspartate	10.1 g/L
Glutamate	11.0 g/L
Final concentration after 4:1 mix with blood	
Glucose	350 mg/dL
Potassium	14 mEq/L
Ionic Ca^{2+}	~1.0 mmol/L
Magnesium	1–1.5 mmol/L

TABLE 2.8. Warm blood cardioplegic solution.[105]

Crystalloid component	
Glucose	1 L of 5% dextrose solution
Potassium	High: 100 mEq/L
	Low: 30 mEq/L
Tham	12 mmol/L
Magnesium	18 mEq/L
Citrate Phosphate Dextrose (CPD)	20 mL
Final concentration after 4:1 mix with blood	
Glucose	50 mmol/L
Potassium	High: 22 mEq/L
	Low: 9 mEq/L
Ionic Ca^{2+}	0.7 mmol/L
Magnesium	3 mmol/L

required for the cardioplegic infusion circuit. Moderate systemic hypothermia and local cold irrigation are useful adjuncts to cold blood cardioplegia as one attempts to achieve homogeneous cooling of the myocardium.

Continuous Warm Blood Cardioplegia

Warm blood cardioplegia, a relatively recently popularized technique of myocardial protection,[54,64,103-105] has several theoretical advantages. First, most of the reduction of metabolic rate with cardioplegic techniques is achieved by chemical arrest of the heart (Figure 2.3). The warm blood cardioplegic technique utilizes chemical arrest, thereby greatly reducing the need for myocardial blood flow. Second, by maintaining the heart in a warm condition, its metabolic integrity is preserved. The heart arrested with warm blood cardioplegia is a metabolically intact heart, and the chemical processes necessary for maintenance of cellular integrity are in balance. Since the heart is perfused in a warm, arrested state, this technique is particularly applicable when the heart has been damaged by ischemia prior to the arrest interval. The entire arrest interval represents a period of myocardial resuscitation, when continuous warm blood cardioplegia is used. With cold blood techniques, the interval of myocardial resuscitation is limited, because hypothermia compromises the chemical processes necessary for cellular resuscitation.

Warm blood cardioplegia is administered by mixing blood from the arterial line of the pump oxygenator with a crystalloid cardioplegic solution, usually in approximately a 4:1 mixture, and infusing this mixture into the ascending aorta after aortic crossclamping (Table 2.8). Cardioplegic arrest is usually achieved with a high-potassium solution (final potassium concentration of approximately 30 mEq/L) infused at approximately 300 mL/min (ascending aortic pressure of approximately 70 mm Hg). Cardioplegic arrest is then maintained by continuing both antegrade and retrograde infusions of a low-potassium solution (final potassium concentration of approximately 11 mEq/L) into the ascending aorta (at approximately 200 mL/min) or into the coronary sinus (maintaining a coronary sinus pressure of approximately 40 mm Hg, at approximately 150 mL/min flow). Occasionally, cardioplegic arrest is not maintained by the low-potassium solution, and an additional dose of high-potassium solution is necessary. The warm blood technique usually leads to excellent recovery of myocardial function if nutrient flow has been adequate. If nutrient flow is inadequate (for example, if the surgeon does not notice a dislodged coronary sinus catheter), the heart may suffer a potentially catastrophic warm ischemic interval. A very hypertrophied heart may be susceptible to relative hypoperfusion when a warm blood protection technique is used. Intramyocardial muscle tone is maintained and the inner layers of the heart may be hypoperfused, resulting in an interval of warm ischemia.

A major problem with the continuous warm blood technique is difficulty in visualization of distal coronary anastomoses. Some surgeons use a carbon dioxide gas jet, and others discontinue cardioplegic infusion during critical portions of distal anastomoses.[106] This is obviously a threat to the heart, since it suffers short intervals of warm ischemia while the cardioplegic solution is not being infused. These short intervals are generally well tolerated (for 2 to 10 minutes), but the margin of safety for this modification of the continuous warm technique has not been well defined. (Warm blood cardioplegia is discussed in Chapter 34.)

Adaptation of Myocardial Protection Techniques to Cardiac Pathology

The remainder of this chapter will present specific clinical problems and appropriate strategies for clinical myocardial protection using the basic concepts and clinical systems described above.

Coronary Artery Disease

With Good Left Ventricular Function

The patient with coronary artery disease and good left ventricular function challenges myocardial protection techniques. This situation is challenging, not because results are poor, but because expectations are so high. The surgeon and the patient expect close to 100% survival and close to 100% preservation of myocardial function. Because ventricular function is good, the margin of safety is enhanced and simple systems of myocardial protection may be safely utilized.

Oxygenated Crystalloid Cardioplegia

The basic crystalloid technique involves systemic cooling to 25°C, local irrigation of the pericardium, infusion of a cold (2° to 4°C) oxygenated crystalloid solution (1 L in volume at 70 mm Hg pressure) into the aortic root after crossclamping, and reinfusion of 200 mL of this solution down each vein graft as the distal anastomosis is completed. Reinfusion of cardioplegic solution into the ascending aorta may be accomplished every 15 to 20 minutes. Venting of the left heart is usually not necessary. Proximal anastomoses are accomplished after the crossclamp interval, using a side-biting clamp. Visualization of distal coronary anastomoses is excellent, and this technique is consistent with a simple, rapid, and safe operation. It should be emphasized that much of the margin of safety with this technique is provided by the fact that preoperative left ventricular function is good.

Cold Blood Cardioplegia

Cold blood cardioplegia may be utilized in this clinical setting with systemic cooling to 25°C, local irrigation of the pericardium, infusion of 1 L of cold blood solution into the ascending aorta after aortic crossclamping, infusion of blood cardioplegic solution down each vein graft after the completion of each anastomosis, and reinfusion into the aortic root every 15 to 20 minutes. Proximal anastomoses are constructed using a side-biting clamp after the aortic crossclamp interval. Infusion of warm blood cardioplegic solution ("hot shot") at the termination of the crossclamp interval is optional.

Warm Blood Cardioplegia

The use of warm blood cardioplegia in the circumstance of coronary artery disease with good left ventricular function is somewhat cumbersome. Continuous warm blood cardioplegic techniques lead to difficulty in visualization of distal anastomoses. Temporary cessation of cardioplegic infusion or local coronary isolation (for example, with tourniquets or soft clamps on the coronary arteries) may aid in visualization of the distal anastomoses. Warm blood cardioplegic solution, in this circumstance, ordinarily should be infused in both an antegrade and a retrograde manner, since simple antegrade infusion may lead to maldistribution in patients with coronary disease. Warm blood cardioplegia is discussed thoroughly in Chapter 34.

With Poor Left Ventricular Function

Patients with poor left ventricular function require more sophisticated systems of myocardial protection to provide an adequate margin of safety. Generally, it is best to have a standard system of myocardial protection such as one of the systems outlined above. This standard system may then be enhanced to increase the margin of safety. The extent of enhancement may be varied to fit the individual patient.

Oxygenated Crystalloid Cardioplegia

Oxygenated crystalloid cardioplegia has been safely and effectively used for patients with poor left ventricular function. Careful attention to pharmacologic preparation of the heart (as described above), with adequate glucose loading and appropriate drug therapies is essential. If the heart rate is fast, β-blockade is appropriate just as CPB is initiated. The standard system outlined above may be enhanced by systemic cooling to 22° or even 20°C. Careful attention should be given to local cooling of the heart. A "phrenic pad" (a sheet of insulating material placed inside the pericardium) may be used to protect the phrenic nerves, while saline slush is used around the heart, or a cooling pad may be used to enhance local cooling.

After initiation of CPB, left ventricular venting should be considered. The most critical time for venting is before and after cardioplegic arrest; while the heart is arrested, the adverse metabolic sequelae of ventricular distention are minimized. On the other hand, an interval of ventricular distention (which is often accompanied by hypotension and either tachycardia or ventricular fibrillation) just prior to the crossclamp interval is very harmful. Recalling the example of the swimmer who is required to swim through a tunnel from one lake to another, an interval of ventricular distention with hypotension just prior to the crossclamp interval is equivalent to forcing our swimmer to exhale vigorously just prior to taking his underwater swim!

There are several venting techniques. These are categorized as *active* or *passive*, as described earlier. The most popular active venting technique is the placement of a suction catheter via the right superior pulmonary vein and the mitral valve into the left ventricle. A second technique of left ventricular venting is the placement of a catheter directly into the left ventricular apex. Both techniques provide very effective left ventricular decompression. Suction catheters may also be placed in the pulmonary artery or in the aorta (the aortic cardioplegia catheter is often placed on suction, by a siphon technique). The aortic suction technique is effective only during the crossclamp interval, and the pulmonary artery suction technique is relatively ineffective (compared to venting a left heart chamber) for left ventricular decompression. *All active venting techniques that involve suction on a cardiac chamber may lead to the introduction of intracardiac air. Even pulmonary artery suction can lead to the introduction of air into the left heart chambers. For this reason, meticulous de-airing of the heart is necessary if active venting techniques are used.* The potentially catastrophic complications of air embolism are discussed further in Chapter 18.

Passive venting techniques do not involve suction on the cardiac chambers. The most effective technique of passive venting is amputation of the tip of the left atrial appendage. This is easily accomplished, and leaves the left atrial appendage as a flap valve to discourage introduction of air (the left atrial appendage is also submerged during much of the cardiac operation). The left atrial appendage is usually repaired by a purse-string suture placed during the crossclamp interval. This purse-string suture is left untied until the heart is fully recovered and is in an empty, beating state. The heart is then lifted and the purse-string suture is tied. This technique is easily utilized both before and after the crossclamp interval. A less effective passive venting technique entails placing a hole, or a catheter open to air, in the pulmonary artery. Other techniques include passively allowing the aortic cardioplegic cannula to vent during the crossclamp interval, or punching holes in the ascending aorta for proximal anastomoses early in the crossclamp interval, thus allowing blood to passively flow from the ascending aorta. Obviously, aortic venting techniques may be used only during the crossclamp interval.

The oxygenated crystalloid technique may be enhanced further by using retrograde as well as antegrade infusions of cardioplegic solutions. A very important enhancement of the oxygenated crystalloid technique is the completion of all anastomoses (both distal and proximal) during a single crossclamp interval.[107] This allows the heart to be completely reperfused at the time of removal of the crossclamp, without an interval of partial reperfusion while proximal anastomoses are being constructed. A reperfusion modification may be included with a cold oxygenated crystalloid technique by dosing the heart with cardioplegic solution just prior to crossclamp removal. This leaves the heart in a homogeneously arrested state at the time of crossclamp removal. The heart remains arrested during the early interval of blood reperfusion, and then slowly begins to beat. An alternative method of reperfusion modification with the cold oxygenated crystalloid technique is to partially remove the aortic crossclamp while oxygenated crystalloid solution is infused into the ascending aorta. This provides a mixture of blood and cardioplegic solution in the ascending aorta during the first 3 minutes of cardiac reperfusion, allowing the heart to be empty and asystolic during the first few minutes of reperfusion.

Cold Blood Cardioplegia

Most of the myocardial protection enhancements listed above for cold, oxygenated crystalloid techniques are also applicable to a cold blood technique: metabolic and hemodynamic preparation of the heart prior to crossclamp, active and/or passive venting, antegrade and retrograde reinfusion of cardioplegia, construction of all anastomoses under a single crossclamp, further systemic cooling, and enhanced local cooling. The blood technique offers the additional advantage of warm induction of cardioplegia. With this technique, warm blood cardioplegic solution is infused into the ascending aorta immediately after placement of the crossclamp; this prepares the heart metabolically for the cold interval. The blood technique also facilitates a reperfusion modification, since warm blood cardioplegic solution may be infused into the ascending aorta for the 5 to 10 minutes prior to crossclamp removal, ensuring that the heart is reperfused in an empty, asystolic state. Substrate enhancement (particularly with glutamate and aspartate) is also thought to be useful during the reperfusion interval.

Warm Blood Cardioplegia

Warm blood cardioplegia is an excellent myocardial protective technique for patients with poor left ventricular function. The heart is metabolically invigorated during the crossclamp interval. It is important, in patients with severe coronary disease, to use retrograde infusion of cardioplegic solution. As mentioned earlier, the warm blood cardioplegic technique does lead to some difficulty in visualization of distal anastomoses. With poor left ventricular function, one should not turn off the cardioplegia infusion for extended intervals, since the margin of safety in patients with poor left ventricular function is limited. It is certainly clear that warm ischemia is hazardous and multiple intervals of warm ischemia have cumulative damaging effects (see Chapter 34).

Acute Ischemia

Surgical myocardial revascularization offers unique advantages in the treatment of acute myocardial ischemia. By modifying myocardial reperfusion conditions, the surgeon may salvage myocardium to a greater extent than is possible with either thrombolytic therapy or percutaneous transluminal coronary angioplasty. These myocardial salvage techniques have been experimentally defined and employed successfully in the clinical setting. Multiple studies have demonstrated that blood cardioplegic techniques are superior to crystalloid techniques for the salvage of infarcting myocardium.[66]

As discussed in Chapter 22, a patient in acute infarction should be taken to the operating room and placed on CPB as rapidly as possible. Decreasing the metabolic requirements of the myocardium by the use of CPB stops the progression of a myocardial infarction if the left ventricle is vented. A passive venting technique is preferable in order to avoid introduction of air into the left heart chambers.

If a cold blood technique is utilized, retrograde and antegrade infusion of cardioplegic solution should be employed. A reperfusion modification—warm blood cardioplegic solution infused into the aortic root at the termination of the crossclamp interval—should be used. Substrate enhancement (glutamate and aspartate) is also an integral part of this technique of myocardial salvage, although its relative importance has not been determined.

Warm blood cardioplegic techniques provide an opportunity for an extended period of myocardial resuscitation, as the resuscitation interval extends throughout the crossclamp interval. For this reason, acute ischemia may be the most compelling reason for the use of warm blood cardioplegic methods. Experimentally, the warm blood technique is superior to crystalloid techniques and is probably more effective than cold blood methods in this situation.

Coronary Artery Reoperations

Coronary artery reoperations pose special problems. Old vein grafts make aortic crossclamping difficult, and the presence of a patent internal mammary graft may make antegrade infusion of cardioplegic solution into some myocardial regions especially difficult. For this reason, hypothermic myocardial protection, without chemical asystole (discussed earlier in this chapter) is particularly applicable in patients undergoing coronary artery reoperations, especially patients with intact internal mammary artery grafts. However, the surgeon should keep in mind that retraction and manipulation of the heart may cause atherosclerotic embolism from dislodged plaques within the vein grafts; such embolization to the distal myocardium is often a catastrophic complication.

Crystalloid, cold blood, and warm blood techniques may be used for coronary artery reoperations. Retrograde infusion of the cardioplegic solution is particularly useful during coronary reoperations, as it may flush out from the distal coronary bed debris from old vein grafts which has embolized. Retrograde cardioplegic techniques may also be combined with occlusion of patent internal mammary grafts to allow infusion of cardioplegic solution into regions of myocardium supplied by these grafts. All anastomoses, distal and proximal, should be constructed during a single crossclamp interval. When old vein grafts are present, placement of a side-biting clamp on the ascending aorta is hazardous, since it unnecessarily manipulates the old grafts, which can cause atherosclerotic embolism. Some authors advocate the early removal of all old grafts to prevent embolism, but most surgeons do not automatically remove these grafts.

Valve Operations

Aortic Stenosis and Regurgitation

In general, the heart with aortic stenosis and/or regurgitation is hypertrophied and enlarged. Particular attention should be paid to the metabolic and hemodynamic preparation (as described earlier in this chapter) of this vulnerable heart. β-Blockade is an especially useful adjunct. Indeed, the prevention of the "stone heart" by β-blockade was originally described for patients with hypertrophied hearts.[23] If the patient has aortic regurgitation, special care must be taken to prevent myocardial distention during the interval of systemic cooling on CPB prior to placement of the aortic crossclamp. *As soon as the heart begins to distend*, the aortic crossclamp should be placed and cardioplegic solution infused. Cardioplegic arrest may be accomplished by antegrade infusion into the aortic root. If the aortic valve is competent, adequate antegrade flow of cardioplegic solution is achieved; if the aortic valve is incompetent, it is necessary to manually massage the left ventricle to achieve antegrade flow of cardioplegic solution, or to open the aorta and infuse cardioplegic solution directly into the coronary ostia. With the latter technique, a soft-tipped infusion cannula is used to avoid direct damage to the coronary ostia. Finally, retrograde techniques are particularly useful in patients with aortic valve disease. Cardioplegic solution may be reinfused at intervals (or, in the case of warm blood cardioplegia, continuously) during the crossclamp interval without disrupting the conduct of the valve replacement. Local irrigation and systemic cooling should be used to augment cold techniques, ensuring that the heart remains cold during the crossclamp interval. If retrograde warm blood cardioplegic techniques are utilized, care must be taken that adequate flow *and pressures* are provided. These very large hearts may require flows as high as 250 mL/min in order to achieve coronary sinus pressures of 35 to 40 mm Hg. If lower coronary sinus pressures are utilized, it is possible that retrograde flow may be shunted to some regions of the myocardium, and other regions (particularly the endocardium in those hearts with near normal myocardial tone) may be hypoperfused and suffer warm ischemic damage.

Mitral Valve Disease

In patients with mitral valve disease, there are three major techniques for myocardial protection. The first two depend on systemic hypothermia and antegrade, coronary ostia blood flow. The third and most commonly employed method depends on chemically induced myocardial arrest. The patient with a competent aortic valve is simply placed on CPB and cooled. When ventricular fibrillation occurs, the left atrium is opened and the mitral valve is replaced or repaired without aortic crossclamping. Exposure is sometimes difficult because of the tense aorta and normal myocardial tone, but this technique provides adequate myocardial protection, provided perfusion pressure (aortic root pressure) is maintained.

Another myocardial protection technique used extensively for myocardial repair is intermittent aortic crossclamping with hypothermia but without chemical asystole. The patient is placed on CPB and cooled to 20°C. The aorta is crossclamped to facilitate exposure for intervals of 10 to 12 minutes. The aortic crossclamp is intermittently removed, allowing reperfusion and resuscitation of the heart. This technique tends to maintain myocardial tone, which is especially important for complex myocardial repair.

Cardioplegic techniques of myocardial protection are the ones most commonly used in the presence of mitral valve disease. Cold oxygenated crystalloid or cold blood is infused, providing a flaccid heart and excellent exposure of the mitral valve. Ordinarily, antegrade infusion of cardioplegic solution is performed initially. If a second dose of antegrade cardioplegic solution is required, the aorta must be de-aired carefully to prevent air embolism (the myocardium supplied by the right coronary artery is especially vulnerable), as the aortic root is usually completely filled with air at this point. Retrograde infusion of cold cardioplegic solution is an excellent alternative if an extended crossclamp interval is necessary.

Continuous warm blood cardioplegia may be the optimal myocardial protection technique for mitral valve operations. Antegrade infusion of cardioplegic solution achieves arrest and retrograde cardioplegia ensures continuing myocardial protection (continuous antegrade infusion may be utilized, but retrograde techniques are more convenient). Myocardial tone is maintained to a sufficient extent to allow mitral valve repair. When the aortic crossclamp is removed, the heart recovers quickly for testing of the repair. Rearrest is accomplished easily if further repair is necessary.

Congenital Heart Disease

For decades, hypothermia has been the mainstay of myocardial protection in congenital heart disease. As cardioplegic protection was added to hypothermia in adult cardiac operations, cardioplegic arrest was extended to surgery for congenital disease—usually performed in infants and neonates—as well.[108] But the immature heart is different in structure and function from the mature heart, and pediatric cardioplegic solutions are also likely to be different.[109,110] In neonatal lambs, neither blood nor crystalloid cardioplegia exhibited any additive protective effect to hypothermia alone.[111] In rabbits, some popular cardioplegic solutions seemed to actually damage hypothermic myocardium, while the same solutions were beneficial in pig hearts.[112-115]

Rapid cooling of the infant heart may occur because of the small body mass of infants and may lead to contracture, an indication that warm induction blood cardioplegia may be useful in infants.[116] Retrograde techniques may be useful in some types of congenital heart disease, but these techniques are only beginning to be clinically applied.

Transplantation

Cardiac transplantation offers unique opportunities and challenges for myocardial protection. Noncoronary collateral flow is absent and washout of cardioplegic solutions does not occur. Prolonged intervals of myocardial ischemia are obviously present, and very cold myocardial temperatures are possible. Because of these unique conditions, the solutions that are appropriate for the conduct of nontransplant cardiac operations are not likely to be similar to the solutions that are optimal for cardiac transplantation.[117] Indeed, it appears that solutions appropriate for nontransplant cardiac operations should be similar to extracellular fluid or to blood, while the solutions appropriate for cardiac transplantation should more nearly approximate intracellular fluid.[118] The goal of transplantation is generally a state of suspended metabolic activity with profound hypothermia (approximately 4°C), a metabolic milieu that prevents passive flow of intracellular electrolytes and proteins out of the cell and prevents intracellular swelling. Therefore, the solution should be generally intracellular in composition, with a relatively high osmotic and oncotic pressure.

The University of Wisconsin solution has been tested extensively for transplantation.[118-120] This solution contains high-molecular-weight compounds that prevent intracellular water accumulation. Experimental studies have confirmed that the University of Wisconsin solution and other solutions which are similar to intracellular fluids, such as the Stanford cardioplegic solution, are superior to extracellular crystalloid solutions for transplantation.[117,118] Despite this experimental evidence, extracellular solutions are utilized by a number of institutions. As long as the ischemic interval is relatively short, the margin of safety is adequate with either extracellular or intracellular solutions, but there is no question that the intracellular solutions provide a greater margin of safety for transplantation.

Summary

Myocardial protection must be customized to the individual patient's pathology, as well as to the talents, temperaments, and preferences of the surgical team. Myocardial protection for transplantation is distinctly different from that for triple-vessel coronary disease. Myocardial protection for infants is not the same as that for octogenarians. A patient with good left ventricular function and two-vessel coronary disease should not receive the same system of myocardial protection as a patient with poor ventricular function, mitral regurgitation, and coronary disease. In the former instance, a simple, streamlined system of myocardial protection affords a rapid operation with a short crossclamp interval and, perhaps most importantly, a very short CPB time. In the latter instance, a complex system of myocardial protection is necessary to give the myocardium the best chance for recovery.

One might reasonably ask, why not use the most complex system, which gives the best chance for myocardial recovery in all patients? Complexity, unfortunately, always raises the possibility of technical or pathophysiologic misadventure. In a patient with a good ventricle and coronary artery disease, a simple system of myocardial protection should provide an adequate margin of safety for virtually complete myocardial recovery in 99.5% of cases. If one uses a more complex system of myocardial protection, then each component of that system adds its own small risk. For example, venting of the heart, particularly active venting, involves a 0.2% chance of some complication related to intracardiac air. Extensive cooling to 20°C with prolonged use of ice slush is associated with a 0.2% chance of phrenic nerve damage or myocardial damage from freezing. Use of a retrograde technique carries a 0.5% risk of damage to coronary sinus, inadequate protection, or an inadequately constructed distal anastomosis because of poor visualization. As these very small risks are combined, one sees that a complex system of cardioplegic protection poses an unreasonable and unnecessary risk for a simple operation.

This, then, is the challenge in myocardial protection: customization of the myocardial protection technique to provide a sufficient margin of safety for the particular patient without additional risk to the patient because of the complexity of the protection technique. One seeks the gentlest, smoothest, shortest operation consistent with an adequate margin of safety. This challenge can be met if one is familiar with a number of different methods of myocardial protection and has a thorough knowledge of the advantages and disadvantages of each method.

References

1. Guyton RA. Methods and magic in myocardial preservation. In: Hurst JW, ed. *Clinical Essays on the Heart.* New York: McGraw-Hill; 1983;1:183-201.
2. Guyton RA. Cardiopulmonary bypass, cardioplegia, and central nervous system preservation: the surgeon's perspective. In: *Cardiothoracic and Vascular Anesthesia Update.* Philadelphia: W B Saunders Co; 1990:1-13.
3. Lolley DM, Ray JF III, Myers WO, et al. Importance of preoperative myocardial glycogen levels in human cardiac preservation. *J Thorac Cardiovasc Surg* 1979;78:678-687.
4. Salerno TA, Wasan SM, Charrette EJP. Glucose substrate in myocardial protection. *J Thorac Cardiovasc Surg* 1980; 79:59-62.
5. Delva E, Maille JG, Solymoss BC, et al. Evaluation of myocardial damage during coronary artery grafting with serial determinations of serum CPK MB isoenzymes. *J Thorac Cardiovasc Surg* 1978;75:467-475.
6. Guyton RA, McClenathan JH, Newman GE, et al. Significance of subendocardial S-T segment elevation caused by coronary stenosis in the dog. Epicardial S-T segment depression, local ischemia and subsequent necrosis. *Am J Cardiol* 1977;40:373-380.
7. Engleman RM, Spencer FC, Boyd AD, et al. The significance of coronary arterial stenosis during cardiopulmonary bypass. *J Thorac Cardiovasc Surg* 1975;70:869-879.
8. Sink JD, Hill RC, Chitwood WR Jr, et al. Effects of phenylephrine on transmural distribution of myocardial blood

flow in regions supplied by normal and collateral arteries during cardiopulmonary bypass. *J Thorac Cardiovasc Surg* 1979;78:236–243.

9. Miyamoto ATM, Robinson L, Matloff JM, et al. Perioperative infarction. Effects of cardiopulmonary bypass on collateral circulation in an acute canine model. *Circulation* 1978;58(suppl I):I147–155.

10. Kleinman LH, Yarbrough JW, Symmonds JB, et al. Pressure-flow characteristics of the coronary collateral circulation during cardiopulmonary bypass. Effects of hemodilution. *J Thorac Cardiovasc Surg* 1978;75:17–27.

11. Anderson HT, Kessinger JM, McFarland WJ Jr, et al. Response of the hypertrophied heart to acute anemia and coronary stenosis. *Surgery* 1978;84:8–15.

12. Chitwood WR Jr, Sink JD, Hill RC, et al. The effects of hypothermia on myocardial oxygen consumption and transmural coronary blood flow in the potassium-arrested heart. *Ann Surg* 1979;190:106–116.

13. McConnell DH, Brazier JR, Cooper N, et al. Studies of the effects of hypothermia on regional myocardial blood flow and metabolism during cardiopulmonary bypass. II. Ischemia during moderate hypothermia in continually perfused beating hearts. *J Thorac Cardiovasc Surg* 1977;73:95–101.

14. Schaff HV, Ciardullo RC, Flaherty JT, et al. Development of regional myocardial ischemia distal to a critical coronary stenosis during cardiopulmonary bypass: comparison of the fibrillating vs. the beating nonworking states. *Surgery* 1978;83:57–66.

15. Buckberg GD, Hottenrott CE. Ventricular fibrillation. Its effect on myocardial flow, distribution, and performance. *Ann Thorac Surg* 1975;20:76–85.

16. Brazier JR, Cooper N, McConnell DH, et al. Studies of the effects of hypothermia on regional myocardial blood flow and metabolism during cardiopulmonary bypass. III. Effects of temperature, time, and perfusion pressure in fibrillating hearts. *J Thorac Cardiovasc Surg* 1977;73:102–109.

17. Kleinman LH, Wechsler AS. Pressure-flow characteristics of the coronary collateral circulation during cardiopulmonary bypass. Effects of ventricular fibrillation. *Circulation* 1978;58:233–239.

18. Schaff HV, Ciardullo RC, Flaherty JT, et al. Development of regional myocardial ischemia distal to a critical coronary stenosis during cardiopulmonary bypass: comparison of the fibrillating vs. the beating nonworking states. *Surgery* 1978;83:57–66.

19. Ellis AK, Klocke FJ. Effects of preload on the transmural distribution of perfusion and pressure-flow relationships in the canine coronary vascular bed. *Circ Res* 1980;46:68–77.

20. Lucas SK, Gardner TJ, Elmer EB, et al. Comparison of the effects of left ventricular distention during cardioplegic-induced ischemic arrest and ventricular fibrillation. *Circulation* 1980;62(suppl I):I42–49.

21. Little AG, Lin CY, Wernly JA, et al. Use of the pulmonary artery for left ventricular venting during cardiac operations. *J Thorac Cardiovasc Surg* 1984;87:532–538.

22. Robicsek F, Duncan GD. Retrograde air embolization in coronary operations. *J Thorac Cardiovasc Surg* 1987;94:110–114.

23. Cooley DA, Reul GJ, Wukasch DC. Ischemic contracture of the heart: "stone heart." *Am J Cardiol* 1972;29:575–577.

24. Naylor WG, Ferrari R, Williams A. Protective effect of pretreatment with verapamil, nifedipine, and propranolol on mitochondrial function in the ischemic and reperfused myocardium. *Am J Cardiol* 1980;46:242–248.

25. Magee PG, Gardner TJ, Flaherty JT, et al. Improved myocardial protection with propranolol during induced ischemia. *Circulation* 1980;62(suppl I):I49–56.

26. Lochner W, Arnold G, Muller-Ruchholtz ER. Metabolism of the artificially arrested heart and of the gas-perfused heart. *Am J Cardiol* 1966;22:299–311.

27. Komai H, Yamamoto F, Tanaka K, et al. Harmful effects of inotropic agents on myocardial protection. *Ann Thorac Surg* 1991;52:927–933.

28. Weinstein GS, Rao PS, Tyras DH. Reduction of myocardial injury with Verapamil before aortic cross-clamping. *Ann Thorac Surg* 1990;49:419–423.

29. Christakis GT, Fremes SE, Weisel RD, et al. Diltiazem cardioplegia. *J Thorac Cardiovasc Surg* 1986;91:647–661.

30. Krukenkamp IB, Silverman NA, Sorlie D, et al. Temperature-specific effects of adjunct Diltiazem therapy on myocardial energetics following potassium cardioplegic arrest. *Ann Thorac Surg* 1986;42:675–680.

31. Kates RA, Dorsey LM, Kaplan JA, et al. Pretreatment with lidoflazine, a calcium channel blocker. *J Thorac Cardiovasc Surg* 1983;85:278–286.

32. Guyton RA, Dorsey LM, Colgan TK, et al. Calcium-channel blockade as an adjunct to heterogeneous delivery of cardioplegia. *Ann Thorac Surg* 1983;35:626–632.

33. Flameng W, Daenan W, Borgers M, et al. Cardioprotective effects of lidoflazine during 1-hour normothermic global ischemia. *Circulation* 1981;64:796–807.

34. Fiore AC, Naunheim KS, Taug J, et al. Myocardial preservation using Lidocaine blood cardioplegia. *Ann Thorac Surg* 1990;50:771–775.

35. Shumway NE, Lower RR, Stoffer RC. Selective hypothermia of the heart in anoxic cardiac arrest. *Surg Gynecol Obstet* 1959;109:750–754.

36. Boldt J, Kling D, Dapper F, et al. Myocardial temperature during cardiac operations: influence on right ventricular function. *J Thorac Cardiovasc Surg* 1990;100:562–568.

37. Dorsey LM, Colgan TK, Silverstein JI, et al. Alterations in regional myocardial function after heterogeneous cardioplegia. *J Thorac Cardiovasc Surg* 1983;86:70–79.

38. Dailey PO, Pfeffer TA, Wisniewski JB, et al. Clinical comparisons of methods of myocardial protection. *J Thorac Cardiovasc Surg* 1987;93:324–336.

39. Landymore RW, Tice D, Trehan N, et al. Importance of topical hypothermia to ensure uniform myocardial cooling during coronary artery bypass. *J Thorac Cardiovasc Surg* 1981;82:832–836.

40. Daggett WM, Jacocks A, Coleman WS, et al. Myocardial temperature mapping. Improved intraoperative myocardial preservation. *J Thorac Cardiovasc Surg* 1981;82:883–888.

41. Cameron DE, Gardner TJ. Principles of clinical hypothermia. In: Chitwoods WR, ed. *State of the Art Reviews. Myocardial Preservation: Clinical Applications.* Philadelphia: Hanley & Belfus Inc; 1988:xiii–xxv.

42. Buckberg GD, Brazier JR, Nelson RL, et al. Studies of the effects of hypothermia on regional myocardial blood flow

and metabolism during cardiopulmonary bypass. I. The adequately perfused beating, fibrillating, and arrested heart. *J Thorac Cardiovasc Surg* 1977;73:87-94.
43. Mankad PS, Chester AH, Yacoub MH. Role of potassium concentration in cardioplegic solutions in mediating endothelial damage. *Ann Thorac Surg* 1991;51:89-93.
44. Dewar M, Rosengarten MD, Samson CP, et al. Is high potassium solution necessary for reinfusions in "multidose" cold cardioplegia? A randomized prospective study using a computerized Holter system. *Ann Thorac Surg* 1987;93:409-415.
45. Ferguson TB, Smith PK, Lofland GK, et al. The effects of cardioplegic potassium concentration and myocardial temperature on electrical activity in the heart during elective cardioplegic arrest. *J Thorac Cardiovasc Surg* 1986;92:755-765.
46. Carpentier S, Murawsky M, Carpentier A. Cytotoxicity of cardioplegic solutions: evaluation of tissue cultures. *Circulation* 1981;64(suppl II):II90-95.
47. Brazier J, Hottenrott C, Buckberg G. Noncoronary collateral myocardial blood flow. *Ann Thorac Surg* 1975;19:426-435.
48. Rebeyka IM, Axford-Gatley RA, Bush BG, et al. Calcium paradox in an in vivo model of multidose cardioplegia and moderate hypothermia. *J Thorac Cardiovasc Surg* 1990;99:475-483.
49. Kinoshita K, Oe M, Tokunaga K. Superior protective effect of low-calcium, magnesium-free potassium cardioplegic solution on ischemic myocardium. *J Thorac Cardiovasc Surg* 1991;101:695-702.
50. Robinson LA, Harwood DL. Lowering the calcium concentration in St. Thomas' Hospital cardioplegic solution improves protection during hypothermic ischemia. *J Thorac Cardiovasc Surg* 1991;101:314-325.
51. Khuri SF, Marston WA, Josa M, et al. Observations on 100 patients with continuous intraoperative monitoring of intramyocardial pH. *J Thorac Cardiovasc Surg* 1985;89:170-182.
52. Lochner A, Lloyd L, Brits W, et al. Oxygenation of cardioplegic solutions: a note of caution. *Ann Thorac Surg* 1991;51:777-787.
53. von Oppell UO, King LM, DuToit EF, et al. Effect of pH shifts induced by oxygenating crystalloid cardioplegic solutions. *Ann Thorac Surg* 1991;52:903-907.
54. Lichtenstein SV, Abel JG, Panos A, et al. Warm heart surgery: experience with long cross-clamp times. *Ann Thorac Surg* 1991;52:1009-1013.
55. de Nido PJ, Wilson GJ, Mickle DAG, et al. The role of cardioplegic solution buffering in myocardial protection. *J Thorac Cardiovasc Surg* 1985;89:689-699.
56. Buckberg GD. A proposed "solution" to the cardioplegic controversy. *J Thorac Cardiovasc Surg* 1979;77:809-815.
57. Vinten-Johansen J, Julian S, Yokoyama H, et al. Efficacy of myocardial protection with hypothermic blood cardioplegia depends on oxygen. *Ann Thorac Surg* 1991;52:939-948.
58. Oguma F, Imai S, Eguchi S. Role played by oxygen in myocardial protection with crystalloid cardioplegic solution. *Ann Thorac Surg* 1986;42:172-179.
59. Hendren WG, O'Keefe DD, Geffin GA, et al. Maximal oxygenation of dilute blood cardioplegic solution. *Ann Thorac Surg* 1987;44:48-52.
60. Ledingham SJM, Braimbridge MV, Hearse DJ. Improved myocardial protection by oxygenation of the St. Thomas' Hospital cardioplegic solutions. *J Thorac Cardiovasc Surg* 1988;95:103-111.
61. Guyton RA, Dorsey LMA, Craver JM, et al. Improved myocardial recovery after cardioplegic arrest with an oxygenated crystalloid solution. *J Thorac Cardiovasc Surg* 1985;89:877-887.
62. Tabayashi K, McKeown PP, Miyamoto M, et al. Ischemic myocardial protection. Comparison of nonoxygenated crystalloid, oxygenated crystalloid, and oxygenated fluorocarbon cardioplegic solutions. *J Thorac Cardiovasc Surg* 1988;95:239-246.
63. Steinberg JB, Doherty NE, Munfakh NA, et al. Oxygenated cardioplegia: the metabolic and functional effects of glucose and insulin. *Ann Thorac Surg* 1991;51:620-629.
64. Yau TM, Weisel RD, Mickel DAG, et al. Optimal delivery of blood cardioplegia. *Circulation* 1991;84(suppl III):III380-388.
65. Doherty NE III, Turocy JF, Geffin GA, et al. Benefits of glucose and oxygen in multidose cold cardioplegia. *J Thorac Cardiovasc Surg* 1992;103:219-229.
66. Barner HB. Blood cardioplegia: a review and comparison with crystalloid cardioplegia. *Ann Thorac Surg* 1991;52:1354-1367.
67. Illes RW, Silverman NA, Krukenkamp IB, et al. The efficacy of blood cardioplegia is not due to oxygen delivery. *J Thorac Cardiovasc Surg* 1989;98:1051-1056.
68. Vinten-Johansen J, Buckberg GD, Okamoto F, et al. Studies of controlled reperfusion after ischemia. V. Superiority of surgical versus medical reperfusion after regional ischemia. *J Thorac Cardiovasc Surg* 1986;92:525-534.
69. Allen BS, Okamoto F, Buckberg GD, et al. Studies of controlled reperfusion after ischemia. XV. Immediate functional recovery after six hours of regional ischemia by careful control of conditions of reperfusion and composition of reperfusate. *J Thorac Cardiovasc Surg* 1986;92:621-635.
70. Cheung EH, Arcidi JM Jr, Dorsey LMA, et al. Reperfusion of infarcting myocardium: benefit of surgical reperfusion in a chronic model. *Ann Thorac Surg* 1989;48:331-338.
71. Bottner RK, Wallace RB, Visner MS, et al. Reduction of myocardial infarction after emergency coronary artery bypass grafting for failed coronary angioplasty with use of a normothermic reperfusion cardioplegia protocol. *J Thorac Cardiovasc Surg* 1991;101:1069-1075.
72. Julia PL, Buckberg GD, Acar C, et al. Studies of controlled reperfusion after ischemia. XXI. Reperfusate composition: superiority of blood cardioplegia over crystalloid cardioplegia in limiting reperfusion damage. Importance of endogenous oxygen free radical scavengers in red blood cells. *J Thorac Cardiovasc Surg* 1991;303-313.
73. Quillen J, Kofsky ER, Buckberg GD, et al. Studies of controlled reperfusion after ischemia. XXIII. Deleterious effects of simulated thrombolysis preceding simulated coronary artery bypass grafting with controlled blood cardioplegic reperfusion. *J Thorac Cardiovasc Surg* 1991;101:455-464.

74. Schaff HV, Goldman RA, Bulkley BH, et al. Hyperosmolar reperfusion following ischemic cardiac arrest. *Surgery* 1981;89:141-150.
75. Lazar HL, Buckberg GD, Manganaro AM, et al. Myocardial energy replenishment and reversal of ischemic damage by substrate enhancement of secondary blood cardioplegia with amino acids during reperfusion. *J Thorac Cardiovasc Surg* 1980;80:350-359.
76. Mills SA, Hansen K, Vinten-Johansen J, et al. Enhanced functional recovery with venting during cardioplegic arrest in chronically damaged hearts. *Ann Thorac Surg* 1985;40:566-573.
77. Lucas SK, Schaff HV, Flaherty JT, et al. The harmful effects of ventricular distention during postischemic reperfusion. *Ann Thorac Surg* 1981;32:486-494.
78. Bolling SF, Bies LE, Bove EL, et al. Augmenting intracellular adenosine improves myocardial recovery. *J Thorac Cardiovasc Surg* 1990;99:469-474.
79. Haas GS, DeBoer LWV, O'Keefe DD, et al. Reduction of postischemic myocardial dysfunction by substrate repletion during reperfusion. *Circulation* 1984;70(suppl I):I65-74.
80. Svedjeholm R, Ekroth R, Joachimsson PO, et al. Myocardial uptake of amino acids and other substrates in relation to myocardial oxygen consumption four hours after cardiac operations. *J Thorac Cardiovasc Surg* 1991;101:688-694.
81. Rosenkranz ER, Okamoto F, Buckberg GD, et al. Safety of prolonged aortic clamping with blood cardioplegia. II. Glutamate enrichment in energy-depleted hearts. *J Thorac Cardiovasc Surg* 1984;88:402-410.
82. Engelman RM, Rousou JA, Flack JE III, et al. Reduction of infarct size by systemic amino acid supplementation during reperfusion. *J Thorac Cardiovasc Surg* 1991;101:855-859.
83. Rosenkranz ER, Okamoto F, Buckberg GD, et al. Safety of prolonged aortic clamping with blood cardioplegia. III. Aspartate enrichment of glutamate-blood cardioplegia in energy-depleted hearts after ischemic and reperfusion injury. *J Thorac Cardiovasc Surg* 1986;91:428-435.
84. Ferreira R, Burgos M, Milei J, et al. Effect of supplementing cardioplegic solution with deferoxamine on reperfused human myocardium. *J Thorac Cardiovasc Surg* 1990;100:708-714.
85. Chambers DJ, Braimbridge, MV, Hearse DJ. Free radicals and cardioplegia: Allopurinol and Oxypurinol reduce myocardial injury following ischemic arrest. *Ann Thorac Surg* 1987;44:291-297.
86. Shlafer M, Kane PF, Kirsh MM. Superoxide dismutase plus catalase enhances the efficacy of hypothermic cardioplegia to protect the globally ischemic, reperfused heart. *J Thorac Cardiovasc Surg* 1982;83:830-839.
87. Magovern GJ, Bolling SF, Casale AS, et al. The mechanism of mannitol in reducing ischemic injury: hyperosmolarity or hydroxyl scavenger? *Circulation* 1984;70(suppl I):I91-95.
88. Guyton RA, Arcidi JM Jr, Langford DA, et al. Emergency coronary bypass for cardiogenic shock. *Circulation* 1987;76(suppl V):V22-27.
89. Akins CW. Noncardioplegic myocardial preservation for coronary revascularization. *J Thorac Cardiovasc Surg* 1984;88:174-181.
90. Akins CW, Carroll DL. Event-free survival following nonemergency myocardial revascularization during hypothermic fibrillatory arrest. *Ann Thorac Surg* 1987;43:628-633.
91. Bonchek LI, Burlingame MW, Vazales BE, et al. Applicability of noncardioplegic coronary bypass to high-risk patients. Selection of patients, technique, and clinical experience in 3000 patients. *J Thorac Cardiovasc Surg* 1992;103:230-237.
92. Coetzee A, Boussouw G, Fourie P, et al. Preservation of myocardial function and biochemistry after blood and oxygenated crystalloid cardioplegia during cardiac arrest. *Ann Thorac Surg* 1990;50:230-237.
93. Guyton RA, Dorsey LM, Craver JM, et al. Improved myocardial recovery after cardioplegic arrest with an oxygenated crystalloid solution. *J Thorac Cardiovasc Surg* 1985;89:877-887.
94. Robinson LA, Braimbridge MV, Hearse DJ. Comparison of the protective properties of four clinical crystalloid cardioplegic solutions in the rat heart. *Ann Thorac Surg* 1984;38:268-274.
95. Aldea GS, Austin RE Jr, Flynn AE, et al. Heterogeneous delivery of cardioplegic solution in the absence of coronary artery disease. *J Thorac Cardiovasc Surg* 1990;99:345-353.
96. Johnson RE, Dorsey LM, Moye SJ, et al. Cardioplegia infusion: the safe limits of pressure and temperature. *J Thorac Cardiovasc Surg* 1982;83:813-823.
97. Menasche P, Subayi JB, Piwnica A. Retrograde coronary sinus cardioplegia for aortic valve operations: a clinical report on 500 patients. *Ann Thorac Surg* 1990;49:556-564.
98. Menasche P, Subayi JB, Veyssie L, et al. Efficacy of coronary sinus cardioplegia in patients with complete coronary artery occlusions. *Ann Thorac Surg* 1991;51:418-423.
99. Bolling SF, Flaherty JT, Bulkley BH, et al. Improved myocardial preservation during global ischemia by continuous retrograde coronary sinus perfusion. *J Thorac Cardiovasc Surg* 1983;86:659-666.
100. Gundry SR, Kirsh MM. A comparison of retrograde cardioplegia versus antegrade cardioplegia in the presence of coronary artery obstruction. *Ann Thorac Surg* 1984;38:124-127.
101. Rosenkranz ER, Vinten-Johanen J, Buckberg GD, et al. Benefits of normothermic induction of blood cardioplegia in energy-depleted hearts with maintenance of arrest by multidose cold blood cardioplegic infusions. *J Thorac Cardiovasc Surg* 1982;84:667-677.
102. Magovern GJ Jr, Flaherty JT, Gott VL, et al. Failure of blood cardioplegia to protect myocardium at lower temperatures. *Circulation* 1982;66(suppl I):I60-67.
103. Salerno TA, Houck JP, Barrozo CAM, et al. Retrograde continuous warm blood cardioplegia: a new concept in myocardial protection. *Ann Thorac Surg* 1991;51:245-247.
104. Lichtenstein SV, Abel JG, Salerno TA. Warm heart surgery and results of operation for recent myocardial infarction. *Ann Thorac Surg* 1991;52:455-460.
105. Lichtenstein SV, Abel JG. Warm heart surgery: theory and

current practice. In: Karp RB, Laks H, Wechsler AS, eds. *Advances in Cardiac Surgery*. St. Louis: Mosby Year Book; 1992:135-154.
106. Teoh KHT, Panos AL, Harmantas AA, et al. Optimal visualization of coronary artery anastomoses by gas jet. *Ann Thorac Surg* 1991;52:564.
107. Weisel RD, Hoy FBY, Baird RJ, et al. Comparison of alternative cardioplegic techniques. *J Thorac Cardiovasc Surg* 1983;86:97-107.
108. Konishi T, Apstein CS. Comparison of three cardioplegic solutions during hypothermic ischemic arrest in neonatal blood-perfused rabbit hearts. *J Thorac Cardiovasc Surg* 1989;98:1132-1137.
109. Yano Y, Braimbridge MV, Hearse DJ. Protection of the pediatric myocardium. Differential susceptibility to ischemic injury of the neonatal rat heart. *J Thorac Cardiovasc Surg* 1987;94:887-896.
110. Bove EL, Stammers AH. Recovery of left ventricular function after hypothermic global ischemia. Age-related differences in the isolated working rabbit heart. *J Thorac Cardiovasc Surg* 1986;91:115-122.
111. Fujiwara T, Heinle J, Britton L, et al. Myocardial preservation in neonatal lambs. *J Thorac Cardiovasc Surg* 1991;101:703-712.
112. Baker JE, Boerboom LE, Olinger GN. Cardioplegia-induced damage to ischemic immature myocardium is independent of oxygen availability. *Ann Thorac Surg* 1990;50:934-939.
113. Kempsford RD, Hearse DJ. Protection of the immature heart. *J Thorac Cardiovasc Surg* 1990;99:269-279.
114. Baker JE, Boerboom LE, Olinger GN. Is protection of ischemic neonatal myocardium by cardioplegia species dependent? *J Thorac Cardiovasc Surg* 1990;99:280-287.
115. Baker EJ IV, Olinger GN, Baker JE. Calcium content of St. Thomas' II cardioplegic solution damages ischemic immature myocardium. *Ann Thorac Surg* 1991;52:993-999.
116. Williams WG, Rebeyka IM, Tibshirani RJ, et al. Warm induction blood cardioplegia in the infant. *J Thorac Cardiovasc Surg* 1990;100:869-901.
117. Foreman J, Pegg DE, Armitage WJ. Solutions for preservation of the heart at 0°C. *J Thorac Cardiovasc Surg* 1985;89:867-871.
118. Gott JP, Pan-Chih, Dorsey LMA, et al. Cardioplegia for transplantation: failure of extracellular solution compared with Stanford or UW solution. *Ann Thorac Surg* 1990;50:348-354.
119. Yeh T Jr, Hanan SA, Johnson DE, et al. Superior myocardial preservation with modified UW solution after prolonged ischemia in the rat heart. *Ann Thorac Surg* 1990;49:932-939.
120. Stein DG, Drinkwater DC, Laks H, et al. Cardiac preservation in patients undergoing transplantation. A clinical trial comparing University of Wisconsin solution and Stanford solution. *J Thorac Cardiovasc Surg* 1991;102:657-665.

3
Hypothermia, Cardiac Surgery, and Cardiopulmonary Bypass

Willis H. Williams, Hakob G. Davtyan, and Milada Drazanova

Introduction

The ability to control a patient's body temperature within a very wide range is one of the most important therapeutic modalities available to the cardiac surgeon, anesthesiologist, and perfusionist. Hypothermia facilitates coronary arterial bypass surgery, heart valve repair or replacement, and the correction of congenital cardiac defects. Furthermore, precise anatomic correction of complex congenital heart defects, in a bloodless and motionless surgical field, is possible even in tiny premature infants during profoundly hypothermic total circulatory arrest. The technology of deep hypothermia and total circulatory arrest also is useful in operations on the thoracic aorta, the aortic arch, the brachiocephalic vessels, and the brain, during which cerebral or spinal cord blood flow is compromised or interrupted. Therapeutic clinical hypothermia, usually used for support of the patient during operation on or within the heart, requires uniform cooling of the entire body.

This chapter discusses definitions relevant to clinical hypothermia as it is employed today, with consideration of some historical milestones on which modern methods are founded. After review of the pathophysiology of ischemia, we will consider the effects of hypothermia on metabolism and the physiologic consequences for pH homeostasis and cerebral blood flow. Finally, we will examine clinical applications and available methods for induction of, and recovery from, hypothermia, including cardiopulmonary bypass (CPB), core cooling, surface cooling, surface cooling with supplementary partial CPB, deep hypothermic total circulatory arrest, and low-flow, profoundly hypothermic perfusion.

Definitions

For clinical purposes, either accidental or deliberately induced hypothermia in the human is defined as a body temperature below 35°C[1,2] or "a state in which the body temperature of a homeothermic mammal is below normal."[3] Discussion of induction, treatment, clinical application, and complications of this continuous biophysiologic variable of hypothermia (lower than normal body temperature) is facilitated by further definition based on the degree of cooling. The four generally accepted categorical definitions include *mild* hypothermia (32° to 35°C), *moderate* hypothermia (26° to 31°C), *deep* hypothermia (20° to 25°C), and *profound* hypothermia (14° to 19°C, or below 20°C) (Table 3.1).[1]

History of the Development of Clinical Hypothermia

The application of cold to wounds of the head and to the infected or ulcerated breast was recommended in one of the earliest known written records in medicine, the Edwin Smith papyrus (circa 1650 BC).[4] From antiquity through the centuries, therapeutic total body hypothermia has been one of medicine's most dramatic and effective technologies.

In 1973, Henry Swan, a pioneer in the clinical application of hypothermia in cardiovascular surgery, published an intriguing and colorful review[5] of deliberate therapeutic hypothermia, the historical details of which are summarized in Table 3.2. Swan concluded that "a poorly understood and badly practiced modality [hypothermia], ancient in lore but in its scientific infancy, needed a pur-

TABLE 3.1. Four categories of hypothermia.[a]

Mild hypothermia	32° to 35°C
Moderate hypothermia	26° to 31°C
Deep hypothermia	20° to 25°C
Profound hypothermia	<20°C

[a]From Taylor.[1]

TABLE 3.2. Summary of interesting and important historical milestones in the clinical application of hypothermia, based upon Swan's fascinating review.[5] The reader is referred to Swan's original paper for details and references.

Date	Contributor	Contribution
Ca. 1650 BC	Edwin Smith papyrus	Cold applications recommended for head injuries and for breast infections
4th century BC	Hippocratic School on Cos	Cold used to treat infections, head injuries, seizures, tetanus, gout, sprains, and broken bones, and to stop bleeding
1st century AD	Aretalus	Cold applications to the chest to treat and prevent hemoptysis
	Celsus	Plunging head under cold water to treat various forms of "madness" including hydrophobia
2nd century AD	Galen	Drug treatment of fever, cold baths for malaria and erysipelas
	Hua T'O and Chang Chung-Ching in China	Total body cooling to control fever
Ca. 600 AD	Alexander of Tralles	Cold packs to treat quartan fever
Dark Ages	Avicenna	Used ice and snow as a narcotic
	Sultan Saladin	Packed Richard the Lion-Hearted in snow from distant mountains to save him from a desert illness, then traded him for ransom!
17th century AD	Mercurialis Forli (Italy)	Treated his own and his patients' renal colic by squatting in the cold springs of the Arnus river
	Savonarola	Treatment of fever and other diseases with cold baths
	Sanctorius	Invented the thermometer and the "balneotorium," a device for administration of cold water to and around the entire body
1661	Bartholin	Published *The Medical Uses of Snow*
1680	Pennsylvania Indians	Alternating hot baths with plunges into the cold river
18th century AD	John Hunter	Developed usable clinical thermometer
	James Currie	Documented clinical experience with hypothermia as a mode of treatment for many diseases
	Napoleon's Surgeon General	Used snow and ice to induce anesthesia for amputations
19th century AD	*US Medical and Surgical Journal*	Paper published recommending application of cold packs to the hypogastrium to treat "nymphomania (furor uterinus)"
	Arnott, Blundell, Cahill, Perrin, Lallemand, and many others	Advocated topical cold as an anesthetic agent for surgery, safer than chloroform or ether and quite effective
1866	Corbiere	Published major review of therapeutic uses of cold
Early 20th century	The "Ice Doctor" of Maharashtra	Applied ice all over the body of Mahatma Mohandas Gandhi to treat his severe dysentery during World War I as he "lay thus, ever expectant of death."

pose and a cause before it could grow.... These soon appeared. The purpose: lowered metabolism; the cause: direct-vision open-heart surgery."[5]

The potential usefulness of systemic hypothermia to facilitate direct surgical exposure within the heart was proposed in 1950 by Bigelow and colleagues.[6] During the early 1950s, several different methods were evaluated and advocated to facilitate exposure and repair of defects inside the heart. Brief periods of vena caval inflow occlusion and normothermic circulatory arrest were used to expose and permit closure of atrial septal defects. Systemic or total body hypothermia of only modest degree (30° to 33°C), induced by surface cooling, extended the duration of apparent safety for interruption of cerebral blood flow, allowing the surgeon more time for intracardiac exposure and repair of simple intracardiac defects. In subsequent experiments, Bigelow again cooled dogs to 20°C, using surface cooling, with recovery after 15 minutes of total circulatory arrest.[7,8]

The efficacy of hypothermic total circulatory arrest was suggested by Boerema and associates[9] in 1951, after demonstrating that dogs perfused with cold blood tolerated and survived 15 minutes with absolutely no cardiac output and no extracorporeal circulatory support. Table 3.3 summarizes the clinical application that followed shortly after the successful use of hypothermia in experimental animal studies.[23]

Sir Brian Barratt-Boyes[22,24] and his colleagues at the Green Lane Hospital in Auckland, New Zealand, developed and popularized the techniques most widely used today for the correction of complex congenital heart defects in neonates, infants, and small children. In their 1970 re-

TABLE 3.3. Historically significant clinical experience in the evolution of hypothermia, with and without total circulatory arrest, for repair of intracardiac defects.

Date	Contributor	Contribution
1950	Bigelow et al	First proposal of the potential usefulness of systemic hypothermia to facilitate direct exposure within the heart
1950	Bigelow et al	Used brief periods of vena caval inflow occlusion at normothermia to visualize and close atrial septal defects in experimental animals; minimal surface cooling extended duration of apparent safety for interruption of cerebral blood flow
1950	Bigelow et al	Cooled dogs to 20°C using surface cooling, with recovery after 15 minutes of total circulatory arrest
1951	Boerema et al	Demonstrated that dogs perfused with cold blood tolerated and survived 15 minutes of total circulatory arrest
1953	Lewis and Taufic	Successfully closed an atrial septal defect in a 5-year-old girl using surface cooling
1953	Swan	Reported successful clinical results using methods similar to Lewis and Taufic's
1954	Lillehei et al at the University of Minnesota	Demonstrated the practical reality of repairing complex intracardiac defects using controlled cross circulation with another human as the "pump oxygenator"
1958	Sealy, Brown, and Young at Duke University	Reported successful repairs of heart defects in humans using hypothermia combined with cardiopulmonary bypass
1959	Drew et al	Reported experimental studies in which cardiopulmonary bypass was combined with the use of the patients' own lungs as the oxygenator, at 15°C
1960	Dubost et al	Used profound hypothermia with total circulatory arrest for intracardiac surgery
1961	Kirklin et al	At the Mayo Clinic used profound hypothermia and total circulatory arrest for repair of intracardiac defects in 52 patients
1963	Horiuchi et al	Described 16 survivors following repair of ventricular septal defect in 18 infants less than 1 year of age using surface cooling to 25°C and total circulatory arrest
1967	Hikasa et al at Kyoto University	Repaired numerous intracardiac malformations using surface cooling to 20°C with periods of total circulatory arrest of 15 to 75 minutes followed by cardiopulmonary bypass for rewarming and resuscitation
1967	Dillard et al at the University of Washington in Seattle	Corrected total anomalous pulmonary venous drainage during infancy utilizing deep hypothermia with total circulatory arrest, using *both surface cooling and surface rewarming*
1968	Wakusawa et al	Reported good results in 525 patients operated upon using essentially the Kyoto technique (see above)
1970	Barratt-Boyes et al at Green Lane Hospital in Auckland, New Zealand	Described repair of a variety of complex congenital cardiac defects in infancy using profound hypothermia and total circulatory arrest in 34 infants weighing less than 10 kg, with surface cooling to 22°–27°C followed by a brief period of CPB to below 20°C and rewarming after the repair using CPB exclusively
1973	Hamilton et al	Eliminated surface cooling, relying entirely upon core cooling using CPB in 18 infants to establish profound hypothermia to below 20°C prior to total circulatory arrest for repair with rewarming using CPB alone

port,[22] they described repair of a variety of defects using profound hypothermia with total circulatory arrest in 34 infants weighing less than 10 kg. They used surface cooling down to 22° to 27°C, followed by a brief period of CPB to lower the temperature further to below 20°C. Rewarming was accomplished, after repair, using CPB exclusively. Hamilton[23] eliminated surface cooling, relying entirely on core cooling with CPB in 18 infants to establish profound hypothermia (usually below 20°C) prior to a period of total circulatory arrest, during which repair was accomplished. CPB was then reinstituted for rewarming to normothermia.

These two methods—(1) initial surface cooling[22] plus a brief period of CPB for additional cooling to below 20°C, total circulatory arrest for repair, and rewarming on CPB; or (2) core cooling alone on CPB[23] to profoundly hypothermic levels (below 20°C), total circulatory arrest for repair, and rewarming on CPB—are in common use today for the repair of complex congenital heart defects, even in neonates weighing less than 2 kg. For larger and older infants and children, and in adults requiring prolonged intracardiac operations, mild to moderate systemic hypothermia induced by core cooling on CPB is the current standard of care, although some surgical groups are advocating the use of normothermic CPB.[25,26]

Pathophysiology of Ischemia

Ischemia—inadequate oxygen delivery to cells—damages all living tissue. Cardiac ischemia, cerebral ischemia, renal or hepatic ischemia, and total body ischemia are all potential complications of extracorporeal perfusion. The causes of ischemic injury are complex, multifactorial, and interactive. In some cases, these ischemic insults are at least partially related to the pathology prompting the operation itself: atherosclerotic coronary arterial occlusive disease or cyanotic congenital heart disease. In other cases, the ischemic injury is a consequence of associated secondary pathology: atherosclerotic cerebrovascular disease, chronic hypertension, renal arterial occlusive disease, peripheral vascular arterial occlusive disease, or diabetic microangiopathy.

Diffuse or focal ischemia can occur as a consequence of CPB itself, caused by low-flow perfusion without adequately protective hypothermia, inadequate systemic arterial blood flow due to excessive "runoff" through aortopulmonary collateral vessels or systemic arterial-to-pulmonary arterial shunts (including a patent ductus arteriosus or a Blalock-Taussig shunt), nonpulsatile flow from the rotary pump head, macroembolization, microembolization, air embolization, intravascular thrombosis, equipment malfunction, inadequate monitoring, excessive hemodilution, hemorrhage caused by anticoagulation or postperfusion coagulopathy, systemic inflammatory responses to CPB, or excessive total circulatory arrest beyond the safe limits of hypothermic protection.[27]

More often, diffuse or organ-specific ischemia complicating CPB is multifactorial, in part the primary disease for which the operation is being performed, complicated by secondary or associated conditions to which the potential iatrogenic insults of extracorporeal perfusion are added. Prevention of ischemia—focal, organ-specific, or generalized—is the goal of effective CPB.

In general, ischemic damage to tissue can be reduced by (1) minimizing the duration of the ischemic insult, (2) reducing metabolic activity within the preischemic or ischemic tissue while high-energy phosphate stores and intracellular organization remain intact, (3) modulating the biochemical events induced by ischemia, and (4) assuring the integrity of the macrovascular and microvascular beds so that the toxic end products of ischemic metabolism can be quickly removed and oxygen and metabolic substrate supplies restored to the individual cells, the organs, and the body as a whole, after termination of the ischemic insult. Hypothermia attenuates the effects of ischemia primarily by mechanisms 2 and 3.

Life itself depends upon preservation of the integrity of phospholipid cell membranes across which a gradient is maintained between extracellular sodium ions and intracellular potassium ions. This ionic gradient is maintained by the energy-consumptive "sodium-potassium pump." High-energy adenine nucleotides—adenosine triphosphate (ATP) and adenosine diphosphate (ADP)—synthesized primarily (95%) in the mitochondria by oxidative phosphorylation, constitute the repository of energy required to sustain virtually all other metabolic processes and cellular functions. Oxygen is obviously an essential component in the energetics and metabolism of oxidative phosphorylation, on which all other intracellular processes depend. These basic biochemical reactions are simply yet elegantly explained and illustrated by Guyton,[28,29] to whom the reader is referred for details.

Although brief periods of anaerobiosis can be tolerated with subsequent recovery, "ATP is essential for operation of the sodium pump in the cell membrane, and ischaemia thus results in a loss of normal intracellular homeostasis because the tendency for ions to diffuse across the membrane can no longer be balanced by active transport processes. Sodium ions diffuse into, and potassium ions diffuse out of, the cell."[30]

Ischemia causes a reduction of intracellular pH and an alteration of ionic composition, releases autolytic enzymes from lysozomes, and causes abnormal enzymatic transformations by disorganization of biochemical and spatial intracellular relationships. Consequently, the cells release free radicals that react autocatalytically, degradatively, and destructively with cell membrane lipids. The end result is tissue that is destroyed beyond the point of recovery. Normal cellular function and homeostasis do not then return, even after restoration of normal blood supply, oxygen, and nutrient substrates. In fact, microvascular consequences of ischemic injury, including swelling of the endothelial cells lining small arterioles and capillaries, may preclude restoration of a normal blood supply with its resources to the cell.[30]

Rationale for Hypothermia During Cardiac Surgery

Since chemical reactions are slower at lower temperatures, it is entirely reasonable to assume that the rate of consumption of intracellular high-energy phosphate stores will be slower at lower temperatures. Likewise, it is equally reasonable to assume that ischemic damage to the oxygen-carrying vehicles (red blood cells), the "superhighways" (the vascular endothelium), the loading docks (cellular membranes), and, indeed, the energy-producing factories themselves (the mitochondria) will be slowed by cooling.

Ideal protection from an ischemic insult should temporarily and reversibly reduce metabolic activity in all cells and subcellular organelles, and hence slow the depletion or degradation of all important metabolites, including cofactors and high-energy adenine nucleotides. It should then be possible to resume a normal supply of oxygen to the cells through undamaged vascular endothelium and smooth muscle with, at the appropriate physiologic temperature, restoration of normal transmembrane transport, synthetic processes, and mechanical work.

Total body (systemic) hypothermia slows all biochemical reactions. With lowering of metabolic activity, there is a marked reduction in the consumption of metabolic substrates and oxygen. The production of carbon dioxide and water—the end products of metabolism—diminishes proportionately. Oxygen consumption can thus be used as an indicator of overall tissue metabolic activity, assuming no limitation of other metabolic substrates. Hypothermia thus offers a vital adjunct to extracorporeal perfusion, creating a metabolic state that prevents cellular ischemia while allowing a marked reduction in blood flow rate even to the point of temporary total circulatory arrest or very low-flow perfusion.

Michenfelder and Theyer,[31] in 1968, demonstrated that moderate hypothermia (28°C) lowered tissue oxygen consumption to about half that at normothermia. At 25°C, oxygen consumption was lowered further to about 33% of normothermic consumption. Normothermic total body oxygen consumption is about 150 mL/min/m². As a simple approximation, one can assume that oxygen consumption diminishes exponentially at about 9% for each Celsius degree reduction in temperature, although Michenfelder and Milde[32] have recently challenged the existence of either an exponential or a linear relationship between temperature and the cerebral metabolic rate of oxygen consumption ($CMRO_2$) (Figure 3.1). In fact, their experimental data, derived in a canine model, demonstrated that Q_{10} varied from 2.23 between 27° and 37°C, to more than 5 between 14° and 22°C. Q_{10} is a unit-free ratio describing $CMRO_2$ at a given temperature divided by the $CMRO_2$ 10°C *lower*, or:

$$Q_{10} = (CMRO_2 \text{ at } T°C / CMRO_2 \text{ at } [T\text{-}10°C])$$

Michenfelder and Milde's[32] data thus suggest that whereas cooling to 27°C reduces cerebral oxygen consumption to less than half of cerebral oxygen consumption at 37°C, similar 10°C temperature decrements around 20°C result in a much greater reduction in cerebral oxygen consumption per degree cooled. In fact, based on these data, cerebral oxygen consumption at 15°C would be only about 20% of that measured at 25°C, consistent with the very low incidence of neurologic complications that we have experienced when we have cooled patients to 15° to 18°C during 30 minutes prior to a period of 60 minutes of total circulatory arrest. Indeed, Norwood and Norwood[33] emphasize that, in the clinical setting, central nervous system damage would be expected to decrease fivefold at 20°C *if* the Q_{10} were 2.2 and linearly related to temperature. In fact, clinical experience with profound hypothermia and total circulatory arrest at 20°C indicates that it provides 20 to 30 times the protection from neurologic complications of normothermia, suggesting a nonlinear Q_{10} of far more than 2.0 to 2.5 (see discussion of total circulatory arrest below [Techniques to Induce Hypothermia for

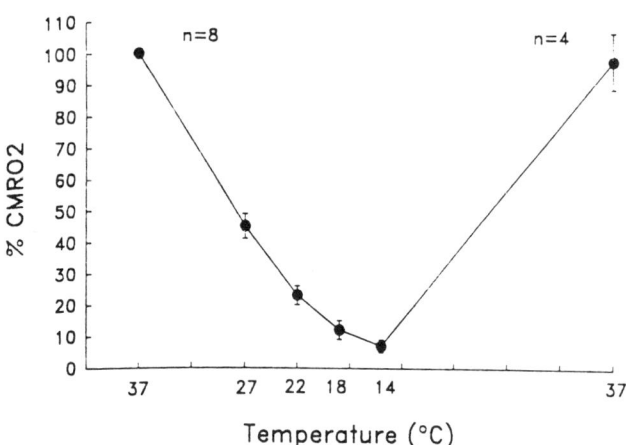

FIGURE 3.1. Effect of temperature on $CMRO_2$. The change in $CMRO_2$ with change in temperature is plotted as a percent of control (±SD). The relationship is neither linear nor exponential. With rewarming, $CMRO_2$ returned to control. Each temperature interval on the abscissa equals 5°C. (From Michenfelder, JD, and Milde, JN,[32] by permission of *Anesthesiology*.)

Cardiac Surgery]). Of note, however, is the fact that a hypothermia-induced reduction in oxygen consumption alone does not necessarily justify a proportional reduction in blood flow rate.[34] Other factors are also involved, including the hemoglobin concentration, the oxyhemoglobin dissociation curve, rheological considerations, non-temperature-related pharmacologic and metabolic inhibitors, microvascular tone, vasoactive substances, and the critical opening pressure of the microvascular capillary bed.

Tolerance of ischemia before tissue damage occurs is also variable from organ to organ. For example, the mammalian kidney will tolerate about 60 minutes of ischemia at 37°C[30,35,36]; the liver will tolerate about 30 minutes of normothermic ischemia; while the brain, of course, is far more sensitive, tolerating no more than 2 to 4 minutes of normothermic ischemia without irreversible injury. The consequences of ischemic injury are also quite variable, depending on the yardstick used to measure those consequences. For example, survival of the patient remains likely even when there has been significant ischemic renal or hepatic injury; the kidneys and liver have an enormous reserve capacity and regenerative capability. This luxury of reserve and regeneration does not exist in the central nervous system. Both survival and quality of life are dependent first on preservation of the brain and spinal cord, without which preservation of the heart, liver, and kidneys is of little consequence.

From a biochemical point of view, the influence of temperature on enzymatic metabolic reactions, and hence on oxygen consumption, can be described quantitatively by consideration, within a physiologic temperature range, of van't Hoff's law indicating the exponential effect of temperature where $\log(V_{O_2}) = kT$ or, otherwise stated, $V_{O_2} = 10^{kT}$ in which V_{O_2} is oxygen consumption, T is temperature (degrees Celsius), and k is a constant.[37,38] However, as noted above, Michenfelder and colleagues have recently challenged these assumptions in regard to cerebral metabolism,[32] and Norwood et al[33,39] have emphasized that the clinically protective effects of hypothermia are "incompletely accounted for by the known temperature-dependent reduction in metabolic rate."

The important interdependence of temperature and intracellular hydrogen ion concentration (pH) was emphasized by Norwood and Norwood[33] in their demonstration that intracellular pH fell more rapidly in the brain than in the liver during a 30-minute anoxic insult, but in both brain and liver, the accumulation of hydrogen ions was markedly attenuated, during the 30 minutes of anoxia, by cooling to 20°C. No fall in intracellular pH could be demonstrated at 20°C in this model, suggesting also a role for the physical chemical properties of intracellular water itself, and of the imidazole-buffering radicals, the dissociation of both being strongly temperature dependent. Water has a pH of 6.8 at a temperature of 37°C; at 20°C it is less dissociated (fewer hydrogen ions) and therefore its pH is 7.2. The imidazole system of intracellular proteins behaves in a similar manner, shifting toward a higher pH at lower temperatures. Intracellular pH is thus maintained in a more normal range in spite of anoxia or ischemia, during which hydrogen ions generated by glycolysis are no longer removed from the mitochondria by oxidation, remaining to inhibit phosphofructokinase activity (glycolysis) at an intracellular pH of around 6.0. The myriad of biochemical interactions and their microstructural consequences contributing to ischemic injury, reversible and irreversible, are beyond the scope of this discussion; excellent reviews are available.[30,40–42] The pathophysiology of central nervous system ischemia is discussed in Chapter 6.

Grout and Morris[30] were not optimistic about the prospects for "perfect" organ preservation during hypothermia and ischemia, stating that "the problem of differential disorganization of metabolic pathways under such conditions may limit the duration of hypothermic storage." In other words, not all organs, cells, subcellular structures, and biochemical or biophysical processes are altered at the same rate, or linearly by alteration in temperature. Simply stated, there is more involved than mere physical chemical constants determining the rate of biochemical reactions.

The relationships among temperature, metabolic activity, organ and cell viability, oxygen consumption, oxygen delivery, substrate availability, end product elimination, enzyme kinetics, endothelial synthetic functions, vasomotor reactivity, and intracellular pH and the data available from models, including cellular and subcellular preparations, thin tissue slices, isolated perfused organs, and intact perfused animals or humans, are complex, sometimes seemingly inconsistent, and deserve detailed analysis of the multiple factors involved in each. Some, for example, assume unlimited oxygen availability while temperature is changed. Others, probably more realistically for clinical extrapolation, assume that oxygen is limited. Still other models, particularly those involving long ischemic times in isolated perfused organs or the whole body perfused model equivalent to CPB, introduce the variables of so-called reperfusion injury, the no-reflow phenomenon, or luxury perfusion, where oxygen supply exceeds oxygen demand.

In 1982, Norwood and Norwood[33] described the role of hypothermia in protection from ischemia: "... neither the reason for organ-specific susceptibility to ischemia or anoxia, nor, more importantly, those biochemical events that prevent tissue recovery following deprivation have been clarified. Hypothermia is widely used clinically for its *empirically established, yet poorly understood* [emphasis mine], attenuation of the process or processes leading to irreversible loss of cellular function during ischemia."

Adverse Effects of Hypothermia

Hypothermia, while relatively benign, is not entirely without its own morbidity. Most notable among these are the deleterious effect of hypothermia on platelet function and potentiation of citrate toxicity, with subsequent reduction in serum ionized calcium, leading to reversible coagulopathy and depression of myocardial contractility.[43-45] Hypothermic perfusion requires hemodilution to reduce blood viscosity. Hypothermia, with hemodilution, affects proteins of the coagulation cascade and prolongs the activated clotting time.[27,43] The coagulopathy is usually reversible with rewarming to normothermia, but when duration of CPB is prolonged due to cooling and rewarming, coagulopathy can be quite severe. Generous transfusion of fresh frozen plasma, cryoprecipitate concentrates of clotting factors, platelets, packed red blood cells, and even fresh whole blood may be required to control such posthypothermic extended perfusion coagulopathy.

Other potential complications of therapeutic hypothermia include ventricular fibrillation, other dysrhythmias, alterations of calcium-mediated excitation-contraction coupling, vasoconstriction, endovascular stasis, hypervolemia, hemoconcentration, myocardial depression, attenuation of the adrenal medullary humoral response to stress, hyperglycemia and other endocrine responses, and altered pharmacokinetics, all of which can be prevented or endured without harmful sequelae during properly managed CPB.[27,46] Importantly, the advantages of hypothermia as an adjunct to CPB far exceed the manageable disadvantages.

Techniques to Induce Hypothermia for Cardiac Surgery

The decision to use hypothermia as an adjunct to CPB during a specific operation, the degree of hypothermia, the method of induction and maintenance of hypothermia, the use of total circulatory arrest with profound hypothermia, the use and route of supplementary cardioplegic or topical hypothermic myocardial protection, and the timing of rewarming are all based on the complexity of the anatomy and pathophysiology of the defect to be corrected during the planned operation, the anticipated duration of aortic occlusion with interruption of coronary arterial perfusion and subsequent myocardial ischemia, the age, weight, and hemodynamic stability of the patient, and the extent to which cerebral and/or spinal cord blood flow is in jeopardy. As in the case of cannulation for CPB itself, the surgeon's preferences and prejudices play a major role in these decisions. Communication is essential. Choice of anesthetic technique, administration of neuroprotective medications, degree of hemodilution, initial temperature of the perfusate, heparinization and maintenance of systemic anticoagulation, administration of α-adrenergic antagonists, management of acid-base balance and blood glucose, and the administration of diuretics all depend upon the degree of hypothermia desired and the method(s) chosen for achieving and maintaining both total body and local myocardial hypothermia. Several methods exist for cooling the patient, and they are listed in Table 3.4.

A few generalizations serve as guidelines. Surface cooling is used only for very small infants (less than 2.5 to 3.0 kg). Profound hypothermia with total circulatory arrest is used for repair of complex congenital heart defects in small infants and children, and for operations involving the aortic arch, in which cerebral blood flow must be interrupted (atresia of the aortic tract or hypoplastic left heart syndrome, aneurysms involving the transverse aortic arch or brachiocephalic arteries) or in which maintenance of venous drainage back to the pump oxygenator would be difficult (anomalies of systemic venous drainage or total anomalous pulmonary venous connections).

Multiple periods of total circulatory arrest interrupted by brief periods of hypothermic reperfusion are preferable to a single long (more than 60 minutes) period of total circulatory arrest.[47] Most operations can be accomplished in a single period of total circulatory arrest lasting less than 60 minutes. Low-flow hypothermic perfusion is safer, when possible, than total circulatory arrest,[36] assuming adequate and unobstructed venous drainage back to the heart-lung machine. The desire to avoid heterologous blood and blood product transfusion in selected larger patients may influence the degree of hypothermia and the perfusion technique.

Surface Cooling

Infants and small children can be cooled relatively quickly by exposure in the cold operating room, use of a water-perfused cooling mattress, and vasodilation accompanying the induction of general anesthesia. When cooling to deep or profound levels of around 20°C is desired, the child can be covered from head to toe with plastic bags filled with crushed ice, after the induction of general anesthesia and the establishment of appropriate intravascular access and monitors (Figure 3.2A-D). A thin plastic surgical drape or one layer of cloth surgical towel separating

TABLE 3.4. Methods of inducing and reversing hypothermia.

Total extracorporeal circulation ("core cooling")
Surface cooling
Surface cooling with supplementary partial CPB
Deep hypothermic total circulatory arrest
Low-flow, profoundly hypothermic perfusion

3. Hypothermia

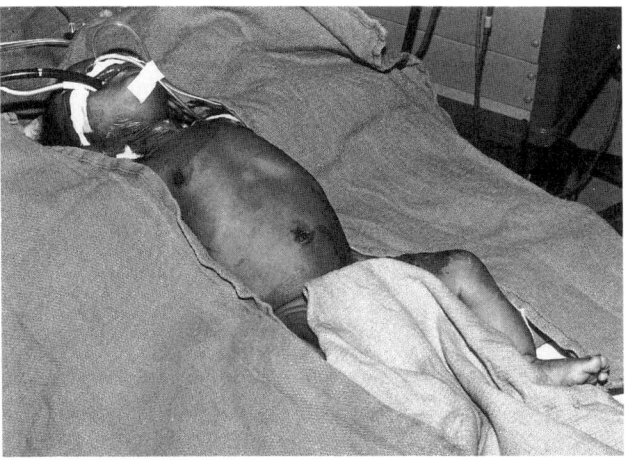

A

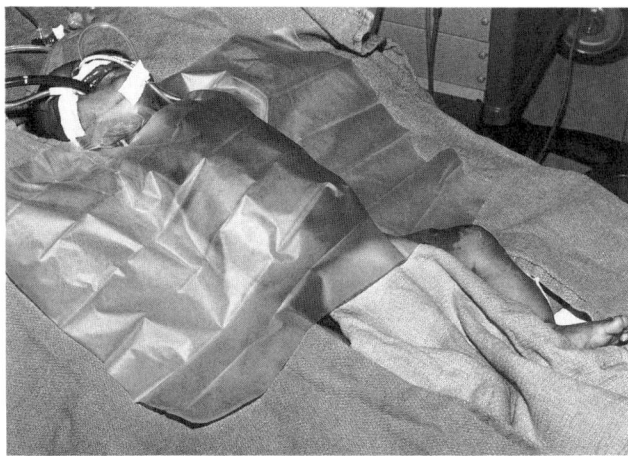

B

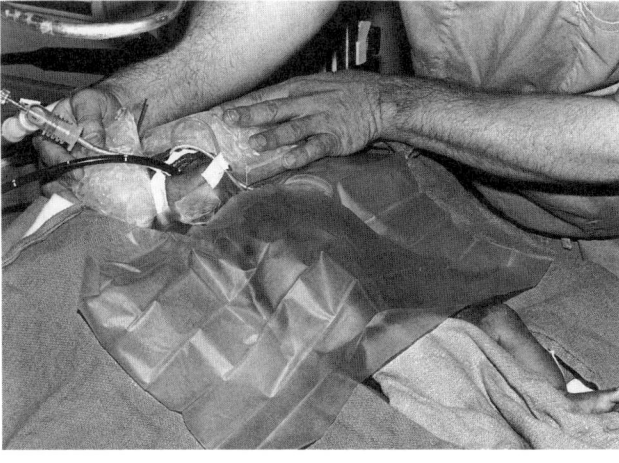

C

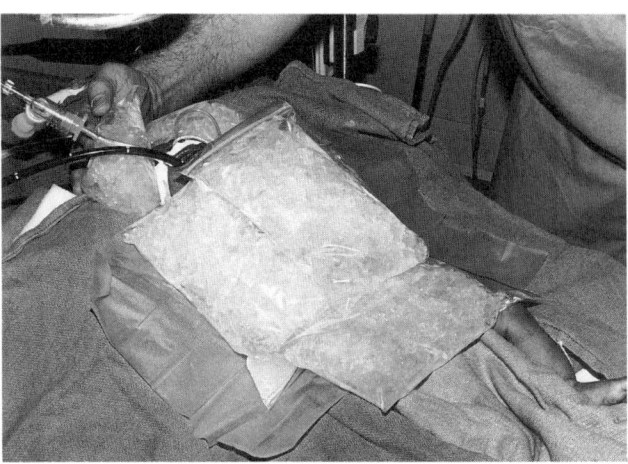

D

FIGURE 3.2. (A) Anesthetized infant exposed in cool operating room prior to application of ice for surface-induced hypothermia. (B) Infant covered with thin plastic surgical drape to avoid thermal injury during cooling with ice in plastic bags. (C) Crushed ice in sealed plastic bags applied around the head and over all exposed surfaces of the infant's body. (D) All exposed surfaces are covered by the ice-filled plastic bags until the body temperature reaches 20° to 24°C. Those bags over the anterior chest wall are then removed to allow sterile surgical skin preparation, draping, and the median sternotomy incision. The ice around the head is left in place to further facilitate cerebral cooling.

the ice bags from the child's skin will protect the skin from frostbite (although we have never seen any skin injury during the relatively short periods of exposure to ice in plastic bags used in this manner). This dramatic, seemingly archaic method remains quite effective in reducing the total duration of CPB perfusion and facilitates cannulation of the very small ascending aorta in the tiny infant. When the infant's temperature falls to 22° to 24°C, or when there is no more than 25 mm Hg difference between the mean arterial blood pressure and the mean right atrial blood pressure, the ice bags are removed, the infant's anterior chest wall is prepared with antiseptic solution, surgical drapes are applied, and the operation continues in a routine manner. Sodium heparin, 4 mg/kg, is administered intravenously through a central vascular catheter when the infant's temperature falls to 30°C, so that anticoagulation will be complete and confirmed well before the likelihood of ventricular fibrillation, which might force a quick median sternotomy, cannulation, and institution of CPB. Such urgent sternal entry is rare indeed, even in the most critically ill infants. On the contrary, the heart typically beats more and more slowly, usually falling to about 40 beats per minute before the median sternotomy is performed. Should ventricular fibrillation occur under these circumstances, there is no reason for panic. One or two attempts at defibrillation, if unsuccessful, should prompt sternotomy and cannulation of the ascending aorta for arterial inflow, and cannulation of the right atrium (with a single cannula in the right atrial appendage) for venous drainage. The 2 or 3 minutes required for cannulation are well tolerated under these hypothermic conditions.

Our methods are similar to those of the Brompton Hospital in London, where surface cooling to 25°C (nasopharyngeal) has been used for infants weighing less than 8 kg. When the chest is opened, the aorta and right atrium are cannulated, and further cooling to 15°C on partial CPB is completed. In recent years, we have reserved this method of surface cooling for infants weighing less than about 2.5 kg and those having a very small ascending aorta, in whom initial aortic cannulation might be technically difficult with consequent compromise of cerebral blood flow.

Partial CPB and Circulatory Arrest with Surface Cooling

When a period of total circulatory arrest under profoundly hypothermic conditions (below 20°C) is planned, 5 to 10 *additional* minutes of perfusion on partial CPB, after surface cooling as described above, assures adequate and uniform cooling. The prime temperature of the heart-lung machine is kept about 10°C below the patient's temperature, down to a lowest prime temperature of about 12°C. There have been suggestions, based solely on clinical anecdotes, that cooling below 15°C can be neurologically harmful. We have not seen evidence to support these observations, but, nonetheless, we rarely cool below 15°C even for the longest and most complex operations, and for elective total circulatory arrest of up to 60 minutes. When essential, we have continued total circulatory arrest even longer—up to as much as 90 minutes—but we certainly do not do this electively, and we do not advise it. In fact, we try to plan all operations so that they can be accomplished in less than 60 minutes of total circulatory arrest, and where necessary, we try to divide the operation into two periods of total circulatory arrest, each period well under 60 minutes, if we do not feel that the entire operation can be accomplished in less than a single 60-minute period of total circulatory arrest. We also prefer low-flow hypothermic perfusion over total circulatory arrest whenever possible, believing empirically as well as experimentally that some flow is better than no flow.[48-51] Cerebral blood flow autoregulation appears to remain intact over a wide range of extracorporeal perfusion flow rates if the alpha-stat strategy of acid-base management is practiced.[47] Certainly the likelihood of cerebral air embolization is less if even minimal positive blood pressure is maintained within the aorta and carotid arteries during low-flow perfusion, rather than the atmospheric pressure present during total circulatory arrest with its increased possibility for air entrainment.

Griepp and Griepp,[47] in 1992, published an extensive collective review of clinical and experimental data concerning the cerebral consequences of hypothermic circulatory arrest in adults in which they discussed other potentially useful monitoring methods, including intraoperative electroencephalography (EEG) and measurement of jugular venous oxygen content. The authors, experienced in both clinical and experimental laboratory settings, advocate a strategy of pretreatment with barbiturates and steroids, use of alpha-stat pH management during both cooling and rewarming, intraoperative EEG monitoring, slow and adequate cooling, packing the patient's head in ice even with core cooling on CPB, monitoring of internal jugular venous oxygen content, hemodilution, and avoidance of hyperglycemia. Within their strategy, the use of barbiturates is perhaps the most controversial issue, substantial data having been reviewed by Weir[52] in support of the thiopentone administration prior to an anticipated ischemic insult. Siegman and colleagues,[53] to the contrary, demonstrated that thiopental prevented the increase in cerebral energy state normally observed with hypothermia and actually resulted in a decrease in the energy state of the brain during and after hypothermic circulatory arrest. These experimental observations in sheep were interpreted as suggestive that thiopental administration before hypothermic circulatory arrest might, in fact, be detrimental to the preservation of the energy state of the brain; many clinicians do not agree, and continue to administer barbiturates before circulatory arrest. (Cerebral protection with barbiturates during CPB is discussed further in Chapter 6.)

Regardless of the cooling method—surface cooling alone, surface cooling plus additional core cooling on CPB, or core cooling alone—we always cool the patient for at least 30 minutes before discontinuing CPB to establish a period of total circulatory arrest. This obligatory 30-minute cooling interval helps assure uniform cooling of all vascular beds and organs, especially the brain, and avoids potential temperature measurement errors and dangerous assumptions regarding the cerebral protection that one can justifiably expect.

Uniform cooling is important. Weiss and colleagues[16,54] have demonstrated that EEG activity persists in the white matter and cerebellum of patients who have undergone uneven cooling, with subsequent choreoathetosis. This reflection of continuing metabolic activity is thought to be the principal cause of choreoathetosis.[55] The incidence of this complication may be reduced by the use of surface cooling, followed by a short period of final core cooling, producing a more even cooling of the cerebral structures than with core cooling by CPB perfusion alone.[56]

Profound Hypothermia and Low-Flow CPB

For longer and more complex operations, even in small infants, two vena caval cannulas can be used, with periods of total circulatory arrest being interspersed with periods of low-flow CPB, as used successfully and reported by Rossi and colleagues[57,58] in 1989.

Fearing caval obstruction, dangerously inadequate venous drainage, and consequent cerebral edema or total body edema, which so often complicate long periods of total CPB in the infant, we prefer to use low-flow arterial perfusion through the ascending aorta, but we sometimes provide venous return to the cardiotomy reservoir, using two small, multiholed, right-angled ventricular sump catheters connected by a Y-connector to the cardiotomy suction pump to assure excellent venous decompression. Alternatively, we have also had good results with the more widely practiced direct cannulation of the superior vena cava and the inferior vena cava using two small, right-angled, metal-tipped Pacifico (DLP) cannulas.

In slightly larger infants (3 to 5 kg), venous drainage can be satisfactorily provided through two small, tapered, flexible-wired, plastic cannulas—one in each tourniquet-occluded vena cava through the opened right atrium. The cannulas are simply allowed to drain directly into an open glass "asepto" syringe, to the tip of which is attached the tubing from the cardiotomy suction pump. The minimal positive pressure in each vena cava forces blood through the cannulas into the open syringe, preventing caval collapse and cannula occlusion by avoidance of excessive negative pressure or suction created by the usual gravity drainage system of siphonage. We have found both of these modified methods of venous drainage to be quite useful in allowing us to maintain a low-flow perfusion state—thus avoiding total circulatory arrest—during repair of complex atrioventricular septal defects, transposition of the great arteries, and truncus arteriosus in the tiny infant. In infants weighing more than 3 kg, simple standard gravity siphonage drainage is sufficient, with both venous cannulas connected by way of a Y-adapter in the venous drainage of the CPB circuit. Venous blood thus drains directly to the venous reservoir in the usual manner without cardiotomy suction. Trauma to the cellular and noncellular blood components is thus minimized.

When low-flow CPB is used, it seems important that some parameter be established and monitored to assure that the flow being delivered is adequate to meet the metabolic requirements of even the most sensitive organs, usually assumed to be the brain, kidney, and liver. Unfortunately, no such specific parameter exists. There is no method of continuously assessing brain function during CPB in the anesthetized patient, and multiple factors contribute to cerebral injury that may only become obvious several hours after completion of CPB and the patient's awakening from general anesthesia.[56] Therefore, such parameters as there are should be monitored to ensure that oxygen delivery to the body as a whole is adequate to meet overall metabolic demands.

Kirklin and Kirklin,[59] in 1981, studied mixed venous oxygen levels during CPB as a reflection of oxygen delivery and consumption. They reported that a mixed venous oxygen level of 30 mm Hg, corresponding to a mixed venous oxygen saturation of 60%, was associated with a normal recovery from CPB.[56] The availability of in-line oxygen saturation monitors has made it possible to follow continuously this important parameter, which we have found clinically useful. The mixed venous oxygen saturation must be interpreted with some caution, however. Obviously, if the arterial blood does not reach the metabolically active tissue itself, bypassing the capillaries through larger arteriovenous shunts, little or no oxygen will be extracted and the mixed venous oxygen saturation will remain high, suggesting that more than enough oxygen is being delivered to meet demands, when, in fact, such may not be the case at all. We also do not know that blood flow is distributed equally or appropriately to all vascular beds, in proportion to need, when blood flow, pressure, and temperature are all far below normal levels. Much remains to be learned about autoregulation of blood flow under these conditions. Empirically, the logically interpreted mixed venous oxygen saturation, when maintained above 60%, has served us well as an indicator of the adequacy of perfusion, even during hypothermic and low-flow perfusion.

Profound Hypothermia with Total Circulatory Arrest Versus Low-Flow Hypothermic Perfusion

Recent clinical and experimental data convincingly favor low-flow hypothermic perfusion as a safer method that is virtually as convenient as total circulatory arrest at temperatures below 20°C.[48-52] Newburger and colleagues[48] found a higher incidence of clinical and EEG seizure activity, a longer time to the recovery of normal brain activity by EEG, and a greater release of the BB isoenzyme of creatine kinase during the first 6 hours after operation in infants managed primarily by a strategy of total circulatory arrest compared to infants treated with low-flow hypothermic perfusion. Additionally, the probability of a postoperative seizure or EEG evidence of ictal activity was directly related to the duration of circulatory arrest (Figure 3.3). On the other hand, by the time of discharge from the hospital, these infants were similar in overall incidence of abnormalities on neurologic examination and EEG to those from a group managed by a strategy of low-flow hypothermic perfusion (50 mL/kg/min). The use of low-flow perfusion prolongs the duration of CPB and complicates, to some degree, the otherwise ideal bloodless, motionless, and uncluttered operative field of total circulatory arrest.[60,61] The long-term implications and comparative prognoses of infants and children operated on using these two minimally different strategies of low-flow hypothermic perfusion versus profound hypothermia with total circulatory arrest must await longitudinal follow-up studies, now under way.[48] Certainly, one can conclude

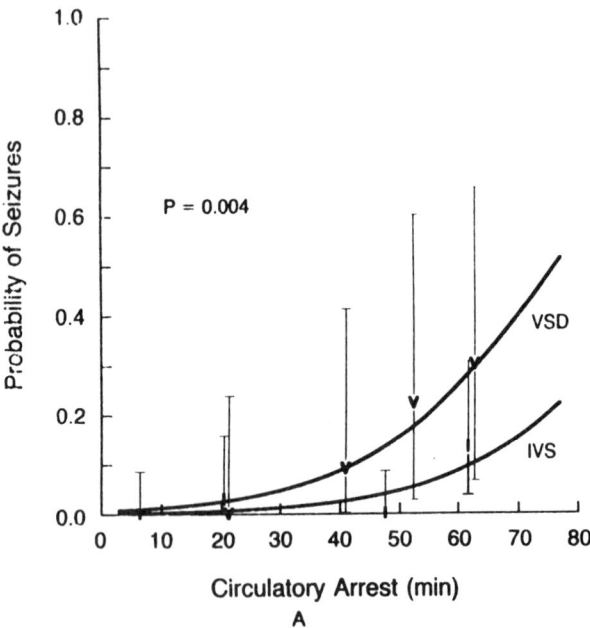 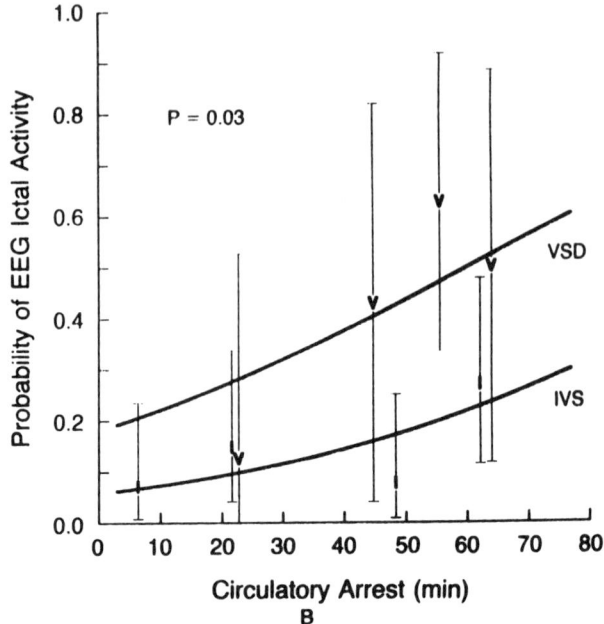

FIGURE 3.3. Estimated probabilities of definite seizures in infants following repair of transposition of the great arteries with ventricular septal defect (VSD) or intact ventricular septum (IVS) in the first week after surgery (A) and of ictal activity on continuous video EEG in the first 48 hours after surgery (B), as a function of the duration of total circulatory arrest. (Reprinted with permission from *The New England Journal of Medicine* 329:1057–1064, 1993.[48])

that when a strategy of total circulatory arrest *is* used, the patient should be cooled long enough to assure uniform cooling (probably about 30 minutes) to well below 20°C, the head should be packed in ice throughout the operation until rewarming commences, care should be exercised to avoid air embolization, and the total circulatory arrest time should be kept to an absolute minimum. Less than 30 minutes of interrupted cerebral perfusion under these conditions is safe. Up to 60 minutes of circulatory arrest is usually tolerated when the temperature is about 15°C, but if a longer period of arrest is required for the operation, low-flow perfusion should be used or a period of reperfusion should separate two deliberately shorter periods of total circulatory arrest.

Rewarming During Extracorporeal Circulation

During rewarming, one should not exceed a 10° to 12°C temperature gradient between the venous blood temperature and the water temperature in the heat exchanger, or a similar 10° to 12°C gradient between the temperature of the arterial blood returning to the patient and the patient's own core temperature. The temperature of the water perfusing the heat exchanger should not exceed 42°C, nor should the arterial blood temperature or the patient's core temperature exceed 38°C. We usually maintain the patient on CPB until the bladder temperature is 36° to 37°C, to assure uniform and complete rewarming, reperfusion, and resuscitation of the heart. This prolongs the duration of CPB somewhat, but we believe it is preferable to weaning the patient from CPB too soon, in which case the body temperature is likely to drift downward again with associated deterioration of cardiac performance and development of a clinically significant coagulopathy. Importantly, rewarming should not result in *hyperthermia*; even a 1° to 2°C increase in brain temperature can exacerbate ischemic cerebral damage.

Lack of uniformity and adequacy of cooling can result in even more complex interactions and variability during ischemia itself and during rewarming. Oxygen is more tightly bound to hemoglobin at low temperatures; therefore, less oxygen is available to meet the metabolic needs of the tissue. Carbon dioxide production is reduced at low temperatures, worsening the problem of respiratory alkalosis (excessive elimination of carbon dioxide) associated with some oxygenators. Accumulation of vasodilator substances—inorganic phosphate, adenosine monophosphate (AMP), and adenosine diphosphate (ADP)—as the adenosine triphosphate (ATP) and creatine phosphate (CP) high-energy phosphate stores are consumed in metabolically active but hypoperfused tissue creates a state of hyperemia and vasodilatation with a "washout" systemic acidosis during reperfusion of the previously underperfused tissue beds. This must be differentiated from the true metabolic acidosis of continuing hypoperfusion or low cardiac output.

Temperature Monitoring Sites

The duration and uniformity of cooling, the duration of ischemia and circulatory arrest, and the temperature of the body and brain all influence outcome following perfusion, low-flow perfusion, and total circulatory arrest. Accurate measurement of temperature is certainly one of the most important parameters followed during hypothermic perfusion and rewarming. Neither cooling nor rewarming is uniform throughout the body. The vascularity of the organ (low in skin, fat, and muscle; high in kidney, liver, heart, and brain), the intrinsic metabolic activity of the organ (high in liver and heart), and neuroendocrine factors[62] play a role in organ temperature gradients within the body and the core (central aortic) temperature itself.

Heidenreich et al[63] studied noninvasive measures of temperature to predict core temperature in 25 severely hypothermic patients, in whom core temperature was determined by measurement of pulmonary arterial, bladder, and esophageal temperatures. Less invasive tympanic membrane thermometers, oral and axillary electronic thermometers, and a forehead surface temperature indicator appeared to be valid indicators of core temperature in these hypothermic patients. We have found the bladder temperature,[64,65] as monitored by a thermistor incorporated into the urinary drainage catheter, to be an excellent determinant of core temperature, not influenced by the cold saline or ice slush often flooding the mediastinum during open-heart operations. Likewise, the bladder temperature is not influenced by warm gases in the endotracheal tube or the presence of transesophageal echocardiographic probes. The nasopharyngeal temperature and the tympanic membrane temperature, preferred by many because of their proximity to the brain, have not been as dependable in our experience, influenced as they are by multiple environmental variables. Likewise, the rectal temperature tends to lag far behind the bladder and nasopharyngeal temperatures in response to temperature changes in the hypothermic patient, probably due to vasoconstriction and diminished perfusion of the rectal mucosa. (Temperature monitoring sites and methods are also discussed in Chapter 22.)

Management of pH During CPB

The management of blood pH during CPB remains a source of controversy and the subject of considerable recent clinical and laboratory investigation. Issues of concern include the effects of blood pH and carbon dioxide on cerebral blood flow, oxygen availability and the oxyhemoglobin dissociation curve, the effects of pH on 2,3-diphosphoglyceric acid (2,3-DPG) activity, and the increased transmembrane diffusibility of lipophilic substrates in a more alkaline environment (in contrast to the relatively less diffusible hydrophilic substrates in a more acidic environment).

The solubility of both oxygen and carbon dioxide increases as the temperature falls; hence, the measured partial pressure of each gas will decrease as the temperature decreases and more gas dissolves or "goes into solution." When blood samples are drawn at low temperature but analyzed at 37°C, corrections must be made if one is to know the true pH at the actual patient body temperature during hypothermic perfusion. To "correct" pH, add 0.0147 to the pH reading at 37°C for each degree Celsius below 37°C. The P_{O_2} decreases 7.2% and the P_{CO_2} decreases 4.4% for each degree of cooling below 37°C.[27]

The pH of water at 37°C is 6.8; at 20°C the pH is 7.4. In the more alkaline intracellular environment of hypothermia, intermediate metabolites exist to a greater degree in the ionized, hydrophilic, relatively entrapped state, able to escape from the cell only through specific channels. Alkalinization of the intracellular environment creates more lipophilic intermediate metabolites capable of passive diffusion through cell membranes, with consequent loss of substrate from within the cell.[66] Norwood and colleagues[39] have investigated the effects of these pH-related phenomena and of hypothermia on cerebral anoxia.

The activity of 2,3-DPG is depressed by hypothermia and by alkalinity, and 2,3-DPG is, to some extent, responsible for the dissociation of oxygen from hemoglobin. After prolonged storage of banked blood and resulting depletion of 2,3-DPG activity, hypothermia and alkalosis may interact to inhibit oxygen *release* into perfused tissue even from otherwise well-oxygenated blood.[35]

Hypothermia shifts the oxygen-hemoglobin dissociation curve to the left. Alkalosis also shifts the curve to the left. Hence the combination of hypothermia and alkalosis would be expected to decrease the availability of oxygen at the tissue level due to the relatively smaller amount of dissociated, or free, oxygen.

This concept of the oxyhemoglobin dissociation curve suggests one possible advantage of the so-called pH-stat management of hypothermic CPB perfusion (by the addition of carbon dioxide to the oxygenator to maintain a normal pH of 7.4 when the pH is corrected to the temperature of the patient); that is, it creates an apparent mild acidosis when the blood pH measurement is corrected to, or measured at, 37°C in the blood-gas analyzer. Likewise, the relative acidosis produced by the addition of carbon dioxide—"pH-stat" management—would be expected to increase cerebral blood flow by cerebral vasodilation.

On the other hand, total body oxygen consumption has been shown to be greater when CO_2 is *not* added to correct the pH when measured at 37°C, permitting the actual pH during hypothermia, corrected to the patient's actual temperature at the time rather than to 37°C, to rise to moderately alkaline levels consistent with the rise in the pH of water caused by the change in its dissociation constant as a function of temperature. This so-called alpha-stat pH management during hypothermic perfusion—allowing the *ratio* or "alpha" of dissociated to nondissociated imidazole groups of the histidine buffer system to remain constant during cooling—probably facilitates enzyme function and hence increases metabolic activity and total body oxygen consumption under hypothermic conditions.[66] This would not, in fact, seem advantageous, since most methods of protecting from ischemia aim at *reduction* of metabolic activity and, consequently, reduction in oxygen consumption.

Limited available clinical evidence suggests better protection of the brain when a "pH-stat" protocol is used,[66] but these differences might well be overcome if a longer prearrest perfusion time had been used to assure uniform cerebral cooling in the absence of additional carbon dioxide in the oxygenator to increase cerebral vasodilation.

Stephan and colleagues,[67] in 1992, compared the effects of blood-gas management on cerebral blood flow, metabolism, and neurologic outcome after hypothermic CPB in 65 adult patients undergoing coronary artery bypass surgery, allocated randomly to either a pH-stat (temperature-corrected blood-gas management) or an alpha-stat (temperature-uncorrected blood-gas management) group. They concluded that acid-base management did *not* affect cerebral metabolism, despite its influence on blood flow. After rewarming, cerebral blood flow and cerebral metabolism normalized independently of acid-base management during hypothermia. Nevertheless, neurologic dysfunction occurred more often in the pH-stat group ($p = 0.036$). Cerebral blood flow increased by 191% in the pH-stat group during hypothermia, in contrast to an 18% reduction in cerebral blood flow in the alpha-stat group. Hence, neurologic dysfunction appeared to be associated with *increased* rather than decreased cerebral blood flow during hypothermia—a seemingly paradoxical but provocative observation that may be related to embolic load. It is probably not justifiable to extrapolate from this "model" to the very different circumstances of profound hypothermia and total circulatory arrest, with a quite different cellular insult and reperfusion environment.

While the debate concerning alpha-stat versus pH-stat acid-base management during various degrees of systemic hypothermic CPB, with or without total circulatory arrest, continues,[48,66,68] most centers in which profound hypothermia with total circulatory arrest is commonly used in both children and adults employ an alpha-stat strategy.[47,69] This strategic decision is based on the assumption that maximizing cerebral blood flow by the addition of carbon dioxide to the oxygenator gas mixture during hypothermic CPB may, in fact, be harmful[70,71]; preservation of cerebral blood flow autoregulation via alpha-stat strategy is believed to be more physiologically rational.[47]

Summary

Hypothermia, either accidental or therapeutically induced, is an important biologic, biochemical, and biophysiologic concept demanding consideration and understanding from virtually every clinical specialist: from neonatologist to geriatrician, from emergency room physician to cardiothoracic surgeon, from sports medicine physician to internist. The concepts of induced hypothermia and its management are central to the practice of cardiothoracic surgery and anesthesiology and to extracorporeal perfusion technology. Contemporary primary repair of complex congenital cardiac defects in tiny infants and children and predictable resection and replacement of the aortic arch simply would *not* be possible without profound hypothermia and either low-flow perfusion or total circulatory arrest. Swain suggests that "Hypothermia is the current mainstay of cerebral protection."[72] Even in the more routine and predictable coronary artery bypass graft operations and in heart valve replacement or reconstruction in the adult, hypothermia is an important adjunct to CPB for preservation of cerebral, myocardial, renal, and hepatic function. Optimal preservation, however, remains a provocative challenge. Hypothermia alone does not *yet* assure complete neurologic recovery in the adult or normal neurologic and intellectual development in the infant after prolonged extracorporeal perfusion.

References

1. Taylor CA. Surgical hypothermia. *Pharmac Ther* 1988;38:169-200.
2. Reuler JB. Hypothermia: pathophysiology, clinical settings, and management. *Ann Intern Med* 1978;89:519-527.
3. Virtue RW. *Hypothermic Anesthesia*. Springfield, Ill: Charles C Thomas; 1955:vii.
4. Breasted JH. *The Edwin Smith Surgical Papyrus. Vol. I.* Chicago: University of Chicago Press; 1930.
5. Swan H. Clinical hypothermia: a lady with a past and some promise for the future. *Surgery* 1973;73:736-758.
6. Bigelow WG, Lindsay WK, Greenwood WF. Hypothermia—its possible role in cardiac surgery: an investigation of factors governing survival in dogs at low body temperatures. *Ann Surg* 1950;132:849-864.
7. Bigelow WG, Lindsay WK, Harrison RC, et al. Oxygen transport and utilization in dogs at low body temperatures. *Am J Physiol* 1950;160:125-137.
8. Bigelow WG, Callaghan JC, Hopps JA. General hypothermia for experimental intracardiac surgery. *Ann Surg* 1950;132:531-539.
9. Boerema I, Wildschut A, Schmidt WJH, et al. Experimental researches into hypothermia as an aid in the surgery of the heart. *Arch Chirurg Neerl* 1951;3:25.
10. Lewis FS, Taufic M. Closure of atrial septal defects with the aid of hypothermia: experimental accomplishments and the report of one successful case. *Surgery* 1953;33:52.

11. Swan H, Seavin I, Blount SG, et al. Surgery by direct vision in the open heart during hypothermia. *JAMA* 1953;153:1081.
12. Lillehei CW. Controlled cross circulation for direct-vision intracardiac surgery; correction of ventricular septal defects, atrioventricularis communis and tetralogy of Fallot. *Post Grad Med* 1955;17:388–396.
13. Warden HE, Cohen M, Read RC, et al. Controlled cross circulation for open intracardiac surgery. *J Thorac Surg* 1954;28:331.
14. Sealy WC, Brown IW, Young WG. A report on the use of both extracorporeal circulation and hypothermia for open heart surgery. *Ann Surg* 1958;147:603.
15. Drew CE, Keen G, Benazon BB. Profound hypothermia. *Lancet* 1959;1:745.
16. Weiss M, Piwnica A, Lenfant C, et al. Deep hypothermia with total circulatory arrest. *Trans Am Soc Artif Intern Organs* 1960;6:227.
17. Kirklin JW, Dawson B, Devloo RA, et al. Open intracardiac operations: use of circulatory arrest during hypothermia induced by blood cooling. *Ann Surg* 1961;154:769.
18. Horiuchi T, Koyamada K, Matano I, et al. Radical operation for ventricular septal defect in infancy. *J Thorac Cardiovasc Surg* 1963;46:180.
19. Hikasa Y, Shirotani H, Satomura K, et al. Open heart surgery in infants with the aid of hypothermic anesthesia. *Arch Jpn Chir* 1967;36:495–508.
20. Dillard DH, Mohri H, Hessel EA, et al. Correction of total anomalous pulmonary venous drainage in infants utilizing deep hypothermia with total circulatory arrest. *Circulation* 1967;36(suppl I):I-105.
21. Wakusawa R, Shibata S, Sata H, et al. Clinical experience in 525 cases of open-heart surgery under simple profound hypothermia. *Jpn J Anesth* 1968;18:240.
22. Barratt-Boyes BG, Simpson MM, Neutze JM. Intracardiac surgery in neonates and infants using deep hypothermia. *Circulation* 1970;61–62(suppl III):III-73.
23. Hamilton DI, Shackleton J, Rees GJ, et al. Experience with deep hypothermia in infancy using core cooling. In: Barratt-Boyes BG, Neutze JM, Harris EA, eds. *Heart Disease in Infancy*. Baltimore: Williams & Wilkins; 1973:52.
24. Barratt-Boyes BG, Simpson M, Neutze JM. Intracardiac surgery in neonates and infants using deep hypothermia. *Circulation* 1971;43(suppl 1:25; suppl 1:30).
25. Christakis GT, Weisel RD, Fremes SE, et al. Coronary artery bypass grafting in patients with poor ventricular function. *J Thorac Cardiovasc Surg* 1992;103:1083–1091.
26. Christakis GT, Koch JP, Deemar KA, et al. A randomized study of the systemic effects of warm heart surgery. *Ann Thorac Surg* 1992;54:449–457.
27. *Systemic Effects of Cardiopulmonary Bypass*. New York: Cahners Healthcare Communications; 1993:1–28.
28. Guyton AC. The cell and its function. In: *Textbook of Medical Physiology*. 8th ed. Philadelphia: W B Saunders Company, Harcourt Brace Jovanovich Inc; 1991:9–23.
29. Guyton AC. Metabolism of carbohydrates and formation of adenosine triphosphate. In: *Textbook of Medical Physiology*. 8th ed. Philadelphia: W B Saunders Company, Harcourt Brace Jovanovich Inc; 1991:744–753.
30. Grout BWW, Morris GJ, eds. *The Effects of Low Temperatures on Biological Systems*. London: Edward Arnold; 1987.
31. Michenfelder JD, Theyer RA. Hypothermia: effect on canine brain and whole-body metabolism. *Anesthesiology* 1968;29:1107–1112.
32. Michenfelder JD, Milde JH. The relationship among canine brain temperature, metabolism, and function during hypothermia. *Anesthesiology* 1991;75:130–136.
33. Norwood WI, Norwood CR. Influence of hypothermia on intracellular pH during anoxia. *Am J Physiol* 1982;243:C62–C65.
34. Berger EC. *The Physiology of Adequate Perfusion*. St. Louis: C V Mosby Company; 1979.
35. Abouna GM, Pashley DH, Ginsbury JM, et al. Kidney preservation by hypothermic perfusion with albumin versus plasma and with pulsatile versus non-pulsatile flow. *Br J Surg* 1974;61:555–561.
36. Abouna GM, Delong TG, Pashley DH, et al. Proceedings: critical evaluation of viability assays in renal preservation. *Br J Surg* 1974;61:325.
37. Harris EA, Seelye ER, Squire AW. Oxygen consumption during cardiopulmonary bypass with moderate hypothermia in man. *Br J Anaesth* 1971;43:1113–1120.
38. Evans PJD, Ruygrok P, Seelye ER, et al. Does sodium nitroprusside improve tissue oxygenation during cardiopulmonary bypass? *Br J Anaesth* 1977;40:799–803.
39. Norwood WI, Norwood CR, Castaneda AR. Cerebral anoxia: effect of deep hypothermia and pH. *Surgery* 1979;86:203–209.
40. Rangel DM, Stevens GH, Yakeishi Y, et al. Physiologic evaluation of canine lung allografts from cadaver donors. *Surgery* 1969;66:863–870.
41. Fonkalsrud EW, Rangel DM, Byfield J, et al. Hepatic preservation with chlorpromazine and phenoxygenzamine. *Surgery* 1969;66:23–33.
42. Thaw C, Wittlin SD, Gershengorn MC. Tetracaine, propranolol and trifluoperazine inhibit thyrotropin releasing hormone-induced prolactin secretion from GH3 cells by displacing membrane calcium: further evidence that TRH acts to mobilize cellular calcium. *Endocrinology* 1982;111:2138–2140.
43. Khuri SF, Michelson AD, Valeri CR. The effect of cardiopulmonary bypass on hemostasis and coagulation. In: Loscalzo J, Schafer AI, eds. *Thrombosis and Hemorrhage*. Cambridge, Mass: Blackwell; 1993.
44. Valeri CR, Feingold H, Cassidy G, et al. Hypothermia-induced reversible platelet dysfunction. *Ann Surg* 1987;205:175–181.
45. Valeri CR, MacGregor H, Pompei F, et al. Acquired abnormalities of platelet function. *N Engl J Med* 1991;324:1670.
46. Endoh M. Regulation of intracellular Ca^{2+} transients of myocardial cell. In: Tada M, ed. *Molecular Biology of the Myocardium*. Tokyo: Japan Scientific Societies Press & CRC Press; 1992:203–218.
47. Griepp EB, Griepp RB. Cerebral consequences of hypothermic circulatory arrest in adults. *J Cardiac Surg* 1992;7:134–155.
48. Newburger JW, Jonas RA, Wernovsky G, et al. A comparison of the perioperative neurologic effects of hypothermic circulatory arrest versus low-flow cardiopulmonary bypass in infant heart surgery. *N Engl J Med* 1993;329:1057–1064.
49. Rebeyka IM, Coles JG, Wilson GJ, et al. The effect of low-flow cardiopulmonary bypass on cerebral function: an ex-

perimental and clinical study. *Ann Thorac Surg* 1987;43: 391-396.
50. Swain JA, McDonald TJ Jr, Griffith PK, et al. Low-flow hypothermic cardiopulmonary bypass protects the brain. *J Thorac Cardiovasc Surg* 1991;102:76-83.
51. Wilson GJ, Rebeyka IM, Coles JG, et al. Loss of the somatosensory evoked response as an indicator of reversible cerebral ischemia during hypothermic, low-flow cardiopulmonary bypass. *Ann Thorac Surg* 1988;45:206-209.
52. Weir DL, The use of thiopentone and propofol. In: Smith P, Taylor K, eds. *Cardiac Surgery and the Brain*. London: Edward Arnold; 1993:245-251.
53. Siegman MG, Anderson RV, Balaban RS, et al. Barbiturates impair cerebral metabolism during hypothermic circulatory arrest. *Ann Thorac Surg* 1992;54:1131-1136.
54. Weiss M, Weiss J, Cotton J, et al. A study of the electroencephalogram during surgery with deep hypothermia and circulatory arrest in infants. *J Thorac Cardiovasc Surg* 1975; 70:316-329.
55. Reilly El, Brunberg JA, Doty DB. The effect of deep hypothermia and total circulatory arrest on the electroencephalogram in children. *Electroencephalogr Clin Neurophysiol* 1974;36:661-667.
56. Kay PH. Low flow and circulatory arrest. In: Kay PH, ed. *Techniques in Extracorporeal Circulation*. 3rd ed. Oxford: Butterworth-Heinemann Ltd; 1992:230-235.
57. Rossi R, van der Linden J, Ekroth R, et al. No flow or low flow? A study of the ischemic marker creatine kinase BB after deep hypothermic procedures. *J Thorac Cardiosvasc Surg* 1989;98:193-199.
58. Ekroth R, Thompson RJ, Lincoln C, et al. Elective deep hypothermia with total circulatory arrest: changes in plasma creatine kinase BB, blood glucose, and clinical variables. *J Thorac Cardiovasc Surg* 1989;97:30-35.
59. Kirklin JK, Kirklin JW. Management of the cardiovascular system after cardiac surgery. *Ann Thorac Surg* 1981;32:311-319.
60. Greeley WJ, Ungerleider RM. Assessing the effect of cardiopulmonary bypass on the brain. *Ann Thorac Surg* 1991;52: 417-419.
61. Kirklin JW, Barratt-Boyes BG, Hypothermia, circulatory arrest, and cardiopulmonary bypass. In: *Cardiac Surgery*. 2nd ed. New York: Churchill Livingstone; 1993:61-128.
62. Stupful M, Severinghaus JW. Internal body temperature gradients during anesthesia and hypothermia and effect of vagotomy. *J Appl Physiol* 1956;9:380.
63. Heidenreich T, Guiffre M, Doorley J. Temperature and temperature measurement after induced hypothermia. *Nurs Res* 1992;41:296-300.
64. Bone ME, Feneck RO. Bladder temperature as an estimate of body temperature during cardiopulmonary bypass. *Anaesthesia* 1988;43:181-185.
65. Horrow JC, Rosenberg H. Does urinary catheter temperature reflect core temperature during cardiac surgery? *Anesthesiology* 1988;69:986-989.
66. Jonas RA. Problems of deep hypothermic circulatory arrest and low-flow perfusion: with particular reference to the paediatric population. In: Smith P, Taylor K, eds. *Cardiac Surgery and the Brain*. London: Edward Arnold, Hodder & Stoughton; 1993:95-107.
67. Stephan H, Weyland A, Kazmaier S, et al. Acid-base management during hypothermic cardiopulmonary bypass does not affect cerebral metabolism but does affect blood flow and neurological outcome. *Br J Anaesth* 1992;69:51-57.
68. Jonas RA, Bellinger DC, Rappaport LA, et al. Relation of pH strategy and developmental outcome after hypothermic circulatory arrest. *J Thorac Cardiovasc Surg* 1993;106:362-368.
69. Tan PS. The anaesthetic management of circulatory arrest. *Br J Hosp Med* 1990;43:36-41.
70. Watanabe T, Orita H, Kobayashi M, et al. Brain tissue pH, oxygen tension, and carbon dioxide tension in profoundly hypothermic cardiopulmonary bypass. Comparative study of circulatory arrest, nonpulsatile low-flow perfusion, and pulsatile low-flow perfusion [see comments]. *J Thorac Cardiovasc Surg* 1989;97:396-401.
71. Watanabe T, Miura M, Orita H, et al. Brain tissue pH, oxygen tension, and carbon dioxide tension in profoundly hypothermic cardiopulmonary bypass. Pulsatile assistance for circulatory arrest, low-flow perfusion, and moderate-flow perfusion. *J Thorac Cardiovasc Surg* 1990;100:274-280.
72. Swain JA. Cardiac surgery and the brain (editorial). *N Engl J Med* 1993;329:1119-1120.

4
Pharmacokinetics and Pharmacodynamics During Cardiac Surgery and Cardiopulmonary Bypass

Richard I. Hall, Brian L. Thomas, and Carl C. Hug, Jr.

Introduction

The physiologic trespasses produced by cardiac surgery and cardiopulmonary bypass (CPB) profoundly affect the concentrations of drugs within the body and its ultimate response to these agents. The application of systemic hypothermia precipitates significant changes in regional blood flow and the eventual metabolism and elimination of these compounds. The effects of hypothermia and CPB on drug levels and receptor dynamics will be examined in this chapter, as well as the effects of bypass on individual compounds. To fully grasp the changes produced during cardiac surgery, however, a basic understanding of the principles of pharmacokinetics and pharmacodynamics is imperative.

Basic Principles of Pharmacokinetics and Pharmacodynamics

Drugs introduced into the body must be absorbed and delivered to a target site in order to exert their effect. The study of the way in which the body processes a particular drug, including its eventual metabolism and excretion, is termed *pharmacokinetics*. Once available at the cellular level, drugs interact with specific membrane receptor sites to initiate a sequence of intracellular events leading to a pharmacologic effect. The study of how an individual drug interacts with a cell to produce this effect is termed *pharmacodynamics*. Related classes of drugs, such as inotropic agents, share common pharmacokinetic and pharmacodynamic properties. We shall first examine the pharmacokinetic forces that determine the plasma concentration of drug available in the body at a given time.

Determinants of Drug Concentration in Plasma[1-4]

Measurement of Drug Concentration in Plasma

The study of pharmacokinetics depends upon the precise quantification of drug levels within the body. Levels are usually reported as the concentration of unaltered drug in the plasma or whole blood. This value, however, may be composed of the concentrations of up to three different forms of a compound. A large percentage of drug may be bound to carrier plasma proteins, such as albumin or α-1-acid glycoprotein. The protein-bound fraction of the drug is generally inactive, but is measured as part of the total plasma concentration. The drug may exist in its free, unbound state, which generally accounts for the active fraction of the drug. If drug levels in whole blood are measured, a portion may also be sequestered by the red blood cells.[5,6] The free concentration may be determined by measuring the amount of drug in a protein-free ultrafiltrate of plasma, using techniques of ultrafiltration or equilibrium dialysis.[7,8]

The metabolic products of a drug (which may frequently produce pharmacodynamic effects) are generally not reported as a component of the measured drug concentration. The analytical procedure employed for measurement of a drug must thus be specific for active drug and not its metabolites.[9-12]

Single IV Dose

The majority of medications given during cardiac surgery are administered as single IV bolus injections. Following an IV bolus of a drug, a number of processes occur that ultimately determine the concentration of drug to be found in plasma over time. Following a rapid injection, the drug will be diluted in the blood, achieving its peak concentration within 1 to 2 minutes after administration.

Drug within the bloodstream will then be delivered to and taken up by tissues within the body, a process known as *distribution*. The drug concentration in plasma rapidly equilibrates with a group of highly perfused tissues, known as the vessel-rich group, during this initial distribution phase. Uptake of drug by the brain, heart, lungs, liver, and kidneys results in a rapid decline in blood levels measured shortly after administration, especially for those drugs that are highly lipid soluble. Drug concentrations in plasma are reduced further by a gradual uptake into less well-perfused tissues, such as muscle and fat, which serve as a large peripheral compartment where the drug may accumulate. Elimination by biotransformation and excretion ultimately removes the drug from the blood and the tissue reservoirs in the body. Elimination of most drugs follows *first-order* kinetics, whereby a constant fraction of the drug remaining in the body is eliminated per each unit of time.

A two-compartment model may be constructed to describe the distribution of a drug within a central compartment (blood) and peripheral compartment(s) (tissues), and the ultimate biotransformation of drug and its elimination from the body (Figure 4.1). The rate of transfer between the blood, tissues, and elimination sites can be described by a series of rate constants:

K_{10} or K_e: elimination rate constant representing the sum of all first-order elimination processes (such as biotransformation and excretion) that occur from the central compartment.

K_{12}: first-order rate constant for diffusion or transfer of drug from the central to peripheral compartment.

K_{21}: first-order rate constant for transfer of drug from the peripheral compartment back to the central compartment.

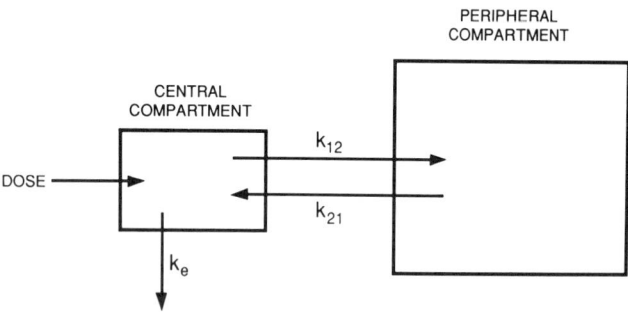

FIGURE 4.1. Two-compartment pharmacokinetic model illustrating the distribution of a drug within a central compartment (blood) and peripheral compartment (tissues), and its ultimate biotransformation and elimination from the body. K_{12} and K_{21} represent first-order rate constants for transfer of drug between the peripheral and central compartments, while K_e represents the elimination rate constant.

Measurement of drug levels in plasma after a single IV dose allows the construction of a concentration versus time curve depicting the respective contributions of the distribution and elimination processes to the logarithmic decline in plasma drug concentrations (Figure 4.2). Pharmacokinetic models may then be constructed based on the mathematical equations describing this log concentration versus time curve. The concentration of the drug in plasma (C_p) at any time may be calculated from the equation:

$$C_p = Ae^{-at} + Be^{-\beta t}$$

where:

C_p = concentration of drug in plasma

A = constant determined from the Y-axis intercept (time = 0) of the distribution portion of the log concentration versus time curve, derived by subtracting the contribution of the (constant, first-order) elimination phase of the curve

a = slope of the log concentration versus time curve of the distribution phase, derived by subtracting the contribution due to elimination

B = constant determined from the Y-axis intercept (time = 0) of the elimination phase of the log concentration versus time curve

β = slope of the log concentration versus time curve of the elimination phase

A three-compartment model incorporates two phases of distribution (fast, to *highly perfused* tissues, and slow, to *less highly perfused* tissues), as well as an elimination phase.

The plasma concentration versus time curve for the three-compartment model is described by the equation:

$$C_p = Pe^{-pt} + AE^{-at} + Be^{-\beta t}$$

where A, B, a, and β are the same as for a two-compartment model, and:

P = Y-axis intercept (time = 0) for the log concentration versus time curve derived after subtracting the contributions of the slow distribution and elimination phases

p = slope of the log concentration versus time curve for the rapid distribution phase

Other models may be constructed,[13] but two- and three-compartment models are sufficient for the vast majority of drugs.

The concentration of a drug in plasma may be predicted once an estimation of the *volume of distribution* (V_d) into which the dose will be introduced can be made. This theoretical volume does not correspond directly to actual tissue compartments within the body (such as blood, brain, extracellular fluid, etc.) but is useful in predicting drug

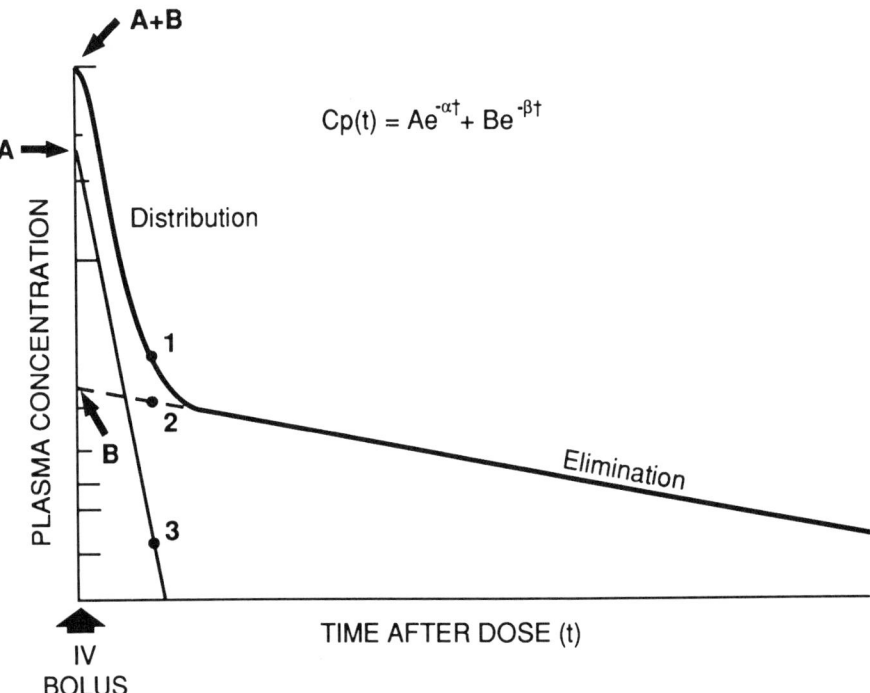

FIGURE 4.2. Plasma [log] concentration versus time curve for a hypothetical drug after a single IV dose. The curve (A + B) is the sum of the contributions from the rapid distribution (A) phase, and the slow elimination (B) phase to the logarithmic decline in concentration following a bolus dose. See text for explanation of the mathematical equations describing this log concentration versus time curve ($C_p = Ae^{-\alpha t} + Be^{-\beta t}$).

levels based on distinct pharmacokinetic parameters. Volume of distribution may be described by either:

V_d: total volume of distribution (including all compartments), or

V_c: volume of the central compartment, or the initial volume of distribution, (also termed V_i)

V_c will determine the concentration of drug immediately after injection, where the predicted level (in mg/mL) will be total dose (in milligrams) divided by the volume of distribution (in milliliters). V_d is useful in calculating maintenance doses of long-term medications, and in quantifying clearance of drugs from the body.

Clearance refers to the removal of drug from the body, usually by way of the central compartment, by first-order processes including biotransformation and excretion. Clearance is customarily expressed as milliliters of blood cleared of drug per minute. The rate of removal of a drug from the bloodstream may be more conveniently gauged by the *elimination half-life* ($t_{1/2}\beta$). The elimination half-life (or half-time) is the time required for the concentration of a drug to decrease by one-half. The $t_{1/2}\beta$ is represented graphically by the terminal, linear portion of the log concentration (C_p) versus time curve. The $t_{1/2}\beta$ may be expressed by the equation:

$$t_{1/2}\beta = \frac{0.693}{\beta}$$

where 0.693 is the natural logarithm of 2, and β again equals the slope of the log concentration versus time curve of the elimination phase.

The $t_{1/2}\beta$ may also be expressed as a function of clearance and volume of distribution, where:

$$t_{1/2}\beta = \frac{0.693 * V_d}{Cl}$$

V_d is the volume of distribution and Cl represents clearance; $t_{1/2}\beta$ is therefore brief when the distribution volume is small and the rate of drug clearance is rapid. Highly lipid-soluble drugs distribute widely throughout the body (large V_d), and their rate of return from peripheral compartments to the central compartment can be slow. As clearance generally occurs from the central compartment, a slow return to the bloodstream from a large V_d is the rate-limiting step in the ultimate elimination of highly soluble drugs from the body; hence their long $t_{1/2}\beta$. The $t_{1/2}p$ and $t_{1/2}\alpha$ represent the distribution phase half-time(s) represented by the initial phases (rapid and slow distribution) of the C_p versus time curve.[14-18]

Continuous IV Administration

To sustain a particular drug effect, it may be necessary to readminister the agent following an initial bolus. This may be accomplished by multiple IV doses,[19,20] continuous infusion,[21-23] use of a loading dose followed by a variable-rate continuous infusion, or by use of computer-controlled infusion pumps.[24-30] Administration of a "loading dose" of drug enables the practitioner to rapidly attain serum drug levels within the desired therapeutic range. Initiation of an infusion as the concentration ebbs during the distribution phase allows maintenance of drug levels within the therapeutic window for an indefinite time, while minimizing the potential toxicity of repetitive bolus doses.

Non-IV Drug Administration

Although the majority of drugs administered during CPB are given by vein, it may not always be possible or desirable to administer drugs intravenously. Other sites (and examples) of non-IV drug administration include transcutaneous (nitroglycerin),[31,32] subcutaneous (insulins),[33,34] intramuscular (analgesics),[35] nasal (narcotic premedicants),[36] buccal,[37] oral,[38] rectal,[39] epidural,[40] and spinal[41] routes. Absorption of drug into the blood from non-IV sites is dependent upon the dose of drug administered, the blood flow to the site of administration, the proximity and permeability of the capillaries to the drug, the degree of tissue binding at the administration site, the local pH of the tissues, and the acid-base status of the drug.[4,38,42]

Drug Elimination

Termination of drug effect occurs predominantly by drug elimination from the body. While several routes of elimination are possible (eg, lungs, transdermal), the primary routes of elimination are via hepatic and renal mechanisms. Clearance for any drug can be defined as the number of milliliters of blood from which the drug is completely removed per unit time.[43]

Hepatic Elimination[44]

In the liver, lipophilic compounds are metabolized into more polar configurations, which are ultimately excreted from the body. These metabolites are usually inactive, although active metabolites are formed in certain instances (eg, enalapril). The enzymatic reactions leading to degradation of a drug can be classified as either Phase I or Phase II reactions. *Phase I* reactions convert the parent compound to a more hydrophilic one by an oxidation, reduction, or hydrolytic reaction. *Phase II* reactions couple the drug (or its metabolite) to an endogenous substrate, such as glucuronate, sulfate, acetate, or amino acid, through a conjugation reaction, forming a highly polar compound. Factors known to affect hepatic drug metabolism include coexisting liver disease, the presence of liver enzyme inducers (phenobarbital) or inhibitors (cimetidine), age (tendency towards decreased liver function with increasing age), and genetic predisposition (heterogeneity exists in the cytochrome P_{450} enzyme system, so that there are slow or fast metabolizers).

Intrinsic hepatic clearance (Cl_i) describes the ability of the liver to remove drug from the bloodstream in the absence of limitations imposed by hepatic blood flow or drug-protein binding. The rate and extent to which drugs are metabolized by the liver may likewise be expressed by the *hepatic extraction ratio*. The hepatic extraction ratio is the fraction of drug contained in hepatic arterial blood that is removed as it passes through the liver. If a drug has a hepatic extraction ratio of 1, essentially all drug is removed from the blood as it flows through the liver. The relationship between intrinsic clearance and hepatic extraction ratio may be illustrated by the following equations:

$$Cl_{\text{hepatic}} = Q * \frac{Cl_i}{(Q + Cl_i)} = \frac{Q*(C_a - C_v)}{C_a} = Q*E$$

where:

Cl_{hepatic} = hepatic clearance rate of a drug
Q = liver blood flow
Cl_i = intrinsic hepatic clearance
C_a = arterial drug concentration
C_v = venous drug concentration
E = hepatic extraction ratio

As the intrinsic clearance of a drug becomes very high (many times liver blood flow), total hepatic clearance approaches hepatic blood flow. Drugs that have a *high* hepatic extraction ratio (eg, fentanyl and lidocaine) are critically dependent on liver blood flow for their elimination and are said to possess blood-flow-dependent clearance. Factors that reduce liver blood flow (rather than liver function per se) will reduce the elimination of these medications from the body. Drugs with a *low* hepatic extraction ratio (eg, diazepam and thiopental) are dependent on intrahepatic cellular processes for their elimination, and are said to possess a restricted intrinsic clearance. The clearance of these drugs is not strictly related to blood flow. The presence or absence of hepatic disease, the degree of drug-protein binding, and the level of activity of specific liver enzymes will exert a much greater impact on the clearance of these drugs than will changes in hepatic flow. The impact of these factors may be represented by the following equation:[4]

$$\text{Intrinsic clearance} = Cl_i = Cl_\mu \times f_\mu$$

where:

Cl_μ = clearance term based on the concentration of *un*bound drug in plasma and a measure of hepatic cellular activity
f_μ = fraction of *un*bound drug in plasma

Renal Elimination[4,43]

Renal excretion of a drug is dependent on renal blood flow, glomerular filtration rate, and tubular secretion and reabsorption rates. Filtration, which is a passive process, increases directly with higher renal blood flow and plasma drug concentrations. Tubular secretion and reabsorption are active processes, and these transport systems can become saturated. Clearance may thus decrease once plasma concentrations increase beyond a certain point. The majority of drugs must be in their free (unbound) state before they will be eliminated by the kidney. The rate of clearance for drugs with a *high* renal extraction ratio depends on renal blood flow rather than the degree of protein binding. As in the liver, changes in protein binding may have profound effects on clearance for drugs with a *low* renal extraction ratio. Intrinsic renal disease may affect the clearance of drugs regardless of their extraction ratios, as changes in blood flow and filtration often accompany alterations in cellular function in patients with renal insufficiency. Changes in urinary pH may greatly influence the reabsorption of weak acids and bases. With regard to weak acids, alkalinization of the urine promotes renal excretion by increasing the proportion of ionized (charged) drug in the renal tubules, which is less readily reabsorbed into the blood. Clearance of weak acids (such as salicylates and phenobarbital) may be enhanced by systemic administration of bicarbonate following overdose of these drugs. Alkalinization of the urine has also been advocated to increase the solubility and excretion of myoglobin in the urine following trauma.

Theoretical Effects of Hypothermia on Pharmacokinetics and Pharmacodynamics

Temperature affects virtually all physical and chemical processes in the body. Hypothermia depresses metabolism and thereby decreases the myocardial and cerebral metabolic rates for oxygen. Hypothermia alters tissue and organ perfusion directly, by increasing blood viscosity, and indirectly, by reflex autonomic and endocrine vasoconstruction. A variety of processes affecting drug disposition are thus altered by hypothermia. Deliberate, controlled hypothermia produced in association with CPB could logically be expected to produce a number of changes in pharmacokinetics and pharmacodynamics.

Decreased absorption rate: The absorption of nonintravenously administered drugs is slowed by hypothermia.[45]

Slowed distribution rate: Transfer from central to peripheral compartments declines (decreased k_{12}, Figure 4.1). The extent of distribution throughout the body may also be reduced (decreased volume of distribution, V_d). Hypothermia alone reduces the volume of distribution and clearance of fentanyl[46] and propranolol.[47]

Altered drug penetration into the CNS: The penetration of a number of drugs into the brain and spinal cord is altered by hypothermia, as reviewed by Ballard.[45]

Slowed reuptake of drug from peripheral tissues (decreased k_{21}, Figure 4.1): The rate of drug delivery to sites of metabolism and excretion is also reduced (decreased k_e, Figure 4.1), with decreased clearance and increased elimination half-time.[14,48,49]

Slowed rate of biotransformation: Leading to decreased k_e, (Figure 4.1), decreased clearance, and increased elimination half-time.[46,50-54]

Altered renal excretion: Decreased renal perfusion, decreased glomerular filtration rate, and decreased tubular secretion would slow excretion. Decreased tubular reabsorption could increase the rate of loss of some compounds.[49]

Altered membrane and receptor function: Alterations in membrane characteristics, receptor interaction, and receptor transduction may greatly modify a wide range of pharmacodynamic responses (See Drug-Receptor Interaction, below).[55-62]

The ultimate effects of hypothermia on drug levels during cardiac surgery will depend on the timing of drug administration relative to the onset of hypothermia, the depth of hypothermia, and the rate and extent of rewarming near the termination of CPB. Hyperthermia would be expected to alter regional perfusion and increase the rate of biotransformation and other metabolically dependent processes.[45]

Theoretical Effects of CPB on Pharmacokinetics[63,64]

The initiation and maintenance of CPB, with or without systemic hypothermia, would logically be expected to produce a number of changes in the pharmacokinetic profiles of drugs administered during (or before) this phase of the procedure. Cardiopulmonary bypass implies hemodilution and altered perfusion with modifications of autonomic and endocrine reflexes, all of which may produce significant pharmacokinetic changes.

Changes Due to Hemodilution

Most centers employ a crystalloid solution to prime the CPB apparatus, and deliberately seek to reduce the hematocrit into the range of 20% to 25%. Hemodilution produces numerous physiologic alterations that may have important effects on the way drugs are handled by the body:

Decreased plasma protein concentration: Decreased levels of albumin and α-1-acid glycoprotein may lead to changes in the level of free drug, through shifts in the bound to free drug ratio.[65-68]

Reduced red blood cell concentration: Hemodilution may produce a reduction in total drug content for compounds that are sequestered within the red blood cells to a significant degree.[69-72]

Reduction in free concentration with acute hemodilution at the onset of CPB: The decrease in free drug levels at the initiation of CPB appears to be a very transient phenomenon.[65,68] The rapid movement of free drug out of tissues (especially from the capacious peripheral stores of drugs with a large V_d) expeditiously restores the concentration equilibrium. Hemodilution during CPB has not been shown to significantly reduce the free drug concentration of alfentanil,[73] thiopental, or methohexital.[74,75]

Altered Perfusion: Pulsatile Versus Nonpulsatile Flow

Although pulsatile flow during bypass is technically possible, most cardiac centers continue to perform surgery using nonpulsatile CPB. Nonpulsatile CPB is associated with alterations in tissue perfusion, including reductions in peripheral[76] and renal[77,78] flows. Pulsatile flow may provide improved renal, cerebral, and peripheral perfusion. Pulsatile CPB has also been found to improve oxygen extraction while reducing total peripheral resistance, mean arterial pressure, metabolic acidosis, and edema formation.[79,80]

The effects of pulsatile CPB perfusion on drug distribution and elimination remain largely unstudied. No differences in the pharmacokinetics of thiopental could be detected between pulsatile and nonpulsatile CPB.[81] In another study, tissue concentrations of cefamandole were higher and the elimination half-time was prolonged in patients undergoing pulsatile perfusion as compared to conventional CPB.[82]

Changes in Autonomic and Endocrine Axis During CPB

Cardiopulmonary bypass is associated with a number of changes in autonomic and endocrine function. Catecholamine levels are elevated.[23,83-85] Levels of β-endorphin, glucagon, aldosterone, renin, and cortisol are likewise increased.[86] Changes in levels of vasopressin,[77,87,88] free fatty acids,[83] serotonin,[84,89] kinins, thromboxane, and complement[90-94] have also been described. The exact influence of these changes on the processing of drugs by the body is largely unknown, but they probably affect regional tissue perfusion characteristics as well as distribution and elimination processes.[95,96]

Drug-Receptor Interaction

The pharmacologic effect exerted by a drug depends upon the eventual interaction between that agent and a receptor specific for it. For example, the autonomic nervous system contains several types of catecholamine receptors associated with the cell membrane. A drug may bind to and activate more than one of these typical receptors, and a receptor may be activated by a variety of similar compounds. Binding of a drug or neurotransmitter to a receptor initiates a conformational change that is transduced to a series of membrane-bound proteins. For catecholamine receptors, "G proteins" activate or inactivate second messengers within the cell, such as cyclic AMP or cyclic GMP. Second messengers may cause activation or inactivation of intracellular enzymes, such as the protein kinases. Second messengers catalyze modifications of a wide variety of cellular parameters, including conductance through ion channels. The influx of calcium as a third messenger may then initiate a host of intracellular events, such as interaction of actin and myosin, resulting in augmented muscle contractility.[97]

Factors Affecting Free Drug Concentration at Receptor Sites

Distribution of Drug to Receptor Area

Drugs within the body will exert a pharmacologic effect only if they are delivered to, and are able to interact with, specific receptor sites in the cell membrane. Distribution of drug to the receptor area may be influenced by a number of factors (Figure 4.3).[98]

Protein Binding

The majority of drugs employed during cardiac surgery are transported through the blood bound to serum proteins, predominantly albumin and α-1-acid glycoprotein. α-1-Acid glycoprotein is an acute phase reactant that binds basic drugs, including fentanyl and lidocaine. The amount of free (unbound) drug may thus be significantly altered by changes in protein binding.[99-101] This is of clinical significance primarily for drugs that are highly protein bound, or when extreme changes in the levels of serum proteins occur. The degree of drug-protein binding depends on the total drug concentration, the available protein concentration, the affinity of the protein for the drug, and the presence of other substances that may compete with the drug or alter the drug binding site.[5] Measurement of total drug concentration in plasma (both free and bound) may thus be deceiving if the concentration of serum proteins fluctuates widely, as it does during CPB.[74,100]

The degree of protein binding and resulting free drug concentrations may also be affected by a vast array of pathologic conditions. Renal failure and liver disease decrease stores of albumin available for drug binding, potentially elevating the level of free drug in the body. The affinity of albumin for drugs such as phenytoin or thiopental may also be reduced in chronic disease states.[6,102] Concentrations of α-1-acid glycoprotein may be increased with chronic disease or following myocardial infarction and surgery. Drugs that are highly bound to this protein (such as narcotics and local anesthetics) may have a lower free fraction available under these conditions.[103,104]

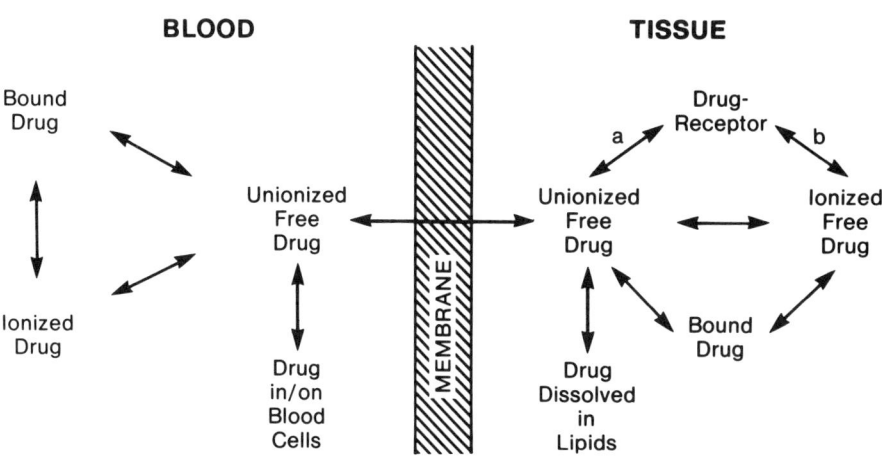

FIGURE 4.3. Reversible processes affecting the total amount of drug on either side of a biologic membrane. The membrane is typically permeable only to the un-ionized (free) form of the drug. Both ionized and un-ionized drug may bind to carrier proteins, though one form of the compound tends to be preferentially bound in the plasma. One form of the drug, frequently the free, un-ionized form, is pharmacologically active when bound at the receptor site, while the other moiety may prove to be essentially inert. Extensive partitioning in peripheral tissues and binding to inactive sites creates a large volume of distribution, limiting the amount of agent available to form drug-receptor complexes. (From Hug,[98] by permission of *Anesthesiology*.)

Tissue Binding

Tissues may serve as a reservoir for drug, depending on the relative affinity of the tissue for that particular drug.[105-108] Digitalis is found in much higher concentrations in myocardial tissue than in plasma. The lungs may serve as a reservoir for fentanyl during CPB.[109] Changes in free drug concentration induced by shifts in protein binding are, to a large extent, buffered by equilibration between drug available in the vast peripheral tissue stores and that circulating in the blood.

Age

The aging process is associated with a variety of physiologic changes that influence the drug levels eventually attained in plasma, independent of any pathologic state. Cardiac index declines as age progresses, while systemic vascular resistance is slightly increased. Renal, hepatic, and skeletal blood flow may likewise be reduced.[110-112] This decline in regional blood flow may cause a decrease in renal and hepatic clearance rates, as well as a reduction in the efficiency of metabolism by these two organs.[113] Older patients have a larger proportion of adipose tissue; thus, the volume of distribution for lipid-soluble drugs may be increased. The elderly typically have lower serum albumin levels, which may lead to higher free drug concentrations when a standard dose is administered. These changes have clear implications in terms of free drug availability at peripheral receptor sites.[114,115] There are several difficulties, however, with interpreting studies addressing the question of pharmacologic changes with age. Most investigations have involved small numbers of patients, and there has been great variability in the pharmacokinetic parameters obtained. Chronological age does not necessarily correspond to physiologic age, which is obviously impossible to quantify.[116]

Variable changes in central nervous system (CNS) sensitivities to sedative compounds have been reported among older patients. Brain sensitivity (ie, the pharmacodynamic response) to barbiturates is not altered with aging.[114] Reductions in thiopental dose requirements with increasing age may be ascribed to a delay in return of drug to the central compartment (the blood) from the rapidly equilibrating compartment (the brain or effect site)—a pharmacokinetic difference.[117,118]

Increased CNS sensitivity to fentanyl and alfentanil, as measured by electroencephalographic (EEG) effect, has also been demonstrated among the elderly. A greater hysteresis (lag) is seen between the rise of serum opioid levels and the onset of EEG effect.[119] Dosages of many drugs, especially the opioids and hypnotic agents, should be adjusted downward in older patients to avoid untoward reactions associated with high free drug levels.

Rate of Free Drug Uptake from Plasma and Delivery to Receptor Sites

Free drug must migrate from the plasma to a receptor site for its effect to be exerted. The peak pharmacologic effect of a drug, however, does not necessarily coincide with its peak plasma concentration. A hysteresis between peak drug levels in serum and maximum pharmacologic response has been shown for a significant number of compounds. A clear hysteresis occurs between peak fentanyl concentrations and shift in the spectral edge frequency of the EEG, a measure of narcotic effect in the brain. The hysteresis for alfentanil is considerably shorter, and return of the EEG to baseline occurs more rapidly than with fentanyl.[120] A lag is also seen as plasma concentrations of both drugs fall; return of the spectral edge frequency to normal trails the decline in plasma levels. Several factors may account for the hysteresis between changing plasma narcotic concentration and effect (eg, interaction with the opioid receptor). Delivery of drug to the receptor site is dependent on regional perfusion, which may not be equal in all tissue beds. The drug must also diffuse across capillary and supporting tissue membranes (such as the blood-brain barrier) to reach the receptor site. Partitioning, or nonspecific binding of the opioid to pharmacologically inactive tissue components, may also delay the appearance of peak pharmacologic effect. Once drug is delivered to the receptor, complex interactions between the drug and the receptor must occur before an effect is clinically observed. Both fentanyl and alfentanil have rapid receptor association and dissociation constants. Differences at the receptor level would thus be an unlikely explanation for any variation in the onset of narcotic effect. Fentanyl is concentrated in brain tissue lipids, however, and this partitioning may prevent concentrations from rising at the opioid receptor sites, prolonging the time to maximal drug effect. Alfentanil is not concentrated in the brain to the same extent that fentanyl is. Fentanyl is optimally administered 5 to 10 minutes before an anticipated stimulus, whereas alfentanil will produce its maximum effect within 1 to 2 minutes and may be more effective in treating acute responses to painful or noxious stimuli.[98]

Comparisons between fentanyl and sufentanil show no meaningful differences with respect to hysteresis or other pharmacodynamic variables. The IC_{50} of sufentanil (concentration required to produce a 50% reduction in spectral edge frequency) is much lower than the IC_{50} of fentanyl.[121] Although the potency of sufentanil is indeed 5 to 10 times greater, its onset of action is no different from that of fentanyl. Similar methods have been employed to compare the pharmacodynamics of midazolam and diazepam. Results from these experiments suggest that the lag to peak effect for midazolam is slightly longer than that of diazepam. Midazolam has also been shown to be five times more potent than diazepam in these early models.[122-125]

Using pharmacokinetic models from single-dose studies, alfentanil has been shown to possess a short elimination half-time (1.6 hour versus 3.1 hours for fentanyl).[15] Alfentanil has thus frequently been championed for use as a short-acting opioid. The manner in which a drug is administered, however, may affect its clinical duration, regardless of elimination half-life. A computer model designed by Shafer and Varvel[16] simulates changes in the effect-site concentration (at the receptor) over time following administration of fentanyl, alfentanil, and sufentanil.[16] Following bolus administration, alfentanil, as expected, produces a higher peak effect-site concentration (37% of the concentration in plasma) at an earlier time (1.4 minutes) with a more rapid recovery than either fentanyl or sufentanil. When the peak effect-site concentration is maintained for 10 minutes by an infusion, alfentanil no longer demonstrates this rapid recovery profile. For infusions lasting less than 30 minutes, shifts in the effect-site concentration (receptor level) are indistinguishable among the three narcotics. For infusions lasting less than 8 hours, the effect-site concentration of sufentanil decreases 50% more rapidly after discontinuation than does the effect-site concentration of alfentanil. In all cases, reduction in the effect-site concentration of fentanyl is prolonged relative to either sufentanil or alfentanil. Alfentanil may be an appropriate agent for situations where a single dose is administered, or for infusions lasting longer than 8 hours if rapid termination of effect is desired. Sufentanil may be more efficacious for infusions shorter than 8 hours (eg, most cardiac surgery procedures), despite its longer elimination half-time.[15,16]

Equilibration Across Plasma Membranes

The rate of drug delivery to the receptor by way of the bloodstream generally determines its rate of onset, while the rate of drug removal from the receptor site determines the duration of drug action. There are several factors besides drug delivery that may modify the onset, intensity, and duration of drug effect. It is generally true that the more lipid soluble the drug, the more rapid its onset of action. Highly lipid-soluble drugs show closer relationships between plasma and brain concentrations, and between plasma concentrations and the intensity of pharmacologic effect.[98,126-128] As noted above, however, lipid portions of the brain serve as a sink for lipophilic agents, slowing the rise in free drug concentration at the receptor and thus prolonging the time to maximum drug effect. There are indeed differences between fentanyl and its congeners with regard to onset of peak effect, and in recovery times from a single bolus dose, despite the similarities of their plasma disposition curves over the first 90 minutes.[16,98] It is the free, unchanged form of a drug that equilibrates across the capillary membranes separating plasma from the drug receptor site (see Figure 4.3).[98-100] Alterations in protein binding may thus have considerable effects on the onset and intensity of drug response.

Termination of pharmacologic effect is contingent on redistribution of drug from the active (receptor) site to other tissues as well as its eventual elimination by intrinsic clearance mechanisms. Redistribution of opioid analgesics depends on the rate of drug dissociation from receptor (rapid for alfentanil, slow for lofentanil), the rate of diffusion across plasma membranes and out of the CNS (slow for morphine), and the capacity of peripheral tissues for accumulating the drug (large V_d for lipid-soluble drugs). Clearance of drug may be affected by a myriad of factors, including temperature, coexisting disease states, alterations in regional blood flow, and the presence of other compounds that may modify enzymatic activity or drug-protein binding. Knowledge of events at the membrane receptor level has allowed sophisticated computer models to correlate changes in plasma drug levels with changes in concentration at the effector site,[122,123,129] providing rational guidelines for IV anesthetic drug administration.[24]

Factors Affecting Receptor-Mediated Events

The interaction of a drug with its receptor and the subsequent generation of intracellular events may be affected by many factors, including fluctuations in temperature, pH, and electrolyte concentrations. There are thus significant perturbations in pharmacodynamic response during cardiac surgery and CPB, as wide fluctuations occur in the aforementioned parameters. The presence of anesthetic agents may likewise alter the body's response to other medications. The effect of each of these factors on pharmacodynamics is reviewed in the following sections.

Temperature

Systemic hypothermia is employed during the vast majority of adult cardiac surgical procedures. Hypothermia may dramatically alter receptor function by several distinct mechanisms. Changes in ion pump function at lower temperatures may alter intracellular ionic composition, affecting the response of second messengers to receptor stimulation. Hypothermia may also lead to change in phase of the lipid and protein components of the cell membrane, thus altering the milieu of the membrane-bound receptors. Changes in the hydration state of specific molecules with changing temperature may also affect receptor dynamics.[130]

Transformation of receptor subtypes occurs with fluctuations in temperature. Conversion of β-receptor function at normothermia to α-receptor function under systemic hypothermia has been demonstrated by several investigators,[55,131] while Benfey could not confirm the conversion of cardiac adrenoreceptor function at low temperature.[56] Hypothermia may also lead to conversion of histamine receptors from type H_1 to type H_2.[57]

Alterations in receptor affinity also take place with changes in body temperature. Brain membranes incubated with sodium at 37°C exhibit increased opiate receptor binding of ^{3}H-dihydromorphine when compared to membranes at 0°C. This may be secondary to dissociation of an endogenous inhibitor of opiate receptor binding from the receptor site at normothermia.[58] In a guinea pig myenteric plexus model, opiate potency is reduced as temperature decreases from 37° to 30°C. This may result from a reduced affinity of the receptor for the agonist under hypothermic conditions.[59]

Dramatic changes in neuromuscular transmission are seen with both moderate and profound hypothermia. The ability of d-tubocurarine to induce muscle relaxation in rats is reduced as temperature declines to 26°C. This appears due to changes in receptor affinity rather than changes in receptor density. Below 26°C, spontaneous paralysis of the muscle occurs, potentiating the effect of d-tubocurarine.[132] Although hypothermia decreases the efficacy of d-tubocurarine, the duration of the block does not appear to be affected.[133] Hypothermia may sensitize the postjunctional membrane to acetylcholine, thus increasing the amount of nondepolarizing agent required to produce a constant level of neuromuscular blockade. Hypothermia increases the amount of d-tubocurarine required to induce twitch depression (a measure of neuromuscular blockade) in a rat hemidiaphragm preparation, but does not change the amount of pancuronium required to depress neuromuscular transmission.[134] Miller and Roderick have reported that decreased amounts of pancuronium are required under hypothermic conditions. Pancuronium concentrations were not measured in their study, however, and the effects of active metabolites were not considered. Pharmacokinetic changes (ie, variations in the amount of drug available to the receptor) may in fact explain their findings, rather than alterations in the pharmacodynamics of the receptor per se.[135] Initiation of CPB in patients receiving d-tubocurarine or pancuronium is associated with a rapid increase in twitch height (reduced neuromuscular blockade), due in large part to dilution of drug by the pump prime. Cooling the patient is associated with a reduction in twitch height, and rewarming is associated with recovery of neuromuscular function. It may be concluded that hypothermia enhances the effect of both curare and pancuronium during CPB.[136] Farrell[137] has found that temperature reduces the requirements for d-tubocurarine and pancuronium in a rat diaphragm model, though the magnitude of temperature-induced change, while statistically significant, is small. The conflicting data summarized above may be a result of hypothermia-induced changes in pharmacokinetics superimposed upon pharmacodynamic alterations. Interspecies variations must also be considered. Although the dosage of neuromuscular blockers based upon changes in twitch response may be optimal, many anesthesiologists empirically dose these agents at specific intervals during the cardiac procedure. The reductions in twitch height observed with hypothermia, combined with the practice of empiric dosing, generally result in concentrations of neuromuscular blockers well in excess of those necessary to prevent patient movement. When one considers the wide variability in dose requirements for neuromuscular blockers in vivo, small alterations in pharmacodynamics due to temperature are unlikely to be clinically important.

pH Effects

Acidosis secondary to ischemia (relative or absolute) may lead to significant changes in intracellular enzyme function. Xanthine oxidase is converted to xanthine hydrogenase under acidotic conditions, leading to formation of oxygen free radicals and tissue damage.[138,139] Metabolic acidosis diminishes the body's response to endogenous and exogenous catecholamines,[140] and pH affects the degree of ionization of drugs that are weak acids or bases. The activity of local anesthetics (which are weak bases) is critically dependent on pH. Local anesthetics are ineffective in acidic environments such as sites of infection, as only a small percentage of the drug is in its active, unionized form.[141] Variations in pH alter the protein binding of fentanyl and alfentanil, thus changing the amount of free drug available to bind to opiate receptors.[142] These alterations in protein binding and ionization may affect many of the drugs employed in cardiac surgery.

Electrolytes

Changes in the electrolyte environment may also have profound effects on physiologic function and drug action. Acute electrolyte changes are extremely common during cardiac surgery. Calcium, magnesium, and potassium levels may decline during CPB. Muscle weakness, arrhythmias, and enhanced digitalis toxicity may ensue, depending on the magnitude of electrolyte flux.[143-146] Use of continuous retrograde cardioplegia, on the other hand, may produce alarming levels of hyperkalemia near the end of the bypass run. Calcium availability is a major determinant of catecholamine receptor response. Acidosis may increase available ionized calcium by decreasing the amount of calcium-protein binding.[147]

Anesthetic Agents

A variety of anesthetic agents have been safely applied during cardiac surgery and CPB. These compounds, however, may profoundly affect the autonomic nervous system and global myocardial function. Halothane (but not enflurane or isoflurane) sensitizes the myocardium to the arrhythmogenic effects of epinephrine. This sensitization may be mediated through increased α-adrenergic receptor sensitivity.[148] Volatile anesthetics produce dose-dependent myocardial depression, which may be significantly augmented by verapamil. Volatile agents also have been shown to alter the pharmacokinetics of verapamil so that higher plasma levels are attained than in the awake state.[149] Volatile agents may also disrupt intracellular transduction mechanisms.[150-153] Since one hypothesis to explain the mechanism of general anesthesia produced by volatile agents involves the dissolution of agents into the protein-phospholipid membrane, it is not surprising that these anesthetics would affect receptor-mediated events.

The role played by changes in pharmacodynamics in altering the body's response to drugs employed during cardiac surgery is only beginning to be explored. In dogs receiving enflurane, the minimum alveolar concentration, or MAC (essentially the ED_{50} of an agent), is significantly reduced following normothermic CPB. The cause of the reduction cannot be attributed to anemia, alterations in acid-base status, or conduct of bypass (ie, aorto-atrial versus femoral artery-vein). This suggests that some alteration in brain function itself, perhaps at the receptor level, must occur to explain the observed variations in sensitivity to enflurane.[154] Further investigations of specific changes in receptor affinity may help to explain the variations in pharmacodynamic response observed during hypothermia and CPB.

Factors Affecting Receptor Density

The number of specific receptors available to combine with a drug will determine the number of drug-receptor complexes that ultimately may be formed. The number of complexes formed should, in theory, determine the intensity of effect of an individual drug. In patients with congestive heart failure, there is a significant reduction in cellular levels of cyclic AMP. This is associated with a decrease in the number of β_1-adrenergic receptors, a phenomenon termed *down-regulation*. Defects in receptor transduction, as well as impairment of synthesis and reuptake of norepinephrine, may also contribute to this decreased sympathetic response.[155-158] Use of β-adrenergic agonists in heart failure has met with very limited success, and is associated with further reductions in the number of β-receptors and eventual loss of hemodynamic efficacy.[159,160]

Removal of β-adrenergic blockade in patients treated for angina pectoris has been associated with exacerbations in symptomatology, and several deaths have been reported. It is speculated that β-adrenergic receptor blockade is accompanied by an up-regulation (increase) in the number of β-receptors, resulting in increased adrenergic responsiveness. Increases in heart rate and contractility thus lead to increased myocardial oxygen demand and worsened symptomatology.[161]

Factors Determining Free Drug Concentration During Cardiac Surgery

The entire spectrum of factors delineated above may influence the quantity of free drug that is ultimately available to interact with a receptor during cardiac surgery and CPB. Though many of these forces exist in any pharmacologic situation, several are unique to the process of CPB, and are discussed in some detail below.

Dose and Rate of Administration

Increasing the dose or rate of drug administration should theoretically increase the concentration of free drug available to penetrate to the receptor site. This concept has been employed to establish the effective dose and rate of administration of neuromuscular blocking agents.[162] Timing the dosage of prophylactic antibiotics before cardiac surgery must also be done with an understanding of this concept to avoid inadequate antimicrobial concentrations at the time of incision.[163,164]

Binding to Plasma Proteins

Drugs exist in plasma in two distinct forms: bound to plasma proteins such as albumin (acidic drugs) or α-1-acid glycoprotein (basic drugs), and in their free or unbound state.[99,100] The equilibrium between bound and free drug is predicated on the total drug concentration, the concentration of the protein in plasma, the number of available binding sites on the protein molecule, and the affinities of plasma protein binding sites for that drug.[5,6] For the vast majority of drugs, the rate of drug association and dissociation from protein binding sites is quite rapid. In the majority of clinical situations, changes in protein binding have relatively trivial effects on free drug concentrations. The tissues serve as a vast reservoir of free drug in the body. Rapid equilibration of drug between peripheral tissues and plasma suppresses most of the flux resulting from changes in protein binding. In the presence of a second drug competing for protein binding sites, changes in free drug concentration may occur with important clinical results, such as the displacement of warfarin by phenylbutazone.[165] Certain chronic disease states may sufficiently alter α-1-acid glycoprotein levels that meaningful changes in drug–protein binding may occur.[102,104] α-1-Acid glycoprotein is an acute phase reactant protein whose levels rise acutely during stresses such as myocardial ischemia, myocardial infarction, and cardiac surgery. Binding of basic drugs, such as lidocaine, to α-1-acid glycoprotein under these conditions has been shown to increase.[103] Reduced levels of free drug, as a consequence of elevated α-1-acid glycoprotein levels, may have important clinical implications, including breakthrough ectopy during lidocaine administration following myocardial ischemia or infarction.[99,166]

Alterations in protein binding could produce clinically significant changes in free levels of drugs employed during cardiac surgery and CPB. Lipoprotein lipase is an enzyme found in heart, lung, and adipose tissue that clears lipoprotein-bound triglycerides from the plasma.[167] Heparin releases lipoprotein lipase into the plasma, leading to hydrolysis of chylomicrons and release of free fatty acids.[168] These free fatty acids avidly bind to plasma albumin and may displace certain drugs (such as benzodiazepines) from their albumin binding sites.[169] It can be speculated that heparin-induced alterations in the free concentrations of anesthetic agents may, in part, explain the transient hypotension commonly observed after bolus heparin administration.

Dilution and Volume of Distribution

The level of drug in the body may be critically altered during situations where the blood volume is rapidly diluted, as occurs upon initiation of CPB.[63,64] As discussed above, it is the free, unbound portion of the total drug concentration that is generally the active moiety.[170] The degree of change in drug concentration will be determined by the ability of tissue stores to release free drug and re-establish a plasma-tissue equilibrium. Despite significant reductions in total drug levels, little change in free drug concentration occurs upon initiation of CPB, perhaps due in part to the acute decrease in plasma proteins observed with rapid hemodilution.[65,73-75] Alterations in drug requirements for neuromuscular blockers have been reported during CPB, but the role of hypothermia per se in these observations has not been well characterized.[171-180]

Uptake by Blood Cells

Anemia may influence the level of available free drug, should binding to or uptake by red blood cells play a significant part in the transport of that particular compound. In vitro alfentanil levels are higher with addition of blood to the CPB priming solution, as opposed to cases where a nonhemic prime is employed. A similar difference between fentanyl levels, however, has not been observed. Alfentanil may undergo a greater degree of protein binding while remaining less subject to uptake by red blood cells. Free drug levels under these conditions have not been measured.[69,181]

The Lungs as a Reservoir for Drug

The lungs may serve as a sink that can sequester certain drugs. This effect is most pronounced during cardiac surgery when the lungs are removed from the perfusion circuit during CPB. Lung sequestration is responsible for a secondary peak in plasma fentanyl levels following resumption of ventilation at the termination of CPB. A common clinical observation is that anesthetic requirements are reduced following CPB; indeed, drug washout from the lungs may be a partial explanation for this phenomenon. These changes in drug concentration during ventilation and reperfusion, though, are quite transient in nature.[182-186]

Changes in Blood Flow During CPB

Blood flow to organs may be altered during CPB, and hence, drug delivery to both receptor sites and clearance sites may vary. Renal blood flow is reduced during CPB secondary to afferent arteriolar vasoconstriction.[187] Handling of sodium and potassium by the kidney during CPB is normal, although a diuresis induced by the priming solution usually occurs.[188] Renal function tends to deteriorate postoperatively in older patients with prolonged (>60 minutes) duration of bypass.[189] Reductions in glomerular filtration rate and renal blood flow, as well as tubular reabsorptive and secretive processes, lead to increased sodium excretion during CPB.[190] Blood flow to liver and muscle is also reduced during CPB.[76,191] These reductions in blood flow to clearance organs should prolong the duration of action of drugs dependent upon these organs for elimination. Cerebral blood flow (CBF) alterations during CPB have also been described. The use of a temperature-corrected method of adjusting blood gases during CPB (pH-stat) results in a relative hyperperfusion of the brain with loss of cerebral autoregulation. This does not occur when non-temperature-corrected methods (alpha-stat) are employed.[192] Significant alterations in CBF may profoundly affect the delivery of opioids and hypnotics to their effector sites in the CNS.

Binding to CPB Apparatus

Binding of drugs by apparatus such as the CPB oxygenator, blood scavenging equipment, and hemoconcentrators would be expected to reduce free drug levels. Although such binding has been demonstrated for drugs such as fentanyl and alfentanil in vitro,[69,142] it is unlikely to play a major role in vivo due to the large tissue stores available to replace drug lost to this equipment.[193-197] (See further discussion in Opioids under Specific Drugs, below.)

Clearance from Plasma During CPB

The free drug concentration attained in plasma at any given time depends upon the distribution of drug to tissues and its rate of elimination from the body. Disease states such as chronic liver disease may increase distribution volumes, while they may be reduced in patients with congestive heart failure and renal impairment.[198] Volumes of distribution may also be influenced by hemorrhage and concurrent drug administration.[199,200] Drug elimination may be slowed by hypothermia,[50-52] lung sequestration,[182] decreased hepatic blood flow,[199] and impaired renal function.[198,201] Elimination may, of course, also be modified by CPB itself.[177,189,191,202]

Specific Drugs

NB: Unless otherwise specified, all concentrations of drugs referred to below represent the total drug concentration in plasma.

Anesthetic Agents

Opioids

Opioids are either natural or synthetic substances that bind at specific receptors in the CNS to produce intense analgesia and, at very high doses, loss of consciousness. Opioids are frequently chosen as the primary anesthetic agent for cardiac surgery, particularly in patients with impaired cardiac function. Opioids provide hemodynamic stability during periods of maximal stimulation and assure that some degree of analgesia will be present during the early postoperative period.

Hypothermic CPB is associated with a prolonged elimination half-time and an increased volume of distribution for fentanyl[203] and alfentanil.[21,22,204] Clearance of fentanyl (which has a high hepatic extraction ratio) is reduced during CPB, presumably due to changes in liver blood.[191] The more restricted clearance of alfentanil, though, is not altered. However, CPB patients compared to patients not exposed to extracorporeal circulation have an increase in alfentanil elimination half-time, central distribution volume, and total volume of distribution after CPB.[204]

Using computer-controlled infusion and pharmacokinetic data derived from a general surgical population, Flezzani[28] was able to achieve and maintain stable plasma sufentanil levels before CPB in a group of patients undergoing coronary artery revascularization. Stable plasma sufentanil levels were also attained by Okutani[205] using conventional drug administration techniques. These studies suggest that in otherwise healthy adults, opioid administration employing pharmacokinetic data obtained from noncardiac patients will result in stable plasma concentrations during cardiac surgery. The level attained may be different from the target level, however, on the basis of hemodilution, altered clearance, and changes in volumes of distribution. It remains unclear whether these assumptions may be extended to patients with severely impaired myocardial function. Clearance of fentanyl is reduced during profound hypothermia (18° to 25°C) lasting 100–140 minutes, although total plasma fentanyl levels remain unchanged (Figure 4.4).[46]

Administration of fentanyl to children with congenital heart disease using infusion regimens derived from adults has resulted in plasma fentanyl levels up to 300% higher than predicted.[206] These higher plasma levels may, in part, result from smaller volumes of distribution in pediatric patients than in adults. This may also be a disease-related

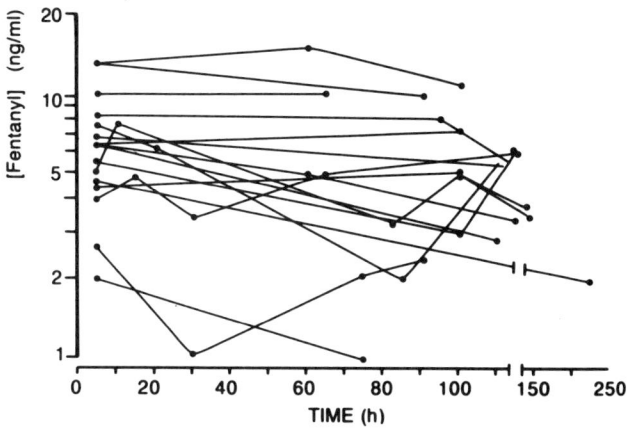

FIGURE 4.4. Fentanyl plasma concentrations in 18 children during profound hypothermia (18° to 25°C). Time zero is the initiation of CPB. Total plasma fentanyl levels remain essentially unchanged. (From Koren, Barker, Goresky et al,[46] by permission of *Eur J Clin Pharmacol*.)

phenomenon, as the highest opioid levels were observed in children with tetralogy of Fallot in severe congestive heart failure.[207] As mentioned previously, heart failure may cause significant reduction in volume of distribution. Younger children and infants also show reduced clearance of fentanyl when compared to older patients, and these severely ill children were operated on at an earlier age than those with less severe symptoms. Younger children also have a higher sufentanil clearance than older children, with a smaller volume of distribution. Elimination halftime for sufentanil is prolonged in children who undergo surface cooling during cardiac surgery, whereas children who remain normothermic show no changes in elimination.[208] Hypothermia indeed appears to have significant effects on opioid pharmacokinetics during cardiac surgery.

Hemodilution also may alter plasma opioid concentrations during CPB. Total plasma alfentanil levels fall with hemodilution at the initiation of CPB, while the free drug concentration remains unchanged (Figure 4.5). These changes are the result of an increase in the unbound fraction of alfentanil (ie, ratio of free drug to total drug concentration).[73]

Sequestration of fentanyl in the lungs during CPB has been demonstrated by Bentley[186] (Figure 4.6). Washout of fentanyl from the lungs occurs following resumption of ventilation and cardiac ejection prior to separation from CPB. This effect is likely very transient and appears to exert little effect upon the depth of anesthesia postbypass. Pulmonary sequestration of sufentanil is comparable to that of fentanyl.[205]

A number of investigators have demonstrated in vitro binding of fentanyl to the CPB apparatus (Figure 4.7).

Binding of alfentanil to the bypass equipment, however, appears to be much less avid.[193-196] Differences in binding between fentanyl and alfentanil may occur as a result of dissimilarities in the ionization of these drugs with changes in pH (Figure 4.8).[142] Total plasma concentrations of both fentanyl and alfentanil are reduced upon the initiation of CPB. This is preventable by the addition of opioid to the CPB priming solution. Regardless of supplementation, plasma levels are found to reach a new, stable level within 2.5 minutes of the onset of bypass (Figure 4.9).[69] Free drug levels, however, have not been measured. It appears that minimal reductions in plasma opioid concentrations may be anticipated following the use of autotransfusion devices, hemoconcentrators, or cell savers.[193] It is unlikely that binding of opioids to the CPB apparatus and other nonbiologic equipment would exert an observable clinical effect, due to the tremendous reservoir of drug available in the peripheral tissues of the body. Opioids will diffuse down their concentration gradient to replace any drug that is lost to the CPB apparatus.

To summarize, opioid infusions administered before CPB that are based on pharmacokinetic parameters gleaned from noncardiac populations appear to approximate the desired target concentrations in adult cardiac patients with preserved ventricular function. Changes in clearance and volumes of distribution in children, especially infants and those patients with severe hemodynamic disruptions, render these assumptions untenable. Initiation of CPB may be expected to produce a reduction in total plasma opioid levels, while changes in free drug levels may indeed be minimal. Sequestration of opioid in the lungs and CPB apparatus does occur, although the clinical significance of these processes is likely minimal. Elimination half-times for opioids appear to be prolonged following hypothermic CPB. Repeated doses of narcotic after CPB may thus lead to drug accumulation. The effects of hypothermic CPB on opioid pharmacokinetics have been recently reviewed in detail by Hall.[209]

Barbiturates

Barbiturates are derivatives of barbituric acid that possess sedative and hypnotic properties. Barbiturates may be administered as induction agents for cardiac surgery patients and can be used to deepen anesthesia prior to stimuli such as aortic cannulation. The role of barbiturates as cerebral protective agents during cardiac surgery remains controversial.[210]

When thiopental is administered at a continuous rate by infusion, plasma levels fall by 50% at the onset of bypass, then rise to 70% of the prebypass level during the hypothermic pump run. Free thiopental levels, however, decline only 25% at the onset of bypass and subsequently return to 100% of the prebypass level (Figure 4.10). This

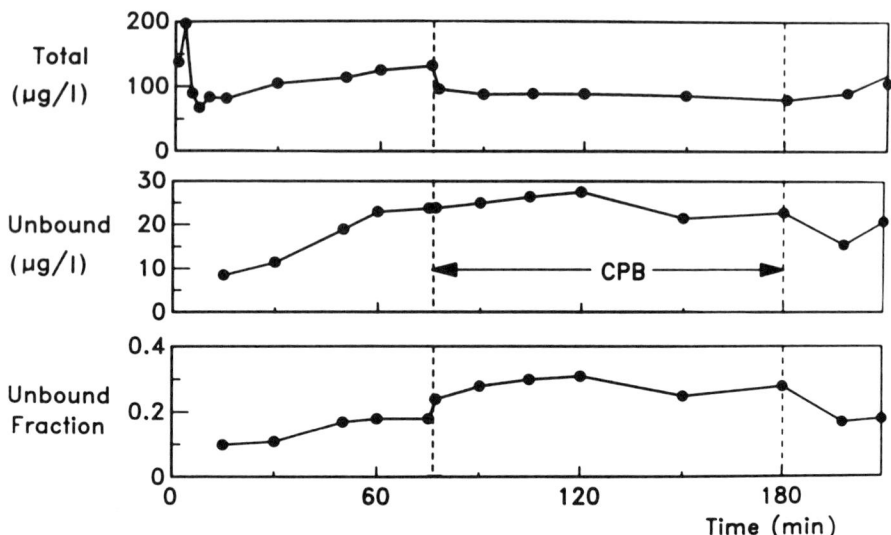

FIGURE 4.5. Total and unbound plasma alfentanil levels and unbound (free) fraction of drug in a patient receiving a continuous infusion of alfentanil during cardiac surgery. The horizontal arrows between the dotted lines indicate the time of initiation and termination of bypass. The decline in total alfentanil concentration at the onset of CPB is offset by an increase in unbound fraction, such that free drug levels do not change. (By permission of *Eur J Clin Pharmacol* 1988;35:47–52.)

results in an increase in the free (unbound) fraction from 16.6% to 29.3% during CPB. The binding ratio of thiopental is strongly correlated with the plasma albumin concentration. Changes in thiopental-protein binding during CPB are likely due to hemodilution. Clearance of thiopental, eliminated by the liver with a hepatic extraction ratio of 25% to 30%, is unaltered by the shifts produced during CPB. The authors who performed this study recommend against adjustments in thiopental dosage during cardiac surgery employing CPB.[65] A follow-up study from the same group confirmed their observations for thiopental and described similar findings for methohexital (Figure 4.11).[74] No differences in thiopental pharmacokinetics have been detected between groups receiving pulsatile or nonpulsatile perfusion during hypothermic CPB (Figure 4.12).[81] Although thiopental is not sequestered in the lungs, up to 50% uptake by the CPB apparatus has been detected in vitro. Although changes in plasma concentrations of barbiturates may be observed during CPB, no dosing adjustments should be necessary, as very little change in free drug level occurs.

Benzodiazepines

Benzodiazepines are frequently used in cardiac surgery patients for their sedative and amnestic properties. These drugs are customarily employed as premedicants and may be used for induction or maintenance of general anesthesia.

Boscoe has examined the relationship between timing of lorazepam dosage and maintenance of blood levels considered sufficient for amnesia (≥ 30 ng/mL) during cardiac surgery. Lorazepam was administered the night before surgery (group 1), at induction (group 2), or 10 minutes before CPB (group 3). Satisfactory "amnestic levels" of lorazepam were sustained only in group 3.[211] Plasma concentrations fell below 20 ng/mL in group 1 and below 30 ng/mL in group 2, while remaining above 45 ng/mL in group 3. Plasma concentrations declined 27% upon initiation of CPB, rising 17% at the time of separation. The pharmacokinetics of lorazepam do not appear to vary with age, nor does elimination half-time change during hypothermic CPB. A drop in total plasma lorazepam concentration may be detected at the initiation

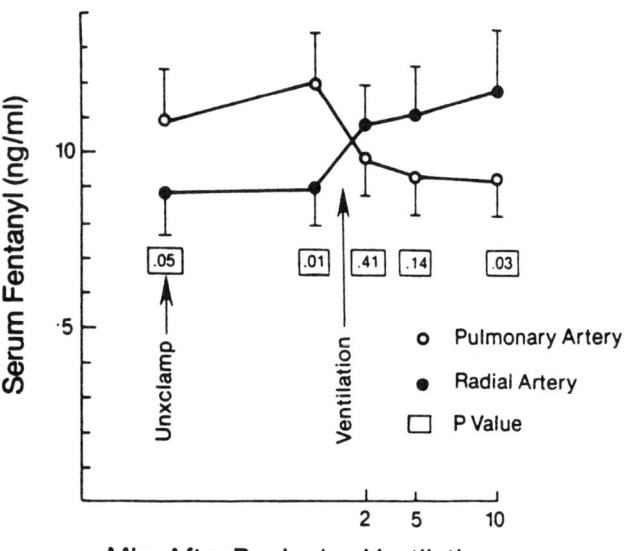

FIGURE 4.6. Mean fentanyl levels in 7 cardiac surgery patients as ventilation and perfusion to the lung are resumed near the end of cardiopulmonary bypass. Systemic fentanyl concentrations rise with ventilation while levels in the pulmonary artery fall, suggesting washout of fentanyl sequestered in the lungs during CPB. (Unxclamp = removal of aortic crossclamp.) (From Bentley, Conahan, and Cork,[184] by permission of *Clin Pharmacol Ther.*)

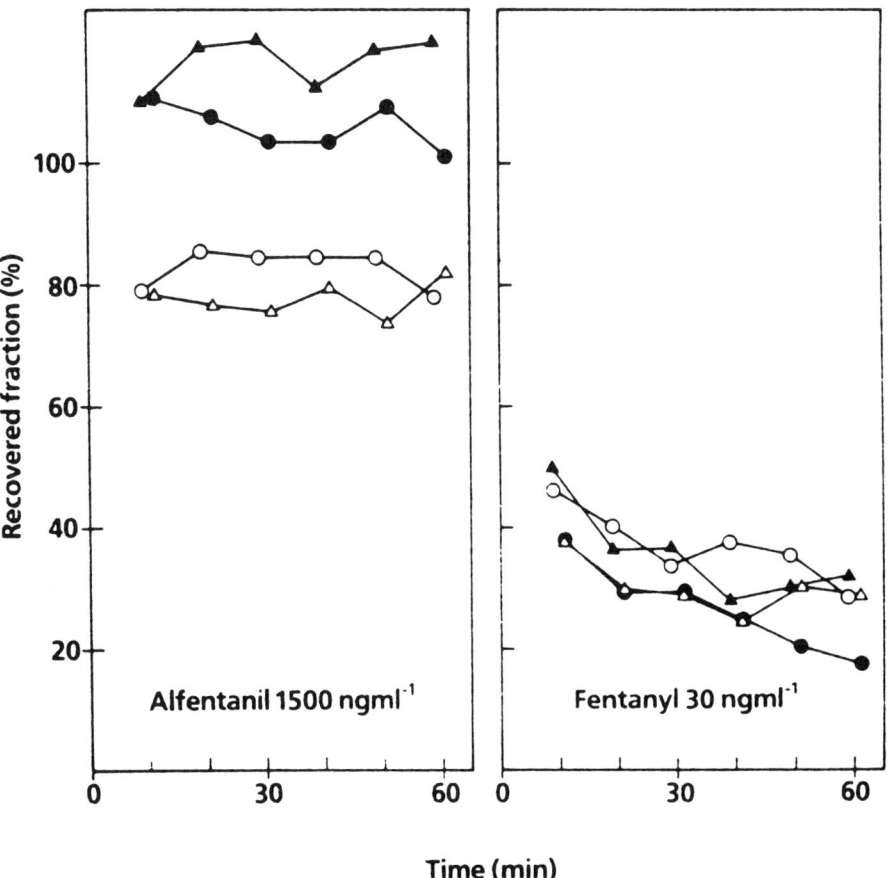

FIGURE 4.7. Fractions of the calculated concentrations of alfentanil (after a dose of 1500 ng/mL) and fentanyl (after a dose of 30 ng/mL) recovered from prime solutions during a 60-minute circulation through a closed CPB system. Each line represents a single experiment. The *circles* represent trials with a bubble oxygenator, while the *triangles* show data from a membrane oxygenator. Blood-containing primes are represented by *filled data points* (●,▲), while nonhemic primes are designated by *data points* (○,△). The binding of alfentanil to the CPB apparatus is much less avid than that of fentanyl. (From Hynynen,[69] by permission of *Acta Anaesthesiol Scand*.)

of CPB, while free drug concentrations rise (ie, the free fraction increases), accompanying the hemodilution of plasma proteins. Following termination of bypass, total lorazepam levels increase secondary to redistribution in the post-CPB period.[212]

Kanto administered midazolam, 0.075 mg/kg (low dose) or 0.15 mg/kg (high dose), in combination with fentanyl (75 μg/kg) to males undergoing coronary bypass surgery. As described for lorazepam above, plasma midazolam levels fall upon initiation of CPB, stabilize during bypass, and rise following its discontinuation. The elimination half-time for midazolam was prolonged to 281 minutes (in the high-dose group), versus 120 minutes in normal, healthy subjects. Plasma levels were undetectable in the low-dose group after 240 minutes. Precise definition of the terminal elimination half-time of midazolam, however, would require measurement of plasma levels over at least 3 half-times. Concentrations were followed only to 360 minutes in this study, as limited by the sensitivity of the assay methods employed.[213] The prolongation of elimination half-time of midazolam during bypass may be secondary to alterations in hepatic metabolism induced by CPB. Lorazepam depends solely on hepatic glucuronidation for its elimination, whereas midazolam requires metabolism by mixed function oxidases as well as glucuronidation prior to its clearance from plasma.

Midazolam has gained widespread acceptance as a postoperative sedative in the cardiac care unit. Clearance, volumes of distribution, and elimination half-times for midazolam are all increased following cardiac surgery when compared to age-matched patients undergoing minor operations.[214] When administered on a schedule every 2 hours, diazepam (5 mg) has been shown to accumulate in the blood, whereas midazolam (5 mg) is associated with stable levels after the initial 4 hours.[215] Midazolam levels fall quickly after discontinuation and are undetectable after 24 hours, whereas plasma levels of diazepam remain elevated. Plasma levels of midazolam may be quite variable, however, and frequently fall below the level felt to be necessary for adequate sedation (40 ng/mL), particularly at the start of a constant-dose regimen. It has been suggested that higher "loading" doses be employed at the initiation of therapy to assure adequate sedation.

To achieve adequate "amnestic" levels of benzodiazepine prior to CPB, it would seem that dosing should be in proximity to the initiation of bypass. Midazolam appears to be an excellent choice for postoperative sedation, while

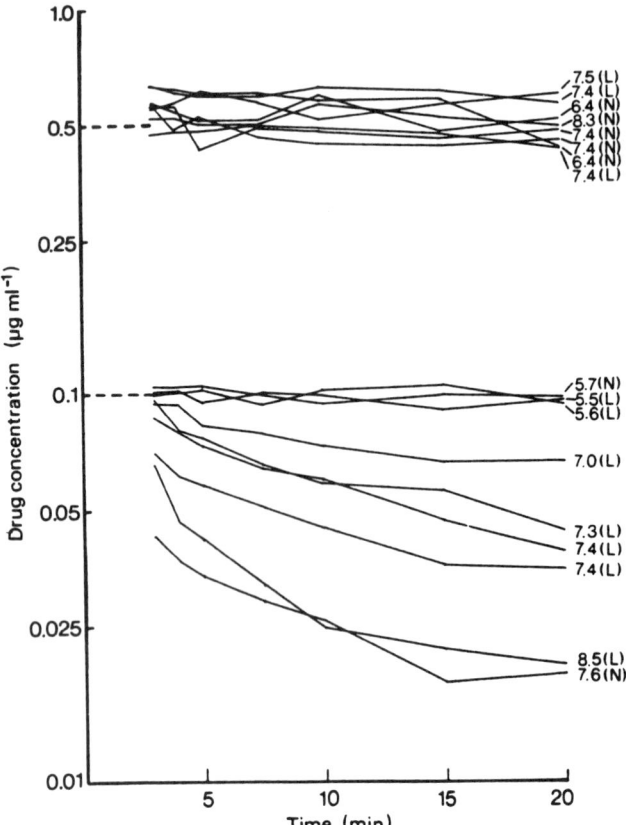

FIGURE 4.8. Changes in concentrations of alfentanil (top) and fentanyl (bottom) in extracorporeal circuit prime over time. Drug concentrations are shown on the vertical axis using the same logarithmic scale. Dotted lines represent predicted concentrations based on the loading dose. Numbers to the right of each line represent the pH values of individual priming solutions. (L) = Low temperature (24.4–25.7°C); (N) = normothermia (34.1–37°C). Differences in binding to the CPB apparatus may occur as a result of dissimilarities in the ionization of the two drugs with changes in pH. (From Skacel, Knott, Reynolds et al,[142] by permission of *Br J Anaesth*.)

accumulation of diazepam can be anticipated if frequent dosing is employed in the postoperative period.

Propofol

Propofol is a short-acting sedative-hypnotic recently released for use in the United States. It is a hydrophobic derivative of phenol, formulated as a distinctive "milky" emulsion of soybean oil, glycerol, and egg phosphatide. Propofol may be used for both induction and maintenance of anesthesia. The use of propofol during cardiac surgery is in the preliminary stages of investigation, as is its use as a postoperative sedative in the intensive care unit. The volume of distribution, clearance, and terminal elimination half-time of propofol in cardiac surgery patients do not differ significantly from those reported in a noncardiac population.[216] Stable plasma propofol concentrations may be maintained in patients with preserved ventricular function before CPB through use of a continuous infusion. Total plasma propofol concentration falls at the onset of CPB, while the free propofol fraction rises. Application of hypothermia is associated with an increase in plasma propofol levels, which return to prebypass levels following rewarming.[217] In patients undergoing coronary bypass grafting following a propofol dose of 2 mg/kg, total clearance of the drug is high (averaging 2390 mL/min), with an initial hepatic extraction ratio of 82%. Over a 60-minute observation period, the hepatic extraction rises to 92%. Within that hour, however, only 44% of the administered dose is removed by the liver. This suggests that the change in hepatic extraction ratio may be secondary to the slow release of propofol from its soybean emulsion. The potential for drug accumulation may exist if repeated doses of propofol are administered.[218] Hall has compared a sufentanil-propofol technique to a sufentanil-enflurane anesthetic in patients with preserved ventricular function undergoing cardiac surgery with CPB. There is no increase in either the degree or the incidence of myocardial ischemia, nor are there significant differences in myocardial lactate extraction, perioperative hemodynamics, or electrocardiographic data.[25]

Propofol has also been studied for its potential as a sedative in the intensive care unit following cardiac surgery. The elimination half-time of propofol is prolonged (470 minutes) and clearance is reduced (1140 mL/min) in postoperative patients who have undergone CPB. When compared to patients sedated with midazolam, however, propofol-treated patients were extubated significantly earlier. This difference may be due in part to the rapid redistribution of propofol (average redistribution half-time, 13.4 minutes). Redistribution in postoperative patients is prolonged, however, when compared to noncardiac patients, where redistribution half-time averages 2 to 4 minutes. These initial studies suggest that changes in free propofol concentrations are similar to those reported for other drugs administered during CPB. Hepatic clearance of propofol may be affected by CPB, and there is a risk of prolonged drug effects if repetitive dosing is employed. The rapid reawakening characteristic of propofol in noncardiac subjects may be delayed in postoperative cardiac patients due to reductions in hepatic clearance and prolongation of distribution half-times associated with altered tissue perfusion.[219]

Volatile Anesthetic Agents

Volatile anesthetic agents are frequently employed during cardiac surgery to increase the depth of anesthesia and provide amnesia during the procedure. These compounds are halogenated hydrocarbons, and enflurane and isoflur-

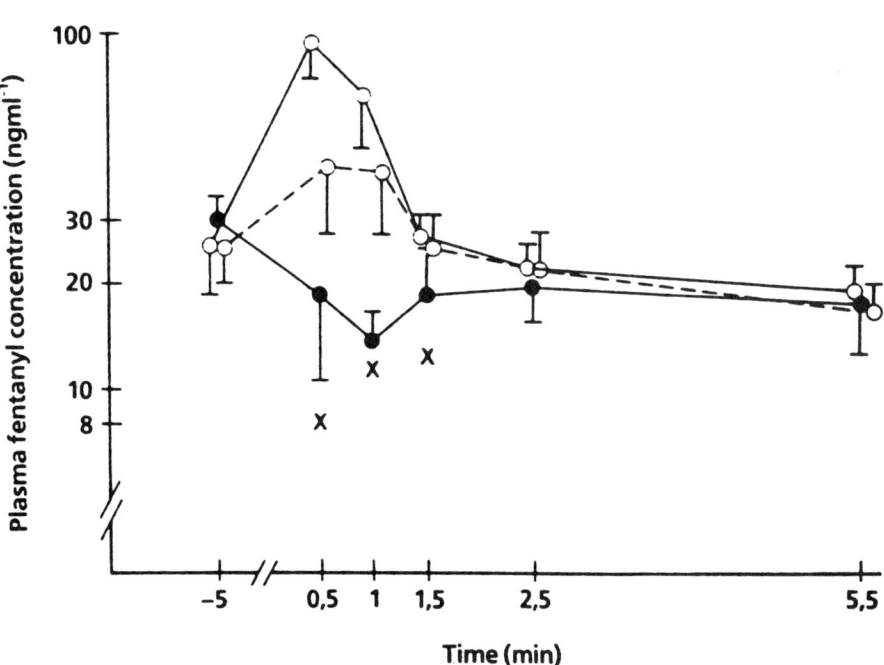

FIGURE 4.9. Plasma fentanyl concentrations (mean values ± SD) in patients measured at the initiation of CPB. Individual lines represent primes containing no fentanyl (●-●), a calculated fentanyl concentration of 140 ng mL (○---○), or a calculated fentanyl concentration of 280 ng mL (○-○). X indicates the lowest fentanyl level measured during the initial 1.5 minutes of the study in patients not receiving fentanyl in the pump prime. Regardless of supplementation, plasma fentanyl levels reach a new, stable level within 2.5 minutes of the onset of CPB. (From Hynynen,[69] by permission of *Acta Anaesthesiol Scand.*)

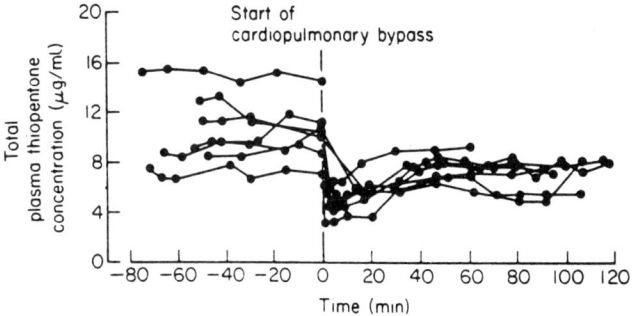

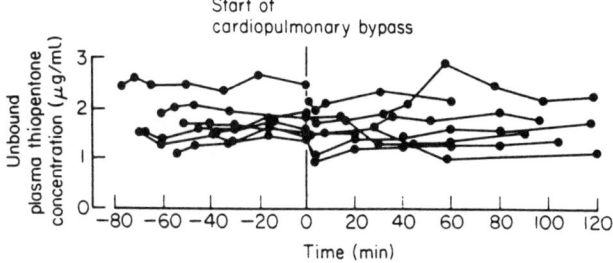

FIGURE 4.10. *Top*: *Total* plasma thiopentone (thiopental) concentrations in cardiac surgery patients receiving a continuous IV infusion. Time = 0 is taken as the start of bypass. *Bottom*: *Unbound* (free) plasma thiopentone (thiopental) concentrations from the same cardiac patients. Total pentothal levels fall dramatically at the onset of CPB, while free pentothal levels decline only slightly before returning to the prebypass level. (From Morgan, Crankshaw, Brideaux et al,[65] by permission of *Anaesthesia.*)

ane (the most commonly used agents in adult cardiac surgery) are derivatives of diethyl ether. They are administered through complex vaporizer systems to assure that a constant percentage of drug is delivered regardless of gas flows. Prior to CPB, these agents are delivered through the anesthesia machine to the lungs; while the patient is on bypass, volatile anesthetics may be administered through the oxygenator apparatus.

EEG burst suppression (a standard of anesthetic depth) occurs after administration of isoflurane at a mean vaporizer setting of 2.2% for an average of 27 minutes at 26°C. Removal of isoflurane from the blood is rapid, with a mean elimination half-time of 19 minutes.[220] The concentration of isoflurane required to produce burst suppression during hypothermic CPB is below that previously reported in patients not undergoing CPB.[221] These reduced requirements for isoflurane may be due to differences in anesthetic uptake by the membrane oxygenator versus the lungs, or a change in blood/gas partitioning of isoflurane at lower temperatures. The solubility of isoflurane in blood would be increased by hemodilution and reduced by hypothermia. The most likely explanation for this phenomenon, however, may be a reduction in anesthetic requirements secondary to the application of hypothermia per se.[62] Hypothermia has been consistently shown to reduce requirements for halothane, isoflurane, and enflurane during general anesthesia, although the exact mechanisms have not been precisely elucidated.[60-62] The possibility that the pharmacodynamics of enflurane may be altered by CPB has also been raised by Hall[154] in a study on dogs.

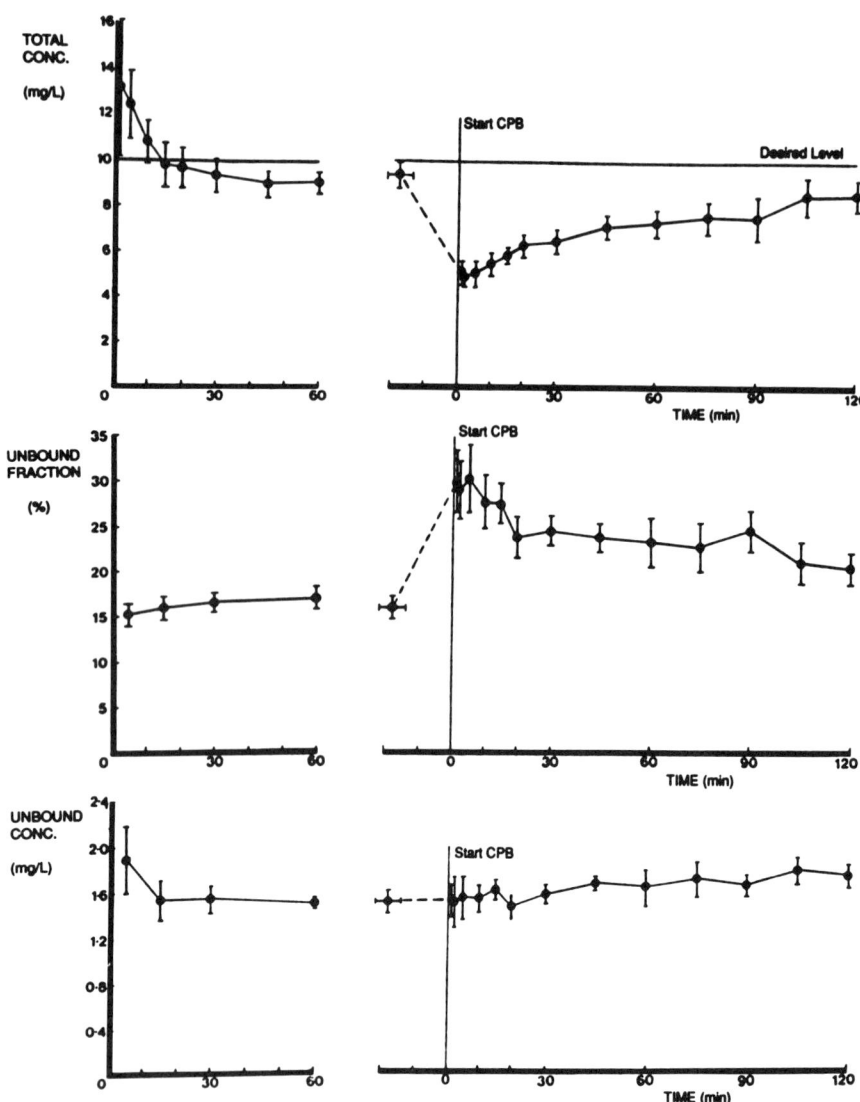

FIGURE 4.11. Total plasma concentration, unbound fraction, and unbound plasma concentrations of methohexital as a function of time for the prebypass period (*left*), and after the initiation of CPB (*right*). The data point to the left of time = 0 in each CPB graph represents the mean of the prebypass samples from each patient plotted at the mean time, before CPB, at which they were measured. Vertical bars: ±SD. Total methohexital levels fall at the onset of CPB, while the unbound drug fraction rises. The net result is little, if any, change in the free methohexital concentration. (From Bjorksten, Crankshaw, Morgan et al,[74] by permission of author *J Cardiothorac Anesth*.)

The in vitro blood/gas partition coefficients of isoflurane, enflurane, and halothane in hemodiluted blood at 25°C (hemoglobin concentrations 9 g/dL) are similar to those measured in undiluted blood at normothermia. In vitro washin of isoflurane through a Ben-10® bubble oxygenator is rapid (>50% equilibration by 4 minutes, >90% by 16 minutes) at all gas inflow rates (Figure 4.13). Isoflurane washout is also rapid (<25% of peak concentration remaining by 4 minutes, <10% 16 minutes after discontinuing administration). Washin and washout are significantly increased at higher gas inflow rates but are not affected by variations in pump flow. When washin and washout curves for three concurrently administered volatile agents (enflurane, isoflurane, and halothane) are examined, it can be seen that equilibration is similarly rapid (Figure 4.14). The rates of washin and washout of these agents differ as a function of their blood/gas solubilities. Agents with lower solubility (isoflurane and enflurane) equilibrate more rapidly than does halothane (which has a higher solubility in blood). It appears that the CPB oxygenator imposes insignificant limitations to volatile anesthetic diffusion in vitro.[70] Whether these observations apply to other types of oxygenators, however, remains to be seen.

The blood/gas partition coefficient of isoflurane in patients undergoing cardiac surgery also does not vary with hypothermia (23°C) or hemodilution (hematocrit 23%). The rate of washin of isoflurane during hypothermic CPB is considerably slower than that found in normothermic patients not undergoing CPB. The duration of isoflurane washin averages 43 (±17) minutes, during which time the arterial partial pressure of isoflurane rises toward the inlet gas partial pressure, with 57% equilibration at 48 minutes. During washout (the rewarming phase), the arterial

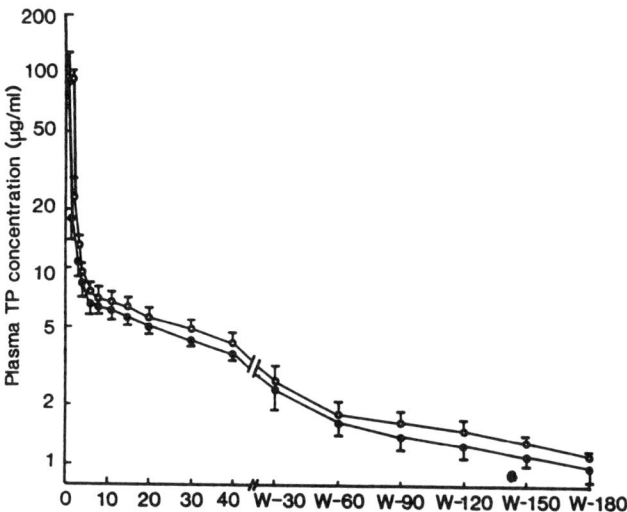

FIGURE 4.12. Plasma thiopental (TP) concentrations (mean values ± SD) in patients undergoing CPB with a nonpulsatile (○, n = 8) or pulsatile (●, n = 9) flow. The codes on the horizontal axis denote minutes after the administration (0–40) of thiopental (6 mg/kg), and minutes after the start of rewarming (W30-W180). No differences in thiopental pharmacokinetics are seen between groups receiving pulsatile or nonpulsatile perfusion during hypothermic CPB. (From Hynynen, Olkkola, Naveri et al,[81] by permission of *Acta Anaesthesiol Scand*.)

concentration falls to 36% of its peak after 8 minutes and 13% of peak after 32 minutes. Washout of this volatile agent occurs much more rapidly than washin.[71] The slower rate of wash-in may be attributable to higher isoflurane solubility in peripheral tissues under conditions of hypothermia, which would delay the rate of rise in arterial concentration while decreasing average tissue perfusion. Isoflurane washout approaches that reported in normothermic patients. Any effects of hypothermic CPB during washout are likely offset by the reduced total amount of agent present in the body at equilibrium or changes in blood/gas partitioning during rewarming. Washin and washout curves in vitro are faster than those seen in vivo, demonstrating the significant role that tissue uptake plays in limiting the rise in anesthetic concentration in the hypothermic patient. The washin of isoflurane remains comparatively rapid, however, and does not likely impair the ability to adjust anesthetic depth during hypothermic CPB (Figure 4.15).[67]

Following discontinuation of isoflurane during hypothermic CPB, in vivo exhaust gas concentrations from a Bentley Ben-10® bubble oxygenator decline rapidly in a manner best described by a single-compartment pharmacokinetic model with a time constant of 1.94 minutes (ie, 95% washout within 5 minutes).[222] It appears that discontinuation of isoflurane can indeed be delayed until very near the anticipated time of separation from CPB due to this rapid washout. Isoflurane equilibration during hypothermic CPB using either a Terumo Capiox® membrane or a Bentley Bro® bubble oxygenator will not be achieved during the usual washin period. Following discontinuation of isoflurane, a very rapid initial washout phase occurs (50.5% to 71.4% eliminated within 2 minutes), followed by a slower washout phase with an elimination half-time of 9 to 15 minutes (mean of 13 minutes). Within 15 minutes, 75% of the isoflurane will be removed. No differences in washout have been detected between membrane and bubble oxygenators.[223]

CPB may alter the metabolism of halothane in patients undergoing surgical correction of either cyanotic or noncyanotic congenital heart disease.[224] Higher serum fluoride levels are seen in children with cyanotic congenital heart disease following separation from CPB than in comparable acyanotic patients. This increase in metabolism may be on the basis of enhanced reductive metabolism of halothane in patients with cyanotic disease. Alterations in liver function are evidenced only by increases in blood urea nitrogen and direct bilirubin in the cyanotic children. The clinical significance of this increased reductive metabolism in the setting of CPB, though, remains unclear.

It is difficult to summarize the results of the studies cited above, as different surgical procedures, oxygenators, and measuring techniques were applied. It appears, however, that the administration of volatile anesthetic agents during CPB is comparatively unrestricted by the oxygenator apparatus itself. Effective agent concentrations may be most expeditiously achieved by using higher gas inflow rates to the oxygenator during washin. Washout certainly occurs more rapidly than washin, yet firm guidelines regarding the timing of discontinuation of volatile agents before separation from CPB do not currently exist. It would seem prudent to discontinue volatile agents relatively early during the rewarming phase to minimize potential myocardial depression at separation from CPB.

Neuromuscular Blocking Agents

Neuromuscular blocking agents are universally employed during cardiac surgery to facilitate intubation of the trachea and ensure patient immobility during the operative procedure. A number of studies have documented changes in pharmacokinetics of various muscle relaxants employed during cardiac surgery.[171-179,225]

Administration of heparin before CPB does not appear to influence plasma concentrations of *d*-tubocurarine (a preparation of curare), the oldest of the neuromuscular blocking agents. At the onset of CPB, the free fraction of curare rises from 58% to 69% (secondary to protein hemodilution), while total curare concentrations also in-

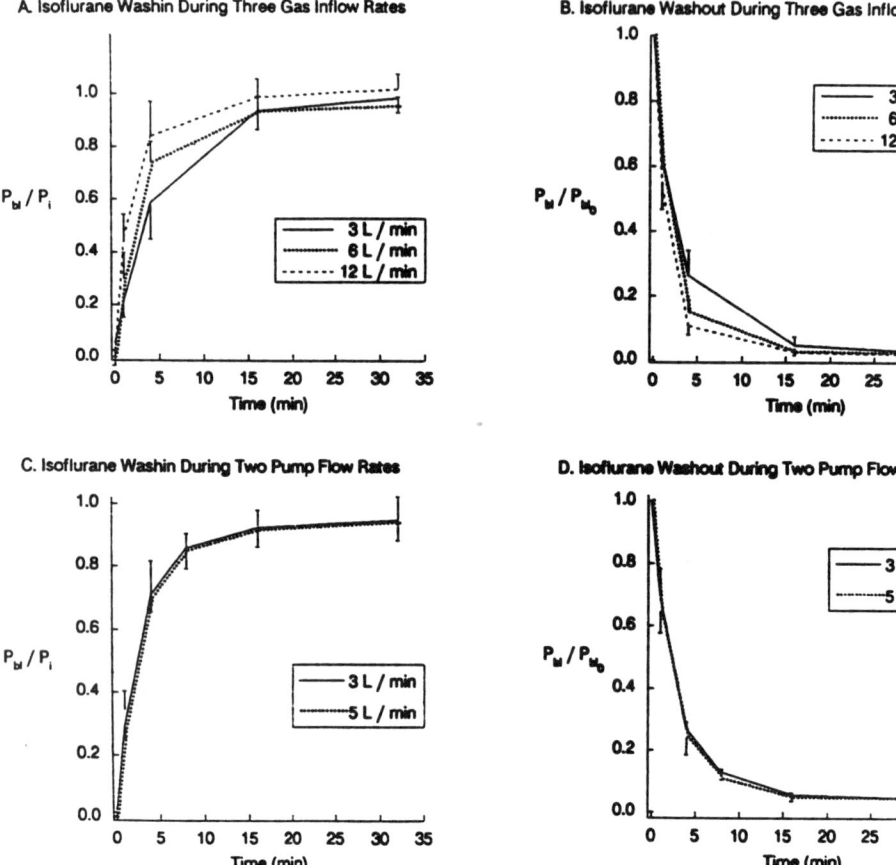

FIGURE 4.13. Washin and washout curves for isoflurane at various gas inflow rates (A and B) and pump flow rates (C and D) through a Ben-10® bubble oxygenator. The partial pressure of isoflurane in blood (P_{bl}) is expressed on the vertical axis as a ratio; the denominator is the simultaneously obtained inlet gas partial pressure (P_i) during washin (A and C) and the peak partial pressure in the blood sample obtained just before discontinuing anesthetic administration (P_{bl_o}) during washout (B and D). Washin of isoflurane is rapid at all gas inflow rates, increasing significantly with higher flows. Isoflurane washout is also rapid but is not substantially affected by variations in pump flow. (From Nussmeier, Moskowitz, Weiskopf et al,[70] by permission of *Anesth Analg.*)

crease. Clearance is reduced (0.60 versus 2.7 mL/kg/min), elimination half-time increases (633 versus 172 minutes), and volume of distribution remains unchanged when compared to noncardiac surgery patients.[174] The rise in curare concentrations during bypass may be due to either a decrease in effective blood volume or a reduction in distribution of the drug to highly perfused tissues (ie, the lungs excluded from the CPB circuit). Alterations in renal clearance may also be responsible for a portion of these changes.

Pancuronium requirements (as measured by reduction in twitch height) are increased at the initiation of bypass because of hemodilution yet are reduced during the remainder of hypothermic CPB. This reduction in pancuronium requirements may be secondary to altered function of the neuromuscular junction caused by hypothermia.[177]
Futter[172] has also found that pancuronium requirements are reduced during hypothermic CPB when compared to the prebypass period. Pancuronium requirements increase during rewarming, then decline again following separation from CPB secondary to incomplete rewarming of the muscle bed and decreased hepatic and renal clearances.

The elimination half-time of alcuronium (which is structurally similar to pancuronium) increases in cardiac surgery patients (532 versus 199 minutes in noncardiac "controls"). Clearance of alcuronium is reduced (0.8 versus 1.3 mL/kg/min), and no change in volume of distribution is seen. The elevation of alcuronium concentrations during CPB may also be due to reductions in effective blood volume caused by the exclusion of the lungs from the bypass circuit. Reduction of alcuronium clearance likely stems from changes in protein binding associated with hemodilution and hypothermia.[176]

The infusion rate of atracurium must be reduced during hypothermic CPB to maintain a constant level of neuro-

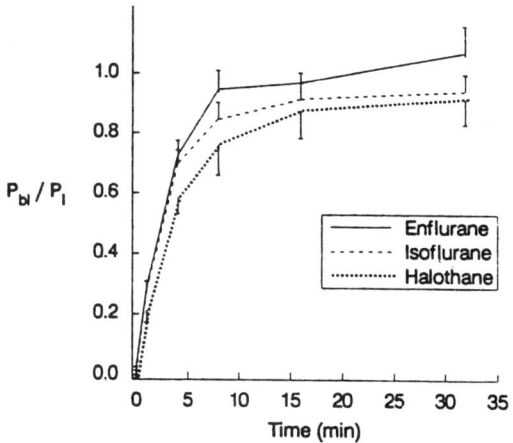

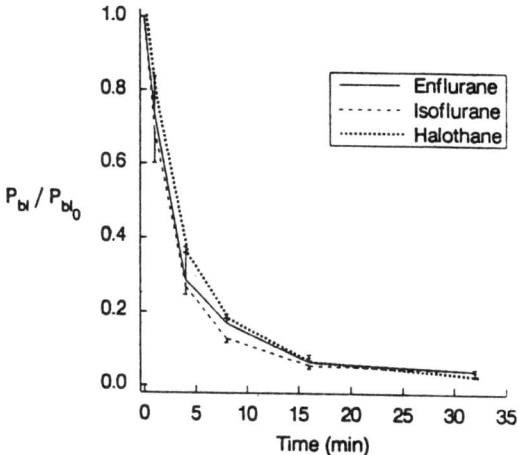

FIGURE 4.14. Washin and washout curves for three volatile anesthetic agents: isoflurane, enflurane, and halothane. The partial pressure of each anesthetic in blood (P_{bl}) is expressed on the vertical axis as a ratio; the denominator is the simultaneously obtained inlet gas partial pressure (P_i) during washin (A) and the peak partial pressure in the blood sample obtained just before discontinuing anesthetic administration (P_{bl_o}) during washout (B). Equilibration of these volatile agents is rapid. The rates of washin and washout differ as a function of blood/gas solubilities. Agents that are *less soluble* in blood (isoflurane and enflurane), *equilibrate more rapidly* than do agents with higher solubility (eg, halothane). (From Nussmeier, Moskowitz, Weiskopf et al,[70] by permission of *Anesth Analg.*)

muscular blockade.[173] Atracurium undergoes Hoffman degradation; its metabolism is thus independent of hepatic function. Hoffman degradation is temperature sensitive, however, which would explain the clinically observed reductions in atracurium requirements.

Some resistance to the effect of metocurine is seen during hypothermic CPB, with plasma concentrations of 0.67 µg/mL producing a 69% paralysis during bypass versus an 87% paralysis at the end of the procedure. No change in measurable pharmacokinetic parameters occurs. Indeed, there is little variation in the pharmacokinetics of metocurine when comparing cardiac surgery patients to similar subjects undergoing total hip replacement.[171] The lack of observable pharmacokinetic changes may be related to the rapid initiation of CPB (over a 30-second period) in this particular study and the more gradual induction of hypothermia. The pharmacokinetics of pipecuronium are likewise unaffected by hypothermic CPB.[225] Outside the setting of CPB, hypothermia per se is associated with a reduction in efficacy of some neuromuscular blocking agents.

In the absence of neuromuscular blocking agents, the onset of hypothermic CPB facilitates neuromuscular transmission as measured by EMG response. Mechanical performance of the muscle, however, is attenuated by hypothermia.[179] These effects are reversed during rewarming. Hypothermia appears to play a significant role in altering requirements for neuromuscular blockers, and this is a pharmacodynamic rather than a pharmacokinetic effect. A similar conclusion has been reached by Buzello[175] in a study examining requirements for pancuronium and vecuronium.

To summarize, hypothermic CPB has not been associated with significant changes in volumes of distribution for most neuromuscular blocking agents. Changes in clearance and elimination half-times will vary depending on the specific agent employed and its primary method of elimination. Reduced infusion rates of atracurium and pancuronium are required to produce a constant level of relaxation during hypothermic CPB. Increased infusion rates during bypass may be required for alcuronium, *d*-tubocurarine, and metocurine. It appears that both pharmacokinetic and pharmacodynamic factors interact to alter the requirements for neuromuscular blockade during hypothermia and CPB. The pharmacodynamic changes, which are predominantly due to systemic hypothermia, may result from changes in the relative sensitivities of pre- and postjunctional receptors during bypass. The relative sensitivities of these receptors, however, have not been specifically investigated in the setting of CPB. Monitoring of neuromuscular blockade with a peripheral nerve stimulator or similar device will facilitate the optimal administration of these agents during cardiac surgery.

Antibiotics

Prophylactic antibiotics are administered before cardiac surgery to reduce the incidence of postoperative infection. A number of studies have investigated whether therapeutic antibiotic concentrations are achieved or maintained during cardiac surgery employing CPB.

When cephalexin (1 g p.o.) was given to 12 cardiac pa-

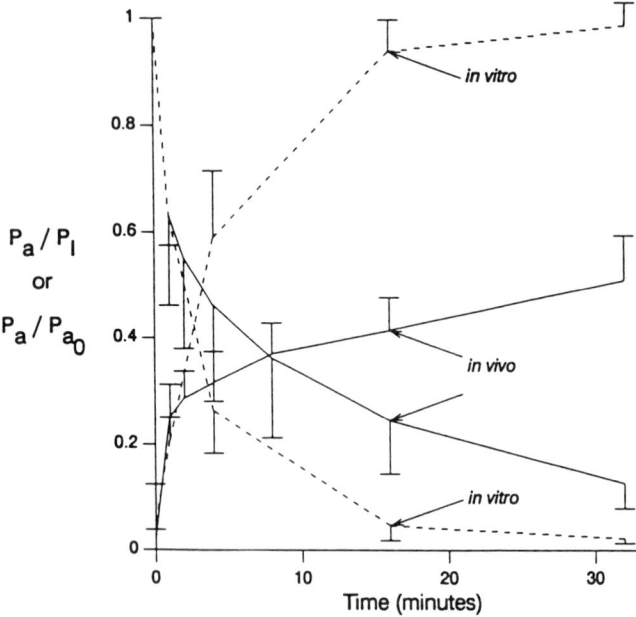

FIGURE 4.15. Washin and washout of isoflurane via bubble oxygenators in vitro are more rapid than observed in patients undergoing cardiac surgery employing CPB. P_a = partial pressure of agent measured in arterial blood; P_i = partial pressure measured in inlet gas; P_{a_o} = partial pressure measured in arterial blood just before discontinuing anesthetic administration. Washin and washout curves in vitro are faster than those seen in vivo, illustrating the role that tissue uptake plays in delaying the rise of arterial anesthetic concentrations. Washout of this volatile agent occurs more rapidly than does washin. (From Nussmeier, Lambert, Moskowitz et al,[71] by permission of *Anesthesiology*.)

tients at midnight prior to their surgery, no cephalosporin activity was detectable in plasma just before induction of anesthesia the next morning. This oral cephalexin was supplemented with cephalothin (1 g IV) during induction of anesthesia and upon separation from CPB. Cephalothin levels still fell below the 10 μg/mL concentration felt to be the necessary minimal inhibitory concentration (MIC) in 3 out of 12 patients. Cephalosporin levels fall although clearance of cephalothin is impaired during bypass. The authors of this study recommend that the time interval between drug administration and the onset of CPB (which averaged 52 minutes) should be as brief as possible. Increased dosages are advised for larger patients, and supplementation should be considered if CPB extends beyond 2 hours. Prescribing prophylactic oral antibiotics the night before surgery does not appear to be helpful.[226]

The disposition of cefamandole (20 mg/kg IV at the induction of anesthesia) has been examined in 16 patients undergoing coronary artery revascularization employing CPB with mild hypothermia (32° to 34°C).[227] Plasma levels of cefamandole were well sustained during CPB, which began within 41 ± 12 minutes after completion of the induction dose. The elimination half-time for cefamandole was prolonged during CPB (113 versus 52 minutes in the control group), which suggests impaired elimination or altered distribution of cefamandole during bypass. The authors recommend supplementation of the induction dose of cefamandole if the duration of CPB exceeds 4 hours.

The efficacy of cephalothin (1 g per dose) has been compared to that of cefazolin (500 mg per dose) in cardiac surgery patients. In this study, an IM dose was administered at midnight prior to surgery and 1 hour before induction, followed by an IV dose every 6 hours for the next 5 days. Postoperative infections occurred in 1 of 48 patients given cefazolin, versus 2 of 44 patients in the cephalothin group (one of whom died). Plasma levels of cephalothin were quite variable during bypass, while cefazolin concentrations tended to remain more stable. Only 4 of 31 patients in the cefazolin group and 6 of 38 patients in the cephalothin group had detectable antibiotic concentrations in atrial or papillary muscle samples taken during the procedure.[228] Cephalothin reliably penetrates cardiac tissues, however, as demonstrated by Sato.[229]

The optimal duration of antibiotic prophylaxis following cardiac surgery remains controversial. The trend toward limiting the duration of perioperative antibiotics was enhanced by Goldman's double-blinded comparison of a 2-day and a 6-day regimen employing cephalothin.[230] Cephalothin was given IM "on call" to the operating room (1 g), followed by 2 g IV at the start of the procedure, then 2 g IV every 6 hours for either 48 hours or 6 days postoperatively. Intraoperative cephalothin levels were above the MIC in all patients who were sampled (186 out of 200 subjects). Eleven patients, however, showed no detectable cephalothin activity in serum at the conclusion of surgery, and the rate of infection in this group was increased relative to patients with detectable antibiotic levels. Increased infection rates and declining cephalothin levels were both related to the duration of the procedure. No difference in infection rates was evident between the two antibiotic regimens, apart from the development of earlier and more frequent urinary tract infections in the 2-day group. The authors concluded that a 2-day prophylactic antibiotic course was quite sufficient for cardiac surgery patients.

The disposition of cephalothin has also been examined in cardiac surgery patients undergoing hypothermic (26° to 28°C) CPB. A cephalothin dose of 2 g was administered the day before operation, after induction of anesthesia, then through the day following the procedure. No differences in kinetic parameters could be demonstrated between the preoperative and postoperative periods. At the start of CPB, however, the concentration versus time

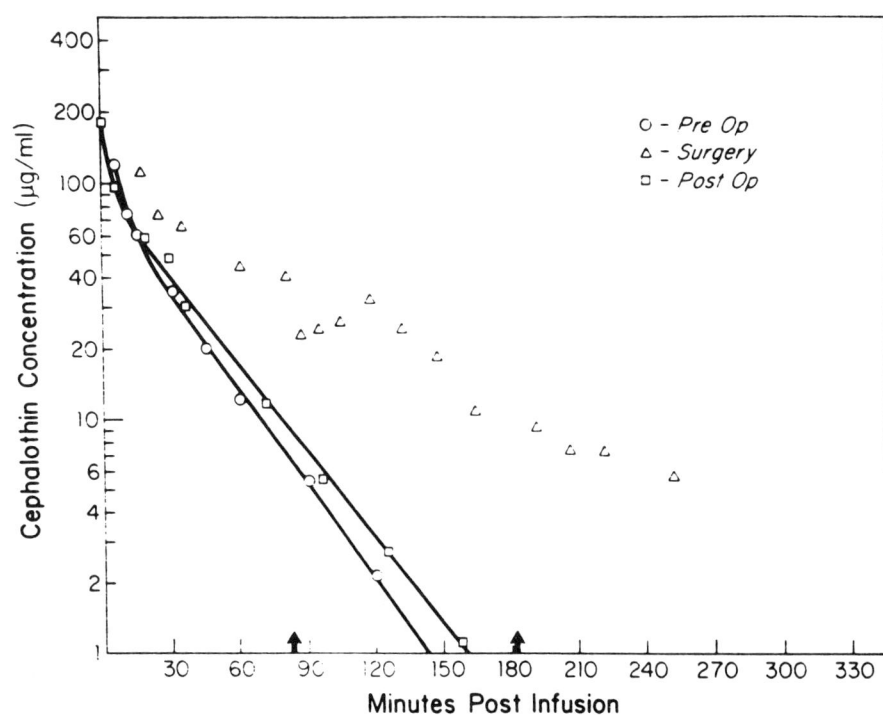

FIGURE 4.16. Cephalothin serum concentrations versus time after infusion in a single patient before, during, and after cardiac surgery. A cephalothin dose of 2 g was administered the day before operation (○), after induction of anesthesia (△), and on the day following the procedure (□). Arrows denote the time of extracorporeal circulation relative to the intraoperative dose. At the start of CPB (first arrow), the concentration versus time curve (○-○) for cephalothin becomes discontinuous. An abrupt fall in plasma levels is followed by either a plateau or a slow increase in concentrations. The elimination half-time for cephalothin during cardiac surgery is prolonged compared to the preoperative and postoperative values, perhaps on the basis of impairment of nonrenal clearance mechanisms. (From Miller, Chan, McCoy et al,[202] by permission of Clin Pharmacol Ther.)

curve for cephalothin becomes discontinuous. An abrupt fall in plasma levels is followed by either a plateau or a slow increase in concentrations (Figure 4.16).[202] The elimination half-time for cephalothin during cardiac surgery is prolonged compared to the preoperative and postoperative values, perhaps on the basis of impairment of nonrenal clearance mechanisms. In a follow-up study designed to clarify whether CPB alters renal cephalosporin clearance (as opposed to nonrenal clearance, demonstrated in the study above), Miller examined the disposition of cefazolin during cardiac surgery employing hypothermic (26° to 30°C) CPB. Cefazolin appears to be eliminated almost wholly unchanged by the kidney. Eight subjects received cefazolin (2 g IV) on the day before surgery, periopera-

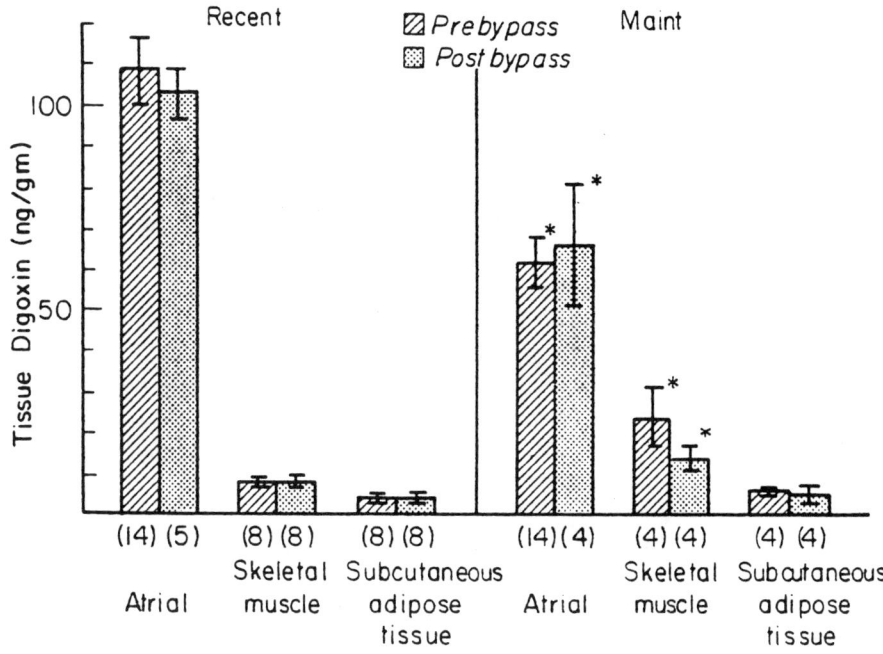

FIGURE 4.17. Concentrations of digoxin in atrial appendage, skeletal muscle, and subcutaneous adipose tissue from pediatric patients undergoing cardiac surgery at the beginning (left bar) and end (right bar) of CPB. The "Recent" group was digitalized acutely for perioperative prophylaxis ($n = 24$), while the "Maint" group received chronic maintenance digoxin therapy ($n = 18$). The "Recent" group had significantly higher atrial digoxin levels than did the "Maint" group (*$p < 0.001$ prebypass, *$p < 0.02$ postbypass). Skeletal muscle levels were higher in the "Maint" group both pre- and post-bypass (*$p < 0.02$). No differences in serum concentrations between the two groups were detected. (Reproduced with permission of Circulation.[240] Copyright 1974 American Heart Association.)

tively, and through the day following surgery. The pharmacokinetic parameters measured postoperatively did not differ from those obtained during the preoperative period. The concentration versus time curve was again discontinuous, with an abrupt fall in cephalosporin concentrations upon initiation of CPB, and either a plateau or a gradual increase in serum levels thereafter. Clearance during bypass was reduced relative to both preoperative and postoperative values, while the volume of distribution during CPB actually increased. Renal clearance of cefazolin was impaired throughout the surgical procedure. The increased volume of distribution was attributed to hemodilution of plasma proteins resulting in higher free cefazolin levels leading to increased uptake of drug by the peripheral tissues.[230,231] Ceftriaxone disposition (14 mg/kg given after induction) was examined in 7 male patients undergoing coronary artery surgery with hypothermic CPB (28°C).[232] Clearance of ceftriaxone decreases during CPB, while the volume of distribution, free drug fraction, and elimination half-time increase.

Comparison of cephalothin, cefazolin, and cefamandole by Eigel[233] in cardiac surgery patients suggests that cefamandole may provide an optimal combination of low toxicity, adequate tissue penetration, and sustained plasma levels during CPB. Sustained cefazolin levels during bypass were found to be higher than those of either cephalothin or cefamandole, raising the potential risk of nephrotoxicity with continued administration.

The effect of pulsatile CPB on cefamandole pharmacokinetics has also been examined. Cefamandole (20 mg/kg) was administered to 13 patients at midnight prior to surgery, at 6:00 AM the day of surgery, and just before initiation of CPB. Cefamandole concentrations exceeded the MIC in all patients studied. Serum levels of cefamandole were statistically higher in the pulsatile group beginning 2 hours after the initiation of CPB. Fat and muscle levels were greater in the pulsatile group from 1 hour onward. The elimination half-time of cefamandole is prolonged in the pulsatile group (1.4 versus 0.9 hours), though the volume of distribution does not differ. Supplemental dosing of cefamandole is recommended at 4 hours for nonpulsatile bypass, and at 6 hours during pulsatile perfusion.[82]

To summarize, hypothermic CPB may be expected to prolong the elimination half-times of nearly all the prophylactic antibiotics utilized in cardiac surgery patients. Both increased volumes of distribution and reductions in hepatic and renal clearance contribute to this prolongation of elimination half-life. Administration of the initial cephalosporin dose should occur within 1 to 2 hours of the initiation of bypass to ensure sufficient antimicrobial levels throughout the duration of CPB. If cefamandole, cephalothin, or cefazolin is chosen for prophylaxis, supplemental doses should be considered if CPB extends beyond 4 hours. Recommendations for the duration of antibiotic prophylaxis have been extremely variable, although shorter periods (<48 hours) have been advocated more recently to avoid selection of resistant organisms.

Digitalis Glycosides

Digitalis glycosides (predominantly digoxin preparations) are used in cardiac surgery patients for the management of supraventricular dysrhythmias and congestive heart failure. A great number of studies examining the kinetics of digitalis in cardiac surgery have been published, owing to its longevity in the armamentarium of cardiologists, anesthesiologists, and surgeons.

Heparin administration is associated with an increase in free digitoxin concentrations correlating with equivalent changes in free fatty acid levels. This finding suggests that displacement of glycoside from protein binding sites may increase the free fraction of the drug.[234]

Digoxin levels are reduced 10% to 28% following surgery for congenital heart disease when CPB is used. Digoxin levels remain essentially unchanged in patients undergoing surgery for congenital heart disease not employing bypass. No correlation between the duration of CPB and the degree of reduction in myocardial digoxin levels has been found.[235] A portion of radiolabeled digoxin administered to patients presenting for congenital cardiac surgery is subsequently detectable in the oxygenator, indicating adsorption by the CPB apparatus. Although serum levels are reduced, myocardial digoxin concentrations remain unchanged. The amount of digoxin taken up by the oxygenator (about 1 μg) appears clinically insignificant.[236] Similar data have been reported by Koren.[194] There is no meaningful washout of radiolabeled digoxin from myocardial tissues during bypass, prompting Hernandez[237] to suggest that administration of digoxin in the postoperative period be approached with great caution.

Serum digoxin concentrations are transiently reduced following CPB in patients receiving chronic digoxin therapy prior to repair of congenital cardiac lesions. Digoxin levels return to baseline within 16 hours of surgery, however. The initial fall in digoxin levels may be secondary to hemodilution with loss of the glycoside. The increased sensitivity to digoxin observed after cardiac surgery might be due to such factors as changes in potassium levels and urinary clearance, rather than changes in digoxin concentrations per se.[238]

A group of 34 patients receiving chronic digoxin or digitoxin therapy was studied by Morrison and Killip.[239] Glycoside was discontinued the day before surgery and was not restarted until 24 hours postoperatively. Digitalis levels fell after the initiation of CPB, and rose after bypass to levels exceeding the pre-CPB concentrations. Two groups of patients were identified based on the presence ($n = 8$) or absence of arrhythmias in the postoperative period. Patients with arrhythmias (attributed to digitalis toxicity) showed higher digitalis levels than the group in whom no arrhythmias occurred, though all concentrations were within the "normal therapeutic range." The arrhythmias did not appear to be related to the patient's age, duration of bypass, blood-gas values, or potassium and magnesium concentrations. The authors concur that sensitivity to digitalis may be increased following CPB.

Krasula[240] examined changes in serum digoxin levels during cardiac surgery in two groups of pediatric patients. The first set received chronic maintenance digoxin therapy ($n = 18$), while the other was digitalized acutely for perioperative prophylaxis ($n = 24$). Serum digoxin concentrations fell in both groups following the initiation of bypass. Digoxin levels returned to prebypass levels within 2 hours following termination of CPB, and fell again within 10 hours after separation from bypass. No differences in serum concentrations between the two groups were detected. The group receiving digoxin acutely had significantly higher atrial digoxin levels than did the chronic group (109 ± 9 versus 62 ± 6 ng/mL) (Figure 4.17). The reductions in serum digoxin levels were attributed to hemodilution. No explanation was offered for the increased myocardial digoxin concentrations seen in the acutely treated group.

Although changes in serum digoxin levels may occur during CPB, they are not reliably correlated with changes in myocardial digoxin levels. This may be in part related to whether the drug is administered chronically before surgery or given as an acute loading dose during the preoperative period. More thorough tissue equilibration may be attained with chronic glycoside dosing, rendering more total drug available for release from tissue stores. Clinically significant binding of digoxin to the CPB apparatus does not appear to occur. Digoxin is cleared predominantly (at least 75%) by the kidney. Patients frequently exhibit increased sensitivity to the effects of digoxin during the postoperative period. Alterations in renal clearance, electrolyte ratios, or the pharmacodynamics of these glycosides may contribute to this increased susceptibility. The risk of digitalis toxicity in the perioperative period appears to be enhanced by larger doses of glycoside, acute preoperative administration, and dosing in proximity to the surgical procedure. Alterations in glomerular filtration and electrolyte balance associated with CPB would mandate caution any time administration of digoxin after cardiac surgery is considered.

Vasodilators

Papaverine

Papaverine is used during myocardial revascularization surgery to reverse or prevent spasm of the internal mammary artery after its harvest for coronary grafting. Papaverine is a powerful systemic vasodilator, and may cause a drop in perfusion pressure during bypass if returned to the CPB circuit via the cardiotomy suction. Papaverine is cleared almost exclusively by the liver, with a hepatic extraction ratio approaching 1. The elimination half-time of papaverine is prolonged in cardiac bypass patients when compared to matched subjects undergoing major vascular surgery (2.77 ± 0.28 versus 1.39 ± 0.25 hours).[241] Drugs with high hepatic extraction ratios are essentially dependent on the liver for their clearance. Alterations in the pharmacokinetics of papaverine during CPB are likely due to changes in hepatic blood flow.

Nitroprusside

Sodium nitroprusside is a systemic and pulmonary vasodilator that may be used during cardiac surgery to treat hypertension and reduce left ventricular afterload. Clearance of nitroprusside involves a nonenzymatic interaction between nitroprusside and hemoglobin, leading to liberation of free cyanide (CN^-) ion. This release of cyanide is followed by enzymatic conversion of CN^- to thiocyanate, catalyzed by liver rhodanase. The nonenzymatic generation of cyanide ion is unimpaired during CPB.[242] The conversion of free cyanide to thiocyanate, however, is impaired during bypass. This diminished enzymatic activity likely results from the effects of hypothermia on mitochondrial enzyme function. It has been suggested that administration of nitroprusside under hypothermic conditions could lead to cyanide toxicity.

Nitroprusside has been used for blood pressure control over substantial periods of time in postoperative cardiac patients with few apparent deleterious effects. Patients with acute or chronic renal failure may show impaired excretion of the thiocyanate moiety, potentially increasing the possibility of toxicity from this substance. Toxicity is, however, much more likely to result from the cyanide ion itself. Despite these observations, prolonged administration of nitroprusside following cardiac surgery should be undertaken cautiously, and regular monitoring of thiocyanate blood levels appears prudent.

Nitroglycerin

Nitroglycerin (in its various forms) is perhaps the most ubiquitous medication encountered among cardiac surgery patients. Intravenous nitroglycerin is used during cardiac surgery as a remedy for myocardial ischemia or to prevent internal mammary spasm, and may be used to reduce pulmonary artery pressures in the pre- or post-bypass period. There is substantial in vitro adsorption of nitroglycerin to the CPB apparatus, however. Only 18% of an administered nitroglycerin dose can be recovered in the circulating pump fluid after a 60-minute recirculation period. Adsorption of nitroglycerin in the oxygenator (Cobe Optiflo II®) is likewise considerable.[243] Similar in vitro observations have been made by Booth.[244] Patients receiving nitroglycerin as a continuous central vein infusion show substantial variability in arterial nitroglycerin concentrations during cardiac surgery employing CPB. Although there is significant adsorption to the CPB apparatus, actual clearance of nitroglycerin increases 20% during CPB.[245] It is conjectured that the loss of drug to the oxygenator (Bentley Spiraflow BOS-10S® in the investigation above) is offset by reductions in hepatic clearance due to decreased liver blood flow. Temperature-dependent reductions in nitroglycerin metabolism by red blood cells and the peripheral vasculature may also be important. The common clinical observation that requirements for nitroglycerin are increased during CPB may be, in part, explained by these studies.

β-Adrenergic Receptor Blocking Agents

β-Adrenergic blockers are commonly prescribed in cardiac patients to decrease myocardial work in the setting of coronary artery disease. β-Blocker therapy is maintained through the perioperative period by a majority of cardiac anesthesiologists. β-Blockers may be used acutely to treat the manifestations of exaggerated sympathetic activity, including the various tachyarrhythmias and systemic hypertension.

Plasma levels of propranolol in patients undergoing coronary revascularization are reduced at the onset of hypothermic (31°C) CPB, plateau during the rest of bypass, and are elevated after separation from CPB. Elimination half-time of propranolol is notably prolonged by CPB.[246] The fall in plasma propranolol levels during CPB is attributable to hemodilution by the pump prime. Plasma propranolol levels may increase during CPB with deeper levels of hypothermia (27°C).[47] Decreases in drug metabolism with more profound hypothermia, as well as discordant bypass flows, may explain the disparities between these two studies. The rise in plasma propranolol levels following bypass is likely secondary to redistribution from the lungs and peripheral tissue stores. Impaired metabolism resulting from reductions in liver blood flow may also contribute to the increased drug levels observed after bypass. Total propranolol concentrations have been found to decline progressively during the course of cardiac surgery in patients receiving chronic drug therapy. Propranolol concentrations may be restored to the therapeutic range by a sequence of three bolus (1 mg) doses followed by a continuous infusion (0.7 µg/kg/min) in the postoperative period. Not surprisingly, this regimen produces a substantial rightward shift of the isoproterenol versus heart rate response curve.[247]

Studies examining changes in propranolol concentrations during bypass have produced conflicting results. Further investigations incorporating measurements of free drug levels, changes in protein binding, and interactions with other compounds (such as heparin) would be of some interest. Studies of the effects of CPB on the newest β-blockers (such as atenolol and esmolol) are clearly needed.

Lidocaine

Patients with an unstable rhythm during cardiac surgery may require treatment with a bolus or continuous infusion of lidocaine. Lidocaine is sequestered by the lung in normal volunteers (up to 90% following intravenous injection), and this organ may represent an important storage site for the drug during CPB.[183] A lidocaine dose of 2 mg/kg at the time of endotracheal intubation and again following removal of the aortic crossclamp yields a therapeutic concentration (greater than 1.5 µg/mL) for at least 10 minutes following administration during valvular surgery employing hypothermic (25°C) CPB. The handling of IV lidocaine during hypothermic bypass is best described by a three-compartment model. Both the clearance (10.9 versus 14.5 mL/kg/min) and the volume of distribution (308 versus 438 mL/kg) are increased, and the slow distribution half-time is prolonged (2.3 to 5.2 minutes) in cardiac surgery patients. The increase in distribution volume may be attributed to a rise in unbound drug fraction (not yet accurately quantified), resulting from hemodilution by the pump prime. Tissue affinity for lidocaine is also increased during hypothermic CPB.[248] Clearance of lidocaine, however, remains virtually unchanged.[66]

Plasma levels of lidocaine measured 2 minutes after administration of a "low-dose" bolus (1.5 mg/kg) fall below the therapeutic minimum in 40% of patients during hypothermic CPB. Within 4 minutes after the "low-dose" injection, 90% of patients will exhibit subtherapeutic concentrations. Only 10% of patients receiving an "intermediate dose" of 2.5 mg/kg will maintain therapeutic lidocaine levels 30 minutes after their bolus. A "high-dose" lidocaine trial of 3.5 mg/kg had to be abandoned because of hypotensive effects. Satisfactory lidocaine levels during CPB are more consistently obtained after a loading dose of 2.5 mg/kg rather than the standard 1.5 mg/kg. Initiation of a continuous IV infusion after this bolus is also recommended.[67] Lidocaine levels (both free and total) more reliably approach the therapeutic range when a bolus of 1.5 mg/kg (administered 10 seconds before release of the aortic cross clamp) is followed immediately by an infusion of 5 mg/min. This rate should be reduced to 2 mg/min after 1 hour of infusion.[68]

The pharmacokinetics of lidocaine on day 1 after coronary revascularization are unchanged when compared to the same parameters measured immediately before surgery.[166] On postoperative day 3, however, there is a 40% reduction in both the clearance and volume of distribution of lidocaine. These changes are essentially resolved by postoperative day 5. These variations are associated with a doubling of α-1-acid glycoprotein concentrations and a 46% decrease in the free lidocaine fraction. α-1-Acid glycoprotein is an acute phase reactant protein whose concentrations are elevated following cardiac surgery. Measurement of total lidocaine levels may not reflect these changes in free drug concentration if alterations in protein binding following cardiac surgery are not accounted for.[99] Increased tissue-drug binding may be responsible for return of the volume of distribution to control levels by day 7, despite persistent elevations in α-1-acid glycoprotein concentrations.

To summarize, larger initial bolus doses of lidocaine may be required to achieve therapeutic concentrations during cardiac surgery. Free drug levels may decline during the postoperative period despite total drug levels in the "therapeutic" range. It may become necessary to increase the rate of infusion above "normal" to attain acceptable levels of free drug if breakthrough ectopy is observed. Measurement of free drug levels might, in theory, be more helpful, but would require definition of appropriate therapeutic concentrations of free lidocaine in plasma.

Conclusions and Future Directions

It is clear that significant changes may occur in the pharmacokinetics and pharmacodynamics of essentially every drug employed during cardiac surgery and CPB. Factors producing these changes include hemodilution, hypothermia, and variations in organ blood flow, as well as sequestration of drug by the CPB apparatus, lungs, and peripheral tissues throughout the body. Future research may be directed toward clarification of the alterations seen in free drug levels during bypass and a clearer elucidation of the specific role that hypothermia plays in these changes. Further descriptions of changes in drug-protein interaction, as well as additional studies of pharmacodynamic influences, should enhance our ability to make appropriate adjustments in perioperative dosing regimens. An understanding of these factors will allow more precise utilization of hypnotics and narcotics as shorter intensive care unit stays and earlier postoperative tracheal extubation becomes the standard of practice. Further study will indeed be required to improve the efficiency with which we render care to an aging population in a climate of ever-diminishing resources.

References

1. Gibaldi M, Perrier D. *Multicompartment Models in Pharmacokinetics*. 2nd ed. New York: Marcel Dekker Inc; 1982: 45-112.
2. Stanski DR, Watkins WD. *Drug Disposition in Anesthesia*. Toronto: Grune and Stratton Inc; 1982:1-46.
3. Prys-Roberts C, Hug CC Jr, eds. *Pharmacokinetics of Anesthesia*. Boston: Blackwell Scientific Publications; 1984: 1-358.
4. Rowland M, Tozer TN. *Clinical Pharmacokinetics*. Philadelphia: Lea and Febiger; 1980:9-96.
5. Rowland M. Plasma protein binding and therapeutic drug monitoring. *Ther Drug Monitoring* 1980;2:29-37.
6. Wood M. Plasma drug binding: implications for anesthesiologists. *Anesth Analg* 1986;65:786-804.
7. Bowers WF, Fulton S, Thompson J. Ultrafiltration vs equilibrium dialysis for determination of free fraction. *Clin Pharmacokinet* 1984;9 (suppl 1):49-60.
8. Greenblatt DJ, Sellers EM, Koch-Weser J. Importance of protein binding for the interpretation of serum or plasma drug concentrations. *Clin Pharmacol* 1982;22:259-263.
9. Gillespie TJ, Gandolfi AJ, Maiorino RM, et al. Gas chromatographic determination of fentanyl and its analogues in human plasma. *J Analyt Toxicology* 1981;5:133-137.
10. Michiels M, Hendriks R, Heykants J. A sensitive radioimmunoassay for fentanyl: plasma levels in dogs and man. *Eur J Clin Pharmacol* 1977;12:153-158.
11. Michiels M, Hendriks R, Heykants J. Radioimmunoassay of the new opiate analgesics alfentanil and sufentanil. Preliminary pharmacokinetic profile in man. *J Pharm Pharmacol* 1983;35:86-93.
12. Schuttler J, White PF. Optimization of the radioimmunoassay for measuring fentanyl and alfentanil in human serum. *Anesthesiology* 1984;61:315-320.
13. Hull CJ. How far can we go with compartmental models? *Anesthesiology* 1990;72:399-402.
14. Ham J, Miller RD, Benet LZ, et al. Pharmacokinetics and pharmacodynamics of d-tubocurarine during hypothermia in the cat. *Anesthesiology* 1978;49:324-329.
15. Bower S, Hull CJ. Comparative pharmacokinetics of fentanyl and alfentanil. *Br J Anaesth* 1982;54:871-877.
16. Shafer SL, Varvel JR. Pharmacokinetics, pharmacodynamics, and rational opioid selection. *Anesthesiology* 1991;74:53-63.
17. Hull CJ, VanBeem HBH, McLeod K, et al. A pharmacodynamic model for pancuronium. *Br J Anaesth* 1978;50: 1113-1123.
18. Sheiner LB, Stanski DR, Vozeh S, et al. Simultaneous modeling of pharmacokinetics and pharmacodynamics: application to d-tubocurarine. *Clin Pharmacol Ther* 1979; 25:358-371.
19. Hug CC Jr, Hall RI, Angert KC, Reeder DA, Moldenhauer CC. Alfentanil plasma concentration v. effect relationships in cardiac surgical patients. *Br J Anaesth* 1988;61:435-440.
20. Alvis JM, Reves JG, Govier AV, et al. Computer-assisted continuous infusion of fentanyl during cardiac anesthesia: comparison with a manual method. *Anesthesiology* 1985; 63:41-49.
21. Robbins GR, Wynands JE, Whalley DG, et al. Pharmacokinetics of alfentanil and clinical responses during cardiac surgery. *Can J Anaesth* 1990;37:52-57.
22. Hug CC Jr, deLange S, Burm AGL. Alfentanil pharmacokinetics in patients before and after cardiopulmonary bypass (CPB). *Anesth Analg* 1983;62:266.
23. Philbin DM, Rosow CE, Schneider RC, et al. Fentanyl and sufentanil anesthesia revisited: How much is enough? *Anesthesiology* 1990;73:5-11.
24. Jacobs JR, Reves JA, Glass PSA. Continuous infusions for maintaining anesthesia. *Int Anesthesiol Clin* 1991;29:1-85.
25. Hall RI, Murphy JT, Moffitt EA, et al. A comparison

25. study of myocardial metabolic and haemodynamic changes produced by propofol-sufentanil vs enflurane-sufentanil anaesthesia for patients having coronary artery bypass graft surgery. *Can J Anaesth* 1991;38:996-1004.
26. Ausems ME, Hug CC Jr, Stanski DR, et al. Plasma concentrations of alfentanil required to supplement nitrous oxide anesthesia for general surgery. *Anesthesiology* 1986;65:362-373.
27. Kern FH, Ungerleider RM, Jacobs JR, et al. Computerized continuous infusion of intravenous drugs during pediatric cardiac surgery. *Anesth Analg* 1991;72:487-492.
28. Flezzani P, Alvis MJ, Jacobs JR, et al. Sufentanil disposition during cardiopulmonary bypass. *Can J Anaesth* 1987;34:566-569.
29. Raemer DB, Buschman A, Varvel JR, et al. The prospective use of population pharmacokinetics in a computer-driven infusion system for alfentanil. *Anesthesiology* 1990;73:66-72.
30. Ausems ME, Vuyk J, Hug CC Jr, et al. Comparison of a computer-assisted infusion versus intermittent bolus administration of alfentanil as a supplement to nitrous oxide for lower abdominal surgery. *Anesthesiology* 1988;68:851-861.
31. Holley FO, van Steennis C. Postoperative analgesia with fentanyl: pharmacokinetics and pharmacodynamics of constant-rate IV and transdermal delivery. *Br J Anaesth* 1988;60:608-613.
32. Duthie DJR, Rowbotham DJ, Wyld R, et al. Plasma fentanyl concentrations during transdermal delivery of fentanyl to surgical patients. *Br J Anaesth* 1988;60:614-618.
33. Alberti KGMM. Diabetes and surgery. *Anesthesiology* 1991;74:209-211.
34. Hirsch IB, McGill JB, Cryer PE, et al. Perioperative management of surgical patients with diabetes mellitus. *Anesthesiology* 1991;74:346-359.
35. Brose WG, Cohen SE. Oxyhemoglobin saturation following cesarean section in patients receiving epidural morphine, PCA, or IM meperidine analgesia. *Anesthesiology* 1989;70:948-953.
36. Henderson JM, Brodsky DA, Fisher DM, et al. Pre-induction of anesthesia in pediatric patients with nasally administered sufentanil. *Anesthesiology* 1988;68:671-675.
37. Streisand JB, Stanley TH, Hague B, et al. Oral transmucosal fentanyl citrate premedication in children. *Anesth Analg* 1989;69:28-34.
38. Goldstein-Dresner MC, Davis PJ, Kretchman E, et al. Double-blind comparison of oral transmucosal fentanyl citrate with oral meperidine, diazepam and atropine as preanesthetic medication in children with congenital heart disease. *Anesthesiology* 1991;74:28-33.
39. Saint-Maurice C, Laguenine G, Couturier C, et al. Rectal ketamine in pediatric anesthesia. *Br J Anaesth* 1979;51:573-574.
40. Cousins MJ, Mather LE. Intrathecal and epidural administration of opioids. *Anesthesiology* 1984;61:276-310.
41. Maurette P, Tauzin-Fin P, Vincon G, et al. Arterial and ventricular CSF pharmacokinetics after intrathecal meperidine in humans. *Anesthesiology* 1989;70:961-966.
42. Varvel JR, Shafer SL, Hwang SS, et al. Absorption characteristics of transdermally administered fentanyl. *Anesthesiology* 1989;70:928-934.
43. Benet LZ, Mitchell JR, Sheiner LB. Pharmacokinetics: the dynamics of drug absorption, distribution, and elimination. In: Gilman AG, Rall TW, Nies AS, et al, eds. *The Pharmacological Basis of Therapeutics*. Toronto: Pergamon Press; 1990:3-32.
44. Wilkinson G, Shand DG. A physiological approach to hepatic drug clearance. *Clin Pharmacol Ther* 1975;18:377-390.
45. Ballard BE. Pharmacokinetics and temperature. *J Pharm Sci* 1974;63:1345-1358.
46. Koren G, Barker C, Goresky G, et al. The influence of hypothermia on the disposition of fentanyl—human and animal studies. *Eur J Clin Pharmacol* 1987;32:373-376.
47. McAllister RG Jr, Bourne DW, Tan TT, et al. Effects of hypothermia on propranolol kinetics. *Clin Pharmacol Ther* 1979;25:1-7.
48. Miller RD, Agoston S, vanderPol F, et al. Hypothermia and the pharmacokinetics and pharmacodynamics of pancuronium in the cat. *J Pharmacol Exp Ther* 1978;207:532-538.
49. Koren G, Barker C, Bohn D, et al. Influence of hypothermia on the pharmacokinetics of gentamicin and theophylline in piglets. *Crit Care Med* 1985;13:844-847.
50. Kalser SC, Kelvington EJ, Randolph MM, et al. Drug metabolism in hypothermia. 1. Biliary excretion of C^{14}-atropine metabolites in the intact and nephrectomized rat. *J Pharmacol Exp Ther* 1965;147:252-259.
51. Kalser SC, Kelvington EJ, Randolph MM. Drug metabolism in hypothermia. Uptake, metabolism, and excretion of S^{35}-sulfanilamide by the isolated, perfused rat liver. *J Pharmacol Exp Ther* 1968;159:389-398.
52. Kalser SC, Kelvington EJ, Kunig R, et al. Drug metabolism in hypothermia. Uptake, metabolism, and excretion of C^{14}-procaine by the isolated, perfused rat liver. *J Pharmacol Exp Ther* 1968;164:396-404.
53. Larsen JA. The effect of cooling on liver function in cats. *Acta Physiol Scand* 1971;81:197-207.
54. McAllister RG Jr, Tan TG. Effects of hypothermia on drug metabolism. *Pharmacology* 1980;20:95-100.
55. Ahlquist RP. Adrenoceptor sensitivity in disease as assessed through response to temperature alteration. *Fed Proc* 1977;36:2572-2574.
56. Benfey BG. Cardiac adrenoceptors at low temperature: what is the experimental evidence for the adrenoceptor interconversion hypothesis? *Fred Proc* 1977;36:2575-2579.
57. Cook DA, Kenakin TP, Krueger CA. Alterations in temperature and histamine receptor function. *Fed Proc* 1977;36:2584-2589.
58. Simantov R, Snowman AM, Snyder SH. Temperature and ionic influences on opiate receptor binding. *Mol Pharmacol* 1976;12:977-986.
59. Puig MM, Warner W, Tang CK, et al. Effects of temperature on the interaction of morphine with opioid receptors. *Br J Anaesth* 1987;59:1459-1464.
60. Regan MJ, Eger EI II. Effect of hypothermia in dogs on anesthetizing and apneic doses of inhalation agents. *Anesthesiology* 1967;28:689-700.
61. Steffey EP, Eger EI II. Hyperthermia and halothane MAC in the dog. *Anesthesiology* 1974;41:392-396.
62. Vitez TS, White PF, Eger EI II. Effects of hypothermia on halothane MAC and isoflurane MAC in the rat. *Anesthesiology* 1974;41:80-81.

63. Holley FO, Ponganis KV, Stanski DR. Effect of cardiopulmonary bypass on the pharmacokinetics of drugs. *Clin Pharmacokinet* 1982;7:234-251.
64. Buylaert WA, Herregods LL, Mortier EP, et al. Cardiopulmonary bypass and the pharmacokinetics of drugs: an update. *Clin Pharmacokinet* 1989;17:10-26.
65. Morgan DJ, Crankshaw DP, Prideaux PR, et al. Thiopentone levels during cardiopulmonary bypass. Changes in plasma protein binding during continuous infusion. *Anaesthesia* 1986;41:4-10.
66. Morrell DF, Harrison GG. Lignocaine kinetics during cardiopulmonary bypass: optimum dosage and the effects of haemodilution. *Br J Anaesth* 1983;55:1173-1177.
67. Landow L, Wilson J, Heard SO, et al. Free and total lidocaine levels in cardiac surgical patients. *J Cardiothorac Anesth* 1990;4:340-347.
68. Landow L, Wilson J. An improved lidocaine infusion protocol for cardiac surgical patients. *J Cardiothorac Vasc Anesth* 1991;5:209-213.
69. Hynynen M. Binding of fentanyl and alfentanil to the extracorporeal circuit. *Acta Anaesthesiol Scand* 1987;31:706-710.
70. Nussmeier NA, Moskowitz GJ, Weiskopf RB, et al. In vitro anesthetic washin and washout via bubble oxygenators: influence of anesthetic solubility and rates of carrier gas inflow and pump blood flow. *Anesth Analg* 1988;67:982-987.
71. Nussmeier NA, Lambert ML, Moskowitz GJ, et al. Washin and washout of isoflurane administered via bubble oxygenators during hypothermic cardiopulmonary bypass. *Anesthesiology* 1989;71:519-525.
72. Nazari A, Sheikh H, Sterns LP, et al. Experimental blood volume studies during extracorporal circulation. *Int Surg* 1970;54:11-17.
73. Kumar K, Crankshaw DP, Prideaux PR, et al. Thiopentone levels during cardiopulmonary bypass. *Clin Pharmacol* 1983;34:703-706.
74. Bjorksten AR, Crankshaw DP, Morgan DJ, et al. The effects of cardiopulmonary bypass on plasma concentrations and protein binding of methohexital and thiopental. *J Cardiothorac Anesth* 1988;2:281-289.
75. Morgan DJ, Crankshaw DP, Prideaux PR, et al. Thiopentone levels during cardiopulmonary bypass. *Clin Pharmacol* 1983;34:703-706.
76. Stanley TH. Arterial pressure and deltoid muscle gas tensions during cardiopulmonary bypass in man. *Can Anaesth Soc J* 1978;25:286-290.
77. Philbin DM, Levine FH, Emerson CW, et al. Plasma vasopressin levels and urinary flow during cardiopulmonary bypass in patients with valvular heart disease. Effect of pulsatile flow. *J Thorac Cardiovasc Surg* 1979;78:779-783.
78. Maney M, Soroff HS, Birtwell WC, et al. The physiologic role of pulsatile and nonpulsatile blood flow. *Arch Surg* 1968;97:917-923.
79. Mavroudis C. To pulse or not to pulse. *Ann Thorac Surg* 1978;25:259-271.
80. Shepard RB, Kirklin JW. Relation of pulsatile flow to oxygen consumption and other variables during cardiopulmonary bypass. *J Thorac Cardiovasc Surg* 1969;58:694-701.
81. Hynynen M, Olkkola KT, Naveri E, et al. Thiopentone pharmacokinetics during cardiopulmonary bypass with a nonpulsatile or pulsatile flow. *Acta Anaesthesiol Scand* 1989;33:554-560.
82. Weiner B, Melby MJ, Faraci PA, et al. Cefamandole pharmacokinetics during standard and pulsatile cardiopulmonary bypass. *J Clin Pharmacol* 1988;28:655-659.
83. Hirvoven J, Huttunen P, Nuutinen L, et al. Catecholamines and free fatty acids in plasma of patients undergoing cardiac operations with hypothermia and bypass. *J Clin Pathol* 1978;31:949-955.
84. Replogle R, Levy M, DeWall RA, et al. Catecholamine and serotonin response to cardiopulmonary bypass. *J Thorac Cardiovasc Surg* 1962;44:638-648.
85. Anand KJS, Hansen DD, Hickey PR. Hormonal-metabolic stress responses in neonates undergoing cardiac surgery. *Anesthesiology* 190;73:661-670.
86. Bailey PL, Stanley TH. Narcotic intravenous anesthetics. In: Miller RD, ed. Anesthesia. 3rd ed. New York: Churchill Livingstone; 1990:281-366.
87. Philbin DM, Coggins CH, Wilson N, et al. Antidiuretic hormone levels during cardiopulmonary bypass. *J Thorac Cardiovasc Surg* 1977;73:145-148.
88. Philbin DM, Coggins CH. Plasma vasopressin levels during cardiopulmonary bypass with and without profound hemodilution. *Can Anaesth Soc J* 1978;25:282-285.
89. Martin DS, DelCastillo J, Martinez M, et al. Beneficial influence of a serotonin-histamine antagonist on perfusion sequelae. *Surgery* 1964;56:1064-1066.
90. Kluft C, Dooijewaard G, Emeis J. Role of the contact system in fibrinolysis. *Semin Thrombosis Hemostasis* 1987;13:50-66.
91. Blauhut B, Gross C, Necek S, et al. Effects of high-dose aprotinin on blood loss, platelet function, fibrinolysis, complement, and renal function after cardiopulmonary bypass. *J Thorac Cardiovasc Surg* 1991;101:958-967.
92. Tanaka K, Takao M, Yada I, et al. Alterations in coagulation and fibrinolysis associated with cardiopulmonary bypass during open heart surgery. *J Cardiothorac Anesth* 1989;3:181-188.
93. van Oeveren W, Jansen NJG, Bidstrup BP, et al. Effects of aprotinin on hemostatic mechanisms during cardiopulmonary bypass. *Ann Thorac Surg* 1987;44:640-645.
94. Nagaoka H, Yamada T, Hatano R, et al. Clinical significance of bradykinin liberation during cardiopulmonary bypass and its prevention by a kallikrein inhibitor. *Jpn J Surg* 1975;5:222-233.
95. Mirenda JV, Grissom TE. Anesthetic implications of the renin-angiotensin system and angiotensin-converting enzyme inhibitors. *Anesth Analg* 1991;72:667-683.
96. Johnson MD, Park CS, Malvin RL. Antidiuretic hormone and the distribution of renal cortical blood flow. *Am J Physiol* 1977;232:F111-F1116.
97. Ross EM. Pharmacodynamics: mechanisms of drug action and the relationship between drug concentration and effect. In: Gilman AG, Rall TW, Nies AS, et al., eds. *The Pharmacological Basis of Therapeutics*. Toronto: Pergamon Press; 1990:33-48.
98. Hug CC Jr. Lipid solubility, pharmacokinetics, and the EEG: are you better off today than you were four years ago? *Anesthesiology* 1985;62:221-226.
99. Marathe PH, Shen DD, Artru AA, et al. Effect of serum protein binding on the entry of lidocaine into brain and ce-

rebrospinal fluid in dogs. *Anesthesiology* 1991;75:804–812.
100. Wood M. Plasma binding and limitation of drug access to site of action. *Anesthesiology* 1991;75:721–723.
101. Anton AH. The relation between the binding of sulfonamides to albumin and their antibacterial efficacy. *J Pharmacol Exp Ther* 1960;129:282–290.
102. Piafsky KM. Disease-induced changes in the plasma binding of basic drugs. *Clin Pharmacokinet* 1980;5:246–262.
103. Routledge PA, Stargel WW, Wagner GS, et al. Increased alpha-1-acid glycoprotein and lidocaine disposition in myocardial infarction. *Ann Intern Med* 1980;93:701–704.
104. Piafsky KM, Borga O, Odar-Cederlof I, et al. Increased plasma protein binding of propranolol and chlorpromazine mediated by disease-induced elevations of plasma α-1-acid glycoprotein. *N Engl J Med* 1978;299:1435–1439.
105. Coltart J, Howard M, Chamberlain D. Myocardial and skeletal muscle concentrations of digoxin in patients on long-term therapy. *Br Med J* 1972;2:318–319.
106. Carruthers SG, Cleland J, Kelly JG, et al. Plasma and tissue digoxin concentrations in patients undergoing cardiopulmonary bypass. *Br Heart J* 1975;37:313–320.
107. Carroll PR, Gelbart A, O'Rourke MF, et al. Digoxin concentrations in the serum and myocardium of digitalised patients. *Aust NZ J Med* 1973;3:400–403.
108. Binnion PF, Morgan LM, Stevenson HM, et al. Plasma and myocardial digoxin concentrations in patients on oral therapy. *Br Heart J* 1969;31:636–640.
109. Roerig DL, Kotrly KJ, Ahlf SB, et al. Effect of propranolol on the first pass uptake of fentanyl in the human and rat lung. *Anesthesiology* 1989;71:62–68.
110. Bender AD. The effect of increasing age on the distribution of peripheral blood flow in man. *J Am Ger Soc* 1965;13:192–198.
111. Leithe ME, Hermiller JB, Magorien RD, et al. The effect of age on central and regional hemodynamics. *Gerontology* 1984;30:240–246.
112. Brandfonbrener M, Landowne M, Shock NW. Changes in cardiac output with age. *Circulation* 1955;12:557–566.
113. Greenblatt DJ, Sellers EM, Shader RI. Drug disposition in old age. *N Engl J Med* 1982;306:1081.
114. Homer T, Stanski DR. The effect of increasing age on thiopental disposition and anesthetic requirement. *Anesthesiology* 1985;62:714–724.
115. Crooks J, O'Malley K, Stevenson IH. Pharmacokinetics in the elderly. *Clin Pharmacokinet* 1976;1:280–296.
116. Maitre PO, Ausems ME, Vozeh S, et al. Evaluating the accuracy of using population pharmacokinetic data to predict plasma concentrations of alfentanil. *Anesthesiology* 1988;68:59–67.
117. Stanski DR, Maitre PO. Population pharmacokinetics and pharmacodynamics of thiopental: the effect of age revisited. *Anesthesiology* 1990;72:412–422.
118. Avram MJ, Krejcie TC, Henthorn TK. The relationship of age to the pharmacokinetics of early drug distribution: the concurrent disposition of thiopental and indocyanine green. *Anesthesiology* 1990;72:403–411.
119. Scott JC, Stanski DR. Decreased fentanyl and alfentanil dose requirements with age. A simultaneous pharmacokinetic and pharmacodynamic evaluation. *J Pharmacol Exp Ter* 1987;240:159–166.
120. Scott JC, Ponganis KV, Stanski DR. EEG quantitation of narcotic effect: the comparative pharmacodynamics of fentanyl and alfentanil. *Anesthesiology* 1985;62:234–241.
121. Scott JC, Cooke JE, Stanski DR. Electroencephalographic quantitation of opioid effect: comparative pharmacodynamics of fentanyl and sufentanil. *Anesthesiology* 1991;74:34–42.
122. Hughes MA, Glass PSA, Jacobs JR. Context-sensitive half-time in multi-compartment pharmacokinetic models for intravenous anesthetic drugs. *Anesthesiology* 1992;76:334–341.
123. Shafer SL, Stanski DR. Improving the clinical utility of anesthetic drug pharmacokinetics. *Anesthesiology* 1992;76:331–333.
124. Buhrer M, Maitre PO, Hung O, et al. Electroencephalographic effects of benzodiazepines. I. Choosing an electroencephalographic parameter to measure the effect of midazolam on the central nervous system. *Clin Pharmacol Ther* 1990;48:544–554.
125. Buhrer M, Maitre PO, Crevoisier C, et al. Electroencephalographic effects of benzodiazepines. II. Pharmacodynamic modeling of the electroencephalographic effects of midazolam and diazepam. *Clin Pharmacol Ther* 1990;48:555–567.
126. Hug CC Jr, Murphy MR. Tissue redistribution of fentanyl and termination of its effects in rats. *Anesthesiology* 1981;55:369–375.
127. Hug CC Jr, Murphy MR. Fentanyl disposition in cerebrospinal fluid and plasma and its relationship to ventilatory depression in the dog. *Anesthesiology* 1979;50:342–349.
128. Hug CC Jr, Murphy MR, Rigel EP, et al. Pharmacokinetics of morphine injected intravenously into the anesthetized dog. *Anesthesiology* 1981;54:38–47.
129. Ebling WF, Lee EN, Stanski DR. Understanding pharmacokinetics and pharmacodynamics through computer simulation: 1. The comparative clinical profiles of fentanyl and alfentanil. *Anesthesiology* 1990;72:650–658.
130. Karow AM Jr. Drugs and hypothermia—who cares? *Fed Proc* 1977;36:2569–2571.
131. Nickerson M, Kunos G. Discussion of evidence regarding induced changes in adrenoceptors. *Fed Proc* 1977;36:2580–2583.
132. Holmes PEB, Jenden DJ, Taylor DB. The analysis of the mode of action of curare on neuromuscular transmission; the effect of temperature changes. *J Pharmacol* 1951;103:382–402.
133. Bigland B, Goetzee B, Maclagan J, et al. The effect of lowered muscle temperature on the action of neuromuscular blocking drugs. *J Physiol* 1958;141:425–434.
134. Horrow JC, Bartkowski RR. Pancuronium, unlike other non-depolarizing relaxants, retains potency at hypothermia. *Anesthesiology* 1983;58:357–361.
135. Miller RD, Roderick LL. Pancuronium-induced neuromuscular blockade, and its antagonism by neostigmine, at 29, 37, and 41°C. *Anesthesiology* 1977;46:333–335.
136. Park WY, Macnamara TE. Temperature change and neuromuscular blockade by d-tubocurarine or pancuronium in man. *Anesthesiology* 1979;50:161–163.
137. Farrell L, Dempsey MJ, Waud BE, et al. Temperature and

potency of d-tubocurarine and pancuronium in vitro. *Anesth Analg* 1981;60:18–20.
138. Murdoch J, Hall RI. Brain protection: physiological and pharmacological considerations. Part I: The physiology of brain injury. *Can J Anaesth* 1990;37:663–671.
139. Odeh M. The role of reperfusion-induced injury in the pathogenesis of the crush syndrome. *N Engl J Med* 1991; 324:1417–1422.
140. Hindman BJ. Sodium bicarbonate in the treatment of subtypes of acute lactic acidosis: physiologic considerations. *Anesthesiology* 1990;72:1064–1066.
141. Stoelting RK. Local anesthetics. In: *Pharmacology and Physiology in Anesthetic Practice*. Philadelphia: JB Lippincott; 1991:148–168.
142. Skacel M, Knott C, Reynolds F, et al. Extracorporeal circuit sequestration of fentanyl and alfentanil. *Br J Anaesth* 1986;58:947–949.
143. Lockey E, Longmore DB, Ross DN, et al. Potassium and open-heart surgery. *Lancet* 1966;1:671–675.
144. Dieter RA, Neville WE, Pifarre R. Hypokalemia following hemodilution cardiopulmonary bypass. *Ann Surg* 1970; 171:17–23.
145. Scheinman MM, Sullivan RW, Hyatt KH. Magnesium metabolism in patients undergoing cardiopulmonary bypass. *Circulation* 1969 (supp 1);39:I235–I241.
146. Romero EG, Castillo-Olivares JL, O'Connor F, et al. The importance of calcium and magnesium ions in serum and cerebrospinal fluid during cardiopulmonary bypass. *J Thorac Cardiovasc Surg* 1973;66:668–672.
147. Maze M. Clinical implications of membrane receptor function in anesthesia. *Anesthesiology* 1981;55:160.
148. Spiss CK, Maze M, Smith CM. Alpha-adrenergic responsiveness correlates with epinephrine dose for arrhythmias during halothane anesthesia in dogs. *Anesth Analg* 1984; 63:297.
149. Chelly JE, Rogers K, Hysing ES, et al. Cardiovascular effects and interaction between calcium blocking drugs and anesthetics in chronically instrumented dogs. I. Verapamil and halothane. *Anesthesiology* 1986;64:560.
150. Kress HG, Muller J, Eisert A, et al. Effects of volatile anesthetics on cytoplasmic Ca^{2+} signaling and transmitter release in a neural cell line. *Anesthesiology* 1991;74:309–319.
151. Maze M. Transmembrane signalling and the holy grail of anesthesia. *Anesthesiology* 1990;72:959–961.
152. Eskinder H, Rusch NJ, Supan FD, et al. The effects of volatile anesthetics on L- and T-type calcium channel currents in canine cardiac purkinje cells. *Anesthesiology* 1991;74: 919–926.
153. Robinson-White AJ, Muldoon SM, Elson L, et al. Evidence that barbiturates inhibit antigen-induced responses through interactions with a GTP-binding protein in rat basophilic leukemia (RBL-2H3) cells. *Anesthesiology* 1990; 72:996–1010.
154. Hall RI, Sullivan JA. Does cardiopulmonary bypass alter enflurane requirements for anesthesia? *Anesthesiology* 1990;73:249–255.
155. Cohn JN, Levine TB, Francis GS, et al. Neurohumoral control mechanisms in congestive heart failure. *Am Heart J* 1981;102:509–514.
156. Packer M. Neurohormonal interactions and adaptations in congestive heart failure. *Circulation* 1988;77:721–730.
157. Fowler MB, Laser JA, Hopkins GL, et al. Assessment of the β-adrenergic receptor pathway in the intact failing heart: progressive receptor down-regulation and subsensitivity to agonist response. *Circulation* 1986;74:1290–1302.
158. Spann JF, Chidsey CA, Pool PE, et al. Mechanism of norepinephrine depletion in experimental heart failure produced by aortic constriction in the guinea pig. *Circ Res* 1965;17:312–321.
159. Colucci WS, Alexander RW, Williams GH, et al. Decreased lymphocyte beta-adrenergic-receptor density in patients with heart failure and tolerance to the beta-adrenergic agonist pirbuterol. *N Engl J Med* 1981;305:185–190.
160. Francis GS, Cohn JN. The autonomic nervous system in congestive heart failure. *Annu Rev Med* 1986;37:235–247.
161. Alderman EL, Coltart DJ, Wettach GE, et al. Coronary artery syndromes after sudden propranolol withdrawal. *Ann Intern Med* 1974;81:625–627.
162. Shanks CA. Pharmacokinetics of the nondepolarising neuromuscular relaxants applied to calculation of bolus and infusion dosage regimens. *Anesthesiology* 1986;64:72–86.
163. Kluge RM, Calia FM, McLaughlin JS, et al. Serum antibiotic concentrations pre and post cardiopulmonary bypass. *Antimicrob Agents Chemother* 1973;4:270–276.
164. Austin TW, Coles JC, Finley R, et al. Prophylactic antibiotic therapy and heart valve replacement. *Can J Surg* 1976; 19:349–352.
165. O'Reilly RA. The binding of sodium warfarin to plasma albumin and its displacement by phenylbutazone. *Ann NY Acad Sci* 1973;226:293–308.
166. Holley FO, Ponganis KV, Stanski DR. Effects of cardiac surgery with cardiopulmonary bypass on lidocaine disposition. *Clin Pharmacol Ther* 1984;35:617–626.
167. LaRosa JC, Levy RI, Windmueller HG, et al. Comparison of the triglyceride lipase of liver, adipose tissue, and postheparin plasma. *J Lipid Res* 1972;13:356–363.
168. Krauss RM, Levy RI, Fredrickson DS. Selective measurement of two lipase activities in postheparin plasma from normal subjects and patients with hyperlipoproteinemia. *J Clin Invest* 1974;54:1107–1124.
169. Desmond PV, Roberts RK, Wood AJJ, et al. Effect of heparin administration on plasma binding of benzodiazepines. *Br J Clin Pharmacol* 1980;9:171–175.
170. Svensson CK, Woodruff MN, Baxter JG, et al. Free drug concentration monitoring in clinical practice. Rationale and current status. *Clin Pharmacokinet* 1986;11:450–469.
171. Avram MJ, Shanks CA, Henthorn TK, et al. Metocurine kinetics in patients undergoing operations during cardiopulmonary bypass. *Clin Pharmacol Ther* 1987;42:576–581.
172. Futter ME, Whalley DG, Wynands JE, et al. Pancuronium requirements during hypothermic cardiopulmonary bypass in man. *Anaesth Intens Care* 1983;11:216–219.
173. Flynn PJ, Hughes R, Walton B. Use of atracurium in cardiac surgery involving cardiopulmonary bypass with induced hypothermia. *Br J Anaesth* 1984;56:967–971.
174. Walker JS, Shanks CA, Brown KF. Altered d-tubocurarine disposition during cardiopulmonary bypass. *Clin Pharmacol Ther* 1984;35:686–694.

175. Buzello W, Schluermann D, Schindler M, et al. Hypothermic cardiopulmonary bypass and neuromuscular blockade by pancuronium and vecuronium. *Anesthesiology* 1985;62: 201-204.
176. Walker JS, Brown KF, Shanks CA. Alcuronium kinetics in patients undergoing cardiopulmonary bypass surgery. *Br J Clin Pharmacol* 1983;15:237-244.
177. d'Hollander AA, Duvaldesten P, Henzel D, et al. Variations in pancuronium requirement, plasma concentration, and urinary excretion induced by cardiopulmonary bypass with hypothermia. *Anesthesiology* 1983;58:505-509.
178. Shanks CA, Ramzan IM, Walker JS, et al. Gallamine disposition in open-heart surgery involving cardiopulmonary bypass. *Clin Pharmacol Ther* 1983;33:792-799.
179. Buzello W, Pollmaecher T, Schluermann D, et al. The influence of hypothermic cardiopulmonary bypass on neuromuscular transmission in the absence of muscle relaxants. *Anesthesiology* 1986;64:279-281.
180. Feldman SA. Hypothermia and neuromuscular blockade. *Anesthesiology* 1979;51:369-370.
181. Meuldermans WEG, Hurkmans RMA, Heykants JJP. Plasma protein binding and distribution of fentanyl, sufentanil, alfentanil, and lofentanil in blood. *Arch Int Pharmacodyn* 1982;257:4-19.
182. Roerig DL, Kotrly KJ, Vucins EJ, et al. First pass uptake of fentanyl, meperidine, and morphine in the human lung. *Anesthesiology* 1987;67:466-472.
183. Roth RA, Wiersma DA. Role of the lung in total body clearance of circulating drugs. *Clin Pharmacokinet* 1979;4: 355-367.
184. Bentley JB, Conahan TJ III, Cork RC. Fentanyl sequestration in lungs during cardiopulmonary bypass. *Clin Pharmacol Ther* 1983;34:703-706.
185. Taeger K, Weninger E, Schmelzer F, et al. Pulmonary kinetics of fentanyl and alfentanil in surgical patients. *Br J Anaesth* 1988;61:425-434.
186. Jorfeldt L, Lewis DH, Lofstrom JB, et al. Lung uptake of lidocaine in healthy volunteers. *Acta Anaesth Scand* 1979; 23:567-574.
187. Porter GA, Kloster FE, Herr RJ, et al. Relationship between alterations in renal hemodynamics during cardiopulmonary bypass and postoperative renal function. *Circulation* 1966;34:1005-1021.
188. Mielke JE, Maher FT, Hunt JC, et al. Renal performance in patients undergoing replacement of the aortic valve. *Circulation* 1965;32:394-405.
189. Nuutinen L, Hollmen A. Cardiopulmonary bypass time and renal function. *Ann Chir Gyn* 1976;65:191-199.
190. Lundberg S. Renal function during anaesthesia and open-heart surgery in man. *Acta Anaesth Scand* 1967 (supp. 27): 5-82.
191. Koska AJ III, Romagnoli A, Kramer WG. Effect of cardiopulmonary bypass on fentanyl distribution and elimination. *Clin Pharmacol Ther* 1981;29:100-105.
192. Murkin JM, Farrar JK, Tweed WA, et al. Cerebral autoregulation and flow/metabolism coupling during cardiopulmonary bypass: the influence of $Paco_2$. *Anesth Analg* 1987;66:825-832.
193. Stone JG, Damask MC, Khambatta HJ. Is sufentanil removed by blood conservation devices? *J Cardiothorac Anesth* 1988;2:615-618.
194. Koren G, Crean P, Klein J, et al. Sequestration of fentanyl by the cardiopulmonary bypass (CPBP). *Eur J Clin Pharmacol* 1984;27:51-56.
195. Rosen D, Rosen K, Davidson B, et al. Fentanyl uptake by the Scimed membrane oxygenator. *J Cardiothorac Anesth* 1988;2:619-626.
196. Hanowell LH, Eisele JH, Erskine EV. Autotransfusor removal of fentanyl by blood. *Anesth Analg* 1989;69:239-241.
197. Shanks CA, Avram MJ, Ronai AK, et al. The pharmacokinetics of d-tubocurarine with surgery involving salvaged autologous blood. *Anesthesiology* 1985;62:161-165.
198. Klotz U. Pathophysiological and disease-induced changes in drug distribution volume: pharmacokinetic implications. *Clin Pharmacokinet* 1976;1:204-218.
199. Pentel P, Benowitz N. Pharmacokinetic and pharmacodynamic considerations in drug therapy of cardiac emergencies. *Clin Pharmacokinet* 1984;9:273-308.
200. Benowitz N, Forsyth RP, Melmon KL, et al. Lidocaine disposition kinetics in monkey and man. II. Effects of hemorrhage and sympathomimetic drug administration. *Clin Pharmacol Ther* 1974;16:99-109.
201. Caldwell JE, Canfell PC, Castagnoli KP, et al. The influence of renal failure on the pharmacokinetics and duration of action of pipecuronium bromide in patients anesthetized with halothane and nitrous oxide. *Anesthesiology* 1989;70: 7-12.
202. Miller KW, Chan KKH, McCoy HG, et al. Cephalothin kinetics: before, during, and after cardiopulmonary bypass surgery. *Clin Pharmacol Ther* 1979;26:54-62.
203. Bovill JG, Sebel PS. Pharmacokinetics of high-dose fentanyl. A study in patients undergoing cardiac surgery. *Br J. Anaesth* 1980;52:795-801.
204. Hug CC Jr, Burm AGL, de Lange S. Alfentanil pharmacokinetics in cardiac surgical patients. *Anesth Analg* 1994;78: 231-239.
205. Okutani R, Philbin DM, Rosow CE, et al. Effect of hypothermic hemodilutional cardiopulmonary bypass on plasma sufentanil and catecholamine concentrations in humans. *Anesth Analg* 1988;67:667-670.
206. Koren G, Goresky G, Crean P, et al. Pediatric fentanyl dosing based on pharmacokinetics during cardiac surgery. *Anesth Analg* 1984;63:577-582.
207. Koren G, Goresky G, Crean P, et al. Unexpected alterations in fentanyl pharmacokinetics in children undergoing cardiac surgery: age related or disease related? *Dev Pharmacol Ther* 1986;9:183-191.
208. Davis PJ, Cook DR, Stiller RL, et al. Pharmacodynamics and pharmacokinetics of high-dose sufentanil in infants and children undergoing cardiac surgery. *Anesth Analg* 1987;66:203-208.
209. Hall RI. The pharmacokinetic behaviour of opioids administered during cardiac surgery. *Can J Anaesth* 1991;38:747-756.
210. Zaidan JR, Klochany A, Martin WM, et al. Effect of thiopental on neurologic outcome following coronary artery bypass surgery. *Anesthesiology* 1991;74:406-411.
211. Boscoe MJ, Dawling S, Thompson MA, et al. Lorazepam in open-heart surgery—plasma concentrations before, during and after bypass following different dose regimens. *Anaesth Intens Care* 1984;12:9-13.

212. Aaltonen L, Kanto J, Arola M, et al. Effect of age and cardiopulmonary bypass on the pharmacokinetics of lorazepam. *Acta Pharmacol Toxicol* 1982;51:126-131.
213. Kanto J, Himberg JJ, Heikkila H, et al. Midazolam kinetics before, during and after cardiopulmonary bypass surgery. *Int J Clin Pharm Res* 1985;5:123-126.
214. Harper KW, Collier PS, Dundee JW, et al. Age and nature of operation influence the pharmacokinetics of midazolam. *Br J Anaesth* 1985;57:866-871.
215. Lowry KG, Dundee JW, McClean E, et al. Pharmacokinetics of diazepam and midazolam when used for sedation following cardiopulmonary bypass. *Br J Anaesth* 1985;57:883-885.
216. Massey NJ, Sherry KM, Oldroyd S, et al. Pharmacokinetics of an infusion of propofol during cardiac surgery. *Br J Anaesth* 1990;65:475-479.
217. Russell GN, Wright EL, Fox MA, et al. Propofol-fentanyl anaesthesia for coronary artery surgery and cardiopulmonary bypass. *Anaesthesia* 1989;44:205-208.
218. Lange H, Stephan H, Rieke H, et al. Hepatic and extrahepatic disposition of propofol in patients undergoing coronary bypass graft surgery. *Br J Anaesth* 1990;64:563-570.
219. McMurray TJ, Collier PS, Carson IW, et al. Propofol sedation after open heart surgery. A clinical and pharmacokinetic study. *Anaesthesia* 1990;45:322-326.
220. Loomis CW, Brunet D, Milne B, et al. Arterial isoflurane concentration and EEG burst suppression during cardiopulmonary bypass. *Clin Pharmacol Ther* 1986;40:304-313.
221. Homi J, Konchigeri HN, Eckenhoff JE, et al. A new anesthetic agent—Forane: preliminary observations in man. *Anesth Analg* 1972;51:439-447.
222. Price SL, Brown DL, Carpenter RL, et al. Isoflurane elimination via a bubble oxygenator during extracorporeal circulation. *J Cardiothorac Anesth* 1988;2:41-44.
223. Henderson JM, Nathan HJ, Lalande M, et al. Washin and washout of isoflurane during cardiopulmonary bypass. *Can J Anaesth* 1988;35:587-590.
224. Moore RA, McNicholas KW, Gallagher JD, et al. Halothane metabolism in acyanotic and cyanotic patients undergoing open heart surgery. *Anesth Analg* 1986;65:1257-1262.
225. Wierda JMKH, Karliczek GF, Vandenbrom RHG, et al. Pharmacokinetics and cardiovascular dynamics of pipecuronium bromide during coronary artery surgery. *Can J Anaesth* 1990;37:183-191.
226. Williams DJ, Steele TW. Cephalothin prophylaxis assay during cardiopulmonary bypass. *J Thorac Cardiovasc Surg* 1976;71:207-211.
227. Polk RE, Archer GL, Lower R. Cefamandole kinetics during cardiopulmonary bypass. *Clin Pharmacol Ther* 1978;23:473-480.
228. Kini PM, Fernandez J, Causay RS, et al. Double-blind comparison of cefazolin and cephalothin in open-heart surgery. *J Thorac Cardiovasc Surg* 1978;76:506-509.
229. Sato Y, Kanazawa H, Okazaki H, et al. A comparison of the penetration characteristics of latamoxef and cephalothin into right atrial appendage and pericardial fluid of adult patient undergoing open-heart surgery. *Jpn J Antibiotics* 1984;37:678-679.
230. Goldmann DA, Hopkins CC, Karchmer AW, et al. Cephalothin prophylaxis in cardiac valve surgery. A prospective, double-blind comparison of two-day and six-day regimens. *J Thorac Cardiovasc Surg* 1977;73:470-479.
231. Miller KW, McCoy HG, Chan KKH, et al. Effect of cardiopulmonary bypass on cefazolin disposition. *Clin Pharmacol Ther* 1980;27:550-556.
232. Jungbluth GL, Pasko MT, Beam TR, et al. Ceftriaxone disposition in open-heart surgery patients. *Antimicrob Agents Chemother* 1989;33:850-856.
233. Eigel P, Tschirkov A, Satter P, et al. Assays of cephalosporin antibiotics administered prophylactically in open heart surgery. *Infection* 1978;6:23-28.
234. Storstein L, Nitter-Hauge S, Fjeld N. Effect of cardiopulmonary bypass with heparin administration on digitoxin pharmacokinetics, serum electrolytes, free fatty acids, and renal function. *J Cardiovasc Pharmacol* 1979;1:191-204.
235. Austen WG, Ebert PA, Greenfield LJ, et al. The effect of cardiopulmonary bypass on tissue digoxin concentrations in the dog. *J Surg Res* 1962;2:85-89.
236. Beall AC Jr, Johnson PC, Driscoll T, et al. Effect of total cardiopulmonary bypass on myocardial and blood digoxin concentration in man. *Am J Cardiol* 1963;11:194-200.
237. Hernandez A Jr, Kouchoukos N, Burton RM, et al. The effect of extracorporeal circulation upon the tissue concentration of digoxin-H^3. *Pediatrics* 1963;31:952-957.
238. Coltart DJ, Chamberlain DA, Howard MR, et al. Effect of cardiopulmonary bypass on plasma digoxin concentrations. *Br Heart J* 1971;33:334-338.
239. Morrison J, Killip T. Serum digitalis and arrhythmia in patients undergoing cardiopulmonary bypass. *Circulation* 1973;47:341-352.
240. Krasula RW, Hastreiter AR, Levitsky S, et al. Serum, atrial, and urinary digoxin levels during cardiopulmonary bypass in children. *Circulation* 1974;49:1047-1052.
241. Kramer WG, Romagnoli A. Papaverine disposition in cardiac surgery patients and the effect of cardiopulmonary bypass. *Eur J Clin Pharmacol* 1984;27:127-130.
242. Moore RA, Geller EA, Gallagher JD, et al. Effect of hypothermic cardiopulmonary bypass on nitroprusside metabolism. *Clin Pharmacol Ther* 1985;37:680-683.
243. Dasta JF, Jacobi J, Wu LS, et al. Loss of nitroglycerin to cardiopulmonary bypass apparatus. *Crit Care Med* 1983;11:50-52.
244. Booth BP, Henderson M, Milne B, et al. Sequestration of glyceryl trinitrate (nitroglycerin) by cardiopulmonary bypass oxygenators. *Anesth Analg* 1991;72:493-497.
245. Dasta JF, Weber RJ, Wu LS, et al. Influence of cardiopulmonary bypass on nitroglycerin clearance. *J Clin Pharmacol* 1986;26:165-168.
246. Plachetka JR, Salomon NW, Copeland JG. Plasma propranolol before, during, and after cardiopulmonary bypass. *Clin Pharmacol Ther* 1981;30:745-751.
247. McDonald DH, Hug CC Jr, Kaplan JA. Continuous propranolol infusion: Isoproterenol response. *Anesthesiology* 1982;57:A69.
248. Schiavello R, Mezza A, Feo L, et al. Compartmental analysis of lidocaine kinetics during extracorporeal circulation. *J Cardiothorac Anesth* 1988;2:290-296.

5
Hemostasis and Cardiopulmonary Bypass

Markku T. Salmenperä, Jerrold H. Levy, and Laurence A. Harker

In the early days of open-heart surgery, it was routine to transfuse several units of donor blood during each operation. In contrast, in the 1990s, adults undergoing primary cardiac surgery commonly receive no donor blood. The change in the use of transfused blood products is the result of multiple alterations in perioperative patient management, including: (1) autologous blood salvage, (2) the acceptance of transiently reduced hemoglobin values, (3) improved surgical procedures, and (4) the use of more compatible biomaterials in the extracorporeal circuit (ECC). Despite these advances, between 10% and 20% of patients undergoing cardiopulmonary bypass (CPB) bleed excessively, as defined by the need for multiple transfusions of blood products in the perioperative period. Between 3% and 5% of these patients will undergo re-exploration mandated by abnormal bleeding.[1-4] In about half of these cases, a distinct bleeding site will be identified, while in the others the bleeding will be attributed to acquired hemostatic defects. These bleeding complications may lead to serious consequences, including reoperation, delayed chest closure, and increased risk of mediastinitis or other infections.[5] In addition, hypovolemia, due to excessive bleeding, and the constricting effects of blood accumulating in the pericardium, may give rise to biventricular cardiac dysfunction. Each unit of donor blood also carries a small risk of transmitting infectious diseases. For example, the frequency of nosocomial non-A, non-B hepatitis among cardiac surgery patients is between 1.6% and 11.6%, a disturbing indication of serious risk.[6,7] Blood products may also result in untoward immunologic effects, including anaphylaxis, transfusion-related acute lung injury, and graft versus host disease.[8] Finally, excessive and inappropriate use of blood products may threaten the supply, since cardiac surgery uses about 25% of all blood resources.[9]

The mechanisms underlying hemostatic defects during CPB are multiple. The effect of exposing blood to biomaterial surfaces of the ECC apparatus is primarily responsible for the platelet hemostatic abnormalities. Other factors associated with cardiac surgery also contribute to the alterations in hemostasis, including hemodilution, hypothermia, endocrine stress response, extensive surgery, and drugs administered intraoperatively. Since the relative influence of these factors on hemostasis produced by CPB is not well defined, a multidisciplinary approach to cardiac surgery, anesthesiology, perfusion technology, hematology, and transfusion medicine is needed to facilitate identification of those patients at risk for bleeding and development of appropriate therapeutic approaches when bleeding occurs.

Anticoagulation During Bypass

The massive clotting of the entire CPB circuit that occurs if anticoagulation is not instituted prior to CPB illustrates the inherent thrombogenicity of the system. The nonendothelialized biomaterial surface is largely responsible for initiating thrombus formation. Intact vascular endothelium exhibits both passive and active antithrombotic properties, including release of prostacyclin and endothelium-derived relaxing factor, which prevent platelet aggregation and promote flow; activation of the physiologic anticoagulant protein C; and inactivation of thrombin. ECC surfaces directly activate platelets and initiate the sequence of serine proteases comprising the coagulation and fibrinolytic cascades (Figure 5.1).

Cardiac surgery also activates the hemostatic apparatus leading to thrombus formation. Median sternotomy liberates tissue thromboplastin and activates platelets, giving rise to activated coagulation products in the circulating blood, via cardiotomy suction, from the operative field during CPB. Hemodilution decreases the concentration of coagulation factors, platelets, and the physiologic anticoagulant factors protein C, protein S, and antithrombin-III.

Patient anticoagulation is achieved and maintained during CPB most frequently with heparin. Understanding heparin's mechanism of action, and where it acts in the hemostatic cascade, is important in understanding the limi-

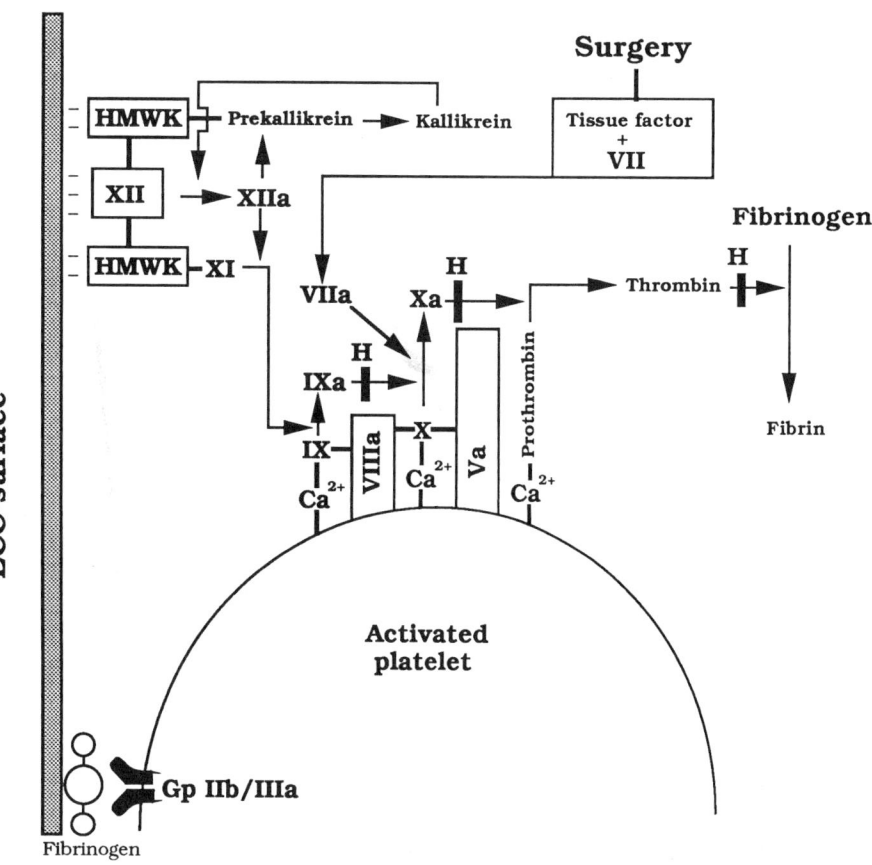

FIGURE 5.1. Hypothetical and schematic presentation of hemostatic activation and pathways during CPB. Note that the extracorporeal artificial surface can cause activation of the intrinsic coagulation cascade via surface activation of factor XII–high-molecular-weight kininogen–prekallikrein complex and direct activation of platelets. Extrinsic loop of the coagulation is also activated during CPB by tissue phopholipids liberated during surgery. ECC-surface, extracorporeal surface; Gp IIb/IIIa, platelet surface receptor for fibrinogen; HMWK, high-molecular-weight kininogen; H, site of action of heparin–AT-III complex: Procoagulants and their activated forms (-a) designated by their roman numerals.

tations of heparin as an antagonist of hemostatic activation during CPB.

In 1939, 26 years after the discovery of heparin, a plasma factor was shown to be required for heparin to exert its anticoagulant effect.[10,11] This factor, named antithrombin-III (AT-III), was identified as the principal physiologic inhibitor protein of the coagulant serine proteases in the early 1970s.[12,13] Standard heparin is a mixture of mucopolysaccharides with a molecular weight ranging from 3000 to 30,000 daltons (mean MW, 15,000) with a repetitive pentasaccharide-glucosamine sequence that is required for its binding to AT-III.[14] Heparin molecules are highly negatively charged polyanions. As heparin is the main proteoglycan of the mast cell granule, tissues rich in mast cells—porcine intestinal mucosa or beef lung—are the main source of clinically used heparin. There are differences in chemical structure and biologic activity between heparins from these two sources (Table 5.1); these differences may be important during the use of heparin for CPB anticoagulation.[15] Since the specific anticoagulant activity of heparin varies among different preparations, heparin activity should be expressed in units of biological activity, rather than in milligrams. To reduce the possibility of serious dosing errors, only those preparations that contain the standard amount of heparin (eg, 1000 U/mL) should be available in the cardiac operating room.

Heparin Pharmacokinetics and Pharmacodynamics

After an intravenous bolus injection of heparin, there is a rapid initial fall in concentration, due to redistribution, followed by a slower constant elimination. The redistribution is saturated by the "maxidoses" of heparin usually used during CPB.[16] Consequently, the dose-response duration is not linear; on average, the half-life of heparin is prolonged from 56 to 152 minutes when the dose is increased from 100 to 400 U/kg.[17] Clearance kinetics are further complicated by the fact that heparin binds with many plasma proteins, causing variable and unpredictable molecule inactivation. For example, elevated levels of his-

TABLE 5.1. Differences between heparins extracted from bovine lung (BLH) and porcine intestinal mucosa (PMH).

Sulfate residues are more abundant in BLH
Specific activity (USP unit/mg) is higher in BLH
More protamine is needed to neutralize 1 USP unit of BLH
Incidence of thrombocytopenia is higher after BLH
Variability of activity mg (USP units/mg) is higher in PMH
BLH is more expensive

---

tidine-rich glycoprotein,[18] vitronectin,[19] platelet factor 4,[20] and von Willebrand factor (vWF) may cause relative and variable heparin resistance, particularly in malignant and inflammatory disorders. Endothelial cells remove and depolymerize heparin in a process that involves glycosaminoglycans and platelet factor 4.[21] The final elimination routes of heparin are not well defined, but they are probably not affected by impaired renal function. The effects on heparin pharmacokinetics caused by CPB and/or hypothermia have not been characterized. However, substantial amounts of heparin may be removed with hemofiltration or with cell savers, requiring additional heparin monitoring.

The pentasaccharide sequence of heparin binds to lysine sites of AT-III, producing a conformational change in its arginine-reactive center, increasing its capacity to inhibit thrombin by 2000- to 10,000-fold.[22] Heparin–AT-III complexes also inactivate other serine proteases in the coagulation cascade, including factor Xa and factor IXa (Figure 5.1). AT-III is not a major inhibitor of contact factors XIIa, XIa, or kallikrein, and heparin–AT-III does not appreciably accelerate this inhibition.[23] As a result of the accelerated inhibition of activated coagulation factors in the final common and distal intrinsic pathway, a nearly complete hemostatic inactivation is obtained with heparin concentrations of 2 to 4 U/mL, typical levels used during CPB. Marked reductions of plasma AT-III may decrease anticoagulation response to heparin. Importantly, an inverse correlation between preoperative AT-III activity and cumulative heparin dose is needed to keep activated clotting time above 400 seconds.[24] Reductions of AT-III can occur in patients with intravascular coagulation[25] and ongoing heparin therapy.[26] A qualitative alteration in the AT-III molecule has been proposed as the explanation for the decreased heparin sensitivity brought about by nitroglycerin infusion.[27]

The side effects of rapid IV heparin administration are minor. Occasional small decreases in arterial pressure may be caused by a sudden increase in free drug levels of intravenous anesthetic agents due to their displacement, by heparin, from the common binding sites on the plasma proteins.[28] Heparin also binds to platelets and may either inhibit platelet aggregation or function as a platelet-aggregating agonist.[29] These effects may be important with high doses and blood levels of heparin. A heparin concentration of 5 U/mL, which is within the range found during routine CPB, caused a profound inhibition of platelet function as assessed by hemostatometry, a recently developed technique that measures platelet plug formation after shear-induced activation in vitro.[30] High-molecular-weight heparin fractions, abundant in the heparin preparations used clinically, have greater platelet effects than low-molecular-weight fractions.[29] The interaction of heparin with platelets may contribute to heparin-induced bleeding, by a mechanism that is independent of its anticoagulant effects. The side effect of greatest concern in the setting of cardiac surgery is heparin-induced thrombocytopenia in patients previously exposed to heparin or those on "chronic" heparin therapy.[31] Although this is usually mild and of no great clinical concern, it may occasionally occur as a form of potentially lethal thrombosis associated with the thrombocytopenia.[32]

Heparin Monitoring

Before heparin monitoring systems became widely available, empirical fixed-dose protocols of heparin anticoagulation were used for CPB. Larger doses of heparin were administered routinely, since an effective antidote, protamine, was available. Today, with the advent of user-friendly portable devices for measuring both heparin concentration and activity, which are feasible for operating room use, anticoagulation is routinely monitored by activated clotting time (ACT) devices, and in some institutions by heparin levels.

Heparin Activity Tests

As noted above, the heparin–AT-III complex inhibits multiple serine proteases in the intrinsic and common coagulation pathway. Thus, those tests measuring the activity of these combined pathways can be used as a functional assay to detect heparin activity.

Whole blood clotting time (WBCT) was the first test to be used in the operating room to monitor heparin effect. The main problem with this test is that clotting times are prolonged over an unmeasurable range, with the high concentrations of heparin occurring during bypass. WBCT can be used to detect successful reversal of heparin with protamine, and it is a more sensitive indicator than ACT.[33]

Activated partial thromboplastin time (PTT) is a standard monitor for chronic heparin therapy. This test is not suitable for heparin monitoring during CPB, however, since plasma preparation requires centrifugation, and because, in the heparin concentrations used during cardiac surgery, the linear dose-response relationship is lost and clotting is easily prolonged over the sensitive range. PTT is more sensitive than ACT at low levels of heparin, which might be seen after protamine administration.[33,34] PTT measurements using portable devices and whole blood have been introduced recently; their usefulness after cardiac surgery is, however, unproved. Thrombin time (TT) is too sensitive to use as a routine test of heparin activity. Moreover, TT may also be prolonged by fibrinogen deficiency or fibrinogen degradation products. An abnormal TT coupled with normal reptilase time signifies the pres-

5. Hemostasis and Cardiopulmonary Bypass

TABLE 5.2. Factors affecting activated clotting time (ACT) besides heparin.

ACT shortened	Operative stress (ACT shorter after sternotomy than after induction)
ACT prolonged	Hereditary deficiency in contact factors (factor XII, high-molecular-weight kininogen, prekallikrein)
	Hemodilution and severe anemia
	Thrombocytopenia
	Factor VIII deficiency
	Hypofibrinogenemia
	Coumadin therapy or severe hepatic dysfunction

ence of heparin, and these tests are helpful when complex coagulopathies are evaluated after cardiac surgery.[35]

Activated clotting time, the mainstay of heparin monitoring during cardiac surgery, was introduced in 1966.[36] The ACT uses large surface areas provided by diatomaceous earth (celite) or kaolin to initiate contact activation. There are also automated ACT methods using celite (Hemochron) or kaolin (Hemotec). The end point of clotting is detected by the displacement of the rotatory magnet bar by the clot (Hemochron) or by the decrease in the drop rate of the plunger (Hemotec). Since temperature is critical for consistent results, the devices warm the blood to 37°C. Most of the documentary studies on ACT have been made with Hemochron systems, but the smaller sample size used in the Hemotec systems (0.2 mL) may be particularly attractive for use in the pediatric patient, since less blood is lost to sampling, and the smaller sample is more rapidly heated to 37°C from extreme hypothermia. ACT systems represent useful monitoring devices in the setting of cardiac surgery, since minimum experience is needed to obtain reproducible results. In addition, tests are done using whole blood, reagents are stable without refrigeration, and the results are available immediately. Results from the two systems should not be used interchangeably, since they will be consistently different. The Hemotec system, for example, gives slightly shorter clotting times. This is not surprising because sample volume, mode of clot detection, and activators are all different.

ACT is a heparin activity test. It should not be used to assess coagulation either before or after surgery, since it gives a crude, nonspecific assessment of the complete intrinsic coagulation cascade. Only severe deficiencies in the contact factors, factor VIII, and thrombocytopenia cause increases in ACT.[35] Various other factors shown to affect ACT, besides heparin, are listed in Table 5.2. Apparently, the control ACT value cannot be assumed to be stable during the whole cardiac operation, and prolongation of ACT postoperatively is often due to factors other than heparin.

An ACT value of 400 seconds has been considered a *sine qua non* of adequate anticoagulation during CPB. This "magical" value is based on a monkey experiment of Young et al,[37] who detected fibrin monomers in six of nine monkeys after 30 minutes of CPB, five of which had ACT values under 400 seconds. Since the accuracy of the ACT determination is not good, with a coefficient of variation approaching 10%, the requirement of an ACT of 480 seconds, as was originally proposed by Bull,[38] may add a reasonable margin of safety in preventing the occurrence of heparin levels incompatible with the prevention of subclinical coagulation activity.

A gaussian distribution of heparin dose/ACT response is observed when a standard dose of heparin of 300 to 400 U/kg is given to those patients about to be cannulated for CPB. Distribution of the observed ACT response is flat, with greater than threefold variation in the normal cardiac surgical patient.[39] Those patients showing ACT less than or greater than the 95% confidence limit have been designated as "heparin resistant" or "heparin sensitive," respectively. Increased heparin sensitivity may not be a clinically important problem, since it is usually related to a relative "overdose" in those patients whose lean body mass (and corresponding blood volume) is clearly lower than what might be assumed from their actual body weight (Table 5.3). Also, increased heparin sensitivity may be due to a preexisting deficiency in the coagulation factors or to thrombocytopenia. Heparin resistance may be of greater concern, since underdosing heparin may lead to subclinical coagulation with the consumption of the coagulation factors.[24] The proposed etiologies are presented in Table 5.3. It is essential that errors in administration be excluded, preferably by documenting adequate heparin levels in these cases. Relative heparin resistance occurs most commonly in patients who have been receiving IV heparin prior to surgery[39,40] and therefore have a decreased ACT responsiveness to standard heparin administration.

Heparin Level

Plasma heparin measurements, used intraoperatively, rely on measuring heparin's biologic activity. Protamime neutralizes heparin's effects in a dose ratio of 1 mg of prota-

TABLE 5.3. Etiologies of altered heparin dose-ACT response.

Heparin sensitivity	Obese patients (relative overdose)
	Aprotinin therapy
	Deficiency in contact factors, factor VIII, and fibrinogen
Heparin resistance	AT-III deficiency (hereditary or acquired)
	Intravascular coagulation (intracardiac thrombus)
	Preoperative heparin therapy
	Inflammatory diseases (endocarditis)
	Preoperative nitroglycerin therapy?
	Advanced age

mine sulfate to 100 U of heparin. Using the series of known protamine concentrations, heparin concentrations can be determined. This test has been automated in devices using cartridges that contain, in addition to a series of protamine concentrations, tissue thromboplastin for extrinsic and common pathway activation. The change in light transmission in the test tubes indicates clotting by the retention of the formed clot in nylon mesh after air bubbling (Hepcon/System A-10, Hemotec), or by the decreased drop rate of the plunger-and-flag system (Hepcon/Heparin Monitoring System [HMS]). Cartridges sensitive to a variety of different high-dose heparin concentrations, or low doses appropriate for measurements during CPB and after heparin reversal, respectively, should be selected before running the assay.

More exact and sensitive determination of heparin is possible using chromogenic assays with added AT-III and known amounts of thrombin. The thrombin activity, measured as the liberation of a fluorescent probe, is inversely proportional to the amount of heparin in the sample. The problem with the fluorometric assay systems is that plasma must be prepared. Although an instrument that will perform this function and measure heparin concentration in 5 minutes is available and has been used to guide intraoperative anticoagulation, this methodology is primarily used for research applications.[41,42]

In normal patients, heparin levels between 2.0 and 4.0 U/mL are probably adequate for anticoagulation. After protamine neutralization, however, no free heparin should be measurable, and the weakness of protamine titration is that, due to inaccuracies in the methodology, only relatively high concentrations of heparin (ie, >0.4 U/mL) are detected reliably. Since plasma heparin levels do not take into account the variability of the heparin dose-response, this indicator should be used in conjunction with heparin activity tests like ACT.

Heparin Administration Protocol for Cardiac Surgery

Inadequate heparinization continues to be one of the most common iatrogenic complications during CPB.[43] Consequently, institutions and cardiac surgical teams should develop their own heparin administration protocols. Anesthesiologists, surgeons, and perfusionists should be thoroughly familiar with these protocols and should follow them rigorously. A representative protocol is shown in Figure 5.2. Heparin should be administered in a consistent manner, from a labeled syringe via a central vein, before CPB. Importantly, appropriate prolongation of the ACT should document the effects of heparin before proceeding with CPB.

Bull[38] originally proposed to calculate heparin dose-ACT responses in vivo in each patient to reach individualized bolus and maintenance doses. Although some clinicians follow this practice, most do not construct the curves before the institution of CPB. An in vitro technique to determine heparin dose-responses is available (Hemotec). This may enable identification of a patient who is heparin resistant prior to anesthesia induction and allow time for appropriate therapeutic maneuvers, such as ordering and thawing fresh frozen plasma (FFP).

The need to maintain ACT values over 400 seconds has been challenged.[44] Metz and Keats[45] reported no differences in postoperative chest-tube drainage when ACT varied from 300 to over 750 seconds. Macroscopically, no clotting was detected in the oxygenator, even in the four patients with ACTs of less than 300 seconds. In another study, thrombin activity during CPB did not change from baseline, measured before heparin administration, when ACT values were maintained at more than 350 seconds.[46] A significant positive correlation between heparin concentration during CPB and postoperative blood loss was observed. These data suggest that acceptance of a lower critical value of ACT of 350 seconds is permissible in a patient with heparin resistance, once heparin has been given in a dose of up to 400 to 600 U/kg and a heparin level of >2.5 U/mL has been ascertained. The most common explanations for relative heparin resistance are (1) heparin binding with endothelial glycosaminoglycans or plasma proteins, increasing fibronectin, vitronectin, vWF, and heparin cofactor II, and (2) acquired AT-III deficiency (following heparin administration).[40] Increasing heparin doses potentially increases the risk of postoperative bleeding due to the platelet effects of high heparin levels and heparin rebound. Occasionally, heparin sensitivity may be achieved by restoring AT-III levels with transfused FFP[47] (or AT-III concentrates,[48] not currently available in the United States). Also, ACT alone may not always be an adequate measurement of anticoagulation during bypass. ACT is critically dependent on contact activation factors, which may decrease more than the other coagulation factors during bypass and elevate ACT values.[49] Also, coagulation may still be activated via the extrinsic pathway and various bypass routes distal to the contact factors in the intrinsic pathway. This is illustrated by studies in factor XII–deficient patients who require normal heparin concentrations during bypass for their anticoagulation, despite baseline ACT values exceeding 400 seconds before heparin administration.[50] Consequently, maintaining both ACT over 350 seconds and heparin concentrations of ≥2.5 U/mL is sound policy during CPB, based on previous studies.

Heparin-Induced Thrombocytopenia

A transient decrease in platelet count is usually observed after the bolus doses of heparin required for CPB anticoagulation. This is thought to be secondary to platelet agglutination and sequestration and is of trivial clinical consequence.[51] Between 2% and 5% of the patients on heparin therapy for longer than 6 days develop significant

FIGURE 5.2. A suggested protocol for CPB anticoagulation and its reversal.

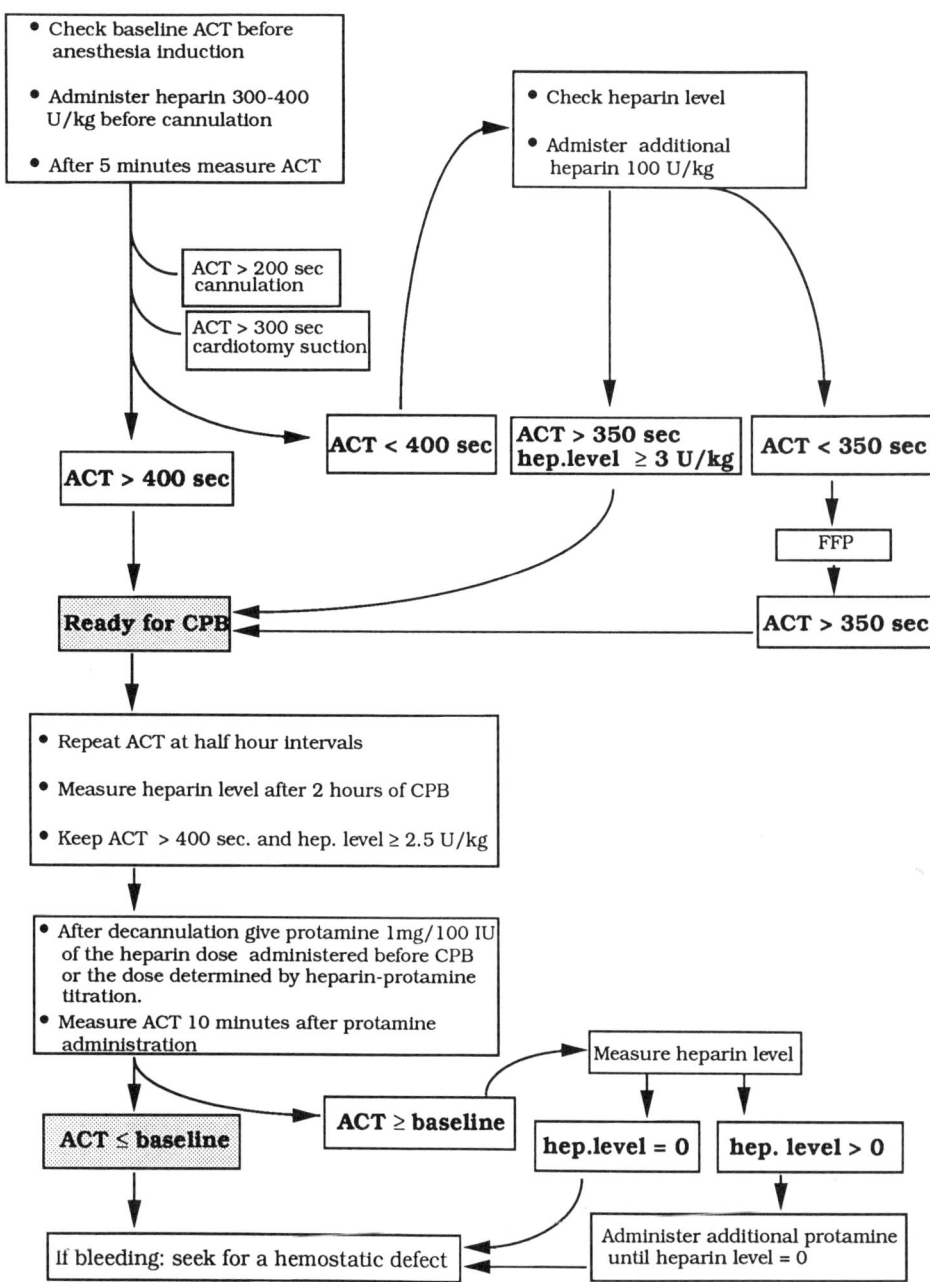

thrombocytopenia,[31] and in about 0.4%, therapy may be complicated by associated arterial thrombosis, including strokes, myocardial infarctions, and limb ischemia.[52] In heparin-induced thrombocytopenia, an anti-heparin immunoglobulin G (IgG) is present in plasma, and binds to repeating antigenic determinants of heparin and to the platelet surface epitopes most likely to be Fc-receptors.[31,53] Following IgG binding, a platelet-release reaction and subsequent aggregation may contribute to both thrombosis and profound thrombocytopenia.[54] Assays detecting serotonin release from platelets, at subtherapeutic (0.1 U/mL) and high (100 U/mL) concentrations in the platelet-rich plasma, are reported to be the most reliable detectors of heparin-induced thrombocytopenia.[55] In the postoperative period, heparin-induced thrombocytopenia must be considered if a patient who has been receiving heparin therapy develops severe thrombocytopenia, and other causes have been ruled out. If heparin-induced thrombocytopenia is diagnosed, any form of patient-heparin contact, including use of heparin-bonded catheters and heparin-flush, must be discontinued immediately. Platelet transfusions are contraindicated because they may precipitate additional thrombotic events.

Since standard anticoagulation with heparin in patients with documented previous heparin-induced thrombocytopenia may be life-threatening, sugery should be postponed until the status of the heparin-specific IgG antibody is defined.[56] Substitution of porcine heparin for bovine heparin may also obviate the recurrence of heparin-induced thrombocytopenia.[31] Alternatives to heparin anticoagulation in the presence of heparin-induced thrombocytopenia include a defibrinogenating agent (ancrod; Arvin®)[57] and synthetic heparinoid (ORG 10172).[58] Alternatively, successful management has been achieved with the concomitant administration of porcine heparin and continuous infusion of a prostacyclin analog, Iloprost®.[59] By elevating intraplatelet cAMP levels, this prostanoid prevents heparin- and heparin-antibody-induced aggregation of platelets in vitro, and presumably also in vivo, since perioperative bleeding, bleeding times, and transfusion requirement in heparin-induced thrombocytopenia patients managed with this protocol were comparable to those of historical controls.

Future Trends in CPB Anticoagulation

To date, heparin remains the only practical anticoagulant. Advantages of its use include predictable response, opportunity to monitor effects, low incidence of side effects, availability of reliable reversal agent, and cost-effectiveness. The investigational heparin alternatives, such as hirudin (an AT-III–independent antithrombin), are not likely to replace heparin in the near future, but may be considered in occasional patients with heparin-induced thrombocytopenia, hereditary AT-III deficiency, or protamine allergy (Table 5.4).

Despite heparin's widespread use for CPB, it is a poor inhibitor of contact activation factors, and does not prevent platelet activation induced by ECC and circulating agonists[23] (Figure 5.1). Activation of these additional pathways may result in acquired bleeding syndromes after CPB. The combined use of inhibitors of contact activation, along with heparin, may be more feasible in the near future. Aprotinin (currently available in most parts of the world), when given in high doses during cardiac surgery, prevents factor XII–mediated and kallikrein effects, as well as dramatically reducing postoperative bleeding and potentiating the prolongation of ACT with heparin.[60,61] This last noted effect should not be considered as a heparin-sparing effect of aprotinin, since it is probably only an in vitro effect; a normal anticoagulation dose and concentration of heparin should be used to prevent coagulation in vivo. Prostacyclin (PGI_2) and its analog Iloprost protect platelets reversibly during in vitro and animal models of CPB.[62] However, clinical trials to decrease bleeding and, hence, transfusion requirements have been negative.[63-66]

The development of new blood/circuit interfacing biomaterials may reduce thrombogenicity of the CPB apparatus. The heparin-coated surfaces for CPB are the subject of current research.[67,68] Systemic heparin doses during CPB can probably be reduced when heparin-bonded circuits are used. Although bonding may help to reduce local thrombosis and improve catheter patency, it may also increase the electronegativity of the surface, making it potentially more hostile to contact factors and platelets. Thus, this approach is unlikely to solve hemostatic problems and contact activation associated with CPB. The use of heparin-bonded tubing and centrifugal pumps (without a reservoir and oxygenator) with reduced systemic heparinization may, however, decrease intraoperative blood loss when used for the repair of thoracic aneurysms.[69] Studies with a small number of patients also seem to demonstrate decreases in blood loss and donor blood requirements with heparin-coated circuits coupled with low-dose systemic heparin, as compared with standard circuits and high systemic doses of heparin.[70]

Reversal of Heparin Anticoagulation

Protamine, the only currently available reversal agent for heparin, is a strong basic protein with a molecular weight of 4300. The positive charge of the protein is due to abundant arginine residues. Protamine, a polycation, binds to heparin, a polyanion, forming a noncovalent complex in a dose ratio of 1 mg to 100 U. The resulting complex binds to other plasma proteins, including AT-III, and heparin's

TABLE 5.4. Potential alternatives to heparin and protamine.

	Substitute	Drawback
Heparin	Low-molecular-weight heparin, heparinoids	No reversal agent, unavailability of suitable monitoring method.
	Defibrinogenation (ancrod)	Exogenous fibrinogen needed for reversal, anticoagulant monitoring demanding, long time (12 h) to induce anticoagulation
Protamine	Hexadimethrine	Anapyhlactoid reactions, renal toxicity
	Heparinase or immobilized protamine filters	Still in development, require recirculation of blood through the filter, do not entirely remove heparin

anticoagulant properties are neutralized.[71] Intravenous protamine is available in two salt forms, sulfate and chloride. The latter is used extensively in Europe, and has been shown to be more resistant to breakdown by peptidases in plasma.[72] There seems to be no advantage in this difference, demonstrated in vitro, in terms of heparin rebound, in patients.[33] After IV injection, protamine, due to its low molecular weight, is rapidly distributed to the extracellular space. The pharmacokinetics are poorly described, but its clearance from plasma is several orders faster than that of heparin.[73] In a clinical setting, elimination of free protamine from the circulation is even more rapid, since heparin-protamine complexes form at a rate that depends on the relative intravascular concentrations.

Large amounts of protamine may inhibit coagulation in vitro. A concentration in excess of 10 μg/mL prolongs WBCT and ACT.[74] A very large dose of 10 mg/kg given to nonheparinized volunteers caused a modest increase in WBCT.[75] These effects may be mediated via protamine's effects on platelets and clotting proteins. Potentially by nonimmunologic complement activation, protamine has been shown to cause thrombocytopenia in animals[76] and humans,[77] and heparin-protamine complexes decrease platelet function.[78] Protamine also binds and inhibits thrombin in vitro.[79] These anticoagulant effects of protamine in vitro are of questionable clinical significance, since free protamine concentrations remaining after heparin neutralization are likely to be small and rapidly cleared.

Adverse Reactions to Protamine

Rapid protamine infusion is known to cause hypotension. This rate- or free-concentration-dependent hypotension may result from one or several diverse causes. Proposed explanations include: stimulation of endothelium-derived relaxing factor release,[80] inhibition of plasma carboxypeptidase N,[81] inactivation of various vasoactive peptides, and nonimmunologic release of histamine from mast cells. Histamine can be released by protamine from isolated human cutaneous mast cells at high concentrations, but not from lung mast cells.[82] Some protamine reactions may be associated with complement activation via the classical pathway, either through protamine-heparin complexes or through protamine and anti-IgG-antibody interaction.[83] The generation of anaphylatoxins may induce mediator release from mast cells and can also stimulate the generation of new mediators, such as thromboxane A_2, from membrane phospholipids of activated leukocytes. Other reactions probably represent classical immunoglobulin E (IgE)-mediated allergy and appear as classical anaphylactic reactions with rash, urticaria, bronchospasm, and systemic vasodilation.[84] Some patients show a very pronounced increase in pulmonary artery pressure from pulmonary vasoconstriction with right heart failure. This reaction is mediated by release of thromboxane A_2 into the plasma, since concentrations of thromboxane B_2 (its metabolite) have been shown to correlate with pulmonary vasoconstriction.[83,85]

Prior exposure to protamine from protamine-containing insulin preparations increases the risk of severe protamine reaction during CPB. While the frequency of protamine reactions in patients never exposed to protamine-containing insulin preparations has been suggested to be 0.06%,[86] there is a 10- to 30-fold increased risk in neutral protamine Hagedorn (NPH) insulin-dependent diabetics,[87] suggesting that prior exposure to IV protamine may potentially increase the risk of protamine reaction. The presence of cross-reacting antibodies in patients with fish allergy and vasectomies has also been implicated as a risk factor for severe protamine reaction, but the evidence is limited to case reports.[88,89] Levy et al[86] did not observe any clinical reactions to protamine reversal of heparin in 16 vasectomized and 6 fish-allergic patients, or in inpatients after repeat cardiac surgical procedures. Diabetes, valvular surgery, and existing pulmonary hypertension have been suggested to be risk factors for pulmonary vasoconstriction, but the data do not support these suggestions.[86,87] In patients who have received NPH insulin previously, the presence of anti-protamine IgE- or IgG-antibodies may help to identify those at high risk for protamine reaction, and prescreening them might be worthwhile to delineate appropriate strategy for reversal of heparin anticoagulation.

Several possible methods have been proposed to prevent protamine reactions in susceptible patients (Table 5.5). Although the infusion rate may not affect IgG- or IgE- mediated anaphylactic reactions, it will attenuate responses that may depend on the concentration of free protamine and circulating heparin-protamine complexes. Therefore, a slow infusion of protamine (≤ 25 mg/min) is always advisable. The most logical approach in patients

TABLE 5.5. Approaches to prevent protamine reactions.

Established	Slow diluted infusion (<25 mg/min)
Sometimes indicated	Spontaneous decay of heparin activity
	Reheparinization (treatment of ongoing reaction)
Questionable significance, not proven, or not feasible	Prophylaxis with steroids and antihistamines
	Defibrinogenation (ancrod) instead of heparin
	Hexadimethrine
	Heparinase or immobilized protamine filters
	Left-sided injection (aorta, left atrial line)
	Prostaglandin inhibitors

with a known allergy would be to omit protamine and allow heparin to be cleared spontaneously.[90] The disadvantage of this approach is the greatly prolonged time required for chest closure and the additional blood loss, requiring potential transfusion of coagulation factors. Several groups have attempted to attenuate protamine reactions by infusing it through the left atrial line[91] or the aorta.[92,93] The results have been inconclusive, and it appears that the site of infusion is irrelevant as long as the drug is given slowly and in dilute form. Furthermore, if the patient has an antibody to protamine, the reaction will occur irrespective of how the drug is given.[94] Attempts to protect the patient pharmacologically with steroids, histamine-receptor blockers, or prostaglandin inhibitors are either not effective or have not been tested clinically.[95-97] If there is a known protamine allergy, alternatives to protamine, such as hexadrimethrine, can be considered. Heparin removal devices placed in ECC, and heparinase filters, are being developed.[98]

Protamine Dose and Administration

The most commonly used protamine protocols determine the reversal dose of protamine based on the total dose of heparin given during bypass, using a reversal ratio of 1 to 1.5 mg protamine to 100 U heparin. These methods do not account for the elimination of heparin during bypass and may result in substantial overdose of protamine. The protamine doses calculated from the heparin dose-ACT response curve,[44] heparin level measurement (heparin-protamine titration [Hemotec]),[99] or protamine dose-ACT response in vitro (Hemochron) all result in lower heparin doses.[100] Although initial neutralization of heparin with all these methods is adequate, small amounts of free heparin can be detected with chromogenic substrate assay or repeat protamine titration between 1 and 5 hours after neutralization.[33] Reduced-dose protamine protocols should be used, since they have been shown to be associated with less bleeding.[101] Heparin level measurement at the end of the bypass may be the most practical of these protocols. In the absence of heparin level measuring devices, a dose of 1 mg protamine for each 100 U heparin given before CPB will almost invariably result in complete reversal of heparin. If the blood left in the CPB circuit after decannulation is reinfused using bags, 20 to 30 mg additional protamine should be administered upon completion of the infusion to neutralize the 1000 to 2000 U of heparin present in the perfusate bags. If perfusate is washed with a cell saver, heparin should be mostly eliminated, but this method is unpredictable. Therefore, additional small protamine doses may be warranted when washed red cells from the CPB circuit are returned to the patient.

After CPB, protamine should always be administered as a dilute solution, at a rate no faster than 25 g/min. Peripheral IV infusion may further dilute free protamine and decrease the level of heparin-protamine complexes reaching the lung capillaries, and this should prevent untoward responses. As is the case with heparin administration, all members of the cardiac surgical team should be fully aware that protamine has been started. It is very important that no blood be returned from the operative field to the CPB machine after the start of protamine infusion, since only small amounts of protamine are needed to cause clotting in the oxygenator. A femoral arterial cannula can be left in place during the first minutes of protamine administration if instability and diffuse blood loss not controllable with surgical hemostasis is anticipated. If a femoral arterial cannula has not been used, inflow may be switched to the venous cannula to provide volume support in the potentially labile patient.

The completeness of heparin reversal is assessed 5 to 10 minutes after the end of the infusion, by measuring ACT. If the ACT has not returned to baseline, heparin level measurement can also be useful in ascertaining if the dose of protamine has been sufficient. Obviously, no free heparin should be detected after protamine administration, but the sensitivity of the automated heparin level measuring device is low (>0.4 U/mL). Also, ACT will be consistently prolonged only after heparin concentrations exceeding 0.1 U/mL, and a normal ACT does not preclude the presence of a significant amount of heparin. In addition, prolongation of ACT may be caused by factors other than heparin. Heparinase, an enzyme extracted from *Heparinum falciparum*, has recently been added in lyophilized forms to ACT tubes. This will destroy all free heparin in the sample without affecting the clotting cascade. Heparinase coupled to ACT methodology seems to be a promising and practical way to uncover residual unneutralized heparin.[102]

Heparin Rebound

Heparin rebound is defined as a resurgence of anticoagulant activity in a patient who has been adequately neutralized with protamine. Variations in the reported incidence of heparin rebound may result from differences in methods used to assess heparin's effects, and widely varying protamine reversal protocols. Studies that use sensitive and specific measurement of heparin usually demonstrate increases in free heparin concentration from 1 to 5 hours after protamine administration.[33] Although various theories have been proposed, heparin rebound can probably be explained by differences in the disposition kinetics of the two drugs (Table 5.6). At the time of protamine administration, heparin is undergoing slow elimination, and protamine is rapidly distributed, degraded by proteases, and bound to the accessible heparin. The rapid disappearance of protamine will leave small amounts of heparin reappearing unbound in the circulation. Low levels of free

TABLE 5.6. Proposed mechanisms of heparin rebound.

Difference in the phase of the disposition kinetics of heparin and protamine

Heparin release from postulated storage and binding sites (red cells, connective tissue, endothelium)

Temporary neutralization of heparin with endogenous antagonists which subsequently are cleared, leaving free heparin uncovered

A naturally occurring protaminase (carboxypeptidase N) may degrade protamine

heparin that have been measured may not affect ACT; however, the thrombin time and APTT are more sensitive to low heparin levels than is the ACT.[33] On the other hand, low levels of free rebound heparin are unlikely to cause bleeding, since no convincing correlation has been demonstrated between unneutralized heparin and postoperative bleeding. In occasional patients, increased chest tube output and prolongation of ACT 2 to 3 hours after bypass may respond to additional protamine administration. It seems prudent not to withhold additional protamine in order to rule out unneutralized heparin, providing that the previously administered protamine dose does not exceed the 1 mg/100 U heparin given during the procedure. The only problem with this approach is that the search for more likely causes of bleeding may be delayed.

Effect of CPB on Hemostasis

Exposure of blood to large, foreign, nonendothelialized surfaces of the CPB circuit is the major trigger for the hemostatic derangements seen in cardiac surgical patients. Other factors, however, including hemodilution, a multitude of drugs, and hypothermia, inherently associated with cardiac surgery, undoubtedly modify the hemostatic outcome.[103] Basic understanding of primary and secondary hemostasis and the alterations in platelets and procoagulants induced by CPB (Figures 5.1 and 5.3) is essential to the appropriate management of bleeding complications after cardiac surgery. The mechanisms by which normal hemostasis is altered to produce postoperative bleeding complications will be discussed.

Hemodilution

The ECC prime and cardioplegia administration result in about 50% hemodilution, as assessed from the decrease in hematocrit and total protein content, and platelets and coagulation factor proteins are usually decreased to the same degree[104] (Figure 5.4). This reduction is compatible with normal hemostasis, since all clotting factors remain well above 30% and platelets rarely drop below 60,000/μL. Stress-related coagulation factor VIII:c and vWF may remain within normal limits, or even significantly increase, during CPB.[104-106] The other labile coagulation factor, factor V, seems to decrease more than is explained by dilution, but it remains above the stated critical value of 15% during and after CPB. Usually, all the hemostatic factors normalize within 12 hours after CPB, but the platelet count takes several days to normalize. Dilutional coagulopathy can contribute to a bleeding diathesis in a subset of patients after CPB. In pediatric patients, or in small individuals, the larger prime-to-blood-volume ratio may result in critical decreases in platelets and coagulation factors, requiring transfusions to correct the deficiencies. In addition to passive dilutional effects, prime composition may also impact hemostasis. Accordingly, after high-molecular-weight hydroxyethyl starch (HMW-HES) was used in the CPB prime, factor VIII:c and vWF were significantly lower than after plain Ringer's solution was used in the prime. There were also signs of decreased coagulability, as assessed by thromboelastogram, and increased need for reoperations because of bleeding after HMW-HES priming.[107]

Activation of Hemostatic Cascades on ECC Surfaces

Platelets

When blood interfaces with artificial surfaces of the ECC, proteins are absorbed on the blood-surface interface.[108] This protein film consists largely of conformationally altered fibrinogen that increases platelet adhesion to the surface. Once the shear forces are overcome and platelet surface contact is established, the activation sequence of platelets is initiated (Figure 5.3). As bypass continues, albumin partly displaces fibrinogen, and platelet affinity to the surface is reduced.[109] In a simulated CPB model, albumin precoating of the circuit preserved platelet function.[110] In addition to circuit-blood interface, heparin in the high concentrations needed to suppress coagulation during CPB may be responsible for the loss of platelet function (heparin-induced thrombocytopenia [HIT]).[30]

Multiple factors, and circulating agonists that include thrombin, adenosine disphosphate (ADP), and epinephrine may contribute to the observed platelet activation during CPB. Thrombin activity that is heparin resistant can be measured during CPB.[111] ADP concentration in the plasma may be increased because of hemolysis.[112] Epinephrine concentrations increase when the stress response is exacerbated by hypothermia and nonpulsatile flow.[113] Hypothermia alone can also activate platelets, as shown in experimental baboon models.[104] The mechanism may be related to impaired thromboxane A_2 synthesis in hypothermia.[114]

Platelets undergo morphologic changes consistent with activation during CPB, as demonstrated by elevated levels of the biochemical indicators of platelet activation, includ-

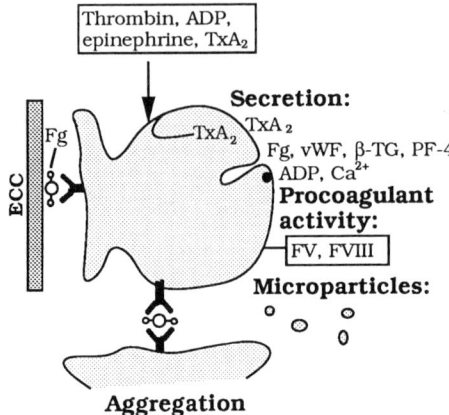

FIGURE 5.3. Schematic drawing of platelet activation during CPB. Artificial surfaces and the conformationally altered macromolecules deposited on them can directly activate platelets. The constitutive glycoprotein receptors for fibrinogen on platelet surface exposed with platelet activation may facilitate platelet immobilization. Circulating agonists may amplify platelet activation. When activated, platelets are changed from discoid to spherical shape with pseudopods. Thromboxane A_2 is generated from membrane phopholipids and diffuses out of platelets and amplifies platelet activation. The contents of the platelet specific granules are released and platelets bind procoagulants on their surface, greatly accelerating the conversion of factor X to factor Xa and prothrombin to thrombin. GpIIb/IIIa, fibrinogen receptor; GbIb, von Willebrand receptor; ECC, extracorporeal circuit; TxA_2, thromboxane A_2; Fg, fibrinogen; vWF, von Willebrandt factor; β-TG, β-thromboglobulin; PF-4, platelet factor 4; ADP, adenosine diphosphate; FV and FVIII, factors V and VIII.

ing platelet factor 4 (PF-4), β-thromboglobulin (β-TG), and thromboxane B_2 in plasma and/or urine.[104,114] Although the exact mechanism(s) of reversible platelet dysfunction after CPB has not been elucidated, platelets may be in a "refractory state" similar to that observed after ADP stimulation in vitro.[112] Studies that include nonhuman primates, in vitro ECC circuits with human blood, and clinical CPB also suggest that prevention of platelet activation by the infusion of prostaglandin E_1, prostacyclin, or Iloprost preserves platelet function.[115-119]

The oxygenator, a large blood-to-surface area, represents a major site of the platelet activation that occurs during bypass.[109,120] Other sites with large contact areas and stagnant, nonlaminar flow areas, including the venous reservoir and the arterial line filter, may also contribute to platelet activation.[121,122] In vitro comparisons suggest a difference in the way platelets are handled in membrane oxygenators as compared to bubble oxygenators.[109,123,124] In vivo with membrane oxygenators, the initial rapid decrease in the platelet count is partially reversed with time; however, with bubble oxygenators, no recovery is observed, but a constant slow decrease in platelet count occurs throughout CPB.[125-127] Attempts to prevent platelet activation with prostaglandin E_1 were only partially effective using bubble oxygenators, suggesting that platelets undergo direct injury by blood-air interfaces.[124] Clinical studies that compare membrane and bubble oxygenators largely have failed to demonstrate differences in postoperative blood loss and bleeding.[127-129] These comparative studies have evaluated only the patients with relatively short CPB times; the difference between the oxygenators in terms of blood loss and bleeding may become relevant during longer CPB runs, as suggested by one study.[130]

CPB-induced platelet dysfunction has also been attributed to the temporary depletion of the constitutive glycoproteins (Gp) that form the receptors on the platelet surface.[131] Platelet glycoproteins are responsible for bridging platelets to the site of the injury (adhesion), binding to each other (cohesion or aggregation), and binding circulating platelet agonists. The decrease in GpIb (von Willebrand receptors),[132,133] GpIIb/IIIa (fibrinogen receptors),[134] and α_2-adrenergic receptors[135] has been documented. Mechanical factors, such as shear stress, surface adherence, and turbulence, may explain the fragmentation of platelet membranes.[131] The activation sequence of platelets includes conformational changes in their membranes, allowing expression of Gp receptor activity. Using monoclonal antibodies with fluorescent probes directed

5. Hemostasis and Cardiopulmonary Bypass

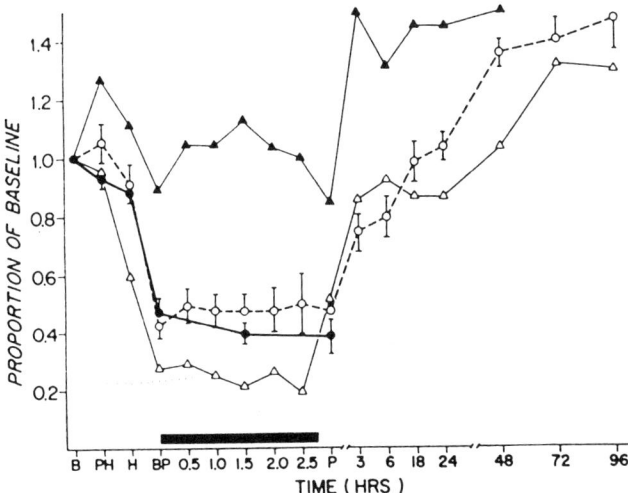

FIGURE 5.4. Changes in coagulation during cardiopulmonary bubble oxygenator bypass. Nonblood prime in the extracorporeal oxygenator bypass dilutes the red cells and albumin to about half (●). Circulating fibrinogen levels (○) are similarly decreased by dilution. Coagulation factor V (△) is reduced in excess of dilution, and factor VIII (▲) levels are relatively unaffected by dilution. Clotting factor levels return to baseline values or above 12 h after CPB. Horizontal solid bar indicates period of bypass. (From Harker LA et al,[104] by permission of *Blood*.)

against GpIIb/IIIa receptors, flow cytometry receptor binding was detected after 1 hour of CPB in both platelets and in platelet-derived microparticles.[136] The importance of GpIIb/IIIa receptor in mediating CPB-induced platelet dysfunction is suggested by a recent observation that the glycoprotein antagonist of this receptor (Ro 44-9883) was shown to reverse the decrease in platelet count and prolongation of bleeding time in a canine CPB model.[137]

Platelet-derived GpIIIa can also be recovered from detergent washings of the CPB circuit.[134] After fragmentation and adherence, following CPB, platelets may re-enter the circulation with reduced quantities of surface receptors. Proteolytic activity after plasmin generation and leukocyte activation has also been proposed as a mechanism for loss of these receptor proteins. Circulating levels of either plasmin or plasmin–α_2-antiplasmin complex have not been measured in plasma during CPB, but platelets have been shown to bind plasminogen, which could generate plasmin to degrade or redistribute GpIb receptors.[138,139]

Although platelets are consistently activated by CPB, the correlation between clinical bleeding and in vitro markers of platelet activation or platelet membrane abnormalities is yet to be established. The bleeding time, as an in vivo test of platelet function, also has been shown to be a good indicator of CPB-induced platelet dysfunction[104] (Figure 5.5). Bleeding times disproportionately prolonged beyond that predicted for the decrease in platelet count develop within minutes after starting CPB. After 2 hours of CPB, bleeding times are longer than 30 minutes; after discontinuation of CPB, bleeding times usually normalize about 15 minutes after protamine administration. Heparin is not responsible for these changes, since it causes only a modest increase in bleeding time at high doses. Bleeding time usually normalizes by 2 to 4 hours after CPB. Persistent prolongation indicates platelet dysfunction.

Contact Factors

Factor XII undergoes autocatalytic activation after it has been adsorbed on artificial surfaces of the EEC (Figure 5.1). Activated factor XII, a serine protease, in association with its cofactor, high-molecular-weight kininogen (HMWK), activates two zymogens, factor XI and prekallikrein. Activated factor XI initiates the intrinsic coagulation cascade. Kallikrein has the potential to activate kinin, fibrinolytic, and complement systems. Contact activation during CPB is only partially inhibited by heparin, which may explain the increased rate of formation of thrombin–AT-III complexes when CPB is started.[24,111] It has been shown that 70% of factor XII is converted to factor XIIa during CPB.[49] The consumptive decrease of factor XII may not be clinically significant after CPB, since alternative modes of intrinsic system activation distal to factor XII and extrinsic cascades can bypass this defect in vivo. The potential for fibrinolysis by contact activation complex will be discussed below.

Release of Procoagulants by CPB

During CPB, not all the coagulation factors are decreased by hemodilution; both factor VIII (procoagulant component factor VIII:c) and von Willebrand factor (vWF) tend to stay at or above the level measured before CPB.[104-106] An increase in the proportion of vWF high-molecular-weight multimers has also been demonstrated during CPB, further suggesting release from platelet α-granules or endothelial cells.[140] vWF promotes hemostasis by several mechanisms that include promoting platelet adhesion at endothelial surfaces to overcome the high shear stress between platelets and site of injury. It also facilitates platelet-to-platelet interaction (Figure 5.6) and protects factor VIII:c from proteolytic activity to prolong its half-life.

The ability of vWF to increase platelet adhesion may be beneficial when the concentrations increase above those known to be critical. Patients with vWF level less than 1.8 U/mL preoperatively and 1.2 U/mL postoperatively have a reported tendency toward excessive postoperative bleeding.[140] Also, Bagge et al[105] reported a statistically signifi-

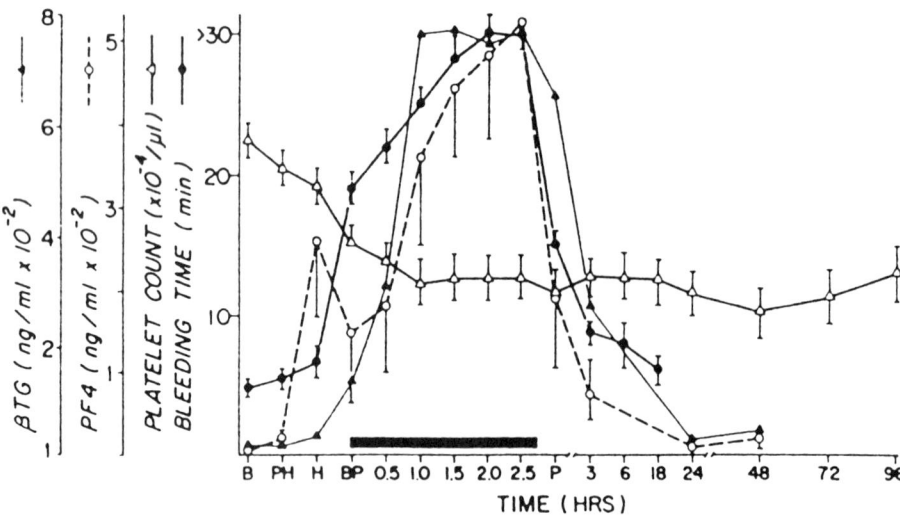

FIGURE 5.5. Changes in platelet behavior during cardiopulmonary bubble oxygenator bypass. Platelet count (△) falls progressively during the initial operative and bypass period in part due to dilution of nonblood priming solutions. Thereafter, the platelet count remains about half baseline throughout the 4-day period of observation. Bleeding time (●) is unaffected by heparinization but increases abruptly following the initiation of bypass and lengthens progressively during the first 2 h of bypass. Plasma platelet factor 4 (PF4) (○) peaks sharply after heparinization followed by a progressive rise throughout the remainder of bypass. β-Thromboglobulin (β-TG) (▲) levels rise rapidly following the initiation of bypass. Bleeding time measurements, PF4, and β-TG fall quickly after bypass. Horizontal solid bar indicates period of bypass. Means ± SEM are indicated. (From Harker LA et al,[104] by permission of *Blood*.)

cantly greater increase of vWF level after CPB and after the first 16 hours in a group of patients with "minor bleeding" (<500 mL/16 h) compared to patients with "heavy bleeding" (>800 mL/16 h). High-dose opioid anesthesia during CPB may also affect the observed vWF and factor VIII:c responses[106] (Figure 5.7). The mechanism for coagulant factor release during CPB could be triggered by hypophyseal arginine vasopressin (AVP), since it is increased in a dose-dependent manner with exogenous AVP,[141] and since the stress response of CPB releases AVP, if it is not blocked by opioids.[106] In addition to quantitative changes in vWF levels, a deficiency in high-molecular-weight monomers may be important in subgroups of cardiac surgical patients. Mechanical damage due to turbulence and proteolysis may be responsible for their reported decrease in association with aortic stenosis and in children with noncyanotic congenital heart disease.[142,143]

Consumptive Coagulopathy and Fibrinolysis

Adequate heparinization during CPB prevents clinically significant conversion of fibrinogen to fibrin. Except for factors V and XII, hemodilution explains the decreases observed in clotting factors and their inhibitors.[104,143] Other perioperative complications, such as septic or cardiogenic shock, or use of thrombolytic drugs, may cause thrombocytopenia or hypofibrinogenemia by consumptive mechanisms.

CPB can initiate fibrinolysis by different mechanisms that include contact activation of factor XII or kallikrein to generate plasmin, and stress- or surgery-mediated release of tissue-type plasminogen activator (TPA) from endothelium[144] (Figure 5.8). Both of these mechanisms may convert sufficient plasminogen to plasmin to produce systemic fibrinolysis. The capacity of endogenous fibrinolysis inhibitors seems to be exceeded during CPB because significant increases in fibrin degradation products are also observed during this time.[105,111,145] However, the peak of fibrinolysis, as assessed by euglobulin lysis time or t-PA levels, is observed within the first hour of CPB.

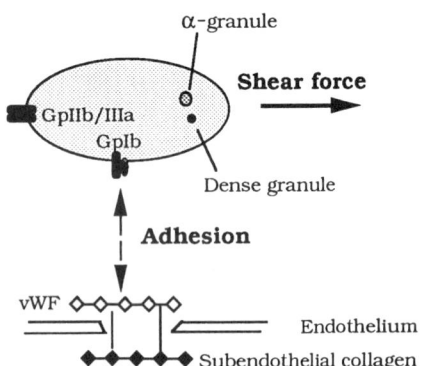

FIGURE 5.6. Role of von Willebrand factor (vWF) in promoting adhesion of platelets via glycoprotein Ib (GpIb) surface receptor on subendothelial collagen at the site of endothelial injury.

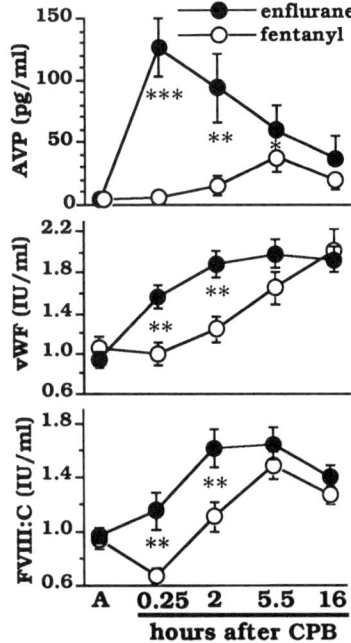

FIGURE 5.7. Plasma arginine vasopressin (AVP), von Willebrand (vWF) and procoagulant (FVIII:C) component of factor VIII after induction of anesthesia (A) and after cardiopulmonary bypass (CPB) in patients anesthesized with enflurane or fentanyl ($n = 15$ each). Anesthetics were discontinued within 2 hours after CPB. *$p < 0.05$; **$p < 0.01$; ***$p < 0.001$ enflurane vs fentanyl groups. Mean ± SEM are indicated. (By permission of Salmenpera M et al, *Anesthesiology* 1991;75: A74.)

Once the stimulus bypass run has been discontinued, fibrinolysis should rapidly subside, and fibrin degradation products should be cleared, depending on hepatic and renal function.

Current evidence suggests that *persistent* fibrinolysis is rarely the cause of bleeding after CPB. In fact, the presence of fibrin degradation products after CPB has been shown to be less than 50% predictive of which patients will hemorrhage.[146,147] Fibrinolysis during CPB, however, may inhibit platelet hemostatic function. It has been postulated, on the basis of in vitro studies, that plasminogen can bind to platelets, which may in turn act as sources of plasmin that cleaves platelet surface proteins responsible for platelet adhesion and aggregation.[139]

Abnormal Bleeding After CPB

The reported average chest drain output varies greatly from institution to institution, but upper limits reported for 16 hours (up to the first postoperative morning) in patients with primary cardiac surgery are between 800 and 1000 mL, with a hemoglobin loss of about 60 g. The drainage should decrease with time, but in the first 3 hours, anything exceeding 3 mL/kg/h should cause concern, and, after that, values over 1.5 mL/kg/h should be considered excessive. The typical chest drainage hemoglobin values should be less than 5 g/100 mL, while higher values suggest active bleeding. Chest tube output exceeding 10 mL/kg/h during the first hour and 5 mL/kg/h after that, any sudden bleeding, or signs of cardiac tamponade are all indications for a return to the operating room to locate and stop the bleeding.[148] The reoperation rate is currently

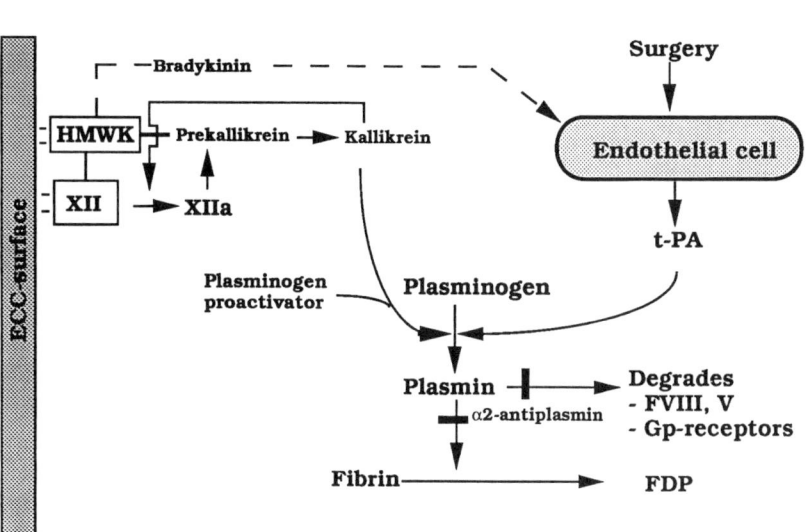

FIGURE 5.8. Scheme for fibrinolytic activation during CPB. ECC-surface, extracorporeal circuit surface; XII and XIIa, nonactivated and activated forms of factor XII; HMWK, high-molecular-weight kininogen; t-PA: tissue-type plasminogen activator; FVIII and V, factor VIII and V; Gp-receptors, glycoprotein receptors; FDP, fibrin degradation products.

reported to be about 5%.[2,3] The anatomic site of bleeding is usually found in at least half of these patients, whereas in the others, hemostatic failure is presumed to be the cause. However, if the preoperative red cell mass, based on body size, and hematocrit are not in the lower percentile ranges, and a bleeding complication does not develop, then transfusion with donor blood can often be avoided. The putative causes of bleeding after CPB are indicated in Table 5.7. The most difficult bedside diagnosis is between surgical and nonsurgical bleeding. Sudden increases in chest tube output and clotting within the drains suggest a surgical cause, whereas continuous moderate output associated with oozing from the wounds or bleeding from cutaneous sites suggest hemostatic dysfunction. The treatment should be aimed at the most likely cause. Laboratory diagnosis is likely to be of limited value, partly because of the long turnover time required. Routine clinical coagulation assays can now be performed with on-site methods using whole blood, thus circumventing the time-consuming plasma separation, but the clinical utility of these methods remains to be demonstrated.[149] The tests that might be helpful and their interpretation are listed in Table 5.8. Small deviations from normal values are almost always present after CPB, and only significant changes from baseline identify the actual cause of bleeding. Because platelet dysfunction is the most likely cause of nonsurgical bleeding, a bleeding time determination is the most informative test to be considered in cases of bleeding after CPB. It has been suggested that bleeding times will be prolonged up to 2 hours after CPB but should normalize (<9 min) after that.[104] Values exceeding 15 minutes with clinically significant bleeding call for platelet transfusions. Platelet counts should also be determined, since these will also affect bleeding times once the count falls below 100,000/μL.

Recent research in coagulation monitoring has assessed devices that measure viscoelastic changes in the clotting blood in vitro. The thromboelastogram (TEG) was developed during World War II and was introduced as an intraoperative monitor to assess the rapidly changing coagulation profile during liver transplantation.[150] Its use to detect developing hemostatic defects during surgical hemorrhage and rapid blood replacement and after CPB has also been recommended.[146,147,151,152] Routine laboratory coagulation tests examine the activity of the individual hemostatic components or their combinations in centrifuged blood fractions. Viscoelastic measurements have been used to evaluate the interaction of the coagulation cascades and platelet surfaces and may provide information about decreasing clot strength over time, a phenomenon that may be associated with fibrinolysis in vivo. The viscoelastic changes in the forming clot are detected by impedance caused by a clot either on a rapidly oscillating probe (Sonoclot^R) or between the rotatory cuvette and a piston (thromboelastography). In both systems, the impedance is transformed to an analog pattern to form a characteristic viscoelastic "signature," indicating the beginning of clot formation, maximum clot strength, and possible dissolution over time.

Data demonstrating the usefulness of viscoelastic monitoring in cardiac surgical patients are limited. Increased bleeding (>1 mL/kg/h) and abnormal TEG profile were shown to be associated in 80% of the bleeding episodes.[147] The predictive accuracy of routine coagulation tests, including ACT, prothrombin time (PT), PTT, platelet count, and fibrinogen concentration, was about 50%. Unfortunately, bleeding time determinations were not included because "standard" coagulation tests are already known to be of very limited value in diagnostic or therapeutic decisions, and therefore no definitive conclusions as to the role of the usefulness of TEG in the diagnostic evaluation of surgical or nonsurgical bleeding can be made. Although characteristic TEG patterns can be produced in nonsurgical patients with coagulation abnormalities that include hemophilia, thrombocytopenia, and fibrinolysis, these data cannot be directly extrapolated to a very different hemostatic defect induced by CPB. Current attempts to direct therapy with specific blood fractions and hemostatic agents, using information provided by viscoelastic signatures, lack scientific grounding.

Patients at Risk for Bleeding After CPB

The frequency of detecting a previously unrecognized inherited factor or platelet defect before cardiac surgery is low, but the catastrophic consequences of bleeding in these patients mandate the recording of a careful bleeding history in every patient scheduled for open-heart surgery. Frequent nosebleeds and easy bruisability are nonspecific complaints that have a very low predictive value. However, adequate hemostasis after common surgical procedures, such as tooth extraction or tonsillectomy, virtually excludes a significant inherited hemostatic defect. Platelet

TABLE 5.7. Causes of excessive bleeding after CPB.

Probable
    Local bleeding site
    Acquired platelet dysfunction
Possible
    Preoperative drug-induced hemostatic dysfunction (aspirin, warfarin)
    Preoperative hemostatic dysfunction attributable to associated disease (uremia, hepatic failure)
    Inherited hemostatic dysfunction (von Willebrand disease, platelet defect)
    DIC (sepsis, low-output state)
    Primary fibrino(geno)lysis
    Dilutional coagulopathy and thrombocytopenia
Unlikely
    Free heparin (unneutralized and rebound)
    Protamine overdose

TABLE 5.8. Common laboratory tests for hemostatic function after cardiac surgery.

Test	Abnormal value (after CPB)	Comment
Platelets		
Platelet count	$<60,000/\mu L$	Very low values: DIC, HIT?
Bleeding time	>15 min	Not feasible in the operating room; unreliable in hypothermic and poorly perfused skin sites
Coagulation system		
ACT (activated clotting time)	$>$ baseline	Heparin effect?; very insensitive to hemostatic defects
PTT (partial thromboplastin time)	$>1.5 \times$ baseline	Heparin effect?; intrinsic or common pathway defect
PT (prothrombin time)	$>1.5 \times$ baseline	Extrinsic or common pathway defect
TT (thrombin time)	>17 s	Heparin effect, hypofibrinogenemia
Fibrinogen	<100 mg/dL	DIC, fibrinolysis?
Fibrinolytic system		
D-dimers	>200 μg/mL	Trend important: persistently high or increasing values suggest ongoing fibrinolysis
Euglobulin lysis time	<2 h	Low values may be common immediately after CPB

count, PT, PTT, and template bleeding time are usually ordered as a preoperative evaluation of hemostasis. Although the yield of these tests is likely to be low, they can detect major coagulation disorders and provide baseline values in the event of postoperative bleeding complications. In patients with a previous history of a bleeding disorder, hematologic consultation is mandatory, and additional tests, such as urea clot lysis (factor XIII screen), whole blood clot lysis, α_2-antiplasmin determination, factor VIII-IX assays, and platelet aggregation, may be needed. With appropriate replacement therapy planned, CPB can be successfully performed in most patients with hemophilias or other inherited deficiencies of hemostasis.[103] A carefully planned strategy and full support of hematology and transfusion medicine is essential for successful patient management.

Preoperative cardiac status, associated diseases, and drug therapies may also produce an acquired hemostatic defect in the cardiac surgical patient. Severe congestion of the liver, produced by biventricular failure, may result in a deficiency of prothrombin complex production. Preoperative coumadin therapy also decreases the vitamin K-dependent factors. Uremia is associated with multiple defects in hemostasis.[153] The list of drugs affecting platelet function is long, and although many of these drugs are administered during the perioperative period, they are of minimal concern at the concentrations likely to be used in vivo.[109] Aspirin irreversibly acetylates platelet cyclooxygenase-blocking thromboxane A_2 formation from platelet membrane and endothelial cell phospholipids. Thromboxane A_2 acts as an intracellular mediator of the events associated with platelet release reaction, and also acts as a powerful agonist for platelet aggregation and promotes local vasoconstriction. Inhibiting thromboxane A_2 generation produces a defect in primary hemostasis. Platelets, unlike endothelial cells, cannot synthesize cyclooxygenase to generate thromboxane A_2 de novo, and the effect on cyclooxygenase persists for the life span of the affected platelets. Most, but not all, of the existing clinical studies show that preoperative aspirin therapy significantly increases blood loss and transfusion requirements in cardiac surgery.[154-159] If possible, aspirin therapy should be discontinued at least 5 days before the planned operation, although postponing the surgery is often not feasible due to the presence of unstable angina.

Patients receiving thrombolytic therapy are also at increased risk for postoperative bleeding. Reocclusion and/or cardiogenic shock may complicate thrombolytic therapy for acute evolving myocardial infarction in about 15% of patients.[160,161] Thus, a significant number of these patients may require emergency coronary artery bypass graft (CABG). Besides the effects on fibrin clot, thrombolysis causes proteolytic destruction of factor V, factor VIII, and fibrinogen.[162] Also, high levels of fibrin degradation products interfere with fibrin polymerization and decrease platelet function. It has also been suggested that circulating plasmin may impair platelet function by destroying GpIb and GpIIb/IIIa receptors on platelet surfaces.[162] In patients who have had thrombolytic therapy, the added insult of CPB can increase bleeding. In a series of patients receiving streptokinase therapy and requiring emergency CABG, all need FFP and platelets.[160] In the postoperative period, fibrinogen level and fibrin degradation products were already normalized in most of the patients, suggesting that the hemostatic defect was primarily a sequela of fibrinolysis before and during CPB. Perioperative bleeding may be less of a problem after thrombolysis with fibrin-specific recombinant TPA (r-TPA) than after streptokinase, based on preliminary reports.[161] Excessive bleeding and increased transfusion requirements were observed in two of 24 patients undergoing emergency CABG after unsuccessful thrombolysis with r-TPA. Since, in the postoperative period, fibrinolysis has already subsided, therapy with coagulation factors may be the rational therapy for bleeding after CABG and failed thrombolysis.

Not all cardiac surgical procedures carry the same risk of bleeding. Repeat sternotomies are associated with increased bleeding because of dissection of vascularized adhesions. Although one-sided internal mammary artery use has not been shown to cause increased bleeding, bilateral implantations do increase transfusion requirements.[163]

Treatment of Bleeding

Although the therapeutic options overlap, attempts to prevent and to treat bleeding and hemostatic defect after bypass should be considered separately. Prophylactic therapy should not be used in uncomplicated primary cardiac surgery because 50% to 80% of patients having cardiac surgery for the first time can now be managed without autologous transfusions. Proven efficacy of controlled studies to decrease blood loss and transfusion requirements is needed before application of prophylactic hemostatic therapies. The side effects and the costs incurred are factors that should also be considered in the decision to use prophylactic therapies.

Prophylactic Transfusions

Considering the risks of transmittable diseases and allergic complications, there is no rationale for attempts to circumvent bleeding problems with prophylactic transfusions. Prophylactic random administration of donor platelets, FFP, or cryoprecipitate has not been shown to reduce postoperative bleeding significantly.[164,165] Although fresh whole blood transfusions were effective in decreasing bleeding after cardiac surgery in two studies from the same institution,[166,167] their use may be indicated only for special situations, such as pediatric open-heart surgery.[168]

The ability of fresh whole blood and platelets to control bleeding is the rationale for the removal of autologous blood before bypass, and its retransfusion after heparin neutralization, to salvage part of the functional platelet population from the damaging effects of CPB. Two methods of harvesting fresh autologous blood units have been described. Blood can be collected, after anesthesia induction, through central venous cannulas in the standard blood bags containing citrate as anticoagulant,[169] or it may be removed just before CPB from the venous cannulas.[170] Collecting blood after induction of anesthesia may precipitate hemodynamic instability. Also, studies show that platelet count is better augmented when blood is removed just before CPB. Using perioperative autologous blood withdrawal and retransfusion, homologous blood requirements have been shown to be reduced by 20% to 50%.[169-171] However, two studies failed to demonstrate any significant benefit of autologous blood withdrawal.[172,173] Removal of one to two units of autologous blood from the venous line before CPB appears warranted, but only if the patient has an elevated hematocrit and a large body surface area.

Perioperative platelet removal with plasmapheresis has been described recently as an attempt to "rescue" part of the platelet population and coagulation factors from the damaging effects of CPB. Increased platelet numbers after CPB, and small but statistically significant decreases in blood loss, have been demonstrated in two limited clinical studies.[174,175] This technique requires placement of an additional large-bore catheter (7.5 to 8.5F). More extensive clinical studies are needed before definite conclusions can be drawn regarding this technique.

Pharmacologic Prophylaxis of Bleeding

Aprotinin

Aprotinin is a naturally occurring polypeptide of 58 amino acids with a molecular weight of 6512 daltons, which reversibly complexes with the active serine site of multiple plasma proteases to inhibit the serine proteases, trypsin, kallikrein, plasmin, and elastase.[176] It has been used in the treatment of pancreatitis, shock, and fibrinolysis for over 30 years. Initial studies with aprotinin using bolus injections *after* CPB showed no obvious benefit with respect to bleeding.[177,178] Royston[60] designed a technique using loading doses prior to CPB, and in the CPB circuit, with an infusion of aprotinin to maintain kallikrein inhibition in cardiac surgical patients throughout their surgery. This technique, in repeat cardiac surgical patients, produced strikingly reduced postoperative blood loss in 11 aprotinin-treated patients: 286 mL compared to 1509 mL in the 11 control patients.[60] Seven of the 11 aprotinin-treated patients received no banked blood, whereas all control patients had to be transfused with homologous blood. These impressive results have been confirmed in primary and repeat CABG.[133,179-183] Additional results suggest the benefit of aprotinin in certain subgroups at risk for increased bleeding and consequent exposure to donor blood, including patients on aspirin therapy,[184,185] those with ineffective endocarditis[179] or renal failure,[184] and pediatric cardiac surgical patients.[186,187] One practical finding of the aprotinin studies is that oozing from the operative wounds stops more easily after CPB is discontinued, allowing rapid chest closure and a shorter time in the operating room.[187]

The recommended dose of aprotinin is 2 million U administered as a loading dose over 30 minutes, followed by an infusion of 500,000 U/h thereafter throughout the surgery. To compensate for the CPB circuit dilution, a dose of 2 million U is added to the prime. Conspicuous antiprotease activity can be expected for several hours, since the elimination half-life of aprotinin is about 7 hours.[188]

The mechanism by which aprotinin reduces bleeding after CPB remains unclear. Aprotinin is a potent antifibrinolytic agent. Both the propagation of the "intrinsic" fibrinolysis through factor XII–mediated kallikrein activation and the generation of plasmin through "extrinsic" or TPA-mediated activation of plasminogen are effectively inhibited by approximately 4 μmol/L of aprotinin, which is maintained in plasma with the presently recommended infusion regimens.[179]

Although aprotinin therapy was associated with reduced levels of fibrin split products after CPB, transient fibrinolytic activity was still demonstrable after CPB in a similar proportion of aprotinin and control patients.[180] Inhibition of the fibrinolytic digestion of formed fibrin, circulating fibrinogen, or factor VIII may be a contributing, but not the sole, mechanism of the beneficial effect of aprotinin. Aprotinin is reported to attentuate both the increase in bleeding time after CPB[132,179,180] and the loss of platelet membrane GpIb during CPB.[132] These platelet effects theoretically could be mediated by inhibition of plasmin activity on platelet surfaces by aprotinin during CPB. All the above mechanisms remain speculative, but unraveling them could provide important clues to the acquired platelet defect associated with CPB.

Aprotinin accumulates in proximal renal tubular epithelium.[189] Increased potassium-sparing urine output has been found after high-dose aprotinin, but plasma creatinine, urea, and creatinine clearance have been unchanged.[182] Only minimal data are available on the effects of aprotinin on patients with renal failure, but this does not necessarily represent a contraindication for aprotinin.[184] Anaphylaxis after aprotinin administration has been reported almost exclusively in patients with previous exposure.[190] European patients with previous pancreatitis, for example, are likely to have received aprotinin. In *all* patients, however, a small IV test dose must be given before the loading dose is started.

Aprotinin alone does not affect ACT, but it does cause a distinct potential heparin dose–ACT response.[191] This increase in ACT may be related to aprotinin's effects on the initial steps of the intrinsic coagulation cascade, or it may be only an in vitro effect that may be particularly pronounced with celite, but not with kaolin, as an activator.[192] Subclinical coagulation during CPB, as demonstrated by the level of formed thrombin–AT-III complexes, was shown to occur to a similar degree in aprotinin-treated and control patients.[181] Thus, one must be careful not to decrease heparin doses in patients receiving aprotinin. Instead, it may be prudent to dose heparin using heparin level monitoring or a higher than usual ACT target (eg, 750 to 800).[193]

Although the opinion that aprotinin usage in cardiac surgery results in important blood savings is now almost unanimous, its routine use has been hampered by the cost and fears that aprotinin use may result in a prothrombotic state. These fears were sparked by Gosgrove and colleagues[194] who reported an apparent aprotinin dose-related increase (albeit statistically nonsignificant) in Q-wave myocardial infarctions in patients undergoing myocardial revascularizations. Also, an alarming incidence of thrombus formation in multiple organs and renal failure was found in a small retrospective series of patients undergoing aortic surgery using cardiopulmonary bypass and hypothermic circulatory arrest.[195] The interpretation of these studies is complicated by the fact that they both used conventional ACT values for heparin dosing, and this could have led to underheparinization in the patients receiving aprotinin. Murkin and colleagues[185] did not observe an increase in infarction rate attributable to aprotinin in patients receiving aprotinin and undergoing cardiac operations. Two studies seem to refute the speculations that aprotinin use may be associated with a decreased patency rate of bypass grafts.[183,196] The statistical power in these two studies may, however, be insufficient, and larger materials should be available before definitive conclusions.

The currently available data and European experience suggest that aprotinin is indicated in repeat cardiac surgical procedures and in other subsets of patients at high risk for CPB-related bleeding. Its use to minimize exposure to donor blood in primary elective cardiac surgery may prove to be feasible, but the results of studies addressing the effects on aprotinin of graft patency should be on hand before it is incorporated into routine management protocols.

Antifibrinolytic Agents

The synthetic lysine analogue ϵ-aminocaproic acid (EACA; Amicar) inhibits fibrinolysis by attaching to the lysine binding site of the plasmin(ogen) molecule, displacing plasminogen from fibrin. Evidence of the beneficial hemostatic effect of EACA is anecodotal or derived mostly from studies that have been uncontrolled and retrospective.[197] However, three controlled studies using prophylactic administration of EACA during CPB have been performed.[198-200] A significant benefit in terms of blood loss was observed in pediatric cardiac surgical patients with cyanotic defects and in those with CPB times exceeding 60 minutes.[199] Two subsequent studies performed in adult patients undergoing CABG showed a modest (less than 20%) decrease in blood loss.[198,200] Tranexamic acid (AMCA, Cyclocapron), a longer-acting antifibrinolytic, has also been evaluated for CPB-related bleeding in a recent randomized study, with results essentially similar to those described with EACA.[201]

The benefits observed do not support the routine use of prophylactic EACA or AMCA to improve hemostasis after CPB. Although arterial and venous thrombosis are complications associated with antifibrinolytic therapy with EACA, they have not been conclusively identified in patients after CPB, except for two possible cases of EACA-related perioperative myocardial infarctions.[200] The proposed role of fibrinolysis in the development of hemostatic defect during CPB justifies further clinical trials in which EACA or AMCA is administered, maintaining effective blood levels from beginning to end of surgery.

Desmopressin Acetate

1-Deamino-8-D-arginine vasopressin (desmopressin or acetate, DDAVP) administration improves hemostasis in patients with mild hemophilia A and von Willebrand disease.[202] These improvements are mediated by the ability of DDAVP to release vWF from storage sites, presumably in endothelium. Salzman et al[203] were the first to perform a double-blind randomized trial of DDAVP administration in patients undergoing valvular or repeat CABG surgery. They demonstrated a significant reduction in blood loss (900 mL/24 h) but not significantly reduced transfusion requirements. Also, the very high blood loss experienced by the control group has brought into question the general applicability of the results of the study. Another study of prophylactic DDAVP administration showed that intraoperative blood loss before chest closure was reduced, but that overall blood loss was not affected.[204] Subsequently, at least seven other controlled studies with a total of 381 patients have compared DDAVP with placebo in the prophylaxis of bleeding after CPB.[205-211] All failed to show any benefit of DDAVP administration, and there was little effect on the hemostatic parameters. Measured vWF responses to 0.3 μg/kg of DDAVP were either absent or only increased by about 50% as compared with a twofold to threefold increase in vWF concentrations in awake volunteers.[202-205] The attenuated vWF response to DDAVP after CPB may be analogous to that observed after repeated DDAVP administration, and may be related to the storage sites depleted during CPB by endogenous stress mediators. Although the decrease in platelet adhesion represents one part of platelet dysfunction after CPB, the defect may be due more often to the decrease in platelet surface GpIb receptors that bind vWF than to the insufficient level of vWF. Contrary to what was originally believed, the side effects of DDAVP administration can also be significant.

Severe vasodilation producing hypotension requiring vasopressors is observed in many patients, in spite of the recommended slow infusion rate of 0.3 μg/kg for 15 to 20 minutes.[210,211] Hypotension has been suggested to be mediated via vascular vasopressin-2 (V2) receptors or via prostacyclin release. Prophylactic administration of DDAVP is inadvisable after CPB, since the side effects are potentially dangerous and therapeutic benefit is highly unlikely.

Transfusion Therapy

Platelet transfusions are almost always indicated for the treatment of excessive bleeding after bypass when surgical causes have been excluded. The major hemostatic problem after CPB is a platelet functional defect, and this will contribute to bleeding, if it is not solely responsible for it. The response to platelet transfusions should be evaluated by platelet count. The appropriate starting "dose" of platelets is 1 U/10 kg. Platelet counts should be measured before and after transfusion. Typically, one unit of random donor platelets, in the absence of consumption, should increase the platelet count by 5000 to 10,000/μL. Repeated bleeding time determinations and potentially viscoelastic measurements of platelet-fibrin interaction are probably more appropriate as guides to transfusion requirements. Regardless of platelet counts, platelets are indicated for a bleeding patient if bleeding time is prolonged over 15 minutes.[104] Human lymphocyte antigen (HLA)-compatible plateletapheresis units may be needed in patients with alloantibody formation during previous platelet transfusions.

Fresh frozen plasma is not indicated as an initial therapy for bleeding after CPB and should be reserved for patients having specific indications for it. The most commonly encountered problem in the cardiac surgical patient is the acquired deficiency of vitamin K–dependent coagulation factors, caused by preoperative coumadin therapy or liver failure. Substantial blood loss with multiple red cell unit transfusions may, however, require the use of FFP to compensate for the dilutional effect. Cryoprecipitate may be needed as a source of factor VIII and fibrinogen in patients after failed thrombolysis and in those rare cases of disseminated intravascular coagulation (DIC) that develop after cardiac surgery.

Summary

Pharmacologic Therapy of Bleeding

Drugs play a minor role in the therapy of *ongoing* bleeding after CPB. Only anecdotal and uncontrolled clinical data are available. Since blood pressure is a factor promoting diffuse bleeding, its control—or at least an aggressive approach to hypertensive episodes—may be the most reliable way to lessen chest drainage.[212] Some bleeding patients may respond to DDAVP administration. Czer and colleagues[3] used desmopressin in lieu of transfusion therapy in patients with excessive ongoing bleeding after CPB. Although significant reductions in bleeding time, chest drainage, and requirements for red cells and platelets were claimed, comparisons were made to historical controls in the same institution. Consequently, observer and treatment bias is unavoidable, and the extent to which DDAVP was responsible for the beneficial trend is difficult to determine. If the decision to use DDAVP is made, one should be prepared to deal with the hypotension that may be caused by DDAVP-induced vasodilation or hypovolemia in this situation. There are, however, less theoretical grounds for attempting to control bleeding with antifibrinolytics after CPB. Significantly shortened euglobulin lysis time or TEG tracing compatible with fibrinolysis should be documented before the decision is made to use antifibrinolytics after cardiac surgery. If they are used, DIC, although rarely associated with CPB, should be ruled out, since an active fibrinolytic system may be lifesaving in that condition. Since preparation of hemostatic blood fractions always requires significant turnout time, a trial with DDAVP or antifibrinolytics may be considered, but it should not be allowed to delay the institution of effective therapies, which will most likely be surgical re-exploration or infusion of platelet concentrates.

References

1. Ellison N, Jobes DR. *Effective Hemostasis in Cardiac Surgery*. Philadelphia: WB Saunders Company; 1988:195–201.
2. Wasser MNJM, Houbiers JGA, D'Amaro J, et al. The effect of fresh versus stored blood on post-operative bleeding after coronary bypass surgery: a prospective randomized study. *Br J Haematol* 1989;72:81–84.
3. Czer LSC, Bateman TM, Gray RJ, et al. Treatment of severe platelet dysfunction and hemorrhage after cardiopulmonary bypass: reduction in blood product usage with desmopressin. *J Am Coll Cardiol* 1987;9:1139–1147.
4. Cosgrove DM, Loop FD, Lytle BW, et al. Determinants of blood utilization during myocardial revascularization. *Ann Thorac Surg* 1985;40:380–384.
5. Culliford AT, Cunningham JN, Zeff RH, et al. Sternal and costochondral infections following open-heart surgery. *J Thorac Cardiovasc Surg* 1976;72:714–726.
6. Ebeling F, Naukkarinen R, Hanhela R, et al. Post-transfusion hepatitis after open-heart surgery in Finland—a prospective study. *Trans Med* 1991;1:103–108.
7. Hoyos M, Sarrion JV, Perez-Castellanos T, et al. Prospective assessment of donor blood screening for antibody to hepatitis B core antigen as a means of preventing posttransfusion non-A, non-B, hepatitis. *Hepatology* 1989;9:449–451.
8. Walker RH. Special report: transfusion risks. *Am J Clin Pathol* 1987;88:374–378.
9. Czer LSC. Mediastinal bleeding after cardiac surgery: etiologies, diagnostic considerations, and blood conservation methods. *J Cardiothorac Anesth* 1989;6:760–775.
10. McLean J. The thromboblastic action of cephalin. *Am J Physiol* 1916;41:250–257.
11. Brinkhous KM, Smith HP, Warner ED, et al. The inhibition of blood clotting: an unidentified substance which acts in conjunction with heparin to prevent the conversion of prothrombin into thrombin. *Am J Physiol* 1939;125:683–687.
12. Abildgaard U. Highly purified antithrombin III with heparin cofactor activity prepared by disc electrophoresis. *Scand J Clin Lab Invest* 1968;21:89–91.
13. Höök M, Björk I, Hopwood J, et al. Anticoagulant activity of heparin: separation of high-activity and low-activity heparin species by affinity chromatography on immobilized antithrombin. *FEBS Lett* 1976;66:90–93.
14. Choay J, Lormeau J-C, Petitou M, et al. Structural studies on a biologically active hexasaccharide obtained from heparin. *Ann NY Acad Sci* 1981;370:644–649.
15. Boldt J, Zickmann B, Ballesteros M, et al. Does the preparation of heparin influence anticoagulation during cardiopulmonary bypass? *J Cardiothorac Vasc Anesth* 1991;5:449–453.
16. de Swart CAM, Nijmeyer B, Roelofs JMM, et al. Kinetics of intravenously administered heparin in normal humans. *Blood* 1982;60:1251–1258.
17. Olsson P, Lagergren H, Ek S. The elimination from plasma of intravenous heparin: an experimental study on dogs and humans. *Acta Med Scand* 1963;173:619–630.
18. Lijnen HR, Hoylaerts M, Collen D. Heparin binding properties of human histidine-rich glycoprotein: mechanism and role in the neutralization of heparin in plasma. *J Biol Chem* 1983;258:3803–3808.
19. Preissner KT, Müller-Berghaus G. Neutralization and binding of heparin by S protein/vitronectin in the inhibition of factor Xa by antithrombin III. *J Biol Chem* 1987;262:12247–12253.
20. Holt JC, Niewiarowski S. Biochemistry of α granule proteins. *Semin Hematol* 1985;22:151–163.
21. Dawes J, Smith RC, Pepper DS. The release, distribution, and clearance of human β-thromboglobulin and platelet factor 4. *Thrombosis Res* 1978;12:851–861.
22. Rosenberg RD. The heparin-antithrombin system: a natural anticoagulant mechanism. In: Colman RW, Hirsh J, Marder VJ, et al, eds. *Hemostasis and Thrombosis: Basic Principles and Clinical Practice*. 2nd ed. Philadelphia: JB Lippincott; 1987:1373–1392.
23. Pixley RA, Schapira M, Colman RW. Effect of heparin on the inactivation rate of human activated factor XII by antithrombin III. *Blood* 1985;66:198–203.
24. Dietrich W, Spannagl M, Schramm W, et al. The influence of preoperative anticoagulation on heparin response during cardiopulmonary bypass. *J Thorac Cardiovasc Surg* 1991;102:505–514.
25. Rosenberg RD. Actions and interactions of antithrombin and heparin. *N Engl J Med* 1975;292:146–151.
26. Marciniak E, Gockerman JP. Heparin-induced decrease in circulating antithrombin-III. *Lancet* 1977;2:581–584.
27. Becker RC, Corrao JM, Bovill EG, et al. Intravenous nitro-

glycerin-induced heparin resistance: a qualitative antithrombin III abnormality. *Am Heart J* 1990;119:1254–1261.
28. Routledge PA, Kitchell BB, Bjornsson TD, et al. Diazepam and n-desmethyldiazepam redistribution after heparin. *Clin Pharmacol Ther* 1980;27:528–532.
29. Salzman EW, Rosenberg RD, Smith MH, et al. Effect of heparin and heparin fractions on platelet aggregation. *J Clin Invest* 1980;65:64–73.
30. John LCH, Rees GM, Kovacs IB. Inhibition of platelet function by heparin. An etiologic factor in postbypass hemorrhage. *J Thorac Cardiovasc Surg* 1993;105:816–822.
31. King DJ, Kelton JG. Heparin-associated thrombocytopenia. *Ann Int Med* 1984;100:535–540.
32. Cimo PL, Moake JL, Weinger RS, et al. Heparin-induced thrombocytopenia: association with a platelet aggregating factor and arterial thromboses. *Am J Hematol* 1979;6:125–133.
33. Kuitunen AH, Salmenperä MT, Heinonen J, et al. Heparin rebound: a comparative study of protamine chloride and protamine sulfate in patients undergoing coronary artery bypass surgery. *J Cardiothorac Vasc Anesth* 1991;5:221–226.
34. Gravlee G, Goldsmith J, Low J, et al. Heparin sensitivity comparison of the ACT, SCT, and APTT. *Anesthesiology* 1989;71:A4.
35. Kopriva CJ. The activated coagulation time (ACT). In: Ellison N, Jobes DR, eds. *Effective Hemostasis in Cardiac Surgery*. Philadelphia: WB Saunders; 1988:155–161.
36. Hattersley PG. Activated coagulation time of the whole blood. *JAMA* 1966;196:150–154.
37. Young JA, Kisker CT, Doty DB. Adequate anticoagulation during cardiopulmonary bypass determined by activated clotting time and the appearance of fibrin monomer. *Ann Thorac Surg* 1978;26:231–240.
38. Bull BS, Huse WN, Brauer FS, et al. Heparin therapy during extracorporeal circulation. II. The use of a dose-response curve to individualize heparin and protamine dosage. *J Thorac Cardiovasc Surg* 1975;69:685–689.
39. Esposito RA, Culliford AT, Colvin SB, et. Heparin resistance during cardiopulmonary bypass. The role of heparin pretreatment. *J Thorac Cardiovasc Surg* 1983;85:346–353.
40. Cloyd GM, D'Ambra MN, Akins CW. Diminished anticoagulant response to heparin in patients undergoing coronary artery bypass grafting. *J Thorac Cardiovasc Surg* 1987;94:535–538.
41. Umlas J, Taff RH, Gauvin G, et al. Anticoagulant monitoring and neutralization during open heart surgery—a rapid method for measuring heparin and calculating safe reduced protamine doses. *Anesth Analg* 1983;62:1095–1099.
42. Hughes DR, Faust RJ, Didisheim P, et al. Heparin monitoring during cardiopulmonary bypass in man: use of fluorogenic heparin assay to validate activated clotting time. *Anesth Analg* 1982;61:189–190.
43. Stoney WS, Alford WC, Burrus GR, et al. Air embolism and other accidents using pump oxygenators. *Ann Thorac Surg* 1980;29:336–340.
44. Cardoso PFG, Yamazaki F, Keshavjee S, et al. A reevaluation of heparin requirements for cardiopulmonary bypass. *J Thorac Cardiovasc Sug* 1991;101:153–160.
45. Metz S, Keats AS. Low activated coagulation time during cardiopulmonary bypass does not increase postoperative bleeding. *Ann Thorac Surg* 1990;49:440–444.
46. Gravlee GP, Haddon WS, Rothberger HK, et al. Heparin dosing and monitoring for cardiopulmonary bypass. A comparison of techniques with measurement of subclinical plasma coagulation. *J Thorac Cardiovasc Surg* 1990;99:518–527.
47. Sabbagh AH, Chung GKT, Shuttleworth P, et al. Fresh frozen plasma: a solution to heparin resistance during cardiopulmonary bypass. *Ann Thorac Surg* 1984;37:466–468.
48. Dietrich W, Schroll A, Göb E, et al. Improved heparin response by substitution of antithrombin III concentrate during extracorporeal circulation. *Anaesthetist* 1984;33:422–427.
49. Bick RL, Frazier BL, Saudners CR, et al. Alterations of hemostasis during cardiopulmonary bypass: the potential role of Factor XII in inducing primary fibrino(geno)lysis. *Blood* 1984;64:A926.
50. Salmenperä M, Rasi V, Mattila S. Cardiopulmonary bypass in a patient with Factor XII deficiency. *Anesthesiology* 1991;75:539–541.
51. Bell WR, Tomasulo PA, Alving BM, et al. Thrombocytopenia occurring during the administration of heparin. *Ann Int Med* 1976;85:155–160.
52. Warkentin TE, Kelton JG. Heparin-induced thrombocytopenia. *Ann U Rev Med* 1989;40:31–44.
53. Chong BH, Castaldi PA, Berndt MC. Heparin-induced thrombocytopenia: effects of rabbit IgG, and its FAB and Fc fragments on antibody-heparin-platelet interaction. *Thrombosis Res* 1989;55:291–295.
54. Pfueller SL, Weber S, Lüscher EF. Studies of the mechanism of the human platelet release reaction induced by immunologic stimuli. III. Relationship between the binding of soluble IgG aggregates to the Fc receptor and cell response in the presence and absence of plasma. *J Immunol* 1977;118:514–524.
55. Sheridan D, Carter C, Kelton JG. A diagnostic test for heparin-induced thrombocytopenia. *Blood* 1986;67:27–30.
56. Olinger GN, Hussey CV, Olive JA, Malik MI. Cardiopulmonary bypass for patients with previously documented heparin-induced platelet aggregation. *J Thorac Cardiovasc Surg* 1984;87:673–677.
57. Teasdale SJ, Zulys VJ, Mycyk T, et al. Ancrod anticoagulation for cardiopulmonary bypass in heparin-induced thrombocytopenia and thrombosis. *Ann Thorac Surg* 1989;48:712–713.
58. Doherty DC, Ortel TL, de Bruijn N, et al. "Heparin-free" cardiopulmonary bypass: first reported use of heparinoid (Org 10172) to provide anticoagulation for cardiopulmonary bypass. *Anesthesiology* 1990;73:562–565.
59. Kappa JR, Fisher CA, Todd B, et al. Intraoperative management of patients with heparin-induced thrombocytopenia. *Ann Thorac Surg* 1990;49:714–723.
60. Royston D, Bidstrup BP, Taylor KM, et al. Effect of aprotinin on need for blood transfusion after repeat open-heart surgery. *Lancet* 1987;2:1289–1291.
61. de Smet AEA, Joen MCN, van Oeveren W, et al. Increased

anticoagulation during cardiopulmonary bypass by aprotinin. *J Thorac Cardiovasc Surg* 1990;100:520-527.
62. Longmore DB, Bennett G, Gueirrara D, et al. Prostacyclin: a solution to some problems of extracorporeal circulation. Experiments in greyhounds. *Lancet* 1979;1:1002-1005.
63. Walker ID, Davidson JF, Faichney A, et al. A double blind study of prostacyclin in cardiopulmonary bypass surgery. *Br J Haematol* 1981;49:415-423.
64. Aren C, Feddersen K, Ra'degran K. Effects of prostacyclin infusion on platelet activation and postoperative blood loss in coronary bypass. *Ann Thorac Surg* 1983;36:49-54.
65. Malpass TW, Amory DW, Harker LA, et al. The effect of prostacyclin infusion on platelet hemostatic function in patients undergoing cardiopulmonary bypass. *J Thorac Cardiovasc Surg* 1984;87:550-555.
66. Fish KJ, Sarnquist FH, van Steennis C, et al. A prospective, randomized study of the effects of prostacyclin on platelets and blood loss during coronary bypass operations. *J Thorac Cardiovasc Surg* 1986;91:436-442.
67. Bindslev L, Guoda I, Inacio J, et al. Extracorporeal elimination of carbon dioxide using a surface-heparinized venovenous bypass system. *Trans Am Soc Artif Intern Organs* 1986;32:530-533.
68. Videm V, Mollnes TE, Garred P, et al. Biocompatibility of extracorporeal circulation. In vitro comparison of heparin-coated and uncoated oxygenator circuits. *J Thorac Cardiovasc Surg* 1991;101:654-660.
69. Diehl JT, Payne DD, Rastegar H, et al. Arterial bypass of the descending thoracic aorta with the BioMedicus centrifugal pump. *Ann Thorac Surg* 1987;44:422-423.
70. von Segesser LK, Weiss BM, Garcia E, et al. Reduction and elimination of systemic heparinization during cardiopulmonary bypass. *J Thorac Cardiovasc Surg* 1992;103:790-799.
71. Jorpes E, Edman P, Thaning T. Neutralization of action of heparin by protamine. *Lancet* 1939;2:975-976.
72. Benayahu D, Aronson M. Comparative study of protamine chloride and sulphate in relation to the heparin rebound phenomenon. *Thrombosis Res* 1983;32:109-114.
73. Godal HC. A comparison of two heparin-neutralizing agents: protamine and polybrene. *Scand J Clin Lab Invest* 1960;12:446-457.
74. Ellison N, Jobes DR, Schwartz AJ. Heparin therapy during cardiac surgery. In: Ellison N, Jobes DR, eds. *Effective Hemostasis in Cardiac Surgery*. Philadelphia: WB Saunders; 1988:1-14.
75. Ellison N, Ominisky AJ, Wollman H. Is protamine a clinically important anticoagulant? A negative answer. *Anesthesiology* 1971;35:621-629.
76. Jaques LB. A study of the toxicity of the protamine, salmine. *Br J Pharmacol* 1949;4:135-144.
77. Bjoraker DG, Ketcham TR. In vivo platelet response to clinical protamine sulfate infusion. *Anesthesiology* 1982;57:A7.
78. Ellison N, Edmunds LH, Colman RW. Platelet aggregation following heparin and protamine administration. *Anesthesiology* 1978;48:65-68.
79. Cobel-Geard RJ, Hassouna HI. Interaction of protamine sulfate with thrombin. *Am J Hematol* 1983;14:227-233.
80. Akata T, Yoshitake J-I, Nakashima M, et al. Effects of protamine on vascular smooth muscle of rabbit mesenteric artery. *Anesthesiology* 1991;75:833-846.
81. Tan F, Jackman H, Skidgel RA, et al. Protamine inhibits plasma carboxypeptidase N, the inactivator of anaphylatoxins and kinins. *Anesthesiology* 1989;70:267-275.
82. Levy JH, Faraj BA, Zaidan JR, et al. Effects of protamine on histamine release from human lung. *Agents Actions* 1989;28:70-72.
83. Morel DR, Zapol WM, Thomas SJ, et al. C5a and thromboxane generation associated with pulmonary vaso- and broncho-constriction during protamine reversal of heparin. *Anesthesiology* 1987;6:597-604.
84. Weiss ME, Nyhan D, Peng Z, et al. Association of protamine IgE and IgG antibodies with life-threatening reactions to intravenous protamine. *N Engl J Med* 1989;320:886-892.
85. Lowenstein E, Johnston WE, Lappas DG, et al. Catastrophic pulmonary vasoconstriction associated with protamine reversal of heparin. *Anesthesiology* 1983;59:470-473.
86. Levy JH, Schweiger IM, Zaidan JR, et al. Evaluation of patients at risk for protamine reactions. *J Thorac Cardiovasc Surg* 1989;98:200-204.
87. Levy JH, Zaidan JR, Faraj B. Prospective evaluation of risk of protamine reactions in patients with NPH insulin-dependent diabetes. *Anesth Analg* 1986;65:739-742.
88. Knape JTA, Schuller JL, de Haan P, et al. An anaphylactic reaction to protamine in a patient allergic to fish. *Anesthesiology* 1981;55:324-325.
89. Watson RA, Ansbacher R, Barry M, et al. Allergic reaction to protamine: a late complication of elective vasectomy? *Urology* 1983;22:493-496.
90. Castaneda AR. Must heparin be neutralized following open-heart operations? *J Thorac Cardiovasc Surg* 1966;52:716-724.
91. Frater RWM, Oka Y, Hong Y, et al. Protamine-induced circulatory changes. *J Thorac Cardiovasc Surg* 1984;87:687-692.
92. Pauca AL, Graham JE, Hudspeth AS. Hemodynamic effects of intraaortic administration of protamine. *Ann Thorac Surg* 1984;35:637-642.
93. Cherry DA, Chiu RCJ, Wynands JE, et al. Intra-aortic vs. intravenous administration of protamine: a prospective randomized clinical study. *Surg Forum* 1985;36:238-240.
94. Kronenfeld MA, Garguilo R, Weinberg P, et al. Left atrial injection of protamine does not reliably prevent pulmonary hypertension. *Anesthesiology* 1987;67:578-580.
95. Campbell FW, Goldstein MF, Atkins PC. Management of the patient with protamine hypersensitivity for cardiac surgery. *Anesthesiology* 1984;61:761-764.
96. Brauer S. Thoughts on protamine toxicity. *Anesth Analg* 1985;64:1003.
97. Nuttall GA, Murray MJ, Bowie EJW. Protamine-heparin-induced pulmonary hypertension in pigs: effects of treatment with a thromboxane receptor antagonist on hemodynamics and coagulation. *Anesthesiology* 1991;74:138-145.
98. Yang VC, Port FK, Kim J-S, et al. The use of immobilized protamine in removing heparin and preventing protamine-induced complications during extracorporeal blood circulation. *Anesthesiology* 1991;75:288-297.
99. Jobes DR, Schwartz AJ, Ellison N, et al. Monitoring hepa-

rin anticoagulation and its neutralization. *Ann Thorac Surg* 1981;31:161-166.
100. LaDuca F, Mills D, Thompson S, et al. Neutralization of heparin using a protamine titration assay and the activated clotting time test. *J Extracorpor Technol* 1987;19:358-364.
101. Guffin AV, Dunbar RW, Kaplan JA, et al. Successful use of a reduced dose of protamine after cardiopulmonary bypass. *Anesth Analg* 1976;55:110-113.
102. Salmenperä MT, Levy JH, Curling PE. Evaluation of a new heparinase activated clotting time to assess heparin rebound following cardiac surgery. *Abstracts, 1991 Society of Cardiovascular Anesthesiologists*, p 115.
103. Woodman RC, Harker LA. Bleeding complications associated with cardiopulmonary bypass. *Blood* 1990;76:1680-1689.
104. Harker LA, Malpass TW, Branson HE, et al. Mechanism of abnormal bleeding in patients undergoing cardiopulmonary bypass: acquired transient platelet dysfunction associated with selective α-granule release. *Blood* 1980;56:824-834.
105. Bagge L, Lilienberg G, Nyström S-O, et al. Coagulation, fibrinolysis and bleeding after open-heart surgery. *Scand J Thorac Cardiovasc Surg* 1986;20:151-160.
106. Kuitunen A, Hynynen M, Salmenperä M, et al. Anesthesia affects plasma concentrations of vasopressin, von Willebrand factor and coagulation factor VIII in cardiac surgical patients. *Br J Anaesth* 1993;70:173-180.
107. Kuitunen A, Hynynen M, Salmenperä M, et al. Hydroxyethyl starch as a prime for cardiopulmonary bypass: effects of two different solutions on hemostasis. *Acta Anaesth Scand* 1993;37:652-658.
108. Baier RE, Dutton RC. Initial events in interactions of blood with a foreign surface. *J Biomed Mater Res* 1969;3:191-206.
109. Campbell FW, Addonizio VP. Platelet function alterations during cardiac surgery. In: Ellison N, Jobes DR, eds. *Effective Hemostasis in Cardiac Surgery*. Philadelphia: WB Saunders Company; 1988:85-109.
110. Addonizio VP, Macarak EJ, Nicolaou KC, et al. Effects of prostacyclin and albumin on platelet loss during in vitro simulation of extracorporeal circulation. *Blood* 1979;53:1033-1042.
111. Havel M, Teufelsbauer H, Knöbl P, et al. Effect of intraoperative aprotinin administration on postoperative bleeding in patients undergoing cardiopulmonary bypass operation. *J Thorac Cardiovasc Surg* 1991;101:968-972.
112. McKenna R, Bachmann F, Whittaker B, et al. The hemostatic mechanism after open-heart surgery. *J Thorac Cardiovasc Surg* 1975;70:298-308.
113. Reves JG. Adrenergic response to cardiopulmonary bypass. *Mt Sinai J Med* 1985;52:511-515.
114. Addonizio VP, Smith JB, Strauss JF, et al. Thromboxane synthesis and platelet secretion during cardiopulmonary bypass with bubble oxygenator. *J Thorac Cardiovasc Surg* 1980;79:91-96.
115. Malpass TW, Hanson SR, Savage B, et al. Prevention of acquired transient defect in platelet plug formation by infused prostacyclin. *Blood* 1981;57:736-740.
116. Addonizio VP, Strauss JF, Colman RW, Edmunds LH. Effects of prostaglandin E_1 on platelet loss during in vivo and in vitro extracorporeal circulation with a bubble oxygenator. *J Thorac Cardiovasc Surg* 1979;77:119-126.
117. Addonizio VP, Fisher CA, Jenkin BK et al. Iloprost (ZK36374), a stable analogue of prostacyclin, preserves platelets during simulated extracorporeal circulation. *J Thorac Cardiovasc Surg* 1985;89:926-933.
118. Malpass TW, Amory DW, Harker LA, et al. The effect of prostacyclin infusion on platelet hemostatic function in patients undergoing cardiopulmonary bypass. *J Thorac Cardiovasc Surg* 1984;87:550-555.
119. Coppe D, Sobel M, Seamans L, et al. Preservation of platelet function and number by prostacyclin during cardiopulmonary bypass. *J Thorac Cardiovasc Surg* 1981;81:274-278.
120. Nilsson L, Bagge L, Nyström S-O. Blood cell trauma and postoperative bleeding: Comparison of bubble and membrane oxygenators and observations on coronary suction. *Scand J Thorac Cardiovasc Surg* 1990;24:65-69.
121. Edmunds LH, Saxena NC, Hillyer P, Wilson TJ. relationship between platelet count and cardiotomy suction return. *Ann Thorac Surg* 1978;25:306-310.
122. Dutton RC, Edmunds LH, Hutchinson JC, Roe BB. Platelet aggregate emboli produced in patients during cardiopulmonary bypass with membrane and bubble oxygenators and blood filters. *J Thorac Cardiovasc Surg* 1974;67:258-265.
123. Addonizio VP, Macarak EJ, Niewiarowski S, et al. Preservation of human platelets with prostaglandin E_1 during in vitro simulation of cardiopulmonary bypass. *Circ Res* 1979;44:350-357.
124. Addonizio VP, Strauss JF III, Colman RW, Edmunds LH Jr. Effects of prostaglandin E_1 on platelet loss during in vivo and in vitro extracorporeal circulation with a bubble oxygenator. *J Thorac Cardiovasc Sug* 1979;77:119-126.
125. van den Dungen JJAM, Karliczek GF, Brenken U, et al. Clinical study of blood trauma during perfusion with membrane and bubble oxygenators. *J Thorac Cardiovasc Surg* 1982;83:108-116.
126. Peterson KA, Dewanjee MK, Kaye MP. Fate of indium 111-labeled platelets during cardiopulmonary bypass performed with membrane and bubble oxygenators. *J Thorac Cardiovas Surg* 1982;84:39-43.
127. van Oeveren W, Kazatchkine MD, Descamps-Latscha B, et al. Deleterious effects of cardiopulmonary bypass. A prospective study of bubble versus membrane oxygenation. *J Thorac Cardiovasc Surg* 1985;89:888-899.
128. Hessel EA II, Johnson DD, Ivey TD, et al. Membrane versus bubble oxygenator for cardiac operations. A prospective randomized study. *J Thorac Cardiovasc Surg* 1980;80:111-122.
129. Sade RM, Bartles DM, Dearing JP, et al. A prospective randomized study of membrane versus bubble oxygenators in children. *Ann Thorac Surg* 1980;29:502-511.
130. Clark RE, Beauchamp RA, Magrath RA, et al. Comparison of bubble and membrane oxygenators in short and long perfusions. *J Thorac Cardiovasc Surg* 1979;78:655-666.
131. George JN, Pickett EB, Saucerman S, et al. Platelet surface glycoproteins. Studies on resting and activated platelets and platelet membrane microparticles in normal subjects, and observations in patients during adult respiratory distress syndrome and cardiac surgery. *J Clin Invest* 1986;78:340-348.

132. van Oeveren W, Harder MP, Roozendaal KJ, et al. Aprotinin protects platelets against the initial effect of cardiopulmonary bypass. *J Thorac Cardiovasc Surg* 1990;99:788–797.
133. Rinder CS, Mathew JP, Rinder HM. Modulation of platelet surface adhesion receptors during cardiopulmonary bypass. *Anesthesiology* 1991;75:563–570.
134. Wenger RK, Lukasiewicz H, Mikuta BS, et al. Loss of platelet fibrinogen receptors during clinical cardiopulmonary bypass. *J Thorac Cardiovasc Surg* 1989;97:235–239.
135. Wachtfogel YT, Musial J, Jenkin B, et al. Loss of platelet α_2-adrenergic receptors during simulated extracorporeal circulation: prevention with prostaglandin E_1. *J Lab Clin Med* 105;1985:601–607.
136. Abrams CS, Ellison N, Budzynski AZ, et al. Direct detection of activated platelets and platelet-derived microparticles in humans. *Blood* 1990;75:128–138.
137. Carteaux J-P, Roux S, Kuhn H, et al. Ro 44-9883, a new nonpeptide glycoprotein IIb/IIIa antagonist, prevents platelet loss during experimental cardiopulmonary bypass. *J Thorac Cardiovasc Surg* 1993;106:834–841.
138. Miles LA, Ginsberg MH, White JG, et al. Plasminogen interacts with human platelets through two distinct mechanisms. *J Clin Invest* 1986;77:2001–2009.
139. Michelson AD, Barnard MR. Plasmin-induced redistribution of platelet glycoprotein 1b. *Blood* 1990;76:2005–2010.
140. Weinstein M, Ware JA, Troll J, et al. Changes in von Willebrand factor during cardiac surgery: effect of desmopressin acetate. *Blood* 1988;71:1648–1655.
141. Nussey SS, Bevan DH, Ang VTY, et al. Effects of arginine vasopressin (AVP) infusions on circulating concentrations of platelet AVP, Factor VIII:C and von Willebrand factor. *Thrombosis Haemostasis* 1986;55:34–36.
142. Gill JC, Wilson AD, Endres-Brooks J, et al. Loss of the largest von Willebrand factor multimers from the plasma of patients with congenital cardiac defects. *Blood* 1986:67:758–761.
143. Bick RL. Hemostasis defects associated with cardiac surgery, prosthetic devices, and other extracorporeal circuits. *Semin Thrombosis Hemostasis* 1985;11:249–280.
144. Tanaka K, Takao M, Yada I, et al. Alterations in coagulation and fibrinolysis associated with cardiopulmonary bypass during open heart surgery. *J Cardiothorac Ansth* 1989;3:181–188.
145. Marx G, Pokar H, Reuter H, et al. The effects of aprotinin on hemostatic function during cardiac surgery. *J Cardiothorac Vasc Anesth* 1991;5:467–474.
146. Spiess BD, Tuman KJ, McCarthy RJ, et al. Thromboelastography as an indicator of post-cardiopulmonary bypass coagulopathies. *J Clin Monit* 1987;3:25–30.
147. Tuman KJ, Spiess BD, McCarthy RJ, et al. Comparison of viscoelastic measures of coagulation after cardiopulmonary bypass. *Anesth Analg* 1989;69:69–75.
148. Kirklin JW, Barrat-Boyes BG. *Cardiac Surgery*. New York: John Wiley & Sons; 1986:159.
149. Despotis GJ, Santora SA, Spiznagel E, et al. On-site prothrombin time, activated partial thromboblastin time and platelet count. A comparison between whole blood and laboratory assays with coagulation factor analysis in patients presenting for cardiac surgery. *Anesthesiology* 1994;80:338–351.
150. Kang YG, Martin DJ, Marquez J, et al. Intraoperative changes in blood coagulation and thromboelastographic monitoring in liver transplantation. *Anesth Analg* 1985;64:888–896.
151. Franz RC, Coetzee WJC. The thromboelastographic diagnosis of hemostatic defects. *Surg Ann* 1981;13:75–107.
152. Tuman KJ, Spiess BD, McCarthy RJ, et al. Effects of progressive blood loss on coagulation as measured by thromboelastography. *Anesth Analg* 1987;66:856–863.
153. Remuzzi G. Bleeding in renal failure. *Lancet* 1988;1:1205–1207.
154. Torosian M, Michelson EL, Morganroth J, et al. Aspirin- and coumadin-related bleeding after coronary artery bypass graft surgery. *Ann Int Med* 1978;89:325–328.
155. Michelson EL, Morganroth J, Torosian M, et al. Relation of preoperative use of aspirin to increased mediastinal blood loss after coronary artery bypass graft surgery. *J Thorac Cardiovasc Surg* 1978;76:694–697.
156. Ferraris VA, Ferraris SP, Lough FC, et al. Preoperative aspirin ingestion increases operative blood loss after coronary artery bypass grafting. *Ann Thorac Surg* 1988;45:71–74.
157. Goldman S, Copeland J, Moritz T, et al. Improvement in early saphenous venin graft patency after coronary artery bypass surgery with antiplatelet therapy: results of a Veterans Administration Cooperative Study. *Circulation* 1988;77:1324–1332.
158. Taggart DP, Siddiqui A, Wheatley DJ. Low-dose preoperative aspirin therapy, postoperative blood loss, and transfusion requirements. *Ann Thorac Surg* 1990;50:425–428.
159. Karwande SV, Weksler BB, Gay WA Jr, et al. Effect of preoperative antiplatelet drugs on vascular prostacyclin synthesis. *Ann Thorac Surg* 1987;43:318–322.
160. Skinner JR, Phillips SJ, Zeff RH, et al. Immediate coronary bypass following failed streptokinase infusion in evolving myocardial infarction. *J Thorac Cardiovasc Surg* 1984;87:567–570.
161. Kereiakes DJ, Topol EJ, George BS, et al. Emergency coronary artery bypass surgery preserves global and regional left ventricular function after intravenous tissue plasminogen activator therapy for acute myocardial infarction. *J Am Coll Cardiol* 1988;11:899–907.
162. Sane DC, Califf RM, Topol EJ, et al. Bleeding during thrombolytic therapy for acute myocardial infarction: mechanisms and management. *Ann Int Med* 1989;111:1010–1022.
163. Cosgrove DM, Lytle BW, Loop FD, et al. Does bilateral internal mammary artery grafting increase surgical risk? *J Thorac Cardiovasc Surg* 1988;95:850–856.
164. Simon TL, Akl BF, Murphy W. Controlled trial of routine administration of platelet concentrates in cardiopulmonary bypass surgery. *Ann Thorac Surg* 1984;37:359–364.
165. Bernstein MJ. Fresh-frozen plasma. Indications and risks. *JAMA* 1985;253:551–553.
166. Mohr R, Martinowitz U, Lavee J, et al. The hemostatic effect of transfusing fresh whole blood versus platelet concentrates after cardiac operations. *J Thorac Cardiovasc Surg* 1988;96:530–534.
167. Lavee J, Martinowitz U, Mohr R, et al. The effect of trans-

fusion of fresh whole blood versus platelet concentrates after cardiac operations. A scanning electron microscope study of platelet aggregation on extracellular matrix. *J Thorac Cardiovasc Surg* 1989;97:204-212.
168. Manno CS, Hedberg KW, Kim HC, et al. Comparison of the hemostatic effects of fresh whole blood, and components after open heart surgery in children. *Blood* 1991;77:930-936.
169. Wagstaffe JG, Clarke AD, Jackson PW. Reduction of blood loss by restoration of platelet levels using fresh autologous blood after cardiopulmonary bypass. *Thorax* 1972;27:410-414.
170. Kaplan JA, Cannarella C, Jones EL, et al. Autologous blood transfusion during cardiac surgery. A re-evaluation of three methods. *J Thorac Cardiovasc Surg* 1977;74:4-10.
171. Lawson NW, Ochsner JL, Mills NL, et al. The use of hemodilution and fresh autologous blood in open heart surgery. *Anesth Analg* 1974;53:672-683.
172. Pliam MB, McGoon DC, Tarhan S. Failure of transfusion of autologous whole blood to reduce banked-blood requirements in open-heart surgery patients. *J Thorac Cardiovasc Surg* 1975;70:338-343.
173. Sherman MM, Dobnik DB, Dennis RC, et al. Autologous blood transfusion during cardiopulmonary bypass. *Chest* 1976;70:592-595.
174. DelRossi AJ, Cernaianu AC, Vertrees RA, et al. Platelet-rich plasma reduces postoperative blood loss after cardiopulmonary bypass. *J Thorac Cardiovasc Surg* 1990;100:281-286.
175. Boldt J, Kling D, Zickmann B, et al. Acute preoperative plasmapheresis and established blood conservation techniques. *Ann Thorac Surg* 1990;50:62-68.
176. Marder VJ, Butler FO, Barlow GH. Antifibrinolytic therapy. In: Coleman RW, Hirsh J, Marder VJ, Salzman EW, eds. *Hemostasis and Thrombosis*. 2nd ed. Philadelphia: JB Lippincott; 1987:380.
177. Gans H, Castaneda AR, Subramanian V, et al. Problems in hemostasis during open heart surgery: IX. Changes observed in the plasminogen-plasmin system and their significance for therapy. *Ann Surg* 1967;166:980-986.
178. Mammen EF. Natural proteinase inhibitors in extracorporeal circulation. *Ann NY Acad Sci* 1968;146:754-762.
179. Bidstrup BP, Royston D, Sapsford RN, Taylor KM. Reduction in blood loss and blood use after cardiopulmonary bypass with high dose aprotinin (Trasylol). *J Thorac Cardiovasc Surg* 1989;97:364-372.
180. Dietrich W, Spannagl M, Jochum M, et al. Influence of high-dose aprotinin treatment on blood loss and coagulation patterns in patients undergoing myocardial revascularization. *Anesthesiology* 1990;73:1119-1126.
181. Havel M, Teufelsbauer H, Knöbl P, et al. Effect of intraoperative aprotinin administration on postoperative bleeding in patients undergoing cardiopulmonary bypass operation. *J Thorac Cardiovasc Surg* 1991;101:968-972.
182. Blauhut B, Gross C, Necek S, et al. Effects of high-dose aprotinin on blood loss, platelet function, fibrinolysis, complement, and renal function after cardiopulmonary bypass. *J Thorac Cardiovasc Surg* 1991;101:958-967.
183. Lemmer JH Jr, Stanford W, Bonney SL, et al. Aprotinin for coronary bypass operations: efficacy, safety, and influence on early saphenous vein graft patency. A multicenter, randomized, double-blind, placebo-controlled study. *J Thorac Cardiovasc Surg* 1994;107:543-553.
184. Royston D, Bidstrup BP, Taylor KM, et al. Aprotinin (Trasylol) reduces bleeding after open heart surgery in patients taking aspirin and those with renal failure. *Anesthesioloy* 1989;71:A6.
185. Murkin JM, Lux J, Shannon NA, et al. Aprotinin significantly decreases bleeding and transfusion requirements in patients receiving aspirin and undergoing cardiac operations. *J Thorac Cardiosc Surg* 1994;107:554-561.
186. Elliot MJ, Allen A. Aprotinin in pediatric cardiac surgery. *Perfusion* 1990;5:73-76.
187. Dietrich W, Mossinger H, Spannagl M, et al. Hemostatic activation during cardiopulmonary bypass with different aprotinin dosages in pediatric patients having cardiac operations. *J Thorac Cardiovasc Surg* 1993;105:757-760.
188. Kaller H, Patzschke K, Wegner LA, et al. Pharmacokinetic observations following intravenous administration of radioactive labelled aprotinin in volunteers. *Eur J Drug Metab Pharm* 1978;2:79-85.
189. Fritz H, Wunderer G. Biochemistry and applications of aprotinin, the kallikrein inhibitor from bovine organs. *Arzneimittelforschung* 1983;33:479-494.
190. Freeman JG, Turner GA, Venables CW, et al. Serial use of aprotinin and incidence of allergic reactions. *Curr Med Res Opin* 1983;8:559-561.
191. Dietrich W, Barankay A, Dilthry G, et al. Reduction of homologous blood requirement in cardiac surgery by intraoperative aprotinin application—clinical experience in 152 cardiac surgical patients. *Thorac Cardiovasc Surg* 1989;37:92-98.
192. Wang J-S, Lin C-Y, Hung W-T, et al. Monitoring of heparin-induced anticogulation with kaolin-activated clotting time in cardiac surgical patients treated with aprotinin. *Anesthesiology* 1992;77:1080-1084.
193. Hunt BJ, Segal H, Yacoub M. Guidelines for monitoring heparin by the activated clotting time when aprotinin is used during cardiopulmonary bypass. *J Thorac Cardiovasc Surg* 1992;104:211-212.
194. Gosgrove DM III, Heric B, Lytle BW, et al. Aprotinin therapy for preoperative myocardial revascularization: a placebo-controlled study. *Ann Thorac Surg* 1992;54:1031-1038.
195. Sundt TM III, Kouchoukos NT, Saffitz JE, et al. Renal dysfunction and intravascular coagulation with aprotinin and hypothermic circulatory arrest. *Ann Thorac Surg* 1993;55:1418-1424.
196. Bidstrup BP, Underwood SR, Sapsford RN. Effect of aprotinin on aorta-coronary bypass graft patency. *J Thorac Cardiovasc Surg* 1993;105:147-153.
197. Lambert CJ, Marengo-Rowe AJ, Leveson JE, et al. The treatment of postperfusion bleeding using ϵ-aminocaproic acid, cryoprecipitate, fresh-frozen plasma, and protamine sulfate. *Ann Thorac Surg* 1979;28:440-444.
198. DelRossi AJ, Cernaianu AC, Botros S, et al. Prophylactic treatment of postperfusion bleeding using EACA. *Chest* 1989;96:27-30.
199. McClure PD, Izsak J. The use of epsilon-aminocaproic acid to reduce bleeding during cardiac bypass in children

with congenital heart disease. *Anesthesiology* 1974;40:604–608.
200. Vander Salm TJ, Ansell JE, Okike ON, et al. The role of epsilon-aminocaproic acid in reducing bleeding after cardiac operation: a double-blind randomized study. *J Thorac Cardiovasc Surg* 1988;95:538–542.
201. Horrow JC, Hlavacek J, Strong MD, et al. Prophylactic tranexamic acid decreases bleeding after cardiac operations. *J Thorac Cardiovasc Surg* 1990;99:70–74.
202. Mannucci PM. Desmopressin: a nontransfusional form of treatment for congenital and acquired bleeding disorders. *Blood* 1988;72:1449–1455.
203. Salzman EW, Weinstein MJ, Weintraub RM, et al. Treatment with desmopressin acetate to reduce blood loss after cardiac surgery. A double-blind randomized trial. *N Engl J Med* 1986;314:1402–1406.
204. Rocha E, Llorens R, Páramo JA, et al. Does desmopressin acetate reduce blood loss after surgery in patients on cardiopulmonary bypass? *Circulation* 1988;77:1319–1323.
205. Andersson TLG, Solem JO, Tengborn L, et al. Effects of desmopressin acetate on platelet aggregation, von Willebrand factor, and blood loss after cardiac surgery with extracorporeal circulation. *Circulation* 1990;81:872–878.
206. Brown MR, Swygert TH, Whitten CW, et al. Desmopressin acetate following cardiopulmonary bypass: evaluation of coagulation parameters. *J Cardiothorac Anesth* 1989;3:726–729.
207. Hackmann T, Gascoyne RD, Naiman SC, et al. A trial of desmopressin (1-desamino-8-D-arginine vasopressin) to reduce blood loss in uncomplicated cardiac surgery. *N Engl J Med* 1989;321:1437–1443.
208. Hedderich GS, Petsikas DJ, Cooper BA, et al. Desmopressin acetate in uncomplicated coronary artery bypass surgery: a prospective randomized clinical trial. *Can J Surg* 1990;33:33–36.
209. Seear MD, Wadsworth LD, Rogers PC, et al. The effect of desmopressin acetate (DDAVP) on postoperative blood loss after cardiac operations in children. *J Thorac Cardiovasc Surg* 1989;98:217–219.
210. Frankville DD, Harper GB, Lake CL, et al. Hemodynamic consequences of desmopressin administration after cardiopulmonary bypass. *Anesthesiology* 1991;74:988–996.
211. Salmenperä M, Kuitunen A, Hynynen M, et al. Hemodynamic responses to desmopressin acetate after CABG: a double-blind trial. *J Cardiothorac Vasc Anesth* 1991;5:146–149.
212. Cosgrove DM III, Petre JH, Waller JL, et al. Automated control of postoperative hypertension: a prospective, randomized multicenter study. *Ann Thorac Surg* 1989;47:678–683.

6
The Central Nervous System: Responses to Cardiopulmonary Bypass

Christina T. Mora and John M. Murkin

Despite innovative medical treatment regimens involving new classes and types of drugs and interventional cardiology techniques such as intracoronary balloon and laser angioplasty, definitive treatment of refractory ischemic heart disease still necessitates surgical revascularization and cardiopulmonary bypass (CPB). It is estimated that over 300,000 coronary artery bypass graft (CABG) procedures are performed annually in the United States,[1] and over 450,000 such procedures are performed annually worldwide.

In part because the proliferation of techniques and treatment options for the management of ischemic heart disease (IHD) allows patients to be maintained for longer periods prior to surgical intervention, and because continual improvements in technique have decreased operative mortality rates (thus encouraging surgical revascularization in older patients), there has been a progressive rise in the average age of patients presenting for CABG surgery.[2] Because these patients are older, they usually have more concomitant disease and, hence, are more likely to be taking multiple medications and to have more advanced and diffuse atherosclerotic disease. Since advanced age and duration of CPB have been consistently identified as independent risk factors for neurologic and neuropsychologic dysfunction after cardiac surgery, the increase in cardiac operations being performed on an aging population, coupled with a prolonged duration of CPB due to the increasing number of coronary arterial grafts being performed per patient, would be expected to further increase the incidence of postoperative brain dysfunction. A study of 24,672 patients undergoing primary coronary revascularization reported a substantial increase in the proportion of patient deaths causally related to an adverse neurologic event.[3] From 1970 to 1973, 8% of coronary surgery patients died following a neurologic outcome; by 1980 to 1982, 20% of all patient deaths were attributed to neurologic events.[3]

As will be discussed, in most cases, the neurologic and neuropsychologic impairment seen after cardiac surgery is subtle and only apparent on close examination. This problem should not be discounted, however, since the socioeconomic impact of even subtle neurologic dysfunction is heightened by the very large number of cardiac operations being performed annually.

Incidence of Neurologic and Neuropsychologic Dysfunction Following Cardiac Surgery

Neurologic Dysfunction

The incidence of subtle neurologic and neuropsychologic dysfunction in the postoperative period has been repeatedly demonstrated to approach or exceed 50% when assessed in the first 5 to 10 days after CPB.[4-9] This is in contrast to the much lower incidence of clinically obvious stroke, consistently reported as occurring in approximately 2% to 3% of patients undergoing CABG surgery.[10-14]

In large measure, this disparity in incidence reflects both the difference between retrospective and prospective neurologic assessments, and the subtle nature of the majority of observed neurologic deficits. As demonstrated in a study by Sotaneimi,[15] in which the same patient pool was assessed by prospective neurologic examination and later by retrospective chart review, the incidence of neurologic abnormalities detected prospectively was 39%, versus only 4% when hospital records were reviewed retrospectively. A number of subtle neurologic signs were not evident in a review of the patients' hospital records, either because they had not been detected by routine examination, or because they had not been recorded.

In prospective studies investigating neurologic function after cardiac surgery, it is apparent that the types of neurologic dysfunction most frequently being reported are clinically silent. In a prospective study of 312 patients undergoing CABG surgery reported by Shaw et al,[7] 35% of patients demonstrated evidence of neurologic dysfunction

TABLE 6.1. Incidence of new neurological deficits following coronary revascularization procedures.

Author	Year	Incidence of neurologic deficit
Sontaneimi[15]	1983	39%
Breuer[10]	1983	17%
Shaw[7]	1985	61%
Smith[8]	1986	4%
Carella[4]	1988	48%
Strenge[5]	1990	51%
Murkin[6]	1992	38%

preoperatively and 61% manifested new neurologic dysfunction postoperatively. Severe neurologic dysfunction occurred in 1.3% of patients, and 48 patients (12%) with new neurologic dysfunction were mildly disabled in the early postoperative period. Of these patients with new postoperative deficits, fully 35% of the dysfunctions identified involved visual field defects or retinal abnormalities, and a further 38% were hyperreflexias or primitive reflexes.

Similar incidences of subtle neurologic signs have been observed by others. Carella et al,[4] in a prospective study of 91 patients undergoing coronary bypass surgery, reported that over 57% of their patients evidenced abnormal neurologic signs preoperatively. Postoperatively, 48% of patients developed new neurologic signs, including nystagmus, other oculomotor alterations, and primitive reflexes. Five patients (5.7%) had major neurologic complications, including stroke (2.2%) or seizures (1.1%). Strenge et al[5] prospectively assessed 78 patients undergoing CABG surgery and reported a 45% incidence of clinically detectable neurologic abnormalities that were demonstrable preoperatively. Within the first week postoperatively, 51% of patients evidenced new neurologic abnormalities consisting largely of primitive reflexes (65%) or focal signs (62%). No patient demonstrated major neurologic impairment postoperatively. In a prospective assessment of 245 patients undergoing CABG surgery, Murkin et al[6] reported a 38% incidence of new neurologic abnormalities 7 days postoperatively, within domains consisting of cranial nerves, motor and sensory functioning, cerebellar function, gait, and reflexes. A 22% incidence of neurologic impairment was present when assessed 2 months postoperatively. Table 6.1 lists studies reporting the incidence of neurologic impairment following cardiac surgery procedures.[4-8,10,15]

Subtle pathologic neurologic signs are not readily detectable and must be systematically sought out. As reported in the studies discussed above, a high percentage of patients presenting for CABG surgery have preoperative evidence of varying degrees of neurologic dysfunction, which are likely a reflection of the same diffuse atherosclerosis that produced their cardiac symptoms. At the very least, this underscores the importance of a preoperative neurologic assessment to define the etiology of cerebral dysfunction apparent after cardiac surgery, and it may also indicate that atherosclerosis implies a greater susceptibility to post-CPB neurologic impairment.

Neuropsychologic Dysfunction

The incidences of neuropsychologic impairment observed in patients after cardiac surgery are as high as (or, in many cases, even higher than) those reported for neurologic dysfunction. These differences in incidence are likely due to the increased sensitivity, as well as the more readily quantifiable nature, of the neuropsychologic testing employed. Table 6.2 lists reported incidences of neuropsychologic dysfunction following cardiac surgery.[9,16-24]

Shaw and colleagues[19] examined 298 patients undergoing CABG surgery, using a battery of 10 standardized neuropsychologic tests. They demonstrated that 235 patients from this group (79%) exhibited some form of cognitive dysfunction when assessed at day 7 postoperatively, 123 of whom were asymptomatic but 89 of whom (30%) complained of cognitive impairment. Twenty-three patients in this group (8%) were considered overtly disabled. Of the testing employed, the associate learning tests, indicative of auditory memory, new learning ability, and mental control, showed the most consistent pattern of impairment, showing decrements in 36% of patients preoperatively and 33% postoperatively. In addition, performance on the trail-making test, which reflects attention and concentration, psychomotor speed, and visuo-spatial organization, was also impaired in 22% of patients.

Using measures of concentration, psychomotor speed, motor dexterity, and verbal learning, Martzke et al[24] assessed 245 patients undergoing elective CABG surgery preoperatively, 7 days postoperatively, and at follow-up 6

TABLE 6.2. Incidence of neuropsychologic dysfunction following cardiac surgery. Studies reported on both closed- and open-chamber procedures are listed as "mixed." Early incidence refers to the frequency of deficits within 2 weeks of surgery. Late incidence refers to deficts present at 6 weeks or more after operation.

Author	Date	Type of surgery	Incidence	
			Early	Late
Sontaniemi[16]	1981	Valve	—	27%
Savageau[17,18]	1982	Mixed	28%	19%
Shaw[19]	1986	CABG	79%	—
Newman[20]	1987	CABG	73%	37%
Nevin[21]	1987	CABG	20%	—
Mattlar[22]	1988	CABG	—	0%
Hammeke[9]	1988	CABG	54%	—
Newman[23]	1990	CABG	—	35%
Martzke[24]	1992	CABG	68%	22%

to 8 weeks postoperatively. To define abnormal functioning on this series of tests, volunteer control subjects recruited from the community were administered the same neuropsychologic battery, employing an identical protocol, and the cutoff for abnormal functioning was set, as a change score, at or below the fifth percentile for each test. At 7 days postoperatively, the incidence of impairment of motor dexterity was 48% and the incidence of impairment of psychomotor speed was 68%, while the overall incidence of impaired cognitive functioning was 80%. This is very similar to the incidence of 79% shown by Shaw et al.[7] At follow-up, there was a 17% incidence of impairment of psychomotor speed and verbal learning, and an overall incidence of impaired cognitive functioning of 22%. From the tests employed in this screen, the measure of psychomotor speed was the most sensitive indicator of acquired brain dysfunction. When the results of the neuropsychologic screening were combined with measures of neurologic dysfunction, the overall incidence of impairment of either neurologic or neuropsychologic functioning at follow-up was 48%,[6,24] considerably higher than estimates employing either modality separately.

In a prospective study assessing 31 patients undergoing elective CABG surgery, and a control of 16 patients undergoing noncardiac surgical procedures, Raymond et al[25] assessed neuropsychologic performance preoperatively, within 1 to 2 weeks postoperatively, and at 6 to 8 weeks postoperatively. They demonstrated significantly greater declines in neuropsychologic performance in the CABG group, in the early postoperative period, as compared with the control patients. However, at the time of later postoperative follow-up, the level of functioning in both groups was essentially similar and without evidence of significant impairment. A potential confounding factor in this study was the inability to correct for practice effect, a reproducible phenomenon associated with repeated administration of neuropsychologic tests, which could allow the subject to mask subtle impairments in functioning.

Control Group Testing

The increased sensitivity to postoperative cerebral impairment inherent in a standardized prospective neurologic assessment and in appropriately selected neuropsychologic testing allows detection of very subtle abnormalities, as well as diminished cognition and integrative tasking. But it might also allow detection of impairments produced by anesthesia and any type of surgery, rather than by cardiac surgery and CPB specifically. In studies designed to isolate the degree of cerebral dysfunction caused specifically by CPB and cardiac surgery, employment of an appropriate control group undergoing non-CPB surgery is essential.

Although there have been only a few studies in which a control group undergoing non-CPB surgery has been employed, it appears that exposure to CPB is an independent risk factor that significantly increases the incidence of subtle postoperative neurologic dysfunction within the early postoperative period.[8,9,25,26]

Shaw et al[26] investigated 312 patients undergoing CABG surgery and compared their postoperative status to a control group of 50 patients undergoing vascular or thoracic surgery. The incidence of early postoperative neurologic dysfunction and neuropsychologic complications in the CABG patients was 61% (191 of 312) and 79% (235 of 298), respectively, decreasing to 17% and 38% at the time of hospital discharge. In the control group, 18% (9 of 50) developed neurologic complications as a result of trauma to lower limb sensory nerves, and 38% (15 of 48) showed mild neuropsychologic impairment, while none showed moderate or severe impairment, in contrast to the 19% and 5% incidences of moderate and severe impairment noted in the CABG group. The authors speculated that these differences in the incidence and severity of neurologic dysfunction between groups likely reflected cerebral injury occurring as a result of exposure to CPB.

It is not entirely clear that residual dysfunction found at subsequent postoperative assessment (eg, 2 months after surgery) is due entirely to exposure to CPB, since, in some studies, noncardiac surgical control groups have been found to have similar incidences of dysfunction.[8,9,27] Not all investigators have been able to demonstrate higher incidences of neurologic dysfunction as a consequence of cardiac surgery. Hammeke and Hastings[9] prospectively evaluated neuropsychologic performance in 46 CABG patients and 14 patients undergoing peripheral vascular surgery, as well as 26 nonsurgical control patients. They demonstrated significant decrements in performance in both the surgical groups relative to the nonsurgical control group, but no specific morbidity that was associated with the use of CPB. They concluded this implied that nonspecific factors associated with surgery—not CPB—accounted for the decrements in neuropsychological performance. Others have challenged these results. Blauth et al[28] have raised concerns about the susceptibility of certain of the neuropsychologic tests to practice effects, rendering them insensitive upon repeat examination to small decrements in performance. They conclude that the relatively small numbers of patients examined may have produced a type II error, impairing the ability to find differences between the surgical groups.

Smith[27] reported on neuropsychologic dysfunction in 79 patients undergoing coronary bypass surgery, along with a surgical cohort of 30 patients undergoing either major vascular or thoracic surgery. They reported that moderate or severe neuropsychologic deficit was common, occurring in 73% of CABG patients (49 of 67 patients) at 8 days postoperatively and in 37% (25 of 67 patients) at follow-up after 8 weeks. At the time of 1-year follow-up,

35% of patients still exhibited neuropsychologic dysfunction. Prolonged CPB times were associated with greater neuropsychologic dysfunction, but there was no difference in incidence among patients in the noncardiac group, in which incidences of 50% (12 of 24 patients) at 8 days and 46% (11 of 24 patients) at 8 weeks were observed. It was emphasized that the patients undergoing noncardiac surgery were older, manifested more metabolic derangements, and required extensive pharmacologic support; thus, their postoperative dysfunction was considered likely to have been from other causes.

Murkin et al[29] completed detailed neurologic and neuropsychologic assessments of a total of 316 patients undergoing coronary bypass surgery and a surgical cohort of 39 patients undergoing major abdominal vascular surgery or thoracic surgery. They examined patients preoperatively, and at 7 days and 2 months postoperatively, and demonstrated combined incidences of dysfunction of 88% at 7 days, and 45% at 2 months, in the CABG patients. In the surgical cohort, the incidence at 7 days was significantly lower: 65% exhibited either neurologic or neuropsychologic dysfunction. At the time of follow-up, however, the incidence of dysfunction was 44%, virtually identical to that of the CABG group, and strikingly similar to that reported by Smith.[27]

In general, the consensus of investigators working in the area of post-CPB neurologic dysfunction is that cardiac surgery, with the attendant exposure to CPB, produces measurable dysfunction in the immediate postoperative period, over and above that seen in similar patients after general anesthesia and noncardiac surgery.[30] It is similarly apparent that not all of this dysfunction is attributable to exposure to CPB. Interpolating between the relative incidences of postoperative dysfunction in CABG patients versus other surgical patients, it is evident that CPB exerts an additional significant effect in the immediate postoperative period, but that at least half the dysfunction appears to be due to the stresses of anesthesia and surgery. Additionally, the effects of CPB appear to be relatively evanescent, since several groups have demonstrated that, at 2-month follow-up, there is no difference in incidences of dysfunction between groups undergoing major surgery or CABG, both of which exhibit similar and relatively high incidences of subtle neurologic and neuropsychologic impairment.[8,9,27]

Central Nervous System Monitoring

Electroencephalography (EEG)

Although the EEG has been used since the early days of CPB, its value as a routine monitor during extracorporeal circulation is still controversial.[31] Those advocating the use of this monitor point out that central nervous system (CNS) morbidity following cardiac surgery is a significant problem and that there are several reports documenting the utility of this monitoring modality in attenuating the incidence of adverse neurologic events. Additionally, there are several available EEG monitors that process the raw EEG into a readily recognizable signal (Figure 6.1). Two studies have reported improvement in neurologic outcomes following cardiac surgery in CPB through computerized EEG-based intervention during extracorporeal circulation.[32,33] Arom et al[32] reported that modification in either $Paco_2$ or perfusion pressure during CPB in response to EEG changes reduced postoperative neuropsychologic dysfunction from 44% without intervention to 5% with intervention. Similarly, Edmonds and colleagues[33] reported a decrease in the incidence of postoperative disorientation from 29% to 4% when blood pressure was increased in response to EEG evidence of hypoperfusion. There were too few neurologic complications to permit assessment of the effect of EEG-based interventions on major CNS complications.

Others believe that the multiple inherent problems associated with monitoring the EEG during cardiac surgery and CPB limit the usefulness of the EEG. For example, changes in brain temperature and anesthetic concentrations may mimic EEG changes (loss of amplitude or high-frequency activity) associated with cerebral hypoperfusion.[34-36] Additionally, ischemia may produce other types of EEG changes,[37] and even a complete cessation of electrical activity (such as that occurring during profound hypothermia and circulatory arrest) does not necessarily indicate cerebral injury.

Other technical problems confound the interpretation of either the raw or the processed EEG during CPB. Electrical generators, including the electrocautery probe and pacemaker, and/or artifacts produced by the roller-head pump[38] may interfere with EEG interpretation during different phases of the operation. In one study, nearly 40% of EEG recordings were corrupted with electrical noise.[36]

Perhaps the most significant limitation of the EEG monitor is its inability to detect cerebral ischemic changes induced by the most likely source of ischemia during cardiac surgery and CPB: microemboli. The EEG signal is a summation of postsynaptic potentials from several square centimeters of cortical parenchyma. An injury caused by a microembolus would affect only a few square millimeters of cerebral tissue, and the resulting change in electrical activity would be infinitesimally small and therefore not detectable in the summation-EEG signal. Finally, the clinical setting of cardiac surgery and extracorporeal perfusion is in contrast to that of carotid surgery, in which predictable instances of hypoperfusion may be associated with distinct hemisphere changes in the EEG signal.

Bashein and colleagues[36] studied 78 patients undergoing cardiac surgery and hypothermic (28° to 32°C) bypass to assess utility of a two-channel EEG recording to

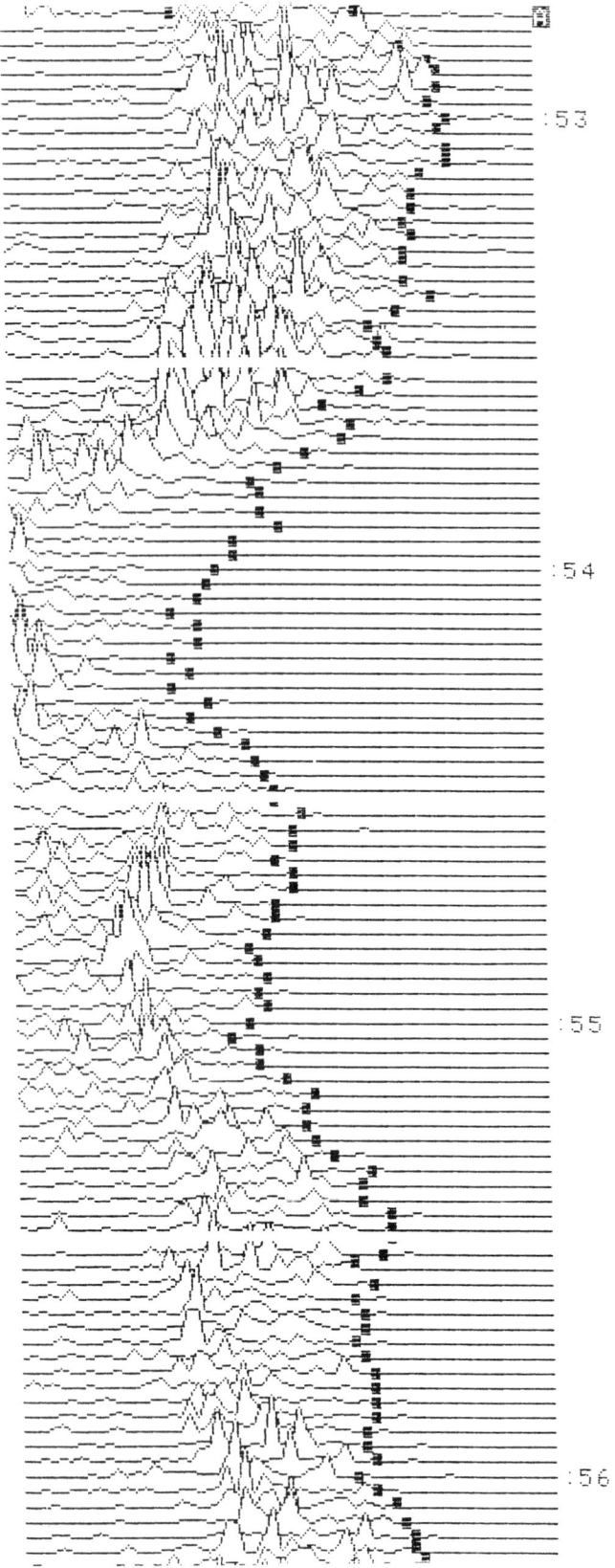

FIGURE 6.1. Eight-channel computerized EEG tracing (compressed spectral array display) during cardiac surgery. (Courtesy of Richard Moberg of Moberg Medical.)

predict CNS injury. Only 58 of the 78 patients had EEG data of acceptable quality, and of the 8 EEG descriptors employed, descriptor shifts were only weakly associated with early neuropsychologic impairment but were not associated with long-term cognitive dysfunction.

In summary, EEG monitoring during CPB may facilitate recognition of episodes of major disruption of cerebral blood flow and will reflect changes in cerebral temperature and anesthetic concentrations. However, more subtle changes in cerebral perfusion are more difficult to identify with the EEG monitor. Because neurologic injury continues to be a significant cause of morbidity and mortality following cardiac surgery, large, randomized, prospective studies on the utility of the EEG monitoring are required.

Doppler Sonography

Transcranial Doppler (TCD) sonography measures blood flow velocity (BFV) in the middle cerebral artery (MCA) and provides a quantitative assessment of cerebral perfusion. Van der Linden and colleagues[39] reported that cerebral blood flow (CBF) and BFV changes correlate during the course of cardiac surgery and hypothermic CPB ($r = 0.77$).

TCD sonography provides continuous data on MCA blood flow and can be used to assess cerebral autoregulation, chemoreactivity, and flow-metabolism coupling. Additionally, embolic events can be detected and quantified with TCD sonography (Figure 6.2). EEG activity has been shown to correlate with BFV. In one study, bursts in EEG activity (during burst suppression) were associated with 21% increase in BFV.[40]

Jugular Venous Oxygen Saturation

A pediatric oximetry catheter may be placed in the jugular bulb to measure continuously cerebral venous oxygen content. Given the increasing number of diabetic patients presenting for CABG surgery (a group in whom impaired cerebral autoregulation has been demonstrated), on-line assessment of the adequacy of cerebral perfusion is becoming increasingly important. Moreover, continuous on-line assessment of cerebral venous oxygen saturation may be one means of assessing the adequacy of cerebral oxygen delivery, particularly in patients felt to be at increased risk of neurologic injury.[41,42]

Cerebral Physiology

In addition to the studies demonstrating high incidences of subtle brain injury after CPB, other investigations have examined directly the effects of CPB on cerebral physiol-

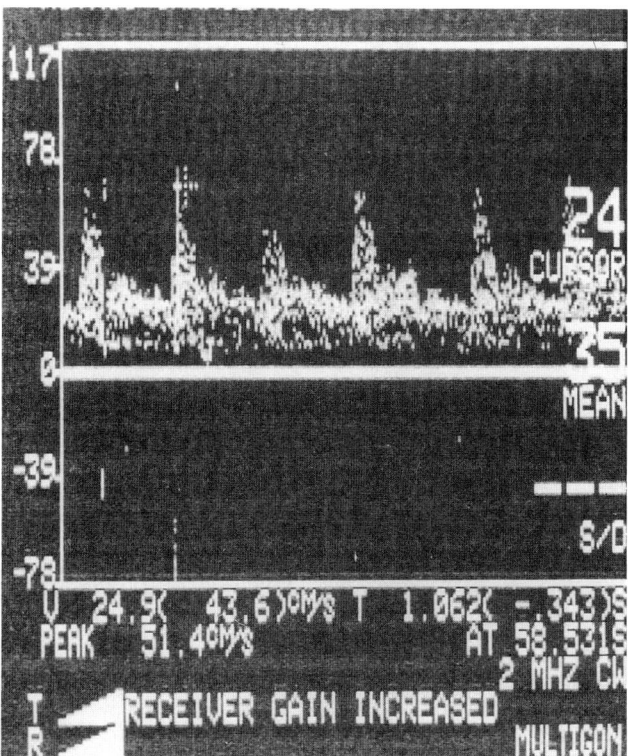

FIGURE 6.2. Transcranial Doppler display of blood flow in the right middle cerebral artery of a patient during aortic cannulation prior to commencement of CPB. A small cluster of signals outside the flow envelope to the left of frame represents cerebral emboli occurring during aortic cannulation. (Courtesy of Dr. J.M. Murkin.)

ogy. Table 6.3 lists normal physiologic parameters for the brain.

Autoregulation of Cerebral Blood Flow

It is well established that blood flow to the brain is tightly coupled to cerebral metabolic demands and that this coupling is exquisitely sensitive to metabolic changes occurring at even a regional level. Using positron emission tomography (PET), selective increases in regional CBF have been observed in areas of cortex associated with incremental motor activity.[43] At a global level, CBF is constant over a wide range of cerebral perfusion pressures (CPP), as demonstrated by Lassen et al.[44] In normotensive awake individuals, CBF is maintained at approximately 50 mL/100 g/min over a range of mean arterial pressure (MAP) from 50 to 150 mm Hg, described as the *autoregulatory plateau*. Concomitant cerebral metabolic rate for oxygen ($CMRO_2$) is approximately 3.0 mL/100 g/min.

The autoregulatory plateau, over which CBF is constant despite a range of MAP, is a reflection of CBF-metabolism coupling. As such, factors that tend to decrease $CMRO_2$ (eg, sedative-hypnotic agents,[45-47] hypothermia[48]) will tend to lower the autoregulatory plateau so that CBF, although reduced, is maintained constant at a lower level as a consequence of the lowered $CMRO_2$ (Figure 6.3). This same principle can be shown to be operative during CPB. Factors that tend to produce cerebral vasodilatation, however, including certain anesthetic agents and direct-acting smooth-muscle relaxants—of which CO_2 is probably the most potent—will alter cerebral autoregulation and tend to disturb this pressure-flow relationship to produce pressure-passive CBF.

Factors Affecting CBF During CPB

Acid-Base Management

The mode of pH management during moderate hypothermia has been shown to profoundly influence cerebral vasodilation and flow-metabolism coupling. Using cerebral clearance of radioisotopic xenon to measure CBF, Prough et al[49] demonstrated that during hypothermic CPB at 28°C with alpha-stat pH management—during which total CO_2 remains constant by keeping non-temperature-corrected Pa_{CO_2} at 40 mm Hg and pH at 7.4—CBF is unaltered despite increases in MAP. Conversely, with pH-stat management—in which total body CO_2 is increased to maintain temperature-corrected values of pH 7.4 and Pa_{CO_2} 40 mm Hg—they observed that CBF varies and is directly proportional to MAP. Using similar radioisotopic clearance techniques, and incorporating a measure of cerebral oxygen extraction to assess $CMRO_2$, these changes in CBF were shown by Murkin et al[50] to be correlated with $CMRO_2$ during alpha-stat acid-base management, but were independent of $CMRO_2$ with pH-stat management (Figure 6.4). Therefore, during alpha-stat acid-base management, it is recognized that CBF is essentially constant over the range of CPP from 20 to 100 mm Hg.[50,51] CBF is also maintained at a much lower level than

TABLE 6.3. Normal physiologic parameters for the brain.

Global CBF	≈ 50 mL/100 g/min
CBF (gray)	≈ 80 mL/100 g/min
CBF (white)	≈ 20 mL/100 g/min
$CMRO_2$	≈ 3.5 mL/100 g/min
$CMR_{glucose}$	≈ 4.5 mL/100 g/min
$CBF/CMRO_2$	≈ 15
ICP	5-12 mm Hg
PV_{O_2}	>35 torr
$S_{JV}O_2$ (awake)	≈ 65-75%

CMR = cerebral metabolic rate
$CMRO_2$ = CMR for oxygen
ICP = intracranial pressure
PV_{O_2} = partial pressure of venous oxygen
$S_{JV}O_2$ = jugular venous oxygen saturation

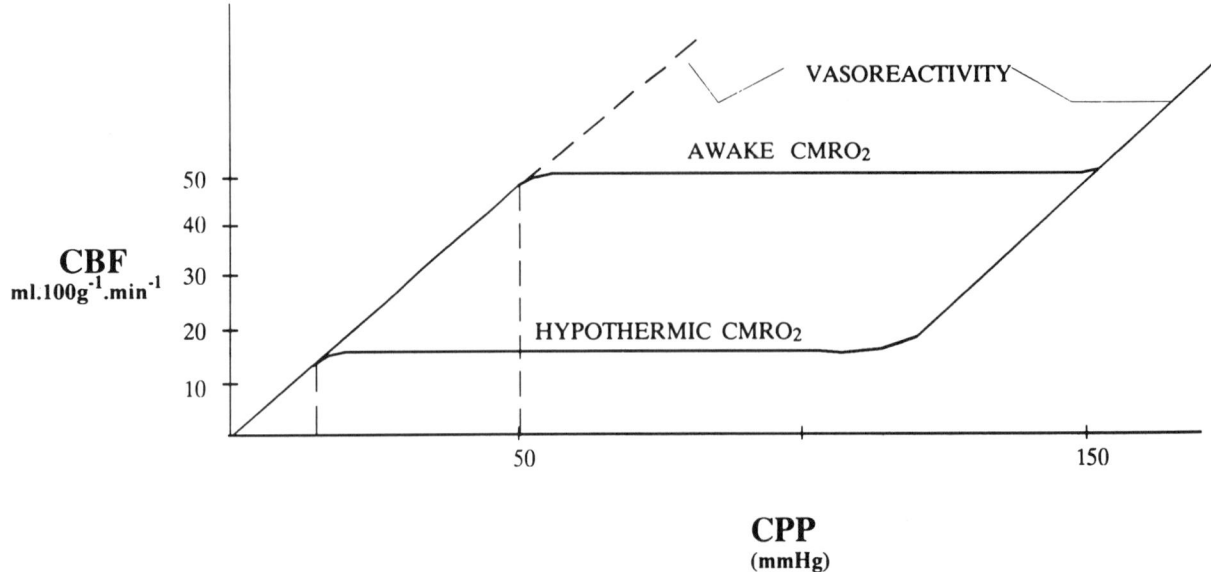

FIGURE 6.3. Cerebral autoregulatory curves during conditions of normal and lowered cerebral metabolic rates ($CMRO_2$), such as occur in the awake state or during hypothermia. The autoregulatory plateau is a reflection of intact cerebral flow/metabolism coupling, such that cerebral blood flow (CBF) is matched to $CMRO_2$. At any given $CMRO_2$, CBF will remain essentially constant over a range of cerebral perfusion pressures (CPP) until the limits of vasoreactivity of the cerebral vasculature are reached. (By permission of J.M. Murkin. Can J Anaesth 36: S41-44 1989.)

in awake individuals, averaging 12 to 15 mL/100 g/min during hypothermic CPB (28°C nasopharyngeal temperature).

Despite the effect of physiologic increases in $PaCO_2$ to produce cerebral vasodilatation and interfere with cerebral autoregulation, there is no evidence that pH-stat acid-base management during moderate hypothermia produces intracerebral steal and cerebral ischemia, even in patients with cerebrovascular disease. Gravlee et al[52] examined CBF in nine such patients undergoing hypothermic CPB and could find no evidence of intracerebral steal when $PaCO_2$ was randomly changed between values required for alpha-stat or pH-stat. It should be noted, however, that in all patients, MAP was over 50 mm Hg during the studies, thus producing a relative cerebral hyperemia during pH-stat management, which could potentially offset any tendency for intracerebral steal to develop.[52]

Profound Hypothermia

Profound hypothermia, with cerebral temperatures less than 22°C, also produces impaired cerebral autoregulation. In pediatric patients, Greeley et al[53] have demonstrated loss of cerebral pressure-flow autoregulation, such that CBF becomes pressure-passive during alpha-stat pH management at these low temperatures. Profound hypothermia thus appears to induce a form of cerebral vasoparesis that impairs cerebral autoregulation, although cerebral responsiveness to changes in CO_2 remains, albeit at a lessened sensitivity.[54]

Deep Hypothermic Circulatory Arrest

After deep hypothermic total circulatory arrest (DHTCA) in infants, CBF has been demonstrated to be significantly lower after re-establishment of flow than that in a group in whom similar temperatures were maintained but circulatory arrest was not employed.[53] In infants after DHTCA, CBF does not recover to prearrest values when assessed after separation from CPB. This is in contrast to patients in whom deep hypothermia has been employed without circulatory arrest, in whom CBF after rewarming returns to pre-CPB levels.[53] Therefore, DHTCA appears to produce a persisting decrease in CBF, the mechanism for which is unclear.

Using a transducer to measure anterior fontanel pressure (AFP) in infants, Burroughs et al[55] have demonstrated a progressive rise in AFP during DHTCA. In these patients, there was a direct correlation between the duration and temperature of DHTCA and the duration of the increase in AFP. They also demonstrated a significant negative correlation between cerebral function, as assessed using cortical evoked potential (EP) monitoring, and AFP. As AFP increased, EP activity decreased, suggesting an impairment of cortical function in the presence of increased AFP. Whether this corresponds to the same mechanism producing persistent decreases in CBF after DHTCA is currently unclear.

Mechanical Factors Affecting CBF

Although it is apparent that, under certain conditions, CBF autoregulation is preserved down to CPP of 20 mm Hg,[50,51] it should be recognized that during CPB, MAP does not necessarily equal CPP. In the presence of a single two-stage venous cannula, in which the inferior vena cava and the right atrium, but not the superior vena cava, are directly drained into the CPB circuit, rotation of the heart for surgical access may produce impaired drainage of the superior vena cava, leading to cerebral venous hypertension with the potential for the development of cerebral edema. In some instances, this may result in cerebral venous pressures that approach MAP, potentially resulting in significant reductions in cerebral perfusion, despite an apparently adequate MAP.

Pulsatile Perfusion

Although the mechanisms responsible for the reported increase in AFP[55] and decrease in CBF after DHTCA are unclear, it is possible that some of these changes may be reversed with the use of pulsatile perfusion. Watanabe et al[56] have shown that, after DHTCA in dogs, the use of pulsatile perfusion during the rewarming phase of CPB enhances metabolic activity of the brain. Pulsatile perfusion has greater kinetic energy than nonpulsatile flow, and this has been shown to decrease vascular resistance[57] and increase the uniformity of tissue perfusion,[58] thus facilitating microcirculatory flow in cerebral and conjunctival

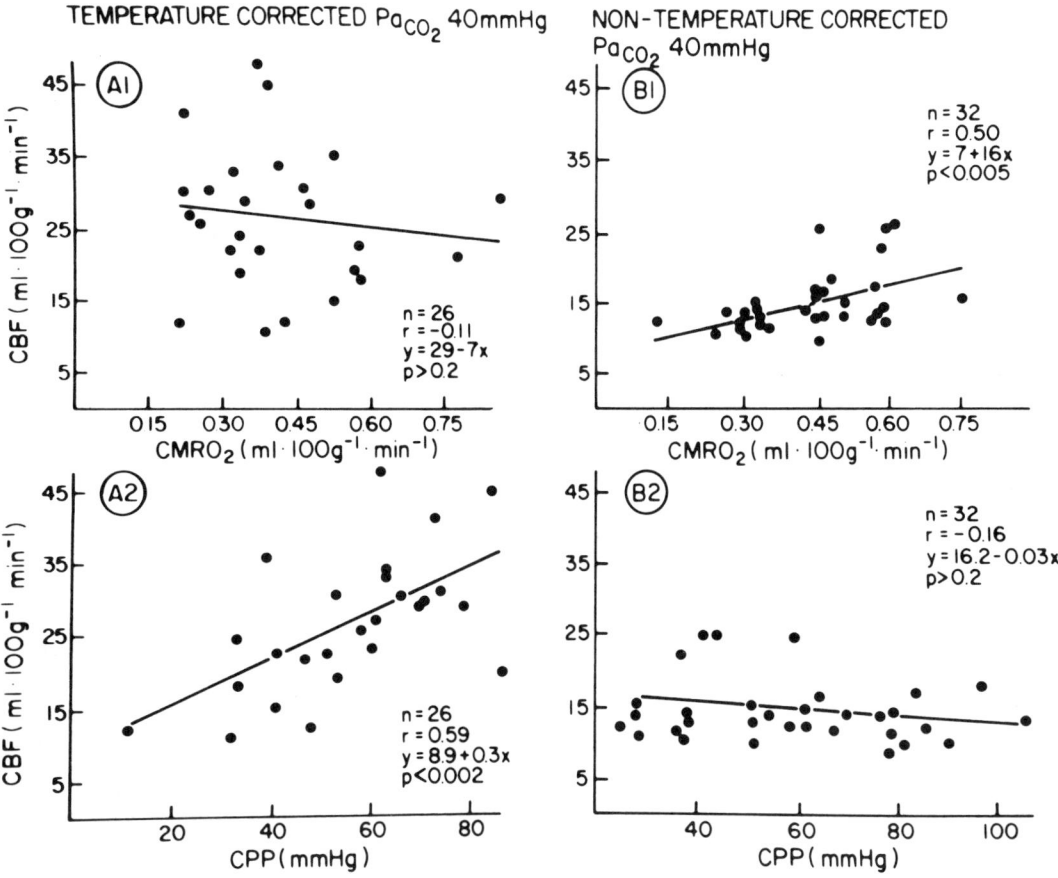

FIGURE 6.4. Correlations between cerebral blood flow and cerebral perfusion pressure, or cerebral blood flow and cerebral oxygen consumption, in a group in whom pH-stat acid-base management was employed during moderate hypothermic CPB (A1 and A2), and a group in whom alpha-stat pH management was used (B1 and B2). With pH-stat, CBF is independent of CMRO$_2$ (A1) and significantly influenced by CPP (A2), reflecting loss of cerebral flow/metabolism coupling and loss of cerebral autoregulation, and development of "pressure-passive" CBF. With alpha-stat, CBF is significantly related to CMRO$_2$ (B1) and independent of CPP (B2) down to 20 mm Hg, demonstrating preservation of cerebral autoregulation and cerebral flow/metabolism coupling. CBF is cerebral blood flow; CMRO$_2$ is cerebral metabolic rate for oxygen; CPP is cerebral perfusion pressure. (From Murkin, et al.[50] by permission of *Anesth Analg*.)

capillaries.[59] Whether this translates into an improved milieu for cerebral functioning is unclear.

Use of a flow interrupter during CPB to produce a cyclical interruption in the action of the roller pump heads can produce a flow pattern that approximates a pulsatile waveform. Although it does not mimic the arterial pressure characteristics of normal ventricular ejection, when assessed using TCD insonation of the MCA during CPB, this pulsatile flow pattern can be shown to be transmitted to the cerebral vasculature.[60] Increases in CBF of 15% over nonpulsatile control values have been produced during hypothermic CPB in man using a flow interrupter to produce pulsatile perfusion.[61] In a control group of dogs placed on normothermic CPB, Tranmer et al[62] demonstrated a 19% increase in CBF with institution of a pulsatile waveform. In this same study, in animals in which cerebral ischemia had been produced by ligation of their MCA, CBF was increased 40% in the ischemic hemisphere with the introduction of pulsatile flow. In contrast, Hindman and colleagues[63] reported that pulsatile perfusion, compared to nonpulsatile blood flow, did not alter either CBF or $CMRO_2$ during hypothermic (27°C) bypass with alpha-stat acid-base management in rabbits.

To date, there have been few clinical evaluations of the effect of pulsatile perfusion during CPB on postoperative organ function or on the incidence of CNS dysfunction. Badner et al[64] were unable to demonstrate any beneficial effects of pulsatile perfusion on postoperative renal function in a study of 100 patients with normal preoperative renal function undergoing elective CABG surgery. In a related study, the incidence of postoperative neurologic and neuropsychologic dysfunction in 316 patients undergoing CABG surgery was not influenced by the use of pulsatile perfusion, although cardiovascular morbidity was significantly lowered in the group receiving pulsatile perfusion.[65] Similarly, in a study of 22 CABG patients randomized to either pulsatile or nonpulsatile perfusion, the method of blood flow did not affect CBF, $CMRO_2$, or neurologic outcome.[66] Whether pulsatile perfusion will be of benefit for patients at increased risk of neurologic dysfunction (eg, elderly or diabetics) is currently unknown.

Hyperoxia and CBF

In addition to the important effects of CO_2, the arterial partial pressure of oxygen also contributes to CBF autoregulation. As part of the homeostatic mechanisms to protect the brain from hypoxemia, cerebral vascular resistance is reduced and CBF is increased with arterial hypoxemia, even when $Paco_2$ is decreased.[67] Similarly, hyperoxia will cause a decrease in CBF secondary to an increase in cerebral vascular resistance.[68] Cerebral Pao_2 also influences CBF during extracorporeal circulation. Rogers and colleagues[69] demonstrated that CBF is reduced by 15% when the Pao_2 is increased from 125 to 300 mm Hg during bypass with alpha-stat acid-base management.

Other Factors Affecting CBF

The effects of pump blood flow, blood pressure, anesthetics, age, and the duration of CPB on CBF during extracorporeal circulation are discussed below.

Mechanisms of Injury

There are three potential mechanisms by which inadequate oxygen delivery to the brain may occur during CPB: (1) global and regional cerebral hypoperfusion, (2) macroembolization, and (3) microembolization. These three processes may result in cerebral ischemia and precipitate the cascade of cellular biochemical events induced by inadequate oxygen delivery. These phenomena and the neurochemistry of ischemia are discussed below.

Etiology of Cerebral Ischemia During CPB and Cardiac Surgery

Cerebral Hypoperfusion

The factors that affect CBF during CPB are incompletely understood, and it is therefore difficult to ensure appropriate global and regional CBF and thus oxygen delivery during CPB. Alterations in blood flow and distribution during the nonphysiologic state of extracorporeal circulation, the attendant reduction in pump flow to facilitate the operative repair, and the individual response to reperfusion all may adversely affect global and regional cerebral perfusion.

Specific areas of the brain are especially vulnerable to cerebral hypoperfusion. A so-called "watershed" infarct may occur in the parieto-occipital lobes in a defined area that is dependent on perfusion from the terminal distributions of the anterior, middle, and posterior cerebral arteries.

Microembolization

The brain is subjected to an almost continuous shower of microparticulate matter during CPB. These microemboli come from a variety of sources and are believed to be factors in the genesis of postoperative cerebral dysfunction.[70,71] The various types and sources of microemboli generated during cardiac surgery and CPB are listed in Table 6.4.

Stump and colleagues,[72] studying elective coronary revascularization patients, reported that the number of emboli delivered to the brain is related to the magnitude of postoperative neuropsychologic dysfunction. The group of patients characterized as having had no significant de-

TABLE 6.4. Types and sources of microemboli generated during CPB.

Type	Source
Air	Oxygenator (bubbler)
	Heart
	Temperature gradients
	Intravenous solutions
	Argerial line filter
Oxygen	Oxygenator
	Temperature gradients
Lipid globules	Operative field cardiotomy suction
Muscle/connective tissue fragments	Muscle/connective tissue Sternotomy site
Platelet/leukocyte fibrin aggregates	Inadequately anticoagulated blood, banked blood
Plastic fragments	CPB circuit
Calcific particles	Aorta
	Major vessels
	Cannulation sites

crease in neuropsychologic functions had approximately half the number of embolic events as those patients who did have a postoperative neuropsychologic deficit.

Moody et al[73] have been able to demonstrate small capillary and arteriolar dilatations (SCADs) in patients dying after cardiac surgery. They observed 15- to 20-mm saccular dilatations that were distributed profusely throughout the cerebral vasculature. In their histologic studies, these lesions were vacuolated, leading to the speculation that they represent either air or fatty deposits that were removed during the staining and fixation procedures. Interestingly, they also observed these same lesions in patients dying after aortography, and therefore speculate that it is proximal aortic instrumentation that is responsible for the production of these emboli (Figures 6.5 and 6.6). In a concomitant series of dog studies, they observed that SCADs were present in dogs in which aortic cannulation and CPB had been employed, but not in dogs subjected to a sham operation.

Macroembolization

Macroembolization of large air bubbles, atheromatous debris from cardiac valvular lesions and/or aortic plaques, and intracardiac thrombi to the cerebral circulation contribute to the neurologic morbidity associated with cardiac surgery and CPB. TCD monitoring of the MCA permits both evaluation of CBF and detection of embolic events. Cerebral embolization may occur at any time, but there is an increase in embolic phenomena during manipulation of the aorta.[74] Further evidence implicating aortic instrumentation in the etiology of cerebral embolization has been obtained by TCD insonation of the MCA (Figure 6.2). Indeed, several investigators have reported that aortic cannulation is associated with a cerebral shower of emboli,[75,76] and it appears that aortic instrumentation and similar procedures associated with CPB account for a significant proportion of the cerebral emboli that do occur. Postmortem studies have demonstrated the presence of atheromatous and calcific debris in the cerebral circulation after open-chamber procedures.[77,78] Similar material has also been observed in the cerebral circulation after closed-chamber coronary artery surgery.[79]

Embolization of unnoticed, moderate amounts of air to the brain is a much more common problem. While air embolism may occur more frequently during open-chamber than in closed-chamber cardiac operations, the problem is substantial in both types of procedures, since there are multiple locations and sources for air trapping and air entrainment in every cardiac operation (Table 6.5).

Neurochemistry of CNS Ischemia

The last two decades have brought an increased understanding of the neurochemistry of stroke. Until the 1980s, ischemic death of cerebral parenchymal cells was believed to be solely secondary to energy failure. Indeed, cellular respiration is necessary to maintain the operation of ion pumps, active transport, and homeostatis of cell organelles, and irreversible ischemia will cause neuronal cell death. But energy failure does not account for all brain cell death induced by ischemia. In 1981, Astrup and colleagues[80] described the *penumbra* region of the ischemic brain. Neuronal cells in the penumbra are thought to lie between the upper threshold of electrical failure and the lower threshold of energy failure. Cells in the penumbra region are adjacent to both normally perfused neuronal tissue and ischemic cerebral parenchyma (Figure 6.7).

The penumbra cells are exposed to a neurochemical milieu produced by the ischemic cells, an environment characterized by an abundance of neuroexcitatory (and inhibitory) amines (glutamate, norepinephrine, dopamine, and γ-aminobutyric acid [GABA]) and multiple chemical mediators of inflammation (bradykinin,[81] serotonin,[82] histamine,[83] arachidonic acid,[84,85] and free radicals[86]) released either by ischemic cells or by sequestered neutrophils and macrophages. Although a thorough discussion of the pathophysiology of stroke is beyond the scope of this chapter, a basic understanding of the cellular consequences of cerebral ischemia is necessary to understand the rationale for potential neuroprotective strategies (see Pharmacologic Strategies for Cerebral Protection During Cardiac Surgery and CPB, below).

As noted above, inadequate delivery of oxygen to the brain tissue threatens two groups of neuronal cells: (1) those that undergo death by energy failure (core cells) and (2) those that are partially perfused but adjacent to ischemic or dying neuronal tissue (penumbra cells). Only rapid restoration of blood and oxygen delivery will prevent the loss of the former type, but cells in the penumbra region

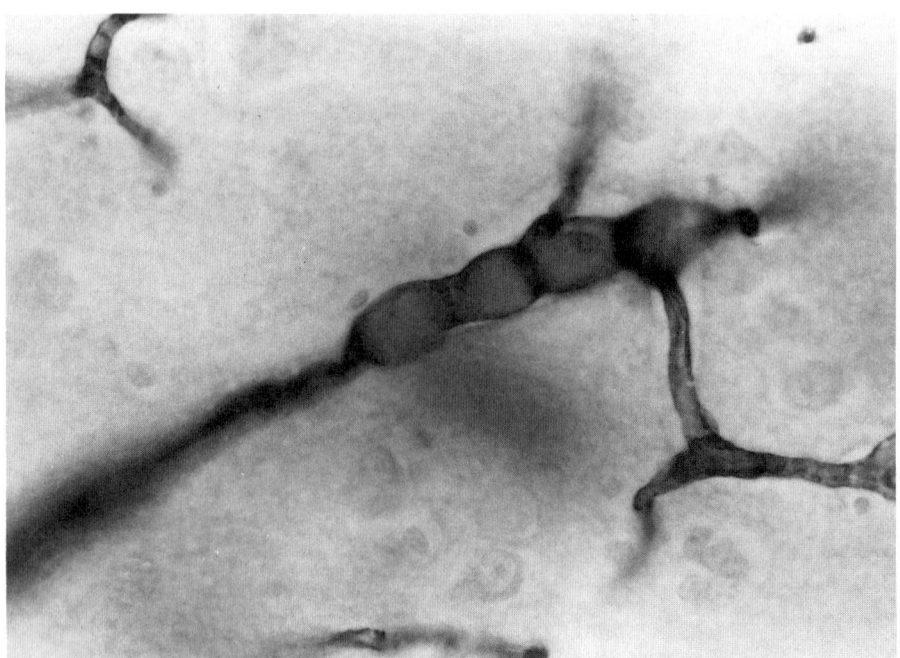

FIGURE 6.5. Photomicrograph demonstrating a cluster of aneurysmal dilatations in a brain capillary from a patient following CPB. The vacuolated appearance suggests these represent lipid emboli after preparation of a 100-μm-thick celloidin section stained for alkaline phosphatase. These lesions were only demonstrated in cerebral capillaries of patients or animals after either CPB or proximal aortic instrumentation. (Reprinted with permission from *Ann Neurol* 28:477–86 1990.)

are theoretically salvageable through modulation of the excitotoxic response (Figure 6.8).

The Excitotoxic Cascade Response

Ischemic cells quickly lose the ability to maintain energy-requiring sodium and potassium pump activity and thus undergo membrane depolarization. This leads to an increase in intracellular calcium and the release of neuroexcitatory amines, especially glutamate.[87] Ten minutes of ischemia will increase glutamate concentrations by a factor of 8.[88] Interestingly, the areas of the brain most vulnerable to ischemia are innervated by glutamatergic[89] neurons, and interruption of these fibers reduces neuronal injury.[90] Normally, excess glutamate is removed from the extracellular space by neuronal and glial cells. But in the absence of oxygen and adenosine triphosphate (ATP) production, these cells are unable to fulfill this function, and glutamate accumulates in the synaptic cleft. Glutamate release appears to be largely triggered by calcium influx via ion-

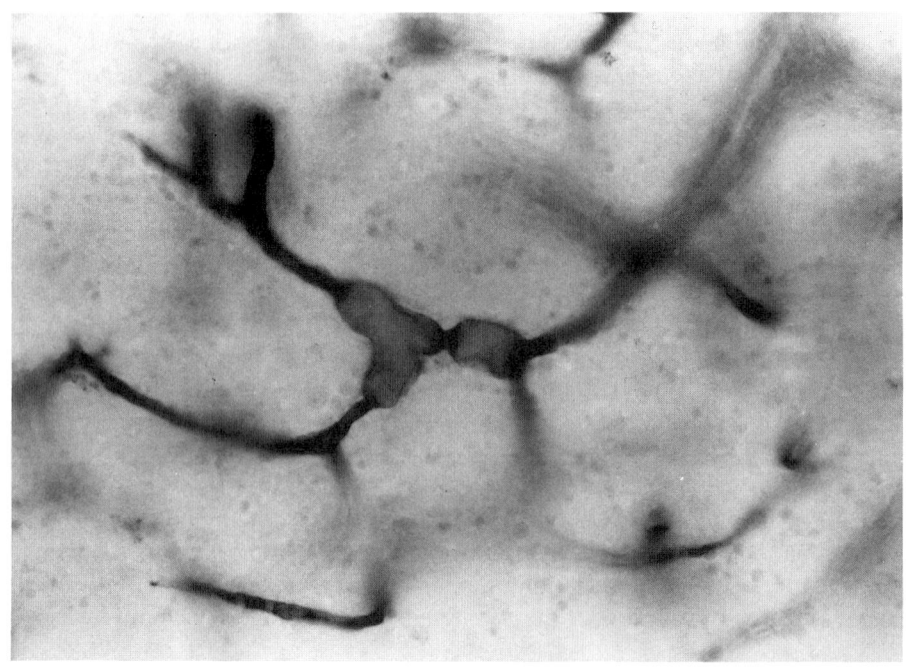

FIGURE 6.6. Photomicrograph of cerebral capillaries from the same series, demonstrating putative embolic material lodged at the bisection of a cerebral capillary of a patient after CPB. (Courtesy of Dr. D. M. Moody.)

TABLE 6.5. Sources and locations of gaseous emboli in cardiac surgery.[a]

Sources
    Aorta, pulmonary vessels, and intracardiac negative pressure vents
    Unexpected resumption of myocardial rhythm
    Open, contracting heart
    Pressured cardiotomy circuit
    Reversal of vent
Locations
    Left arterial appendage
    Ventricular apex
    Spaces between chordae tendineae, papillary muscles, trabeculae carinae
    Cardiac chamber cul-de-sacs
    Aortic root

[a]Sources of massive air emboli are discussed in Chapter 18.

selective L-type calcium channels. Glutamate then stimulates other neurons through several types of postsynaptic receptors (*N*-methyl-D-aspartate [NMDA] kainate, quisqualate/AMPA [α-amino-hydroxymethyl-isoxazole-proprionic acid], metabotrophic receptors) which are permeable to Na^+ and K^+, and of which NMDA receptors also have a high permeability to Ca^{2+}.[91,92] Glycine concentrations also increase after global ischemia and facilitate the neurotoxic effects of glutamate.[93,94] Glutamate stimulation of NMDA and kainate receptors causes the opening of calcium channels (independently of the altered membrane potential) and sodium channels, respectively. Glutamate excitotoxicity has been characterized as a biphasic response to postsynaptic receptor hyperstimulation. The first component results in acute neuronal swelling, largely as a result of NMDA and kainate receptor activation resulting in influx of extracellular Na^+ accompanied by passive Cl^- and water influx. The second component is marked by delayed neuronal disintegration resulting from transmembrane Ca^{2+} influx through NMDA-gated channels or through non-gated voltage-dependent calcium channels. Neuronal cells swell, as sodium (with water and chloride ions) enters the cytoplasm. Stimulation of metabotrophic receptors (such as muscarinic acetylcholine, α-1, histamine H_1, and NMDA) activates phospholipase C (PLC) via the G protein. This enzyme (PLC) cleaves a postsynaptic membrane phospholipid to produce inositol 1,4,5-triphosphate (IP_3) and 1,2 diacylglycerol (DG).[95]

Elevation of intracellular calcium occurs within 60 seconds after the induction of ischemia[96] through multiple mechanisms. IP_3 mobilizes endogenous calcium stores and NMDA-receptor stimulation opens calcium channels. The altered charge distribution across the cell membrane permits movement of calcium into the cell through voltage-gated calcium channels.[97] Finally, excess sodium activates a carrier molecule that exchanges sodium for calcium.

The substantially elevated calcium levels, in combination with DG, activate several enzyme systems. The end result of alteration of these enzymes is an increased sensitivity to excitatory amines. Thus, the response to ischemia is amplified as calcium accumulation continues, and there is further release of glutamate. Ultimately, irreversible cell damage occurs as increased cytosolic calcium activates multiple enzyme systems, which degrade DNA, cellular proteins, and phospholipids. For example, changes in fatty acid composition following 2 minutes of ischemia may be secondary to calcium-induced activation of phospholipase A_2 and other phospholipases.[98] Degradation of ribonucleoside phosphates also occurs, activating cyclic nucleosidase. Phospholipid breakdown leads to the formation of membrane-derived lipid products, such as arachidonic acid and platelet-activating factor (PAF). Me-

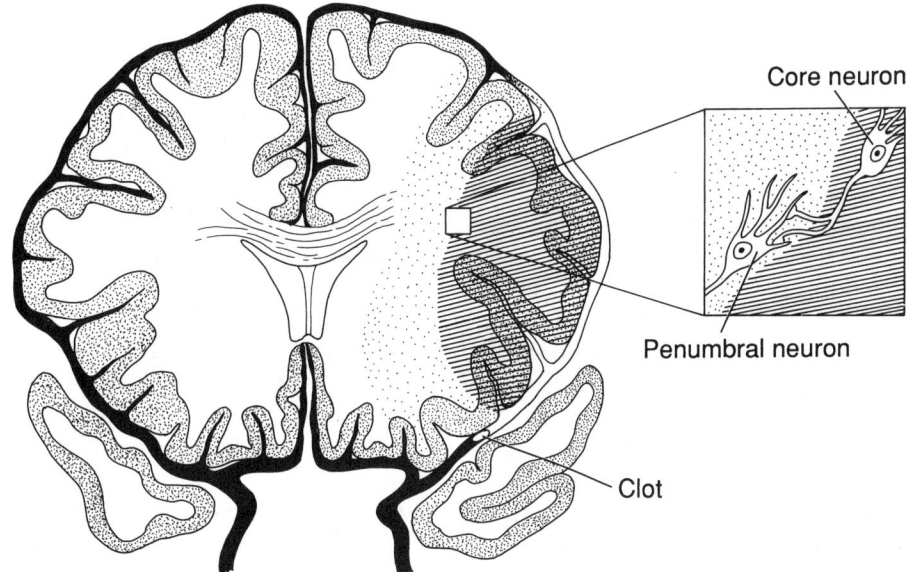

FIGURE 6.7. There are two areas of cerebral tissue that are subject to ischemic damage following occlusion of a cerebral artery. Core cells will die if blood flow and oxygen delivery is not re-established. The penumbral cells receive some blood from other arteries but may be damaged by the excitotoxic cascade induced in the core cells.

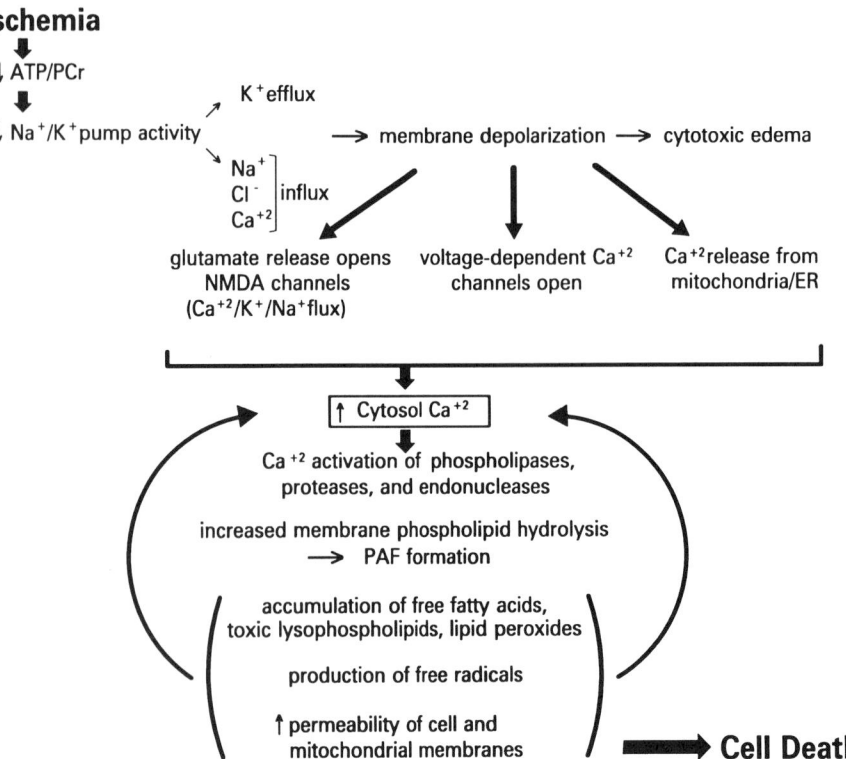

FIGURE 6.8. The excitotoxic cascade. Cerebral ischemia induces a number of biochemical events, including the release of various excitatory amines that cause an increase in intracellular calcium and, ultimately, cell death. (See text for further explanation.)

tabolism of arachidonic acid leads to the formation of oxygen free radicals which can induce lipid peroxidation and subsequent destruction of the cell membrane. Arachidonic acid also facilitates the formation of eicosanoids, which, together with PAF, cause blockage of previously healthy vessels through vasoconstriction and blood cell aggregation.

In summary, cerebral ischemia may cause neuronal death through at least two mechanisms: energy failure and excitotoxicity. The ischemic cell releases a variety of excitatory amines which stimulate a variety of receptors that cause an increase in intracellular calcium and sodium. Simultaneously, glutamate stimulation of metabotrophic receptors causes formation of IP_3 and DG, which will cause a further increase in calcium levels and activation of enzymes that increase the cellular sensitivity to excitatory amines. In the final stage, calcium-activated enzymes degrade ribonucleic acids, proteins, and phospholipids. Arachidonic acid (which will be metabolized to oxygen free radicals and eicosanoid moieties), together with PAF, will cause vasoconstriction, vessel occlusion, and subsequent spreading of ischemia. Although only re-establishment of blood flow to cells subject to energy failure will prevent their loss, there are several potential interventions to attenuate excitotoxic-induced ischemic cell death (see Pharmacologic Strategies for Cerebral Protection During Cardiac Surgery and CPB, below).

Role of Blood-Borne Chemical Mediators

Because attenuation of the putative actions of blood-borne neutrophils and macrophages reduces the amount of brain edema formation associated with cerebral ischemia, these moieties are thought to play an important role in cerebral tissue pannecrosis. For example, Shiga and colleagues[99] reported that the use of antineutrophil monoclonal antibodies reduced the brain water content in rats subjected to transient MCA occlusion.

Brain edema formation is also decreased with the administration of colchicine, a substance that reduces neutrophil sequestration at the site of ischemic tissue, prevents mononuclear cell phagocytosis, and prevents the production of interleukin-1. Presumably, neutrophil depletion and attenuation reduce the release of putative neurotoxic substances, including oxygen free radicals.

Factors Increasing Risk of Neurologic Dysfunction Following Cardiac Surgery

Several preoperative, intraoperative, and postoperative factors have been identified as potential risk factors and/or predictors of adverse neurologic outcomes in patients undergoing cardiac surgery. As noted previously, the methods used to detect neurologic abnormalities greatly

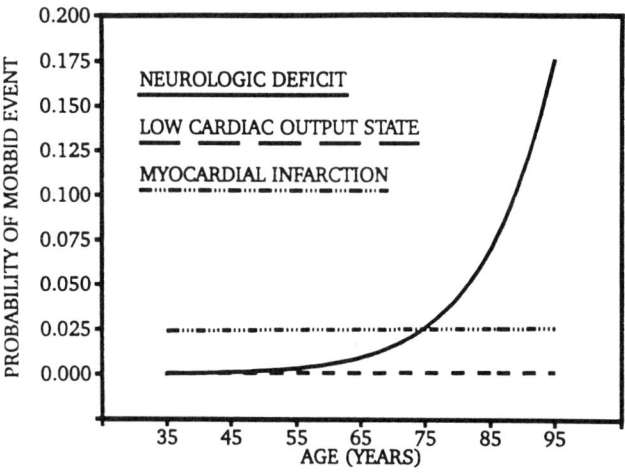

FIGURE 6.9. Effect of advanced age on the predicted probability of neurologic and cardiac morbidity. (From Tuman et al,[108] by permission of *J Thorac Cardiovasc Surg.*)

affect a given study's findings; differences among study designs are therefore critical to their interpretation.

Preoperative or Patient Predictors

Age

Elderly patients have an increased risk of neurologic injury after cardiac surgery.[100-108] In their study of two thousand patients undergoing elective coronary revascularization, Tuman and colleagues[108] reported that advanced age was the most important predictor of an untoward postoperative neurologic event. Patients 75 years of age or older were more than twice as likely to have a neurologic event than patients between the ages of 65 and 74 (8.9% vs 3.6%) and nine times more likely than patients under the age of 65 (0.9%).

There are several potential reasons for this apparent increased risk in older patients. Aged patients are more likely to have preexisting atheromatous cerebrovascular disease and/or atherosclerotic disease of the aorta and other great vessels; both global and regional CBF decreases with advancing age[109,110]; changes in autonomic function may alter CBF autoregulation.[111] However, investigators have failed to document a change in cerebral autoregulation related to age in elderly patients during CPB and alpha-stat acid-base management.[112] The inhomogeneous reduction in gray matter blood flow found in the aged may predispose the elderly patient with compromised cerebrovascular reserve to cerebral hypoperfusion and neurologic injury during CPB.[113]

Importantly, advanced age increases the risk of death from an adverse neurologic event, but not from a postoperative myocardial morbid outcome in elderly patients undergoing cardiac surgery (Figure 6.9).

Diabetes

Shaw and colleagues[114] have reported that diabetes increases the risk of stroke in patients undergoing coronary revascularization procedures. Additionally, a report by Croughwell et al[115] suggests that not all diabetic patients demonstrate intact cerebral autoregulation during hypothermic CPB with alpha-stat pH management. They observed that patients with diabetes mellitus had impaired cerebral autoregulation, with CBF being unrelated to cerebral metabolic rate. In a study of 11 diabetic patients and 12 age-matched controls, there was no change in CBF between hypothermic and normothermic conditions during CPB in the diabetic patients, despite temperature-mediated increases in cerebral oxygen consumption. Cerebral arteriovenous oxygen extraction was significantly increased in the diabetic patients in comparison to the control group, probably to compensate for the impaired oxygen delivery resulting from the lower CBF. CBF-metabolism coupling was absent in the diabetic patients, unlike the control group.

Systemic Hypertension

Earlier studies failed to show a correlation between the presence of systemic hypertension and postoperative adverse neurologic outcome.[13,116] However, a recent prospective study of cardiac surgery patients at the Johns Hopkins University suggests that hypertension may be a predictor of postoperative neurologic dysfunction.[117]

Cerebrovascular Disease

The relationship between cerebrovascular disease (CVD) and postoperative neurologic dysfunction in the cardiac surgery patient is of particular interest. Many studies have assessed the relationship between the signs, symptoms, and laboratory assessments of CVD and adverse neurologic outcome (Table 6.6).[118-126] As the overall incidence of postoperative stroke is small (2% to 7%), it is somewhat difficult to quantify the relationship between CVD and postoperative CNS dysfunction.

Several studies have reported on the positive correlation between a history of stroke or transient ischemia attack (TIA) and perioperative stroke risk.[108,114,118-120,126-128] Although a carotid bruit is a poor measure of the magnitude of carotid disease or of the severity of arterial intimal pathology,[129] several authors have assessed the significance of a cervical bruit as a stroke predictor. Some authors have reported that the presence of an asymptomatic carotid bruit does not appear to increase stroke risk.[118,124] Other investigators have found a positive correlation between carotid bruit (asymptomatic or symptomatic) and postoperative neurologic deficit.[128]

TABLE 6.6. Predictive value of stroke, TIA, cervical bruit, or Doppler signs of carotid disease on perioperative stroke risk.

Author (year)	+Stroke *with* predictor (stroke patients/total patients)	+Stroke *without* predictor (stroke patients/total patients)
TIA OR STROKE		
Turnipseed[118] (1980)	3/108	10/222
Martin[119] (1982)	1/14	7/239
Jones[120] (1984)	6/70	45/5606
CERVICAL BRUIT		
Treiman[121] (1979)	1/70	3/369
Turnipseed[118] (1980)	4/98	9/232
Barnes[122] (1980)	2/44	3/405
Jones[120] (1984)	2/60	49/5616
Taylor[123] (1985)	4/10	16/443
DOPPLER SONOGRAPHY		
Turnipseed[118] (1980)	4/92	9/238
Barnes[122] (1981)	3/63	2/376
Breslau[124] (1981)	0/18	1/84
Brener[125] (1987)	4/64	74/3894

A Doppler study indicative of carotid disease may suggest an increased risk of postoperative stroke (Table 6.6). However, Breslau and colleagues,[124] in a study of 102 patients presenting for cardiac surgery, found no association between postoperative stroke or TIA (2% incidence) and the presence of carotid disease, defined as a 50% or greater reduction in lumen diameter on Doppler sonography. They suggested that the carotid disease is not a specific risk factor per se, but may be a significant marker for susceptibility to CNS dysfunction postoperatively.

Patients with even severe carotid stenosis appear to have intact cerebral autoregulation. In a patient with bilateral carotid stenosis, Brusino et al[130] demonstrated intact cerebral autoregulation over a range of MAP from 35 to 85 mm Hg during alpha-stat acid-base management, implying that, even in the presence of CVD, cerebral autoregulation and CBF-metabolism coupling are preserved using alpha-stat techniques. In 18 patients with severe carotid stenosis and a control group of 37 without apparent CVD, von Reutern et al[131] used TCD ultrasonography to assess cerebral perfusion qualitatively; they were unable to demonstrate any differences in response to hypothermic CPB in either group.

Furlan and colleagues,[132,133] in two separate studies, have reported on the relationship between the severity of angiographically defined carotid stenosis and the risk of postoperative stroke. In one study, they reported that unilateral carotid stenosis (50% to 90%) did not increase the risk of perioperative stroke in coronary revascularization patients who did not have any symptoms of CVD.[132] However, in a later study, patients with 90% or greater carotid stenosis had an increased risk of ipsilateral stroke (1/16) over patients with 50% to 90% occlusion of the carotid artery.[133]

One may conclude from these data that elderly patients, or patients with a history of a stroke or TIA, have an increased risk of perioperative stroke during cardiac surgery. The importance of detectable carotid stenosis, whether by auscultation or laboratory studies, in patients without symptoms of CVD, is unclear. Symptomatic patients, or patients with signs suggestive of cerebrovascular insufficiency, should probably be referred for laboratory assessments of their cerebral circulation. Whereas patients with a recent history of either a TIA or stroke may be referred for elective carotid endarterectomy, the appropriateness of carotid surgery in other groups of patients with CVD is unclear. Because the risk of stroke in a patient with a history of a TIA who undergoes a carotid endarterectomy is 3% to 7%, and the absolute risk of perioperative stroke associated with coronary revascularization, even in the presence of carotid disease, does not exceed 5% to 7%, a decision to perform a prophylactic or simultaneous carotid endarterectomy must be considered carefully.

Intraoperative Predictors

Cardiac Disease: Open vs Closed Procedures

The type and severity of cardiac disease affects the risk of an adverse neurologic outcome following cardiac surgery. Most studies report that patients with cardiac lesions requiring open-chamber procedures are at a higher neurologic risk (eg, 5% to 8%)[70,134,135] than patients undergoing closed procedures (eg, 1% to 2%).[12-14] However, in a study comparing the incidence of neurologic deficits following coronary versus valve procedures (in which bypass time was substantially increased in the coronary group), Kuroda and colleagues[136] reported an increased risk in the closed-procedure group. It is unclear if it is the lesions per se that increase neurologic risk or if it is the operative techniques employed that predispose the open-chamber procedure patient to an adverse neurologic outcome. However, the presence of an intracardiac thrombus[137] or severe aortic or valvular calcification also increases the risk of perioperative stroke.[116] Patients undergoing heart surgery because of a cardioembolic stroke, especially those with infective endocarditis or large infarcts, are at a substantial risk for perioperative cerebral complications. In one study, 29% of these patients were reported to have suffered an adverse postoperative neurologic event.[138]

Preliminary evidence suggests that there are similar incidences of subtle postoperative neuropsychologic dysfunction, regardless of whether open-ventricle procedures, such as valvular surgery, or closed-chamber procedures, such as coronary bypass grafting, are performed.[28] This is not necessarily inconsistent with the observation that the incidence of overt clinical stroke is generally reported as being much higher in open-chamber than in closed-chamber surgery. These observations suggest that there are two different mechanisms producing these disparate results. The subtle abnormalities that are detectable and apparently occur with similar frequency after CPB, regardless of the nature of the surgical procedure, would imply that some mechanism common to CPB is the cause, whereas the generally higher incidence of overt neurologic damage in open-chamber procedures likely indicates macro-particulate emboli.

Aortic Disease

Several investigators have reported on the causal relationship between aortic arch disease and cerebral and peripheral embolic lesions in medical patients.[139-143] Similarly, atheromatous disease of the ascending aorta and aortic arch is emerging as a significant risk factor for the development of postoperative neurologic dysfunction.[13,144-153] As depicted in Figure 6.10, aortic manipulation (including cannulation and crossclamping) is associated with significant cerebral embolization. Presumably, atheromatous debris is dislodged during surgical handling of the aorta or "sand-blasted" off by the high-pressure jet-stream of blood rushing through the tip of the aortic cannula (Figure 6.11).

Older patients (a group at increased risk for an adverse neurologic outcome) are more likely to have atheromatous changes in the ascending aorta or aortic arch. Wareing and colleagues,[152] using intraoperative ultrasonography to assess the ascending aorta, found that 32% of patients over the age of 70 had moderate or severe atherosclerosis. Similarly, Marschall et al[153] reported that increasing age correlates with increasing severity of diseases of the aortic arch and descending thoracic aorta. In this study of 258 patients undergoing different types of car-

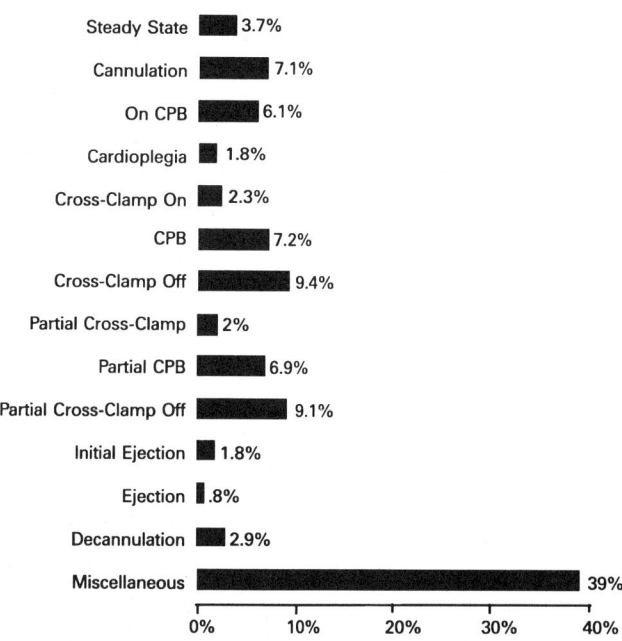

FIGURE 6.10. When cerebral emboli (as measured by transcranial Doppler sonography) occur during cardiac surgery and CPB. Note that a significant percentage of embolic events occur with manipulation of the aorta. (Courtesy of Dr. David A. Stump.)

diac procedures, severe disease (defined as aortic plaques ≥ 5 mm thick or with a mobile component) was not identified in any patient under the age of 50, but was present in approximately 20% of those more than 70 years of age. Katz[142] reported that 18% of 130 patients over the age of 65 had protruding atheromas, the only perioperative variable that was predictive of stroke.

Because the majority of atheromatous lesions are not identifiable by conventional modalities (including chest x-ray and cardiac catherization),[152,153] and intraoperative palpation of the aorta both underpredicts the frequency and location of atheroma and may dislodge atheromatous debris, several investigators[142,152,153] have advocated the use of intraoperative echocardiography to identify patients at significant risk for aortic embolbi. The standard surgical approach used to establish arterial access for extracorporeal circulation can be modified to avoid manipulation of the diseased aorta.

Wareing and colleagues[152] have reported promising results in cardiac surgery patients with a high risk of an adverse postoperative neurologic event. Using intraoperative ultrasonographic scanning, this group modified their operative approach in the 68 patients out of 500 (13.6%) found to have significant atheromatous disease of the aorta. Using the algorithm depicted in Figure 6.12, this group was able to prevent the occurrence of a postoperative neurologic deficit in this high-risk group of patients.

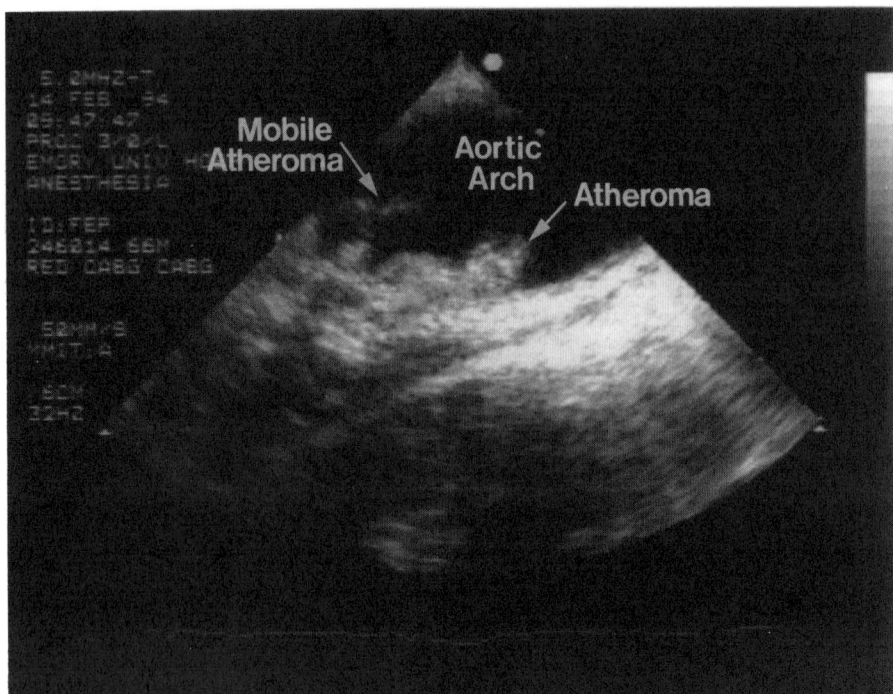

FIGURE 6.11. Ultrasonic image obtained with a transesophageal echocardiographic (TEE) examination of the aortic arch during cardiac surgery demonstrating moderate atherosclerosis and a mobile atheroma. (Courtesy of Dr. Jack S. Shanewise.)

Hypotension

Multiple studies have investigated the relationship between intraoperative hypotension and perioperative neurologic dysfunction (Table 6.7).[18,32,49,70,100,103,154-162] Because *earlier* studies tended to report the intraoperative hypotension placed cardiac surgery patients, undergoing either closed or open procedures, at an increased risk for an adverse CNS outcome, these early investigators recommended that the mean arterial blood pressure be maintained above 50 mm Hg.[105,160] Since the early 1970s, the severity of intraoperative hypotension has been quantified by several investigators using Stockard's hypotension index, TM^{50}.[105,160] This measure is defined as the product of the duration and degree during which the MAP is less than 50 mm Hg. Significant or substantial hypotension is defined as $TM^{-50} < 100$ mm Hg/min. Importantly, *more recent* studies have failed to find a causal relationship between intraoperative hypotension and neurologic morbidity. For example, Fish and colleagues,[161] in their study assessing the effect of prostacyclin on postoperative neuropsychologic dysfunction in coronary revasculariza-

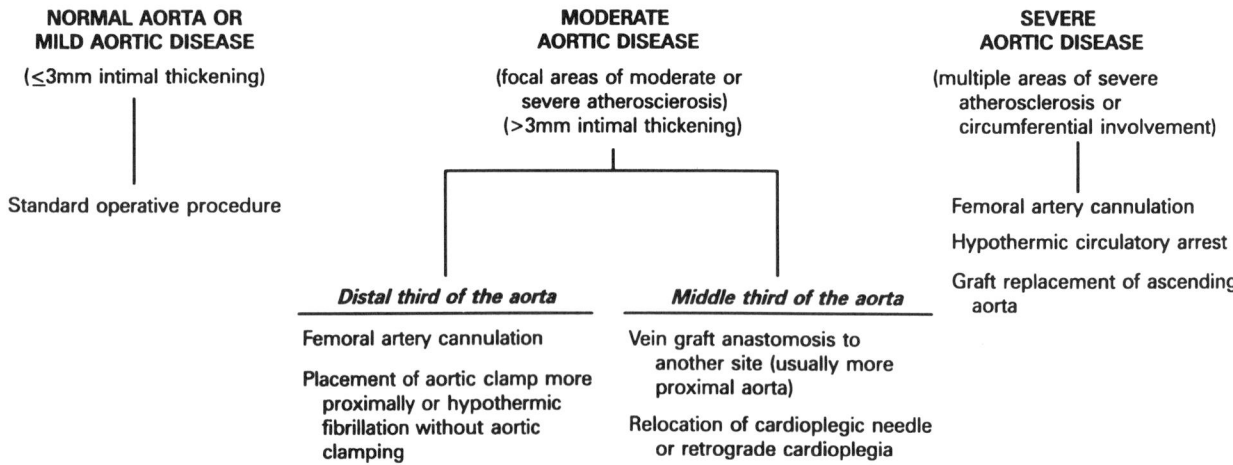

FIGURE 6.12. Algorithm for management of the atheroslcerotic ascending aorta based on ultrasonography. (Adapted from Wareing et al[152] by permission of *J Thorac Cardiovasc Surg*.)

tion patients, reported that the twofold increase in TM^{-50} among the prostacyclin-treated versus the control patients did not substantially affect postoperative neuropsychologic testing. Although there are several potential reasons for the dichotomous findings of early and late investigators with regard to the relationship between hypotension and neurologic outcome (arterial filter use, improved biocompatible materials, increased use of membrane oxygenators), the evolution of acid-base management during CPB from pH-stat to alpha-stat may have had the most significant effect on cerebral perfusion in the face of substantial intraoperative hypotension. As noted above, cerebral autoregulation is maintained with alpha-stat acid-base management, but CBF is pressure dependent when pH-stat techniques are employed. Thus, patients managed with pH-stat techniques may be more likely to have inadequate cerebral perfusion with hypotension. However, Bashein and colleagues[162] were unable to demonstrate any significant differences in neuropsychologic outcomes between patients managed with alpha-stat or pH-stat techniques. There was an equal number of hypotensive patients in each treatment group, but this study did not assess CBF in either of the treatment groups. Thus, the effect of hypotension on CBF in either treatment group is unknown.

Pump Flow

To date, there are no studies defining the optimal pump flow during CPB for patients undergoing either closed or open cardiac procedures. Clearly, the "perfect" pump flow would be that which provides adequate oxygen delivery without excess cerebral perfusion and the attendant increased embolic load.

Govier and colleagues[153] reported that, under CPB conditions of moderate hypothermia, normocapnia (determined with temperature-uncorrected blood-gas measurements), nonpulsatile blood flow, and an MAP between 45 and 70 mm Hg, variation of pump flow between 1.0 and 2.0 L/min/per m^2 did not affect CBF (Figure 6.13).

Both temperature and blood gas management will greatly affect both cerebral oxygen requirements and coupling of $CMRO_2$ and CBF. As discussed in Chapter 3, both low-flow bypass with hypothermia and deep hypothermic circulatory arrest are well tolerated. Swain and colleagues[163] demonstrated that low-flow hypothermic CPB in sheep is neuroprotective.

Equipment (Oxygenators, Arterial Filters)

In addition to emboli generated during aortic instrumentation, the type of CPB equipment can also affect the embolic load delivered to the brain. Use of membrane instead of bubble oxygenators has been shown to produce greater volumes of microparticulate air measured using ultrasonic transducers placed over the arterial inflow cannula. Padayachee and colleagues[164] have shown that delivery of emboli into the cerebral microcirculation, as assessed by TCD sonography, is much greater with the bubble than with the membrane oxygenator. Use of an arterial line filter is effective in decreasing the embolic load, with a 20-μm type being more effective than a 40-μm filter.[165] Pugsley et al[75] have been able to show that employment of an arterial line filter decreases embolic load during CPB but does not influence emboli associated with aortic instrumentation and initiation of CPB. This is again consistent with the aorta as a primary site for embolus generation that cannot be influenced by oxygenator type, but may be remedied by modifications of aortic cannulation sites and strategies. In this same study, this group also presented preliminary evidence that neuropsychologic outcome is related to embolic load, and that it can be improved with the use of arterial line filtration during CPB.[75] In the canine model, the use of arterial filters during CPB eliminates the rise in cerebral spinal fluid creatinine phosphokinase-B (CPK-B) that normally occurs

TABLE 6.7. Intraoperative hypotension as a predictor of perioperative neurologic morbidity.

Refuted		Supported	
Author	No. patients	Author	No. patients
Kolkka (1980)[102]	204	Gilman (1965)[157]	35
Ellis (1980)[103]	30	Javid (1969)[100]	100
Sotaniemi (1981)[16]	49	Tufo (1970)[134]	85
Slogoff (1982)[70]	204	Lee (1971)[158]	71
Govier (1984)[51]	17	Stockard (1973)[105]	25
Gardner (1985)[13]	168	Stockard (1974)[160]	75
Nussmeier (1986)[135]	187	Brainthwaite (1975)[126]	528
Fish (1987)[161]	100	Savageau (1982)[17]	227
Townes (1989)[156]	90		
Bashein (1990)[162]	78		
Stanley (1990)[159]	19		
Kramer (1994)[155]	230		

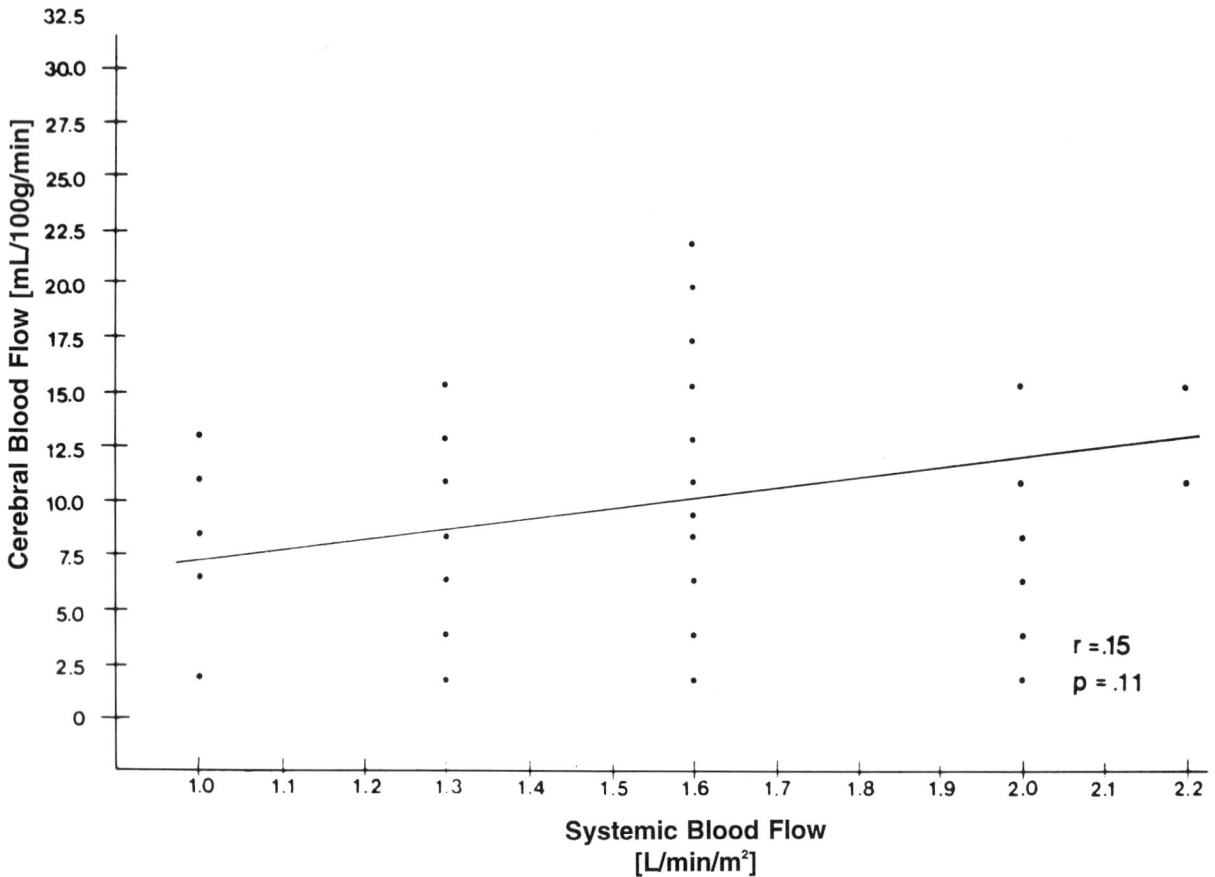

FIGURE 6.13. Relationship between cerebral blood flow and systemic blood flow during CPB. The line represents an average regression line over all patients. There are 44 hidden observations. Note that cerebral blood flow is relatively constant over a wide range of pump blood flow. (Reprinted with permission from the Society of Thoracic Surgeons [*The Annals of Thoracic Surgery*, 1984;38:592–600].)

after CPB.[166] Presumably, arterial filtration reduces the number of microemboli and the attendant brain cell damage.

Using fluorescein retinal angiography, Blauth et al.[167] have shown that progressive retinal microvascular embolization occurs during CPB. Since the retinal vasculature is essentially an extension of the cerebral microcirculation, presumably a similar process occurs throughout the brain during CPB. Whether these retinal microemboli are similar in nature to the SCADs observed by Moody et al is unknown, but they are a manifestation of the same process. Blauth et al were also able to demonstrate a significant reduction of retinal microemboli with employment of a 20-μm arterial line filter on the aortic inflow cannula.

Temperature Management

The influence of hypothermia in decreasing $CMRO_2$, and thus prolonging tolerance for ischemia, has been felt to provide some measure of protection for the brain during CPB. Importantly, hypothermia may attenuate the effect of cerebral ischemia either by decreasing $CMRO_2$ or by attenuating the excitotoxic response to ischemia (see Neurochemistry of CNS Ischemia, above). The salutary effect of hypothermia on $CMRO_2$ may be a less important effect of temperature on cerebral protection during ischemia. The log-linear relationship between temperature and $CMRO_2$ does not correlate with the magnitude of cerebral protection provided by hypothermia: brain injury, as quantified by histologic changes, has a sigmoid relationship with temperature. The degree of metabolic depression does not predict the magnitude of hypothermic protection from ischemic injury.

For example, the tolerance for cerebral ischemia has been shown to be prolonged disproportionately during mild hypothermia to 34°C.[168] In rats subjected to four-vessel occlusion of the cerebral circulation, despite severe depletion of brain energy metabolites during ischemia at all temperatures, small increments of intraischemic brain temperature markedly accentuated histopathologic changes following 3 days' survival, so that ischemic neurons within the central zone of striatum were not observed in any rats treated at 34°C but were present in all rats maintained at 36°C. Natale and colleagues[169] reported

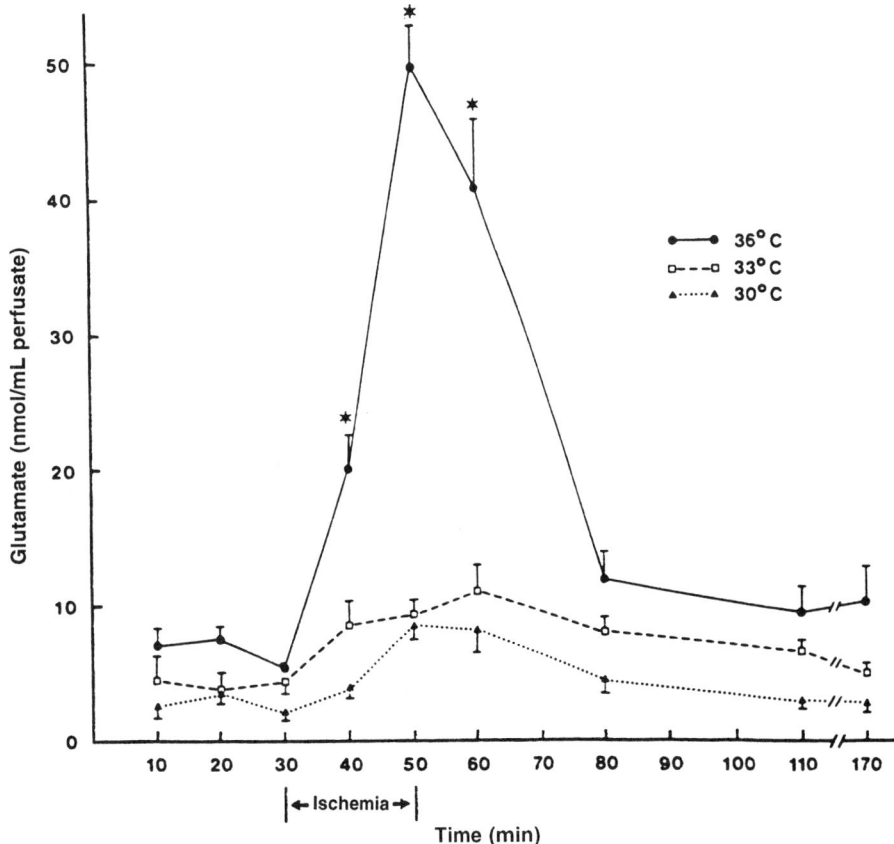

FIGURE 6.14. Line plot of time-course changes in the perfusate levels of glutamate (nmol/mL) in animals whose intraischemic brain temperature was maintained at 36°C ($n = 10$) (●–●), 33°C ($n = 4$) (□---□), and 30°C ($n = 8$) (▲···▲). The data presented are mean ± SEM. Statistical significance was assessed by two-way ANOVA. In animals whose intraischemic brain temperature was maintained at 36°C, a massive increase in extracellular glutamate was demonstrated (*significantly higher than control values, $p < 0.01$). No significant changes were found in animals whose intraischemic brain temperature was maintained at 33° or 30°C. (From Busto et al[170] by permission of *Stroke*.)

that hypothermia provides cerebral protection even in the *absence* of apparent metabolic depression. This group subjected dogs to 10 minutes of ventricular fibrillation at hyperthermic (27°–39°C) or hypothermic (33°–34°C) temperature. Although there was no difference in brain lactate tissue levels (suggesting a similar depletion of ATP levels among the group), only the hypothermic dogs survived for 24 hours after fibrillation. As discussed in the section, Neurochemistry of CNS Ischemia, energy failure induces a cascade of excitotoxic events. During normothermic ischemia, glutamate and other excitatory amines are released into the synaptic cleft (Figure 6.8). Moderate hypothermia (30° to 33°C) abolishes the release of glutamate and greatly attenuates the release of dopamine (Figure 6.14).[170]

In contrast to the salutary effect of mild hypothermia, normothermia or hyperthermia to 40.6°C has been demonstrated to decrease markedly the tolerance to ischemia and impair metabolic recovery after transient global cerebral ischemia.[171,172] Dietrich and colleagues[172] demonstrated that 20 minutes of forebrain ischemia at 39°C, compared to a similar insult at 37°C, augmented brain-injury-increased mortality and accelerated histologic evidence of injury. Hyperthermia has an especially harmful effect on the blood-brain barrier, causing multifocal breakdown at thalamic, hippocampal, and striatal sites.[173,174]

The issue of the effect of temperature on protection from ischemic cerebral insult is of particular interest in view of the resurgence of interest in normothermic bypass techniques. If the cerebral injury associated with cardiac surgery and CPB is caused by atheromatous debris dislodged from the aorta prior to or after bypass, then temperature management during extracorporeal circulation should not affect cerebral outcome, since the brain is normothermic during the atheromatous embolic insult. Although laboratory evidence suggests that hypothermia is protective during *temporary ischemia*, it is less clear if reduced brain temperatures will attenuate brain injury following permanent lesions (eg, atheroemboli). Ridenour and colleagues[175] reported that mild hypothermia (33°C) did not improve histologic evidence of cerebral infarction following permanent focal ischemia. However, Onesti[176] found deep hypothermia (24°C) to offer protection from permanent ischemic insults, while Morikawa and colleagues[177] observed a trend toward cerebral protection with moderate hypothermic (27° to 28°C) extracorporeal circulation.

Alternatively, if the cerebral injury associated with cardiac surgery and CPB is induced principally by cerebral hypoperfusion and/or gaseous or microparticulate emboli occurring during CPB, then the mode of temperature management may affect neurologic outcome. To date, studies have reported seemingly conflicting results on the effect of temperature on neurologic outcome following coronary revascularization procedures. Wong and colleagues[178] assessed the effect of temperature on cognitive function following coronary procedures. Thirty-four patients were randomly assigned to undergo either normothermic (34.7 ± 0.5°C) or hypothermic (27.8 ± 2.0°C) bypass after preoperative cognitive function testing. There were no significant differences in the neuropsychologic test scores of the two groups, and no patient suffered a postoperative stroke. Although this study suggests that hypothermia did not protect against neurologic injury, as manifested by cognitive dysfunction, the small number of patients studied precludes any assessment of the effect of temperature during bypass on focal neurologic injury or stroke. Martin and colleagues[179] at Emory University randomly assigned 1001 patients undergoing elective coronary revascularization procedures to normothermic (with temperature *maintained* at 37°C) or hypothermic (28°C) bypass. Although there was no difference between the treatment groups in myocardial outcomes as measured by death, Q-wave MI, or need for intraaortic balloon pump counterpulsation, warm bypass did appear to increase the risk of an adverse neurologic event. There was a statistically significant difference in total neurologic deficits (cold 1.4%, warm 4.5%, $p \leq 0.005$) and focal neurologic lesions (cold 1.0%, warm, 3.1%, $p \leq 0.02$). Importantly, preoperative neurologic assessments were not done in the 1001-patient study, and therefore the overall incidence of stroke was most likely underestimated. However, a companion study by Mora and colleagues[180] included both preoperative and postoperative neurologic assessments in a 140-patient subset of the 1001-patient study group. Again, the adverse effect of normothermic techniques during CPB was noted. Of the seven new focal deficits noted in the 140-patient study group, all were identified in the warm bypass treatment group ($p \leq 0.006$).

It is important to note the differences among the techniques employed in the Wong, Martin, and Mora studies. In the Wong investigation, patient temperatures were allowed to "drift" during CPB. Thus, the "normothermic" group in the Wong study had mean temperatures of 34.7 ± 0.5°C during bypass. This is contrary to the techniques employed in the Martin and Mora studies, in which patients were actively warmed to maintain temperature at 37°C and therefore did not drift below 35°C. These patients may have been exposed to *hyperthermic* temperatures during bypass, since the blood perfusing the brain through the aorta cannula is actively warmed in a water bath maintained at 40° to 42°C.

In summary, there is substantial laboratory and clinical evidence that hyperthermia increases the neurologic risk associated with temporary, and probably permanent, cerebral ischemia. The clinical studies by Martin and Mora suggest that active warming and maintenance of normothermic temperatures during bypass should not be employed because of the significant neurologic threat associated with these techniques. Further clinical studies are required to delineate the optimal temperature during CPB.

Glucose Management

Glucose management during CPB is highly controversial. Metz and Slogoff[181] have demonstrated that fluid balance is less positive in patients who are infused with 5% dextrose in lactated Ringer's solution (D_5LR) (blood glucose during CPB = 600-800 mg/dL) during CPB, and that gross neurologic dysfunction is no different in patients managed with or without (blood glucose = 200-300 mg/dL) glucose supplementation. However, the overall incidence of neurologic injury in this study was very low (1/107), and the methods used to quantify neurologic injury were not well defined. Similarly, others have been unable to demonstrate any relationship between blood glucose concentrations and neuropsychologic outcome.[182] Investigators at Duke University[182] assessed the effect of blood glucose on neurologic and neuropsychologic function in 60 patients undergoing cardiac surgery. Blood glucose concentrations during CPB ranged from 103 to 379 mg/dL, and glucose concentrations greater than 250 mg/dL were treated with insulin. Overall, there was a significant decrement in cognitive function, but changes in 10 of the 12 neuropsychologic tests were not related to mean blood glucose concentrations during CPB.

As pointed out in a comprehensive editorial overview,[183] there is, however, a large body of literature, from human and animal studies, in which a direct correlation has been shown between hyperglycemia and worsened neurologic outcome. This likely reflects the phenomenon of anaerobic conversion of glucose to lactate, resulting in a decrease in intracellular pH, and subsequent impairment of cellular metabolic processes. Ultimately, this metabolic impairment leads to a decreased cellular tolerance for ischemic insult. Importantly, studies reporting a worsening of neurologic injury in the presence of hyperglycemia include *normothermic* conditions. In the human studies noted above, hyperglycemia occurred during *hypothermic* bypass. Hypothermia has been shown to attenuate the detrimental effects of hyperglycemia during cerebral ischemia.[184,185] Dietrich and colleagues[185] reported that moderate hypothermia (30°C) attenuates the disruptive effect of hyperglycemia on blood-brain barrier integrity, while others have demonstrated the desirable effect of hypothermia (32° to 33°C) on both neurologic and histologic outcomes following brain ischemia with hyperglycemia. Therefore, the lack of conclusive evidence for a causal relationship between hyperglycemia and adverse neurologic outcome following cardiac surgery may be due to the use of hypothermia. Therefore, it is currently recommended that no glucose be administered during CPB and that blood glucose levels be maintained within the euglycemic range.

Blood Gas Management

The type of acid-base management during CPB (alpha-stat or pH-stat) greatly affects CBF during extracorporeal circulation. During pH-stat management, the relative hypercarbia causes cerebral vasodilation and a concomitant increase in CBF and loss of cerebral autoregulation.[29] Because $CMRO_2$ is minimally affected by the type of blood-gas management during hypothermic (27°C) CPB, pH-stat management causes a mismatch of CBF and $CMRO_2$, a so-called *luxury perfusion*. This luxury perfusion is potentially advantageous during bypass, as it may provide a margin of safety during hypotension, or it may be disadvantageous, because it increases the embolic load to the brain. Two studies have assessed the effect of blood-gas management on neurologic and neuropsychologic outcomes following cardiac surgery and CPB. Bashein and colleagues[162] compared the effects of alpha-stat and pH-stat acid-base management during CPB on neuropsychologic outcomes. Eighty-six adults undergoing cardiac surgery were randomized to either alpha-stat or pH-stat management during hypothermic (30°C) bypass that included an unfiltered bubble oxygenator and a MAP ranging from 50 to 60 mm Hg. The cognitive testing administered preoperatively and at 7 days and 6 months after surgery failed to demonstrate any differences in short- or long-term neuropsychologic function of patients in the two treatment groups. Whereas Bashein and colleagues did not include measurements of CBF or $CMRO_2$ in their study, Stephan et al[186] assessed the effect of blood-gas management on neurologic outcomes and on CBF and $CMRO_2$ during CPB. Similar to the patient study by Murkin et al,[50] and the animal study by Hindman et al,[187] CBF was greater in the pH-stat group, but $CMRO_2$ was not affected by the type of blood-gas management. Importantly, neurologic deficits were detected more commonly in patients managed with pH-stat techniques (10/35) than in patients managed with alpha-stat techniques (2/30) ($p = 0.04$). Because there are no apparent disadvantages to alpha-stat management techniques during CPB with moderate hypothermia and there is a potential disadvantage with pH-stat techniques, temperature-uncorrected blood-gas management techniques are preferable in adult patients undergoing hypothermic CPB.

Duration of Bypass

There are now tentative data that prolonged CPB duration may be a greater risk factor for overt neurologic dysfunction than the nature of the surgery itself.[188] Based on a retrospective review of 983 patients, one report has indicated that the incidence of stroke was 11% in patients undergoing CABG surgery versus 7% in patients undergoing valvular surgery.[136] It is notable that the average duration of CPB in the CABG group was 230 minutes, significantly longer than the 130 minutes in the group undergoing valvular surgery, and again markedly longer than CPB durations in most North American cardiac centers.

Pharmacologic Strategies for Cerebral Protection During Cardiac Surgery and CPB

Anesthetics and Cerebral Protection

Various pharmacologic strategies have been employed in an attempt to decrease the neurologic and neuropsychologic impairment associated with cardiac surgery and CPB. Most potentially protective anesthetics either maintain coupling of $CMRO_2$ and CBF or increase (or maintain) CBF while markedly decreasing $CMRO_2$. Volatile anesthetics, including enflurane, halothane, isoflurane, and sevoflurane, belong to the latter group, while barbiturates, propofol, etomidate, and benzodiazepines belong to the former group. The disassociative anesthetics, ketamine and phencyclidine, increase $CMRO_2$ but may provide cerebral protection by attenuating the excitotoxic cascade effects of ischemia (see neurochemistry of stroke). Dexmedetomidine, an α_2-receptor agonist, may offer some protection by enhancing neuronal inhibitory transmission.

There are three separate phases of ischemic injury, and different pharmacologic therapies may be differentially effective at each of these phases. In the first phase of ischemic insult, oxygen supply is inadequate but ATP and phosphocreatinine stores are not depleted. Therapies that slow $CMRO_2$ thus retarding the loss of high-energy phosphates, provide 1 to 3 minutes of "protection" before complete cell energy failure occurs and the excitotoxic cascade is initiated. Therefore, drugs that decrease $CMRO_2$ (potent volatile anesthetics, barbiturates, propofol) may provide protection from cerebral ischemia (though relatively short-lived) through this mechanism. To be effective in the second phase of cerebral ischemia, a pharmologic intervention must ameliorate or attenuate the excitotoxic events associated with brain tissue ATP depletion. A study by Illievich et al[189] has reported preliminary evidence that halothane or burst-suppression doses of isoflurane, pentobarbital, or propofol do not attenuate ischemia-induced increases in glutamate concentrations (Figure 6.15). The third phase of injury occurs when the ischemia area is reperfused. The renewed availability of oxygen enhances the release of oxygen free radicals which cause further membrane damage. Because post-ischemic hypermetabolism (in the absence of seizure activity) does

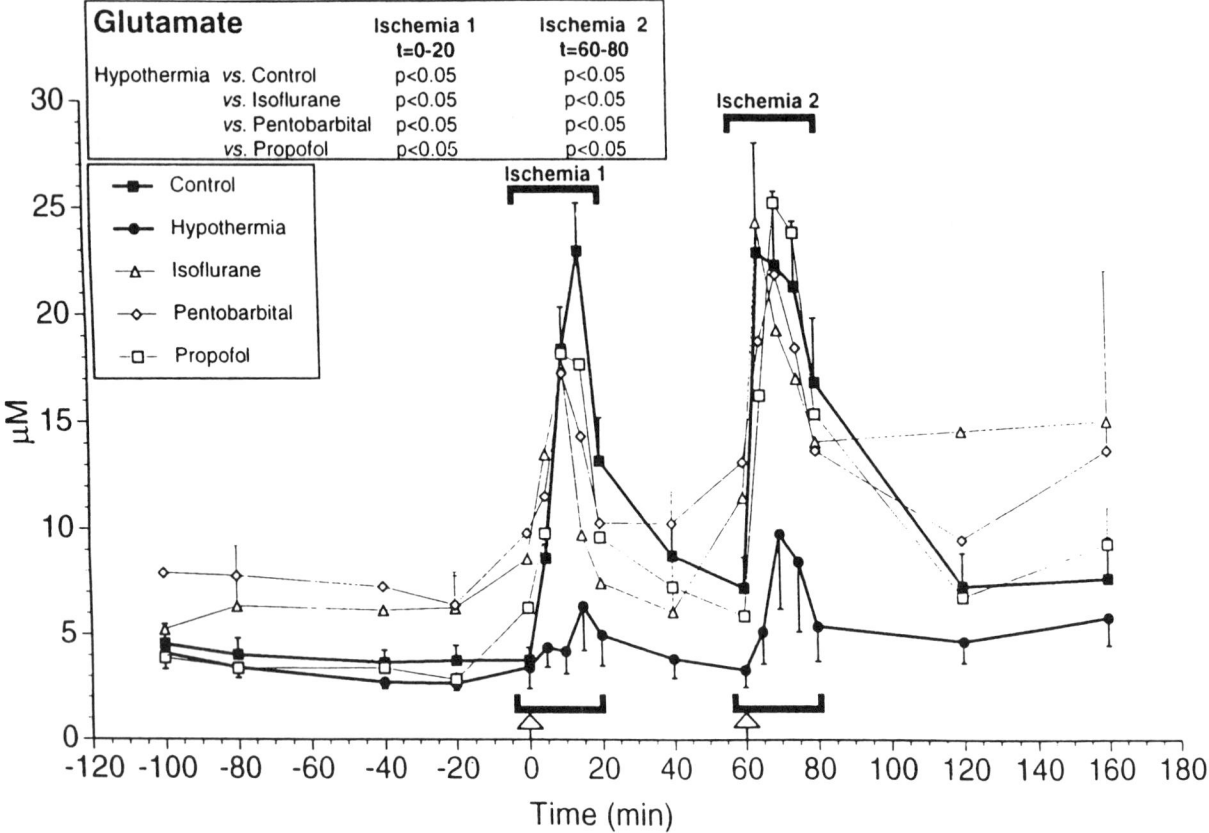

FIGURE 6.15. Ischemia-induced glutamate increase (mean ± SEM; some error bars have been removed to increase the legibility of the graph). Note that only hypothermia attenuates the increase in glutamate following the ischemic events. Arrows = onset of ischemic episodes; brackets = time periods over which analysis of variance was performed. (From Illievich et al[189] by permission of *Anesthesiology*.)

not occur, and because most anesthetics are poor scavengers of oxygen free radicals, the role of anesthetics in attenuating the effects of reperfusion ischemic injury is unclear.[190]

Although relatively few anesthetics have been assessed in the clinical setting of cardiac surgery and CPB, there is a substantial body of literature concerning the effects of anesthetics on cerebral ischemia. However, the potential cerebroprotective effect of barbiturates has been extensively studied in the cardiac surgery patient. These barbiturate studies and the animal and human studies evaluating potent volatile anesthetics as neuroprotectants are discussed below.

Barbiturates

There are several potential mechanisms by which barbiturates may limit cerebral ischemic injury. First, barbiturates reduce $CMRO_2$, producing an isoelectric EEG pattern. Importantly, as is the case with other anesthetics, the isoelectric EEG reflects reduced oxygen consumption associated with suppression of metabolic processes involved with synaptic transmission (about 60% in the awake state), but not in those responsible for maintaining cell homeostasis (about 40%).[191] Thus, thiopental helps maintain high-energy phosphates in the face of decreased oxygen availability and anaerobic metabolism.[192] However, as noted above, this decrease in $CMRO_2$ will provide protection for only a short time (1–3 minutes), and ischemic injury will ensue if oxygen delivery is not re-established quickly. Barbiturates also may provide cerebroprotection during incomplete global ischemia by facilitating the restoration of pH homeostasis.[193] Although barbiturate-induced reduction of the release of glutamate and other excitotoxic amines could attenuate the adverse effects of the excitotoxic cascade,[194] one study has failed to demonstrate a decrease in ischemia-induced hippocampal glutamate release with pentobarbital.[189] In vitro studies suggest that thiopental reduces lipid peroxidation and therefore may act as a free radical scavenger.[195] Finally, because barbiturates maintain coupling of $CMRO_2$ and CBF, regional perfusion to ischemic tissue may be enhanced during focal cerebral ischemia through an inverse steal phenomenon.

Several animal studies have demonstrated that barbiturates are more effective in protecting the brain from temporary focal ischemia than from permanent lesions. For example, in a study assessing the effects of temporary versus permanent MCA occlusion in baboons, animals *not* administered barbiturates and subjected to *permanent* MCA occlusion had a better neurologic outcome than those undergoing *temporary* occlusion (reperfusion injury is the likely causal factor for the increased morbidity in the temporary occlusion group).[196] However, barbiturate-treated animals subjected to *temporary* focal ischemia had almost complete neurologic protection and a superior neurologic outcome than animals not given barbiturates. Importantly, barbiturate treatment did not prevent neuronal damage in baboons subjected to permanent MCA occlusion. In fact, the latter group had the worst neurologic outcome of any of the treatment groups.

Encouraged by the number of animal studies suggesting that thiopental is neuroprotective in focal temporary ischemia, Slogoff and colleagues[70] sought to determine the effect of thiopental on neurologic outcome in patients undergoing either closed or open cardiac procedures. Because gas micro- and macroemboli from the CPB circuit or open cardiac chamber are significant sources of temporary focal ischemia, barbiturates may be expected to be cerebroprotective in the clinical setting of bypass and cardiac surgery, especially in open-chamber procedures. In Slogoff's first study assessing the effect of thiopental on neurologic outcomes following either closed- or open-chamber cardiac surgery, thiopental, 15 mg/kg, given 15 minutes prior to the initiation of CPB, did not improve neurologic or neuropsychologic outcomes compared to diazepam, 0.15 mg/kg. Using data from this initial study, Slogoff, in collaboration with Nussmeier,[135] studied the effect of thiopental on cardiac patients at the highest risk of an adverse neurologic outcome (ie, open-ventricle procedure patients). In this second study, thiopental was titrated to maintain an EEG burst-suppression pattern from just prior to aortic cannulation until the completion of weaning from bypass. A substantial dose of thiopental was required to achieve this EEG end point (mean dose = 40 ± 8 mg/kg). Although the incidence of neuropsychiatric changes was similar in thiopental and control groups (enflurane/fentanyl) (5.6% versus 8.6%), patients given thiopental had a statistically significant decreased incidence of frank stroke (0 of 89) compared to the control group (6 of 93 or 6.5%). Adverse effects of high-dose thiopental treatment included an increased requirement for inotropic support (7% versus 1%) and prolonged mechanical ventilation (19 ± 8 versus 14 ± 5 hours). An accompanying editorial suggested that thiopental protection had been demonstrated, and it advocated, as did the authors, the use of thiopental in this clinical setting.[197] It is important to recognize that the clinical conditions in which this study was conducted do not mirror common clinical practice. This study included bubble oxygenators, normothermic (34°C) bypass, and a glucose CPB-circuit prime but did not include an arterial line filter. Thus, the general applicability of Nussmeier findings to clinical practice is questionable. The clinical circumstances of this study (open-chamber procedure, bubble oxygenator, absence of arterial line filter) maximize the likelihood of gas micro- and macroemboli to the brain (which could be expected to be reabsorbed in a few minutes) causing temporary focal ischemia and, therefore, create a model that would most likely demonstrate thiopental cerebral protection.

In a follow-up study, Slogoff and Metz[198] tested the hypothesis that a single bolus of thiopental given at the time of aortic crossclamp removal would be as effective as a continuous infusion of thiopental. Additionally, they postulated that the bolus technique would ameliorate all the undesirable side effects associated with a continuous infusion of thiopental. Patients in the bolus-treatment group received thiopental, 15 mg/kg, while those managed with continuous infusion received a total dose of thiopental of 36 ± 10 mg/kg. There were no significant differences between the two groups in neurologic or neuropsychiatric outcomes, but the thiopental-bolus group was extubated sooner than patients given a continuous infusion (16 ± 5 versus 18 ± 6 hours). Criticisms of this study included the insufficient power to detect a significant difference between the two treatment groups, given the low incidence of adverse neurologic events (less than 2% in each treatment group), as well as the absence of an untreated control group. An implicit assumption of the study design is that neurologic injury occurs primarily at the time of crossclamp removal. Other studies suggest that embolic phenomena occur with any manipulation of the aorta (Figures 6.2 and 6.10), and that the duration of bypass is directly correlated with the incidence of neurologic injury.

In contrast with the findings of Nussmeier and Slogoff, Zaidan et al[199] were unable to demonstrate thiopental cerebroprotection in cardiac surgery patients. Zaidan's group employed a thiopental regimen similar to that used by Nussmeier et al, but in a somewhat different clinical setting: coronary artery patients were studied (instead of patients undergoing open-chamber procedures), and bypass management included hypothermia (28°C), arterial filters, and membrane oxygenators in the bypass circuit. The importance of these variables for neurologic outcome is discussed elsewhere in this chapter (see Factors Increasing Risk of Neurologic Dysfunction Following Cardiac Surgery). In Zaidan's coronary study, two of 151 (1.3%) control patients, compared with 5 of 149 (3.3%) of patients given thiopental, had new postoperative neurologic deficits. As in the Nussmeier study, patients in this study treated with high-dose thiopental had an increased requirement for inotropes and vasopressors and were intubated longer than patients in the control group (22 ± 18

versus 17 ± 10 hours). In contrast to the patients in the Nussmeier study, patients in the coronary study were at a low risk for cerebral gas emboli (closed cardiac procedure, membrane oxygenator, and arterial filter) and had the neurologic benefit of hypothermia. Importantly, those patients found to have focal injury were noted to have computed tomographic (CT) scan evidence of a permanent focal lesion. Thus, barbiturate therapy is unlikely to have been of any benefit in Zaidan's study, in which patients had radiologic evidence of a *permanent* focal lesion.

Potent Inhalational Anesthetics

Of all the clinically used potent inhalational anesthetics (enflurane, halothane, isoflurane, sevoflurane, and desflurane), isoflurane and sevoflurane have the most profound effect on $CMRO_2$; in a dose-related manner, both drugs cause up to a 50% reduction in cerebral metabolism.[200] Because of this effect on metabolism, the effectiveness of isoflurane in attenuating neurologic injury following an ischemic insult has been extensively evaluated. However, investigators studying different species and varying models of ischemia have reported conflicting results regarding the efficacy of isoflurane in attenuating cerebral ischemic damage. Michenfelder,[201] in an retrospective review of 2196 carotid surgery patients, reported that isoflurane, compared to enflurane and halothane, decreased the critical CBF (the blood flow at which the majority of patients developed ipsilateral EEG changes) and that isoflurane anesthesia during carotid surgery was associated with fewer adverse EEG changes (18%) than enflurane (26%) or halothane (25%). However, neurologic outcomes among the treatment groups were similar. Other studies have demonstrated that isoflurane prolongs survival in hypotensive dogs[202,203] and maintains cerebral tissue ATP and phosphocreatine levels during ischemia. Baughman and colleagues,[204] using a model of incomplete cerebral ischemia, reported that isoflurane, compared to N_2O and methohexital, was as effective as the barbiturate in attenuating neuronal injury following *moderate* cerebral ischemia, and was more effective than either of the other two treatments in preventing neuronal damage following *severe* ischemia. In contrast, Nehls et al[205] reported that isoflurane is *not* cerebroprotective and does not compare favorably to barbiturates, despite causing similar reductions in $CMRO_2$. Gelb and colleagues[206] concluded that isoflurane was not cerebroprotective in rats subjected to hypotension and severe temporary focal ischemia.

Although many investigators have postulated that it is the decrease in $CMRO_2$ associated with the barbiturates and volatile anesthetics that confers cerebroprotection during ischemia, other studies challenge this assumption. For example, Baughman and colleagues[207] compared the cerebroprotective effects of halothane and isoflurane to N_2O in rats undergoing incomplete cerebral ischemia. Both halothane and isoflurane similarly improved neurologic outcome compared to N_2O in a non-dose-related manner. Thus, the reduction in $CMRO_2$ (which was most substantial in the high-dose isoflurane group) did not correlate with the magnitude of cerebroprotection. This study is consistent with a substantial number of reports showing that changes in $CMRO_2$ do not predict the cerebroprotective effects of volatile anesthetics.[205,206,208-211]

The important effect of temperature, compared to that of volatile anesthetics, on neurologic outcome has been highlighted in a number of studies. Sano et al[210] assessed the cerebroprotective effects of isoflurane (1.3 minimum alveolar concentration [MAC]) and halothane (1.3 MAC) at normothermia (38°C) and halothane at 35°C, in a model of incomplete forebrain ischemia in the rat. There were no significant differences in the neurologic damage in the normothermic groups. However, the modest reduction in temperature (3°C) in the animals anesthetized with halothane was associated with a reduction in cerebral injury. A report by Warner and colleagues[211] provides provocative, but inconclusive, evidence for an anesthetic cerebroprotective effect that is *not* related to $CMRO_2$. In a study designed to compare the effects of halothane versus isoflurane, and the anesthetized versus the awake state, on neurologic outcome following temporary focal ischemia, they observed that an increase in pericranial temperature from 38° to 39.2°C in halothane-anesthetized rats resulted in increased neurologic damage, similar to that observed in the awake animals. Because other unpublished studies by these investigators suggested that cerebral temperature increases in response to an ischemic insult, they postulated (but did not prove) that volatile anesthetics may be cerebroprotective because of their ability to attenuate the cerebral hyperthermic response to ischemia. Another study evaluating the effects of various anesthetics (pentobarbital, isoflurane, and propofol) and hypothermia (32°C) on hippocampal glutamate and glycine concentrations after transient global cerebral ischemia underscores the important effect of temperature on biochemical markers of ischemic insult.[189] Only hypothermia was noted to attenuate the ischemia-induced increase in both glutamate and glycine concentrations, whereas propofol (1.2–1.6 mg/kg/hour) titrated to burst suppression modified increases in glycine concentrations (Figure 6.16).

Propofol

Propofol is a short-acting intravenous anesthetic that has cerebral effects similar to those of the barbiturates.[212] Propofol reduces $CMRO_2$ and CBF in a dose-dependent manner without affecting cerebral autoregulation.[213,214] It also favorably affects intracranial pressure (ICP), reducing ICP in humans with intracranial hypertension.[215] Be-

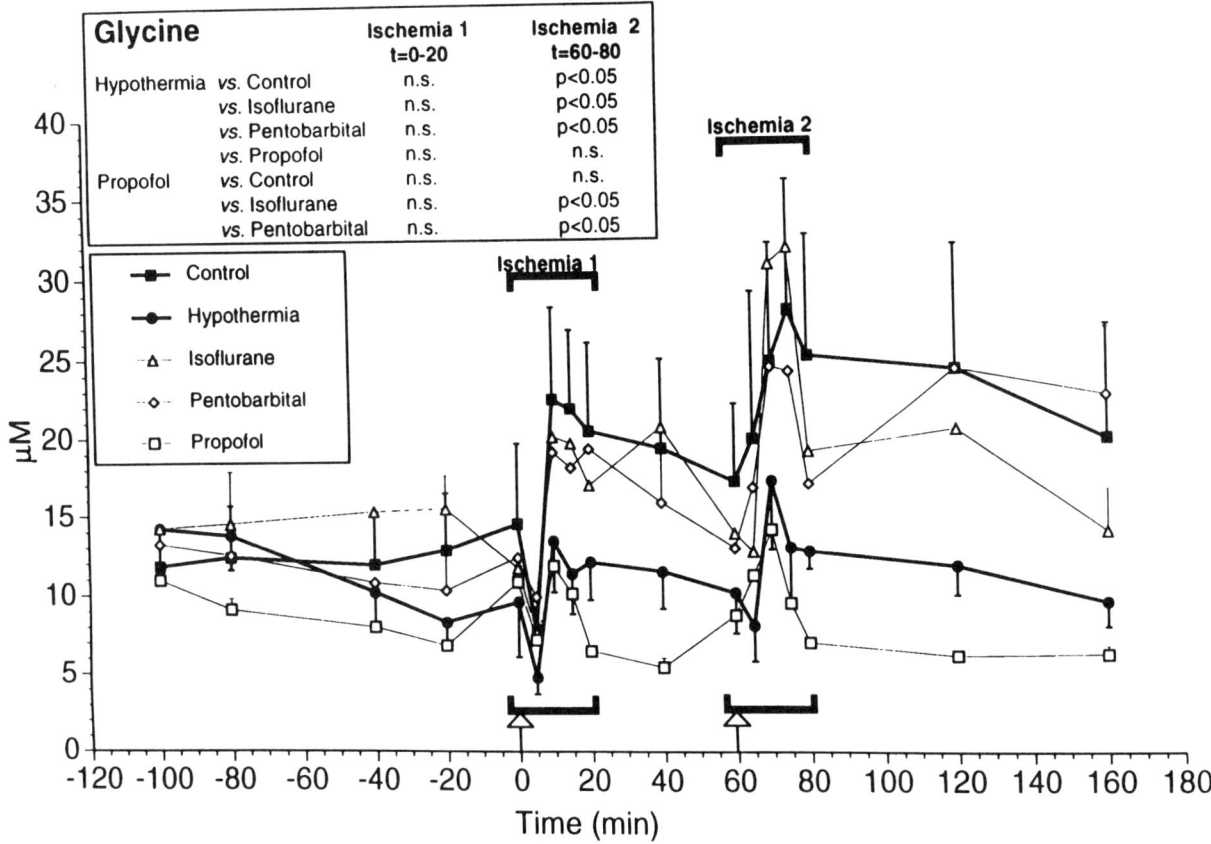

FIGURE 6.16. Ischemia-induced glycine increase (mean ± SEM; some error bars have been removed to increase the legibility of the graph.) Note that only hypothermia and propofol attenuate the increase in glycine following the ischemic events. Arrows = onset of ischemic episodes; brackets = time periods over which analysis of variance was performed. (From Illievich et al,[189] by permission of *Anesthesiology*.)

cause of these cerebral effects and other desirable pharmacokinetic and pharmodynamic characteristics of propofol, several studies have assessed the potential of propofol to provide cerebroprotection during ischemia. Kochs and colleagues[216] compared the effects of propofol and fentanyl/N_2O on neurologic outcome and EEG activity in rats undergoing incomplete cerebral ischemia. Propofol-anesthetized rats had a significantly better neurologic outcome than those anesthetized with fentanyl/N_2O. These investigators concluded that propofol, compared to fentanyl/N_2O anesthesia, administered in doses to produce EEG burst suppression, improves neurologic outcome and decreases neuronal death following incomplete ischemia. In contrast, Ridenour and colleagues[209] were unable to demonstrate any propofol cerebroprotection effects from focal cerebral ischemia. Spontaneously hypertensive rats were anesthetized with either halothane (0.5%–0.7%) or propofol, in doses sufficient to initiate and maintain EEG burst suppression, and subjected to reversible ligation of the MCA. Neurologic deficits at 24 and 95 hours postischemia were similar in the two groups, as were the total cerebral infarct volumes. As no control group was included in this study, it is not possible to ascertain the magnitude, if any, of the cerebroprotective effects of either propofol or halothane. However, if these effects did exist, it is unlikely that they would be related to reduction in $CMRO_2$.

A prospective, randomized study assessing the effects of propofol on neuropsychologic and neurologic outcomes following valvular heart surgery is being conducted by the Multicenter Study of Perioperative Ischemia (McSPI) Research Group.

Pharmacologic Agents

Calcium Channel Blockers

A preliminary report demonstrating some efficacy of nimodipine in improving cognitive function after CPB, in contrast to an untreated control group, suggests that biochemical effects, particularly those associated with transmembrane calcium flux and suppression of excitatory amino acids, may be especially important.[217]

Cerebroplegia

Various approaches have been taken in an attempt to decrease the potential for neurologic injury, particularly after deep hypothermic circulatory arrest. The use of selective cerebral perfusion and regional cooling has been investigated. Using a large-animal model, selective cannulation of bilateral internal carotid arteries was used for anterograde infusion of hypothermic oxygenated asanguinous cardioplegic solution (cerebroplegia) during 2 hours of DHTCA at 12° to 15°C.[218] Phosphorus nuclear magnetic resonance (NMR) spectroscopy was employed to assess changes in cerebral intracellular pH, ATP, and creatine phosphate (CP) in a control group and a group in which cerebroplegia was employed. During rewarming after DHTCA, EEG activity returned after 36 minutes in the animals receiving cerebroplegia but not until 117 minutes in the control group. Cerebral high-energy phosphates and intracellular pH also remained higher in the cerebroplegia-treated group. Using a similar DHTCA sheep model, the effects of anterograde and retrograde cerebroplegia, and external cranial cooling, were compared with a control group, and all animals were assessed postoperatively for degree of neurologic recovery. Animals were then sacrificed at 7 days for the additional determination of cerebral histologic appearance.[219] Animals subjected to anterograde cerebroplegia tended to have better preservation of neurologic functioning (5 of 7 animals survived, all free of deficit) than all other groups, although statistically they did not fare better than the externally cooled group (3 of 5 animals survived, 1 free of deficit). Diffuse histologic evidence of neuronal degeneration was seen in every animal in all groups, regardless of neurologic status. The authors concluded that infusion of cerebroplegia or external cranial cooling conferred distinct cerebroprotective effects after prolonged DHTCA. These results are not dissimilar to those obtained by Wolfson et al[220] in primates using saline cerebral perfusion during hypothermic circulatory arrest. In that study, trained animals were able to retain previously conditioned responses when cold (0°C) saline cerebral perfusion was employed, in marked contrast to an untreated control group. It would thus appear that, independently of the substrate composition of such cerebroplegic solutions, the washout of toxic metabolites and the prevention of early rewarming of the brain are likely the factors of paramount importance in the provision of cerebroprotective measures during DHTCA.

In clinical practice, a similar approach has been described by one group. In a series of 54 patients, moderate hypothermic CPB and total circulatory arrest with continuous selective carotid perfusion using blood cooled to 6° to 12°C was employed for aortic arch surgery between 1984 and 1989.[221] These authors reported that such a technique was associated with a low incidence of neurologic complications (1 neurologic death and 2 transient hemianopia) and did not limit the time necessary to perform the aortic repair, although it must be recognized that this was not a comparative or randomized trial. Whether the use of cerebroplegic solutions or selective carotid perfusion has any clinically relevant beneficial effects during cardiac surgery remains to be proven.

References

1. Rimm AA. Trends in cardiac surgery in the United States. *N Engl J Med* 1985;312:119-120.
2. Jones EL, Weintraub WS, Craver JM, et al. Coronary bypass surgery: is the operation different today? *J Thorac Cardiovasc Surg* 1991;101:108-115.
3. Cosgrove DM, Loop FD, Lytle BW, et al. Primary myocardial revascularization. *J Thorac Cardiovasc Surg* 1984;88:677-684.
4. Carella F, Travaini G, Contri P, et al. Cerebral complications of bypass surgery; a prospective study. *Acta Neurol Scand* 1988;77:158-163.
5. Strenge H, Lindner V, Paulsen G, et al. Early neurological abnormalities following coronary artery bypass surgery. A prospective study. *J Arch Psychiatry Neurol Sci* 1990;239:277-281.
6. Murkin JM, Martzke JS, Buchan AM, et al. Cognitive and neurological function after coronary artery surgery: a prospective study. *Anesth Analg* 1992;74:S215.
7. Shaw PG, Bates D, Cartlidge NEF, et al. Early neurological complication of cardiopulmonary bypass surgery. *Br Med J* 1985;291:1384-1387.
8. Smith PCC, Treasure T, Newman SP, et al. Cerebral consequences of cardiopulmonary bypass. *Lancet* 1986;1:823-825.
9. Hammeke TA, Hastings JE. Neuropsychologic alterations after cardiac operations. *J Thorac Cardiovasc Surg* 1988;96:326-331.
10. Breuer AC, Furlan AJ, Hanson MR, et al. Central nervous system complications of coronary artery bypass graft surgery: prospective analysis of 421 patients. *Stroke* 1983;14:682-687.
11. Gonzalez-Scarano F, Hurtig HI. Neurologic complications of coronary artery bypass grafting: case-control study. *Neurology* 1981;31:1032-1035.
12. Bojar RM, Najafi H, DeLaria GA, et al. Neurological complications of coronary revascularization. *Ann Thorac Surg* 1983;36:427-432.
13. Gardner TJ, Horneffer PJ, Manolio TA, et al. Stoke following coronary artery bypass grafting: a ten-year study. *Ann Thorac Surg* 1985;40:574-581.
14. Martin WRW, Hashimoto SA. Stroke in coronary bypass surgery. *Can J Neurol Sci* 1982;9:21-26.
15. Sotaniemi KA. Cerebral outcome after extracorporeal circulation. Comparison between prospective and retrospective evaluations. *Arch Neurol* 1983;40:75-77.
16. Sotaniemi KA, Juolasmaa A, Hokkanen ET. Neuropsychologic outcome after open-heart surgery. *Arch Neurol* 1981;38:2-8.
17. Savageau JA, Stanton B, Jenkins CD, et al. Neuropsychological dysfunction following elective cardiac operation—

early assessment-I. *J Thorac Cardiovasc Surg* 1982;84:585-594.
18. Savageau JA, Stanton B, Jenkins CD, et al. Neuropsychological dysfunction following elective cardiac operation-II. A six month reassessment. *J Thorac Cardiovasc Surg* 1982;84:595-600.
19. Shaw PA, Bates D, Cartlidge NEF, et al. Early intellectual dysfunction following coronary bypass surgery. *Q J Med* 1986;58:59-86.
20. Newman S, Smith P, Treasure T, et al. Acute neuropsychological consequences of coronary artery bypass surgery. *Curr Psychol Res Rev* 1987;6:115-124.
21. Nevin M, Adams S, Colchester ACF, et al. Evidence for involvement of hypocapnia and hypoperfusion in etiology of neurological deficit after cardiopulmonary bypass. *Lancet* 1987;2:1493-1495.
22. Mattler CE, Engblom E, Vanttinen E, et al. Neuropsychological findings and personality structural associated with coronary artery bypass surgery (CABS). *J Clin Exp Neuropsych* 1988;10:329.
23. Newman S, Klinger L, Venn G, et al. The persistence of neuropsychological deficits twelve months after coronary artery bypass surgery. In: Wilner A, Rodewald G, eds. *Impart of Cardiac Surgery on the Quality of Life*. New York: Plenum Press, 1990:173-179.
24. Martzke JS, Murkin JM, Buchan AM, et al. A prospective survey of cognitive function following coronary artery bypass (CAB). *J Clin Exp Neuropsych* 1992;14:A60.
25. Raymond M, Conklin C, Schaeffer J, et al. Coping with transient intellectual dysfunction after coronary bypass surgery. *Heart Lung* 1984;13:531-539.
26. Shaw PJ, Bates D, Cartlidge NEF, et al. Neurologic and neuropsychological morbidity following major surgery: comparison of coronary artery bypass and peripheral vascular surgery. *Stroke* 1987;18:700-707.
27. Smith PL. The cerebral complications of coronary artery bypass surgery. *Ann R Coll Surg Engl* 1988;70:212-216.
28. Blauth C, Griffin S, Klinger L, et al. Neuropsychological alterations after cardiac operation. (letter) *J Thorac Cardiovasc Surg* 1989;98:454-455.
29. Murkin JM, Martzke JS, Buchan AM, et al. pH management during prolonged hypothermic cardiopulmonary bypass significantly influences the incidence of postoperative neuropsychological dysfunction. *Can J Anaesth* 1993;40:A46.
30. Smith PS. Conference report—the brain and cardiac surgery. *Intens Crit Care Dig* 1990;9:13-14.
31. Theye RA, Patrick R, Kirklin JW. The electroencephalogram in patients undergoing open intracardiac operations with the aid of extracorporeal circulation. *J Thorac Surg* 1957;34:709-717.
32. Arom KV, Cohen DE, Strobl FT. Effect of intraoperative intervention on neurological outcome based on electroencephalographic monitoring during cardiopulmonary bypass. *Ann Thorac Surg* 1989;48:476-483.
33. Edmonds HL Jr, Griffiths LK, Van der Laken J, et al. Quantitative electroencephalographic monitoring during myocardial revascularization predicts postoperative disorientation and improves outcome. *J Thorac Cardiovasc Surg* 1992;103:555-563.
34. Russ W, Kling D, Sauerwein G, et al. Spectral analysis of the EEG during hypothermic cardiopulmonary bypass. *Acta Anaesthesiol Scand* 1987;31:111-116.
35. Levy WJ. Quantitative analysis of EEG changes during hypothermia. *Anesthesiology* 1984;60:291-297.
36. Bashein G, Nessly ML, Bledsoe SW, et al. Electroencephalography during surgery with cardiopulmonary bypass and hypothermia. *Anesthesiology* 1992;76:878-891.
37. Clute HL, Levy WJ. Electroencephalographic changes during brief cardiac arrest in humans. *Anesthesiology* 1990;73:821-825.
38. Levy WJ, Shapiro HM, Meathe E. The identification of rhythmic EEG artifacts by power spectrum analysis. *Anesthesiology* 1980;53:505-507.
39. van der Linden J, Wesslen O, Ekroth R, et al. Transcranial Doppler-estimated versus thermodilution-estimated cerebral blood flow during cardiac operations. *J Thorac Cardiovasc Surg* 1991;102:95-102.
40. Walker DA, Isley MR, Lucas WJ, et al. Cerebral blood flow velocity is coupled to EEG activity during hypothermic cardiopulmonary bypass. *Anesthesiology* 1991;75:A177.
41. Schell RM, Kern FH, Reves JG. The role of continuous jugular venous saturation monitoring during cardiac surgery with cardiopulmonary bypass. *Anesth Analg* 1992;74:627-629.
42. Nakajima T, Kuro M, Hayashi Y, et al. Clinical evaluation of cerebral oxygen balance during cardiopulmonary bypass: on-line continuous monitoring of jugular venous oxyhemoglobin saturation. *Anesth Analg* 1992;74:630-635.
43. Lassen NA, Henriksen L, Paulson O. Regional cerebral blood flow in stroke by 133-Xenon inhalation and emission tomography. *Stroke* 1981;12:284-289.
44. Lassen NA, Christensen MS. Physiology of cerebral blood flow. *Br J Anaesth* 1976;48:719-734.
45. Strandgaard S, Paulson OB. Cerebral autoregulation. *Stroke* 1984;15:413-416.
46. Astrup J, Rosenorn J, Cold GE, et al. Minimum cerebral blood flow and metabolism during craniotomy. Effect of thiopental loading. *Acta Anaesthesiol Scand* 1984;28:478-481.
47. Forster A, Juge O, Morel D. Effects of midazolam on cerebral blood flow in human volunteers. *Anesthesiology* 1982;56:453-455.
48. Michenfelder JD. The hypothermic brain. In: Michenfelder JD, ed. *Anesthesia and the Brain*. New York: Churchill Livingstone Inc; 1988:23-34.
49. Prough DS, Stump DA, Boy RC, et al. Response of cerebral blood flow to changes in carbon dioxide tension during hypothermic cardiopulmonary bypass. *Anesthesiology* 1986;64:576-581.
50. Murkin JM, Farrar JK, Tweed WA, et al. Cerebral autoregulation and flow/metabolism coupling during cardiopulmonary bypass: the influence of Pa_{CO_2}. *Anesth Analg* 1987;66:825-832.
51. Govier AV, Reves JG, McKay RD, et al. Factors and their influence on regional cerebral blood flow during nonpulsatile cardiopulmonary bypass. *Ann Thorac Surg* 1984;38:592-600.
52. Gravlee GP, Roy RC, Stump DA, et al. Regional cerebrovascular reactivity to carbon dioxide during cardiopulmonary bypass in patients with cerebrovascular disease. *J Thorac Cardiovasc Surg* 1990;99:1022-1029.

53. Greeley WJ, Ungerleider RM, Smith R, et al. The effects of deep hypothermic cardiopulmonary bypass and total circulatory arrest on cerebral blood flow in infants and children. *J Thorac Cardiovasc Surg* 1989;97:737–745.
54. Kern FH, Ungerleider RM, Quill TJ, et al. Cerebral blood flow response to changes in arterial carbon dioxide tension during hypothermic cardiopulmonary bypass in children. *J Thorac Cardiovasc Surg* 1991;101:618–622.
55. Burrows FA, Hillier SC, McLeod ME, et al. Anterior fontanel pressure and visual evoked potentials in neonates and infants undergoing profound hypothermic circulatory arrest. *Anesthesiology* 1990;73:632–636.
56. Watanabe T, Miura M, Orita H, et al. Brain tissue pH, oxygen tension, and carbon dioxide tension in profoundly hypothermic cardiopulmonary bypass. *J Thorac Cardiovasc Surg* 1990;100:272–280.
57. Raj JU, Kaapa P, Anderson J. Effect of pulsatile flow on microvascular resistance in adult rabbit lungs. *J Appl Physiol* 1992;72:73–81.
58. Williams GD, Seifen AB, Lawson NW, et al. Pulsatile perfusion versus conventional high-flow non-pulsatile perfusion for rapid core cooling and rewarming of infants for circulatory arrest in cardiac operations. *J Thorac Cardiovasc Surg* 1979;78:667–677.
59. Matsumoto T, Wolferth CC, Perlman MH. Effects of pulsatile and non-pulsatile perfusion upon cerebral and conjunctival microcirculation in dogs. *Am Surg* 1971;37:61–64.
60. Murkin JM, Lee DH. Transcranial doppler verification of pulsatile cerebral blood flow during cardiopulmonary bypass. *Anesth Analg* 1991;72:S194.
61. Murkin JM, Farrar JK. The influence of pulsatile vs nonpulsatile cardiopulmonary bypass on cerebral blood flow and cerebral metabolism. *Anesthesiology* 1989;71:A41.
62. Tranmer BI, Gross CE, Kindt GW, et al. Pulsatile versus nonpulsatile blood flow in the treatment of acute cerebral ischemia. *Neurosurgery* 1986;19;5:724–731.
63. Hindman BJ, Dexter F, Ryu KH, et al. Pulsatile versus non-pulsatile cardiopulmonary bypass. *Anesthesiology* 1994;80:1137–1147.
64. Badner NH, Murkin JM, Lok P. Differences in pH management and pulsatile/nonpulsatile perfusion during cardiopulmonary bypass do not influence renal function. *Anesth Analg* 1992;75:696–701.
65. Murkin JM, Martzke JS, Buchan AM, et al. Pulsatile perfusion during hypothermic cardiopulmonary bypass significantly influences morbidity and mortality after coronary artery bypass surgery. *Anesth Analg* 1993;76:S280.
66. Henze T, Stephan H, Sonntag H. Cerebral dysfunction following extracorporeal circulation for aortocoronary bypass surgery: no differences in neuropsychological outcome after pulsatile versus non-pulsatile flow. *Thorac Cardiovasc Surg* 1990;38:65–68.
67. Nunn JF. Hypoxia. In: *Applied Respiratory Physiology*. 3rd ed. Cambridge: Butterworth and Company, University Press; 1987:471–477.
68. Turner JE, Lambertsen CJ, Owen SG, et al. Effects of 0.08 and 0.8 atmospheres of inspired P_{O_2} upon cerebral hemodynamics at a 'constant' alveolar P_{CO_2} of 43 mm Hg. *Fed Proc* 1957;16:A565:130.
69. Rogers AT, Stump DA, Prough DS, et al. Cerebrovascular responsiveness to Pa_{O_2} is preserved during hypothermic cardiopulmonary bypass. *Anesthesiology* 1987;67(suppl):A12.
70. Slogoff S, Girgis KZ, Keats AS. Etiologic factors in neuropsychiatric complications associated with cardiopulmonary bypass. *Anesth Analg* 1982;61:903–911.
71. Pugsley W, Klinger L, Paschalis B, et al. Microemboli and cerebral impairment during cardiac surgery. *Vasc Surg* 1990;22:34–43.
72. Stump DA, Tegeler CH, Rogers AT, et al. Neuropsychologic deficits are associated with the number of emboli detected during cardiac surgery. *Stroke* 1993;24(3):A509.
73. Moody DM, Bell MA, Challa VR, et al. Brain microemboli during cardiac surgery or aortography. *Ann Neurol* 1990;28:477–486.
74. Stump DA, Rogers AT, Kahn ND, et al. When emboli occur during coronary artery bypass graft surgery. *Anesthesiology* 1993;79(suppl 3A):A49.
75. Pugsley W, Klinger L, Paschalis C, et al. Microemboli and cerebral impairment during cardiac surgery. *Vasc Surg* 1990;1:34–43.
76. Albin MS, Hantler C, Bunegin L, et al. Intracranial air embolism is detected by transcranial Doppler (TCD) during cardiopulmonary bypass procedures. *Anesthesiology* 1990;73:A458.
77. Brierley JB. Neuropathological findings in patients dying after open-heart surgery. *Thorax* 1963;18:291–304.
78. Aguilar MJ, Gerbode F, Hill JD. Neuropathologic complications of cardiac surgery. *J Thorac Cardiovasc Surg* 1971;61:676–685.
79. Brennan RW, Patterson RH, Kessler J. Cerebral blood flow and metabolism during cardiopulmonary bypass: evidence of microembolic encephalopathy. *Neurology* 1971;21:665–672.
80. Astrup J, Siesjo BK, Symon L. Thresholds in cerebral ischemia: the ischemic penumbra. *Stroke* 1981;12:723–725.
81. Unterberg A, Baethmann A. The kallikrein-kinin system as mediator in vasogenic brain edema. Cerebral exposure to bradykinin and plasma. *J Neurosurg* 1984;61:87.
82. Westergaard E. The blood-brain barrier to horseradish peroxidase under normal and experimental conditions. *Acta Neuropathol* 1977;39:181–187.
83. Domer FR, Bortje SB, Bing EG, et al. Histamine- and acetylcholine-induced changes in the permeability of the blood-brain barrier of normotensive and spontaneously hypertensive rats. *Neuropharmacology* 1983;22:615–619.
84. Black KL, Hoff JT. Leukotrienes increase blood-brain barrier permeability following intra-parenchymal injection in rats. *Ann Neurol* 1985;18:349–351.
85. Unterberg A, Wahl M, Hammersen F, et al. Permeability and vasomotor response of cerebral vessels during exposure to arachidonic acid. *Acta Neuropathol* 1987;73:209–219.
86. Olsen SP. Free oxygen radicals decrease electrical resistance of microvascular endothelium in the brain. *Acta Physiol Scand* 1987;129:181–187.
87. Rothman SM, Olney JW. Glutamate and the pathophysiology of hypoxic-ischemic brain damage. *Ann Neurol* 1986;19:105–111.
88. Benveniste H, Drejer J, Schousboe A, et al. Elevation of

88. the extracellular concentration of glutamate and aspartate in rat hippocampus during transient cerebral ischemia monitored by intracerebral microdialysis. *J Neurochem* 1984;43:1369-1374.
89. Fagg GE, Foster AC. Amino acid neurotransmitters and their pathways in the mammalian central nervous system. *Neuroscience* 1983;9:701-719.
90. Benveniste H, Jorgensen MB, Sandberg M, et al. Ischemic damage in hippocampal CA1 is dependent on glutamate release and intact innervation from CA3. *J Cereb Blood Flow Metab* 1989;9:629-639.
91. Choi DW, Maulucci-Gedde M, Kriegstein AR. Glutamate neurotoxicity in cortical cell culture. *J Neurosci* 1987;7:357-368.
92. Coyle JT, Bird SJ, Evans RH, et al. Excitatory amino-acid neurotoxins: selectivity, specificity, and mechanisms of action. Based on an NRP one-day conference held June 30, 1980. *Neurosci Res Prog Bull* 1981;19:1-427.
93. Dalkara T, Erdemli G, Barun S, et al. Glycine is required for NMDA receptor activations: electrophysiological evidence from intact rat hippocampus. *Brain Res* 1992;576:197-202.
94. Johnson JW, Ascher P. Glycine potentiates the NMDA response in cultured mouse brain neurons. *Nature* 1987;325:529-531.
95. Fisher SK, Agranoff BW. Receptor activation and inositol lipid hydrolysis in neural tissues. *J Neurochem* 1987;48:999-1017.
96. Churn SB, Taft WC, DeLorenzo RJ. Effects of ischemia on multifunctional calcium/calmodulin-dependent protein kinase type II in the gerbil. *Stroke* 1990;21(suppl 3):111-112.
97. Siesjö BK. Historical overview, calcium, ischemia, and death of brain cells. *Ann NY Acad Sci* 1988;522:638-661.
98. Abe K, Kogure K, Yamamoto H, et al. Mechanism of arachidonic acid liberation during ischemia in gerbil cerebral cortex. *J Neurochem* 1987;48:503-509.
99. Shiga Y, Onodera H, Kogure K, et al. Neutrophil as a mediator of ischemic edema formation in the brain. *Neurosci Lett* 1991;125:110-112.
100. Javid H, Tufo HM, Najafi H, et al. Neurologic abnormalities following open-heart surgery. *J Thorac Cardiovasc Surg* 1969;58:502-509.
101. Branthwaite MA. Neurologic damage related to open-heart surgery. A clinical survey. *Thorax* 1972;27:738-753.
102. Kolkka R, Hilbermann M. Neurologic dysfunction following cardiac operation with low-flow, low-pressure cardiopulmonary bypass. *J Thorac Cardiovasc Surg* 1980;79:432-437.
103. Ellis RJ, Wigniewski A, Potts R, et al. Reduction of flow rate and arterial pressure at moderate hypothermia does not result in cerebral dysfunction. *J Thorac Cardiovasc Surg* 1980;79:173-180.
104. Aberg T, Kihlgran M, Johnson I, et al. Improved cerebral protection during open heart surgery. In: Becker R, Katz J, Polonius M-J, eds. *Psychopathological and Neurological Dysfunctions Following Open-Heart Surgery*. Heidelberg: Springer; 1982:343-351.
105. Stockard JJ, Bickford RG, Schauble JF. Pressure-dependent cerebral ischemia during cardiopulmonary bypass. *Neurology* 1973;23:521-529.
106. Sotaniemi KA. Brain damage and neurological outcome after open-heart surgery. *J Neurol Neurosurg Psychiatry* 1980;43:127-135.
107. Bergdahl L, Bkork VO, Jonasson R. Aortic valve replacement in patients over 70 years. *Scand J Thorac Cardiovasc Surg* 1981;15:123-128.
108. Tuman KJ, McCarthy RJ, Najafi H, et al. Differential effects of advanced age on neurologic and cardiac risks of coronary artery operations. *J Thorac Cardiovasc Surg* 1992;104:1510-1517.
109. Shaw TG, Mortel KF, Meyer JS, et al. Cerebral blood flow changes in benign aging and cerebrovascular disease. *Neurology* 1984;34:855-862.
110. Rogers RL, Meyer JS, Mortel KF, et al. Age-related reductions in cerebral vasomotor reactivity and the law of initial value: a 4-year prospective longitudinal study. *J Cereb Blood Flow Metab* 1985;5:79-85.
111. Collins KJ, Exton-Smith AN, James MH, et al. Functional changes in autonomic nervous system responses with aging. *Age Ageing* 1980;9:17-24.
112. Brusino FG, Reves JG, Smith LR, et al. The effect of age on cerebral blood flow during hypothermic cardiopulmonary bypass. *J Thorac Cardiovasc Surg* 1989;97:541-547.
113. Naritomi H, Meyer JS, Sakai F, et al. Effects of advancing age on regional cerebral blood studies in normal subjects and subjects with risk factors for atherothrombotic stroke. *Arch Neurol* 1979;36:410-416.
114. Shaw PG, Bates D, Cartlidge NEF, et al. An analysis of factors predisposing to neurological injury in patients undergoing coronary bypass operations. *Q J Med* 1989;72:633-646.
115. Croughwell N, Lyth M, Quill TJ, et al. Diabetic patients have abnormal cerebral autoregulation during cardiopulmonary bypass. *Circulation* 1990;82(suppl IV):IV-407-412.
116. Slogoff S, Reul GJ, Keats AS, et al. Role of perfusion pressure and flow in major organ dysfunction after cardiopulmonary bypass. *Ann Thorac Surg* 1990;50:911-918.
117. Personal Communication, Guy McKhann, MD.
118. Turnipseed WD, Berkoff HA, Belzer OF. Postoperative stroke in cardiac and peripheral vascular disease. *Ann Surg* 1980;192:365-368.
119. Martin WRW, Hashimoto SA. Stroke in coronary bypass surgery. *Can J Neurosci* 1982;9:21-26.
120. Jones EL, Craver JM, Michalik RA. Combined carotid and coronary operations. *J Thorac Cardiovasc Surg* 1984;87:7-16.
121. Trieman RL, Foran RF, Cohen JL, et al. Carotid bruit: a follow-up report on its significance in patients undergoing cardiovascular surgery. *Arch Surg* 1979;114:1138-1140.
122. Barnes RW, Liebman PR, Marzalek PB, et al. The natural history of asymptomatic carotid disease in patients undergoing cardiovascular surgery. *Surgery* 1981;90:1075-1083.
123. Taylor GJ, Malik SA, Colliver JA, et al. Usefulness of atrial fibrillation as a predictor of stroke after isolated coronary artery bypass grafting. *Am J Cardiol* 1987;60:905-907.
124. Breslau PJ, Fell G, Ivey TD, et al. Carotid arterial disease in patients undergoing coronary artery bypass operations. *J Thorac Cardiovasc Surg* 1981;82:765-767.

125. Brener BJ, Brief DK, Alpert J, et al. The risk of stroke in patients with asymptomatic carotid stenosis undergoing cardiac surgery: a follow-up study. *J Vasc Surg* 1987;5:269-279.
126. Branthwaite MA. Prevention of neurological damage during open heart surgery. *Thorax* 1975;30:258-261.
127. Coffey CE, Massey W, Roberts KB, et al. Natural history of cerebral complications of coronary artery bypass graft surgery. *Neurology* 1983;33:1416-1421.
128. Reed GL, Singer DE, Picard EH, et al. Stroke following coronary artery bypass surgery. A case-control estimate of the risk from carotid bruits. *N Engl J Med* 1988;319:1246-1250.
129. David TE, Humphries AW, Young JR, et al. A correlation of neck bruits and arteriosclerotic carotid arteries. *Arch Surg* 1973;107:729-731.
130. Brusino FG, Reves JG, Prough DS, et al. Cerebral blood flow during cardiopulmonary bypass in a patient with occlusive cerebrovascular disease. *J Cardiothorac Anesth* 1989;3:87-90.
131. von Reutern GM, Hetzel A, Birnbaum D, et al. Transcranial Doppler ultrasonography during cardiopulmonary bypass in patients with severe carotid stenosis or occlusion. *Stroke* 1988;19:674-680.
132. Furlan AJ, Breuer AC. Central nervous system complications of open heart surgery. *Stroke* 1984;15:912-915.
133. Furlan AJ, Cracium AR. Risk of stroke during coronary artery bypass graft surgery in patients with internal carotid disease documented by angiography. *Stroke* 1985;16:797-799.
134. Tufo HM, Ostfeld AM, Shekelle R. Central nervous system dysfunction following open heart surgery. *JAMA* 1970;212:1333-1340.
135. Nussmeier NA, Arlund C, Slogoff S. Neuropsychiatric complications after cardiopolmonary bypass: cerebral protection by a barbiturate. *Anesthesiology* 1986;64:165-170.
136. Kuroda Y, Uchimoto R, Kaieda R, et al. Central nervous system complications after cardiac surgery: a comparison between coronary artery bypass grafting and valve surgery. *Anesth Analg* 1993;76:222-227.
137. Breuer AC, Franco I, Marzewski D, et al. Left ventricular thrombi seen by ventriculography are a significant risk factor for stroke in open-heart surgery. *Ann Neurol* 1981;10:103-104.
138. Maruyama M, Kuriyama Y, Sawada T, et al. Brain damage after open heart surgery in patients with acute cardioembolic stroke. *Stroke* 1989;20:1305-1310.
139. Tunick PA, Culliford AT, Lamparello PJ, et al. Atheromatosis of the aortic arch as an occult source of multiple systemic emboli. *Ann Intern Med* 1991;114:391-392.
140. Amarenco P, Cohen A, Baudrimont M, et al. Transesophageal echocardiographic detection of aortic arch disease in patients with cerebral infarction. *Stroke* 1992;23:1005-1009.
141. Rubin DC, Plotnick GD, Hawke MW. Intra-aortic debris as a potential source of embolic stroke. *Am J Cardiol* 1992;69:819-820.
142. Katz ES, Tunick PA, Rusinek H, et al. Protruding aortic atheromas predict stroke in elderly patients undergoing cardiopulmonary bypass: experience with intraoperative transesophageal echocardiography. *J Am Coll Cardiol* 1992;20:70-77.
143. Amarenco P, Duyckaerts C, Tzourio C, et al. The prevalence of ulcerated plaques in the aortic arch in patients with stroke. *N Engl J Med* 1992;326:221-225.
144. Lynn GM, Stefanko K, Reed JF 3d, et al. Risk factors for stroke after coronary artery bypass. *J Thorac Cardiovasc Surg* 1992;104:1518-1523.
145. Mills NL, Everson CT. Atherosclerosis of the ascending aorta and coronary artery bypass. *J Thorac Cardiovasc Surg* 1991;102:546-553.
146. Blauth CI, Cosgrove DM, Webb BW, et al. Atheroembolism from the ascending aorta. An emerging problem in cardiac surgery. *J Thorac Cardiovasc Surg* 1992;103:1104-1112.
147. Marshall WG, Barzilai B, Kouchoukos NT, et al. Intraoperative ultrasonic imaging of the ascending aorta. *Ann Thorac Surg* 1989;48:339-344.
148. Ohteki H, Tsuyoshi I, Natsuaki M, et al. Intraoperative ultrasonic imaging of the ascending aorta in ischemic heart disease. *Ann Thorac Surg* 1990;50:539-542.
149. Barzilai B, Saffitz JE, Miller JG, et al. Quantitative ultrasonic characterization of the nature of atherosclerotic plaques in human aorta. *Circ Res* 1988;60:459-463.
150. Barzilai B, Marshall WG Jr, Saffitz JE, et al. Avoidance of embolic complications by ultrasonic characterization of the ascending aorta. *Circulation* 1989;80:1275-1279.
151. Hosoda Y, Watanabe M, Hirooka Y, et al. Significance of atherosclerotic changes of the ascending aorta during coronary bypass surgery with intraoperative detection by echocardiography. *J Cardiovasc Surg* 1991;32:301-306.
152. Wareing TH, Davila-Roman VG, Barzilai B, et al. Management of the severely atherosclerotic ascending aorta during cardiac operations: a strategy for detection and treatment. *J Thorac Cardiovasc Surg* 1992;103:453-462.
153. Marschall K, Kanchuger M, Kessler BE, et al. Superiority of transesophageal echocardiography in detecting aortic arch atheromatous disease: identification of patients at increased risk of stroke during cardiac surgery. *J Cardiothorac Vasc Anesth* 1994;8:5-13.
154. Aberg T, Tonquist G, Tyden H, et al. Adverse effects on the brain in cardiac operations as assessed by biochemical, psychometric, and radiologic methods. *J Thorac Cardiovasc Surg* 1984;87:99-105.
155. Kramer DC, Stanley TE, Sanderson I, et al. Failure to demonstrate relationship between mean arterial pressure during cardiopulmonary bypass and postoperative cognitive function. Presented at the Society of Cardiovascular Anesthesiologists, Montreal, Canada, April 1994. p. 211.
156. Townes BD, Bashein G, Hornbein TF, et al. Neurobehavioral outcome in cardiac operations. A prospective controlled study. *J Thorac Cardiovasc Surg* 1989;98:774-782.
157. Gilman S. Cerebral disorders after open-heart operations. *N Engl J Med* 1965:272:489-498.
158. Lee WH Jr, Brady MP, Rowe JM, et al. Effects of extracorporeal circulation upon behavior, personality, and brain function. II. Hemodynamic, metabolic, and psychometric correlations. *Ann Surg* 1971;173:1013-1023.
159. Stanley TE, Smith LR, White WD, et al. Effect of cerebral perfusion pressure during cardiopulmonary bypass on neu-

160. Stockard JJ, Bickford RG, Myers RR, et al. Hypotension-induced changes in cerebral function during cardiac surgery. *Stroke* 1974:5:730–746.
161. Fist KJ, Helms KN, Sarnquist FH, et al. A prospective, randomized study of the effects of prostacyclin on neuropsychologic dysfunction after coronary artery operation. *J Thorac Cardiovasc Surg* 1987;93:609–615.
162. Bashein G, Townes BD, Nessle ML, et al. A randomized study of carbon dioxide management during hypothermic cardiopulmonary bypass. *Anesthesiology* 1990;72:7–15.
163. Swain JA, Griffith PK, Balabal RS, et al. Low-flow hypothermic cardiopulmonary bypass protects the brain. *J Thorac Cardiovasc Surg* 1991;102:76–83.
164. Padayachee TS, Parsons S, Theobold R, et al. The detection of microemboli in the middle cerebral artery during cardiopulmonary bypass: a transcranial Doppler ultrasound investigation using membrane and bubble oxygenators. *Ann Thorac Surg* 1987;44:298–302.
165. Padayachee TS, Parsons S, Theobold R, et al. The effect of arterial filtration on reduction of gaseous microemboli in the middle cerebral artery during cardiopulmonary bypass. *Ann Thorac Surg* 1988;45:647–649.
166. Taylor KM, Devlin BJ, Mittra SM, et al. Assessment of cerebral damage during open heart surgery: a new experimental model. *Scand J Thorac and Cardiovas Surg* 1980;14:197–203.
167. Blauth CI, Smith PL, Arnold JV, et al. Influence of oxygenator type on the prevalence and extent of microembolic retinal ischemia during cardiopulmonary bypass. *J Thorac Cardiovasc Surg* 1990;99:61–69.
168. Busto R, Dietrich WD, Globus MY-T, et al. Small differences in intra-ischemic brain temperature critically determine the extent of ischemic neuronal injury. *J Cereb Blood Flow Metab* 1987;7:729–738.
169. Natale JA, D'Alecy LG. Protection from cerebral ischemia by brain cooling without reduced lactate accumulation in dogs. *Stroke* 1989;20:770–777.
170. Busto R, Globus MY-T, Dietrich WD, et al. Effect of mild hypothermia on ischemia-induced release of neurotransmitters and free fatty acids in rat brain. *Stroke* 1989;20:904–910.
171. Chopp M, Welch KMA, Tidwell CD, et al. Effect of mild hyperthermia on recovery of metabolic function after global cerebral ischemia in cats. *Stroke* 1988;19:1521–1525.
172. Dietrich WD, Busto R, Valdes I, et al. Effects of normothermic versus mild hyperthermic forebrain ischemia in rats. *Stroke* 1990;21:1318–1325.
173. Dietrich WD, Busto R, Halley M, et al. The importance of brain temperature in alterations of the blood-brain barrier following cerebral ischemia. *J Neuropathol Exp Neurol* 1990;49:486–497.
174. Dietrich WD, Halley M, Valdes I, et al. Interrelationships between increased vascular permeability and acute neuronal damage following temperature-controlled brain ischemia in rats. *Acta Neuropathol* 1991;86:615–625.
175. Ridenour TR, Warner DS, Todd MM, et al. Mild hypothermia reduces infarct size resulting from temporary but not permanent focal ischemia in rats. *Stroke* 1992;23:733–738.
176. Onesti ST, Baker CJ, Sun PP, et al. Transient hypothermia reduces focal ischemic brain injury in the rat. *Neurosurgery* 1991;29:369–373.
177. Morikawa E, Ginsberg MD, Dietrich WD, et al. The significance of brain temperature in focal cerebral ischemia: histopathological consequences of middle cerebral artery occlusion in the rat. *J Cereb Blood Flow Metab* 1992;12:380–389.
178. Wong BI, McLean RF, Naylor CD, et al. Central nervous system dysfunction following warm and hypothermic cardiopulmonary bypass. *Lancet* 1992;339:1383–1384.
179. Martin TC, Craver JM, Gott JP, et al. Prospective, randomized trial of retrograde warm-blood cardioplegia: myocardial benefit and neurologic threat. *Ann Thorac Surg* 1994;57:298–304.
180. Mora CT, Weintraub WS, Martin TC, et al. A prospective randomized study comparing normothermic and hypothermic extracorporeal circulation on neurologic and neuropsychologic outcomes in coronary revascularization. In press.
181. Metz S, Keats AS. Benefits of a glucose-containing priming solution for cardiopulmonary bypass. *Anesth Analg* 1991;72:428–434.
182. Frasco P, Croughwell N, Blumenthal J, et al. Association between blood glucose level during cardiopulmonary bypass and neuropsychiatric outcome. *Anesthesiology* 1991;75:A55.
183. Lanier W. Glucose management during cardiopulmonary bypass: cardiovascular and neurologic implications. *Anesth Analg* 1991;72:423–427.
184. Lundgren J, Smith ML, Siesjo BK. Influence of moderate hypothermia on ischemic brain damage incurred under hyperglycemic conditions. *Exp Brain Res* 1991;84:91–101.
185. Dietrich WD, Alonso O, Busto R. Moderate hyperglycemia worsens acute blood-brain barrier injury after forebrain ischemia in rats. *Stroke* 1993;24:111–116.
186. Stephan H, Weyland A, Kazmaier S, et al. Acid-base management during hypothermic cardiopulmonary bypass does not affect cerebral metabolism but does affect blood flow and neurological outcome. *Br J Anaesth* 1992;69:51–57.
187. Hindman BJ, Dexter F, Cutkamp J, et al. Hypothermic acid-base management does not affect cerebral metabolic rate for oxygen at 27°C. *Anesthesiology* 1993;79:580–587.
188. Murkin JM. Neurological dysfunction after CAB or valvular surgery: is the medium the miscreant? *Anesth Analg* 1993;76:213–214.
189. Illievich UM, Zornow MH, Choi KT, et al. Effects of hypothermia or anesthetics on hippocampal glutamate and glycine concentrations after repeated transient global cerebral ischemia. *Anesthesiology* 1994;80:177–186.
190. Todd MM, Warner DS. Cerebral metabolic depression and brain protection during ischemia. *Anesthesiology* 1992;76:161–164.
191. Michenfelder JD. Hypothermia plus barbiturates: apples plus oranges? *Anesthesiology* 1978;49:157–158.
192. Michenfelder JD. The interdependency of cerebral functional and metabolic effects following massive doses of thiopental in the dog. *Anesthesiology* 1994;41:231–236.
193. Weir DL, Goodchild CS. Cortical extracellular fluid activities of K^+, Ca^{++} and pH in severe hypotension: effects of thiopentone, isoflurane and propofol. *J Cereb Blood Flow Metab* 1987;7(suppl I):S119–123.

194. Pocock G, Richards CD. Cellular mechanisms in general anaesthesia. *Br J Anaesth* 1991;66:116-128.
195. Smith DS, Rehncrona S, Siesjo BK. Inhibitory effects of different barbiturates on lipid peroxidation in brain tissue in vitro. *Anesthesiology* 1980;53:186-194.
196. Selman WR, Spetzler RF, Roessmann UR, et al. Barbiturate-induced coma therapy for focal cerebral ischemia: effect after temporary and permanent MCA occlusion. *J Neurosurg* 1981;55:220-226.
197. Michenfelder JD. A valid demonstration of barbiturate-induced brain protection in man—at last. *Anesthesiology* 1986;64:140-142.
198. Metz S, Slogoff S. Thiopental sodium by single bolus dose compared to infusion for cerebral protection during cardiopulmonary bypass. *J Clin Anesth* 1990;2:226-231.
199. Zaidan JR, Klochany A, Martin W, et al. Effect of thiopental on neurologic outcome following coronary artery bypass grafting. *Anesthesiology* 1991;74:406-411.
200. Scheller MS, Tateishi A, Drummond JC, et al. The effects of sevoflurane on cerebral blood-flow, cerebral metabolic rate for oxygen, intracranial pressure, and the electroencephalogram are similar to those of isoflurane in the rabbit. *Anesthesiology* 1988;68:548-551.
201. Michenfelder JD, Sundt TM, Fode N, et al. Isoflurane when compared to enflurane and halothane decreases the frequency of cerebral ischemia during carotid endarterectomy. *Anesthesiology* 1987;67:336-340.
202. Newberg LA, Michenfelder JD. Cerebral protection by isoflurane during hypoxemia or ischemia. *Anesthesiology* 1983;59:29-35.
203. Newberg LA, Milde JH, Michenfelder JD. The cerebral metabolic effects of isoflurane at and above concentrations that suppress cortical electrical activity. *Anesthesiology* 1983;59:23-28.
204. Baughman VL, Hoffman WE, Thomas C, et al. Comparison of methohexital and isoflurane on neurologic outcome and histopathology following incomplete ischemia in rats. *Anesthesiology* 1990;72:85-94.
205. Nehls DG, Major MC, Todd MM, et al. A comparison of the cerebral protective effects of isoflurane and barbiturates during temporary focal ischemia in primates. *Anesthesiology* 1987;66:453-464.
206. Gelb AW, Boisvert DP, Tang C, et al. Primate brain tolerance to temporary focal cerebral ischemia during isoflurane or sodium nitroprusside induced hypotension. *Anesthesiology* 1989;70:678.
207. Baughman VL, Haffman WE, Miletich DJ, et a. Neurologic outcome in rats following incomplete cerebral ischemia during halothane isoflurane, or N_2O. *Anesthesiology* 1988;69:192-198.
208. Warner D, Zhou J, Ramani R, et al. Reversible focal ischemia in the rat: effects of halothane, isoflurane and methohexital anesthesia. *J Cereb Blood Flow Metab* 1991;11:794-802.
209. Ridenour T, Warner D, Todd M, et al. Comparative effects of propofol and halothane on outcome from temporary middle cerebral artery occlusion in the rat. *Anesthesiology* 1992;76:807-812.
210. Sano T, Drummond JC, Patel PM, et al. A comparison of the cerebral protective effects of isoflurane and mild hypothermia in a model of incomplete forebrain ischemia in the rat. *Anesthesiology* 1992;76:221-228.
211. Warner DS, McFarlane C, Todd MM, et al. Sevoflurane and halothane reduce focal ischemic brain damage in the rat. Possible influence of thermoregulation. *Anesthesiology* 1993;79:985-992.
212. Sebel P, Lowdon J. Propofol: a new intravenous anesthetic. *Anesthesiology* 1989;73:499-505.
213. Van Hemelrijck J, Fitch W, Mattheussen M, et al. Effect of propofol on cerebral circulation and autoregulation in the baboon. *Anesth Analg* 1990;71:49-54.
214. Werner C, Hoffman W, Miletich D, et al. Propofol decreases cerebral and spinal cord blood-flow and maintains autoregulation in rats. *J Neurosurg Anesth* 1990;2:220. Abstract.
215. Herregods L, Verbeke J, Rolly G, et al. Effect of propofol on elevated intracranial pressure: preliminary results. *Anaesthesia* 1988;43:107-109.
216. Kochs E, Hoffman WE, Werner C, et al. The effects of propofol on brain electrical activity, neurologic outcome, and neuronal damage following incomplete ischemia in rats. *Anesthesiology* 1992;76:245-252.
217. Forsman M, Olsnes BT, Semb G, et al. Effects of nimodipine on cerebral blood flow and neuropsychological outcome after cardiac surgery. *Br J Anaesth* 1990;65:514-520.
218. Robbins RC, Balaban RS, Swain JA. Intermittent hypothermic asanguinous cerebral perfusion (cerebroplegia) protects the brain during prolonged circulatory arrest. *J Thorac Cardiovasc Surg* 1990;99:878-884.
219. Crittenden MD, Roberts CS, Rosa L, et al. Brain protection during circulatory arrest. *Ann Thorac Surg* 1991;51:942-947.
220. Wolfson SK Jr, Icoz MV, Luber S. Preservation of conditioned responses in primates after total circulatory arrest with preferential cerebral hypothermia. *Surg Forum* 1965;16:409-411.
221. Bachet J, Guilmet D, Goudot B, et al. Cold cerebroplegia. *J Thorac Cardiovasc Surg* 1991;102:85-94.

7
The Respiratory, Renal, and Hepatic Systems: Effects of Cardiac Surgery and Cardiopulmonary Bypass

James G. Ramsay

The Respiratory System

The pathophysiology of cardiopulmonary bypass (CPB), as described in the preceding chapters, includes hemodilution (both red cells and plasma proteins), fluid accumulation, hypothermia, and the response of blood components to artificial surfaces. Superimposed on these processes are the mechanical complications inherent in cardiac surgery, and the consequences of inadequate organ perfusion secondary to myocardial failure in the perioperative period. Particularly in the respiratory system, it is often difficult to ascribe changes in function to any one of these aspects of the procedure. This section of the chapter delineates the effects of cardiac surgery and CPB on the individual components of the respiratory system. Additionally, the "postperfusion lung" and possible causes for this syndrome are described and potential prophylactic therapies discussed.

Expected Respiratory Changes After Cardiac Surgery

The various components of the respiratory system—airway, lungs, chest wall, intercostal muscles, diaphragm, and neural pathways to and from these various components—are subject to damage caused by a variety of processes associated with cardiac surgery and CPB. Cardiac surgery, through either a sternotomy or thoracotomy, has deleterious effects on the functioning of the muscle pump and the chest wall. Additionally, phrenic nerve damage and/or diaphragm dysfunction, resulting from cold topical solutions applied inside the pericardium, may cause mechanical problems. Physical handling of the lungs, fluid collections, and pain, due to both the surgery and the presence of chest tube drains, may all interfere with normal respiratory function. Left-sided cardiac distension or elevated pressures may cause alveolar edema, and transfusion reactions or allergic reactions to drugs (eg, protamine) may increase capillary permeability, leading to alveolar flooding. Thus, it is doubtful that "pump lung," the postperfusion syndrome described in the early years of CPB,[1] was simply a consequence of extracorporeal perfusion. Table 7.1 summarizes changes in the respiratory system found after cardiac surgery and CPB. These changes are discussed individually below.

Mechanics

A number of investigators have documented changes in pulmonary mechanics and gas exchange after thoracotomy and cardiac surgery, with or without CPB. In many respects, these changes parallel those occurring after upper abdominal procedures, and appear to be secondary to surgical factors other than CPB. The mechanical properties of the respiratory system are usually referred to in terms of compliance (pressure change for a given volume change, either static or dynamic), elastance (the reciprocal of compliance), and resistance (pressure change related to gas flow rate). After thoracotomy, either lateral or midline (ie, sternotomy), both lung and chest wall compliance decrease significantly.[2] The maximum decrease (30%) occurs at 3 days, although a significant decrease in compliance (approximately 25%) is still present 6 days after sternotomy and myocardial revasculariza-

TABLE 7.1. Respiratory sequelae of CPB.

Reduced respiratory system compliance
Increased respiratory system resistance
Reduced lung volumes and gas flow rates
Impaired gas exchange (worsened oxygenation)
Atelectasis
Phrenic nerve dysfunction/damage
Reduced "pump" function (muscle weakness)
Cardiogenic pulmonary edema
Noncardiogenic pulmonary edema ("ARDS" or "pump lung")

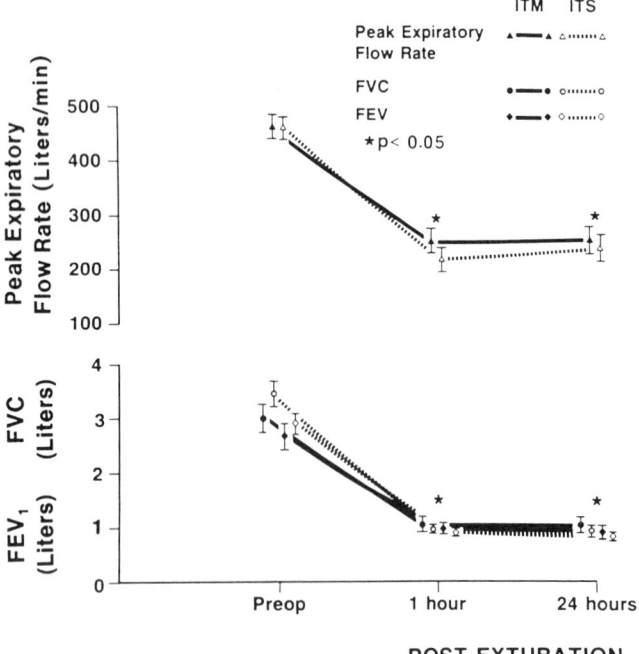

FIGURE 7.1. Mean (±SEM) peak expiratory flow rate, forced vital capacity (FVC), and forced expired volume in 1 second (FEV$_1$) before and after CABG in a study of intrathecal morphine ($n = 19$, ITM) vs saline ($n = 21$, ITS). Measurements were not different between groups but showed significant (*$p < 0.05$) postoperative decreases in lung volume and gas flow rates (extubation occurred approximately 22 hours after the preoperative intrathecal injection). (Modified from Casey WF, Wynands JE, Ralley FE, et al,[5] by permission of *J Cardiothorac Anesth*.)

tion.[3] Although chest wall resistance increases significantly, airway resistance is unaltered after uncomplicated coronary revascularization procedures.[4] (However, airway resistance is reduced after mitral valve replacement for valvular stenosis.) Associated with these changes are significant decreases in lung volumes and flow rates. Forced expiratory volume (FEV$_1$) is decreased immediately after coronary bypass surgery[5] (Figure 7.1). These changes persist in the first 6 postoperative weeks.[6,7] Functional residual capacity (FRC) is reduced by 40% to 50% immediately after extubation, with only a modest recovery (5% to 25%) in the next 72 hours.[8] Opening of the pleural space does not affect the postoperative change in respiratory volumes. These restrictive changes in volumes and flow rates are probably due to alterations in chest wall mechanics, since similar changes are seen after upper abdominal surgery.[9,10] In addition to the changes in flows and volumes, both reduced inspiratory strength[11] and reduced or uncoordinated rib cage expansion occur.[12] These alterations lead to an increase in respiratory rate and a decrease in tidal volume, decreasing respiratory "efficiency" and increasing the oxygen cost of breathing.[13] Indeed, the percentage of total body oxygen consumption attributed to the respiratory system after coronary bypass surgery (approximately 20%) is similar to that seen in medical patients recovering from respiratory failure.[14] Factors leading to diminished effectiveness of the breathing effort after cardiac surgery and CPB are summarized in Table 7.2.

Phrenic Nerve Damage

Phrenic nerve damage or dysfunction secondary to trauma or extreme cold (ie, exposure to topical slush) may result in significant postoperative loss of lung volume. The "frostbitten phrenic nerve" was originally described in 1963,[15] but despite recognition of this morbid phenomenon, the problem of phrenic nerve damage persists. With the use of topical ice "slush" to maintain cardiac hypothermia, Esposito and Spencer[16] found that 73% of 70 studied patients developed an elevated hemidiaphragm if a pericardial insulating pad was not used, versus 17% when the pad was used. In another study in which conduction of the phrenic nerve was measured, prolonged left phrenic nerve dysfunction occurred in 3 of 17 patients in the absence of an insulating pad, but only transient dysfunction (less than 1 week) occurred in 2 of 40 patients when the pad was used.[17] An important finding in this latter study was the high incidence of left lung atelactasis (50 of 57, or 88% of patients studied). The authors concluded that atelectasis was not related to phrenic nerve damage in the majority of patients (Figure 7.2). In a study in which a pericardial insulating pad was employed, ultrasound evaluation of the diaphragm documented a 15% incidence of significantly diminished left diaphragmatic motion.[18] The consequences of bilateral phrenic nerve cold-induced injury, or unilateral injury in a patient with preexisting pulmonary disease, may include ventilator dependence for a

TABLE 7.2. Factors leading to diminished effectiveness of breathing effort after cardiac surgery and CPB.

Chest wall motion
    Majority of patients show discoordination between airflow and rib cage motion at 1 week, improving at 3 months[12]
Maximum inspiratory pressure
    30% decrease 10 days postop[11]
Breathing pattern
    Reduced tidal volume and increased frequency
Work of breathing
    Significantly increased[2]
    Oxygen cost of breathing 20% of whole body VO$_2$[13]
Lung volumes
    FRC 15% decreased at chest closure
        40–50% decrease immediately postextubation
        Still down 25–40% at 72 hours[8]
        Still down 20% at 2 weeks[6]
    FEV$_1$ 50% decrease in first 3 days[5]
        At 6–8 weeks recovered to 75% of preop[7]

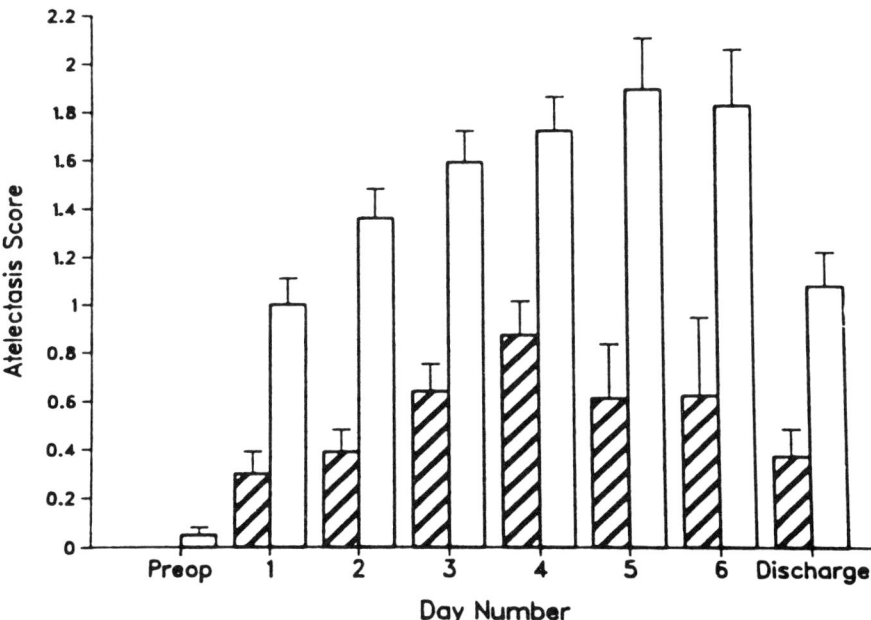

FIGURE 7.2. Radiological atelectasis scores for right (*hatched bars*) and left (*open bars*) lungs before (Preop), and on postoperative days 1–6 and at discharge after elective CABG surgery. On the preoperative and discharge days and days 1, 2, and 3, $n = 57$; on days 4, 5, and 6, $n = 46$, 18, and 8, respectively. Bars are ±SEM. (From Wilcox P, Baile EM, Hards J, et al,[17] by permission of *Chest*.)

period of months. In a recent report, severe postoperative diaphragmatic dysfunction was found in 13 of 13 patients with an otherwise unexplained need for prolonged mechanical ventilation.[19]

Surfactant

Another proposed mechanism of pulmonary dysfunction after CPB is the depletion of surfactant, which may lead to atelectasis. However, evidence for this proposed mechanism is lacking. A laboratory study in 1968 suggested that surfactant changes occurred only *after* significant microvascular damage was apparent.[20] A more recent human study failed to demonstrate inhibition of surfactant activity after CPB in either adults or children.[21]

Gas Exchange

In 1978, Rea et al[22] demonstrated that the alveolar-to-arterial oxygen gradient (A-a O_2 gradient) increases immediately after cardiac surgery and stays significantly elevated for weeks. The decrease in arterial Po_2 appears to be due to the mechanical changes described above: atelectasis and a decrease in lung volume, leading to an increase in ventilation:perfusion mismatching and shunt.[23]

Internal mammary artery (IMA) dissection does not necessarily worsen the increase in postoperative A-a O_2 gradient. Singh et al[24] documented similar changes in postoperative A-a O_2 gradients and Pao_2 values in patients with and without IMA dissections (Table 7.3). However, the magnitude of Po_2 decrease was greater in the presence of radiographic evidence of a pleural effusion and/or pleural thickening, and greater still if an IMA graft had been placed.[3]

CPB-Induced Hemodilution and Postoperative Lung Function

Hemodilution during CPB results from the nonhemic prime of the bypass circuitry, crystalloid cardioplegic solution infused during the bypass run, and fluids administered by the anesthesiologist. It is not uncommon for cardiac surgery patients to gain 3 to 5 kg from perioperative fluid administration. Not surprisingly, a number of investigations have addressed the possibility that some of the pulmonary changes described above are the result of interstitial or alveolar edema.

The Starling equation, which relates capillary permeability factors to hydrostatic and colloid osmotic pressures, describes the tendency for a capillary to transudate fluid.[25]

Starling Equation

Net fluid flux $(J) = K_F [(P_{IV} - P_{EV}) - \sigma(\tau_{IV} - \tau_{EV})]$

where:

K_F = filtration coefficient (product of permeability to water and surface area)
P_{IV} = intravascular hydrostatic pressure
P_{EV} = extravascular (interstitial) hydrostatic pressure
σ = reflection coefficient for albumin (protein permeability factor)

TABLE 7.3. Mean values (±SD) for PaO_2 (mm Hg) and $P(A-a)O_2$ (mm Hg) (with patients breathing room air) preoperatively and postoperatively after elective CABG[a].

Group Day	n	Vein grafts only		n	Internal mammary artery and vein grafts	
		PaO_2	$P(A-a)O_2$		PaO_2	$P(A-a)O_2$
Preoperative	55	75.4 ± 8.3	21.8 ± 7.5	70	74.9 ± 7.3	20.8 ± 7.6
Postoperative						
1	50	58.1 ± 8.7	36.9 ± 9.9	67	59.1 ± 8.2	35.5 ± 9.8
2	51	55.1 ± 6.2	42.4 ± 6.9	68	55.8 ± 6.8	40.2 ± 8.8
4	52	59.7 ± 7.4	40.0 ± 8.5	70	58.9 ± 6.1	40.2 ± 8.0
6	51	64.4 ± 7.0	34.2 ± 7.6	66	62.6 ± 6.3	36.5 ± 9.0
8	37	67.4 ± 7.7	30.8 ± 9.8	43	64.2 ± 6.7	34.6 ± 8.7

[a]Differences between groups did not reach statistical significance, although recovery between the 2nd and 8th postoperative days was greater in the SVG group ($p < 0.05$). The decrease in PaO_2 and increase in $P(A-a)O_2$ gradient did not correlate with pump time or duration of intubation. (From Singh NP, Vargas FS, Cukier A, et al,[24] by permission of *Chest*.)

τ_{IV} = intravascular colloid osmotic pressure
τ_{EV} = extravascular (interstitial) colloid osmotic pressure

Examination of this equation reveals that the term ($P_{IV} - P_{EV}$), or the net hydrostatic gradient driving fluid from the capillary, should be balanced by the term $\sigma(T_{IV} - T_{EV})$, the net colloid pressure gradient that tends to hold fluid in the capillary. This latter term is dependent on permeability to protein (σ). Usually, the value for the entire equation is slightly positive due to the magnitude of intravascular hydrostatic pressure compared to the other factors; an increase in capillary hydrostatic pressure or a reduction in colloid osmotic pressure should promote fluid transudation from the capillary. An increase in protein permeability is expressed as a reduction in σ; this will reduce the effect of any change in colloid osmotic pressure.

Although the Starling equation is conceptually sound, its application to clinical medicine is made difficult by the inability to measure many of the equation factors, and by the fact that changes in one factor often lead to, or result from, changes in another. Perhaps the most important limitation of the Starling equation is that it only considers the tendency to transudate fluid from the capillary; it does *not* describe the tendency of a tissue to develop edema.

In a classic study, Zarins et al[26] demonstrated that pulmonary interstitial colloid oncotic pressure may fall along with the plasma oncotic pressure, illustrating how changes in one factor of the Starling equation induce changes in another. In this baboon study, plasmapheresis produced very low plasma oncotic pressures (76% reduction of normal values) while normal intravascular hydrostatic pressures were maintained, and pulmonary lymphatic flow and gas exchange were measured. Large increases (six- to sevenfold) in lymphatic drainage occurred, indicating fluid transudation, but there was no increase in the shunt fraction and no pulmonary edema. Both interstitial colloid and plasma oncotic pressures fell. Many investigations in the setting of cardiopulmonary resuscitation have demonstrated that administration of large amounts of crystalloid is not associated with pulmonary edema, provided intravascular hydrostatic pressures are not elevated. This is true in the presence[27] and absence[28] of increased capillary permeability. Therefore, it seems unlikely that hemodilution alone, which results in net fluid accumulation and a reduced plasma oncotic pressure, can be considered responsible for gas exchange abnormalities after heart surgery and CPB.

If transcapillary fluid transudation is so rapid or excessive that the lymphatics are overwhelmed, then interstitial and alveolar edema will develop. This situation is likely to occur when the capillary hydrostatic pressure is elevated, and/or in the presence of an increase in the capillary permeability associated with elevated hydrostatic pressure. Clearly, the potential for increased capillary hydrostatic pressure exists during all phases of cardiac surgery: pre- or postbypass left ventricular failure may expose the pulmonary capillaries to high pressures; left ventricular distension during bypass has the same effect. A recent report by Louagie et al[29] found postoperative ventricular dysfunction to be one of two risk factors for development of lung edema after CPB.

Scientific evidence for an increase in capillary permeability after uneventful CPB is not conclusive, although there are many reasons to suspect that such should be the case. Investigations in dogs suggest that increased vascular permeability and lung edema occur after 90 to 120 minutes of CPB,[30] and that microvascular permeability to proteins in the small intestine is increased after 120 minutes of bypass.[31] In one human study (9 patients), increased clearance of a radioactive tracer from the lungs into the blood was demonstrated after a mean CPB time of 100 min.[32] In another study, 4 of 12 patients exhibited similar findings, and all had prolonged CPB times (mean

156 minutes).[33] Tennenberg et al[34] were, however, unable to demonstrate an increase in pulmonary capillary permeability after uneventful coronary bypass procedures.

Few prospective studies have measured pulmonary fluid accumulation in cardiac surgical patients. One of the difficulties in interpreting existing studies is the difference in techniques used to measure lung water, while another difficulty is interpreting the clinical relevance. For example, while one study demonstrated an increase in lung water 1 and 2 days after coronary bypass, the increase was in the range of 1 to 2 mL/kg (ie, 70 to 140 mL in a 70-kg man).[35] In the one patient with a significant increase in lung water immediately after surgery, pulmonary hypertension occurred during bypass. In another study, an increase in extravascular lung water was demonstrated 30 minutes postbypass if operative fluid balance was >1500 mL, but not if balance was less than this.[36] This same group of investigators found that patients who received cardiopulmonary resuscitation in the preoperative period demonstrated significantly increased extravascular lung water 5 hours postoperatively, while a matched group of patients, not requiring resuscitation, did not have any increase in lung water at this time.[37] Other studies have failed to demonstrate any increase in lung water after uncomplicated cardiac surgery.[38-40]

As in other settings, there is debate over the importance of colloid oncotic pressure (generated by plasma proteins) in preventing pulmonary fluid accumulation during cardiac surgery. Klancke et al[41] suggested that reduction in protein concentration is a major factor in the development of edema, but examination of their data reveals that pulmonary hydrostatic pressure (pulmonary artery occlusion pressure) was significantly elevated in the group of patients with pulmonary edema.

The differential effects of various factors on postoperative lung water accumulation have been assessed. The use of colloid to maintain plasma colloid osmotic pressure either during,[42,43] or immediately after, bypass[38] does not reduce postoperative shunt or lung water accumulation, although overall fluid accumulation may be reduced.[44] Byrick et al[45] reported that bubble, but not membrane, oxygenators may cause postoperative extravascular lung water accumulation. However, in the study by Tennenberg[34] in which no increase in pulmonary capillary permeability was found, bubble oxygenators were used. Finally, several case reports on small series of patients have documented the association of elevated capillary permeability with massive pulmonary edema after bypass. Pre-existing pulmonary edema is one such condition,[46] as is the occurrence of a protamine reaction[47] or the presence of an antigranulocyte antibody in the recipient of a blood transfusion.[48]

In summary, there is little evidence supporting the concept that there is a significant increase in lung water after routine CPB. Similarly, the type of fluids used periopera-

tively and the decrease in colloid oncotic pressure do not appear to independently cause lung water accumulation. Rather, it appears that an elevated pulmonary capillary pressure, induced by elevated cardiac filling pressures, is the most important factor in pulmonary edema formation. It may be, however, that when associated with decreased colloid osmotic pressure, modest increases in capillary hydrostatic pressure will be of greater significance. There is conflicting evidence as to whether pulmonary capillary permeability is affected after routine CPB; when there is a definite increase in permeability, there is likely to be severe postoperative pulmonary edema. Table 7.4 summarizes the importance of the various factors in the Starling equation in the cardiac surgical patient.

The Postperfusion Lung Syndrome ("Pump Lung")

In the classic treatise *Extracorporeal Circulation*,[49] published in 1958 (before the era of intensive care units and routine postoperative ventilation), postoperative pulmonary failure was estimated to occur after 15% to 25% of perfusions and was usually fatal. Histologic studies of lung tissue from patients with "pump lung" demonstrated nonsegmental atelectasis and abnormal elastic fibers, but no edema or cellular infiltrate, leading the author to conclude that "an injury to the pulmonary alveolar membrane has been produced." Focal or diffuse pulmonary hemorrhages were described in this early study and in a similar report a few years later.[1] Lung biopsies taken before and after CPB have documented a variety of nonspecific changes, including patchy atelectasis[50] and cellular (endothelial and pneumocyte) swelling and vacuolization.[51] Sequestration of leukocytes, in association with interstitial edema, and damage to cellular components appear, especially with increasing bypass times.[52,53] All of these pathologic changes also describe the lung histology associated with the adult respiratory distress syndrome (ARDS).

TABLE 7.4. Lung water, capillary permeability, and oncotic pressure after uncomplicated CPB.

Extravascular lung water
  One study showed 1–2 mL/kg on first 2 days after CABG[35]
  One study found 3 mL/kg increase 30 min post CPB if fluid gain >1500 mL[36]; same group showed no increase 5 hours post CPB[37]
  Two studies failed to show increase[39,40]
Capillary permeability
  Animal study showed slight increase in lung[30] and gut[31] permeability
  Human studies are conflicting[32-34]
Maintenance of colloid oncotic pressure
  One study suggested increased pulmonary edema related to reduction in protein concentration[41]
  Other studies suggest reduced fluid requirement if albumin given, but no pulmonary benefit[42-44]

Adult Respiratory Distress Syndrome (ARDS)

The similar pathology and clinical course of what has been called the postperfusion syndrome and ARDS have led most authors to consider the former as simply one expression of the latter. ARDS has been defined as the presence of widespread bilateral pulmonary infiltrates of less than 7 days' duration associated with a $PaO_2/FiO_2 < 150$ off positive end expiratory pressure (PEEP) or <200 on PEEP, and a pulmonary artery occlusion pressure (PAOP) <18 mm Hg.[54] The latter criterion implies low-pressure pulmonary edema or "capillary leak," and all conditions in which capillary leak occurs may also lead to ARDS. However, the majority of patients developing ARDS (75%) have sepsis, acid aspiration, or trauma, or have had massive transfusions[54] (10 units of packed cells or whole blood given within 24 hours). In one review, 15% of all ARDS cases occurred after CPB[55]; however, recent reports suggest that a much lower proportion of all ARDS patients come from the postcardiac surgery population. In a series from the University of Colorado, ARDS after bypass was estimated to occur at a rate of 1.7%,[56] accounting for about 6% of all cases of ARDS. In the same report, a series from the University of Washington included no cases of ARDS after bypass; similarly, the estimate from Massachusetts General Hospital is "vanishingly small" (only two cases over several years).[57] A report from Great Britain suggests an incidence of 1.3%.[58] Since the development of ARDS after bypass often occurs in a setting where other inciting causes, such as massive transfusion or low-grade sepsis, also occur, it is usually not clear that the bypass run has "caused" the ARDS. For example, in an intensive care unit setting, a patient receiving 15 units of blood products in 24 hours has a 34% risk of developing ARDS, independent of any other risk factors.[56] In coronary artery bypass graft (CABG) patients, left ventricular dysfunction and blood product transfusions are clearly associated with postoperative pulmonary edema[29] (Figure 7.3).

The exact etiology of ARDS—including the mediators, mechanisms, and pathophysiology of lung injury—is not fully understood. Table 7.5 lists endogenous substances that have been proposed either as actual mediators or as markers of injury in ARDS.[59] The injury causes an increase in capillary permeability resulting in alveolar and interstitial fluid accumulation, capillary congestion, and infiltration of the interstitium by erythrocytes and leukocytes. Type I alveolar cells show a variable degree of degeneration, and hyaline membranes appear in areas of severe damage. Microthrombi and capillary plugging by leukocytes are also visible. All of these changes are similar to those seen in the lung studies after CPB.[50,51] Over days, this histologic picture progresses to include thickened endothelium (generated by the Type II cells), expansion and infiltration of the interstitial space with leukocytes and fibroblasts, and a decreased number of capillaries. Eventually, widespread fibrosis occurs. High inspired oxygen concentrations and high levels of PEEP are required to attain acceptable oxygenation, and death occurs in 50% to 75% of patients, usually as a result of multisystem organ

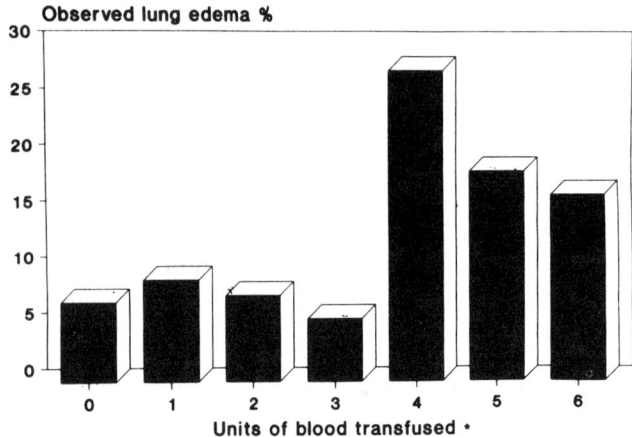

FIGURE 7.3. Incidence of lung edema (Y axis) after elective CABG surgery ($n = 100$) increased sharply in relation to the number of transfusions of blood collected in mobile units (X axis). Lung edema was defined as the presence of diffuse bilateral pulmonary infiltrates, with or without the need for prolonged ventilatory support. (From Louagie Y, Gonzales E, Jamart J, et al,[29] by permission of *Chest*.)

TABLE 7.5. Circulating mediators or markers of acute lung injury.

Formed blood elements
   Neutrophils
   Platelets
Chemoattractants
   Complement fragments
   Lipoxygenase products
   Platelet-activating factor
   Bacterial peptides
Mediators of cell damage
   Toxic oxygen intermediates
   Proteolytic enzymes
   Phospholipase products
Markers of cell damage
   Prostacylcin
   Factor VIII
Miscellaneous markers
   Angiotensin-converting enzyme
   Fibronectin
   Fibrin degradation products
   Phospholipase A_2

(From Maunder RJ, and Hudson LD,[59] by permission of Marcel Dekker Inc.)

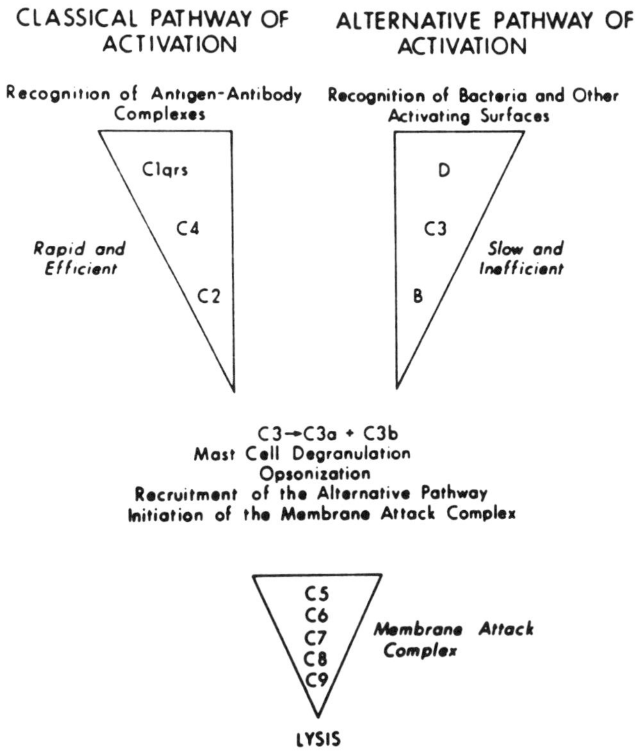

7. Respiratory, Renal, and Hepatic Systems

FIGURE 7.4. Simplified components of the complement system. (From Haynes BF, Fauci AS,[60] by permission of McGraw-Hill.)

failure (MSOF) and/or sepsis rather than inability to oxygenate the blood.

Once ARDS, sepsis, or MSOF has intervened in the cardiac surgical patient, the course and outcome resemble that of any disease that progresses to these syndromes. The mediators of lung injury in ARDS (and probably MSOF) are of particular interest in the CPB patient, since many of the mediators listed in Table 7.5 have been found in this population.

Possible Mediators of Lung Injury Associated with CPB

Complement

The complement system is a "cascading" series of enzymes (analogous to the coagulation cascade) that is activated by foreign substances (Figure 7.4). The various complement components have activities that include: (1) opsonization and cell lysis; (2) cell activation (release of histamine, serotonin); (3) chemoattraction (monocytes and leukocytes)[60]; and (4) leukocyte sequestration in the lung that results in endothelial damage.[61]

Complement fragments C3a and C5a are called "anaphylotoxins"; fragments C5b-9, the "membrane attack complex," cause formation of cell pores and eventually cytolysis.[62] The C5a fragment and its degradation product C5a desArg cause neutrophil aggregation and release of lysosomal enzymes. A summary of the biological actions of complement fragments ("split-products") is given in Table 7.6. Further discussion of the complement system is found in Chapter 5.

Similar to the coagulation cascade, there is a classical pathway of complement activation and an "alternate" pathway. The former appears to be initiated by antigen-antibody complexes, while the alternate pathway is initiated by bacteria and foreign surfaces. Studies with hemodialysis and leukapheresis membranes in the late 1970s determined that certain coatings are potent activators of the alternate pathway and are associated with a postperfusion syndrome similar to that seen after CPB.[63,64] Chenowith et al[65] demonstrated that C3a is generated during routine coronary bypass procedures (Figure 7.5) and inferred that C5a is released (C5a is rapidly taken up by neutrophils). As nylon fiber appeared to be the surface causing complement activation during leukapheresis,[64] this group studied the nylon mesh liner of the bubble oxygenator and demonstrated that this surface did indeed cause C5a liberation. In the same investigation, they demonstrated that bubble oxygenators alone released C3a. This group also demonstrated the uptake of neutrophils by the lungs when the pulmonary circulation was re-established (Figure 7.6), the degree of which correlated with the duration of aortic crossclamping and total bypass time. A relationship between the degree of leukocyte sequestration and postoperative shunt could not be demonstrated, and no other aspect of patient outcome was described.

Not surprisingly, the findings of Chenowith et al generated much interest, and a series of papers appeared in the 1980s documenting the degree and type of complement activation during bypass.[34,66-74] Investigators determined that both the classical and the alternate pathways are involved, the former predominating with bubble oxygenators and the latter with membrane oxygenators.[65] With

TABLE 7.6. Some biologically significant effects of the various complement-split products.

Biological effect	Complement-split product
Mast-cell degranulation, contraction of smooth muscle, increased vascular permeability	C3a, C5a
Chemotaxis of neutrophils	C5a, C5a des Arg
Neutrophil aggregation	C5a, C5a des Arg
Lysosomal enzyme release	C5a, C3b
Leukocytosis	C3e
Immune adherence/opsonization	C3b, C4b
Membrane lysis	C5b-9 (membrane attack complex)

(From Knudsen F, Anderson LW[62] by permission of *J Cardiothorac Anesth.*)

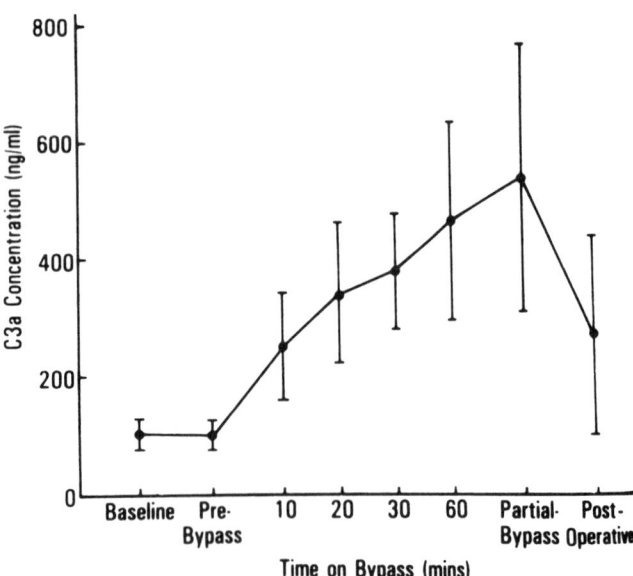

FIGURE 7.5. Plasma levels of C3a in patients undergoing CPB for elective CABG procedures. Levels were unaffected by routine surgical procedures (pre-bypass) but displayed a time-dependent elevation during CPB. Postoperative levels remained elevated. Each point represents the mean (±SEM) of observations in 15 patients. (From Chenowith DE, Cooper SW, Hugli TE, et al,[65] by permission of *N Engl J Med*.)

bubble oxygenators, there is more trauma to formed elements of the blood and denaturing of plasma proteins, both of which result in activation of the classical pathway. Two studies indicate that there is slightly less complement activation with membrane oxygenators,[66,67] while another found no difference.[68] The release of C3a was found in all studies, but due to the difficulty in measuring C5a, it is less frequently documented as elevated. At least two studies, however, have shown increased levels of the "membrane attack complex."[71,73] In one of these studies, this complex was found attached to red and white blood cells, and it correlated with hemolysis.[73]

A report by Kirklin et al[72] demonstrated an association between the C3a level after bypass and pulmonary dysfunction, most evident in pediatric patients who underwent prolonged bypass. Importantly, subsequent studies assessing the relationship between C3a levels and postoperative morbidity either do not report on pulmonary dysfunction or fail to demonstrate that elevated complement degradation product levels are associated with pulmonary injury. Elevated levels of complement degradation products are found in virtually all patients who have had an uneventful perioperative course. Therefore, it seems that complement alone is not the culprit for organ dysfunction after cardiac surgery and CPB.

Other Mediators

There is abundant evidence that other mediators of inflammation, capable of increasing pulmonary capillary permeability or damaging pulmonary endothelium, are released during CPB. Platelet activation and release of histamine and kallikrein/bradykinin occur during CPB and may be important mediators of perioperative inflammation (see Chapter 5). Bacterial endotoxin (or lipopolysaccharide), a potent stimulator of complement and neutrophils, is released into the circulation during bypass.[75,76] The mechanism by which this occurs may be splanchnic

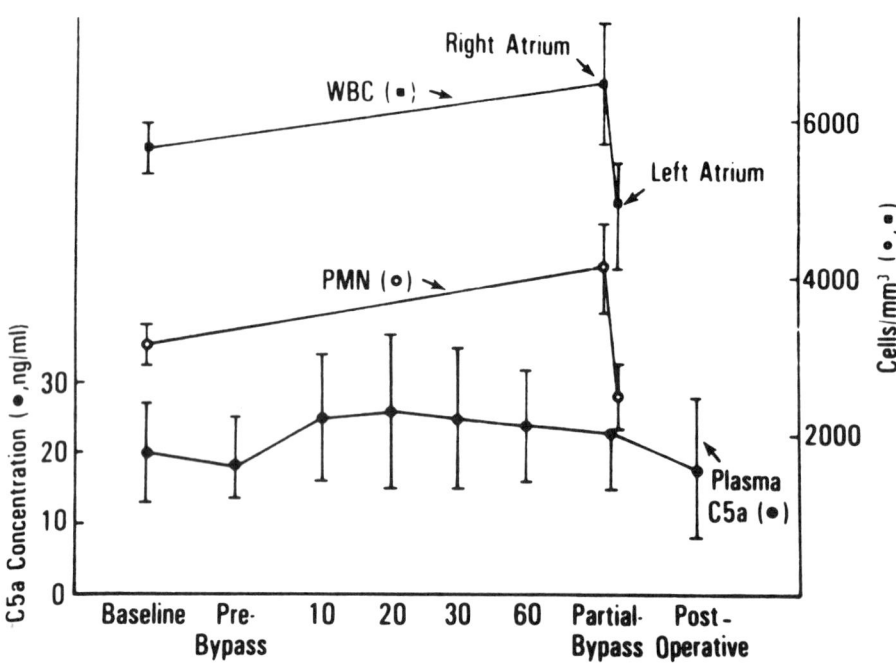

FIGURE 7.6. Plasma levels of C5a and white cell counts in patients undergoing CPB for elective CABG procedures. Levels of C5a did not change significantly during CPB. An increase in white cells (WBC) and polymorphonuclear leukocytes (PMN) was observed, and, when pulmonary circulation was re-established at partial bypass, pulmonary leukosequestration and neutropenia were demonstrable (decrease in WBCs and PMNs from right to left atria). Each point represents the mean (±SEM) of observations in 15 patients. (From Chenowith DE, Cooper WE, Hugli TE, et al,[65] by permission of *N Engl J Med*.)

hypoperfusion, as aortic crossclamping during aortic reconstructive surgery results in absorption of endotoxin from the gut.[77] In animal models, the administration of endotoxin causes pulmonary neutrophil accumulation and activation, resulting in lung injury.[78,79]

Pulmonary Neutrophil Sequestration

Investigators preceding[52,53] and following[67,70,80] Chenowith have described the sequestration of leukocytes in the lung when the pulmonary circulation is re-established after CPB.

Neutrophils possess an array of toxins designed to defend against invading microbes, but depend on other arms of the immune system, including complement, to identify the targets. Nonspecific immune system activation causes neutrophils to unleash their toxins, and host tissues are attacked. The reader is referred to the paper by Weiss[81] for a detailed review of how tissues are destroyed by neutrophils. In brief, neutrophils possess the ability to generate reactive oxygen metabolites ("free radicals") through a membrane-bound NADPH-oxidase, and to release granules containing myeloperoxidase. The interaction of these compounds results in the formation of highly reactive and destructive hypochlorous acid (HOCl), which then can locally inactivate antiprotease systems and allow other destructive enzymes of the neutrophil, such as elastase, gelatinize, and collagenase, to attack host tissues. In patients with ARDS, bronchoalveolar lavage fluid contains large numbers of neutrophils, as well as enzymes indicative of neutrophil activation.[82]

Several investigators have searched for evidence of activated neutrophils during CPB by measuring levels of active enzymes as well as oxygen "free radicals." Both animal and human studies have conclusively demonstrated significant release of myeloperoxidase,[69,83] elastase,[69,83-86] lactoferrin[69,84] (a specific neutrophil granule marker), and an oxygen free radical ("superoxide")[86] during CPB. Figures 7.7 and 7.8 outline these events during uneventful coronary bypass procedures performed with a membrane oxygenator and hypothermia. However, none of these studies included information on postoperative pulmonary morbidity.

Clinical Implications

As is evident from the many studies cited above, it is possible to document the presence of several pathophysiologic processes during bypass, any or all of which may produce pulmonary vascular damage resulting in ARDS or "pump lung." Unfortunately, there are no relevant outcome studies (ie, large numbers of patients), other than that of Kirklin,[72] which document specific relationships between any process and the risk of pulmonary complications. Even this latter study is flawed in that the relationship between C3a levels and pulmonary dysfunction was only strong in the youngest patients. One study has documented significant complement and neutrophil activation with no change in measured pulmonary vascular permeability.[34] It therefore seems likely that some combination of the various processes, in susceptible patients, will eventually result in the 1% to 2% incidence of postbypass ARDS. Far more likely as a cause for postoperative pulmonary edema is the occurrence of elevated pulmonary vascular pressures during the operation. Transient elevation of capillary pressure at a time of low oncotic pressure, as discussed above, may lead to severe postoperative pulmonary edema, although the intravascular pressures may be normal at this (postoperative) time.

Therapies to Attenuate Perioperative Complement and Neutrophil Activation

Several groups of investigators have applied specific therapies to prevent activation of complement or neutrophils. Administration of methylprednisolone, 30 mg/kg, before bypass can reduce complement activation.[87,88] Glucocorticoids also appear to inhibit the neutrophil activation induced by endotoxin.[88] Other therapies shown to reduce complement activation in the setting of bypass include the plasma expander polygeline[89] and heparin bonding of the bypass circuit.[90] Heparin bonding has also been shown to reduce neutrophil activation.[90,91] Release of proteases by neutrophils may be inhibited by prostaglandin E_1,[83,84] lidocaine,[83,84] nifedipine,[69] desferoxamine,[92] and the specific protease inhibitor namfamostat mesilate.[93] Leukocyte depletion with a filter-reduced free-radical formation and lung injury in a dog model.[94] This latter report is virtually the only evidence that a specific therapy to prevent complement or neutrophil activation reduces lung injury. Table 7.7 lists the therapies that have been proposed to reduce complement/neutrophil activation. Application of any of these therapies on a routine basis is therefore not yet warranted, as outcome studies in humans have not been performed, and no therapy is without cost or risk. Large, prospective, and probably multicenter trials of new therapies—such as heparin bonding of circuits, or the pharmacologic agents listed above—will be needed to determine if there is any reduction in the already low incidence of pulmonary injury following CPB.

Postoperative Respiratory Failure (Non-ARDS)

In addition to the small percentage of patients who develop ARDS after bypass, another small percentage will become ventilator-dependent for a variety of reasons. A

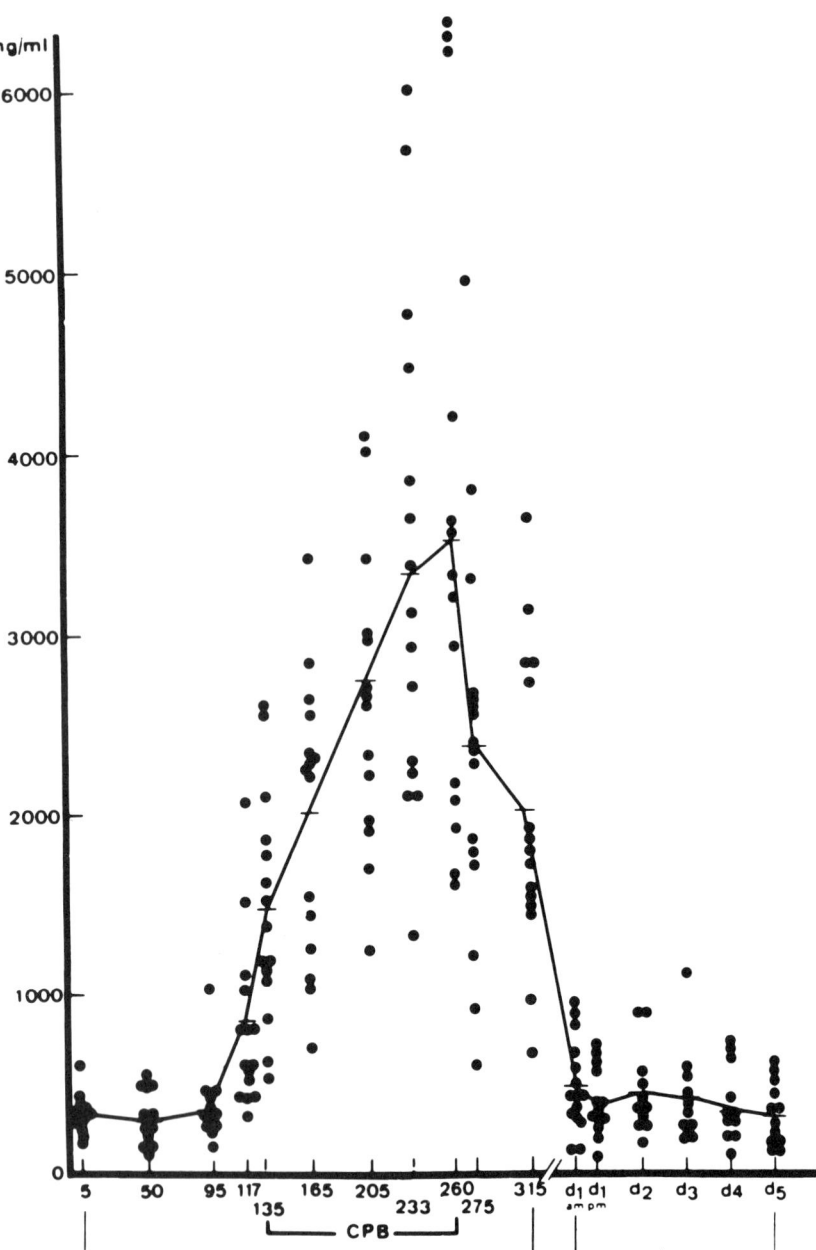

FIGURE 7.7. Individual and mean plasma myeloperoxidase levels in 15 patients undergoing CPB for elective CABG procedures. These results are interpreted as evidence of activation of leukocytes by CPB. (From Faymonville ME, Pincemail J, Duchateau J, et al,[83] by permission of *J Thorac Cardiovasc Surg.*)

recent review of complications from the Cleveland Clinic found the most important risk factor for developing pulmonary complications was congestive heart failure at the time of surgery.[95] Pulmonary vascular congestion or edema present at the time of surgery appears to result in prolonged interstitial or alveolar edema in the postoperative period. This is in keeping with the finding by Ratliff et al[52] that pathologic changes in the lung after bypass were always worse when there were preoperative abnormalities. A decline in pulmonary compliance over and above the usual reduction imposes an intolerable load on the already compromised respiratory system, especially in patients with marginal cardiac status. Other risk factors include emergency surgery or reoperations, chronic obstructive pulmonary disease (COPD) in patients requiring medication, and renal insufficiency.[95]

The usual reduction in lung function and alterations in gas exchange discussed above may be enough to render a patient with severe pulmonary disease ventilator-dependent for an extended period. Similarly, the nutritionally depleted patient may have limited respiratory reserve, and the additional work of breathing in the postoperative period may be intolerable. These causes of postoperative respiratory failure are usually multifactorial, and im-

FIGURE 7.8. Individual and mean plasma concentration curve of elastase-α_1-PI levels in patients undergoing CPB for elective CABG procedures. These results are interpreted as evidence of activation of leukocytes, with the delay in elastase elimination (relative to myeloperoxidase) being due to altered mechanism of elimination such as saturation of antiproteases. (From Faymonville ME, Pincemail J, Duchateau J et al,[83] by permission of *J Thorac Cardiovasc Surg.*)

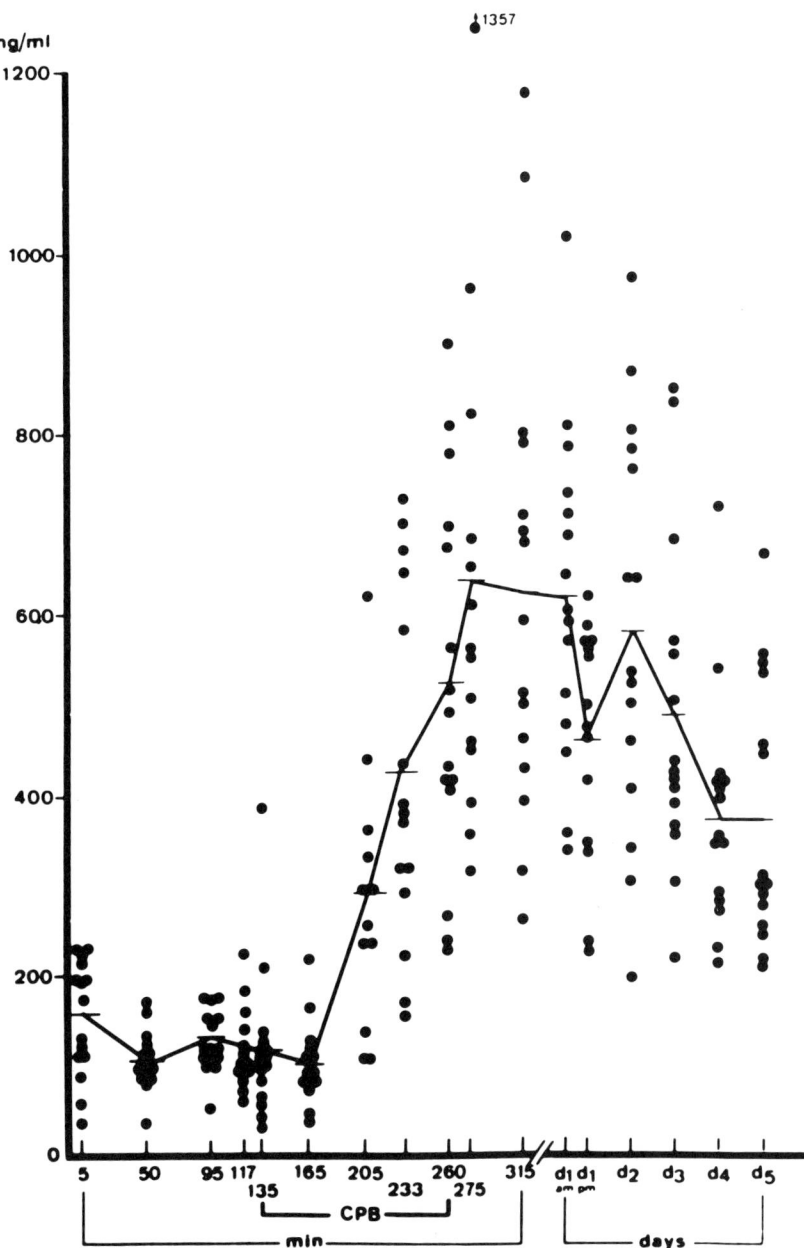

TABLE 7.7. Therapies that may reduce complement/neutrophil activation.

Methylprednisolone pretreatment[87,88]
Polygeline (plasma expander) in pump prime[89]
Heparin bonding of CPB circuit[74,90,91]
Inhibition of neutrophil protease release:
  PGE 1[83,84]
  Lidocaine[83,84]
  Nifedipine[69]
  Desferoxamine[92]
  Namfamostat mesylate[93]
Leukocyte depletion[94]

---

paired cardiac performance may be a limiting factor in overcoming perioperative complications. CPB itself probably has only a small role in this type of postoperative respiratory failure.

The Gastrointestinal System

Although the effect of bypass on the respiratory system has been studied in some detail, there are few studies assessing the effects of CPB on the gastrointestinal (GI) system. This is probably because the frequency of mild to moderate impairment of lung function is high, as discussed above, and because of the high incidence of "pump lung" in the early years of bypass versus a much lower incidence of significant GI complications. Recent reviews of severe GI complications after bypass suggest an overall incidence of approximately 1%.[96-103] Table 7.8 summarizes these studies.

Unlike the usual decreases in respiratory function, there appear to be no "usual" changes in GI function after cardiac surgery with bypass. Indeed, most patients are eating normally 24 to 48 hours after uncomplicated elective procedures. Despite this, investigators have demonstrated transient elevations in liver function tests,[104] hyperamylasemia without overt pancreatitis,[105,106] and (in a piglet model) an increase of 6% to 8% in tissue water in the bowel and pancreas.[40] The latter finding is consistent with the small increase in intestinal permeability to protein found in the canine model referred to above.[30]

Fiddian-Green et al[107] have studied stomach wall pH by tonometry in patients during and after bypass. In the first study, half of the patients developed acidosis of the stomach wall, and all serious complications (8 in 85 patients) had occurred in these patients. Although duration of hypotension was the single best predictor of adverse outcome, the addition of degree and duration of stomach wall acidosis significantly improved predictive ability. This work, and previous work by the same group, suggests stomach wall acidosis is a sensitive indicator of gut hypoperfusion. More recent work by Landow et al,[108,109] using the same technique, has documented a gradual reduction in gastric pH after routine bypass, the degree of which correlates with duration of bypass. Associated with the decrease in gastric pH during bypass is the appearance of endotoxin in the circulation.[75-77,108,110] Although it has been suggested that an important source is "environmental" (eg, the bypass circuitry and fluids),[76] more recent work indicates that the source is endogenous.[108] In these studies, the presence of endotoxin was not associated with systemic infection or other complications, but it did suggest that intestinal barrier function was compromised.

TABLE 7.8. Gastrointestinal complications after CPB.

Ref.	Years	Cases CPB	No. complications (%)[a]	No. deaths (%)
96	1980-88	4473	35 (0.78)	22 (63)
97	1980-84	1686	28 (1.6)	10 (36)
98	1966-81	5682	54 (0.9)	12 (30)
99	1970-75	1000	9 (0.85)	22 (63)
100	1970-81	5080	43 (0.85)	27 (63)
101	1975-85	1596	18 (1.1)	2 (12.5)
102	1976-86	6542	60 (0.9)	30 (59)
103	1980-83	2428	27 (1.1)	22 (17)

[a]In all studies, more than one complication occurred in some patients. In all studies, some patients were managed conservatively, some surgically.

Hampton et al[111] studied hepatic blood flow in 10 patients undergoing routine bypass and found a 19% reduction from control (prebypass). Data from a canine model also demonstrate reduced hepatic and pancreatic blood flow during cooling and rewarming on bypass.[112] In this latter investigation, pulsatile blood flow was associated with greater organ perfusion than nonpulsatile blood flow during CPB, and, in the human study by Huddy et al,[96] GI complications were less likely with pulsatile flow. The elevated levels of angiotensin II associated with nonpulsatile bypass may be a factor in the development of relative splanchnic hypoperfusion.[113] Alternatively, in the presence of relative splanchnic hypoperfusion, there is a benefit associated with the maintenance of pulsatile blood flow.

As the vast majority (99%) of patients do not experience GI complications, decreases in gastric pH, decreased GI organ blood flow, and the appearance of endotoxin appear to be of little importance. However, in this setting of reduced splanchnic blood flow, the subsequent development of low-output state appears to be associated with the development of GI organ damage. Recurring themes in the studies listed in Table 7.8 are the association of low cardiac output and inotropic drug or balloon pump requirement with complications, and the ischemic nature of the complications (bowel infarction, GI bleeding). Kumon et al[114] documented a 22.3% incidence of postoperative low-output syndrome in 3003 cardiac surgical patients; 18.4% developed hepatic failure and 11.1% developed GI bleeding. Table 7.8 reports the mortality of patients developing a GI complication.

Transient elevations in liver function tests occur after bypass, whether or not jaundice develops. In a detailed prospective study of postbypass jaundice, Collins et al[104] demonstrated a high incidence of conjugated hyperbilirubinemia (20% of 248 patients), but were unable to show an association between hypotension and hypoxia (cardiac output was not reported). Jaundice was associated with a 25% mortality (versus 1% in nonjaundiced patients); risk factors included long bypass times, multiple transfusions, and multiple valve replacements. However, patients without these risk factors also developed jaundice. Figure 7.9 demonstrates the changes in bilirubin, transaminases, and alkaline phosphatase in jaundiced versus nonjaundiced patients.

Hyperamylasemia occurs in 32% to 69% of patients after cardiac surgery[105,106,115,116]; the highest incidence is in patients with combined valve and CABG procedures.[105] Although the source appears to be nonpancreatic (salivary, pleural) in some patients, a recent detailed report indicates that 67% of patients with hyperamylasemia have some degree of pancreatic cellular damage, and that mortality is very high in the presence of symptoms of pancreatic injury.[115] Prolonged bypass, postoperative hypotension, and low cardiac output were associated with

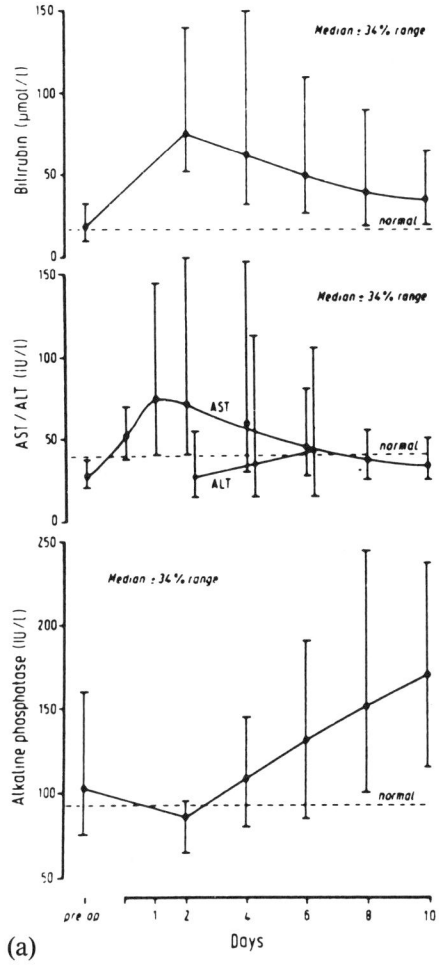

FIGURE 7.9. Liver function tests in 248 consecutive patients (age >16 years) undergoing CPB: (a) 49 patients who developed jaundice; (b) 197 patients who did not develop jaundice. Bilirubin rose to between 17 and 49 μmol/L on day 2 in 140 patients who did not develop jaundice (normal <17 μmol/L). Postoperative mortality was 25% in jaundiced patients, and 1% in patients without jaundice. (From Collins JD, Bassendine MF, Ferner R, et al,[104] Copyright 1983 by *The Lancet Ltd.*)

pancreatic injury, but this recent report also showed a strong association between the dose of calcium chloride administered and the development of pancreatitis. In an accompanying editorial, Reber[117] indicates that, while there are several mechanisms by which calcium could aggravate pancreatic ischemia, ischemia on the basis of hypoperfusion is still likely to be the most important factor in the development of pancreatitis. Murray et al[118] (and others) have shown that there is less amylase release after pulsatile than after nonpulsatile perfusion.

Aziz et al[119] reported an 8.5% incidence of pancreatitis found at autopsy in heart and heart-lung transplant recipients. Unfortunately, it is difficult from their report to determine the onset of pancreatitis, and data about hemodynamic state are not given. The authors quote other work in suggesting that steroid therapy, and possibly azathioprine, may predispose to the development of pancreatitis. Another report of general surgical complications after heart and heart-lung transplantation suggests that early complications are no more frequent than after other types of cardiac surgery.[120]

In summary, the GI consequences of bypass appear to be minimal in most patients, despite studies that have documented reductions in organ flow (directly or indirectly) and blood chemistry indicating abnormal function (increased amylase, bilirubin). When complications occur, they are usually ischemic in nature and are often associated with low-output syndrome. There are some data suggesting a lower incidence of organ dysfunction and a lower incidence of severe complications with the use of pulsatile perfusion.

Renal Consequences of CPB

The effects of CPB on renal function also have been examined in some detail, both in patients and in the labora-

TABLE 7.9. Incidence and outcome of postbypass renal dysfunction.[a]

Ref.	Year of data collection	N	Nondialysis (%)	Mortality (%)	Dialysis (%)	Mortality (%)
Yeboah et al[133]	1968–70	428	26	38	4.7	70
McLeish et al[137]	1969–75	1542	Not reported	Not reported	1.3	35
Bhat et al[122]	1972	490	28.1	10.9	2.2	45
Gailiunas et al[147]	1973–77	752	17	Not reported	1.5	27
Abel et al[136]	1974	500	21.6	13.8	3	100
Hilberman et al[135]	1977	204	2.5	60[b]	2.5	60[b]
Lange et al[123]	1980–83	2959	Not reported	Not reported	1.2	53
Corwin et al[146]	1985	572	6.3	Not reported	1	33

[a]Definitions of renal dysfunction varied from study to study. Mortality was rarely due to renal failure alone.
[b]Mortality is combined for dialysis and nondialysis patients.

tory. Although several investigators have documented a rather high incidence of postoperative "renal failure," as defined by postoperative increases in serum blood urea nitrogen (BUN) or creatinine levels, in reality these studies reveal a substantial incidence of postoperative renal dysfunction (up to 30%) but a relatively low incidence of severe renal impairment necessitating dialysis (1% to 5%). Table 7.9 summarizes several of these studies; a different way of expressing the incidence of renal dysfunction after bypass is according to the postoperative increase in BUN[121] or creatinine[122] (Table 7.10). It is evident from Table 7.9 that there is a very high mortality from renal failure that necessitates dialysis, making this a very serious complication of cardiac surgery and CPB. However, as discussed below, in most cases the renal failure is a consequence of postoperative complications rather than a result of the bypass run itself. The prognosis is worst for those patients with associated respiratory failure, hypotensive episodes, or neurologic dysfunction.[123]

Renal Function During Bypass

In the first two decades of heart surgery, several groups measured renal perfusion with indicator clearance techniques and found that renal blood flow and glomerular filtration rate (GFR) during bypass were reduced by 25% to 75%, with partial but not complete recovery in the first day after bypass.[124–126] Figure 7.10 indicates the changes in inulin clearance as an indicator of GFR, and para-aminohippurate (PAH) extraction as an indicator of renal plasma flow in 32 patients undergoing surgery for valvular or congenital disease from 1963 to 1966.[124] The reasons for this reduction in function were postulated to be renal artery vasoconstriction, hypothermia, and loss of pulsatile perfusion, with these factors being interdependent (eg, vasoconstriction a result of loss of pulsatile perfusion). Two laboratory investigations support a reduction in renal blood flow with bypass: renal arteriograms performed in a canine model demonstrated renal artery vasoconstriction, especially in the first 30 minutes of nonpulsatile bypass,[127] and another canine study using clearance techniques demonstrated a reduced renal blood flow after 2 hours.[128] Comparative studies of the effects of pulsatile versus nonpulsatile flow have been performed for more than 30 years, sometimes with conflicting results. Well-controlled studies performed in mongrel dogs do support the contention that renal blood flow, especially that to the cortex,[112] and renal metabolism[129] are best preserved with physiologic (ie, significant pulse pressure) pulsatile perfusion. Although catecholamine levels do not appear to be affected by the type of flow,[130] angiotensin II levels are higher with nonpulsatile flow.[131] The reader is referred to a comprehensive review of the subject by Hickey et al[132] which concludes that the bulk of evidence does support renal vasoconstriction with the loss of pulsatile perfusion. There are, however, no clinical studies comparing the incidence of postoperative renal dysfunction and renal failure with the use of pulsatile versus nonpulsatile perfusion.

Two factors that might be expected to affect renal perfusion during nonpulsatile bypass are systemic blood pressure and pump flow rate. These factors have been reviewed in many of the studies referenced in Table 7.9, and are not consistently related to the development of postbypass renal dysfunction. Indeed, although Yeboah et al[133] suggested that a perfusion pressure above 80 mm Hg reduced the incidence of renal failure, and Yeh et al[134] found

TABLE 7.10. Expected changes in postoperative BUN and creatinine.

Patients with peak postoperative BUN (209 patients reported, percentage of patients in parentheses)[121]				
BUN (mg%)	<31	31–60	61–100	>100
No. patients/%	117 (56)	68 (32)	18 (9)	6 (3)
Patients with peak postoperative creatinine (490 patients reported)[122]				
Creatinine (mg/dL)	<1.5	1.6–1.9	2–5	>5
No. patients/%	340 (70)	69 (14)	60 (12)	21 (4)

7. Respiratory, Renal, and Hepatic Systems

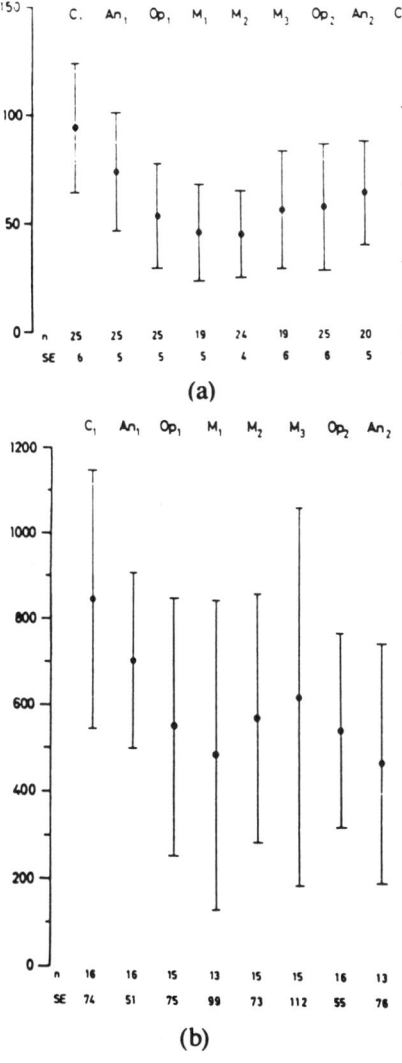

FIGURE 7.10. (a) Insulin clearance and (b) renal blood flow (both expressed in mL × 1.73/min × BSA). Values are the means for 32 patients ± SD. Patients (age 15–55 yr) underwent correction of congenital heart defects, valvular commisurotomy, or valve replacement. C_1 = preoperative control period; An_1 = induction of anesthesia; Op_1 = thoractotomy; M_1 = connection to heart-lung machine and cooling of blood; M_2 = machine with hypothermia (30°C); M_3 = machine with warming of blood; Op_2 = closure of chest; An_2 = completion of anesthesia; C_{24} = control period 24 hours after operation; n = total number of patients; SE = standard error; SD = standard deviation; BSA = body surface area. (From Lundberg S,[126] by permission of *Acta Anaesth Scand*.)

a strong association between low flow (<1.8 L/min/m^2) and renal failure, the lowest combined incidence of renal dysfunction and renal failure was reported by a group which maintained a mean pressure of 65 mm Hg with vasodilators and pump flows at 30–50 mL/kg.[135] Abel et al[136] and McLeish et al[137] could not demonstrate an association between blood pressure and blood flows with renal dysfunction. Koning et al[138] reported that a postoperative increase in creatinine was more likely if low blood flows were delivered to elderly patients with raised creatinine.

Most studies have found a definite relationship between the incidence of postbypass renal dysfunction and the duration of bypass; an example is given in Figure 7.11. Related to the duration of bypass in some studies is the level of plasma hemoglobin, which has also been found to be correlated with postoperative renal dysfunction.[122,134] Free hemoglobin is a nephrotoxin in the setting of low renal perfusion,[139] but modern perfusion techniques have made it unlikely that nephrotoxic plasma hemoglobin levels will occur. More recent studies demonstrate higher plasma hemoglobin levels with prolonged bypass, but it is the duration of bypass, rather than the hemoglobin level, which correlates with renal dysfunction.[140] The importance of duration of bypass may be its association with more complex cardiac procedures that result in poorer cardiac function immediately after surgery, or it may be due simply to the prolonged period of reduced renal perfusion and glomerular filtration.

Renal Function After Bypass

Work done in the late 1970s also suggested that GFR (measured by inulin clearance), and effective renal plasma flow (ERPF, measured by PAH extraction) were

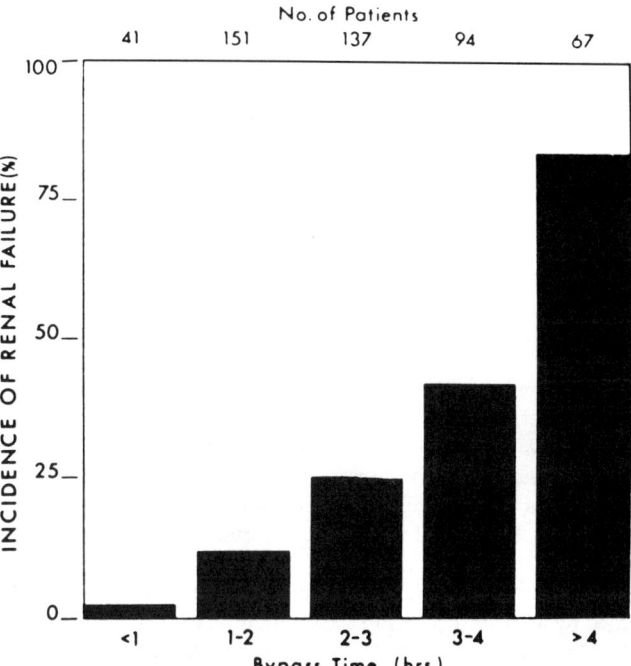

FIGURE 7.11. Bypass time and occurrence of renal failure (defined as increase in creatinine of at least 0.4 mg/dL, and a maximum level of 1.6 mg/dL or greater). (From Bhat JG, Gluck MC, Lowenstein J et al,[122] by permission of *Ann Intern Med*.)

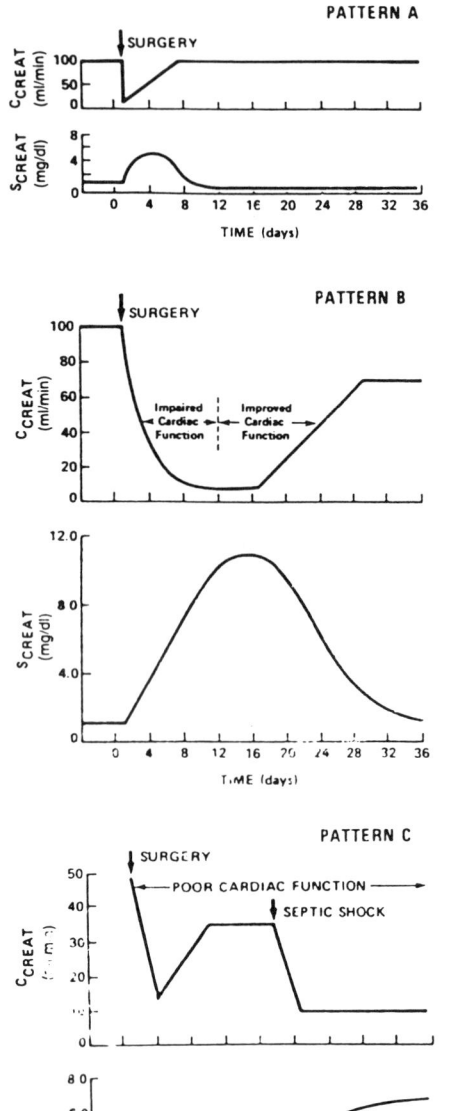

FIGURE 7.12. Three typical courses of acute renal failure after cardiac surgery, illustrated by creatinine clearance (^{C}Creat) and serum levels of creatinine (^{S}Creat) in representative patients who did not undergo dialysis. The upper portion (pattern A) displays a step decrement in clearance that is followed immediately by a ramp increment in serum creatinine typical of abbreviated acute renal failure. The middle portion (pattern B) displays an exponential decrement of clearance that is accompanied by a linear increase in the serum level of creatinine (days 1 to 12). Recovery, which follows improved cardiac performance from day 12, is manifested during days 16 through 30 by a ramp increment in clearance that is accompanied by a sigmoidal decline in the serum level of creatinine. In pattern C (lower portion), successive ramp decrements in clearance (days 1 to 4, and 18 to 21) are accompanied by sigmoid elevation of the serum creatinine level. Recovery of creatinine clearance (ramp increment, days 4 to 7) is seen only after the first episode. A persistent low-cardiac-output state prevents recovery from the second insult. (From Myers BD, Moran MS,[144] by permission of N Engl J Med.)

reduced after cardiac surgery, but only in patients who went on to develop renal dysfunction or overt renal failure.[135,141] In these studies there were no preoperative measurements, however. Using a single-injection clearance technique, Bourgois et al[142] studied 10 children before and 24 to 36 hours after cardiac surgery (8 of 10 had a period of circulatory arrest), and found both GFR and ERPF to be unchanged. Although simultaneously measured creatinine clearance was reduced after surgery, this was explained by artifactually increased plasma creatinine due to plasma chromogens. In a very recent study of 11 adult patients undergoing CABG, "renal functional reserve" was assessed before and after surgery by measuring the increase in creatinine clearance induced by a protein load.[143] Although postoperative creatinine clearance was not significantly decreased, there was a significant loss of "functional reserve," which had been recovered 6 months later. These data were interpreted to demonstrate that bypass "probably causes renal damage that is not sufficient to influence routine renal function parameters." These studies appear to demonstrate that most patients will have little, if any, measurable decline in postoperative renal function, despite the reduction of renal blood flow which occurs on bypass and the possibility that there is a subtle decline in renal functional reserve.

Perhaps the most influential publications on postbypass renal dysfunction are three from the Stanford group.[135,141,144] In the first two studies, data were collected prospectively to determine the incidence of renal dysfunction, with further data collection in a series of patients who did develop renal dysfunction. In the third article,[144] a comprehensive review of the subject of "hemodynamically mediated renal failure" is presented. These authors identify three "typical" courses of renal failure that may occur after cardiac surgery, represented graphically in Figure 7.12. In the first and most common type of renal dysfunction, a brief, isolated ischemic insult occurs intraoperatively, but the effects are moderated by the administration of "protective factors," such as mannitol (see below), before the insult. In addition, postoperative cardiac output and blood pressure are maintained in the normal range. There is rapid recovery of renal function after the ischemic insult, despite a continuing rise in creatinine for several days. In cases where the intraoperative insult is followed by a period of impaired cardiac function postoperatively, renal function may continue to decrease for days, and it may take weeks to recover as cardiac performance improves. If diuretics or mannitol are administered before the initial insult, oliguria may be avoided. In the most severe type of postoperative renal failure, an ischemic insult to the kidneys is followed by a prolonged period of poor cardiac performance, as well as further acute ischemic insults, such as bouts of hypotension or severe cardiac dysrhythmias. This type of renal failure is usually oliguric, progressing to the need for dialysis.

Many other investigators have reported that postoperative renal failure is most common in patients with poor cardiac performance postoperatively.[114,122,124,136,137,140,145] In addition, several investigations have shown that patients with pre-existing renal dysfunction[121,125,133,135,138,146] or poor cardiac performance *before* surgery[135] are at increased risk for postbypass renal failure. It therefore seems that the risk of developing postbypass renal failure is a function of the patient's underlying renal function (also affected by age, as described above) and the perioperative circulatory status, as well as the duration of bypass. Renal failure in this setting is best understood as due to the occurrence of acute renal ischemia superimposed on subacute (ie, caused by bypass) ischemia.

As in other forms of ischemic insult to the kidneys, the histologic changes that accompany severe renal functional impairment after CPB are often characteristic of tubular necrosis.[122,133,147] For reasons that are not completely understood, it appears to be the tubular cells (rather than the glomerular cells) that are the most susceptible to acute reductions in renal perfusion, especially those of the proximal tubule.[144] With ischemia and necrosis of the cells lining the tubules, swelling occurs, with sloughing and tubular obstruction. This further reduces the filtration pressure from its already reduced state and is associated with "back-leak" of tubular fluid into the interstitium of the kidney. In the early stages, it appears to be the tubular injury that is responsible for the impaired renal function, whereas in later stages (ie, after the tubular injury has largely healed), the rate and degree of recovery are determined by restoration of GFR. This in turn depends on maintenance of normal renal perfusion. Although acute tubular necrosis may be identifiable at autopsy, in a significant proportion of patients who develop renal failure there are few, if any, characteristic histologic lesions in the kidneys.[122,133]

Prevention of Renal Failure

Several of the investigations cited above have discussed the use of mannitol during bypass. This drug appears to possess several features that may moderate ischemic insults to the kidney. First, there is some evidence in animal models that renal blood flow during an ischemic insult is preserved or restored with mannitol pretreatment[148,149] and evidence that the same protective effect occurs with mannitol given during bypass.[150,151] Clinical experience (although from the early days of bypass) also suggests that mannitol is of benefit, especially during prolonged pump runs.[121,124] These beneficial effects may be due to volume expansion and hemodilution. In addition to helping maintain renal blood flow, mannitol is a nonreabsorbable compound that may initiate an osmotic diuresis and prevent tubular obstruction, and it is also a free radical scavenger. Furosemide also appears to have a beneficial effect on renal blood flow when given before or during bypass.[152,153] Although it has not been studied during bypass, low-dose dopamine may also help maintain renal blood flow and urine output in a setting of renal ischemia.[154-156] Although dopamine causes renal and mesenteric blood vessels to dilate, increased doses cause α-receptor stimulation and vasoconstriction. A newer dopaminergic agent is fenoldopam, which acts specifically on the renal and mesenteric vessels. This drug has not been used in cardiac surgery, but it may prove to be beneficial. It is possible that one of the beneficial effects of these drugs (mannitol, furosemide, dopaminergic agents) is to preserve urine formation despite the occurrence of severe functional impairment (ie, "nonoliguric" versus "oliguric" renal failure). This might be expected to help avoid the need for dialysis, especially if renal function improves within a few days. However, even with the use of a "renoprotective" drug, the primary approach to prevention of renal failure, or reduction of its severity, is to maintain normal intravascular volume and cardiac output.

Once renal failure has occurred, use of the drugs noted above is unlikely to be of benefit; when renal failure is suspected, the first priority should be given to assessment of the adequacy of volume status and cardiac output. It is possible that large doses of furosemide (or combinations of diuretics) will augment urine production in some patients with acute tubular necrosis, but there is no evidence such therapy will alter the course of the disease. One or two large doses of furosemide (eg, 120 or 240 mg) may be given; if there is no response, then additional doses will only result in ototoxicity. Similarly, if a dose of mannitol (eg, 12.5 to 25 g) is administered without effect, the only result of continued administration will be a hyperosmolar state with hyponatremia, requiring dialysis.

In addition to using "renoprotective" agents and maintaining renal perfusion, it is important to avoid the use of nephrotoxins in the postoperative period; wherever possible, alternative therapies to those associated with nephrotoxicity should be utilized. Some examples include performing radiologic studies without contrast material, choosing nonaminoglycoside antibiotics, and using vasodilators other than angiotensin-converting enzyme (ACE) inhibitors. This latter class of drugs inhibits efferent arteriolar vasoconstriction, which may result in a dramatic decrease in GFR if hypotension occurs. Use of ACE inhibitors should be limited to patients with a stable cardiovascular status, and especially those without hypovolemia.

In summary, as a result of CPB (especially with nonpulsatile flow), subtle impairment of renal function occurs following cardiac surgery. When there is a period of reduced perfusion, as occurs with low post-CPB cardiac output, this subtle impairment may progress to a significant decrease in renal function for several days, with an increase in serum creatinine. This appears to be more likely if there is preexisting renal dysfunction or prolonged bypass. If a reduction in cardiac output is prolonged or repeated, acute renal failure is likely; if dialysis is required, a very high mortality can be expected. Mannitol, furosemide, and possibly dopaminergic agonists, given during bypass, may help maintain renal function or at least urine production in the face of decreased renal perfusion.

References

1. Baer DM, Osborn JJ. The postperfusion pulmonary congestion syndrome. *Am J Clin Pathol* 1960;34:442-445.
2. Peters RM, Wellons HA, Howe TM. Total compliance and work of breathing after thoracotomy. *J Thorac Cardiovasc Surg* 1969;57:348-355.
3. Vargas FS, Cukier A, Terra-Filho M, et al. Relationship between pleural changes after myocardial revascularization and pulmonary mechanics. *Chest* 1992;102:1333-1336.
4. Zin WA, Caldiera MPR, Cardoso WV, et al. Expiratory mechanics before and after uncomplicated cardiac surgery. *Chest* 1989;95:21-28.
5. Casey WF, Wynands JE, Ralley FE, et al. The role of intrathecal morphine in the anesthetic management of patients undergoing coronary artery bypass grafting. *J Cardiothorac Anesth* 1987;1:510-516.
6. Braun SR, Birnbaum ML, Chopra PS. Pre- and postoperative pulmonary function abnormalities in coronary artery revascularization surgery. *Chest* 1978;73:316-320.
7. Berrizbeitia LD, Tessler S, Jacobowitz IJ, et al. Effect of sternotomy and coronary bypass surgery on postoperative pulmonary mechanics. *Chest* 1989;96:873-876.
8. Stock MC, Downs JB, Weaver D, et al. Effect of pleurotomy on pulmonary function after median sternotomy. *Ann Thorac Surg* 1986;42:441-444.
9. Simmoneau G, Viven A, Sartene R, et al. Diaphragm dysfunction induced by upper abdominal surgery. *Am Rev Resp Dis* 1983;128:899-903.
10. Mankikian B, Cantinea U, Bertrand M, et al. Improvement of diaphragmatic function by a thoracic extradural block after upper abdominal surgery. *Anesthesiology* 1988;68:379-386.
11. Estenne M, Yernault JC, De Smet JM, et al. Phrenic and diaphragm function after coronary artery bypass grafting. *Thorax* 1985;40:293-299.
12. Locke TJ, Griffiths TL, Mould H, et al. Rib cage mechanics after median sternotomy. *Thorax* 1990;45:465-468.
13. Wilson RS, Sullivan SF, Malm JR, et al. The oxygen cost of breathing following anesthesia and cardiac surgery. *Anesthesiology* 1973;39:387-393.
14. Field S, Kelly SM, Macklem PT. The oxygen cost of breathing in patients with cardiopulmonary disease. *Am Rev Resp Dis* 1982;126:9-13.
15. Scandell JG, Shaw RS, Burke JF, et al. Operative treatment of aortic stenosis in the adult. *Circulation* 1963;27:772-778.
16. Esposito RA, Spencer FC. The effect of pericardial insulation on hypothermic phrenic nerve injury during open heart surgery. *Ann Thorac Surg* 1987;43:303-308.
17. Wilcox P, Baile EM, Hards J, et al. Phrenic nerve function and its relationship to atelectasis after coronary artery bypass surgery. *Chest* 1988;93:693-698.
18. Fedullo AJ, Lerner RM, Gibson J, et al. Sonographic measurement of diaphragmatic motion after coronary artery bypass surgery. *Chest* 1992;102:1683-1686.
19. Diehl JL, Lofaso F, Deleuze P, et al. Clinically relevant diaphragmatic dysfunction after cardiac operations. *J Thorac Cardiovasc Surg* 1994;107:487-498.
20. Panossian A, Hagstrom JWC, Nehlsen SL, et al. Secondary nature of surfactant changes in postperfusion pulmonary damage. *J Thorac Cardiovasc Surg* 1969;57:628-634.
21. Phang PT, Keough KMW. Inhibition of pulmonary surfactant by plasma from normal adults and from patients having cardiopulmonary bypass. *J Thorac Cardiovasc Surg* 1986;91:248-251.
22. Rea HH, Harris EA, Seelye ER, et al. The effects of cardiopulmonary bypass upon pulmonary gas exchange. *J Thorac Cardiovasc Surg* 1978;75:104-120.
23. Dantzker DR, Cowenhaven WM, Willoughby WJ, et al. Gas exchange alterations associated with weaning from mechanical ventilation following coronary artery bypass grafting. *Chest* 1982;82:674-677.
24. Singh NP, Vargas FS, Cukier A, et al. Arterial blood gases after coronary artery bypass surgery. *Chest* 1992;102:1337-1341.
25. Staub NC. Pulmonary edema. *Physiol Rev* 1974;54:678.
26. Zarins CZ, Rice CL, Peters RM, et al. Lymph and pulmonary response to isobaric reduction in plasma oncotic pressure in baboons. *Circ Res* 1978;43:925-930.
27. Pearl RG, Halperin BD, Mihm F, et al. Pulmonary effects of crystalloid and colloid resuscitation from hemorrhagic shock in the presence of oleic acid-induced pulmonary capillary injury in the dog. *Anesthesiology* 1988;68:12-20.
28. Gallagher J, Banner MJ, Barnes PA. Large volume crystalloid resuscitation does not increase extravascular lung water. *Anesth Analg* 1985;64:323-326.
29. Louagie Y, Gonzalez E, Jamart J, et al. Postcardiopulmonary bypass lung edema: a preventable complication? *Chest* 1993;103:86-95.
30. Braude S, Nolop KB, Fleming JS, et al. Increased pulmonary transvascular protein flux after canine cardiopulmonary bypass: association with lung neutrophil sequestration and tissue peroxidation. *Am Rev Resp Dis* 1986;134:867-872.
31. Smith EEJ, Naftel DC, Blackstone EH, et al. Microvascular permeability after cardiopulmonary bypass; an experimental study. *J Thorac Cardiovasc Surg* 1987;94:225-233.
32. Royston D, Minty BD, Biol MI, et al. The effect of surgery with cardiopulmonary bypass on alveolar-capillary barrier function in human beings. *Ann Thorac Surg* 1985;40:139-143.

33. Raijmakers PGHM, Groeneveld ABJ, Schneider AJ, et al. Transvascular transport of ^{67}Ga in the lungs after cardiopulmonary bypass surgery. *Chest* 1993;104:1825-1832.
34. Tennenberg SD, Clardy DCW, Bailey WW, et al. Complement activation and lung permeability during cardiopulmonary bypass. *Ann Thorac Surg* 1990;50:597-601.
35. Byrick RJ, Kay JC, Noble WH. Extravascular lung water accumulation in patients following coronary artery surgery. *Can Anaesth Soc J* 1977;24:332-345.
36. Boldt J, Bormann BV, Kling D, et al. The influence of extracorporeal circulation on extravascular lung water in coronary surgery patients. *Thorac Cardiovasc Surg* 1986;34:111-115.
37. Boldt J, Kling D, von Bormann B, et al. Reanimation und extravaskulares lungenwasser in der herzchirurgie. *Anesthetist* 1988;37:91-96.
38. Gallagher JD, Moore RA, Kerns D. Effects of colloid or crystalloid administration on pulmonary extravascular water in the postoperative period after coronary artery bypass grafting. *Anesth Analg* 1985;64:753-758.
39. Sivak ED, Starr NJ, Graves JW, et al. Extravascular lung water values in patients undergoing coronary artery bypass surgery. *Crit Care Med* 1982;10:593-596.
40. Brigham KL, Faulkner SL, Fisher D, et al. Lung water and urea indicator dilution studies in cardiac surgery patients. *Circulation* 1976;53:369-376.
41. Klancke KA, Assey ME, Kratz JM, et al. Postoperative pulmonary edema in postcoronary artery bypass graft patients. *Chest* 1983;84:529-534.
42. Yeh, T, Parmar JM, Rebeyka IM, et al. Limiting edema in neonatal cardiopulmonary bypass with narrow-range molecular weight hydroxyethyl starch. *J Thorac Cardiovasc Surg* 1992;104:659-665.
43. Marelli D, Samson R, Edgell D, et al. Does the addition of albumin to the prime solution in cardiopulmonary bypass affect clinical outcome? *J Thorac Cardiovasc Surg* 1989;98:751-756.
44. Hallowell P, Bland JHL, Dalton BC, et al. The effect of hemodilution with albumin or ringer's lactate on water balance and blood use in open-heart surgery. *Ann Thorac Surg* 1978;25:22-29.
45. Byrick RJ, Noble WH. Postperfusion lung syndrome: comparison of travenol bubble and membrane oxygenators. *J Thorac Cardiovasc Surg* 1978;76:685-693.
46. Gould FK, Freeman R, Brown MA. Respiratory complications following cardiac surgery; the role of microbiology in its evaluation. *Anaesthesia* 1985;40:1061-1064.
47. Weiss ME, Nyhan D, Zhikang P, et al. Association of protamine IgE and IgG antibodies with life-threatening reactions to intravenous protamine. *N Engl J Med* 1989;320:886-892.
48. Latson TW, Kickler TS, Baumgartner WA. Pulmonary hypertension and noncardiogenic pulmonary edema following cardiopulmonary bypass associated with an antigranulocyte antibody. *Anesthesiology* 1986;64:106-111.
49. Dodrill FD. The effects of total body perfusion upon the lungs. In: Allen JG, ed. *Extracorporeal Circulation*. Springfield, IL: Charles C Tomas; 1960:327-335.
50. Anyanwu E, Dittrich H, Gieseking R, et al. Ultrastructural changes in the human lung following cardiopulmonary bypass. *Bas Res Cardiol* 1982;77:309-332.
51. Asada S, Yamaguchi M. Fine structural change in the lung following cardiopulmonary bypass; its relation to early postoperative course. *Chest* 1971;59:478-483.
52. Ratliff NB, Young GW, Hackel DB, et al. Pulmonary injury secondary to extracorporeal circulation. *J Thorac Cardiovasc Surg* 1973;65:425-432.
53. Neville WE, Kontaxis A, Gavin T, et al. Postperfusion pulmonary vasculitis. *Arch Surg* 1963;86:126-137.
54. Hyers TM. Adult respiratory distress syndrome: definition, risk factors, and outcome. In: Zapol WM, Lemaire F, eds. *Adult Respiratory Distress Syndrome*. New York: Marcel Dekker Inc; 1991:23-36.
55. Fein AM, Goldbery SK, Lippman ML, et al. Adult respiratory distress syndrome. *Br J Anaesth* 1982;54:723-729.
56. Fowler AA, Hamman RF, Good JT, et al. Adult respiratory distress syndrome: risk with common predispositions. *Ann Intern Med* 1983;98:593-597.
57. Zapol WM, Frikker MJ, Pontoppidan H, et al. The adult respiratory distress syndrome at Massachusetts General Hospital: etiology, progression, and survival rates 1978-1988. In: Zapol WM, Lemaire F, eds. *Adult Respiratory Distress Syndrome*. New York: Marcel Dekker Inc; 1991:367-380.
58. Messent M, Sullivan K, Keogh BF, et al. Adult respiratory distress syndrome following cardiopulmonary bypass: incidence and prediction. *Anesthesia* 1992;47:267-268.
59. Maunder RJ, Hudson LD. Clinical risks associated with the adult respiratory distress syndrome. In: Zapol WM, Lemaire F, eds. *Adult Respiratory Distress Syndrome*. New York: Marcel Dekker Inc; 1991:1-21.
60. Haynes BF, Fauci AS. Introduction to clinical immunology. In: Braunwald E, Isselbacher KJ, Petersdorf RG, et al, eds. *Harrison's Principles of Internal Medicine*. 11th ed. New York: McGraw-Hill; 1987:328-337.
61. Jacob HS. Complement-mediated leucoembolization: a mechanism of tissue damage during extracorporeal perfusions, myocardial infarction, and shock—a review. *Q J Med* 1983;52:289-296.
62. Knudsen F, Andersen LW. Immunological aspects of cardiopulmonary bypass. *J Cardiothorac Anesth* 1990;4:245-258.
63. Craddock PR, Fehr J, Brigham KL, et al. Complement and leukocyte-mediated pulmonary dysfunction in hemodialysis. *N Engl J Med* 1977;296:769-774.
64. Hammerschmidt DE, Craddock PR, McCullough J, et al. Complement activation and pulmonary leukostasis during nylon fiber filtration leukapheresis. *Blood* 1978;51:721-730.
65. Chenowith DE, Cooper SW, Hugli TE, et al. Complement activation during cardiopulmonary bypass, evidence for generation of C3a and C5a anaphylatoxins. *N Engl J Med* 1981;304:497-503.
66. Tamiya T, Yamasaki M, Maeo Y, et al. Complement activation in cardiopulmonary bypass, with special reference to anaphylatoxin production in membrane and bubble oxygenators. *Ann Thorac Surg* 1988;46:47-57.
67. Cavarocchi NC, Pluth JR, Schaff HV, et al. Complement activation during cardiopulmonary bypass: comparison of bubble and membrane oxygenators. *J Thorac Cardiovasc Surg* 1986;91:252-258.
68. van Oeveren W, Kazatchkine MD, Descaps-Latscha B, et

al. Deleterious effects of cardiopulmonary bypass: a prospective study of bubble versus membrane oxygenation. *J Thorac Cardiovasc Surg* 1985;89:888-899.
69. Riegel W, Spillner G, Schlosser V, et al. Plasma levels of main granulocyte components during cardiopulmonary bypass. *J Thorac Cardiovasc Surg* 1988;95:1014-1019.
70. Howard RJ, Crain C, Franzini DA, et al. Effects of cardiopulmonary bypass on pulmonary leukostasis and complement activation. *Arch Surg* 1988;123:1496-1501.
71. Videm V, Fosse E, Mollnes TE, Carred P, et al. Time for new concepts about measurement of complement activation by cardiopulmonary bypass? *Ann Thorac Surg* 1992;54:725-731.
72. Kirklin JK, Westaby S, Blackstone EH, et al. Complement and the damaging effects of cardiopulmonary bypass. *J Thorac Cardiovasc Surg* 1983;86:845-857.
73. Salama A, Hugo F, Heinrich D, et al. Deposition of terminal C5b-9 complement complexes on erythrocytes and leukocytes during cardiopulmonary bypass. *N Engl J Med* 1988;318:408-414.
74. Mollnes TE, Videm V, Gotze O, et al. Formation of C5a during cardiopulmonary bypass: inhibition by precoating with heparin. *Ann Thorac Surg* 1991;52:92-97.
75. Andersen LW, Baek L, Degn H, et al. Presence of circulating endotoxins during cardiac operations. *J Thorac Cardiovasc Surg* 1987;93:115-119.
76. Rocke DA, Gaffin SL, Wells MT, et al. Endotoxinemia associated with cardiopulmonary bypass. *J Thorac Cardiovasc Surg* 1987;93:832-837.
77. Andersen LW, Jensen TH, Jensen FM, et al. Absorption of lipopolysaccharide from the intestine during aortic cross-clamping in humans. *J Cardiothorac Anesth* 1988;2:861-863.
78. Anderson BO, Brown JM, Bensard DD, et al. Reversible lung neutrophil accumulation can cause injury by elastase-mediated mechanisms. *Surgery* 1990;108:262-268.
79. Worthen GS, Haslett C, Rees AJ, et al. Neutrophil-mediated pulmonary vascular injury. *Am Rev Resp Dis* 1987;136:19-28.
80. Royston D, Fleming JS, Desai JB, et al. Increased production of peroxidation products associated with cardiac operations. *J Thorac Cardiovasc Surg* 1986;91:759-766.
81. Weiss SJ. Tissue destruction by neutrophils. *N Engl J Med* 1989;320:365-376.
82. Weiland JE, Davis B, Holter JF, et al. Lung neutrophils in the adult respiratory distress syndrome. Clinical and pathophysiological significances. *Am Rev Resp Dis* 1986;133:218-225.
83. Faymonville ME, Pincemail J, Duchateau J, et al. Myeloperoxidase and elastase as markers of leukocyte activation during cardiopulmonary bypass in humans. *J Thorac Cardiovasc Surg* 1991;102:309-317.
84. Wachtfogel YT, Kucich U, Greenplate J, et al. Human neutrophil degranulation during extracorporeal circulation. *Blood* 1987;69:324-330.
85. Colman RW. Platelet and neutrophil activation in cardiopulmonary bypass. *Ann Thorac Surg* 1990;49:32-34.
86. Stahl RF, Fisher CA, Kucich U, et al. Effects of simulated extracorporeal circulation on human leukocyte elastase release, superoxide generation, and procoagulant activity. *J Thorac Cardiovasc Surg* 1991;101:230-239.
87. Andersen LW, Baek L, Thomsen BS, et al. Effect of methylprednisolone on endotoxemia and complement activation during cardiac surgery. *J Cardiothorac Anesth* 1989;3:544-549.
88. Hart DHL. Polymorphonuclear leukocyte elastase activity is increased by bacterial lipopolysaccharide; a response inhibited by glucocorticoids. *Blood* 1984;63:421-426.
89. Bonser M, Dave JR, Davies ET, et al. Reduction of complement activation during bypass by prime manipulation. *Ann Thorac Surg* 1990;49:279-283.
90. Videm V, Nillson L, Venge P, et al. Reduced granulocyte activation with a heparin-coated device in an in vitro model of cardiopulmonary bypass. *Artif Organs* 1991;15:90-95.
91. Boroweic J, Thelin S, Bagge L, et al. Heparin-coated circuits reduce activation of granulocytes during cardiopulmonary bypass. *J Thorac Cardiovasc Surg* 1992;104:642-647.
92. Menasche P, Pasquier C, Bellucci S, et al. Deferoxamine reduces neutrophil-mediated free radical production during cardiopulmonary bypass in man. *J Thorac Cardiovasc Surg* 1988;96:582-589.
93. Kuratani T, Matsuda H, Sawa Y, et al. Experimental study in a rabbit model of ischemia-reperfusion lung injury during cardiopulmonary bypass. *J Thorac Cardiovasc Surg* 1992;103:564-568.
94. Bando K, Pillai R, Cameron DE, et al. Leukocyte depletion ameliorates free-radical mediated lung injury following cardiopulmonary bypass. *J Thorac Cardiovasc Surg* 1990;99:873-877.
95. Higgins TL, Yared JP, Paranandi L, et al. Risk factors for respiratory complications after cardiac surgery. *Anesthesiology* 1991;75:A258. Abstract.
96. Huddy SPJ, Joyce WP, Pepper JR. Gastrointestinal complications in 4473 patients who underwent cardiopulmonary bypass surgery. *Br J Surg* 1991;78:293-296.
97. Heikkinen LO, Ala-Kulju KV. Abdominal complications following cardiopulmonary bypass in open-heart surgery. *Scand J Thorac Cardiovasc Surg* 1987;21:1-7.
98. Pinson CW, Alberty RE. General surgical complications after cardiopulmonary bypass surgery. *Am J Surg* 1983;146:133-137.
99. Wallwork J, Davidson KG. The acute abdomen following cardiopulmonary bypass surgery. *Br J Surg* 1980;67:410-412.
100. Hanks JB, Curtis SE, Hanks BB, et al. Gastrointestinal complications after cardiopulmonary bypass. *Surgery* 1982;92:394-400.
101. Welling RE, Rath R, Albers JE, et al. Gastrointestinal complications after cardiac surgery. *Arch Surg* 1986;121:1178-1180.
102. Leitman IM, Paull DE, Barie PS, et al. Intraabdominal complications of cardiopulmonary bypass operations. *Surg Gynecol Obstet* 1987;165:251-254.
103. Moneta GL, Misback GA, Ivey TD. Hypoperfusion as a possible factor in the development of gastrointestinal complications after cardiac surgery. *Am J Surg* 1985;149:648-650.
104. Collins JD, Bassendine MF, Ferner R, et al. Incidence and

prognostic importance of jaundice after cardiopulmonary bypass surgery. *Lancet* 1983;1(8334):1119–1123.
105. Rattner DW, Gu Z-Y, Vlahakes GJ, et al. Hyperamylasemia after cardiac surgery. *Ann Surg* 1989;209:279–283.
106. Kazmierczak SC, Van Lente F. Incidence and source of hyperamylasemia after cardiac surgery. *Clin Chem* 1988;34:916–919.
107. Fiddian-Green RG, Baker S. The predictive value of measurements of pH in the wall of the stomach for complications after cardiac surgery: a comparison with other forms of monitoring. *Crit Care Med* 1987;15:153–156.
108. Andersen LW, Landow L, Baek L, et al. Association between gastric intramucosal pH and splanchnic endotoxin, antibody to endotoxin, and tumor necrosis factor-α concentrations in patients undergoing cardiopulmonary bypass. *Crit Care Med* 1993;21:210–217.
109. Landow L, Phillips DA, Heard SO, et al. Gastric tonometry and venous oximetry in cardiac surgery patients. *Crit Care Med* 1991;19:1226–1233.
110. Karlstad MD, Patteson SK, Guszcza JA, et al. Methylprednisolone does not influence endotoxin translocation during cardiopulmonary bypass. *J Cardiothorac Vasc Anesth* 1993;7:23–27.
111. Hampton WW, Townsend MC, Schirmer WJ, et al. Effective hepatic blood flow during cardiopulmonary bypass. *Arch Surg* 1989;124:458–459.
112. Mori A, Watanabe K, Onoe M, et al. Regional blood flow in the liver, pancreas and kidney during pulsatile and nonpulsatile perfusion under profound hypothermia. *Jpn Circ J* 1988;52:219–227.
113. Taylor KM, Bain WH, Morton JJ. The role of angiotensin II in the development of peripheral vasoconstriction during open heart surgery. *Am Heart J* 1980;100:935–937.
114. Kumon K, Tanaka K, Hirata T, et al. Organ failures due to low cardiac output syndrome following open heart surgery. *Jpn Circ J* 1986;50:329–335.
115. Fernandez-del Castillo C, Harringer W, Warshaw AL, et al. Risk factors for pancreatic cellular injury after cardiopulmonary bypass. *N Engl J Med* 1991;325:382–387.
116. Svensson LG, Decker G, Kinsley RB. A prospective study of hyperamylasemia and pancreatitis after cardiopulmonary bypass. *Ann Thorac Surg* 1985;39:409–411.
117. Reber HA. Acute pancreatitis—another piece of the puzzle? *N Engl J Med* 1991;325:423–425.
118. Murray WR, Mittra S, Mittra D, et al. The amylase-creatinine clearance ratio following cardiopulmonary bypass. *J Thorac Cardiovasc Surg* 1981;82:248–253.
119. Aziz S, Bergdahl L, Baldwin JC, et al. Pancreatitis after cardiac and cardiopulmonary transplantation. *Surgery* 1985;97:653–661.
120. Steed DL, Brown B, Reilly JJ, et al. General surgical complications in heart and heart-lung transplantations. *Surgery* 1985;98:739–745.
121. Porter GA, Kloster FE, Herr RJ, et al. Renal complications associated with valve replacement surgery. *J Thorac Cardiovasc Surg* 1967;53:145–152.
122. Bhat JG, Gluck MC, Lowenstein J, et al. Renal failure after open heart surgery. *Ann Intern Med* 1976;84:677–682.
123. Lange HW, Aeppli DM, Brown DC. Survival of patients with acute renal failure requiring dialysis after open heart surgery: early prognostic indicators. *Am Heart J* 1987;113:1138–1143.
124. Porter GA, Kloster FE, Herr RJ, et al. Relationship between alterations in renal hemodynamics during cardiopulmonary bypass and postoperative renal function. *Circulation* 1966;34:1005–1021.
125. Grismer JT, Levy MJ, Lillehei RC, et al. Renal function in acquired valvular heart disease and effects of extracorporeal circulation. *Surgery* 1964;55:24–41.
126. Lundberg S. Renal function during anaesthesia and open-heart surgery in man. *Acta Anaesth Scand (Suppl)* 1967;27:1–82.
127. Finsterbusch W, Long DM, Sellers RD, et al. Renal arteriography during extracorporeal circulation in dogs, with a preliminary report upon the effects of low molecular weight dextran. *J Thorac Cardiovasc Surg* 1961;41:252–262.
128. Moghissi K, MacLell ES, Munday KA. Changes in renal blood flow and PAH extraction during extracorporeal circulation of short and long duration. *Cardiovasc Res* 1969;3:37–44.
129. German JC, Chalmers GS, Hirai J, et al. Comparison of nonpulsatile and pulsatile extracorporeal circulation on renal tissue perfusion. *Chest* 1972;61:65–69.
130. Philbin DM, Levine FH, Kono K, et al. Attenuation of the stress response to cardiopulmonary bypass by the addition of pulsatile flow. *Circulation* 1981;64:808–812.
131. Watkins L Jr, Lucas SK, Gardner TJ, et al. Angiotensin II levels during cardiopulmonary bypass; a comparison of pulsatile and nonpulsatile flow. *Surg Forum* 1979;30:229–235.
132. Hickey PR, Buckley MJ, Philbin DM. Pulsatile and nonpulsatile cardiopulmonary bypass: review of a counterproductive controversy. *Ann Thorac Surg* 1983;36:720–737.
133. Yeboah ED, Petrie A, Pead JL. Acute renal failure and open heart surgery. *Br Med J* 1972;1:415–418.
134. Yeh TJ, Brackney EL, Hall, et al. Renal complications of open-heart surgery: predisposing factors, prevention, and management. *J Thorac Cardiovasc Surg* 1964;47:79–97.
135. Hilberman M, Myers BD, Carrie BJ, et al. Acute renal failure following cardiac surgery. *J Thorac Cardiovasc Surg* 1979;77:880–888.
136. Abel RM, Buckley MJ, Austen WG, et al. Etiology, incidence, and prognosis of renal failure following cardiac operations: results of a prospective analysis of 500 consecutive patients. *J Thorac Cardiovasc Surg* 1976;71:323–333.
137. McLeish KR, Loft FC, Kleit SA. Factors affecting prognosis in acute renal failure following cardiac operations. *Surg Gynecol Obstet* 1977;145:28–32.
138. Koning HM, Koning AJ, Defauw JJ. Optimal perfusion during extra-corporeal circulation. *Scand J Thorac Cardiovasc Surg* 1987;21:207–213.
139. Lowe MB. Effects of nephrotoxins on ischemia in experimental hemoglobinuria. *J Pathol Bacteriol* 1966;92:319–323.
140. Krian A. Incidence, prevention, and treatment of acute renal failure following cardiopulmonary bypass. *Int Anesthesiol Clin* 1976;14:87–101.
141. Hilberman L, Derby GC, Spencer RJ, et al. Sequential pathophysiological changes characterizing the progression

from renal dysfunction to acute renal failure following cardiac operations. *J Thorac Cardiovasc Surg* 1980;79:838–844.
142. Bourgeois BFD, Donath A, Paunier C, et al. Effects of cardiac surgery on renal function in children. *J Thorac Cardiovasc Surg* 1979;77:283–286.
143. Mazzarella V, Gallucci MT, Tozzo C, et al. Renal function in patients undergoing cardiopulmonary bypass operations. *J Thorac Cardiovasc Surg* 1992;104:1625–1627.
144. Myers BD, Moran MS. Hemodynamically mediated acute renal failure. *N Engl J Med* 1986;314:97–105.
145. Doberneck RC, Reiser MP, Lillehei CW. Acute renal failure after open-heart surgery utilizing extracorporeal circulation and total body perfusion. *J Thorac Cardiovasc Surg* 1962;43:441–452.
146. Corwin HL, Sprague SM, DeLaria GA, et al. Acute renal failure associated with cardiac operations; a case control study. *J Thorac Cardiovasc Surg* 1989;98:1107–1112.
147. Gailiunas P Jr, Chalwa R, Lazarus JM, et al. Acute renal failure following cardiac operations. *J Thorac Cardiovasc Surg* 1980;79:241–243.
148. Johnson PA, Bernard DB, Donohoe JF, et al. Effect of volume expansion on hemodynamics of the hypoperfused rat kidney. *J Clin Invest* 1979;64:550–558.
149. Burke TJ, Cronin RE, Duchin KL, et al. Ischemia and tubule obstruction during acute renal failure in dogs; mannitol in protection. *Am J Physiol* 1980;238:F305–314.
150. Schuster SR, Kakvan M, Vawter GF, et al. An experimental study of the effect of mannitol during cardiopulmonary bypass. *Circulation* 1964;29(suppl):72–76.
151. Kahn DR, Cerny JC, Lee RWS, et al. The effect of dextran and mannitol on renal function during open heart surgery. *Surgery* 1965;57:676–679.
152. Hanley MJ, Davidson K. Prior mannitol and furosemide infusion in a model of ischemic acute renal failure. *Am J Physiol* 1981;241:F556–564.
153. Engelman RM, Gouge TH, Smith SJ, et al. The effect of diuretics on renal hemodynamics during cardiopulmonary bypass. *J Surg Res* 1974;16:268–275.
154. Kron IL, Jodb AW, Van Meter C. Acute renal failure in the cardiovascular surgical patient (current review). *Ann Thorac Surg* 1985;39:590–598.
155. Weinberger HD, Anderson RJ. Prevention of acute renal failure. *J Crit Care* 1991;6:95–101.
156. Leuers PB, Mulder AW, Fiers HA, et al. Acute renal failure after cardiovascular surgery. Current concepts in pathophysiology, prevention, and treatment. *Eur Heart J* 1989;10(suppl H):38–42.

8
The Immunologic System: Perturbations Following Cardiopulmonary Bypass and the Problem of Infection in the Cardiac Surgery Patient

Bradley L. Bufkin, John Parker Gott, Christina T. Mora, and Jerrold H. Levy

Cardiopulmonary bypass (CPB) predisposes cardiac surgical patients to postoperative wound infections[1,2] by altering their immunologic host response and increasing their susceptibility to infection, a primary cause of morbidity and mortality following open-heart surgery. The "cost" of infection after cardiac surgery includes human suffering, hospital confinement, loss of productivity, and mortality. There can be a broad range of infectious complications postoperatively (Table 8.1). Mediastinitis, occurring in 1% to 2% of median sternotomies, has a mortality rate of 60% to 70%.[3] Early and late prosthetic valvular endocarditis are associated with mortality rates of 73% and 45%, respectively,[4,5] and occur in approximately 2% to 3% of valvular replacement procedures. An assessment of hospital stay following coronary artery bypass surgery demonstrated that infectious complications prolonged hospitalization fourfold, with infection representing the most important variable for increased length of stay.[6] A 1990 cost assessment of cardiac surgery patients reported that median sternotomy infections produced a median hospital cost of $58,092 (range $19,966 to $408,632), almost triple the cost of an uncomplicated cardiac procedure.[7]

Infection represents an imbalance between the host immune defense mechanisms and microbiologic challenge. Diminished host-defense responses, secondary to pre-existing conditions and/or CPB, combined with multiple portals of entry for bacterial inoculation, places every cardiac surgical patient at risk for serious infection. An understanding of the immunologic changes associated with CPB and recognition of the factors that increase the risk of postoperative infection can help the physician develop strategies to prevent, or at least attenuate, perioperative infection. Additionally, there are numerous advances on the horizon that offer *future* promise of further control of cardiac surgical infections. This chapter will discuss CPB-induced pathophysiologic changes in the immune response, patient risk factors, and strategies to decrease the problem of infection in cardiac surgery.

TABLE 8.1. Potential infectious complications following cardiac surgery.

Wounds
    Superficial sternal
    Sternal osteomyelitis
    Costochondritis
    Mediastinitis
    Saphenous vein harvest site
Cardiac
    Endocarditis—native or prosthetic valves
Pulmonary
    Pneumonia
    Tracheobronchitis
    Empyema
Genitourinary
    Urinary tract infection
Gastrointestinal
    Esophageal candidiasis
    Acalculous cholecystitis
Bacteremia/septicemia
    Intravascular monitoring lines
    Gut bacterial or fungal translocation

Pathophysiologic Changes in the Immune System and Inflammatory Responses During CPB

Normal Immune System Function

In order to appreciate the effects of CPB on the immune system, and the consequences of activation of both the humoral and the cellular components of this system, a fundamental understanding of normal immune function is required. The immune system provides protection from infection and causes destruction of cells and substances detrimental to the host. Immunologic defense includes *innate* and *adaptive* immunity, which provide immunologic protection via different mechanisms.[8] Each of these systems contains humoral and cellular components that activate, mobilize, and direct the host immune response (Figure 8.1).

Innate immunity is a nonspecific type of immunity that is not dependent on prior exposure to a foreign substance. The humoral components responsible for activation of the innate response include complement and the acute phase reactants that participate in microbe opsonization and cellular death. The complement cascade is a series of circulating proteins, like the coagulation cascade (see Chapter 5), that can be activated to produce inflammation (Figure 8.2).[9] Phagocytic cells provide innate protection by directly killing microbes and infected cells. *Adaptive immunity* is acquired following an antigenic stimulus to the immune system. This system provides "immunologic recall" for a specific stimulus and a faster and more profound response with repeated antigen exposures. Following reexposure, there is activation of both the humoral and the cellular systems, resulting in plasma cell-secreted immunoglobulins and specialized T-lymphocyte production.

Normal Inflammatory Processes

Both the humoral and the cellular components of the immune system participate in the activation, amplification, and propagation of most forms of inflammation. Inflammation is a protective response elicited by injury, destruction of tissues, or microbial invasion that serves to provide host defense responses that include fever, leukocytosis, catabolism of host proteins, and release of cytokines, including interleukin-1 (IL-1), interleukin-6 (IL-6), and tumor necrosis factor.[10] The body recognizes surfaces of bacteria, fungi, viruses, and nonendothelialized extracorporeal circuit components as foreign, thus activating humoral and cellular responses. Inflammation occurs when leukocytes try to defend the host from "foreign invaders."

Immunologically mediated or nonimmune activation of host defense systems proceeds through a series of integrated steps. First, the material is recognized as being foreign by immunoglobulins and/or receptors on T lymphocytes that bind to specific determinants (epitopes), or activation of the coagulation, kallikrein, and complement pathways occurs, causing initiation of contact activation.[11] Binding of these components leads to activation of amplification systems initiating the production of proinflammatory substances. These mediators alter blood flow, increase vascular permeability, augment the adherence of circulating leukocytes to vascular endothelium, promote migration of leukocytes into tissues, and activate leukocytes.[11]

Effects of CPB on the Immune System

Immunologic dysfunction following CPB is secondary to the qualitative and quantitative changes in the humoral and cellular components of both the innate and the adaptive immune systems. However, innate immunity is most affected because of the uncontrolled whole-body inflammatory response induced by CPB. During CPB, artificial surfaces and filters coated with plastics, glass, and metal result in many alterations in structure and function of the blood that passes through the extracorporeal circuit and indirectly into the tissues.[12] Currently used extracorporeal systems can never be considered truly physiologic. When

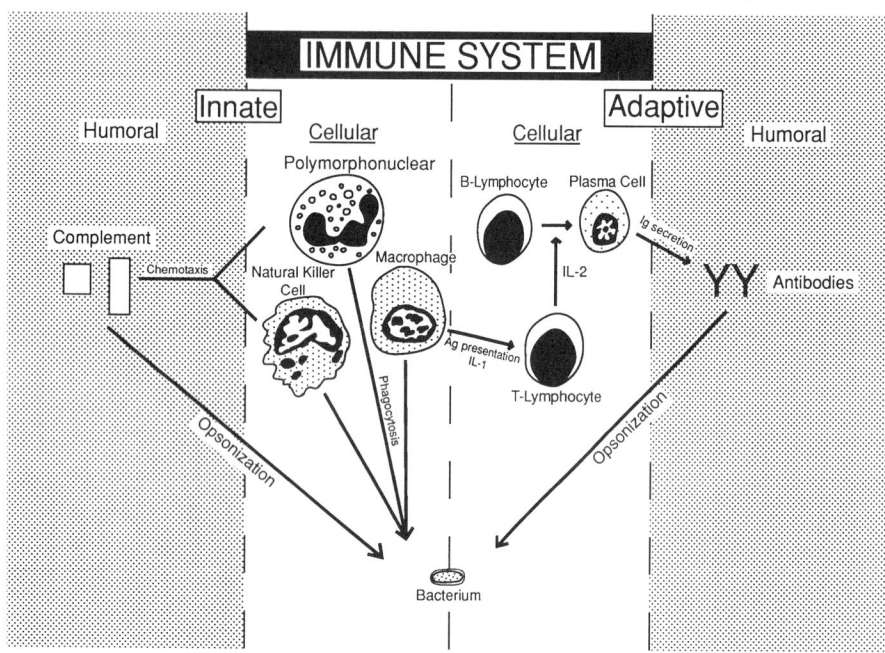

FIGURE 8.1. Components and normal functions of the innate and adaptive arms of the immune system.

FIGURE 8.2. Contact activation of the complement cascade during CPB. Activation of complement occurs primarily through the alternate pathway. (From Ohri SK,[9] by permission of *Perfusion*.)

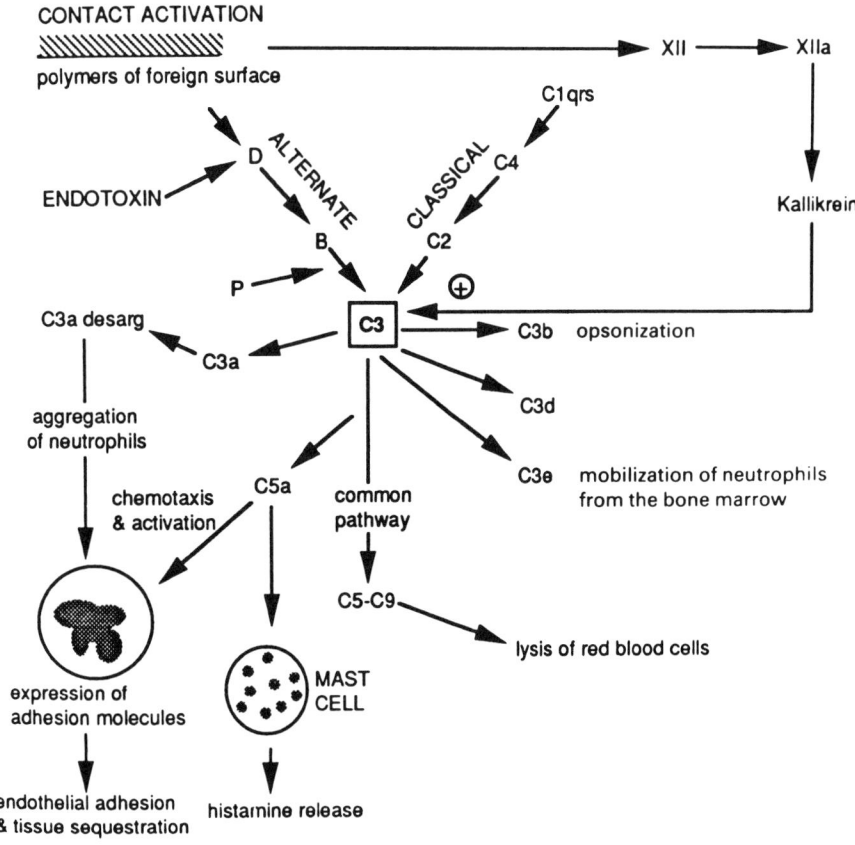

blood first contacts the foreign materials of the extracorporeal circuit, platelets adhere to the surface, and Hageman factor (XII) is activated to initiate clotting[13] (Figure 8.3). (Without the presence of heparin binding to antithrombin III, thrombin would not be inhibited and CPB could not occur.) The humoral cascades of Hageman-factor activation and subsequent activation of kallikrein, the kinin-bradykinin system, and the fibrinolytic and complement cascade are initiated[11] (Table 8.2).

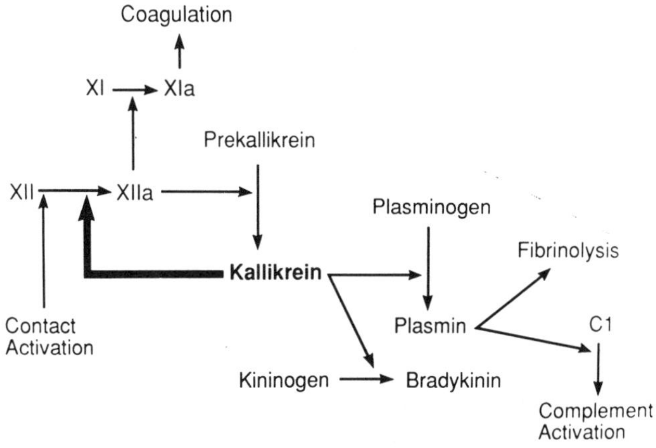

Complement

The complement system may be activated via classical (antibody required) or alternate (independent of antibody) pathways (Figure 8.2). During CPB, activation is primarily through the alternate pathway.[11] Hammerschmidt[14] described pulmonary sequestration of neutrophils and monocytes during CPB; this was direct evidence for complement activation. Chenoweth[15] subsequently demonstrated that C3a appears in the plasma at the onset of CPB and increases until the termination of extracorporeal support. C5a, which is avidly bound to polymorphonuclear leukocytes and platelets, could not be detected. However, neutrophil trapping in the pulmonary circula-

FIGURE 8.3. Relationship between contact activation of Hageman factor (XII) and activation of coagulation, kinin, fibrinolytic, and complement systems. (From Levy JH,[11] by permission of Butterworth-Heinemann.)

TABLE 8.2. Inflammatory cascades activated during CPB.

Coagulation
Fibrinolysis
Complement
Kallikrein-kinin

tion was confirmed by transpulmonary white cell gradients.[15]

Surface contact activation leads to direct activation of the C3 component with production of C3a and C3b. C3b provides further complement activation while covalently bound to foreign surfaces propagating activation via the alternate pathway. Further complement activation via the classical pathway occurs following CPB, with protamine administration.[11] CPB-induced complement activation leads to a significant reduction in serum complement levels.[16,17] Complement depletion reduces the effectiveness of opsonization of bacterial contaminants and disables elimination of foreign substances. Lower values of serum bactericidal activity are displayed following bypass, as compared with baseline, and are directly related to depletion of complement.[18] Widespread complement activation also interferes directly with the function of neutrophils. Inactivation of C3a is associated with expression of C3b receptors by neutrophils.[19] Neutrophil aggregates form with the expression of C3b receptors, rendering this type of white cell ineffective for phagocytosis. Coincidental expression of the C3i receptor produces neutrophil degranulation, increasing serum proteolytic activity.[20,21] Pulmonary sequestration of neutrophil aggregates and degranulation within the pulmonary circulation produce post-CPB pulmonary injury.[22] This topic is discussed in Chapter 7.

Neutrophils

Innate immunity is dependent on the nonspecific function of polymorphonuclear leukocytes for elimination of microbials. Neutrophil immune function requires multiple coordinated cellular functions, including chemotaxis, phagocytosis, and intracellular digestion, for elimination of microbes. CPB disrupts these normal neutrophil antimicrobial functions. Chemotaxis, largely directed by C3a and C5a, is depressed following CPB and remains so for 7 days postoperatively, with longer pump runs producing more profound antichemotactic effects.[23,24] High levels of C5a during CPB attenuate cell chemotaxis by causing internalization of neutrophil C5a receptors, eliminating responsiveness to C5a signaling.[15] Decreased white-cell phagocytic activity is demonstrated experimentally by defective clearance of parenterally administered bacteria following CPB.[25] Intracellular digestion of ingested microbes is diminished by nonspecific release of digestive enzymes (N-acetyl-β-glucosaminidase, β-glucuronidase; lactoferrin, neutrophil elastase, and myeloperoxidase) and oxidative end products secondary to the CPB-induced inflammatory response.[26-33] The premature release of antimicrobial enzymes and other injurious agents (oxygen free radicals) not only reduces antimicrobial effectiveness but produces tissue damage by these mediators of tissue injury.

Macrophages

Macrophages are important components of the innate immune system because they are responsible for consumption of opsonized material and help direct cell-mediated immunity. Macrophages present antigen with major histocompatibility complex class II molecules to T lymphocytes and release IL-1, which activates the T lymphocytes and stimulates the adaptive immune system. Few studies have assessed the effects of CPB on macrophage function, but depression of macrophage bacterial clearance has been noted.[34] Presumably, there is also alteration of the antigen-presenting function that would impair activation of cell-mediated immunity.

Interleukins

IL-1 is a critical mediator of the inflammatory reaction associated with CPB that induces a wide range of clinical and biologic effects.[10] The term *interleukin* was coined for a group of cytokines that represent a means of communication between leukocytes (interleukin). Cytokines are proteinaceous secretory products of various cells that predominantly exert their effect on surrounding cells.[10] The interleukin family of cytokines has been rapidly expanding in number due to the tremendous amount of research on gene cloning. Evidence suggests that cytokines have a pivotal role in the genesis of a whole host of inflammatory responses.

Maximum generation of IL-1 occurs 24 hours after CPB at the same time as increases in body temperature.[35] The peak in IL-1 production is followed 20 hours later by the peak in complement activation, as assessed by C3a and C5a liberation. In addition to the complement peptides, endotoxins and their polysaccharide moieties can induce monocytes to produce IL-1. IL-1 directly mediates multiple aspects of the host inflammatory response, including fever synthesis of acute phase proteins, release of growth factors and immunoregulatory cytokines, changes in endothelial function, increases in capillary permeability, and decreases in vascular resistance.[10,35] IL-1 stimulates nitric oxide (endothelium-derived relaxing factor) in vascular endothelium, which may explain the vasodilation seen clinically during CPB.[36]

IL-6 and α-melanocyte-stimulating hormone (α-MSH) are also important modulators of the immunologic response to tissue injury and antigenic challenge. Whitten et al[37] measured serial changes in the plasma concentrations of these two peptides in 12 patients undergoing heart transplantation. Tissue concentrations of IL-6 in atrial samples from both donor and recipient hearts were also compared. Plasma IL-6 concentration remained stable prior to CPB, initially decreased with onset of CPB, and then increased fourfold over control values at the end of CPB. Plasma IL-6 remained elevated for at least 60 minutes after CPB, and then it returned to control values by 24 hours postoperatively. In contrast to IL-6, plasma α-MSH never increased above control values. These results suggest that CPB and/or perfusion of the newly implanted heart caused a marked increase in IL-6. The return of IL-6 to control values by 24 hours may have been due to immunosuppression, since other studies in surgical patients have shown more persistent postoperative elevations. The absence of a significant change in α-MSH suggests that there is no interaction between these two immunologic modulators under the conditions of Whitten et al's study.

Immunoglobulins and B Lymphocytes

Immunoglobulins (proteins secreted by plasma cells as part of the adaptive immune response) are important for opsonization of microbes and direction of both innate and adaptive immunity. CPB results in decreased immunoglobulin levels and impaired immunoglobulin microbial opsonization through denaturation of the large immunoglobulin moieties, which occurs when these proteins are exposed to the CPB circuit.[38,39] Impaired production of IL-2, a T-lymphocyte product required for B-lymphocyte transformation, decreases the number of B lymphocytes transformed to immunoglobulin-secreting plasma cells.[40] Plasma cells are dysfunctional for several days following bypass, with depressed immunoglobulin production.[41]

T Lymphocytes

T lymphocytes have an important role in both cell-mediated immunity and overall immunocompetence. Specialization of T lymphocytes into T-helper and T-suppressor cells, which are distinguished by specific surface receptors CD4 and CD8, respectively, permits precise control of cell-mediated immunity. T-cell lymphopenia following CPB is largely related to a decline in T-helper cells, with depression of the CD4/CD8 ratio, following CPB. (This change is similar to the ratio observed in the acquired immune deficiency syndrome.[42-44]) As described above, the reduced ability of T lymphocytes to generate IL-2 following CPB results in depressed B-lymphocyte transformation.[45,46] IL-2 is also an important activator of specialized cytotoxic T lymphocytes and natural killer cells, both of which are important in control of viral infections and neoplasia surveillance.[47-49]

Summary

Cardiac surgery and CPB activate a complex network of inflammatory cascades that greatly attenuate normal immune processes (Figure 8.4). Complement and immunoglobulin depletion, and neutrophil, macrophage, and lymphocyte dysfunction, occur following CPB. Propensity for infection is a consequence of these processes, as it creates an imbalance between host defense and inevitable microbiologic contamination in the surgical setting. The problem of microbiologic contamination and methods of attenuating the effects of CPB on the immune system are discussed below.

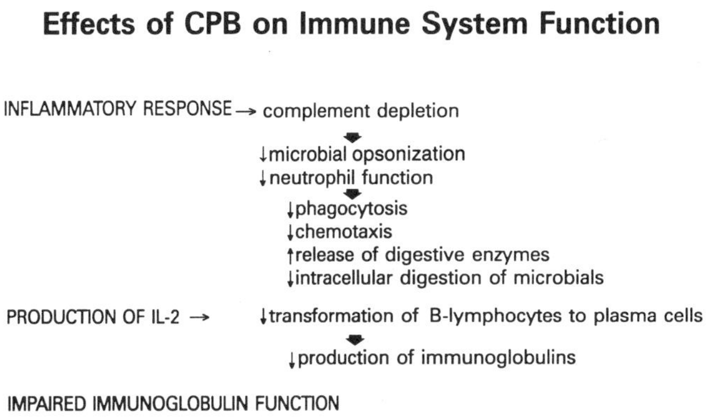

Effects of CPB on Immune System Function

INFLAMMATORY RESPONSE → complement depletion
↓ microbial opsonization
↓ neutrophil function
↓ phagocytosis
↓ chemotaxis
↑ release of digestive enzymes
↓ intracellular digestion of microbials

PRODUCTION OF IL-2 → ↓ transformation of B-lymphocytes to plasma cells
↓ production of immunoglobulins

IMPAIRED IMMUNOGLOBULIN FUNCTION

FIGURE 8.4. Effects of CPB on immune function.

Infection in the Cardiac Surgery Patient: Risk Factors and Prevention

Microbiologic Contamination in Cardiac Surgery

Infection occurs *only* if there is a microbial inoculum. The operating room environment, operating room personnel, patient, and equipment represent sources of microbiologic contamination. Inappropriate ventilation and inadequate filtration systems may increase the number of airborne organisms.[50] Inattention to disinfection of floors, walls, and ceilings can lead to contamination of operating room surfaces by bacterial or spore-forming organisms. Airborne bacteria are an important consideration in longer operations, as 30,000 to 40,000 organisms settle on a 3-m^2 sterile field every hour.[51] In an appropriately ventilated and filtered operating room, airborne bacteria come predominantly from operating room personnel.[52] Contamination of the CPB circuit by bacteria present in ambient air occurs in up to 75% of cases.[52-54] In studies assessing which portals are important CPB-circuit entry points for bacterial pathogens, the highest incidence of positive cultures was from the cardiotomy suction system.[52,55,56] Cardiotomy suction units entrain bacteria that have contaminated the surgical field at the blood-air interface, thus allowing them entrance into the CPB circuit. Intraoperative monitoring devices, such as intravascular catheters and pressure monitoring systems, also provide sources of bacterial contamination.[57,58] Inhalation circuits can be contaminated and produce pulmonary infection. Cell-saver contamination rates of 21% have been reported with cardiac surgical cases.[59]

Despite these multiple sources of bacterial contamination, the patient remains the most frequent source of bacteria that are recovered from postoperative infections following cardiac surgery.[60,61] In epidemiologic studies examining phage types of staphylococci from different sources—operating room personnel, the patient, and organisms isolated from postoperative wound infections—the patient has been identified as the predominant source of organisms producing infection. Therefore, decreasing patient microbial colonization is important for prevention of infection.

Preoperative Considerations

A careful preoperative evaluation of the patient's respiratory system, dentition, urinary tract, and skin, as well as laboratory and radiographic studies, minimizes the risk of an unidentified, occult infection. Identification of risk factors (Table 8.3)[62-64] permits the institution of measures (intensified pulmonary education and physiotherapy for bronchitis, smoking cessation, treatment of urinary tract infection, control of diabetes mellitus, and taper from steroids) that will decrease the likelihood of postoperative infection. Periodontal disease or dental caries suggests the need for oral radiography and a consultation with an oral surgeon, particularly for valvular surgery patients. Brief preoperative hospital stays are associated with less infection, which may be related to changes in skin colonization.[63]

Appropriate skin preparation to decrease skin colonization includes chlorhexidine shower the evening prior to and the morning of the operation. Shaving the evening before an operation is associated with an increased incidence of postoperative wound infection, presumably secondary to contamination of razor abrasions. Hair removal should be postponed until immediately before surgical scrub and preparation of the operative site.[64,66] Mechanical cleansing by vigorous scrubbing with antiseptic soap, followed by the application of antiseptic solution, is appropriate for skin preparation.[67,68] Iodophor agents are the traditional and proven antiseptics for operative site preparation.

TABLE 8.3. Patient factors that increase the risk of infection following cardiac surgery.[62-64]

Occult infection
Chronic obstructive pulmonary disease
Chronic bronchitis
Diabetes mellitus
Obesity
Malnutrition
Chronic corticosteroid therapy
Blood transfusions

Prophylactic antimicrobials are important tools for prevention of infection and are considered in detail below. Inadvertent omission of antimicrobial drugs or mistimed, inappropriate, or incorrect antimicrobial drug dosage may lead to inadequate levels of antimicrobial drugs in the tissues at the time of operation and thus increase the rate of perioperative infection.[69,70] Bacterial contamination of intravascular monitoring lines can be prevented by using meticulous sterile technique. The use of an iodophor-impregnated sterile film during pulmonary artery catheter placement eliminates bacterial contamination of sterile gloves.[71] Methodical and careful preparation of the patient before cardiac surgery with CPB will decrease the problem of perioperative infection.

Intraoperative Considerations

Coordination of strict aseptic techniques during the operation is the surgeon's responsibility and is a critical step in reducing infection risk. Strict precautions must be taken to avoid airborne microbial contamination of the wound, as well as that from direct contact. Cardiac surgical procedures involving CPB require a large sedimentation area with a long sedimentation period; therefore, airborne contamination must be minimized by limiting operating room traffic, thus decreasing outside contamination and the stirring up of airborne bacteria and particles. Specially designed horizontal ventilation systems with high-efficiency particulate filters have been successfully employed to diminish airborne contamination and reduce infection in major orthopedic prosthetic joint replacement surgeries. These ventilation systems have not been widely used during cardiac surgery (presumably due to cost), but are reported to be effective as part of an overall plan of infection prevention in cardiac surgery suites.[72]

An expeditious, technically precise operation, with efficient use of CPB time, is paramount for infection risk reduction. Transfusion of blood products and reentry to stop bleeding are associated with increased infection rates.[62,63,73] Median sternotomy incisions must be closed with orthopedic surgical principles of fracture fixation and plastic surgical principles of soft-tissue management.[74] Precise control of sternal bleeding is necessary to avoid devascularization of the sternum. Electrocautery should be used conservatively over the sternal wound in order to preserve the sternal periosteum and thus avoid devascularization of the bone. Bone wax should be regarded as an undesirable foreign body. Bone wax application can cause direct contamination of the sternum from glove perforation by bone spicules.

Because the internal mammary artery (IMA) is the artery supplying the sternum, some have proposed that the use of bilateral IMAs will result in an avascular sternum and an increased risk of wound infection.[75,76] However, a study by He and colleagues[77] that compared 199 patients

TABLE 8.4. Potential strategies and treatments to attenuate the inflammatory response to CPB.

Use of heparin-coated bypass circuit
Use of membrane (vs bubble) oxygenators
? Aprotinin
? Up-regulation of immune system
    Erythropoietin
    Thyroprotein

who underwent bilateral IMA grafting to patients having saphenous vein or unilateral IMA grafts reported that bilateral IMA grafts did not increase the risk of postoperative wound infection. Sternal infection occurred in 2.5% (5/199) of bilateral IMA graft patients and in 1.32% (13/166) and 1.19% (20/3359) of patients undergoing saphenous vein or unilateral IMA grafting, respectively ($p = 0.27$). Obesity was found to be the only factor increasing the risk of postoperative wound infection after bilateral IMA grafting.

Postoperative Considerations

Careful attention to aseptic technique during postoperative care diminishes the risk of nosocomial infections. Scrupulous handwashing between patient encounters and aseptic wound, pulmonary, and genitourinary care will diminish cross-contamination. Prompt removal of endotracheal tubes, urethral catheters, chest tubes, intravascular catheters, and temporary pacing wires will eliminate portals of entry. These fundamental measures should be combined with a timely transfer from the intensive care unit, as prolonged intensive care unit stay is associated with a greater risk of infection.[73]

Attenuating the Effects of CPB on the Immune System

Depletion of complement and immunoglobulins, and activation of white cells (neutrophils, macrophages, and lymphocytes) during CPB, greatly compromise immune function after cardiac surgery and CPB. Techniques to *prevent* the inflammatory response or *enhance* immunologic function might attenuate the compromising effects of CPB on the immune system and therefore decrease the problem of infection following cardiac surgery and CPB.

Measures to prevent the immunologic consequences of CPB include modification of the CPB circuit and the use of antiinflammatory drugs (Table 8.4). Membrane oxygenators constructed with polypropylene materials cause less activation of leukocytes, platelets, and complement than do bubble oxygenators.[78,79] The use of heparin-coated bypass circuits reduces the activation of blood components and consumption of complement.[80,81] Aprotinin may prevent the consumption of serologic proteins by inhibiting both plasmin and kallikrein activity. This drug, which has already been shown to reduce blood transfusion requirements, may prove to be important in preventing CPB-related immunodepression through its antiinflammatory action.[11]

Pharmacologic treatments to enhance immunologic defenses following the insult of CPB are under investigation. For example, hematogenous growth factors may enhance immune function. Erythropoietin, when administered to increase red cell mass, improves the immunologic function in the early postoperative period.[82] Erythropoietin-treated individuals, compared with controls, have higher levels of total T lymphocytes and T-helper cells. In vitro production of IL-2 is significantly higher in the first postoperative week following erythropoietin administration, suggesting improved immunologic function. Administration of a commercially available leukocyte-stimulating factor, thyroprotein (TP_5) (a pentapeptide similar to thymopoietin, a thymus hormone) also enhances immune system function.[83] TP_5 improves delayed hypersensitivity skin responses in patients undergoing CPB and the in vitro lymphocyte proliferation response to mitogen, and increases in vitro IL-2 synthesis. Although this pharmacotherapy holds promise for the future, trials are necessary to establish the usefulness of these drugs in cardiac surgery patients. Methods to decrease the risk of infection are listed in Table 8.5

Antimicrobial Prophylaxis

Early studies by Burke[84] provide the rationale for antimicrobial prophylaxis. He demonstrated that antimicrobials administered up to 4 hours before bacterial inoculation of abdominal wounds in guinea pigs helped prevent subsequent wound infection, whereas late drug administration had no beneficial effect.

TABLE 8.5. Methods to decrease the incidence of postoperative infection in the cardiac surgery patient.

Preoperative period
    Control occult infection (bronchitis, dental caries, urinary tract infection)
    Treat diabetes mellitus
    Taper steroids
    Administer appropriate antibiotics
    Prepare skin
Intraoperative period[a]
    Strict aseptic technique
    Efficient use of operative time
Postoperative period
    Aseptic techniques
    Prompt removal of indwelling catheters and tubes
    Timely transfer from intensive care unit

[a]Methods to attenuate the effects of CPB on immune function are listed in Table 8.4.

Placebo-controlled studies in coronary bypass procedures have established the benefit of antimicrobial prophylaxis.[69,85,86] Absolute benefit in prosthetic valvular surgery has not been proven in controlled clinical studies, but is presumed.[87] The increased risk of infection with placement of a foreign material, and the devastating consequences of prosthetic valvular endocarditis, provide the rationale for antimicrobial prophylaxis during valvular replacement. The morbidity and mortality of postsurgical infection has resulted in routine use of antimicrobial prophylaxis for cardiac operations requiring CPB.

Antimicrobial Drugs

The type of bacteria responsible for postoperative infections following cardiac surgery dictates the choice of antimicrobial agents to be used for prophylaxis. *Staphylococcus aureus* and *S. epidermidis* are responsible for the majority of cases of early prosthetic valvular endocarditis and mediastinitis.[60,88] The number of postoperative wound infections caused by gram negative bacilli—the second most frequent type of infection in valvular endocarditis and mediastinal wound infections—is increasing in coronary artery bypass patients.[60,89,90] Several reports document the importance of using broad-spectrum antimicrobials in cardiac surgery.

Although many investigators have assessed the effectiveness of different antibiotics in cardiothoracic surgery, most studies have included a limited number of patients. However, Kreter and Woods[86] recently reported their metanalysis of studies of antimicrobial prophylaxis in cardiac surgery during the last 30 years. This study demonstrated that the use of antistaphylococcal penicillins or first-generation cephalosporins decreased wound infection rates by fivefold compared to placebo. Additionally, they reported that the second-generation cephalosporins cefamandole and cefuroxime were associated with reduced wound infection when compared with cefazolin.

Presently, second-generation cephalosporins are considered the most appropriate antimicrobial prophylactic drugs for cardiac surgery. If a patient has a hypersensitivity to penicillin or cephalosporin, vancomycin, with or without an additional drug to cover gram-negative pathogens, is recommended for antibiotic prophylaxis. It is likely that the prophylactic drug of choice will change through the years as new drugs become available and our knowledge of microbiology changes, but adherence to the principles of appropriate drug administration (timing and dose) with appropriate bacterial coverage will remain.

Timing and Duration of Administration of Antimicrobial Prophylaxis

Successful antimicrobial prophylaxis requires correctly timed preoperative drug administration to ensure effective serum and tissue concentrations of the drug before the almost inevitable bacterial inoculation.[84] (The effect of CPB on antibiotic pharmacokinetics and pharmacodynamics is discussed in detail in Chapter 4).

A 48-hour period of antimicrobial administration is usually sufficient coverage. A prospective, double-blind study comparing infection rates in 200 patients undergoing 2- or 6-day courses of cephalothin administration showed no benefit of extended antimicrobial administration.[91] Conte et al[92] compared a single-dose preoperative cephalothin treatment with a regimen that included 5 days of antibiotic therapy. This study demonstrated no significant difference in infection rates between the two groups. Because of the risk of contamination in the immediate postoperative period and the temporary immune system dysfunction induced by CPB, a 48-hour course of antibiotics is a prudent perioperative treatment regimen. During this time, the endotracheal tube, chest tubes, urethral catheter, and monitoring lines are removed, diminishing the number of portals of entry and the risk of contamination. In addition, the immunologic response begins to recover from the effects of CPB, thus improving the host defense.

Prolonged administration of antimicrobials may alter normal bacterial flora and promote the growth of resistant organisms in the host. Injudicious use of antimicrobials may also alter the status of nosocomial contaminants, generating bacteria resistant to available broad-spectrum antibiotics. Antimicrobial administration initiated immediately before surgery and continued for approximately 48 hours postoperatively decreases the risk of postoperative infection and minimizes the impact of broad-spectrum drugs on the host and hospital flora.

Human Immunodeficiency Virus and CPB

The increasing prevalence of human immunodeficiency virus (HIV) infection has resulted in cardiac surgery patients who are HIV infected. The progression of HIV infection to acquired immune deficiency syndrome (AIDS) is 22% at 3 years; serologic markers predictive of progression are available.[93,94] A weighted decision for operation in these patients, based on predicted AIDS-free longevity and prognosis without surgical intervention, selects appropriate patients for operation. The immunologic effects of CPB represent a theoretical concern in individuals with preexisting immunologic compromise. The few reported series do not indicate progression of the AIDS disease state or high rates of postoperative opportunistic infection in these individuals.[95-97] Limited information regarding these circumstances is available at present, and further evaluation is necessary to establish the risk of CPB in these patients. At present, if cardiac surgery is indicated for a patient seropositive for HIV, the operation should be conducted similar to that on a seronegative patient, except for appropriate exposure precautions (double gloves, eyeglasses, impermeable gowns, careful handling of sharp instruments, universal precautions). As of 1993, there have been no reports of transmission of the virus from the patient to the cardiac surgical team.

Summary

CPB-assisted cardiac surgery produces a unique microbiologic challenge to patients. CPB creates multiple portals of entry for environmental microbes, while impairing the host defense system by injuring cellular and humoral components necessary for appropriate immunologic response to bacterial contamination. These factors predispose patients to infection and are amenable to efforts to alter risk. Elimination of preoperative infection, use of strict sterile technique intraoperatively, and aseptic postoperative care all help to diminish patient contamination. Reinforcement of host defense mechanisms with perioperative antimicrobial prophylaxis is an important weapon in the cardiac surgeon's armamentarium. Cephalosporins with half-lives greater than 1 hour, administered immediately prior to operation, provide adequate serum antibacterial concentrations throughout most operations. Short-term prophylaxis is all that is necessary for effective prevention. At present, a knowledge of the host defense alteration by CPB and preoperative, intraoperative, and postoperative strategies for infection prevention, combined with appropriate application of antimicrobial prophylaxis, will minimize the risk of infection following bypass.

In the future, preventing perioperative infection following CPB will focus on technological alterations to minimize deleterious effects. New biocompatible membrane oxygenators and heparin-coated bypass circuits represent early attempts at modifying the host defense alterations. Early evaluation suggests that these adjuncts decrease complement activation during bypass, lessening end-organ complement-mediated injury, while preserving the humoral and cellular elements of host response to microbiologic challenge. Immunologic enhancement via cellular stimulation factors may prove to be valuable postoperatively to bolster host defense mechanisms. Modulation of the immune response to CPB, combined with presently applied preventive measures, should lead to further reduction of cardiac surgical infections.

References

1. Kittle CF, Reed WA. Antibiotics and extracorporeal circulation. *J Thorac Cardiovasc Surg* 1961;41:34-48.
2. Lord JW, Imparato AM, Hackel A, et al. Endocarditis complicating open-heart surgery. *Circulation* 1961;23:489-497.
3. Cheung EH, Craver JM, Jones EL, et al. Mediastinitis after cardiac valve operations. Impact upon survival. *J Thorac Cardiovasc Surg* 1985;90:517-522.
4. Watanakunakorn C. Prosthetic valve infective endocarditis. *Prog Cardiovasc Dis* 1979;22:181-192.
5. Clark RE, Amos WC, Higgins V, et al. Infection control in cardiac surgery. *Surgery* 1976;79:89-96.
6. Weintraub WS, Jones EL, Craver J, et al. Determinants of prolonged length of hospital stay after coronary bypass surgery. *Circulation* 1989;80:276-284.
7. Loop FD, Lytle BW, Cosgrove DM, et al. Sternal wound complications after isolated coronary artery bypass grafting: early and late mortality, morbidity, and cost of care. *Ann Thorac Surg* 1990;49:179-186.
8. Paul WE. The immune system: an introduction. In: Paul WE, ed. *Fundamental Immunology*. New York: Raven Press, 1989:3-19.
9. Ohri SK. The effects of cardiopulmonary bypass on the immune system. *Perfusion* 1993;8:121-137.
10. Stevenson GW, Hall SC, Rudnick S, et al. The effect of anesthetic agents on the human immune response. *Anesthesiology* 1990;72:542-552.
11. Levy JH. *Anaphylatic Reactions in Anesthesia and Intensive Care*. 2nd ed. Boston: Butterworth-Heinemann; 1992.
12. Kirklin JK. Prospects for understanding and eliminating the deleterious effects of cardiopulmonary bypass. *Ann Thorac Surg* 1991;51:529-531.
13. Westaby S. Organ dysfunction after cardiopulmonary bypass. A systemic inflammatory reaction initiated by the extracorporeal circuit. *Int Care Med* 1987;13:89-95.
14. Hammerschmidt DE, Stroncek DF, Bowers TK, et al. Complement activation and neutropenia occurring during cardiopulmonary bypass. *J Thorac Cardiovasc Surg* 1981;81:370-377.
15. Chenoweth DE, Cooper SW, Hughi TE, et al. Complement activation during cardiopulmonary bypass; evidence for generation of C3a and C5a anaphylatoxins. *N Engl J Med* 1981;304:497-503.
16. Collett B, Alhaq A, Abdullah NG, et al. Pathways to complement activation during cardiopulmonary bypass. *Br Med J* 1984;289:1251-1254.
17. Parker DJ, Cantrell JW, Karp RB, et al. Changes in serum complement and immunoglobulins following cardiopulmonary bypass. *Surgery* 1972;71:824-827.
18. Hairston P, Manos JP, Braber CD, et al. Depression of immunologic surveillance by pump-oxygenation perfusion. *J Surg Res* 1969;9:587-593.
19. Moore FD, Warner KG, Assousa S, et al. The effects of complement activation during cardiopulmonary bypass. *Ann Surg* 1988;208:95-103.
20. Todd RF III, Arnaout MA, Rosen RE, et al. Subcellular localisation of the large subunit of Mol, a surface of glycoprotein associated with neutrophil adhesion. *J Clin Invest* 1984;74:1280-1290.
21. O'Shea JJ, Brown EJ, Seligmann BE, et al. Evidence for distinct intracellular pools of receptors for C3b and C3bi in human neutrophils. *J Immunol* 1985;134:2580-2587.
22. Cavarocchi NC, Pluth JR, Schaff HV, et al. Complement activation during cardiopulmonary bypass. *J Thorac Cardiovasc Surg* 1986;91:252-258.
23. Bubeuik O, Meakins JL. Neutrophil chemotaxis in surgical patients: effect of cardiopulmonary bypass. *Surg Forum* 1976;27:267-269.

24. Mayer JE, McCullough J, Weiblen BJ, et al. Effects of cardiopulmonary bypass on neutrophil chemotaxis. *Surg Forum* 1976;27:285-287.
25. Subramanian VA, Gay WA, Dineen PAP. Effect of cardiopulmonary bypass on in vivo clearance of live *Klebsiella* aerogens. *Surg Forum* 1977;28:255-256.
26. Masson PL, Herremans JF, Schonne EJ. Lactoferrin, an iron-binding protein in neutrophil leukocytes. *J Exp Med* 1969;130:643-658.
27. Bos A, Wever R, Roos D. Characterization and quantification of the peroxidase in human monocytes. *Biochem Biophys Acta* 1978;525:37-44.
28. Baehner RL, Johnston RB Jr. Monocyte function in children with neutropenia and chronic infections. *Blood* 1972;40:31-41.
29. Neumann S, Henrich N, Gunzer G, et al. Enzyme-linked immunoassay for human granulocyte elastase in complex with α_1-proteinase inhibitor. In: Horl WH, Heidland A, eds. *Protease, Potential Role in Health and Disease*. New York: Plenum Press, 1984:379-390.
30. Deby-DuPont G, Pincemail J, Thirion A, et al. A radioimmunoassay for polymorphonuclear leukocytes in myeloperoxidase: preliminary results. *Arch Int Physiol Biochem* 1987;95:59.
31. Bakkenist ARJ, Wever R, Vulsma T, et al. Isolation procedure and some properties of myeloperoxidase from human leukocytes. *Biochem Biophys Acta* 1978;524:45-54.
32. Deby-DuPont G, Pincemail J, Reuter AM. Iodination of polymorphonuclear leucocyte myeloperoxidase. *Arch Int Physiol Biochem* 1988;96:B25.
33. Wood WG, Stella G, Muller OA, et al. A rapid and specific method for separation of bound and free antigen in radioimmunoassay systems. *J Clin Chem Clin Biochem* 1979;17:111-114.
34. Benacerraf B, Sebestyen MM, Schlossman JA. A quantitative study of the kinetics of blood clearance of P32 labelled *Escherichia coli* and staphylococci by the reticuloendothelial system. *J Exp Med* 1959;110:27-48.
35. Haeffner-Cavaillon N, Roussellier N, Ponzio O, et al. Induction of interleukin-1 production in patients undergoing cardiopulmonary bypass. *J Thorac Cardiovasc Surg* 1989;98:1100-1106.
36. Kilbourn RG, Belloni P. Endothelial cell production of nitrogen oxides with response to interferon in combination with tumor necrosis factor, interleukin-1, or endotoxin. *J Nat Cancer Inst* 1990;82:772-776.
37. Whitten CW, Latson TW, Allison PM, et al. Does aprotinin inhibit cardiopulmonary bypass-induced inflammation. *Anesthesiology* 1992;77:A266.
38. Hariston P, Manos JP, Gruber CD, et al. Depression of immunologic surveillance by pump-oxygenation perfusion. *J Surg Res* 1969;9:587-593.
39. van Oeveren W, Kazatchkine MD, Descamps-Latscha B, et al. Deleterious effects of cardiopulmonary bypass: a prospective study of bubble versus membrane oxygenation. *J Thorac Cardiovasc Surg* 1985;89:888-899.
40. Hisatomi K, Isamura T, Kawara T, et al. Changes in lymphocyte subsets, mitogen responsiveness and interleukin-2 production after cardiac operations. *J Thorac Cardiovasc Surg* 1989;98:580-591.
41. Eskola J, Salo M, Viljanen MK, et al. Impaired B lymphocyte function during open heart surgery. *Br J Anaesth* 1984;56:333-337.
42. Brody JI, Pickering NJ, Fink GB, et al. Altered lymphocyte subsets during cardiopulmonary bypass. *Am J Clin Pathol* 1987;87:626-628.
43. Pollock R, Ames F, Rubio P, et al. Protracted severe immune dysregulation induced by cardiopulmonary bypass; a predisposing etiologic factor in blood transfusion-related AIDS. *J Clin Lab Immunol* 1987;22:1-5.
44. Nguyen DM, Mulder DS, Shennib H. Effect of cardiopulmonary bypass on circulating lymphocyte function. *Ann Thorac Surg* 1992;53:611-616.
45. Ide H, Matsumoto H, Takayama T, et al. The effect of interleukin-2 and plasma factors in the impaired lymphocyte function after cardiopulmonary bypass. *Eur Surg Res* 1988;20:29-30.
46. Ide H, Kakiuchi T, Ino T, et al. The role of interleukin-2 in the impaired lymphocyte function after open heart surgery. *J Jpn Assoc Thorac Surg* 1989;37:1526-1531.
47. Suzuki R, Hand K, Itoh K, et al. Natural killer (NK) cells as a responder to interleukin-2 (IL-2). I Proliferative response and establishment of cloned cells. *J Immunol* 1983;130:981-987.
48. Palacios R. Mechanisms of T-cell activation; role and functional relationship of HLA-DR antigens and interleukins. *Immunol Rev* 1982;63:73-110.
49. Pauly JL, Russel CW, Planusek JA, et al. Studies of cultured human T lymphocytes. I. Production of the T cell growth promoting lymphokine interleukin-2. *J Immunol Methods* 1982;50:173-178.
50. Verkkala K, Makela P, Ojajarvi J, et al. Air contamination in open heart surgery with disposable coveralls, gowns, and drapes. *Ann Thorac Surg* 1990;50:757-761.
51. Sompolinsky D, Hermann Z, Oeding P, et al. A series of postoperative infections. *J Infect Dis* 1956;100:1-11.
52. Blakemore WS, McGarrity GJ, Thurer RJ, et al. Infection by air borne bacteria with cardiopulmonary bypass. *Surgery* 1971;70:830-838.
53. Geldof WCP, Brom AG. Infections through blood from heart-lung machine. *Thorax* 1972;27:395-397.
54. Kluge RM, Calia FM, McLaughlin JS, et al. Sources of contamination in open heart surgery. *JAMA* 1974;230:1415-1418.
55. Ankeney JL. Discussion of Amoury RA, Bowman FO Jr, Malm JR: Endocarditis associated with intracardiac prosthesis. *J Thorac Cardiovasc Surg* 1966;51:48.
56. Ankeney JL, Parker RF. Staphylococcal endocarditis following open-heart surgery related to positive intraoperative blood cultures. In: Brewer LA III, ed. *Prosthetic Heart Valves*. Springfield, IL: Charles C. Thomas; 1968:719-730.
57. Bentley DW, Lepper MH. Septicemia related to indwelling venous catheter. *JAMA* 1968;206:1749-1752.
58. Weinstein RA, Jones EL, Schwarzmann SW, et al. Sternal osteomyelitis and mediastinitis after open-heart operation: pathogenesis and prevention. *Ann Thorac Surg* 1976;21:442-444.
59. Schwieger IM, Gallagher CJ, Finlayson DC, et al. Incidence of cell-saver contamination during cardiopulmonary bypass. *Ann Thorac Surg* 1989;48:51-53.

60. Beam TR. Perioperative prevention of infection in cardiac surgery. *Antibiot Chemother* 1985;33:114-139.
61. Bernard HR, Cole WR. The epidemiology of postoperative surgical infection. *Surg Clin N Am* 1965;45:509-519.
62. Beyer RH, Mills SA, Hudspeth AS, et al. A prospective study of sternal wound complications. *Ann Thorac Surg* 1984;37:412-416.
63. Nagachinta T, Stephens M, Reitz B, et al. Risk factors for surgical-wound infection following cardiac surgery. *J Infect Dis* 1987;156:967-973.
64. Culliford AT, Cunningham JN, Zeff RH, et al. Sternal and costochondral infections following open-heart surgery. *J Thorac Cardiovasc Surg* 1976;72:714-726.
65. Kaiser AB, Kernodle DS, Barg NL, et al. Influence of preoperative showers on staphylococcal skin colonization: a comparative trial of antiseptic skin cleansers. *Ann Thorac Surg* 1988;45:35-38.
66. Ko W, Lazenby WD, Zelano JA, et al. Effects of shaving methods and intraoperative irrigation on suppurative mediastinitis after bypass operations. *Ann Thorac Surg* 1992;53:301-305.
67. Connell JF, Rousselot LM. Povidone-iodine. Extensive surgical evaluation of a new antiseptic agent. *Am J Surg* 1964;108:849-855.
68. Joress SM. A study of disinfection of the skin: a comparison of povidine-iodine with other agents used for surgical scrubs. *Ann Surg* 1962;155:296-304.
69. Fong IW, Baker CB, McKee DC. The value of prophylactic antibiotics in aorta-coronary bypass operations. *J Thorac Cardiovasc Surg* 1979;78:908-913.
70. Goldman DA, Hopkins CC, Karchmer AW, et al. Cephalothin prophylaxis in cardiac valve surgery. *J Thorac Cardiovasc Surg* 1977;73:470-479.
71. Levy JH, Nagle DM, Curling PE, et al. Contamination reduction during central venous catheterization. *Crit Care Med* 1988;16:165-167.
72. Ferrazzi P, Allen R, Crupi G, et al. Reduction of infection after cardiac surgery: a clinical trial. *Ann Thorac Surg* 1986;42:321-325.
73. Ottino G, DePaulis R, Pansini S, et al. Major sternal wound infection after open-heart surgery: a multivariate analysis of risk factors in 2,579 consecutive operative procedures. *Ann Thorac Surg* 1987;44:173-179.
74. Stoney WS. Median sternotomy. In: Vander Salm TJ, ed. *Cardiac Surgery: State of the Art Reviews*. Philadelphia: Hanley & Belfus Inc., 1988:431-436.
75. Arnold M. The surgical anatomy of sternal blood supply. *J Thorac Cardiovasc Surg* 1972;64:596-610.
76. Seyfer AE, Shriver CD, Miller TR, et al. Sternal blood flow after median sternotomy and mobilization of the internal mammary arteries. *Surgery* 1988;104:899-904.
77. He GW, Ryan WH, Acuff TE, et al. Risk factors for operative mortality and sternal wound infection in bilateral internal mammary artery grafting. *J Thorac Cardiovasc Surg* 1994;107:196-202.
78. Gu YJ, Wanag YS, Chiang BY, et al. Membrane oxygenator prevents lung reperfusion injury in canine cardiopulmonary bypass. *Ann Thorac Surg* 1991;51:573-578.
79. Cavarocchi NC, Pluth JR, Schaff HV, et al. Complement activation during cardiopulmonary bypass. Comparison of bubble and membrane oxygenators. *J Thorac Cardiovasc Surg* 1986;91:252-258.
80. Gu YJ, Oeveren W, Akkerman C, et al. Heparin-coated circuits reduce the inflammatory response to cardiopulmonary bypass. *Ann Thorac Surg* 1993;55:917-922.
81. Videm V, Svennevig JL, Fosse E, et al. Reduced complement activation with heparin-coated oxygenator and tubings in coronary bypass operations. *J Thorac Cardiovasc Surg* 1992;103:806-813.
82. Hisatomi K, Isomura T, Galli SJ, et al. Augmentation of interleukin-2 production after cardiac operations in patients treated with erythropoietin. *J Thorac Cardiovasc Surg* 1992;104:278-283.
83. Faist E, Ertel W, Salem B, et al. The immune-enhancing effect of perioperative thymopentin administration in elderly patients undergoing major surgery. *Arch Surg* 1988;123:1449-1453.
84. Burke JF. the effective period of preventive antibiotic action in experimental incisions and dermal lesions. *Surgery* 1961;50:161-168.
85. Austin TW, Coles JC, Burnett R, et al. Aortocoronary bypass procedures and sternotomy infections: a study of anti-staphylococcal prophylaxis. *Can J Surg* 1980;23:483-485.
86. Kreter B, Woods M. Antibiotic prophylaxis for cardiothoracic operations. *J Thorac Cardiovasc Surg* 1992;104:590-599.
87. Hirschmann JV, Inui TS. Antimicrobial prophylaxis: a critique of recent trials. *Rev Infect Dis* 1980;2:1-23.
88. Sarr MG, Gott VL, Townsend TR. Mediastinal infection after cardiac surgery. *Ann Thorac Surg* 1984;38:415-423.
89. Wells FC, Newsom SWB, Rowlands C. Hospital Practice. Wound infection in cardiothoracic surgery. *Lancet* 1983;1:1209-1210.
90. Farrington M, Webster M, Fenn A, et al. Wound infection in cardiothoracic surgery. *Lancet* 1983;2:395-396.
91. Goldman DA, Hopkins CC, Karchmer AW, et al. Cephalothin prophylaxis in cardiac valve surgery. *J Thorac Cardiovasc Surg* 1977;73:470-479.
92. Conte JE, Cohen SN, Roe BB, et al. Antibiotic prophylaxis and cardiac surgery. *Ann Intern Med* 1972;76:943-949.
93. Moss AR, Cahetti P, Osmond D, et al. Sero-positivity for HIV and the development of AIDS or related condition: three-year follow-up of the San Francisco General Hospital cohort. *Br Med J* 1988;296:745-750.
94. Fahey JL, Taylor JMG, Detels R, et al. The prognostic value of cellular and serologic markers in infection with human immunodeficiency virus type 1. *N Engl J Med* 1990;322:166-172.
95. Uva MS, Jebara VA, Fabiani JN, et al. Cardiac surgery in patients with human immunodeficiency virus infection: indications and results. *J Cardiac Surg* 1992;7:240-244.
96. Frater RWM, Sisto D, Condit D. Cardiac surgery in human immunodeficiency virus (HIV) carriers. *Eur J Cardiothorac Surg* 1989;3:146-150.
97. Nahass RG, Weinstein MP, Bartels J, et al. Infective endocarditis in intravenous drug users: a comparison of human immunodeficiency virus type 1-negative and -positive patients. *J Infect Dis* 1990;162:967-970.

9
The Endocrine System: Effects of Cardiopulmonary Bypass

Carolyn Fleming Bannister and Donald C. Finlayson

Documenting changes in hormone concentrations that accompany hemodynamic fluctuations during cardiac surgery and cardiopulmonary bypass (CPB) has been an important goal of investigators. For, although a causal relationship may not be proven, methods of modifying the associated hormonal changes may lead to improved perioperative hemodynamic control and, thereby, to better patient outcome. Alterations in the endocrine system associated with cardiac surgery and CPB have been evaluated in various ways by numerous investigators. Wide variations in reported plasma hormone and metabolite values are likely due to the multiplicity of interactive and interdependent factors impacting the physiologic response to stress. Some of the factors that make comparisons of patients and study results difficult are outlined in Table 9.1.

This chapter describes normal endocrine function; summarizes the expected changes in the pituitary, thyroid/parathyroid, adrenal, and pancreatic glands during cardiac surgery and CPB; and details the potential influence of patient, surgical, bypass, and anesthetic variables on perioperative endocrine function.

Pituitary Gland Function During Cardiac Surgery and CPB

Posterior Pituitary

Antidiuretic Hormone (ADH) (Vasopressin)

ADH is formed in the supraoptic nuclei of the hypothalamus and is responsible for regulation of the osmotic pressure of extracellular fluid. The most profound stimuli for ADH secretion are hemorrhage and circulatory shock. Drugs such as morphine, nicotine, and tranquilizers increase ADH release.

ADH has several important hemodynamic effects. This hormone is a potent vasoconstrictor with a direct action on smooth muscle. Animal studies have shown a decrease in myocardial performance (decreased cardiac output, increased coronary resistance, decreased dp/dT) and a decrease in blood flow to the coronary arteries and to end organs (liver, kidneys) with vasopressin infusions. In man, single subcutaneous doses of vasopressin, 5–20 µg, have produced angina, myocardial ischemia, and infarcts.[1] Arterial infusions of vasopressin in cirrhotic patients decrease cardiac output.[2]

ADH secretion also increases with trauma and surgical stress, as well as with other normally occurring physiologic stimuli (decreased extracellular volume, anxiety, increased plasma osmolality). In cardiac and noncardiac surgery, ADH secretion increases with surgical incision (Figure 9.1).[3] Patients undergoing coronary revascularization have higher levels of ADH during CPB than those patients having valve replacements, although the levels in both groups during CPB are significantly higher than baseline values.[4]

Several studies have assessed the effect of anesthesia on ADH secretion during cardiac surgery and CPB. Light halothane or morphine anesthesia does not blunt the increase in ADH secretion with skin incision[5]; however, high-dose opioid anesthesia (morphine 1–3 mg/kg, fentanyl 70 µg/kg, or sufentanil 7–23 µg/kg) blunts the ADH release that otherwise occurs with skin incision, up until the time of CPB.[3,6–8] ADH levels increase precipitously in the first 30 minutes of CPB, independent of anesthetic

TABLE 9.1. Variables confounding the assessment of endocrine changes induced by cardiac surgery and CPB.

Patient variables	Age, physical status, primary and coexisting diseases
Surgical variables	Type of procedure performed; use of, and duration of, CPB
CPB variables	Temperature, hemodilution, pulsatile versus nonpulsatile perfusion, various priming solutions
Anesthetic variables	Drugs used and depth of anesthesia

9. Endocrine System

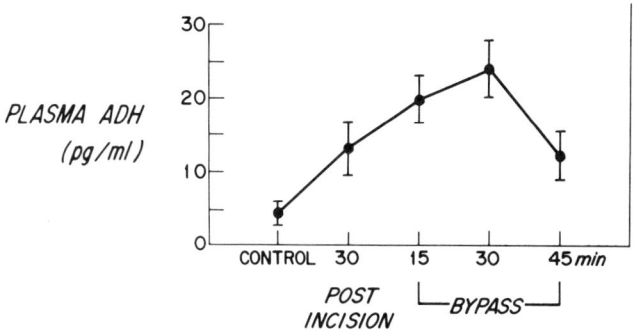

FIGURE 9.1. Graphic representation of the changes in plasma antidiuretic hormone (ADH) levels during cardiac surgery and CPB. (From Philbin et al,[3] by permission of *J Thorac Cardiovasc Surg*.)

technique, although concentrations are greater in patients anesthetized with enflurane or halothane than in those anesthetized with fentanyl (Figure 9.2).[7]

There is no correlation in patients on CPB between ADH levels and plasma or urine osmolality or urine flow; ADH levels at all times exceed those needed for maximum concentration of urine and for control of water excretion. Actually, there is a paradoxical increase in urine flow in the face of high ADH levels. Sodium excretion increases fourfold 15 minutes into CPB, declines for the remainder of CPB, and then peaks 15–30 minutes after CPB.[9] The

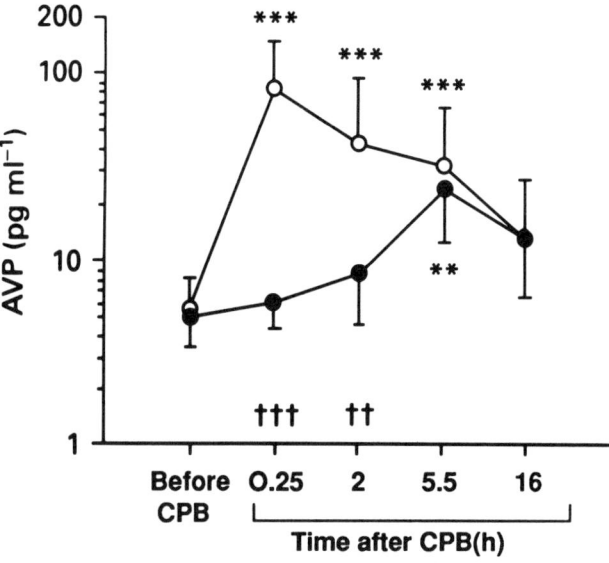

FIGURE 9.2. Changes in plasma concentrations of arginine vasopressin (AVP) (antidiuretic hormone) during cardiac surgery using inhalation anesthetic compared to opioid anesthetic (fentanyl). (○) Enflurane; (●) fentanyl; **$p < 0.01$; ***$p < 0.001$, compared with postinduction values within a group. ††$p < 0.01$, †††$p < 0.001$ between the groups. (From Kuitunen,[7] by permission of *Br J Anaes*.)

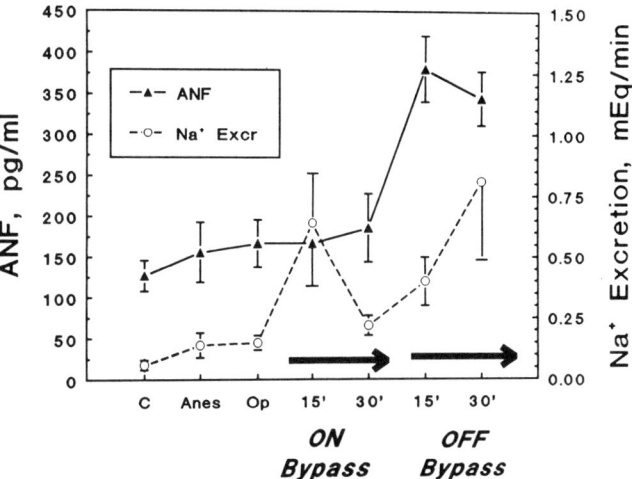

FIGURE 9.3. Changes in atrial natriuretic factor (ANF) and sodium excretion (Na^+ Excr) during CPB. Circulating ANF values, corrected for hemodilution, did not change during CPB but doubled after termination of extracorporeal support. (C is the time control samples were obtained; Anes is the time of anesthesia induction; OP is the time of skin incision.) Data are shown as mean ± SE. (From Schaff HV, Mashburn JP, McCarthy PM et al,[4] by permission of *J Thorac Cardiovasc Surg*.)

late natriuresis parallels elevated levels of atrial natriuretic factor (ANF) that occur after CPB (Figure 9.3), whereas the early natriuresis during CPB occurs while ANF levels are unchanged and aldosterone levels are increasing (Figure 9.4).[4] ADH levels may be significantly increased until

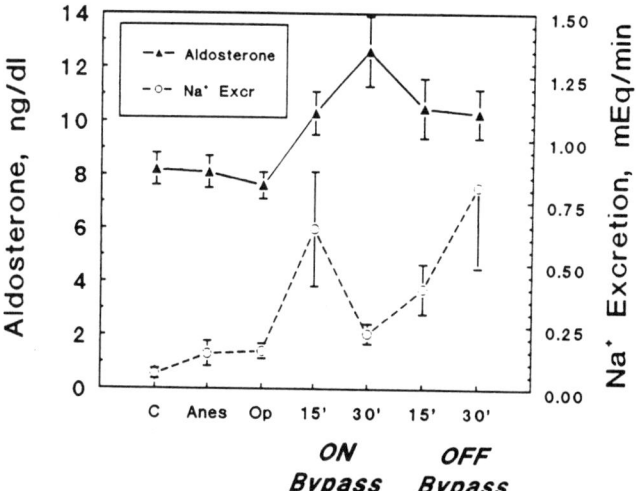

FIGURE 9.4. Serum aldosterone levels and sodium excretion (Na^+ Excr) during CPB. Serum aldosterone level increased during bypass and was highest after 30 minutes of perfusion. Sampling times are the same as in Figure 9.3. Data are shown as mean ± SE. (From Schaff HV, Mashburn JP, McCarthy PM et al,[4] by permission of *J Thorac Cardiovasc Surg*.)

6 hours after CPB but usually approach baseline by the morning of the first postoperative day.

The effects of other variables—the type of blood flow during CPB, the magnitude of hemodilution, and pump prime type—on ADH levels have also been studied. Several studies comparing pulsatile and nonpulsatile blood flow during CPB have reported that pulsatile flow results in lower ADH levels,[9,10] while other studies have reported no difference.[11] Elevated ADH levels during CPB also seem to be independent of the type of pump-priming fluid (blood versus crystalloid) and the magnitude of hemodilution.[12,13]

Anterior Pituitary

Gonadotropic Hormones (Luteinizing Hormone [LH], Follicle-Stimulating Hormone [FSH], and Prolactin)

Three gonadotropic hormones are secreted by the anterior pituitary gland: LH, FSH, and prolactin. LH and FSH are under the control of releasing factors from the hypothalamus and are required for the maturation of male and female reproductive systems. Although secretion of these hormones is affected by CPB, the clinical significance of changes in levels is unknown.

Yokota and colleagues[14] studied male patients undergoing cardiac surgery who were anesthetized with a fentanyl/nitrous oxide technique and managed with hypothermic nonpulsatile CPB. They reported that plasma LH levels were unchanged by the induction of anesthesia, but doubled with skin incision. In this study, LH levels decreased to baseline by the second postoperative day (Figure 9.5).

Prolactin is also known as lactogenic hormone because of its effect on milk secretion by the breasts. Prolactin levels increase significantly after induction of anesthesia and continue to rise with skin incision until the time of CPB. The levels drop precipitously with institution of CPB, increase gradually to 2 hours of CPB, and remain on this plateau until the second postoperative day, when they return to baseline values (Figure 9.5).

Adrenocorticotropic Hormone (ACTH)

ACTH stimulates adrenal gland secretion of glucocorticoid and androgen hormones and has a slight influence on aldosterone release. Small amounts of ACTH are secreted continually, and, within minutes of any type of physiologic stress, ACTH release can increase as much as 20-fold. Cortisol release from the adrenal gland is part of the stress response that affects metabolism of substrates (protein, fat, and carbohydrates), activates the immune system, and supports the aggressive physical response of animals toward insults from the environment.

During cardiac surgery, plasma ACTH levels increase with surgical incision and up to the initiation of CPB. Plasma ACTH levels fall during nonpulsatile CPB and increase above preoperative levels within 1 hour of resumption of normal circulation.[15]

Growth Hormone (GH)

GH release serves a protective function after trauma by decreasing protein catabolism while promoting protein synthesis, increasing fat mobilization, increasing glycogen deposition, and decreasing glucose oxidation.[16] Several types of physiologic perturbations, including surgical stress, heat exposure, hypovolemia, anxiety, exercise, hy-

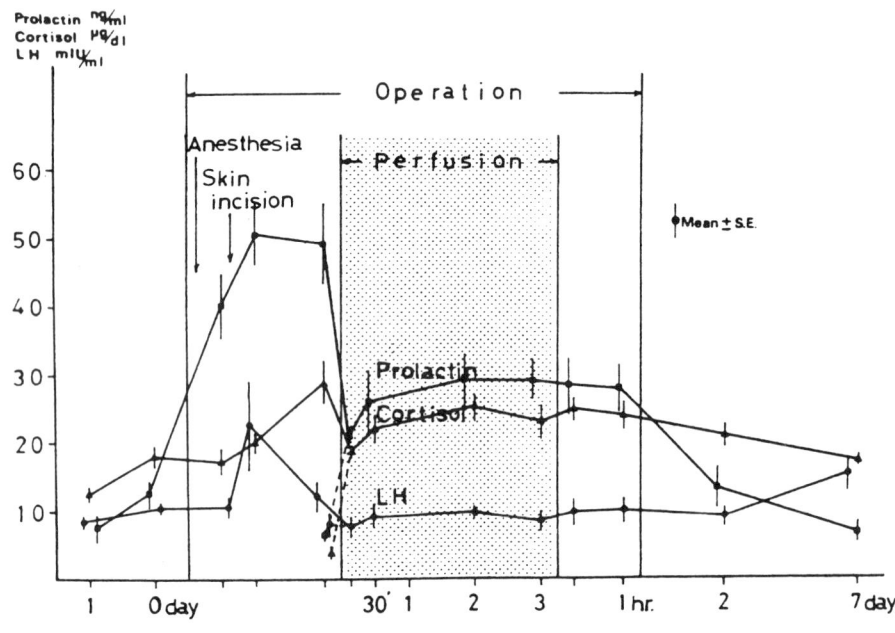

FIGURE 9.5. Fluctuations in plasma cortisol, luteinizing hormone (LH), and prolactin during open-heart surgery. (From Yokota et al,[14] by permission of *J Surg Res*.)

poglycemia, starvation, and myocardial infarction, increase GH levels. α-Adrenergic facilitation of growth hormone-releasing factor (GHRF) secretion appears to cause stress-induced GH release. Patients pretreated with the α-receptor blocker phentolamine do not have an increase in GH levels with surgery.[17]

GH levels increase significantly from skin incision to the initiation of CPB and peak at approximately 120 minutes of CPB.[18,19] Levels decrease rapidly to preoperative levels by 6 hours after CPB and remain normal throughout the postoperative period. Studies comparing the effects of anesthetics on GH release have failed to show significant differences before, during, or after CPB between patients receiving morphine or fentanyl and those anesthetized with halothane.[20,21]

GH secretion increases with decreased glucose utilization.[22] During CPB, glucose utilization decreases secondary to hypothermia, cortisol and catecholamine release, and suppression of insulin secretion. This decreased utilization may account in part for the high GH concentrations observed during CPB, which occur despite the presence of hyperglycemia, hypothermia, and heparinization, all of which, under isolated conditions, would decrease GH secretion.

Pancreatic Function During Cardiac Surgery and CPB

Changes in glucose and insulin concentrations during and after CPB are affected by glucose administration (particularly bypass circuit fluids containing dextrose), patient temperature management during the bypass period, and the presence of pulsatile or nonpulsatile blood flow. The effects of cardiac surgery on pancreatic function and glucose metabolism differ in nondiabetic and diabetic patients; these two types of patients are discussed separately below.

Nondiabetic Patients

Insulin

In nondiabetic patients, plasma insulin levels fall from preoperative concentrations after the induction of anesthesia and the beginning of surgical stimulation. Insulin release during CPB is directly affected by temperature, type of blood flow, and presence (or absence) of glucose in pump-priming solutions.[23-26]

During normothermic and hypothermic CPB (without glucose-containing solutions), there is no significant insulin release, and there is a decrease in plasma insulin levels that persists during CPB, despite mildly increased glucose levels (Figure 9.6). If glucose is administered during *hypothermic* CPB, insulin levels continue to be depressed, reflecting the inhibition of pancreatic function by hypothermia. (However, if insulin levels do increase, it is to an inadequate level for the degree of hyperglycemia present.) With rewarming, insulin concentrations increase severalfold to greater than preoperative fasting levels. If glucose is administered during *normothermic* bypass, there is a substantial increase in blood insulin levels in response to the hyperglycemia that occurs.[23,24] The difference in insulin levels between patients receiving glucose and those not receiving glucose disappears by the second postoperative hour (Figure 9.7). Insulin levels in both groups remain elevated for up to 7 days postoperatively.[25]

The type of blood flow (pulsatile or nonpulsatile) used during extracorporeal circulation may also affect pancreatic function. In one report, insulin levels increased in response to hyperglycemia during hypothermic CPB, and 1 and 5 hours after CPB, when pulsatile perfusion was employed, but no significant increases were noted in the nonpulsatile group, despite elevated glucose levels.[26]

Glucose

During CPB, glucose levels usually increase. In nondiabetic patients, plasma glucose concentrations of 600 mg/dL to greater than 800 mg/dL have been reported. The precise mechanism of hyperglycemia during CPB remains to be elucidated, but a multifactorial etiology is likely. The combined effects of increased hepatic glycogenolysis and gluconeogenesis due to catecholamine, cortisol, and/or glucagon release and the decreased utilization of glucose due to hypothermia and the failure of insulin secretion in response to hyperglycemia may be the primary determinants. Elevated free fatty acid concentrations due to heparin stimulation of lipoprotein lipase may have a glucose-sparing effect by providing alternate substrate to tissues. After CPB and protamine reversal of heparin, glucose levels decrease to preoperative levels by the first or second postoperative day. The reported association of hyperglycemia and poor neurologic recovery following ischemic CNS events, while reported in a different patient population, makes the problem of hyperglycemia during CPB worrisome.[27]

Body temperature during CPB may affect blood glucose values. During normothermic CPB, blood glucose increases steadily from preoperative values after the induction of anesthesia and well into CPB, even without glucose administration.[24] In a study comparing hypothermic and normothermic CPB, blood glucose was elevated during early CPB and remained elevated throughout normothermic CPB. Blood glucose was minimally elevated under hypothermic conditions throughout CPB but increased rapidly with rewarming.[23] At the termination of CPB, glucose levels were similarly elevated in both groups and remained elevated throughout the operative day.[23] Patients administered glucose in pump circuit fluids have

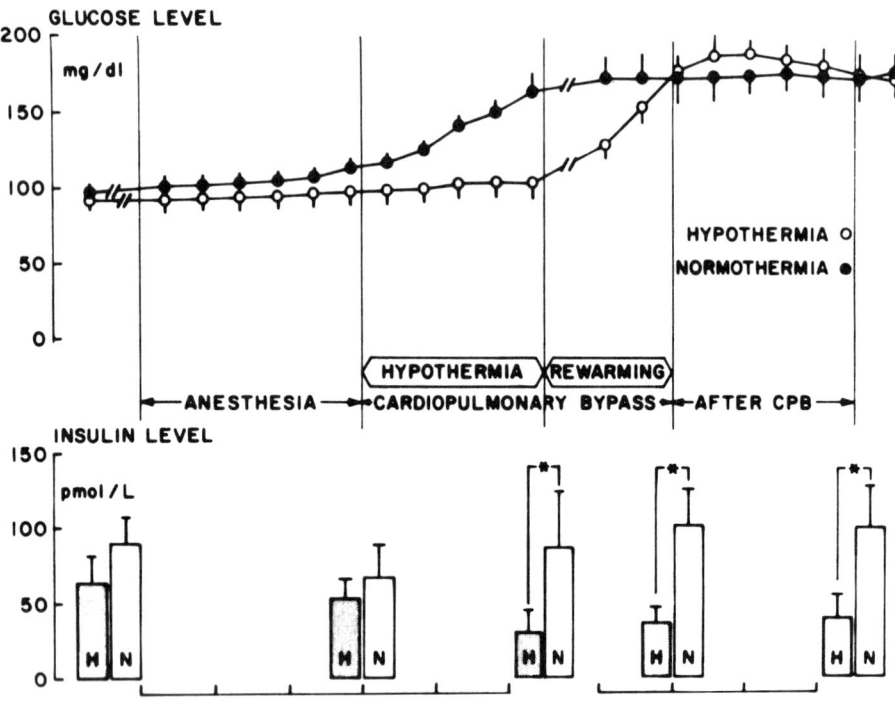

FIGURE 9.6. **Upper Panel.** Changes in mean blood glucose levels (in mg/dL ± SD) in nondiabetic patients during hypothermic CPB compared to changes during normothermic CPB. (Glucose not administered to either group.) **Lower Panel.** Mean plasma insulin levels (in pmol/L with SD) in nondiabetic patients before, during, and after hypothermic (H) versus normothermic (N) CPB. *$p < 0.05$. (From Kuntschen FR, Galletti PM, and Hahn C,[23] by permission of *J Thorac Cardiovasc Surg*.)

a sudden increase in blood glucose at the initiation of bypass, regardless of temperature.[28]

Early attempts to improve myocardial preservation included the use of various combinations of glucose-insulin-potassium (GIK) infusions to improve energy balance in myocardial cells.[29-35] A recent evaluation of this technique reported a wide range of glucose levels and a higher incidence of hypoglycemia (< 50 mg/dL) and hyperglycemia (> 300 mg/dL) in the GIK-treated group when compared to untreated patients. The untreated group did not have glucose levels greater than 250 mg/dL and did not require more inotropic support than the treated patients.[36]

Anesthetic technique may affect blood glucose concentrations during cardiac surgery and CPB. In one study,

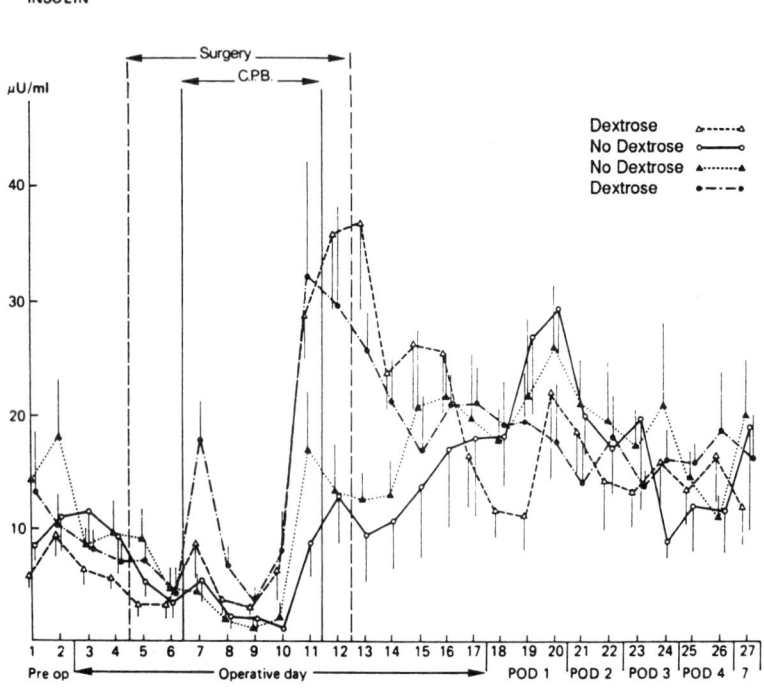

FIGURE 9.7. Effect on serum insulin levels (μU/mL) of using dextrose-containing pump-priming solutions compared to using dextrose-free solutions in nondiabetic patients. POD = postoperative days. Vertical lines at each sample point represent standard errors of the mean. Insulin levels in both groups are elevated for at least 7 days postoperatively, but differences between the two groups disappear within the first few hours after CPB. (Modified from McKnight et al,[25] by permission of *J Thorac Cardiovasc Surg*.)

cardiac surgery patients anesthetized with fentanyl, 60 μg/kg, had no significant change in blood glucose levels, while those anesthetized with nonopioid techniques (halothane/nitrous oxide/oxygen) had significant glucose elevations during aortic cannulation and throughout CPB.[21] In a pediatric study, children administered propofol during CPB tended to have lower glucose levels than those not receiving propofol. However, glucose levels were significantly different between the groups only at the end of CPB, and there were no statistically significant differences in blood glucose levels between the two groups up to 24 hours postoperatively.[37]

CPB and Pancreatic Function in Diabetic Patients

Prior to the initiation of CPB, diabetic patients (compared to nondiabetics) require more insulin to achieve normal plasma glucose levels. During CPB, diabetic patients are insulin deficient, have decreased glucose utilization, and undergo lipolysis and proteolysis. During hypothermic CPB, insulin requirements are minimal in both diabetics and nondiabetics, if glucose levels are normal before the initiation of CPB. With rewarming, insulin requirements increase up to sixfold in both nondiabetic and insulin-dependent diabetic patients. Non-insulin-dependent diabetics have the greatest increase in insulin requirements during rewarming. After CPB, insulin requirements decrease to baseline over the first 3 postoperative days.[38]

The life-threatening condition of hyperosmolar, hyperglycemic, nonketotic coma (HHNC) can occur in non-insulin-dependent diabetics following cardiac surgery and CPB. These patients are at higher risk for hyperglycemia because of severe insulin resistance and the high glucose concentration during CPB. The dehydration accompanying this condition is exacerbated by diuretics given during CPB. Mortality is 42% in patients with HHNC undergoing cardiac surgery, and is directly related to the time elapsed before diagnosis.[39]

Adrenal Gland Function, Cardiac Surgery, and CPB

Adrenal Cortex

Cortisol

Plasma cortisol levels increase during surgical procedures as part of the physiologic response to stress. The magnitude of cortisol release is thought to correlate with the intensity of the stress.[40]

In patients undergoing cardiac surgery and CPB, cortisol levels begin to rise with the surgical incision, fall at the onset of CPB, and then rise steadily to peak values 6 to 24 hours postoperatively, remaining at this higher level until the first postoperative day.[41] After this, cortisol levels fall gradually but may still be significantly higher than preoperative values, even at the 7th postoperative day.[25,42]

Plasma cortisol levels decrease with the initiation of CPB (Figure 9.8), but the active non-protein-bound free fraction increases because of decreased cortisol-binding capacity secondary to the decrease in plasma protein levels during CPB. Early explanations for the decrease in cortisol levels at the onset of CPB included the effect of hemodilution with CPB and the decreased secretion of cortisol due to hypothermia. Subsequent investigation suggests that decreased cortisol secretion may be due to decreased ACTH release from the pituitary rather than to adrenal hyposecretion.[15,43] Synthetic ACTH administered during CPB produces a significant rise in plasma cortisol levels (Figure 9.9).[41,43,44] Surgical patients not managed with CPB have high cortisol levels intraoperatively that do not increase further with ACTH administration.[43]

The effect on adrenal gland function of pulsatile versus nonpulsatile perfusion during CPB is unclear. In one comparative study, plasma cortisol levels rose significantly only if pulsatile flow was used (Figure 9.10).[44] However, in studies using hypothermic CPB, cortisol levels were not affected by the type of blood flow employed during CPB.[11,45] In children, plasma cortisol and ACTH concentrations similarly increase before CPB, and neither hormone decreases during pulsatile or nonpulsatile hypothermic CPB.[46]

The perioperative administration of steroids may affect cortisol levels. Postoperative plasma cortisol levels are lower than preoperative levels for at least 18 hours in patients receiving 1 to 1.5 g of methylprednisolone intraoperatively.[47]

In both children and adults, the type of anesthesia may affect the increase in adrenocortical hormones during cardiac surgery and CPB. In one study, children anesthetized with fentanyl and halothane or enflurane up to the initiation of CPB, and then administered propofol during CPB, had significantly lower cortisol levels during and up to 3 hours after CPB than did those not given propofol (Figure 9.11). In adults, the cortisol response seen after the induction of anesthesia and skin incision, up to the initiation of CPB, can be blunted by fentanyl, 75 μg/kg, or morphine sulfate, 2–4 mg/kg, intravenously.[6,20,42,48,49] In a comparative study assessing the effect of fentanyl and 1% and 2% isoflurane anesthesia during CPB on perioperative cortisol levels, only 2% isoflurane blunted the increase in cortisol release; this effect persisted into the post-CPB period.[50]

Aldosterone/Renin

Aldosterone release from the adrenal cortex controls 95% of sodium reabsorption from the renal tubules. The most important stimuli for aldosterone release, under normal

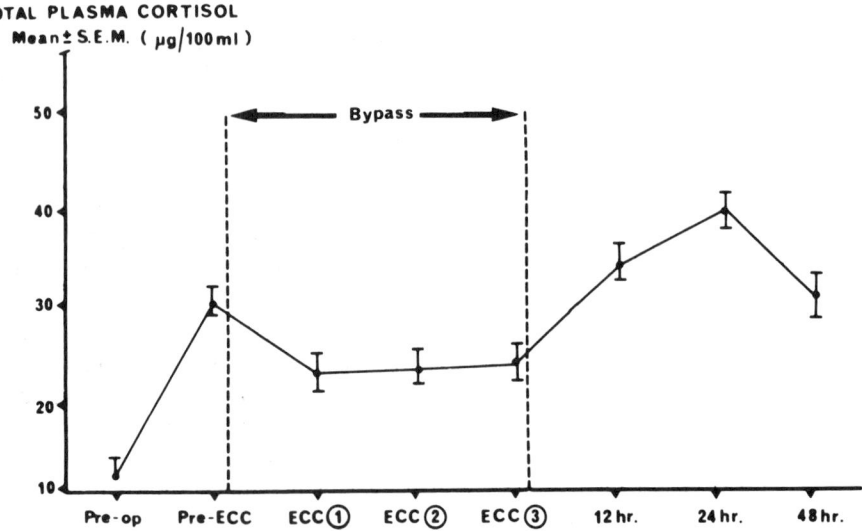

FIGURE 9.8. Mean total plasma cortisol values in 20 patients undergoing CPB. Note the decreased cortisol plasma levels during extracorporeal circulation (ECC). (Reproduced with permission from *Circulation*.[41] Copyright 1976 American Heart Association.)

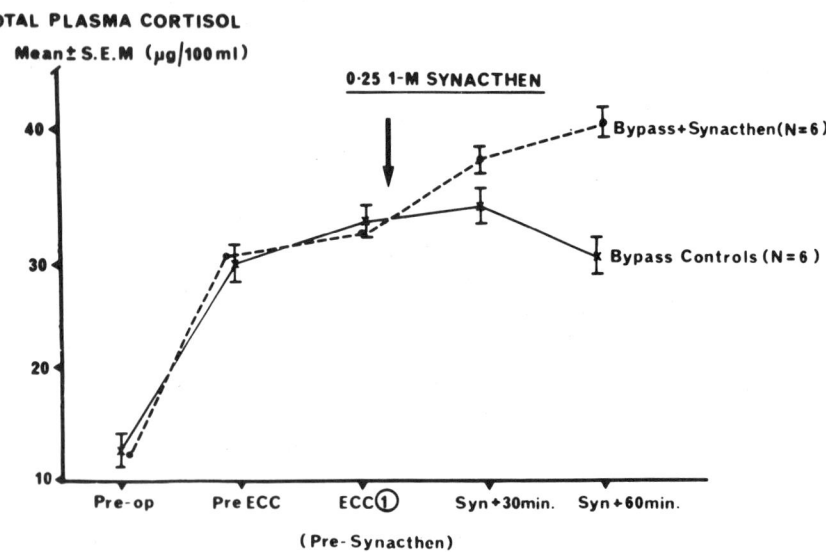

FIGURE 9.9. Mean total plasma cortisol values in six bypass patients given 0.25 mg intramuscular tetracosactrin zinc phosphate (Synacthen; synthetic ACTH) and in six bypass control patients not given Synacthen. The blood samples were obtained at the following times: preoperatively (Pre-op); pre-extracorporeal circulation (PreECC); 30 min after the onset of extracorporeal circulation [ECC 1 (Pre-Synacthen)]; 30 min after injection (Syn + 30 min); 60 min after injection (Syn + 60 min). Synacthen was injected immediately after obtaining the ECC 1 sample. (Reproduced with permission from *Circulation*.[41] Copyright 1976 from American Heart Association.)

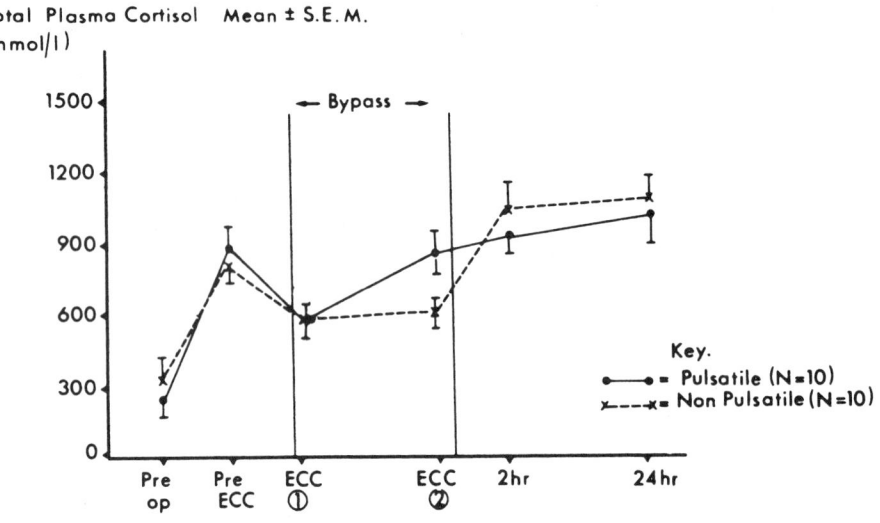

FIGURE 9.10. Mean levels of total plasma cortisol (± SEM) in patients undergoing pulsatile and nonpulsatile extracorporeal circulation (ECC). The ECC 1 and ECC 2 samples were taken 2 minutes after the initiation of bypass and 10 minutes prior to the termination of bypass, respectively. (From Taylor et al,[44] by permission of *J Thorac Cardiovasc Surg*.)

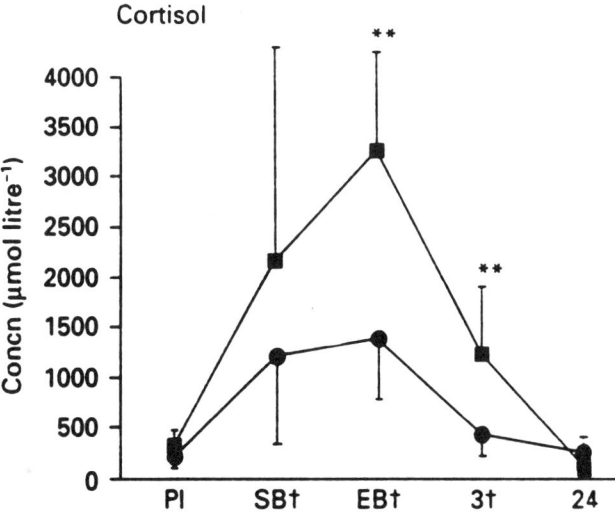

FIGURE 9.11. Change in the concentration of cortisol before, during, and after CPB in children reflecting the effect of different anesthetic techniques. P1 = After induction; SB = start CPB; EB = end CPB; 3 and 24 = 3 and 24 hours, respectively, after CPB. (■) Fentanyl ± halothane, no propofol; (●) fentanyl ± halothane plus propofol infusion; **$p < 0.01$; †corrected for hemodilution. (From Laycock et al,[37] by permission of *Br J Anaesth*.)

Adrenal Medulla

The adrenal medullary response to anesthesia, surgery, and CPB constitutes part of the body's stress response and is affected by numerous factors. Resting plasma catecholamine levels vary with patient physical status and the severity and type of cardiac disease (plasma epinephrine and norepinephrine are found to be higher in some patients requiring valve replacement, when compared to patients with coronary artery disease).[56] Eighty percent of the catecholamine release from the adrenal medulla is epinephrine and 20% is norepinephrine, although the relative proportions change with different physiologic stressers. The short plasma half-life of circulating catecholamines (20 to 60 seconds in vivo) makes quantification of levels very difficult.

Elevated catechloamine levels during CPB contribute to the rise in systemic vascular resistance and the need for vasodilation during and after CPB. These catecholamine levels, in combination with elevated ADH, are likely causes of early postoperative hypertension.[57]

Circulating catecholamines increase at the onset of CPB in patients with both valvular and coronary artery disease. Reves and colleagues[54] reported that epinephrine levels increased ninefold during CPB and norepinephrine levels doubled (Figures 9.13 and 9.14). The observed increase in catecholamines during CPB is likely secondary to both increased production and decreased clearance of epineph-

physiologic conditions, are changes in serum sodium and potassium levels and the release of renin and angiotensin. In patients undergoing noncardiac surgery, general anesthesia causes an increase in aldosterone levels that increases even further with surgical incision.[51] Aldosterone levels initially decline and then increase after 15 minutes of CPB, with a further increase at the end of CPB despite decreased renin activity at this time.[52]

Studies in patients undergoing elective cardiac surgery with CPB report that renin activity increases with surgical stimulus and up to the time of CPB. Renin levels decline approximately 30% during CPB from postanesthesia induction levels but are still higher than baseline levels. These changes correlate with changes in arterial blood pressure (Figure 9.12).[52] Other factors known to affect renin activity, such as serum sodium level or osmotic load, renal blood flow, and mean renal blood pressure, do not correlate with changes in renin levels during CPB; nor do the changes correlate with measured catecholamine levels.[52]

Some investigators have reported that pulsatile blood flow during CPB may attenuate the increases in renin and systemic vascular resistance.[53] Others found decreases in plasma renin levels with pulsatile CPB only in patients undergoing coronary revascularization and mitral valve replacement, and not during aortic valve replacement.[54] These differences have not been noted in other studies.[11,55]

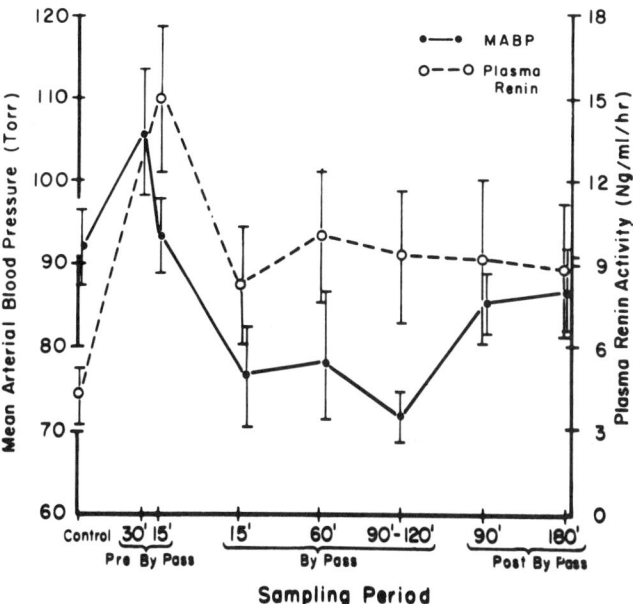

FIGURE 9.12. Changes in mean arterial blood pressure (MABP) closely follow changes in plasma renin activity (ng/mL/h) before, during, and after CPB. Each point represents the mean value for 10 patients (±SE). (From Bailey et al,[52] by permission of *Anesthesiology*.)

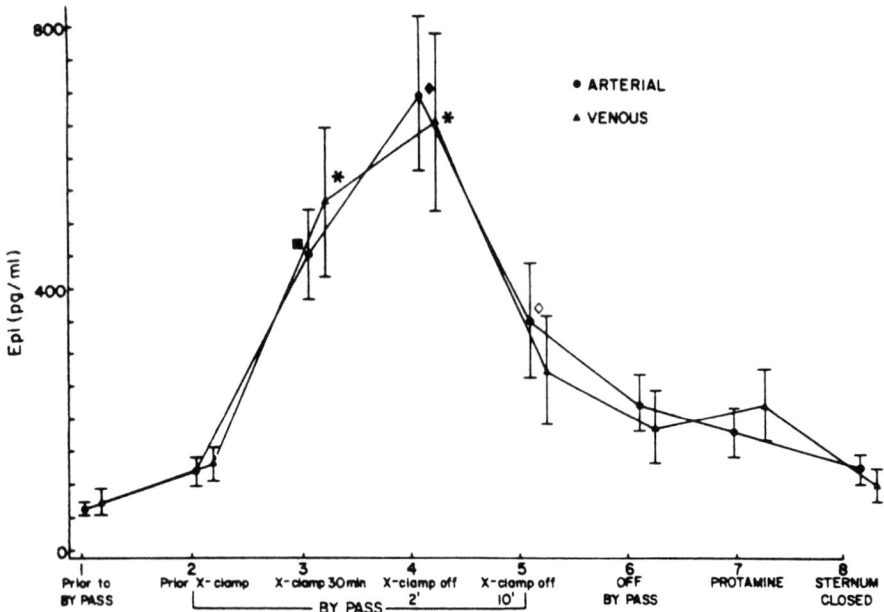

FIGURE 9.13. Arterial and venous plasma levels of epinephrine (Epi) measured during cardiac surgery and bypass. Samples 4 and 5 were measured at 2 minutes (x-clamp off 2′) and 10 minutes (x-clamp off 10′) after the removal of the x-clamp, respectively. Plasma levels of epinephrine rise to 9 times higher than baseline during cardiac surgery. Bars indicate SEM. (Reproduced with permission from *Circulation*.[54] Copyright 1982 American Heart Association.)

rine and norepinephrine. Hypothermia and the exclusion of the heart and lungs from the circulation during bypass decrease metabolism of catecholamines. Levels fall in the immediate post-CPB period in patients undergoing coronary artery revascularization, but they may remain elevated for longer than 24 hours after CPB in patients with combined valvular and coronary artery surgery.[56]

The effect of anesthesia on catecholamines during cardiac surgery and CPB has been studied in multiple investigations.[20,21,58,59] In a study by Sebel et al,[21] fentanyl anesthesia was associated with a slight decrease in plasma catecholamine levels, while levels slightly increased with holathane induction; however, these differences in catecholamines were statistically significant only during aortic cannulation. Elevated catecholamine levels at the initiation of CPB have been demonstrated with both opioid and

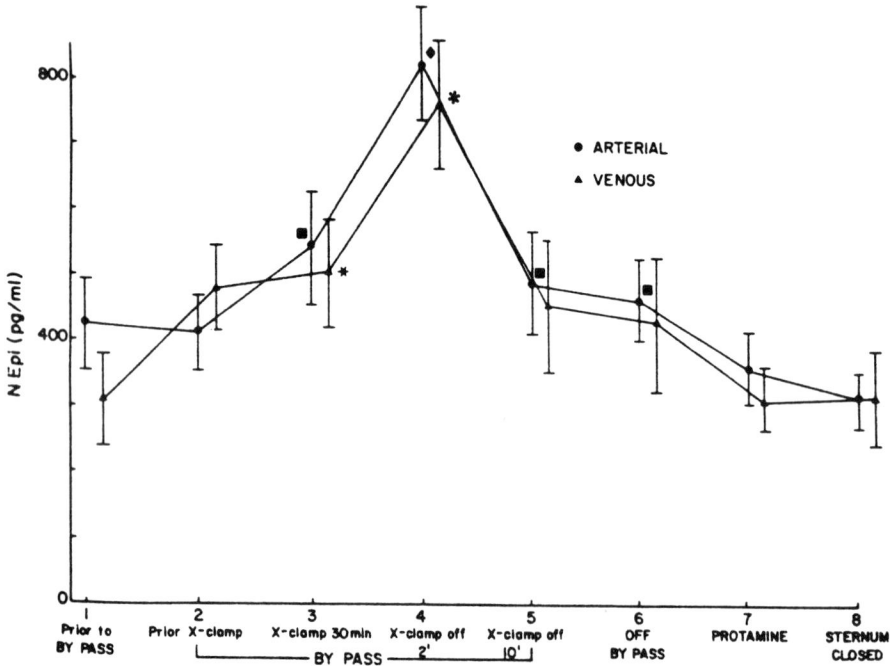

FIGURE 9.14. Arterial and venous plasma levels of norepinephrine (NEpi) measured during cardiac surgery and bypass. Samples 4 and 5 were measured at 2 minutes (x-clamp off 2′) and 10 minutes (x-clamp off 10′) after the removal of the x-clamp, respectively. Plasma levels of norepinephrine twice the baseline values are recorded during cardiac surgery. Bars indicate SEM. (Reproduced with permission from *Circulation*.[54] Copyright 1982 American Heart Association.)

inhalation anesthetic techniques (Figure 9.15).[7] However, in one study, patients anesthetized with halothane for coronary bypass grafting had a decrease in circulating epinephrine and norepinephrine on initiation of CPB that persisted throughout the bypass period.[60] A study in which patients were anesthetized with sodium pentothal, halothane, fentanyl, and nitrous oxide reported that there was no significant change in plasma epinephrine or norepinephrine concentrations throughout the procedure.[59]

Although the use of pulsatile versus nonpulsatile blood flow during CPB is controversial, several studies have reported improved hemodynamics and fewer perioperative problems with the use of pulsatile CPB.[53,61,62] Although plasma catecholamine levels increase during CPB with both techniques, in some studies catecholamine release appears to be attenuated by pulsatile CPB (Figures 9.16 and 9.17). Significantly higher mean arterial pressure, total peripheral resistance, venous capacitance, and positive fluid balance have been reported in patients undergoing nonpulsatile CPB as compared to pulsatile CPB.[61,62] In another study comparing patients with valvular disease and patients with coronary artery disease, nonpulsatile CPB resulted in a significant increase in plasma norepinephrine concentration that was not abolished by pulsatile CPB. In this study, epinephrine release was insignificant during nonpulsatile CPB and was not further reduced with pulsatile CPB.[56]

The "Stress Response"

Anesthesia and surgery, as well as various neural and humoral factors, including anxiety, pain, hypoxemia, and acidosis, activate the stress response, a generalized metabolic outpouring characterized by increased ADH, catecholamine, β-endorphin, renin, and cortisol levels. In healthy patients, this response is a valuable means of dealing with many kinds of stress and is also known as the "fight or flight response." Assuming that the physiologic changes (tachycardia and hypertension) may be harmful to patients with poor cardiac reserve, numerous investigators have focused on ways to blunt the release of stress hormones during surgery.

The stress response is pronounced during CPB, when cortisol, ADH, catecholamines and vasoactive substances, including prostaglandins, are released. For instance, the epinephrine release with CPB is equivalent to that reported in patients with acute myocardial infarction, and norepinephrine levels approach those seen with strenuous exercise.[63,64] Hypothermia, hypovolemia, hemodilution, hypotension, hypoperfusion, and nonpulsatile flow lead to endogenous catecholamine release during CPB. Hypothermia delays enzymatic metabolism of catecholamines, and decreased perfusion to the lungs, liver, and kidneys delays plasma clearance of released catecholamines.[65] Cortisol release rises intraoperatively and peaks during the first postoperative day, indicating that the stress response does not end with the termination of CPB.[25] Prostaglandin release and complement activation are higher in patients requiring CPB than in those having procedures not requiring CPB[65]; this part of the stress response has important pathophysiologic effects on microcirculation, clotting mechanisms, and the immune system. Cortisol and catecholamine release have marked hemody-

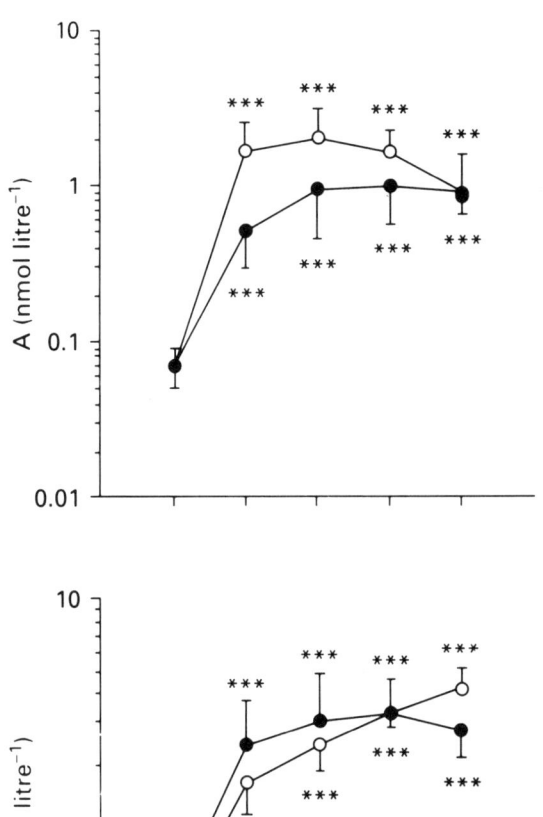

FIGURE 9.15. Changes in plasma concentration of noradrenaline (NA) and adrenaline (A) during cardiac surgery with inhalation compared to opioid anesthetic technique. (○) Enflurane; (●) fentanyl; **$p < 0.01$; ***$p < 0.001$ compared with preoperative (postinduction) value within a group. (From Kuitunen et al,[7] by permission of Br J Anaesth.)

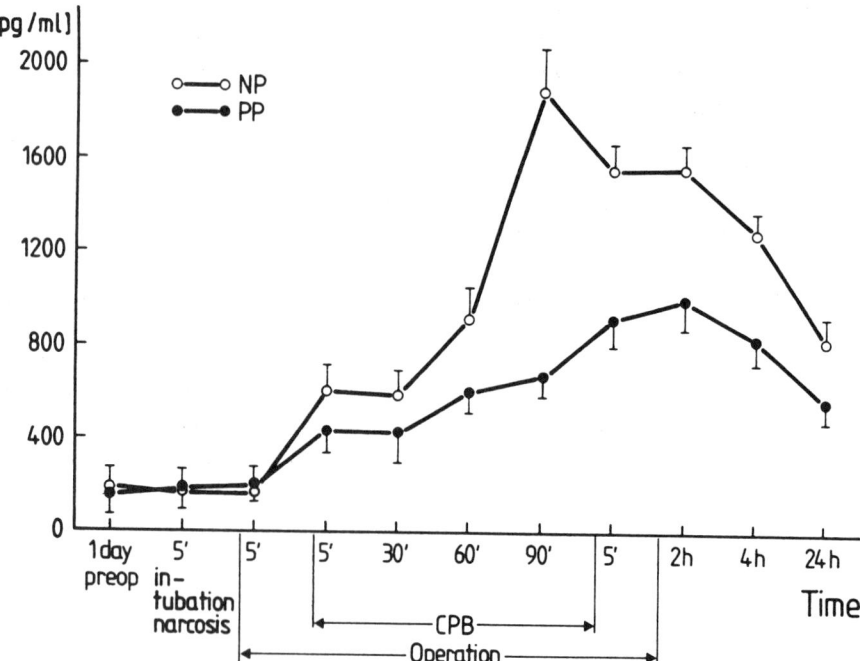

FIGURE 9.16. Differences in plasma epinephrine concentrations (y-axis) during cardiac surgery using nonpulsatile (NP) and pulsatile perfusion (PP). (From Minami et al,[61] by permission of *J Thorac Cardiovasc Surg.*)

namic consequences, manifested by exaggerated α-adrenergic responsiveness, increased systemic vascular resistance (SVR), and elevated perfusion pressure during CPB. Increased SVR during crossclamping of the aorta may lead to washout of cardioplegic solution through collateral circulation and thus impair the myocardial protective effect of cardioplegia.

The use of opioids alone can block the stress response in children prior to CPB.[66] In adults, the stress response can be attenuated, but not completely blocked, during CPB by alfentanil, fentanyl, sufentanil, propofol, enflurane, and isoflurane, and is related to the depth of anesthesia.[37,42,50,67,68] As mentioned in the previous section, results from early studies using halothane anesthesia suggested that halothane inhibited adrenal catecholamine release because of decreased circulating levels of epinephrine and norepinephrine throughout the bypass period. Clonidine, an α-2 agonist that continually inhibits release of adrenergic neurotransmitters, also attenuates the stress response to CPB.[69] Attenuation of vasopressin and catecholamine

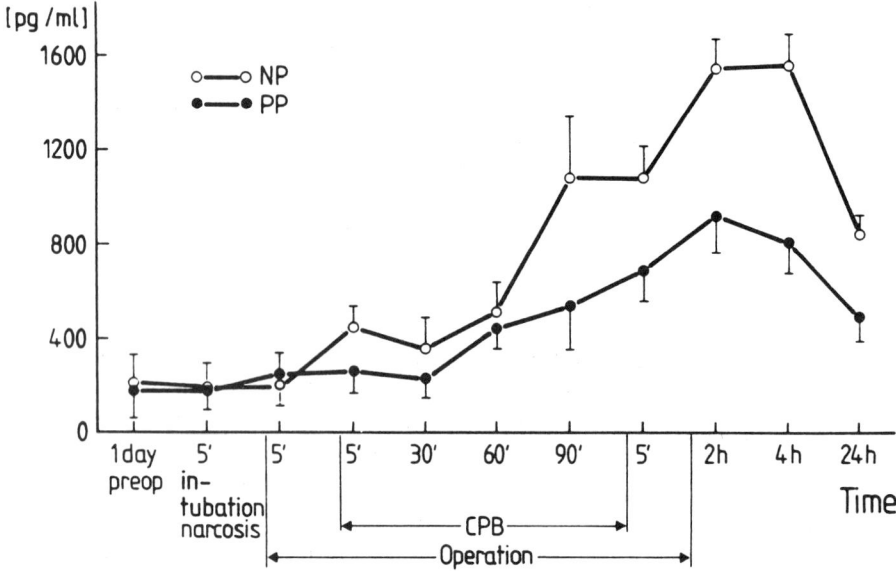

FIGURE 9.17. Differences in plasma norepinephrine concentrations (y-axis) during cardiac surgery using nonpulsatile (NP) and pulsatile perfusion (PP). (From Minami et al,[61] by permission of *J Thorac Cardiovasc Surg.*)

9. Endocrine System

release has been associated with the use of pulsatile flow during CPB.[62] Whether blunting of the stress response protects against the deleterious effects of CPB or reduces morbidity or mortality is still unknown.

Parathyroid and Thyroid Function During CPB

Parathyroid

During hemostatic physiologic conditions, parathyroid hormone (PTH) maintains plasma ionized calcium concentrations within 5% of normal values by effecting a rapid reabsorption of calcium from the bone into extracellular fluids, and by increasing renal tubular reabsorption of calcium and magnesium ions, while decreasing phosphate reabsorption. Calcitriol (the active form of vitamin D) and magnesium enhance the effect of PTH on bone, gastrointestinal, and renal tubular transport of calcium.

CPB routinely results in disturbances in plasma ionized calcium levels. With the onset of CPB, ionized calcium levels decrease and then gradually return toward baseline values by the time of separation from CPB. PTH also decreases on initiation of CPB, remains inappropriately reduced during the early period of CPB, and then gradually increases to maximum values after approximately 90 minutes of bypass. Total calcium and magnesium levels decline at the onset of CPB and remain depressed throughout the procedure. Calcitriol concentrations are unchanged. The low magnesium concentration may delay the PTH response to hypocalcemia. However, magnesium sulfate supplements given during CPB to maintain normal magnesium levels do not result in normal parathyroid secretion of PTH or normal ionized calcium levels during CPB.[70]

The effect of temperature management during CPB on PTH levels is controversial. In one study, no difference in PTH response was found between patients undergoing normothermic or hypothermic CPB.[70] Other investigators report that PTH release is pH- and temperature-dependent during CPB. Chambers and colleagues[71] reported that if the temperature is maintained at or greater than 30°C, a rise in PTH concentration up to 5 times normal occurs during and after CPB, as the pH decreases. In contrast, patients cooled to less than 30°C have no change in PTH levels, even when pH drops to less than 7.3. In this study, PTH levels increased appropriately as these patients were rewarmed.

Thyroid

Thyroid hormone has profound effects on the heart, vascular system, and other major organ systems (Table 9.2).

TABLE 9.2. Actions of thyroid hormone.

↑ Oxygen consumption
↑ Cardiac output
↑ Cardiac contractility
↑ Cardiac mass
↓ Peripheral vascular resistance
↑ Renal blood flow
↑ Renal and hepatic clearance of drug
↑ Hepatic protein synthesis
↑ Skeletal muscle blood flow and oxygen consumption
↑ Myocardial β-adrenergic sensitivity

Triiodothyronine (T_3) is primarily responsible for thyroid hormone effects in the body. Thyroxine (T_4) is extensively protein bound, less available in the circulation, and less active than T_3. Reverse T_3 (rT_3) is the inactive metabolite of T_4 enzymatic conversion in the peripheral circulation. Thyroid stimulating hormone (TSH) from the anterior pituitary gland controls thyroxine release from the thyroid gland.

Several studies have documented the changes in T_3, T_4, rT_3, and TSH levels during cardiac surgery and CPB. Total T_3 and free fraction (unbound) T_3 fall precipitously at the onset of CPB.[72,73] T_3 levels rise to 60% of preoperative values after CPB but remain significantly lower than normal, even at 24 hours postoperatively (Figures 9.18 and

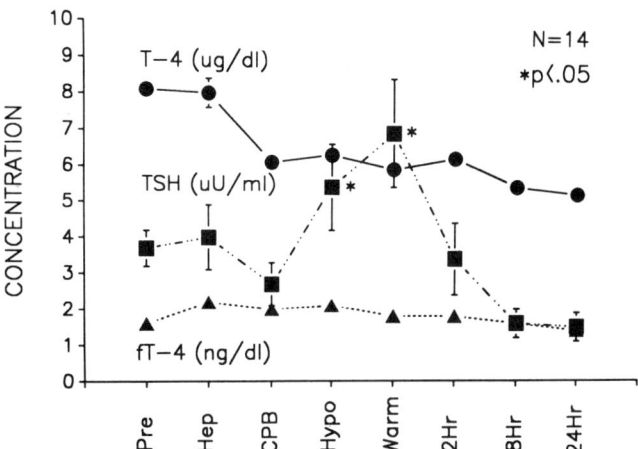

FIGURE 9.18. Concentrations of thyroxine (T-4), free thyroxine (fT-4), and thyroid-stimulating hormone (TSH) before CPB (Pre), after administration of heparin (Hep), after initiation of CPB, at the nadir of hypothermia (Hypo), after rewarming (Warm), and at 2, 8, and 24 hours after CPB. Normal values are as follows: T-4, 64.35-28.7 nmol/L (5-10 μg/dL); fT-4, 12.87-24.45 pmol/L (1.0-1.9 ng/dL); TSH, 0.4-4.6 mU/L (0.4-4.6 μg/dL). [Reprinted with permission from the Society of Thoracic Surgeons (*The Annals of Thoracic Surgery*, 1991, 52:46-50).]

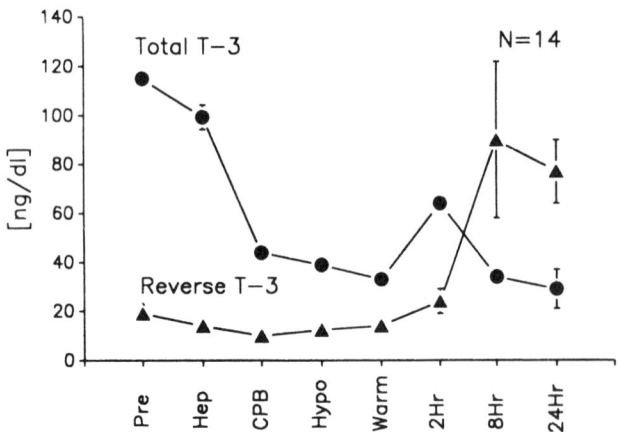

FIGURE 9.19. Concentrations of total triiodothyronine (T-3) and reverse T-3 before CPB (Pre), after administration of heparin (Hep), after initiation of CPB, at the nadir of hypothermia (Hypo), after rewarming (Warm), and at 2, 8, and 24 hours after CPB. Normal values are as follows: T-3, 1.35–2.49 nmol/L (88–162 ng/dL); reverse T-3, 5.0–19.4 ng/dL. [Reprinted with permission from the Society of Thoracic Surgeons (*The Annals of Thoracic Surgery*, 1991, 52:46–50).]

9.19). Total T_4 and TSH are reduced but remain within normal ranges throughout CPB. After CPB, rT_3 increases more than fourfold.[74] Heparin has been shown to increase free T_3 and free T_4 concentrations.[75] The early decrease in TSH is thought to be secondary to the slightly elevated T_4 fraction (FT_4) levels, since cellular T_4 is the major regulator of TSH secretion. Thyrotropin-releasing hormone (TRH), administered intravenously during hypothermic CPB, yields a delayed and blunted TSH response which may be due to slightly elevated FT_4 or to hypothermia.[76]

A syndrome characterized by low T_3, low to normal T_4, high rT_3, and normal TSH follows cardiac surgery and CPB.[74] This set of findings is consistent with the *euthyroid sick syndrome* described in patients with an acute change in thyroid function associated with severe systemic illness. This is in contrast to primary hypothyroidism in which T_3 is normal, T_4 is decreased, and TSH is elevated. The normal increase in TSH and T_4 that should occur in the presence of low T_3 levels does not occur in patients after CPB.[74]

Administration of T_3 to patients having cardiac procedures to correct the profound decrease in T_3 levels has been evaluated in a limited number of trials.[77] In one study, T_3-treated patients with left ventricular ejection fractions of less than 30% required less inotropic support and fewer diuretics than untreated control patients. T_3-treated patients with ejection fractions greater than 40% had improved stroke volumes and cardiac outputs as well as decreased systemic and pulmonary vascular resistances.[78] In animal studies, T_3 has not been shown to improve myocardial performance in normal hearts; however, in ischemic hearts, a marked improvement in left ventricular function may occur.[79,80] Although controversy exists regarding thyroid administration in patients with coronary artery disease (thyroid hormones increase heart rate and myocardial contractility, thereby increasing oxygen consumption and potentially precipitating myocardial ischemia), the potential exists for T_3 to be used for acute augmentation of cardiac function. Studies are in progress to determine the mechanism by which T_3 improves myocar-

TABLE 9.3. Summary of hormonal changes during cardiac surgery and CPB.

Hormone	Induction of anesthesia	Initiation of CPB	End of CPB	Early postoperative period	Return to control levels
ADH	↑ on incision	↑↑	↑	↑	POD 5
ACTH	↑	↓	N	↑	w/in 1^h CPB
Aldosterone	↑	↓then↑	↑(peak)	---	---
Cortisol	↑	↓	↑↑	↑^{a}	POD 2-7
Growth hormone	↑	↑	↑^{b}	↑/N	6^h post CPB
Epinephrine	{slight ↓ with	↑(ninefold)	↑	↑↓	{hours to
Norepinephrine	opioids}	↑(twofold)	↑	↑↓	several days}
Insulin					
Diabetic^c	↑	↓	↑	↓	POD 3-7
Nondiabetic	↓	↓	↑^{d}	↑	POD 7
PTH	N	↓	↑^{e}	N	---
T4	N	±↓/N	±↓/N	±↓/N	---
T3	N	↓↓	↓	↓	POD 5-7
TSH	N	↓	±↑/N	↓/N	---

POD = postoperative day
^{a}Peak 6-24^h postop[41]
^{b}Peak at 120 min of CPB[18,19]
^{c}Values reflect insulin *requirements* since patients are insulin deficient
^{d}Levels increase with rewarming
^{e}Peak at 90 min of CPB[70]

dial performance and whether or not its use decreases patient morbidity and mortality following cardiac surgery.

The effect of CPB on thyroid function in children has also been reported. As in adults, T_3 levels in children decrease during and after CPB. At 24 hours postoperatively, T_3 levels are 35% of the postinduction values and these changes are independent of anesthetic technique.[81] The levels gradually approach normal values at 5 to 7 days after surgery. TSH levels drop with CPB and then rise to 2.5 times normal within 30 minutes of CPB. The levels then fall to a nadir at 12 hours post-CPB, and gradually rise to normal by the third postoperative day.

In infants weighing less than 5 kg, T_3 and T_4 levels fall more than 50% with CPB, slightly increase 3 to 6 hours after CPB, and plummet to 78% below preoperative values at 48 hours postoperatively. In one study, two infants who died, and one other who had an unstable postoperative course, never achieved normal T_3 and T_4 levels.[81]

Summary

Table 9.3 summarizes hormonal changes during cardiac surgery and CPB.

References

1. Slotnick IL, Teigland JP. Cardiac accidents following vasopressin injection. *JAMA* 1951;146:1126-1129.
2. Millette B, Huet PM, Lavoie P, et al. Portal and systemic effects of selective infusion of vasopressin into the superior mesenteric artery in cirrhotic patients. *Gastroenterology* 1975;69:6-12.
3. Philbin DM, Coggins CH, Wilson N, et al. Antidiuretic hormone levels during cardiopulmonary bypass. *J Thorac Cardiovasc Surg* 1977;73:145-148.
4. Schaff HV, Mashburn JP, McCarthy PM, et al. Natriuresis during and early after cardiopulmonary bypass: relationship to atrial natriuretic factor, aldosterone and antidiuretic hormone. *J Thorac Cardiovasc Surg* 1989;98:979-986.
5. Philbin DM, Coggins CH, Emerson SW, et al. Plasma vasopressin levels and urinary sodium excretion during cardiopulmonary bypass. Comparison of halothane and morphine anesthesia. *J Thorac Cardiovasc Surg* 1979;77:582-585.
6. Stanley TH, Philbin DM, Coggins CH. Fentanyl oxygen anesthesia for coronary artery surgery. Cardiovascular and antidiuretic hormone responses. *Can Anaesth Soc J* 1979;26:168-172.
7. Kuitunen A, Hynynen M, Salmenpera M, et al. Anaesthesia affects plasma concentrations of vasopressin, von Willebrand factor and coagulation factor VIII in cardiac surgical patients. *Br J Anaesth* 1993;70:173-180.
8. Boulton AJ, Wilson N, Turnbull KW, et al. Haemodynamic and plasma vasopressin responses during high-dose fentanyl or sufentanil anaesthesia. *Can Anaesth Soc J* 1986;33:475-483.
9. Levine FH, Philbin DM, Coggins CH, et al. Plasma vasopressin levels and urinary Na$^+$ excretion during cardiopulmonary bypass: a comparison of pulsatile and nonpulsatile flow. *Surg Forum* 1978;29:320-322.
10. Levine FH, Philbin DM, Kono K, et al. Plasma vasopressin levels and urinary sodium excretion during cardiopulmonary bypass with and without pulsatile flow. *Ann Thorac Surg* 1981;32:63-67.
11. Frater RWM, Wakayama S, Oka Y, et al. Pulsatile cardiopulmonary bypass: failure to influence hemodynamics or hormones. *Circulation* 1980;62(suppl I):I19-I25.
12. Philbin DM, Coggins CH. Plasma vasopressin levels during cardiopulmonary bypass with and without profound hemodilution. *Can Anaesth Soc J* 1978;25(4):282-285.
13. Wu W, Zbuzek VK, Bellevue C. Vasopressin release during cardiac operation. *J Thorac Cardiovasc Surg* 1980;79:83-90.
14. Yokota H, Kawashima Y, Hashimoto S, et al. Plasma cortisol, luteinizing hormone and prolactin secretory responses to cardiopulmonary bypass. *J Surg Res* 1977;23:196-200.
15. Taylor KM, Bremner WF, Gray CE, et al. Anterior pituitary function during cardiopulmonary bypass. *Br J Surg* 1976;63:161-162.
16. Chevals WJ, Bestrian BR. Role of exogenous growth hormone and insulin-like growth factor I in malnutrition and acute metabolic stress. *Crit Care Med* 1991;19:1317-1322.
17. Vigas M, Malatinsky J, Nemeth S, et al. Alpha adrenergic control of growth hormone release during surgical stress in man. *Metabolism* 1977;26:399-402.
18. Salter CP, Fluck DC, Stimmler L. Effect of open heart surgery on growth hormone levels in man. *Lancet* 1972;2:853-854.
19. Macdonald RG, Buckler JM, Deverall PB, et al. Growth hormone and blood glucose concentrations during cardiopulmonary bypass. *Br J Anaesth* 1975;47:713-718.
20. Brandt MR, Korshen J, Hansen AP, et al. Influence of morphine anaesthesia on the endocrine-metabolic response to open heart surgery. *Acta Anaesth Scand* 1978;22:400-412.
21. Sebel PS, Bovill JG, Schellekers APM, et al. Hormonal responses to high dose fentanyl anaesthesia. A study in patients undergoing cardiac surgery. *Br J Anaesth* 1981;53:941-948.
22. Glick SM, Rota J, Yalow RS, et al. The regulation of growth hormone secretion. *Recent Prog Horm Res* 1963;21:241-242.
23. Kuntschen FR, Galletti PM, Hahn C. Glucose insulin interactions during CPB. *J Thorac Cardiovasc Surg* 1986;91:451-459.
24. Kuntschen FR, Galletti PM, Hahn C, et al. Alterations of insulin and glucose metabolism during CPB under normothermia. *J Thorac Cardiovasc Surg* 1985;89:97-106.
25. McKnight CK, Elliott MJ, Pearson DT, et al. The effects of four different crystalloid bypass pump-priming fluids upon the metabolic response to cardiac operation. *J Thorac Cardiovasc Surg* 1985;90:97-111.
26. Nagaoka H, Innami R, Watanabe M, et al. Preservation of pancreatic beta cell function with pulsatile CPB. *Ann Thorac Surg* 1989;48:798-802.
27. Longstreth WJ Jr, Inill TS. High blood glucose level on hospital admission and poor neurologic recovery after cardiac arrest. *Ann Neurol* 1984;15:59-63.
28. Werb MR, Zinman B, Teasdale SJ, et al. Hormone and met-

abolic responses during coronary artery bypass surgery: role of infused glucose. *J Clin Endocrinol Metab* 1989;69:1010-1018.
29. Jones RM, Knight PR, Hill AB, et al. Termination of CPB facilitated by insulin. *Anaesthesia* 1981;36:394-397.
30. Krukenkamp IB, Sorlie D, Silverman N, et al. Direct effect of high dose insulin on the depressed heart after beta blockade or ischemia. *Thorac Cardiovasc Surg* 1986;34:305-309.
31. Harder W, Benzer H, Schutz W, et al. Improvement of cardiac preservation by preoperative high insulin supply. *J Thorac Cardiovasc Surg* 1984;88:294-300.
32. Oldfield AS, Commerford PJ, Opie LH. Effects of preoperative G-I-K on myocardial glycogen levels and on complications of mitral valve replacement. *J Thorac Cardiovasc Surg* 1986;91:874-878.
33. Sodi-Pallares D, Testille MR, Fishleder BL, et al. Effects of an intravenous infusion of a potassium-glucose-insulin solution on the electrocardiographic signs of myocardial infarction. *Am J Cardiol* 1962;9:166-181.
34. Rackley CE, Russel RO Jr, Rogers WJ, et al. Clinical experience with G-I-K therapy in acute myocardial infarction. *Am Heart J* 1981;102:1038-1049.
35. Krukenkamp IB, Silverman NA, Sorlie D, et al. Direct cardiac effects of supramaximal insulin. *Curr Surg* 1986;43:300-302.
36. Bolt J, Knothe C, Zickmann B, et al. Influence of different glucose-insulin-potassium regimes on glucose homeostasis and hormonal response in cardiac surgery patients. *Anesth Analg* 1993;76:233-238.
37. Laycock GJ, Mitchell IM, Paton RP, et al. EEG burst suppression with propofol during CPB in children. *Br J Anaesth* 1992;69:356-362.
38. Crock PA, Levy CJ, Martin IK, et al. Hormonal and metabolic changes during hypothermic CPB in diabetic and nondiabetic subjects. *Diabetic Med* 1988;5:47-52.
39. Seki S. Clinical features of hyperosmolar hyperglycemic nonketotic coma associated with cardiac operations. *J Thorac Cardiovasc Surg* 1986;91:867-873.
40. Sandberg AD, Eik-Nes K, Samuels LT, et al. The effects of surgery on the blood levels and metabolism of 17-hydroxycorticosteroids in man. *J Clin Invest* 1954;33:1509.
41. Taylor KM, Jones JV, Walker MS, et al. The cortisol response during heart-lung bypass. *Circulation* 1976;54:20-25.
42. Walsh ES, Paterson SL, O'Riordon TBA, et al. Effect of high dose fentanyl anesthesia on the metabolic and endocrine response to cardiac surgery. *Br J Anaesth* 1981;53:1155-1165.
43. Taylor KM, MacIntyre HB, Grant JK, et al. Pituitary-adrenal response patterns during open heart surgery. *J Endocrinol* 1979;81:127P-128P.
44. Taylor KM, Wright GS, Reid JM, et al. Comparative studies of pulsatile and nonpulsatile flow during CPB II. The effects on adrenal secretion of cortisol. *J Thorac Cardiovasc Surg* 1978;75:574-578.
45. Kono K, Philbin DM, Coggins CH, et al. Adrenocortical hormone levels during cardiopulmonary bypass with and without pulsatile flow. *J Thorac Cardiovasc Surg* 1983;85:129-133.
46. Pollock EMM, Pollock JCS, Jamieson MPG, et al. Adrenocortical hormone concentrations in children during cardiopulmonary bypass with and without pulsatile flow. *Br J Anaesth* 1988;60:536-541.
47. Weiskopf M, Braunstein GP, Bateman TM, et al. Adrenal function following coronary bypass surgery. *Am Heart J* 1985;110:71-76.
48. Reier CE, George JM, Kilman JW. Cortisol and growth hormone response to surgical stress during morphine anesthesia. *Anesth Analg* 1973;52:1003-1010.
49. Hasbrouck JD. Morphine anesthesia for open-heart surgery. *Ann Thorac Surg* 1970;10:364-369.
50. Flezzani P, Croughwell DD, McIntyre RW, et al. Isoflurane decreases cortisol response to cardiopulmonary bypass. *Anesth Analg* 1986;65:1117-1122.
51. Oyama T, Taniguichi K, Jin T, et al. Effects of anaesthesia and surgery on plasma aldosterone concentration and renin activity in man. *Br J Anaesth* 1979;51:747-751.
52. Bailey DR, Miller ED Jr, Kaplan JA, et al. The renin-angiotensin-aldosterone system during cardiac surgery with morphine-nitrous oxide anesthesia. *Anesthesiology* 1975;42:538-544.
53. Taylor KM, Bain WH, Russell M, et al. Peripheral vascular resistance and angiotensin II levels during pulsatile and nonpulsatile CPB. *Thorax* 1979;34:594-598.
54. Reves JG, Karp RB, Buttner EE, et al. Neuronal and adrenomedullary catecholamine release in response to cardiopulmonary bypass in man. *Circulation* 1982;66:49-55.
55. Landymore RW, Murphy PA, Kinley CE, et al. Does pulsatile flow influence the incidence of postoperative hypertension? *Ann Thorac Surg* 1979;28:261-268.
56. Balasaraswathi K, Glisson SN, El-Eti AA, et al. Serum epinephrine and norepinephrine during valve replacement and aortocoronary bypass. *Can Anaesth Soc J* 1978;25:198-203.
57. Kaul TK, Sewamenathan R, Chatrath RR, et al. Vasoactive pressure hormones during and after cardiopulmonary bypass. *Int J Artif Organs* 1990;13:293-299.
58. Federsen K, Aurell M, Delin K, et al. Effects of cardiopulmonary bypass and prostacyclin on plasma catecholamines, angiotensin II and arginine-vasopressin. *Acta Anaesthesiol Scand* 1985;29:224-230.
59. Hine IP, Wood WG, Maenwaring-Burton RW, et al. The adrenergic response to surgery involving cardiopulmonary bypass, as measured by plasma and urinary catecholamine concentrations. *Br J Anaesth* 1976;48:355-363.
60. Balasaraswathi K, Glisson SN, El-Eti AA, et al. Effect of priming volume on serum catecholamines during cardiopulmonary bypass. *Can Anaesth Soc J* 1980;27:135-139.
61. Minami K, Korner MM, Vyska K, et al. Effects of pulsatile perfusion on plasma catecholamine levels and hemodynamics during and after cardiac operations with cardiopulmonary bypass. *J Thorac Cardiovasc Surg* 1990;99:82-91.
62. Philbin DM, Levine FH, Kono K, et al. Attenuation of the stress response to cardiopulmonary bypass by the addition of pulsatile flow. *Circulation* 1981;64:808-812.
63. Replogle R, Levy M, DeWall RA, et al. Catecholamine and serotonin response to cardiopulmonary bypass. *J Thorac Cardiovasc Surg* 1962;44:638-639.
64. Nadeau RA, deChamplain J. Plasma catecholamines in acute myocardial infarction. *Am Heart J* 1979;98:548-549.
65. Reves JG, Croughwell N, Jacobs JR, et al. Anesthesia dur-

ing cardiopulmonary bypass: does it matter. In: Tinker JH, ed. *Cardiopulmonary Bypass: Current Concepts and Controversies*. Philadelphia: WB Saunders; 1989:69-93.
66. Morgan P, Lynne AM, Parrot C, et al. Hemodynamic and metabolic effects of two anesthetic techniques in children undergoing surgical repair of acyanotic congenital heart disease. *Anesth Analg* 1987;66:1028-1030.
67. Samuelson PN, Reves JG, Kirklin JK, et al. Comparison of sufentanil and enflurane-nitrous oxide anesthesia for myocardial revascularization. *Anesth Analg* 1986;65:217-226.
68. Hynynen M, Lehtinen AM, Salmenpera M, et al. Continuous infusion of fentanyl or alfentanil for coronary artery surgery. *Br J Anaesth* 1986;58:1260-1266.
69. Flacke JW, Bloor BC, Flacke WE, et al. Reduced narcotic requirement by clonidine with improved hemodynamic and adrenergic stability in patients undergoing coronary bypass surgery. *Anesthesiology* 1987;67:11-19.
70. Robertie PG, Butterworth JF IV, Roysten RL, et al. Normal parathyroid response to hypocalcemia during cardiopulmonary bypass. *Anesthesiology* 1991;75:43-48.
71. Chambers DJ, Dunham J, Braimbridge MV, et al. The effect of ionized calcium, pH and temperature on bioactive parathyroid hormone during and after open-heart operations. *Ann Thorac Surg* 1983;36:306-313.
72. Bremner WF, Taylor KM, Baird S, et al. Hypothalamo-pituitary-thyroid axis function during cardiopulmonary bypass. *J Thorac Cardiovasc Surg* 1978;75:392-399.
73. Robuschi G, Medici D, Fesani F, et al. Cardiopulmonary bypass: a low T_4 and T_3 syndrome with blunted thyrotropin (TSH) response to thyrotropin-releasing hormone (TRH). *Horm Res* 1986;23:151-158.
74. Holland FW II, Brown PS Jr, Weintraub BD, et al. Cardiopulmonary bypass and thyroid function: euthyroid sick syndrome. *Ann Thorac Surg* 1991;52:46-50.
75. Saeed-Uz-Zafar M, Miller MJ, Breneman GM, et al. Observation of the effect of heparin on free and total thyroxine. *J Clin Endocrinol Metab* 1971;32:633-640.
76. Taylor KM, Wright GS, Bremner WF, et al. Anterior pituitary response to thyrotropin-releasing hormone during open heart surgery. *Cardiovasc Res* 1978;12:114-119.
77. Novitzky D, Cooper DKC, Barton CI, et al. Triiodothyronine as an inotropic agent after open heart surgery. *J Thorac Cardiovasc Surg* 1989;98:972-977.
78. Dyke CM, Yeh T Jr, Lehman JD, et al. Triiodothyronine-enhanced left ventricular function after ischemic injury. *Ann Thorac Surg* 1991;52:14-19.
79. Novitzky D, Human PA, Cooper DKC. Inotropic effect of triiodothyronine following myocardial ischemia and cardiopulmonary bypass: an experimental study in pigs. *Ann Thorac Surg* 1988;45:50-55.
80. Novitzky D, Matthews N, Shawly D, et al. Triiodothyronine in the recovery of stunned myocardium in dogs. *Ann Thorac Surg* 1991;51:10-17.
81. Mitchell IM, Pollock JCS, Jameison MPG, et al. The effects of cardiopulmonary bypass on thyroid function in infants weighing less than five kilograms. *J Thorac Cardiovasc Surg* 1992;103:800-805.

Part III
Mechanics and Components of the Heart-Lung Machine

10
Oxygenators for Extracorporeal Circulation

Philip D. Beckley, David W. Holt, and Richard D. Tallman, Jr.

Introduction

It is difficult to single out one development in the science of extracorporeal circulation that made possible the current achievements in cardiac surgery. But the artificial lung, or "oxygenator," is certainly a key component in the performance of cardiopulmonary bypass (CPB). As one reviews the development of the basic components of the bypass apparatus, one can readily see that few have undergone a more dramatic and fascinating course than the oxygenator. However, it is beyond the scope and intent of this chapter to provide a detailed account of its early development or to give proper credit to the many investigators whose work over decades made today's technology possible. For a more detailed survey of the history of oxygenators, the reader is referred to Chapter 1 in this text.[1-5]

Early oxygenating devices utilized the filming concept, that is, bringing a thin layer of blood, supported by screens or disks, into contact with a surrounding oxygen environment. John Gibbon, Jr., credited in 1953 with being the first to use CPB successfully to repair a *human* congenital defect,[6] had provided the first descriptions of a filming oxygenator nearly 15 years earlier.[7-9] These early filming devices were complex, required enormous priming volumes to operate, and caused extensive hemocompatibility problems. The filming oxygenator went through a variety of early modifications, including the familiar disk oxygenator used by Bjork[10] and further modified by Melrose[11] and Cross.[12] Although successfully used in numerous cardiac procedures, the filming oxygenator proved to be an impractical approach to the rapidly growing application of CPB.

The use of bubbles to provide gas transfer was proposed very early in the development of the oxygenator, but all investigators could readily see the hazards of introducing air into the circulatory system. Not until Clark[13] proposed using silicone compounds as defoaming agents did the use of bubbles for gas transfer during CPB become feasible. Dewall and Lillehei[14] developed the helix reservoir as an approach to final defoaming and temperature regulation in the bubble oxygenator. Disposable bag oxygenators incorporating this design quickly followed, as developed by Gott,[15] Hyman,[16] and Rygg and Kyvsgaard.[17,18] This helix design was to become an important feature of many future oxygenators, allowing them to become effective, simple, affordable, and disposable.

In 1944, Kolff had noted that blood was oxygenated as it passed through cellulose dialyzing membranes while patients were on hemodialysis.[19] Shortly after Gibbon's historic surgery, Kolff developed an early polyethylene membrane lung used successfully in numerous experimental trials.[20] Clowes[21] proposed a sandwich-type membrane oxygenator, which was clinically used a few years later.[22] This device became the prototype for more manageable and safer Z-fold sheet-membrane oxygenators. In 1963, Kolobow[23] proposed using silicone rubber in a coiled membrane configuration that remains a respected design today. In that same year, Bodell[24] proposed a silicone rubber, hollow-fiber membrane design, and microporous membrane technology was first proposed by McCaughan in 1969.[25] Further contributions toward the development of membrane lungs were made by Peirce,[26] Lande,[27] and Bramson.[28]

The Ideal Oxygenator

The design objectives of an "ideal" oxygenator (Table 10.1) have not significantly changed since 1962 when Galletti and Brecher described,[29] the "ideal" oxygenator as one that provided:

1. *Oxygenation of venous blood*. There must be a safe and efficient means whereby venous blood is brought into proximity to a source for oxygen transfer. The blood must be a thin film to overcome the barrier to oxygenation posed by large diffusion distances. The device must have sufficient capacity to provide oxygenation over a wide range of venous inlet conditions.

TABLE 10.1. Design objectives of the ideal oxygenator.

Oxygenation of venous blood
Carbon dioxide elimination
Minimum trauma to the blood
Small priming volume
Safety

2. *Carbon dioxide elimination*. There must be a safe and efficient means whereby carbon dioxide can be eliminated in sufficient quantities to avoid arterial hypercarbia or hypocarbia.
3. *Minimum trauma to the blood*. The gas-exchange process must be associated with minimum damage to blood cells, platelets, and protein. This must be accomplished, in part, by careful design of the device to avoid high shear stress, areas of turbulence, and incompatible surfaces. Trauma induced by the direct exposure of gas to blood must be considered.
4. *Small priming volume*. The oxygenator must be able to perform adequate gas exchange with a minimum contribution to the total priming volume of the extracorporeal circuit. This pertains to the impact of hemodilution, not only on oxygen delivery (hemoglobin dilution), but also on protein concentration (eg, proteins responsible for oncotic pressure, immunoglobulins, and procoagulants). Manufacturers should provide devices that can be "sized" to the patient, thereby ensuring adequate oxygen transfer with minimum priming volume.
5. *Safety*. The device must be easily assembled, primed, and operated. It must be designed to allow important components to be highly accessible and visible, and it must be constructed to minimize the possibility of air embolism during normal operation.

Bubble Oxygenators

Design

The bubble oxygenator is constructed to include three primary sections of operation: the bubble column, the debubbling/defoaming area, and the arterial reservoir (Figure 10.1). In all cases, the arterial reservoir should be housed around the debubbling/defoaming area. However, the position of the bubble column may be arranged in one of two designs: sequential or concentric (Figure 10.2). In the sequential design, the bubble column is distinctly separate from, but in series with, the other two sections of operation. In the concentric design, the bubble column is surrounded by the debubbling/defoaming area and the arterial reservoir, respectively. The theoretical advantages of the concentric design include a reduction of the contact between blood and foreign surfaces and a decrease in priming volume and heat loss. The concentric design may have venous blood and gas entering from the bottom of the bubble column with the resulting bubble/blood mixture ascending, or it may have the venous blood and gas entering at the top of the bubble column with the resulting bubble/blood mixture descending. In the sequential design, the venous blood and gas enter from the bottom of the bubble column, with the resulting bubble/blood mixture ascending.

All currently used bubble oxygenators have a number of common features (Table 10.2). Venous inlet and cardiotomy line connection ports are located at the proximal end of the bubble column. A gas dispersion device separates this blood entry point from the gas inlet port. The disperser may be in the form of a polycarbonate plate perforated with holes of precise dimension, or a core of porous silicate. The purpose of the disperser is to break the bulk gas entering the device into small bubbles, allowing gas exchange. Actual bubble size, as determined by the disperser, is a function of orifice diameter, gas flow rate, and blood viscosity and surface tension. The bubble column can be of various dimensions, depending upon the total area required for efficient gas exchange. A venous side heat exchanger is usually located in the path of this bubble column, and allows the venous and cardiotomy blood to be cooled and warmed.

The debubbling/defoaming area is made of polyurethane mesh sponges coated with a silicone compound

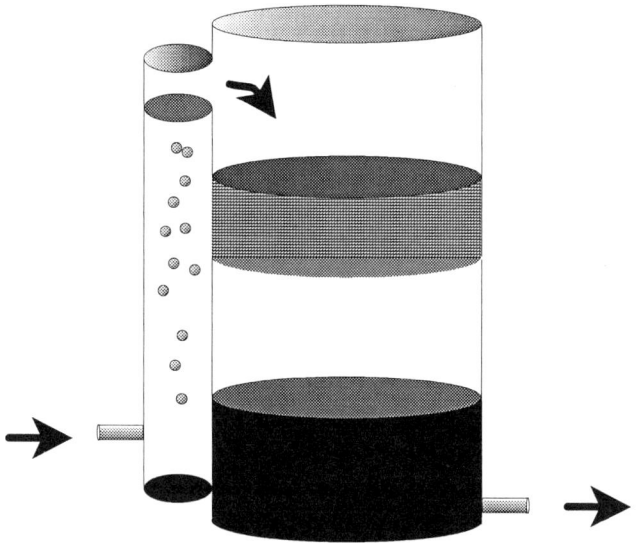

FIGURE 10.1. Diagram showing the three primary sections of operation of the bubble oxygenator: the bubble column followed by the debubbling/defoaming section followed by the arterial reservoir.

FIGURE 10.2. The bubble oxygenator may be configured in a concentric (top) or sequential (bottom) design.

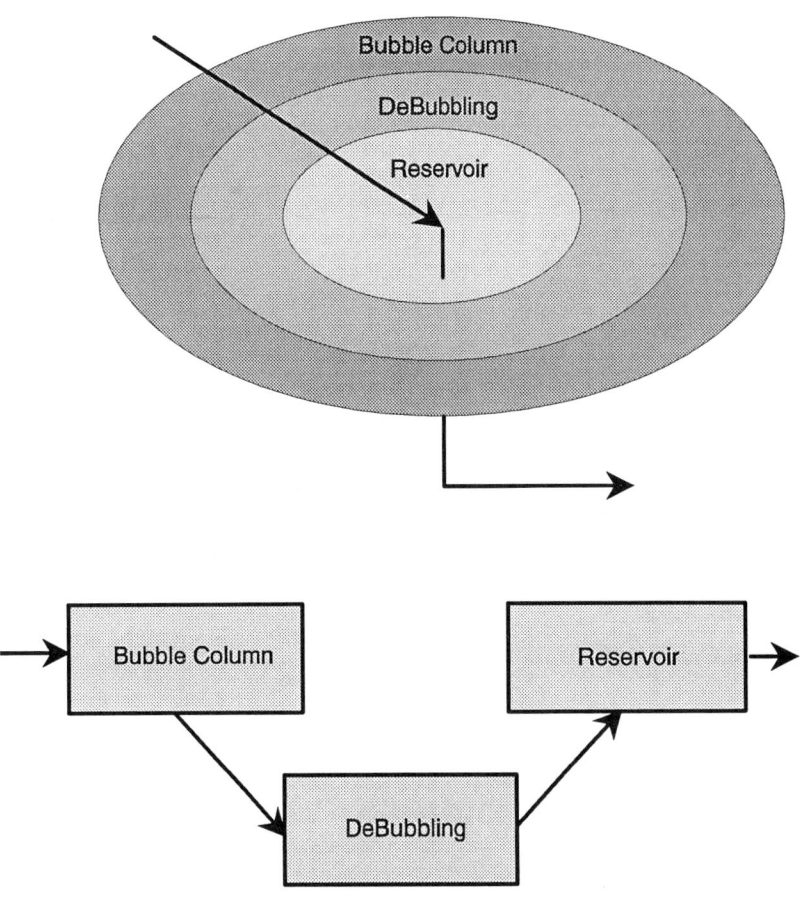

TABLE 10.2. Common features of the bubble oxygenator.

Bubble column
    Venous inlet port
    Cardiotomy inlet port
    Gas dispersion device
    Venous side heat exchanger
    Gas vent
    Fluid/drug administration port(s)
    Venous temperature probe well
Debubbling/defoaming area
    Defoaming sponges
    Antifoam compound
    Polyester fabric
Arterial reservoir
    Arterial outlet port
    Coronary (accessory) port
    Fluid/drug administration port(s)
    Arterial temperature probe well

(Antifoam A, Dow Corning Corporation, Midland, MI 48640). The role of this antifoam compound is to break the surface tension of bubbles coming through the debubbling/defoaming area, causing them to collapse. A polyester fabric surrounds the mesh sponges and functions as a final mechanism for the disruption of bubbles and a filtering medium (typically from 125 to 175 μm) for the blood passing into the arterial reservoir. Efficient bubble elimination by these components and the arterial reservoir is a function of mechanical disruption, surface area of the defoaming section, residence time in the defoaming section, flow pattern, velocity of flow, surface active agents, filtration, volume level, buoyancy, and absorption.[30-33]

An arterial outlet port and a coronary port are located at the bottom of the arterial reservoir. Blood is pumped from the arterial outlet and into the arterial line of the circuit. The arterial outlet must be designed to avoid vortexing of blood when the device is operated at low reservoir volumes (Figure 10.3, Baxter Healthcare Corporation, Bentley Laboratories Division). The coronary port may allow secondary access to arterial blood (Figure 10.4, Bentley Laboratories). This access site may be used for coronary perfusion, blood cardioplegia, cell processing, or any other technique that requires a source of blood.

All bubble oxygenators have a vent provided to allow gas to escape from the device (Figure 10.5, Bentley Laboratories). Some vent ports are designed to allow adaptation to gas-scavenging systems, for use when anesthetic gases are added to the gas source. All scavenging systems must be designed to avoid accidental alteration or obstruction of gas flow through the oxygenator.[34] In addition to the ports described, the devices should also have numerous fluid and drug administration ports as well as sampling ports in both the venous and the arterial paths. Fluids are generally administered into the circuit proximal to the debubbling and defoaming area, to limit entry of entrained air into the arterial reservoir. Drug ports are provided to allow administration of medications proximal to the debubbling/defoaming area or into the arterial reservoir itself. Studies have shown that some drugs (eg, nitroglycerin and fentanyl) are absorbed by polyvinylchloride, polyurethane, and silicone rubber, common materials found in the construction of oxygenators and CPB circuits[35-37] (see Chapter 4 for more discussion). Therefore, although one must understand the risks of administering any fluid with potentially entrained air,[31] adding drugs to the arterial reservoir may decrease the loss of drugs to surfaces and the consequent delay of action. Temperature probe wells are provided in the venous and arterial blood paths to allow monitoring of inlet and outlet temperature, respectively. Ports for blood oxygen saturation measurement may also be provided.

Principles of Gas Transfer

Gas bubbles are dispersed into the venous blood in the bubble column and act as vehicles for the transfer of both oxygen and carbon dioxide (Figure 10.6). Oxygen diffuses from the bubble into the blood film surrounding the bubble. This transfer is limited by the thickness of the blood film surrounding the bubble and the diffusion coefficient of oxygen in plasma. Adequate quantities of oxygen are transferred by diffusion owing to the high partial pressure gradient that exists between the gas in the bubble (potentially 100% oxygen) and the inlet blood Po_2. Carbon dioxide diffuses from the blood film into the bubble, which acts as a vehicle for carbon dioxide transport until the bubble bursts and the gas is released. Although this transport is limited by the low partial pressure gradient of carbon dioxide between the blood film and the bubble, adequate carbon dioxide transfer can occur owing to the high diffusion coefficient of carbon dioxide.

Bubble size is critical to adequate gas transfer. Since the bubble column has fixed dimensions, only a certain volume of bubbles can be accommodated. The surface area of a bubble is a function of the square of the radius, and the volume is a function of the cube of the radius; therefore, doubling the radius of a bubble will increase its surface area by a factor of four and its volume by a factor of

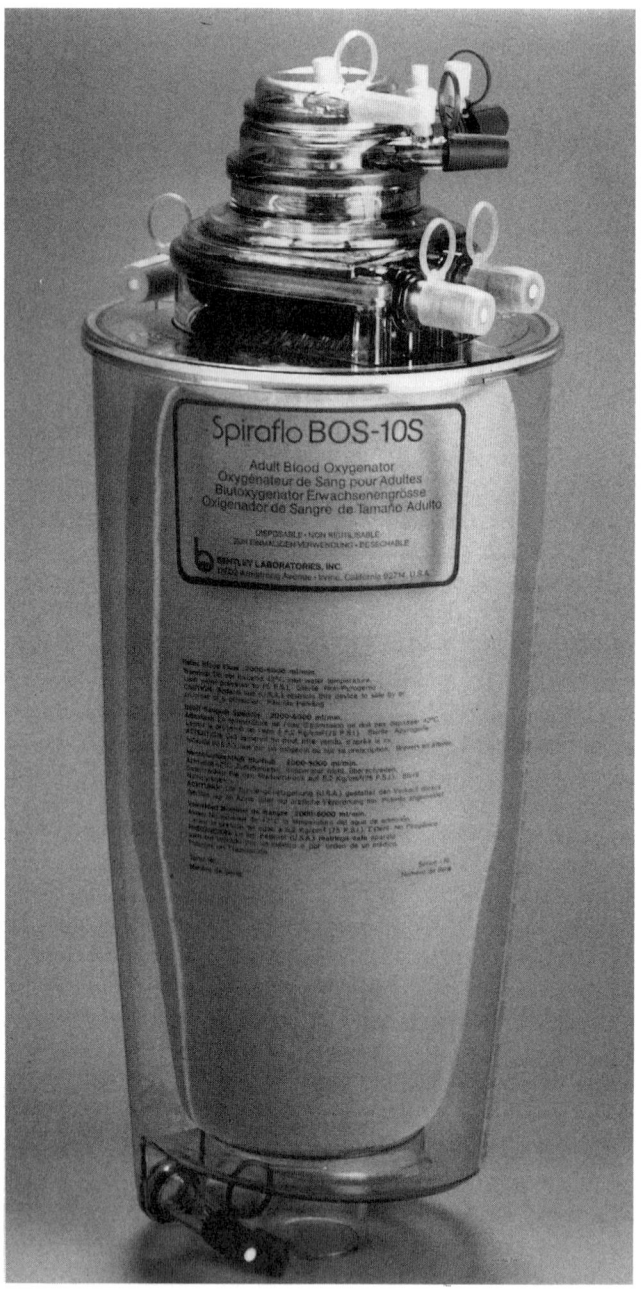

FIGURE 10.3. The arterial outlet of the bubble oxygenator is designed to avoid vortexing of the blood when operating the device at low reservoir volumes (Spiraflo BOS-10S, courtesy of Baxter Healthcare Corporation, Bentley Laboratories Division).

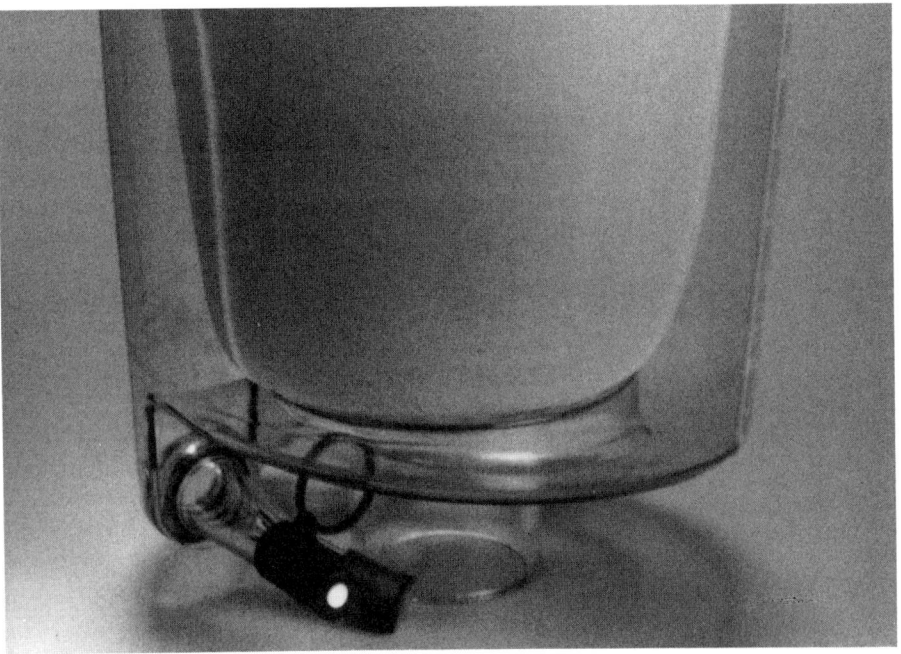

FIGURE 10.4. The coronary port of the bubble oxygenator is an access site which may be used for coronary perfusion, blood cardioplegia, or cell processing (Spiraflo BOS-10S, courtesy of Baxter Healthcare Corporation, Bentley Laboratories Division).

eight. Many small bubbles in a fixed column dimension would provide a large surface area for oxygen transfer (Figure 10.7). However, small bubbles are not efficient for carbon dioxide transfer. As oxygen diffuses from small bubbles to the blood film layer, the bubbles collapse and then are not available for carbon dioxide transfer. If the small bubbles do remain available for transfer, only limited amounts of carbon dioxide can be accommodated before equilibration occurs between the PCO_2 of the blood and that of the bubble. Additionally, small bubbles may be difficult to eliminate in the debubbling/defoaming area. Increasing the size of the bubble will increase carbon dioxide transfer due to the volume capacity available; however, oxygen transfer may be compromised due to a loss in the total surface area available in a fixed column dimension. The bubble size selected must be a compromise between optimal surface area for oxygen transfer and volume for carbon dioxide transfer. A gas dispersion plate is unlikely to produce bubbles of one precise size.[38] Generally, bubble sizes of 3 to 7 mm are used to optimize both oxygen and carbon dioxide gas transfer.[39]

As the bubble/blood mixture moves out of the bubble column and through the debubbling/defoaming area, the bubbles will burst, releasing their contents, which are then vented from the device. This gas environment provides a "secondary" oxygen and carbon dioxide transfer, via a filming process beyond that occurring purely from bubble exchange. If the total area available in the device for secondary oxygenation is decreased, total oxygen transfer may be significantly diminished. One way of compromising this available area is to operate the device with a large volume in the arterial reservoir. The higher the operating level, the smaller the area available outside of the bubble column for secondary oxygenation. For this reason, reservoir levels may be limited by the manufacturer.

It is not recommended that nitrogen be included in the ventilating gas of a bubble oxygenator, and, for this reason, some denitrogenation of the patient will occur. This nitrogen transfer will occur by a process similar to that described for carbon dioxide. Nitrogen diffuses according to its concentration gradient from the film of blood surrounding the bubble into the bubble itself. The nitrogen will be released when the bubble bursts and will be vented from the device. The amount of nitrogen removed from the patient will depend upon the length of the procedure. Much of the denitrogenation occurs both before and after the CPB procedure, due to ventilation of the patient with a high fraction of inlet gas oxygen (F_iO_2) source.

Blood Gas Management of the Bubble Oxygenator

The ventilating gas used with the bubble oxygenator is 100% oxygen or mixtures of oxygen and carbon dioxide. Mixtures that include nitrogen or room air would permit alterations in the F_iO_2 and resultant arterial PO_2, but this is not recommended owing to the instability of nitrogen bubbles. Since the F_iO_2 of the ventilating gas is usually fixed, direct adjustments of arterial PO_2 cannot be made in most bubble oxygenators. The one notable exception to this is the Bentley 10 Plus (Figure 10.8, Bentley Laboratories). This model provides a gas manifold control which allows splitting the gas source between the gas dispersion

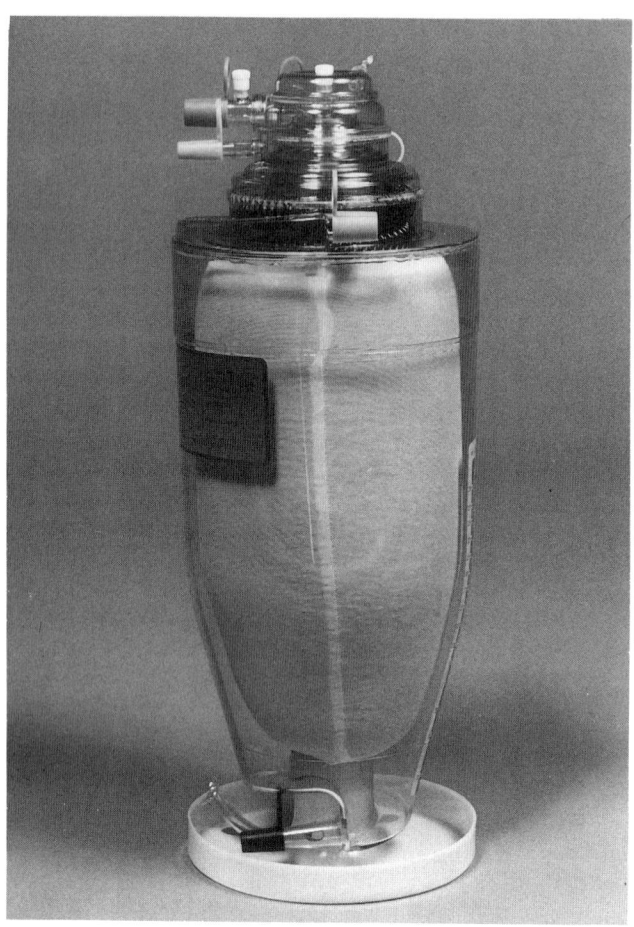

FIGURE 10.5. The bubble oxygenator must have a vent provided to allow gas to escape from the device (Spiraflo BOS-10S, courtesy of Baxter Healthcare Corporation, Bentley Laboratories Division).

device and the debubbling/defoaming area. Gas directed to the disperser forms bubbles for oxygen and carbon dioxide transfer, while gas directed to the debubbling/defoaming area serves to provide carbon dioxide exchange by means of filming. By increasing or decreasing the amount of total gas flow directed to the gas dispersion device, total oxygen transfer can be changed, thus increasing or decreasing arterial Po_2. In this way, independent control of Pao_2 and $Paco_2$ can be accomplished, and more physiologic Pao_2 values can be obtained.[40-43] Although more total gas flow may be necessary to maintain carbon dioxide exchange, this gas flow is not generating bubbles and does not appear to be associated with significantly higher gaseous microemboli release.[41]

Arterial Pco_2 is controlled by adjustments in gas-to-blood-flow ratio (GBFR). If the venous blood flow rate through the device matches the gas flow, the GBFR is 1.0. The GBFR is, in a sense, an indicator of the total bubble volume available for carbon dioxide transfer in any given

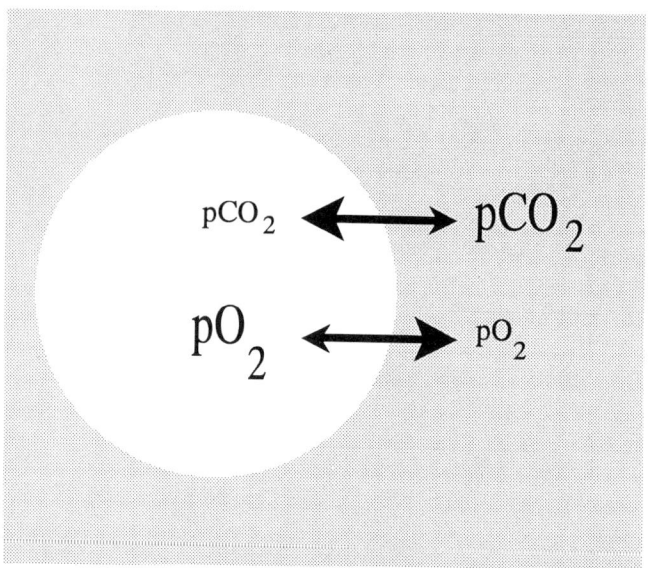

FIGURE 10.6. In the bubble oxygenator, gas bubbles act as vehicles for both oxygen and carbon dioxide transfer. Each gas will transfer according to principles of diffusion gradient and gas solubility.

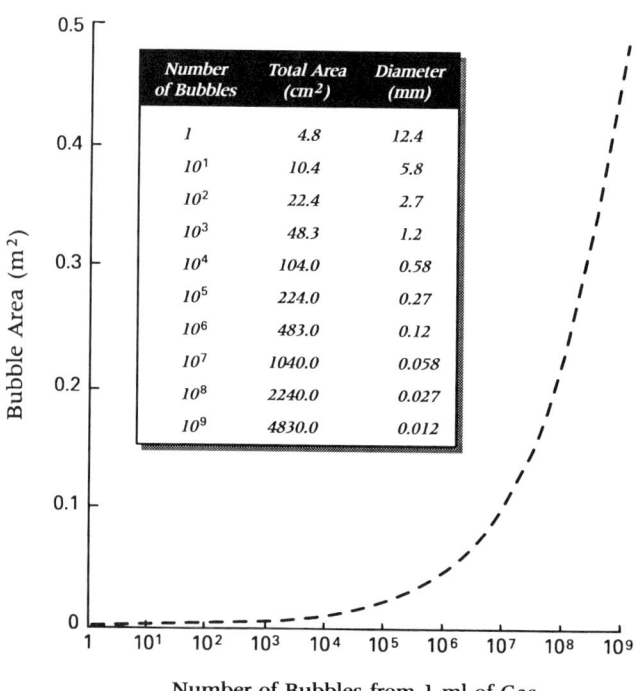

Number of Bubbles	Total Area (cm^2)	Diameter (mm)
1	4.8	12.4
10^1	10.4	5.8
10^2	22.4	2.7
10^3	48.3	1.2
10^4	104.0	0.58
10^5	224.0	0.27
10^6	483.0	0.12
10^7	1040.0	0.058
10^8	2240.0	0.027
10^9	4830.0	0.012

FIGURE 10.7. Tabular and graphic representation of the total surface area produced by 1 mL of gas when it is divided into an increasingly larger number of bubbles of progressively smaller diameter.

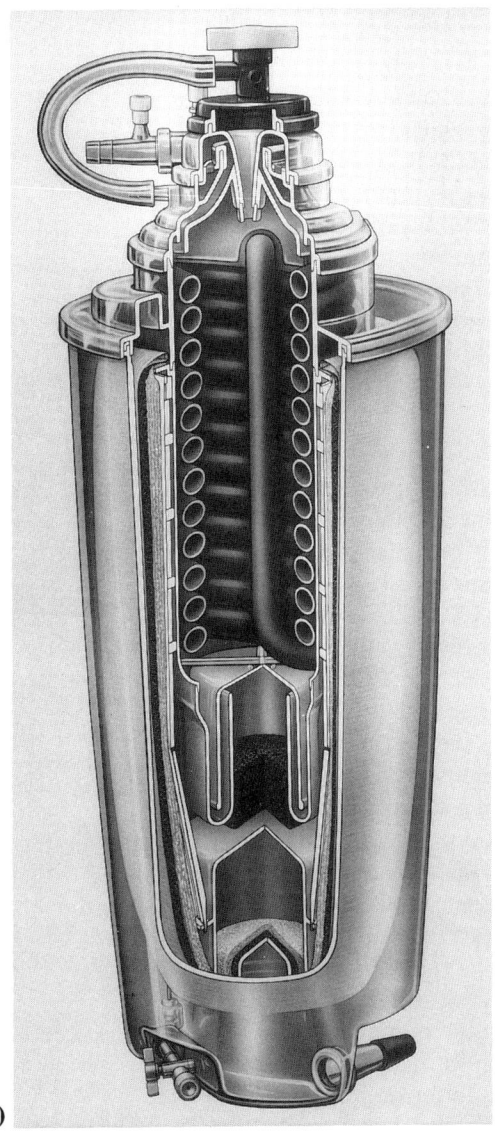

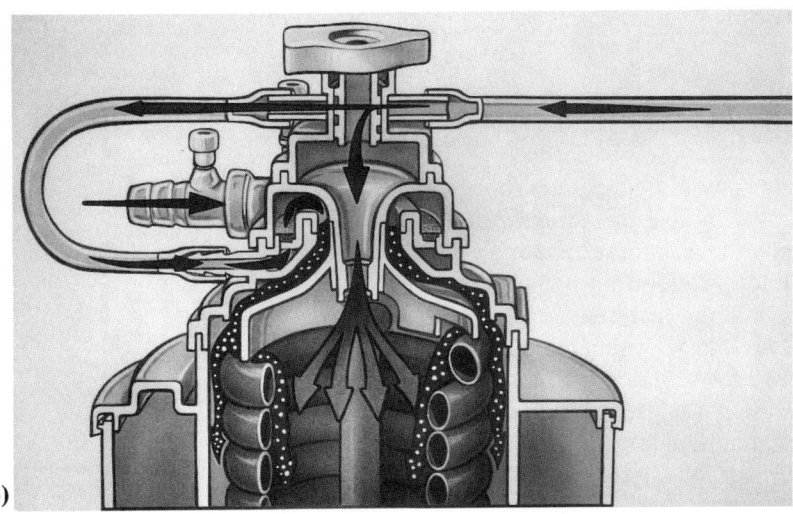

FIGURE 10.8. (a) Bentley 10 PLUS oxygenator; (b) Bentley 10 PLUS gas manifold. This manifold splits gas source to gas dispersion and debubbling/defoaming area. (Courtesy of Baxter Healthcare Corporation, Bentley Laboratories Division.)

blood flow rate. The higher the GBFR, the more volume available for carbon dioxide transfer, which results in a decreased arterial Pco_2. In addition to GBFR, titration of carbon dioxide into the gas source will alter arterial Pco_2. At any given GBFR, addition of carbon dioxide will increase arterial Pco_2. It is essential to operate bubble oxygenators at the lowest possible GBFR, since high GBFRs are associated with high levels of gaseous microemboli, excessive hemolysis, and protein denaturation.[31-33,44-47]

Priming Volumes

Priming volume is important when considering the impact of hemodilution. The priming volume of a bubble oxygenator can be expressed in several ways. "Dynamic" priming volume usually refers to the total volume necessary to operate the device while the patient is on CPB. The dynamic priming volume is composed of two volumes: the reservoir volume and the "hold-up" volume. The reservoir volume is the volume observable in the arterial reservoir and is measured by the level markings on the outside of the reservoir. The "hold-up" volume is that volume held by the oxygenating column and bubbling/defoaming sections of the oxygenator during operation. After priming, recirculating, and stopping the flow in the sequential (and some concentric) bubble oxygenators, much of the hold-up volume of the bubble column and defoaming/debubbling sections of the oxygenator will drain into and become part of the reservoir volume. When bypass is initiated, some of the initial venous return is required to refill these sections before it begins to appear as oxygenated volume in the reservoir. Some moments after stopping bypass, more volume will appear in the reservoir as a result of emptying of the bubble column and debubbling/defoaming sections.

Membrane Oxygenators

Design

The membrane oxygenator physically separates the blood from the gas with a gas-permeable membrane material (Figure 10.9). Historically, the membrane materials chosen have included cellulose, polytetrafluoroethylene, and polyethylene. The two membrane materials currently employed for this purpose are silicone rubber and polypropylene (Table 10.3). The most distinctive difference between these two materials is the fact that the silicone rubber is a homogeneous, nonporous membrane while the polypropylene is a heterogeneous, microporous, hydrophobic membrane.[48] The microporous membranes are developed by stretching the membrane material and forming "rents" in the substance of the membrane that act as "pores" for gas transfer.[49] These pores are 0.03 to 0.07 μm in effective diameter and cover at least 50% of the mem-

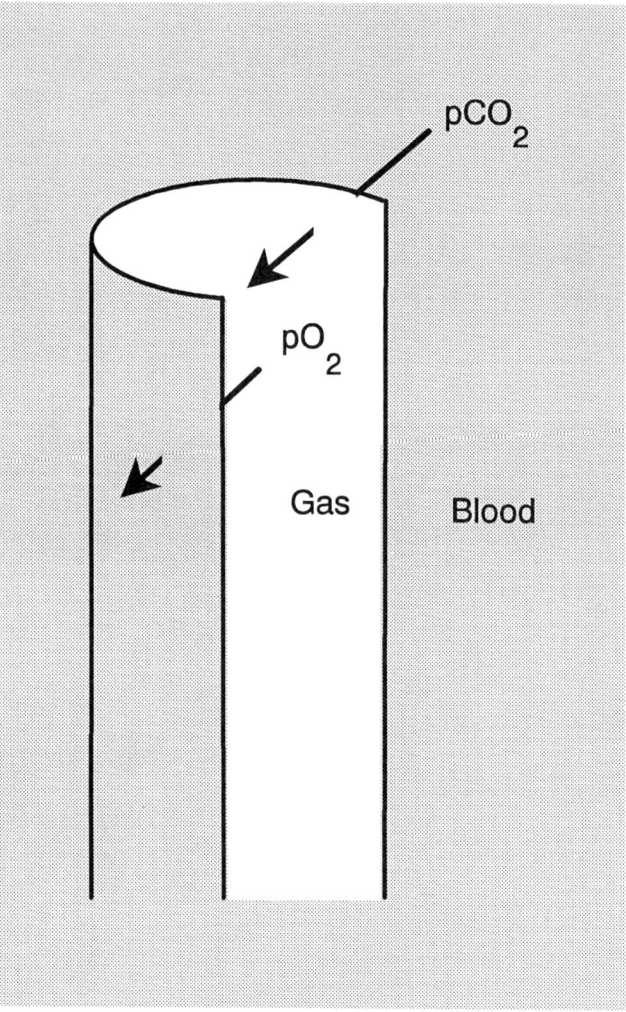

FIGURE 10.9. In the membrane oxygenator, the gas phase is separated from the blood phase by a membrane material. Oxygen and carbon dioxide will transfer according to principles of diffusion gradient and gas solubility.

TABLE 10.3. Membrane oxygenator options.

Membrane material
   Silicone rubber
   Polypropylene
Configuration
   Scrolled envelope
   Parallel plate
   Hollow fiber
      Blood inside fiber
      Blood outside fiber
Venous reservoir
   Closed collapsible bag
   Open hardshell

brane surface. Since the surface is hydrophobic and the pore size is in the submicron range, the microporous membrane does not act as a diafilter.[50] However, gas can be forced into the blood path if the pressure in the gas path exceeds that of the blood path.

Membrane materials are organized into one of three configurations: scrolled envelope, parallel plate, or hollow fiber (Table 10.3) (Figure 10.10). In the scrolled configuration (exclusively AVECOR™ Cardiovascular, Plymouth, MN 55441), an envelope of membrane material is wound onto a core and encased. A gas manifold system is designed to distribute gas into the scrolled envelope while blood is allowed to flow on the outside. A polypropylene screen in the gas path ensures proper gas distribution. In the parallel plate configuration, the membrane material is folded, accordion fashion, and encased. Gas supply is directed to one side of the Z-fold while blood is delivered to the opposite side. Polypropylene screens are placed in the gas and blood paths to ensure appropriate distribution of blood and gas supply. In the hollow-fiber configuration, hollow fibers of membrane material are employed to separate the blood and gas phases. The number of fibers utilized will vary, depending on the total surface area required for gas exchange. Fiber bundles are capped on each end with a polyurethane material. Fiber diameters are typically in the 200- to 300-μm range.

It is possible to design hollow-fiber oxygenators with the blood directed either through the inside or the outside of the fiber and with the gas confined to the opposite side. One consideration in these two designs is possible fiber rupture. If the blood phase is enclosed *inside* the fiber and some of the fibers rupture, blood will spill into the gas phase and may decrease the total surface area available for oxygen transfer. If, however, the blood phase is *outside* the fiber and some of the fibers rupture, blood will spill only into the fibers affected and will not significantly change the total surface area available for oxygen transfer. Additionally, "blood outside" fiber designs may allow visualization of air bubbles in the blood path during priming or operation, whereas "blood inside" fiber designs would not.

Clinical differences between oxygenators of differing membrane composition and configuration have been difficult to determine, analyze, and interpret, but in vitro and in vivo studies have found equivalent performance and blood handling by these devices. Subtle differences between devices seem to be related to oxygenator design rather than to the membrane material or configuration used. Patient studies performed by Bergdahl[51] and Pearson[52,53] found no significant differences in the hemocompatibility of the parallel-plate and hollow-fiber configurations. Additionally, differences in membrane material (polypropylene versus polyethylene) could not be demonstrated. Gourlay[54] also found equivalent hemocompatibility and gas-exchange performance between parallel-plate and hollow-fiber configurations, but variable performance in air trapping. This study suggested substantial differences in how the oxygenators handled gross air removal, based on design. In an in vitro recirculation study, O'Connor[55] found that a polypropylene hollow-fiber oxygenator was associated with less platelet loss, less platelet factor 4 release, and more preservation of platelet reactivity, when compared to a silicone rubber-scroll oxygenator. The study conclusions suggested, however, that the overall oxygenator design, not just the membrane material, was responsible for the differences. Leijala[56] studied

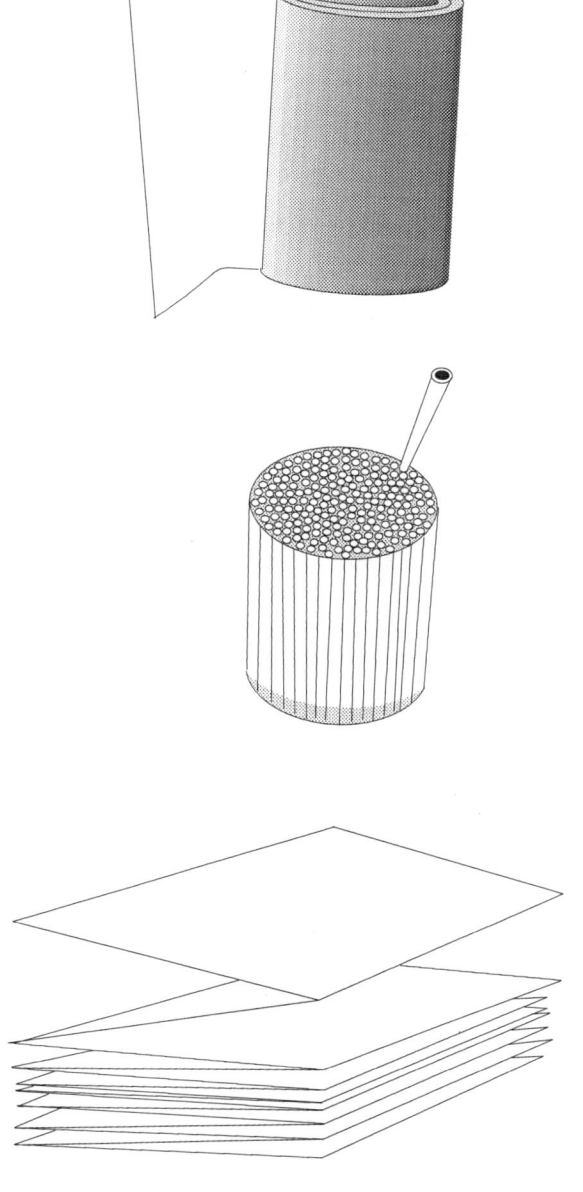

FIGURE 10.10. Membrane oxygenators may be configured as a scrolled envelope (top), hollow fiber (middle), or parallel plate (bottom).

the hemocompatibility of "blood inside" versus "blood outside" hollow-fiber configurations in children, with respect to changes in white blood cells, C3 levels, total hemolytic complement, C-reactive protein, and haptoglobin. Although a trend favored the "blood outside" configuration, the differences were not statistically significant. Hiratzka[57] studied the relationship between oxygenator design/membrane type and patient outcome as reflected in the costs of postoperative care. Although the data tended to favor the scrolled-silicone membrane configuration over a parallel-plate and hollow-fiber design, the differences were not statistically significant.

Membrane oxygenation systems are designed to collect venous return in a reservoir and allow a pump to deliver this volume to the membrane (with one notable exception, to be discussed). The venous reservoirs may be of a collapsible-bag or hardshell-reservoir configuration. The bag reservoir system (made of polyurethane or polyvinylchloride) requires a separate cardiotomy reservoir that can deliver cardiotomy return blood to the bag via a cardiotomy line. The hardshell-reservoir system (made of polycarbonate) may have an integral cardiotomy included in the hardshell venous reservoir. When the cardiotomy is integral, poor mixing and settling of the blood in the reservoir may result, in some designs, if the volume is maintained at a high level and the suction limited.[58] Additionally, high rates of suction into the reservoir with an integral cardiotomy may result in higher levels of gaseous microemboli release from the outlet.[59]

The collapsible-bag configuration (Table 10.3, Figure 10.11) (Bentley Laboratories) is often referred to as a "closed" system, in that the blood volume in the bag is not exposed to room air surrounding the device. As blood volume in the bag increases, the bag expands, and as blood volume decreases, the bag collapses. If the bag expansion is restricted by a volume-limiting device, excess volume coming into the bag is stored either in the cardiotomy or in the patient's veins. Any air collected in the bag from the venous or cardiotomy lines must be removed via the purging ports located at the top of the bag, either manually or by connecting one of these purging ports to suction. Since the bag reservoir does not have direct defoaming capability, significant numbers of gaseous microemboli from venous and cardiotomy air may exit the reservoir if it is not continuously purged. The ability of the bag to trap and eliminate these microemboli is related to the flow pattern through the bag, the size of the microemboli, and the presence of a barrier screen.[60]

The hardshell-reservoir configuration (Figure 10.12) (Bentley Laboratories) is often referred to as an "open" system, since the blood in the reservoir is exposed to air surrounding the device in much the same way as it is in a bubble oxygenator reservoir. As blood volume in the reservoir increases, air is vented out of the reservoir to accommodate it, and as blood volume in the reservoir de-

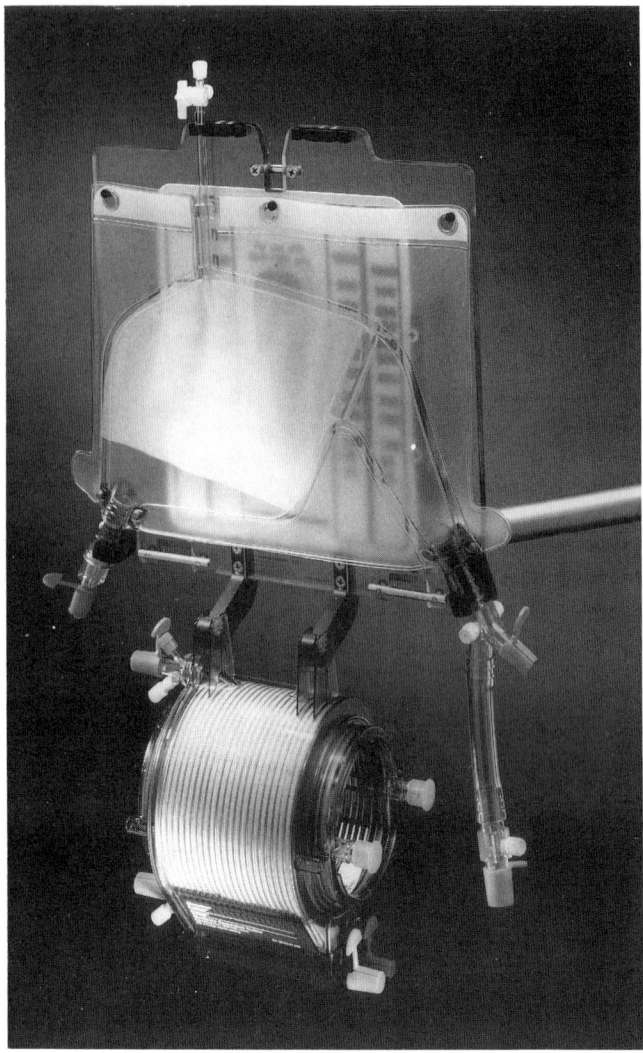

FIGURE 10.11. Univox™ with BMR-800 venous reservoir (courtesy of Baxter Healthcare Corporation, Bentley Laboratories Division).

creases, air is pulled into the reservoir. The closed system is thought to provide an element of safety, in that, if the bag is accidentally emptied during bypass, it collapses and large amounts of air cannot be delivered to the membrane or to the patient. The open system, on the other hand, acts more like a bubble oxygenator reservoir, providing an unlimited source of air that could potentially be delivered to the circuit. Advantages to the open system include better visibility of the reservoir level, a larger volume storage capacity, and an easier passive elimination of air entering from the venous and/or cardiotomy lines.[57,58]

One notable exception to the arterial line membrane oxygenator systems is the Capiox E (Figure 10.13) (Terumo Corporation). In this oxygenator, the venous blood enters a hollow-fiber membrane package, and gas exchange is accomplished prior to accumulation in an arterial reser-

10. Oxygenators for Extracorporeal Circulation

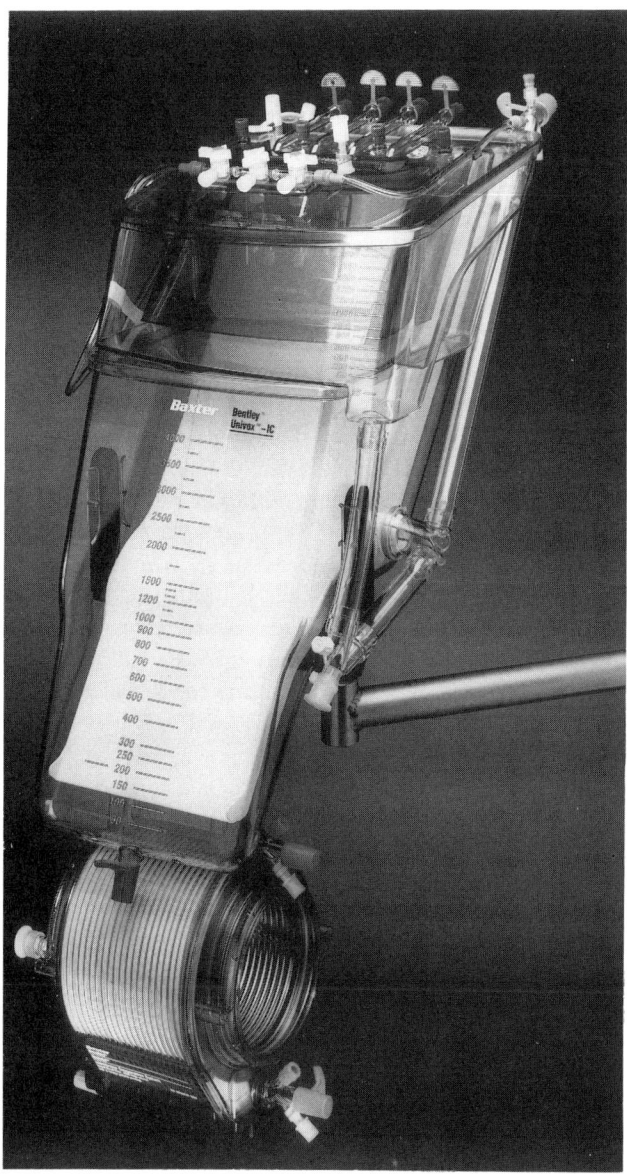

FIGURE 10.12. Univox™-IC reservoir. In this open system, reservoir blood is exposed to air (courtesy of Baxter Healthcare Corporation, Bentley Laboratories Division).

the heat exchanger included in the hardshell venous reservoir prior to the inflow of the oxygenator (see Chapter 14 for more discussion).

The membrane oxygenator circuit is designed to include a recirculation line from the arterial outlet of the oxygenator to the venous reservoir. Although a recirculation line can also be included in a bubbler circuit, this is usually a distinctive feature of the membrane oxygenation system. The recirculation line can be used to: (1) assist in a staged priming procedure; (2) permit continued low-flow circulation of the blood path prior to or after bypass; (3) provide a blood access point for blood cardioplegia or cell processing; (4) eliminate air that may accidentally accumulate in the blood path of the oxygenator; and (5) assist if replacement of the oxygenator is necessary. It is also possible to use the recirculation line to "preoxygenate" the inlet blood by allowing oxygenator arterial outlet blood to mix with the incoming venous blood in the venous reservoir. This may be helpful in situations where the venous blood is excessively desaturated; however, one must consider the fact that the recirculation flow is a shunt flow and decreases the total oxygen delivery to the patient. Therefore, using the recirculation line in this manner is treating a symptom, and other strategies to improve venous inlet saturation are preferred.

Membrane oxygenators are typically flushed with carbon dioxide prior to priming to eliminate poorly soluble nitrogen from the blood path. This facilitates the removal of gas bubbles during the priming procedure. The optimal

voir. As a "gravity flow-through design," it is primed and operated similarly to a bubble oxygenator. Since the blood path is a "blood outside" fiber type, resistance to venous inflow is low and adequate flows can be achieved.[61]

Membrane oxygenator systems provide a heat exchanger to allow the venous and cardiotomy blood to be cooled or warmed. In most membrane oxygenators, the heat exchanger will be included in the inflow path or integrated with the membrane package. The operator then has the choice of using a collapsible bag or hardshell reservoir to serve purely as a venous and cardiotomy blood collection reservoir. It is possible, in the open systems, to have

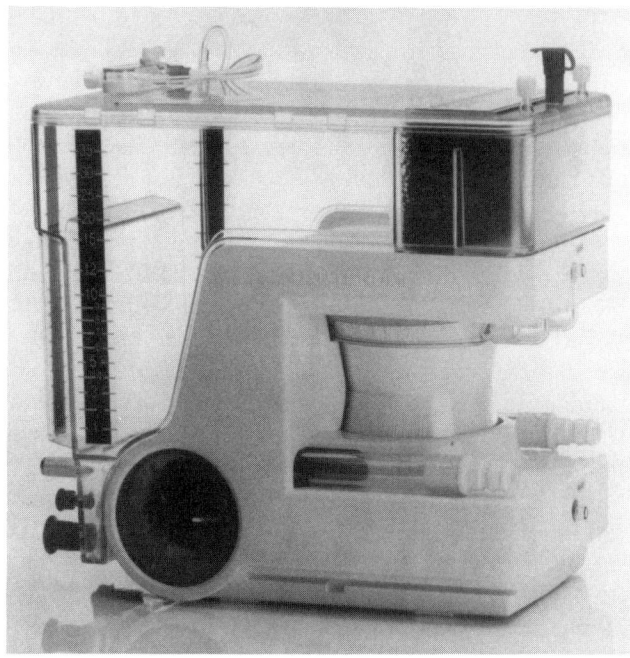

FIGURE 10.13. Capiox E membrane oxygenator. The blood flow is "outside" the membrane fiber (courtesy of Terumo Corporation).

duration, point of entry, and flow rate of this CO_2 flush have not been determined and are subject to individual protocol.[62] The carbon dioxide flush will elevate the P_{CO_2} and decrease the pH of the prime, and it is recommended that the carbon dioxide be eliminated prior to initiating bypass by recirculating the prime through the oxygenator while it is ventilated with an oxygen source.

Principles of Gas Transfer

Oxygen, delivered to the gas path of the membrane oxygenator, diffuses along a concentration gradient through the membrane material to the blood flowing through the device. Oxygen transfer in the membrane oxygenator obeys Fick's law of diffusion and will vary directly with the total surface area of membrane, the oxygen gradient developed across the membrane, and the permeability of the membrane material to oxygen.[4,63,64] It will vary indirectly with the blood film thickness in the blood path of the device. Since the gas phase is physically separated from the blood phase, it is possible to mix the oxygen gas source with nitrogen (most commonly mixed with room air), thus adjusting the fraction of oxygen in the inlet gas (F_iO_2). The oxygen partial pressure gradient between the gas and blood phases, then, can be varied, thus altering the total amount of oxygen transfer. Blood film thickness must be limited in order to have a minimum diffusion distance for oxygen. If blood film thickness cannot be minimized, some means must be provided to augment the primary flow of blood, which increases exposure of the film to the membrane surface.[64] Historically, this was accomplished by providing mechanical turbulence in the blood path (screens), altering the surface of the membrane material, or physically shaking the oxygenator to "vortex" the blood film.[63] Today, although the parallel-plate configuration continues to use blood path screens, the scroll and "blood outside," hollow-fiber configurations use the tightness of the membrane packaging to limit the blood-film thickness. The "blood inside," hollow-fiber configuration uses the internal diameter of the fiber to limit blood-film thickness.

Carbon dioxide delivered in the venous blood diffuses along a concentration gradient through the membrane material to the gas path of the device. Carbon dioxide transfer depends upon the total surface area of membrane, the carbon dioxide gradient developed across the membrane, and the permeability of the membrane material to carbon dioxide.[63,64] In contrast to the bubble oxygenator, which can significantly denitrogenate the patient, nitrogen loss with the membrane oxygenator can be attenuated by using a gas source with high nitrogen content.

Water vapor is also subject to transfer in the membrane oxygenator. This vapor is unique in that its partial pressure varies only with temperature, and it is therefore transferred at greater rates at warm blood temperatures. Water vapor can condense in the cooler gas path of the oxygenator and, if this occurs, can reduce the total membrane surface area available for oxygen and carbon dioxide transfer. The gas path of the oxygenator therefore must be designed to allow condensed water vapor to be eliminated from the device. Gas flow through the device should facilitate this process.

Blood Gas Management of the Membrane Lung

The ventilating gas used with the membrane oxygenator is most commonly a mixture of 100% oxygen and room air, allowing alteration in F_iO_2. This is often accomplished with the use of a mechanical blender that allows the two gas sources (oxygen and room air) to be mixed to achieve F_iO_2 values between 1.0 (100% oxygen) and 0.21 (100% room air). Decreasing the F_iO_2 from 1.0 will decrease the arterial P_{O_2} (Figure 10.14; Sechrist Industries). It is also possible to mix the two gas sources by using a roller pump to deliver the room air and titrate it into a 100% oxygen gas source. The F_iO_2 with this method can be calculated if the two gas flows are known as follows:

$$F_iO_2 = [QO_2 + (QRA \times 0.21)]/QO_2 + QRA$$

where

QO_2 = flow of 100% oxygen (L/min)
QRA = flow of room air (L/min)
0.21 = concentration of oxygen in room air

Oxygen concentration monitoring would be recommended to verify F_iO_2 in either method of gas delivery.

Arterial P_{CO_2} is controlled in much the same way as it is in the bubble oxygenator, ie, with adjustments in GBFR (Figure 10.14). The gas flow through the membrane oxygenator is often referred to as the *sweep rate*. Higher rates of gas flow will eliminate more carbon dioxide from the membrane surface, thus increasing the gradient from the blood-to-gas phase and decreasing the arterial P_{CO_2}.

Priming Volume

As with the bubble oxygenator, the priming volume of the membrane oxygenator will cause hemodilution. The "blood outside" fiber technology has allowed small surface area membranes with correspondingly small priming volumes. "Static" priming volume in the membrane oxygenator is that amount of prime which fills the oxygenator under "no-flow" conditions. "Dynamic" priming volume is flow dependent and is a measure of the membrane compartment compliance. This volume can be found by noting how much volume is lost from the reservoir with each incremental increase in flow and adding it to the static priming volume.

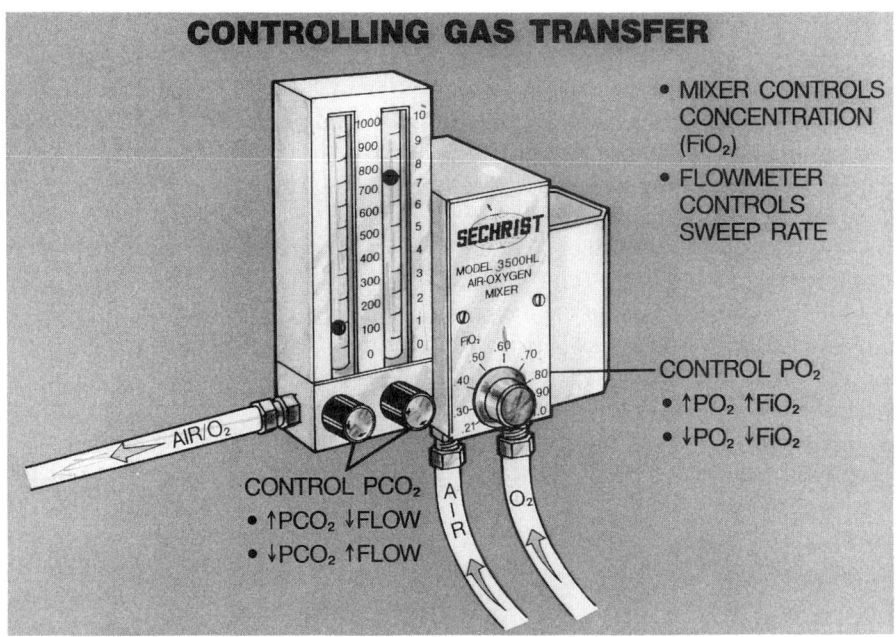

FIGURE 10.14. Manifold used with membrane oxygenator allowing independent control of arterial P_{O_2} and P_{CO_2} (courtesy of Sechrist Industries).

Pressure Drops

It is critical that the pressure within the blood path of the membrane oxygenator always be maintained greater than that of the gas path, to avoid forcing gas into the blood compartment.[65] Although this stipulation may apply more to the microporous membranes, it must be considered as well for the silicone rubber membrane.[64,66] Part of this pressure differential is maintained by keeping the venous reservoir at a higher position in reference to the oxygenator. Additionally, however, one functional advantage of continuous pumping into the membrane is the ability to ensure a constant positive pressure differential in the blood path over the gas path.

Extreme caution must be exercised when using gas scavenging systems on membrane oxygenators for elimination of anesthetic gas added to the gas source. The scavenging system must be designed to avoid accidental kinking which would overpressurize the gas path with respect to the blood path.[67] Also, although the scavenging system must be capable of removing sufficient quantities of exhaust gas to prevent anesthetic gas pollution, scavenging must not be done excessively, to the point that oxygenator performance is altered.[68] It has been demonstrated that excessive scavenging vacuum may decrease oxygen transfer to the point that oxygenator failure is falsely perceived.[69] Justison[67] recommends an optimal scavenge flow : gas flow ratio of 5 : 1.

The pressure drop across the blood path is measured as the difference between the inlet and outlet blood path pressures. The pressure drop will vary with blood flow rate, the resistance to blood flow imposed by the design of the membrane package, and changes in blood viscosity or temperature. High pressure drops may be associated with high shear stresses and blood trauma. High pressure drops in compliant membrane packages may alter blood path dimension and, thus, oxygen transfer efficiency.[70] Blood path pressure drops should be monitored in any long-term use of the membrane oxygenator to assure blood path integrity.

Additional Concepts

Rated Blood Flow

Rated blood flow is the maximum flow at which an oxygenator can receive blood at standard venous inlet conditions and oxygenate it to an arterial oxygen saturation of 95%. The standard venous inlet conditions include an oxygen saturation of 65 ± 5%, a hemoglobin value of 12 ± 1g%, a temperature of 37 ± 2°C, a base excess of 0 + 5 mEq/L, and a P_{CO_2} of 45 ± 5 mm Hg. Rated blood flow is related to the blood residence time in the device, ie, how long the blood is exposed to the oxygenating surface area capacity of the device. In bubble oxygenators, rated blood flow is also related to the capacity of the debubbling and defoaming area to handle the volume of blood that must be processed. Devices (eg, pediatric) that have smaller oxygenating and debubbling/defoaming surface area capacities have correspondingly lower rated blood flows.

Since rated blood flow is based on standard venous blood conditions, the outlet oxygen saturation may change as the venous inlet conditions vary from the standard. During rewarming, the venous inlet P_{O_2} and oxygen saturation are decreased such that more oxygen transfer is required to bring the arterial oxygen saturation to 95%. If venous inlet conditions are depressed below "standard" due to circumstances during rewarming, resulting in increased oxygen consumption, the oxygenator may appear to be failing, when, in actuality, the device simply cannot raise the depressed venous blood conditions to a 95% saturation. One may be tempted to reduce flow at this time to prolong residence time in the oxygenator and improve the outlet blood conditions. This is a time during CPB, however, when high blood flows are desired to provide oxygen and heat delivery. Maneuvers must be implemented to increase oxygen delivery (eg, increase blood flow or hemoglobin concentration) or decrease oxygen consumption (eg, increase depth of anesthesia or muscle paralysis).

Reaction Time

Reaction time is defined as that period of time before the arterial reservoir (in the case of a bubble oxygenator) or venous reservoir (in the case of a membrane oxygenator) completely empties if the venous flow is abruptly stopped. This time period is related to the blood flow through the device and the blood level in the reservoir as follows:

$$RT = (VOL \times 60)/BFR$$

where

RT = reaction time (seconds)
VOL = reservoir level (mL)
BFR = blood flow rate (mL/min)

At any given blood flow rate, a higher reservoir level will be associated with a longer reaction time. Reaction time is prolonged if the venous flow is only partially restricted, eg, with partial venous cannula or venous return line obstruction.

A high operating reservoir level is desirable not only because it will increase reaction time, but also because bubbles that make their way into the arterial or venous reservoir will have a chance to be absorbed or float away if a high level is maintained. Low reservoir levels are associated with a higher bubble count leaving the reservoir.[31,44]

Pulsatile Perfusion

Pulsatile perfusion may be employed with the use of roller or centrifugal pumps designed to periodically vary the velocity of flow. Pulse transmission from the bubble oxygenator, or "gravity flow-through" membrane oxygenator design, is limited by the distal circuit components found in the arterial line (ie, arterial line filter and cannula), the transmission capacity of the arterial line, and the specific operational characteristics of the pulsatile pump itself.

The arterial line membrane oxygenator, on the other hand, can significantly attenuate pulse transmission. In vitro and vivo studies have shown that this attenuation appears to be related to membrane design and compliance.[72-74] Parallel-plate and scroll designs are associated with high compliance and loss of pulse transmission, whereas the hollow-fiber designs better preserve the energy equivalent pressure found at the pump outlet.[75] There does not appear to be a significant difference between the "blood inside" fiber and the "blood outside" fiber design.[74]

Pulsatile pump design allows the operator to stop the pump head completely between pulses, in order to produce an optimal pulse waveform. This practice should not be employed with the microporous arterial line membrane oxygenator, since it may subject the blood path to a negative pressure phase. During this moment of negative pressure, the usual pressure differential between the gas and blood compartments is reversed, with the potential for gas to be pulled into the blood path.[76]

The Bubble Oxygenator Versus the Membrane Oxygenator

Although this chapter has presented the concept, design, and use of both types of oxygenating systems, much of the controversy surrounding the use of bubble oxygenators and membrane oxygenators has abated. Historical objections to the use of membrane oxygenators have included expense, size, and complexity. Early systems, with their two-pump design, closed reservoir, and/or vacuum priming, were indeed more difficult to set up, prime, and operate. At the same time, disadvantages to the bubble oxygenator were well recognized. The lack of independent control of blood gases gave rise to concern over abnormally high P_{O_2} values. Moreover, the direct blood/gas interface increases the damage to cellular elements, protein, and platelets, and results in a higher level of gaseous microemboli. As a compromise (in view of numerous inconclusive studies contrasting the use of bubble oxygenators and membrane oxygenators), most institutions adopted the policy that membrane systems would be reserved for procedures that had an anticipated bypass time of over 2 hours.[77-80]

Currently, however, there is a major shift toward the use of membrane systems for all procedures, regardless of length. Expense, size, and complexity are no longer good arguments for the use of one device over the other. In addition, the use of membrane oxygenators for long-term respiratory support and percutaneous support procedures has been well documented.[81-86] Although membrane oxygenators are now in vogue, the literature continues to be inconclusive on the strict pathophysiologic need for their use. The relative prevalence of disturbances in platelet numbers and function, erythrocyte survival, complement activation, protein denaturation, and gaseous microemboli production should theoretically favor the membrane oxygenator. But studies have been inconclusive due to many confounding variables, including the use of cardiotomy suction, variations in hemocompatibility of the devices used, duration of procedures, variations in the methodology used to correct for the effect of hemodilution, extent of hypothermia employed, use of protamine, and varying sensitivities of the laboratory methods and measurements. Clinical outcome studies have been even less conclusive. Postoperative blood loss, use of transfused blood products, need for inotropic support, incidence of postoperative complications, and neuropsychologic factors have not yet made a case for one oxygenating system over the other. This review offers a brief synopsis of only recent studies within the past decade, specifically addressing the pathophysiologic and clinical results when contrasting the bubble and membrane oxygenators. For a historical review of this topic, the authors refer the reader to more dated sources.[77-80,87-96]

Platelets

Platelet activation and depletion occur as the result of interaction of the blood with artificial and gas surfaces, interaction with surface-adsorbed protein, geometry and velocity of blood flow, and shear-induced trauma.[97-113] Depletion additionally can occur as the result of sequestration in the liver and spleen.[114,115] As a consequence, the patient may experience an impairment in postoperative hemostasis following CPB. Clinically, these patients will have prolonged bleeding times, abnormal clot retraction, increased blood loss, and consequent increased need for blood products.[109] Theoretically, the bubble oxygenator, with its direct blood-gas interface, should cause a greater platelet depletion through lysis than the membrane oxygenator, and many recent clinical studies have shown that platelet depletion is significantly greater in the bubble oxygenator than in the membrane oxygenator.[53,116-119] Levels of plasma β-thromboglobin, a platelet-release product and indicator of platelet activation and damage, have been shown to increase significantly with the bubble oxygenator.[53,115,119-121] Changes in platelet aggregation, as measured by sensitivity to ADP, have been shown either to favor the membrane oxygenator[116,117] or to favor neither oxygenator.[53,122] In a new approach to the problem, Peterson[123] studied indium-111–labeled platelets in dogs perfused with either a bubble oxygenator or silicone rubber membrane oxygenator, and found significant alterations in platelet kinetics in those cases that were less than 2 hours in length. The study found greater platelet destruction, as indicated by release of platelet-bound indium-111, and greater hemodilution-corrected blood loss with the bubble oxygenator, as a result of the direct blood-gas interface.

Complement Activation

Complement activation can occur as a result of the exposure of blood to artificial surfaces, denatured immunoglobulins, cellular debris, substances released from damaged cells, and the interaction of protamine and heparin.[124-135] Complement-derived anaphylatoxins can induce a variety of inflammatory-like reactions that result in increased capillary permeability, interstitial edema, and histamine release.[126-138] Clinical manifestations include pulmonary, cardiac, and renal dysfunction.[127,137-143] Several recent investigations have found little difference in the degree of complement activation occurring with bubble and membrane oxygenators.[120,121,144] Cavarocchi[145] found significantly higher concentrations of C3a in a group of patients perfused with a bubble oxygenator than in a group using a silicone rubber membrane oxygenator, but only after protamine administration. Interestingly, a third group of patients assigned to the bubble oxygenator, with a prebypass dose of methylprednisolone, did not significantly differ from the membrane group. In contrast to this study, Videm[146] found significantly higher C3 activation products at the end of bypass in patients on a silicone rubber membrane when compared to those on a bubbler. The same results were found in an in vitro study[134] contrasting complement activation from six oxygenators, including both bubble and membrane types constructed of various materials (polypropylene, polyethylene, and silicone rubber). It was found that the terminal complement pathway was similarly activated in all oxygenators, but variations in C3 activation still occurred. Since oxygenation was not employed in this in vitro study, the presence or absence of a direct blood-gas interface could not explain the differences in activation. It was concluded that no one oxygenator type or material could be implicated, and that complement activation appears to be a relevant problem in all oxygenator types.

Leukopenia occurs during CPB, probably as a result of complement activation, lung sequestration, surface adhesion, and perhaps shear-induced trauma.[88,122,126,136,138,140,145-157] Although implicated in an impairment of host defense,[121,158-160] this leukopenia is largely transient, and recovery often occurs prior to the termination of bypass, due to the mobilization of a large reserve capacity and the ability for rapid leukopoiesis.[88,126] Recent investigations have found no significant difference between bubble and membrane oxygenators with respect to leukocyte depletion.[53,119,121,122,146] It is suggested that the ability to detect leukopenia as a result of the blood-gas interface of the bubble oxygenator alone is lost with the use of cardiotomy suction.[99,122,161-164] Van Oeveren[165] was able to demonstrate this hypothesis in a controlled canine study. Only mild leukopenia was found with membrane oxygenation that avoided cardiotomy suction, but a more pronounced leukopenia could be induced with membrane oxygenation employing cardiotomy suction. Not only were leukocyte numbers decreased, but polymorphonuclear neutrophil leukocyte (PMN) function, serum bactericidal activity, and opsonizing capacity were also impaired. These results suggest that the blood-gas interface represents a potential weakening of the host defense against infection.

Gaseous Microemboli

Pearson[32] compared the gaseous microemboli production of five bubble oxygenators and one membrane oxygenator. As one would expect, the number of gaseous microemboli detected in the arterial line was significantly lower in the membrane group than in any of the bubble oxygenators studied. When contrasting the gaseous microemboli produced by the bubble oxygenators as a group, greater quantities were associated with higher gas flows, used to control arterial P_{CO_2}, and lower blood levels in the arterial reservoir. This study emphasized, however, that the membrane oxygenator can also, under certain conditions, cause the release of gaseous microemboli. Entrainment of air in the venous line blood, or administered fluids and the use of cardiotomy suction, were the likely cause of observed gaseous microemboli release by the membrane oxygenator.

Padayachee[166] used transcranial Doppler (TCD) ultrasound of the middle cerebral artery in a patient study to detect microemboli released by either a bubble or hollow-fiber membrane oxygenator. The patients assigned to the bubble oxygenator were further perfused either with or without an arterial line filter (see Chapter 6 for more discussion). The results indicated significant elevations in gaseous microemboli in the two bubbler groups when compared to the membrane groups. There was no significant difference in microemboli detection between the two bubble groups. A correlation between gas flow in the bubbler and microemboli detection was demonstrated.

Using a clever new technology, Blauth[167] employed fluorescein angiography to demonstrate microvascular perfusion defects in the retina as the result of microemboli production from a patient series assigned to either a bubble or flat-sheet membrane oxygenator. A 40-μm arterial line screen filter was used in all cases. The patients assigned to the bubble oxygenator had significantly more microvascular occlusions consistent with microemboli than did the patients assigned to the membrane oxygenator. In an extension to this study, patients perfused with the bubble oxygenator were found to have a significantly greater number of occlusion defects than those in the membrane group.[168] Patients with perfusion defects assigned to the membrane group had significantly fewer lesions and less retinal ischemic area than those assigned to the bubble group. The technique is not capable of distinguishing the type of emboli involved in the occlusion (ie, solid debris versus air), but it is suggested that air emboli were included. Although cardiotomy suction and donor blood are sources of emboli, no relationship between cardiotomy blood return and the incidence of retinal ischemia could be demonstrated. Additionally, no correlation could be found between occlusion defects and arterial P_{CO_2} levels, even though the bubbler group had significantly higher maintenance levels of arterial P_{CO_2}. A difference in neuropsychologic test scores between oxygenator groups could not be confirmed. Therefore, a relationship between microvascular occlusion and postoperative functional impairment could not be demonstrated.

Postoperative Blood Loss

If the bubble oxygenator is responsible for a greater degree of blood trauma and impaired hemostasis, one would expect that the postoperative blood loss and transfusion of blood products would be greater in the group of patients perfused with a bubble oxygenator.[103,109,122,137,169] Although several recent studies have found a significantly greater postoperative blood loss and use of blood products in the bubble oxygenator group,[118,122] others have been unable to demonstrate a significant difference.[116,117,121,144,170,171] Again, it must be emphasized that the use of cardiotomy suction with the membrane oxygenator may mask its beneficial effect. It appears that studies are capable of demonstrating clear differences on the cellular and microscopic level, but as yet, firm conclusions have not been drawn in the area of patient outcome.

Summary

The development of the artificial lung or "oxygenator" has had a dramatic impact on the history and science of extracorporeal technology. Initially complex to operate and highly traumatic to the patient, the oxygenator has evolved into an efficient and predictable component of the CPB circuit. Early filming oxygenators gave way to devices that transferred gases into and out of bubbles and through membrane materials. Issues related to safety, simplicity, disposability, and priming volume have driven the technology toward devices that meet the demands of cardiac surgery.

The requirements for an "ideal" oxygenator include the ability to (1) oxygenate the venous blood over a wide range of blood flow rates, (2) eliminate carbon dioxide to avoid hypercarbia or hypocarbia, (3) provide cardiopulmonary bypass with a minimum of trauma to blood components, (4) limit the deleterious effects of hemodilution by providing a small priming volume, and (5) ensure simplicity and safety. All currently used oxygenators fulfill these requirements to varying degrees. Recently, there has been a shift from the dominant use of bubble oxygenators toward the use of membrane oxygenators. Expense, size, and complexity are no longer acceptable arguments against the use of the membrane oxygenator, and its merits should be carefully weighed against those of the bubbler. Although many studies are inconclusive in their results, comparisons of such factors as disturbances in platelet numbers and function, protein denaturation, and gaseous microemboli production favor the use of the membrane oxygenator.

Future developments in the area of oxygenator design are difficult to predict. Research may be concentrated on the development of more efficient membrane materials, which will allow further reductions in priming volume and improved hemocompatibility. Passivation of existing membrane materials with various coatings may attenuate or eliminate the need for heparin, and may obviate other concerns related to the pathophysiology of CPB. In-line monitoring of the variables associated with gas exchange and oxygenator function will likely be refined. Decreasing the cost of the devices and extending their efficiency in long-term use will also be goals for the future.

References

1. Dennis C. A heart-lung machine for open-heart operations. How it came about. *Trans Am Soc Artif Intern Organs* 1989;35:767–777.
2. Drinker PA. Progress in membrane oxygenator design. *Anesthesiology* 1972;37:242–260.
3. Eloessler L. Milestones in chest surgery. *J Thorac Cardiovasc Surg* 1970;60:157–165.
4. Galletti PM, Brecher GA. Principles of extracorporeal gas exchange. In: *Heart Lung Bypass; Principles and Techniques of Extracorporeal Circulation*. New York: Grune and Stratton; 1962:47–60.
5. Peirce EC II. The membrane lung, its excuse, present status, and promise. *J Mt Sinai Hospital New York* 1967;34:437–468.
6. Gibbon JH. Application of a mechanical heart-lung apparatus to cardiac surgery. *Minn Med* 1954;37:171–180.
7. Gibbon JH. Artificial maintenance of circulation during experimental occlusion of pulmonary artery. *Arch Surg* 1937;34:1105–1131.
8. Gibbon JH. The maintenance of life during experimental occlusion of the pulmonary artery followed by survival. *Surg Gyneceol Obstet* 1939;69:602–614.
9. Gibbon JH, Kraul CW. An efficient oxygenator for blood. *J Lab Clin Med* 1941;26:1803–1809.
10. Bjork VO. An artificial heart or cardiopulmonary machine: performance in animals. *Lancet* 1948;255:491–493.
11. Melrose DG. A mechanical heart-lung for use in man. *Br Med J* 1953;2:57–62.
12. Cross FS, Berne KM, Hirose Y, et al. Evaluation of a rotating disc type reservoir oxygenator. *Proc Soc Exp Biol Med* 1956;93:210–214.
13. Clark LC, Gollan F, Gupta VB. The oxygenation of blood by gas dispersion. *Science* 1950;111:85–87.
14. DeWall RA, Warden HE, Read RC, et al. A simple expendable artificial oxygenator for open heart surgery. *Surg Clin North Am* 1956;36:1025–1034.
15. Gott VL, DeWall RA, Paneth M, et al. A self-contained disposable oxygenator of plastic sheet for intra-cardiac surgery. *Thorax* 1957;12:1–9.
16. Hyman ES, Rosenberg D, Hyman AL, et al. A simple artificial heart-lung: an approach to open heart surgery, preliminary report. *J Louisiana St Med Soc* 1956;108:134–136.
17. Rygg IH, Kyvsgaard E. A disposable polyethylene oxygenator system applied in a heart-lung machine. *Acta Chir Scand* 1956;112:433–437.
18. Rygg IH, Kyvsgaard E. Further development of the heart-lung machine with Rygg-Kyvsgaard plastic bag oxygenator. *Minerva Chir* 1958;13:1402–1404.
19. Kolff WJ, Berk HTJ. Artificial kidney: dialyzer with great surface area. *Acta Med Scand* 1944;21:134.
20. Effler DB, Kolff WJ, Groves LK, Sones FN. Disposable membrane oxygenator and its use in experimental surgery. *J Thorac Surg* 1956;32:620–629.
21. Clowes GHA Jr, Hopkins AL, Neville WE. An artificial lung dependent upon the diffusion of oxygen and carbon dioxide through plastic membranes. *J Thorac Surg* 1956;32:630–637.
22. Clowes GHA Jr, Neville W. Membrane oxygenator. In: Allen JG, ed. *Extracorporeal Circulation*. Springfield, IL: Charles C Thomas;1958:81–100.
23. Kolobow T, Bowman RL. Construction and evaluation of an alveolar membrane artificial heart-lung. *Trans Am Soc Artif Intern Organs* 1963;9:238–243.
24. Bodell BR. A capillary membrane oxygenator. *J Thorac Cardiovasc Surg* 1963;46:639–650.
25. McCaughan JS, Weeder RR, Schuder JC, et al. Evaluation of new non-wetable microporous membranes with high permeability coefficients for possible use in a membrane oxygenator. *J Thorac Cardiovasc Surg* 1969;40:574.
26. Peirce EC II, Dibelius NR. The membrane lung: studies with a new high permeability co-polymer membrane. *Trans Am Soc Artif Intern Organs* 1968;14:220.
27. Lande AJ, Edwards L, Bloch JH, et al. Cardiopulmonary support with a practical membrane oxygenator. *Trans Am Soc Artif Intern Organs* 1970;16:352–356.
28. Bramson ML, Osborn JJ, Main FB, et al. A new disposable membrane oxygenator with integral heat exchange. *J Thorac Cardiovasc Surg* 1965;50:391–400.
29. Galletti PM, Brecher GA. Bubble oxygenation and membrane oxygenation. In: *Heart Lung Bypass; Principles and Techniques of Extracorporeal Circulation*. New York: Grune and Stratton; 1962:61–78, 108–120.
30. Butler BD. Biophysical aspects of gas bubbles in blood. *Med Instr* 1985;19:59–62.
31. Pearson DT, Carter RF, Hammo MB, et al. Gaseous microemboli during open heart surgery. In: Longmore DB, ed. *Towards A Safer Cardiac Surgery*. Boston: GK Hall Medical Publ; 1981:325–354.
32. Pearson DT, Holden MP, Poslad SJ, et al. A clinical evalu-

ation of the performance characteristics of one membrane and five bubble oxygenators: gas transfer and gaseous microemboli production. *Perfusion* 1986;1:15-26.
33. Yost G. The bubble oxygenator as a source of gaseous microemboli. *Med Instr* 1985;19:67-69.
34. Muravchick S. Scavenging enflurane from extracorporeal pump oxygenators. *Anesthesiology* 1977;47:468-471.
35. Dasta JF, Jacobi J, Wu LS, et al. Loss of nitroglycerine to cardiopulmonary bypass apparatus. *Crit Care Med* 1983; 11:50-52.
36. Dasta JF, Jacobi J, Sokoloski TD, et al. Extraction of nitroglycerine by a membrane oxygenator. *J Extracorporeal Tech* 1983;15:101-103.
37. Rosen DA, Rosen KR, Silvasi DL. In vitro variability in fentanyl absorption by different membrane oxygenators. *J Cardiothorac Anesth* 1990;4:332-335.
38. Hammond GL, Bowley WW. Bubble mechanics and oxygen transfer. *J Thorac Cardiovasc Surg* 1976;71:422-428.
39. Litwak RS, Giannelli S. Open intracardiac operation employing extracorporeal circulation. In: Litwak RS, Jurado RA, eds. *Care of the Cardiac Surgical Patient*. Norwalk: Appleton-Century-Crofts; 1982;65-117.
40. Basha Jr JW, Sternilieb JJ, Bjork VO, et al. Clinical evaluation of Bentley 10 Plus Bubble Oxygenator. *Proc Am Soc Extracorporeal Tech*, 44-47, 1988.
41. Pearson DT, Clayton R, Murray A, et al. A clinical evaluation of the Bentley 10B and Bentley 10 Plus Bubble Oxygenators. *Perfusion* 1988;3:55-63.
42. Stinkens D, Van den fonteyne F, Alleman J, et al. Clinical evaluation of the gas transfer of the Bentley 10 Plus Bubble Oxygenator during alpha-stat regulated hypothermic cardiopulmonary bypass. *J Extracorporeal Technol* 1988;20: 96-100.
43. Sutherland KM, Pearson DT, Gordon LS. Independent control of blood gas PO_2 and PCO_2 in a bubble oxygenator. *Clin Phys Physiol Meas* 1988;9:97-105.
44. Hatteland K, Pedersen T, Semb BKH. Comparison of bubble release from various types of oxygenators. *Scand J Thorac Cardiovasc Surg* 1985;19:125-130.
45. Lee WH, Krumhaar D, Fonkalsrud EW, et al. Denaturation of plasma proteins as a cause of morbidity and death after intracardiac operations. *Surgery* 1961;50:29-39.
46. Lee WH, Hairston P. Structural effects on blood proteins at the gas-blood interface. *Fed Proc* 1971;30:1615-1620.
47. Pearson DT, Holden MP, Poslad SJ, et al. A clinical evaluation of the gas transfer characteristics and gaseous microemboli production of two bubble oxygenators. *Life Support Syst* 1984;2:252-266.
48. Piskin E, Evren V. Composite membranes for extracorporeal gas exchange. *Life Support Syst* 1986;4(suppl 1):2-17.
49. Sigdell JE. Hollow fiber oxygenators. *Artif Organs* 1983; 7:373-397.
50. Haworth WS. Materials for membrane oxygenators. In: Davids SG, Engell HC, eds. *Physiological and Clinical Aspects of Oxygenator Design*. Amsterdam: Elsevier Scientific Publ; 1976:293-298.
51. Bergdahl MEM, Bergdahl LAL. A comparison of flat-sheet and hollow-fiber membrane oxygenators. *Texas Heart Inst J* 1989;16:27-31.
52. Pearson DT, Clayton R, Murray A, McArdle B. A clinical evaluation of the performance characteristics of six commercially available membrane oxygenators. *Proc Am Acad Cardiovasc Perf* 1988;9:54-62.
53. Pearson DT, McArdle B. Hemocompatibility of membrane and bubble oxygenators. *Perfusion* 1989;4:9-24.
54. Gourlay T, Fleming J, Taylor KM, et al. Evaluation of a range of extracorporeal membrane oxygenators. *Perfusion* 1990;5:117-133.
55. O'Connor C, Stenach N, Fisher CA, et al. Hollow fiber membrane oxygenator reduces platelet loss during simulated extracorporeal circulation. *Proc Am Soc Extracorporeal Tech*, 19-23, 1989.
56. Leijala M, Peltola K, Aronen M, et al. Comparison of hollow fiber membrane oxygenators during cardiopulmonary bypass in children: Dideco Masterflo versus Terumo Capiox II. *Perfusion* 1990;5:33-43.
57. Hiratzka LF, Kenrich D, Laskarewski P, et al. Does oxygenator type affect postoperative care charges? *J Extracorporeal Technol* 1992;23:106-111.
58. Retera EMJ, de Jong DS, Dassen WRM, et al. Poor blood mixing in the Shiley hardshell venous reservoir proven by changes in hematological data on different volume levels. *Proc Am Soc Extracorporeal Tech*, 106-109, 1988.
59. Iatridis A, Jenkins C, Zupkas P. The Shiley hardshell venous reservoir in a membrane oxygenator system. *Proc Am Acad Cardiovasc Perf* 1986;7:39-42.
60. Tyndal CM Jr, Berryessa R, Tornabene SP. An in vitro comparison of micro air passage in the venous reservoir bag. *Proc Am Soc Extracorporeal Tech* 1986;18:101-105.
61. James SA, Kalush SL, Maresca L, et al. Clinical experience with the new Terumo open-type membrane oxygenator (Capiox-E). *Proc Am Acad Cardiovasc Perf* 1988;9:51-53.
62. Hargrove M, McCarthy AP, Fitzpatrick GJ. Carbon dioxide flushing prior to priming the bypass circuit. An experimental derivation of the optimal flow rate and duration of the flushing process. *Perfusion* 1987;2:177-179.
63. Dorson WJ, Voorhees ME. Analysis of oxygen and carbon dioxide transfer in membrane lungs. In: Zapol WM, Qvist J, eds. *Artificial Lungs for Acute Respiratory Failure*. New York: Academic Press; 1976:43-68.
64. Eberhart RC, Dengle SK, Curtis RM. Mathematical and experimental methods for design and evaluation of membrane oxygenators. *Artif Organs* 1978;2:19-34.
65. Servas FM. Product design and its relation to the generation of gaseous microemboli in the extracorporeal circuit. *Med Instr* 1985;19:63-66.
66. Karliczek GF, Tigchelaar I, Dijck L, et al. Clinical comparison between four modern membrane oxygenators. *Life Support Syst* 1986;4(suppl 1):153-166.
67. Justison GA. Anesthetic waste gas management for hollow fiber membrane oxygenators. *Proc Am Soc Extracorporeal Tech* 28-31, 1988.
68. Kurusz M, Andrews JJ, Arens JF, et al. Monitoring oxygen concentration prevents potential adverse patient outcome caused by a scavenging malfunction: case report. *Proc Am Acad Cardiovasc Perf* 1991;12:162-165.
69. Jerabek CF, Walton HG, Doerfler S. The effect of gas scavenging on hollow fiber oxygenator performance. *Proc Am Soc Extracorporeal Tech* 24-29, 1989.
70. Galletti PM, Richardson PD, Snider MT, et al. A standard-

ized method for defining the overall gas transfer performance of artificial lungs. *Trans Am Soc Artif Intern Organs* 1972;18:359-367.
71. AAMI Oxygenator Standard, Association for the Advancement of Medical Instrumentation, 1978.
72. Pearson DT, Holden MP, Poslad SJ. Gaseous microemboli production of bubble and membrane oxygenators. *Life Support Syst* 1986;4(suppl 1):198-208.
73. Gassmann CJ, Galbraith GD, Smith RG. Evaluation of three types of membrane oxygenators and their suitability for use with pulsatile flow. *J Extracorporeal Technol* 1987;19:297-304.
74. Gourlay T, Gibbons M, Taylor KM. Pulsatile flow compatibility of a group of membrane oxygenators. *Perfusion* 1987;2:115-126.
75. Shepard RB, Simpson DC, Sharp JF. Energy equivalent pressure. *Arch Surg* 1966;93:730-740.
76. Riley JA, Winn BA, Justison GA, et al. *The Ability of the Shiley M2000 Membrane Blood Oxygenator to Preserve a Pulsatile Blood Flow Waveform*. Shiley Corporate Publication, 1985.
77. Clark RE, Beauchamp RA, Magrath RA, et al. Comparison of bubble and membrane oxygenators in short and long perfusions. *J Thorac Cardiovasc Surg* 1979;78:655-663.
78. Dancy CM, Townsend ER, Boylett A, et al. Pulmonary dysfunction associated with cardiopulmonary bypass: a comparison of bubble and membrane oxygenators. *Circulation* 1981;64(suppl II):54-57.
79. Hicks GL, Zwart HHJ, DeWall RA. Membrane vs bubble oxygenators: a prospective study of 52 patients. *Arch Surg* 1979;114:1285-1287.
80. Peirce EC II. Is the blood-gas interface of clinical importance? *Ann Thorac Surg* 1974;17:526-529.
81. Allison PL, Kurusz M, Graves DF, et al. Devices and monitoring during neonatal ECMO: survey results. *Perfusion* 1990;5:193-201.
82. Iatridis A, Voorhees M, Miller M. Review of ECMO in adults—North American experience. *Perfusion* 1988;3:37-40.
83. Justison GA, Pelley W. Hemodynamic management during closed circuit percutaneous cardiopulmonary bypass. *Proc Am Soc Extracorporeal Tech*, 88-95, 1989.
84. Litzie K, Roberts CP. Emergency femoro-femoral cardiopulmonary bypass. *Proc Am Acad Cardiovasc Perf* 1987;8:60-65.
85. Lowinger T, Shawl F, Diffee G, Richmond J. Percutaneous cardiopulmonary (bypass) support in the cardiac catheterization laboratory: a new application of perfusion. *Proc Am Soc Extracorporeal Tech*, 9-10, 1989.
86. Sinard JM, Bartlett RH. Extracorporeal membrane oxygenation (ECMO): prolonged bedside cardiopulmonary bypass. *Perfusion* 1990;5:239-249.
87. Dutton RC, Edmunds LH, Hutchinson JC, et al. Platelet aggregate emboli produced in patients during cardiopulmonary bypass with membrane and bubble oxygenators and blood filters. *J Thorac Cardiovasc Surg* 1974;67:258-265.
88. Hammerschmidt DE, Stroncek DF, Bowers TK, et al. Complement activation and neutropenia occurring during cardiopulmonary bypass. *J Thorac Cardiovasc Surg* 1981;81:370-377.
89. Hessell EA II, Johnson DD, Ivey TD, et al. Membrane versus bubble oxygenator for cardiac operations: a prospective randomized study. *J Thorac Surg* 1980;80:111-122.
90. Hill DG, de Lanerolle P, Kosek JC, et al. The pulmonary pathophysiology of membrane and bubble oxygenators. *Trans Am Soc Artif Intern Organs* 1975;21:165-170.
91. Liddicoat JE, Bekassy SM, Beall AC, et al. Membrane vs bubble oxygenator: clinical comparison. *Ann Surg* 1975;181:747-753.
92. Peirce EC II. The membrane versus bubble oxygenator controversy. *Ann Thorac Surg* 1980;29:497-499.
93. Pranger RL, Mook PH, Elstrodt JM, et al. Improved tissue perfusion (PO_2 histograms) in extracorporeal circulation using membrane instead of bubble oxygenators. *J Thorac Cardiovasc Surg* 1980;99:513-522.
94. Sade RM, Bartles DM, Dearing JP, et al. A prospective randomized study of membrane versus bubble oxygenators in children. *Ann Thorac Surg* 1980;29:502-511.
95. Siderys H, Halbrook HH, Pittman JN, et al. A comparison of membrane and bubble oxygenation as used in cardiopulmonary bypass in patients. *J Thorac Cardiovasc Surg* 1975;69:708-712.
96. Trumbull HR, Howe J, Mottl K, et al. A comparison of the effects of membrane and bubble oxygenators on platelet counts and platelet size in elective cardiac operations. *Ann Thorac Surg* 1980;30:52-57.
97. Addonizio VP, Colman RW, Edmunds LH. The effect of blood flow rate and circuit surface area on platelet loss during extracorporeal circulation. *Trans Am Soc Artif Intern Organs* 1978;24:650-655.
98. Baier RE, Cutton RC. Initial events in interaction of blood with a foreign surface. *J Biomed Mater Res* 1969;3:191-206.
99. Brown CH III, Leverett LB, Lewis W, et al. Morphological, biochemical, and functional changes in human platelets subjected to shear stress. *J Lab Clin Med* 1975;86:462-471.
100. Friedman LI, Liem H, Grabowski EF, et al. Inconsequentiality of surface properties for initial platelet adhesion. *Trans Am Soc Artif Intern Organs* 1970;16:63-73.
101. Friedman LI, Leonard EF. Platelet adhesion to artificial surfaces: consequences of flow, exposure time, blood condition, and surface nature. *Fed Proc* 1971;30:1641-1646.
102. Gomes MR, McGoon DC. Bleeding patterns after open-heart surgery. *J Thorac Cardiovasc Surg* 1970;60:87-97.
103. Harker LA, Malpass TW, Branson HE. Mechanism of abnormal bleeding in patients undergoing cardiopulmonary bypass: acquired transient platelet dysfunction associated with selective granule release. *Blood* 1980;56:824-834.
104. Hennessy VL, Hicks RE, Niewiarowski S, et al. Function of human platelets during extracorporeal circulation. *Am J Physiol* 1977;232:H622-H628.
105. Kim SW, Lees RG, Oster H, et al. Platelet adhesion to polymer surfaces. *Trans Am Soc Artif Intern Organs* 1974;20:449-455.
106. Lautier A, Dehe T, Awad J, et al. Deposits on flat plate and hollow fibers oxygenators. *Int J Artif Organs* 1968;9:173-178.
107. Lyman DJ, Brash SW, Chaikin SW, et al. The effect of chemical structure and surface properties of synthetic poly-

mers on the coagulation of blood. *Trans Am Soc Artif Intern Organs* 1968;14:250-255.
108. Lyman DJ, Kim SW. Interactions at the blood-polymer interface. *Fed Proc* 1971;30:1658-1660.
109. McKenna R, Bachmann F, Whittaker B, et al. The hemostatic mechanism after open heart surgery. *J Thorac Cardiovasc Surg* 1975;70:298-308.
110. Packham MA, Evan G, Glynn MG, et al. The effect of plasma proteins on the interaction of platelets with glass surfaces. *J Lab Clin Med* 1969;73:686-697.
111. Salzman EW, Lindon J, Brier D. Surface-induced platelet adhesion, aggregation, and release. *Ann NY Acad Sci* 1977; 283:114-127.
112. Ward CA, Ruegsegger B, Stanga D, et al. Reduction in platelet adhesion to biomaterials by removal of gas nuclei. *Trans Am Soc Artif Intern Organs* 1974;20:77-85.
113. Weiss L. Biophysical aspects of initial cell interactions with solid surfaces. *Fed Proc* 1971;30:1649-1657.
114. De Leval M, Hill JD, Mielke H, et al. Platelet kinetics during extracorporeal circulation. *Trans Am Soc Artif Int Organs* 1972;18:355-358.
115. De Leval MR, Hill JD, Mielke CH, et al. Blood platelets and extracorporeal circulation. *J Thorac Cardiovasc Surg* 1975;69:144-151.
116. Boers M, van den Dungen JJAM, Karliczek GF, et al. Two membrane oxygenators and a bubbler: a clinical comparison. *Ann Thorac Surg* 1983;35:455-462.
117. Boonstra PW, Vermeulen FEE, Leusink JA, et al. Hematological advantage of a membrane oxygenator over a bubble oxygenator in long perfusions. *Ann Thorac Surg* 1986;41: 297-300.
118. Calafiore AM, Glieca F, Marchesani F, et al. A comparative clinical assessment of a hollow-fiber membrane oxygenator (Capiox II) and a bubble oxygenator (Harvey 1500): *J Cardiovasc Surg* 1987;28:633-637.
119. Nilsson L, Bagge L, Nystrom SO. Blood cell trauma and postoperative bleeding: comparison of bubble and membrane oxygenators and observations on coronary suction. *Scand J Thorac Cardiovasc Surg* 1990;24:65-69.
120. Benedetti M, De Caterina R, Bionda A, et al. Blood-artificial surface interactions during cardiopulmonary bypass: a comparative study of four oxygenators. *Int J Artif Organs* 1990;13:488-497.
121. Van Oeveren W, Kazatchkine MD, Descamps-Latscha B, et al. Deleterious effects of cardiopulmonary bypass: a prospective study of bubble versus membrane oxygenation. *J Thorac Cardiovasc Surg* 1985;89:888-899.
122. Van den Dungen JJAM, Karliezek GF, Brenken U, et al. Clinical study of blood trauma during perfusion with membrane and bubble oxygenators. *J Thorac Cardiovasc Surg* 1982;83:108-116.
123. Peterson KA, Dewanjee MK, Kaye MP. Fate of indium 111-labeled platelets during cardiopulmonary bypass performed with membrane and bubble oxygenators. *J Thorac Cardiovasc Surg* 1982;84:39-43.
124. Boralessa H, Shifferli JA, Zaimi F, et al. Perioperative changes in complement associated with cardiopulmonary bypass. *Br J Anaesth* 1982;54:1047-1052.
125. Cavarocchi NC, Schaff HV, Orszulak TA, et al. Evidence for complement activation by protamine-heparin interaction after cardiopulmonary bypass. *Surgery* 1985;98:525-531.
126. Chenoweth DE, Cooper SW, Hugli TE, et al. Complement activation during cardiopulmonary bypass. *N Engl J Med* 1981;304:497-503.
127. Collett B, Alhaq A, Abdullah NB, et al. Pathways to complement activation during cardiopulmonary bypass. *Br Med J* 1984;289:1251-1254.
128. Haslam PL, Townsend PJ, Branthwaite MA. Complement activation during cardiopulmonary bypass. *Anaesthesia* 1980;25:22-26.
129. Heideman M, Kaijer B, Gelin LE. Complement activation by homogenized muscle. *J Surg Res* 1978;25:518-522.
130. Loubser PG. Complement activation during cardiac and thoracic vascular operations. *Texas Heart Inst J* 1987;14: 369-373.
131. Parker DJ, Cantrell JW, Karp RB, et al. Changes in serum complement and immunoglobulins following cardiopulmonary bypass. *Surgery* 1972;71:824-827.
132. Rent R, Ertel N, Eisinstein R, et al. Complement activation by interaction of polyanions and polycations. I. Heparin-protamine induced consumption of complement. *J Immunol* 1975;114:120-124.
133. Tamiya T, Yamasaki M, Yoshinobu M, et al. Complement activation in cardiopulmonary bypass with special reference to anaphylatoxin production in membranes and bubble oxygenators. *Ann Thorac Surg* 1988;46:47-57.
134. Videm V, Fosse E, Mollnes TE, et al. Different oxygenators for cardiopulmonary bypass lead to varying degrees of human complement activation in vitro. *J Thorac Cardiovasc Surg* 1989;97:764-770.
135. White JV. Complement activation during cardiopulmonary bypass. *N Engl J Med* 1981;305:51.
136. Antonsen S, Brandslund I, Clemensen S, et al. Neutrophil lysosomal enzyme release and complement activation during cardiopulmonary bypass. *Scand J Thorac Cardiovasc Surg* 1987;21:47-52.
137. Kirklin JK, Westaby S, Blackstone EH, et al. Complement and the damaging effects of cardiopulmonary bypass. *J Thorac Cardiovasc Surg* 1983;86:845-857.
138. Nilsson L, Brunnkvist S, Nilsson U. Activation of inflammatory systems during cardiopulmonary bypass. *Scand J Thorac Cardiovasc Surg* 1988;22:51-53.
139. Hammerschmidt DE, Weaver LJ, Hudson LD, et al. Association of complement activation and elevated plasma-C5a with adult respiratory distress syndrome: pathological relevance and possible prognostic value. *Lancet* 1980;1:947-949.
140. Jacob HS. Complement-mediated leucoembolization. A mechanism of tissue damage during extracorporeal perfusions, myocardial infarction, and shock. *Q J Med* 1983;52: 289-296.
141. Lew PD, Forster A, Perrin LH. Complement activation in the adult respiratory distress syndrome following cardiopulmonary bypass. *Bull Eur Physiopathol Respir* 1985;21: 231-235.
142. Ratliff NB, Young WG Jr, Hackel DB, et al. Pulmonary injury secondary to extracorporeal circulation. An ultrastructural study. *J Thorac Cardiovasc Surg* 1973;65:425-432.

143. Wilson JW. The pulmonary cellular and subcellular alterations of extracorporeal circulation. *Surg Clin North Am* 1974;54:1204-1221.
144. Nilsson L, Nilsson U, Venge P, et al. Inflammatory system activation during cardiopulmonary bypass as an indicator of biocompatibility: A randomized comparison of bubble and membrane oxygenators. *Scand J Thorac Cardiovasc Surg* 1990;24:53-58.
145. Cavarocchi NC, Pluth JR, Schaff HV, et al. Complement activation during cardiopulmonary bypass. *J Thorac Cardiovasc Surg* 1986;91:252-258.
146. Videm V, Fosse E, Mollnes TE, et al. Complement activation with bubble and membrane oxygenators in aortocoronary bypass grafting. *Ann Thorac Surg* 1990;50:387-391.
147. Baier RE. The organization of blood components near interfaces. *Ann NY Acad Sci* 1977;283:17-36.
148. Chenoweth DE, Hugli TE. Demonstration of specific C5a receptor on intact human polymorphonuclear leukocytes. *Proc Natl Acad Sci USA* 1978;75:3943-3947.
149. Hairston P, Manos JP, Graber CB, et al. Depression of immunologic surveillance by pump-oxygenator perfusion. *J Surg Res* 1969;9:587-593.
150. Hammerschmidt DE, Harnes PE, Wayland JH, et al. Complement-induced granulocyte aggregation in vivo. *Am J Pathol* 1981;102:146-150.
151. Jacob HS, Craddock PR, Hammerschmidt DE, et al. Complement-induced granulocyte aggregation. An unsuspected mechanism of disease. *N Engl J Med* 1980;302:789-794.
152. Mayer JE, McCullough J, Weiblen BJ, et al. Effects of cardiopulmonary bypass on neutrophil chemotaxis. *Surg Forum* 1976;27:285-287.
153. O'Flaherty JT, Kreutzer DL, Ward PA. Neutrophil aggregation and swelling induced by chemotactic agents. *J Immunol* 1977;119:232-239.
154. O'Flaherty JT, Craddock PR, Jacob HS. Effect of intravascular complement activation on granulocyte adhesiveness and distribution. *Blood* 1978;51:731-739.
155. Riegel W, Spillner G, Schlosser V, et al. Plasma levels of main granulocyte components during cardiopulmonary bypass. *J Thorac Cardiovasc Surg* 1988;95:1014-1019.
156. Ryhanen P, Herva E, Hollmen A, et al. Changes in peripheral blood leukocyte counts, lymphocyte subpopulations, and in vitro transformation after heart valve replacement. *J Thorac Cardiovasc Surg* 1979;77:259-264.
157. Wachtfogel YT, Kucich U, Greenplate J. Human neutrophil degranulation during extracorporeal circulation. *Blood* 1987;69:324-330.
158. De Jong JCF, Woltjes J, Paping RHL, et al. Impaired leukocyte function and postoperative infection in extracorporeal circulation. *Proc Eur Soc Artif Organs* 1977;4:523-528.
159. Silva J Jr, Hoeksema H, Fekety FR. Transient defects in phagocytic functions during cardiopulmonary bypass. *J Thorac Cardiovasc Surg* 1974;67:175-183.
160. Van Velzen-Blad H, Dijkstra YJ, Schurink GA. Cardiopulmonary bypass and host defense functions in human beings: I. Serum levels and role of immunoglobulins and complement in phagocytosis. *Ann Thorac Surg* 1985;39:207-211.
161. De Jong JC, Smit Sibinga CT, Wildevuur CR. Platelet behavior in extracorporeal circulation. *Transfusion* 1979;19:72-80.
162. De Jong JC, Ten Duis HJ, Smit Sibinga CT, et al. Hematological aspects of cardiotomy suction in cardiac operations. *J Thorac Cardiovasc Surg* 1980;79:227-236.
163. Edmunds LH Jr, Saxena NC, Hillyer P, et al. Relationship between platelet count and cardiotomy suction return. *Ann Thorac Surg* 1978;25:306-310.
164. Ten Duis HJ, De Jong JCF, Van Asseldonk AGM, et al. Improved hemocompatibility in open heart surgery. *Trans Am Soc Artif Intern Organs*. 1978;24:656-661.
165. Van Oeveren W, Dankert J, Wildevuur CRH. Bubble oxygenation and cardiotomy suction impair the host defence during cardiopulmonary bypass: A study in dogs. *Ann Thorac Surg* 1987;44:523-528.
166. Padayachee TS, Parsons S, Theobold E, et al. The detection of microemboli in the middle cerebral artery during cardiopulmonary bypass: A transcranial Doppler ultrasound investigation using membrane and bubble oxygenators. *Ann Thorac Surg* 1987;44:289-302.
167. Blauth C, Smith P, Newman S, et al. Retinal microembolism and neuropsychological deficit following clinical cardiopulmonary bypass: comparison of a membrane and a bubble oxygenator. *Eur J Cardiothorac Surg* 1989;3:135-139.
168. Blauth CI, Smith PL, Arnold JV, et al. Influence of oxygenator type on the prevalence and extent of microembolic retinal ischemia during cardiopulmonary bypass. *J Thorac Cardiovasc Surg* 1990;99:61-69.
169. Van den Dungen JJAM, Homan van der Heide JN, Karliczek GF, et al. Clinical evaluation of blood damage related to cardiopulmonary bypass. *Proc Eur Soc Artif Organs* 1978;5:238-243.
170. Edmunds LH Jr, Ellison N, Colman RW, et al. Platelet function during cardiac operation: comparison of membrane and bubble oxygenators. *J Thorac Cardiovasc Surg* 1982;83:805-812.
171. Zadeh BJ, Holazo R, Conlon C, et al. A clinical evaluation of three modern blood oxygenators. *Perfusion* 1987;2:263-270.

11
Mechanical Pumps for Extracorporeal Circulation

Christopher R. Trocchio and James O. Sketel

Introduction

Development of a mechanical blood pump intended to replace temporarily the function of the human heart has been the focus of physiologic and engineering research since the early 1900s. The criteria established to define the ideal blood pump during these early developmental stages are still valid.[1-3] The ideal blood pump should have a controllable pulse rate and stroke volume. It should be capable of producing a wide range of outputs which are linearly proportional to the pulse rate, but independent of the resistance to fluid flow in the perfusion circuit, including the resistance in infusion cannulas. Blood handling should occur at low velocities in order to reduce the kinetic energy transferred to the blood and thus reduce hemolysis. The pump should avoid blood stagnation, turbulence, and cavitation, and all pump parts in contact with the blood should be disposable. As a safety feature, the pump, which would be electrically controlled and operated for routine use, should have manual and/or battery operation available in the event of a power failure. Finally, the pump should include a monitoring system which can determine the actual pump speed so that this actual speed can be continuously compared to the desired pump speed set by the speed control. Table 11.1 summarizes the proposed characteristics of the ideal blood pump.

From an engineering standpoint, there are six methods by which fluids can be moved through a circuit: (1) volumetric displacement, either mechanically or with other fluids, (2) action of centrifugal force, (3) mechanical impulse, (4) transfer of momentum from another fluid, (5) electromagnetic force, or (6) gravity.[4] Aside from electromagnetic force (which may find application in future pump designs!), all of these principles can be applied or are being utilized in extracorporeal circuits. The two most common types of blood pumps used clinically are centrifugal pumps and positive displacement roller pumps.

Centrifugal Pumps

Centrifugal pumps produce flow by imparting kinetic energy to fluid in a rotating head. From an engineering point of view, these pumps have a simple transmission and few moving parts; they are compact and efficient.[5] Early attempts to utilize centrifugal pumps with blood yielded unsatisfactory results. In the early 1970s, research efforts related to the development of an artificial heart led to the development of centrifugal pumps suitable for everyday clinical use. In 1973, the Biomedicus Model 600 (Biomedicus, Inc., Minneapolis, MN) became the first disposable centrifugal pump available for clinical procedures (Figure 11.1).[6]

Centrifugal pumps currently in use employ either a cone- or a fin-type design to pump blood. Figure 11.2 shows a cross-sectional view of a cone-type centrifugal pump. Blood enters at point A at the center of the nested cones and exits at point B. The spinning cones create a negative pressure at point A that pulls blood into the pump. Once the blood is inside the pump head, energy is imparted to the blood by the spinning cones, forming a vortex. The vortex is then constrained by the outside plastic housing, generating pressure to pump the blood out at point B. Between the inlet and the outlet there are no occlusive devices in this pump. If the cones were not spinning, fluid could flow through the head in either direction. During operation, the flow generated by this pump is affected both by preload (the pressure at the inlet point A) and afterload (the pressure at the outlet point B). Centrifugal pumps increase flow when the preload increases or when the afterload decreases. Conversely, a decreased preload or an increased afterload will decrease pump flow.[6-8] Centrifugal pumps are therefore pressure sensitive (Figure 11.3).

The disposable pump head is placed in a permanent drive console. A magnet in the drive console spins, causing a magnet in the base of the disposable pump head to

11. Mechanical Pumps for Extracorporeal Circulation

TABLE 11.1. Characteristics of an ideal blood pump.

Controllable stroke volume and pulse rate
Capable of producing a wide range of outputs which are linearly proportional to the pulse rate and independent of afterload
Minimal transfer of kinetic energy to the blood
Parts in contact with blood are disposable, have smooth surface, and are of simple design
Devoid of areas conducive to blood stagnation, turbulence, or cavitation
Calibration easy and reproducible
Automatically controlled and operated for routine use with manual and/or battery operation potential in the event of power failure
Includes a monitor of actual versus predicted pump speed that halts pump flow when the pump speed exceeds the set pump speed by more than a fixed percent

---

spin at an equal rate. Because of this coupling of the permanent drive console magnet and the pump head magnet, the speed (revolutions per minute or rpm) of the drive console equals the speed of the cones in the pump head (Figure 11.4).

Figure 11.5A and B illustrates two other centrifugal pumps (Isoflow, St. Jude Medical, Inc., St. Paul, MN, and the Delphin centrifugal pump, 3M Sarns, Ann Arbor, MI) currently available for clinical use. As shown, the other common type of centrifugal pump uses a finned or vaned impeller instead of nested cones inside the pump housing. These disposable heads are similarly magnetically coupled to a separate drive console. The fins of this impeller still rely on some degree of friction and sheer stress to impart energy to the blood. They also have a direct pushing and lifting effect within the pump housing. The curvature and angle of the fins and their orientation to both the inlet and the outlet of the pump housing have been the focus of much research, attempting to efficiently transport blood while minimizing factors known to cause blood damage. These factors include turbulence, pressure gradients, eddies, cavitation, stagnation points, and foreign surface contact. The fin-type pumps are more efficient at moving fluids at a given speed.[9,10] There are conflicting data as to which pumps are least traumatic to blood.

Because centrifugal pumps are pressure sensitive, they require a separate sensor or flow meter to monitor blood flow out of the pump. Two available monitoring technologies have yielded satisfactory results in the clinical setting. These are based upon either electromagnetic or Doppler principles.[11,12] Electromagnetic flow probes rely on the fact that the flow of blood through an electromagnetic field leads to an alteration in that magnetic field which can be measured. To utilize this technology, a probe needs to be placed in contact with blood. A transducer then relays this information to the pump console which displays an actual blood flow.

Doppler technology does not utilize a probe that is placed in contact with the blood, but rather a probe that wraps around the tubing. The frequency shift in the Doppler signal is related to the velocity of blood flow through the tubing. Since the cross-sectional area of the tube is known, the Doppler shift can then be utilized to determine blood flow.

Centrifugal pumps have two potential advantages over roller pumps. Because centrifugal pumps are sensitive to afterload pressure, a catastrophic pressure buildup in the arterial line (which might happen if the tubing were kinked) cannot occur because flow will decrease through the pump as pressure increases. A second potential advantage is that these pumps have a tendency not to pump air that may be inadvertently introduced into the circuit. In a constrained vortex pump, there is high pressure at the periphery and low pressure at the center of the pump head. Because of this pressure difference, air tends to remain at the center of the pump head and not be expelled from the pump. In the event of a massive introduction of air, the pump can become unprimed, stopping the flow. There are, however, conflicting data on how effectively these types of pumps eliminate the problem of air embolism.[6,9,10,13-16]

In comparing centrifugal and roller pumps, studies examining blood-handling characteristics have produced conflicting results.[17-20] The cost of the disposable centrifu-

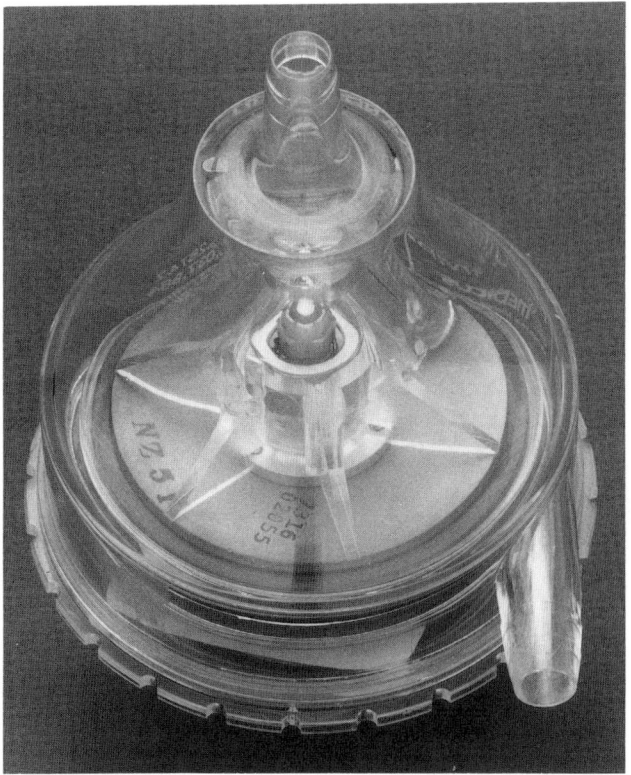

FIGURE 11.1. The Biomedicus model 600, the first disposable centrifugal pump, was available for clinical use in 1973.

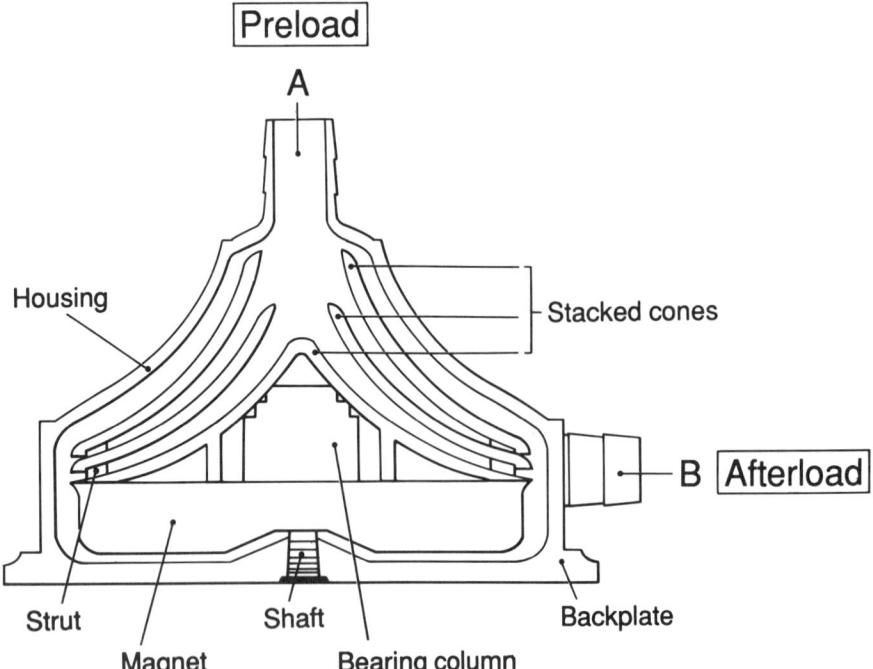

FIGURE 11.2. Cross-sectional view of a cone-type centrifugal pump. Blood enters at point A (preload) and exits at point B (afterload).

gal pump head has always been a concern, but this cost has steadily decreased and more widespread application has resulted. It is estimated that approximately 50% of all CPB procedures now use a disposable centrifugal pump head in the arterial position. Centrifugal pump heads have also found routine use for temporary ventricular assist, mobile emergency CPB circuits, and venovenous bypass for orthotopic liver transplantation.

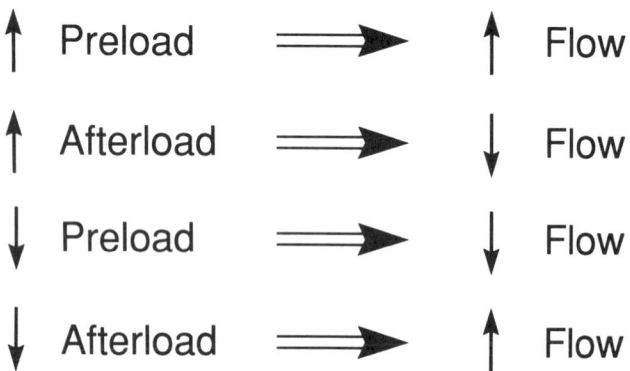

FIGURE 11.3. Relationship of preload, afterload, and centrifugal pump blood flow.

Roller (Rotary) Pumps

Roller or rotary pumps contain mechanical parts that trap a portion of the fluid and propel it forward.[21] They are one type of positive displacement pump. Valves are not required to provide unidirectional flow. The output of the rotary pump depends upon the speed of the pump and the volume displaced with each revolution. Rotary pumps use a roller that compresses a segment of blood-filled resilient tubing against a semicircular backing plate, propelling the blood forward. Depending upon the number of rollers, roller pumps are classified as single, double, and multiple roller pumps (Figure 11.6). The basic design of the roller pump was patented in 1855 by Porter and Bradley.[22] Refinements in pump design and materials engineering (with regard to both the tubing and the pump housing) have led to the efficient and effective roller pumps used today.

In the early years, a well-engineered pump housing and roller did not guarantee efficient blood pumping. The tubing used in the early pumps had a tendency to move vertically up the backing plate and forward through the pumping chamber as the roller passed over it. Several techniques used to prevent vertical movement of the tubing are depicted in Figure 11.7.[21] The forward movement of the tubing has been controlled by having tubing inserts or brushings in the pump head which hold the tubing in place at the inlet and outlet areas of the pump raceway. This provides a constant stroke volume with each pump cycle. The term "pump occlusion" refers to the occlusion of the tubing as the roller presses the tubing against the

11. Mechanical Pumps for Extracorporeal Circulation

FIGURE 11.4. The disposable centrifugal pump head is coupled to the permanent drive console by magnets that spin to effect blood flow.

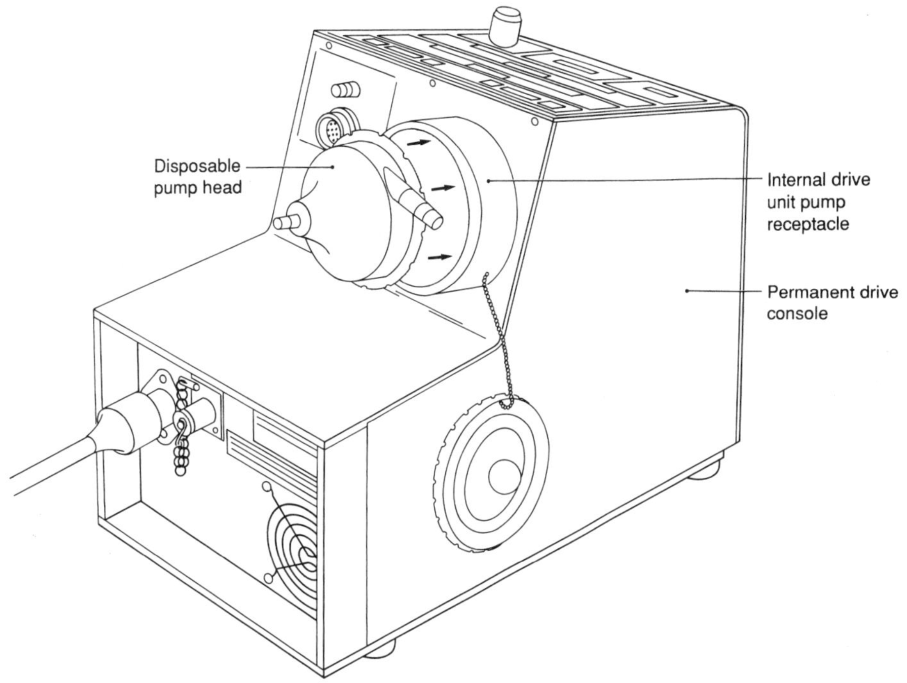

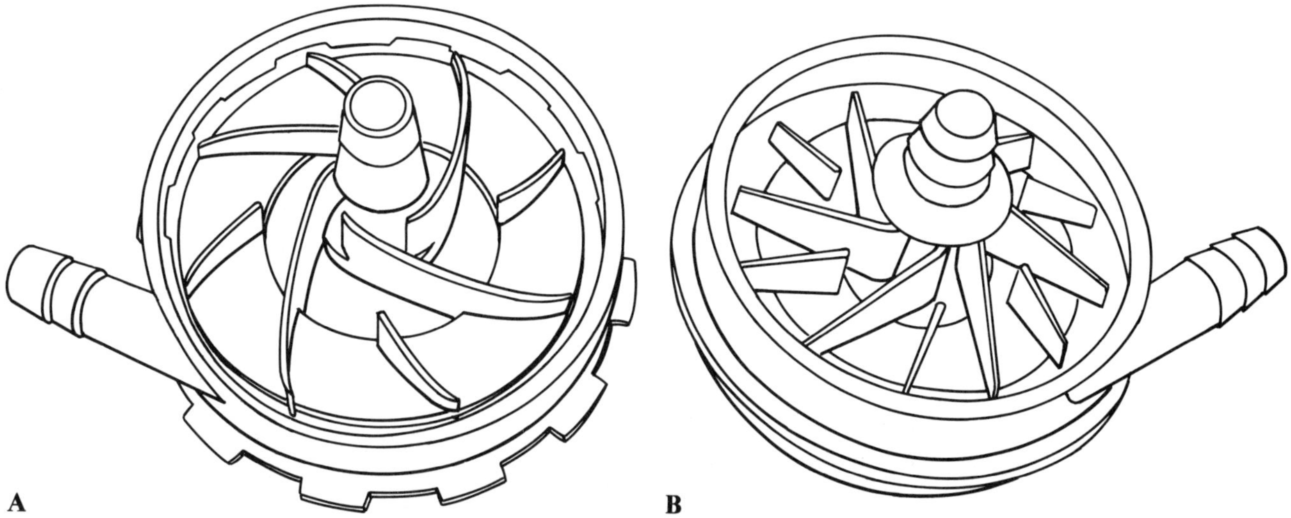

FIGURE 11.5. The Isoflow (A) by St. Jude Medical and the Delphin (B) by 3M Sarns are fin-type centrifugal pumps currently available for clinical use.

FIGURE 11.6. Roller pump classifications: (A) Single-roller pump incorporating a 360° backplate. (B) Double- or twin-roller pump with a 210° backplate and two rollers, 180° out of phase. (C) Triple- or multiple-roller pump, using three roller heads combined with a 120° backplate.

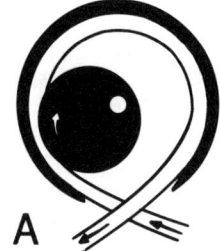
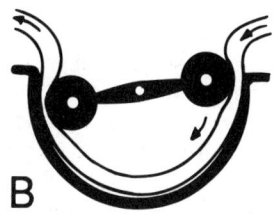
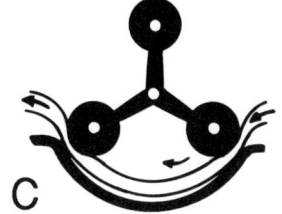

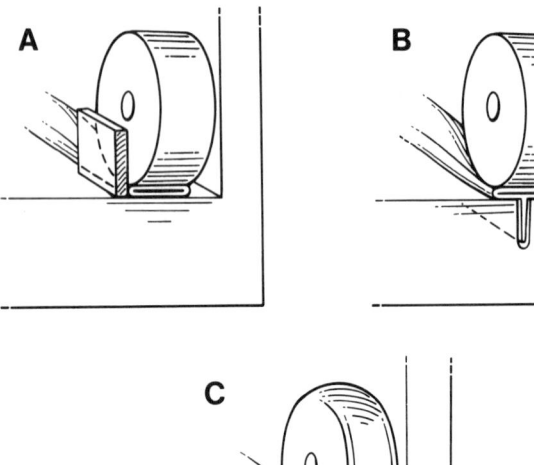

FIGURE 11.7. The different systems employed in roller pumps to keep the tubing in place. The pump housing is in black; the roller is marked by horizontal strips; the tubing shown is compressed between the roller and backplate. (A) Guide rod on the left of the tube prevents lateral movement. (B) Flange inserted into a slot of the backplate keeps the tube straight. (C) Tube compressed between convex roller and grooved backplate.

raceway. Most pumps allow the operator to set the occlusion of each roller separately. The proper tubing occlusion ("just occlusive") can be achieved using the procedure outlined in Table 11.2. The occlusion of each roller should be checked at different areas of the backing plate. It is possible for the backing plate to get "out of round," so that occlusion can vary somewhat at different points of the backplate. If there is a wide discrepancy between different areas on the backplate, the pump should be repaired.

TABLE 11.2. Roller pump occlusion procedure.

Step 1	Load the unprimed tubing in the roller-pump raceway.
Step 2	Introduce the appropriate amount of priming solution into the oxygenator.
Step 3	While holding a segment of tubing on the positive side of the pump vertically, advance a column of crystalloid priming solution approximately 30 cm above the level of the pump.
Step 4	The occlusion of each roller can now be adjusted to allow a 1-cm drop of the priming solution per minute. This 1-cm drop in a 30-cm column of priming solution will mimic the action of blood in a "just occluded" state.

It was initially felt that a nonocclusive pump would cause less hemolysis than an occlusive one. However, it is now felt that a pump which is "just occlusive" causes the lowest hemolysis rates.[23] A nonocclusive pump allows high backflow velocities, increasing the kinetic energy transferred to the blood, thereby increasing hemolysis. A nonocclusive pump also requires more revolutions per minute for any given forward flow rate compared to an occlusive pump.

Roller pump designs have been altered in an attempt to minimize hemolysis. This effort has focused upon the speed required to achieve a desired flow, the number of rollers a pump contains, and the proper occlusion of rollers. It is generally accepted that as the revolutions per minute and the number of rollers are increased, the hemolysis rate increases. This can be attributed to several factors, including mechanical compression, friction heat, and sheer stress. Revolutions per minute can be decreased while maintaining the same flow rate if tubing diameter (and thus stroke volume) is increased and the number of rollers is decreased. Currently, most pumps have two rollers, and tubing of ½ inch or ⅜ inch internal diameter is used in the arterial pump head.

Pump calibration (the relationship between the revolutions per minute of the pump head and the flow per minute generated by the pump) should remain relatively constant over a period of months. Ordinarily, the calibration needs to be checked only at 6-month intervals. Between these checks, the output of the pump should remain within 5% of the original calibration curve. If a change is made in tubing, a new calibration curve should obviously be generated. Because "just occlusive" roller pumps are quite afterload insensitive, the use of the calibration curve in estimating pump flow from revolutions per minute is very accurate.

Single-Roller Pump

The single-roller pump consists of a circular raceway in which a 360° loop of tubing is inserted. The output of a single-roller pump is independent of afterload when the pump is properly occluded. Single-roller pumps were used in heart-lung machines in the 1950s and early 1960s, since the single-roller pump produces more pulsatile flow than the conventional twin-roller pump.[24] For this reason, there is some enthusiasm for the development of new, state-of-the-art, single-roller pumps.

Double- or Twin-Roller Pump

The double- or twin-roller pump has been the most widely used pump in open-heart surgical procedures (Figure 11.8). The design of the twin-roller pump combines a 210° semicircular backing plate and two rollers that are 180° out of phase with one antoher.[21] As one roller ends its occlusive phase, the other has already begun its occlu-

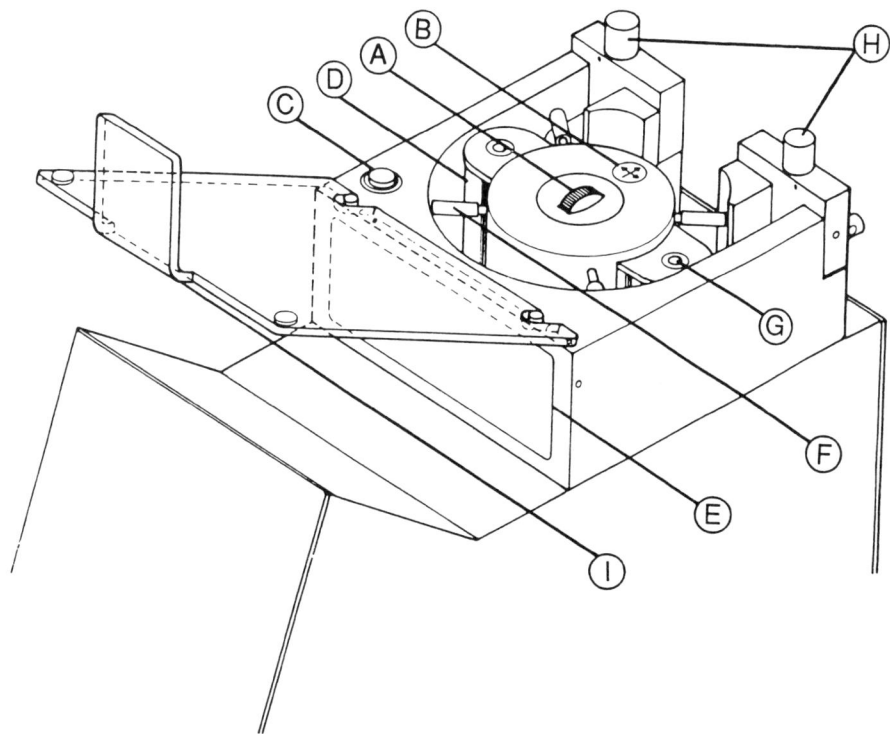

FIGURE 11.8. Roller pump head. (A) Occlusion thumbwheel—moves both tubing rollers (D) inward or outward in unison. (B) Occlusion direction indicator—indicates the direction of thumbwheel motion. (C) Cover switch—is activated when the pump cover (I) is closed. When the cover is opened, the pump head stops. (D) Tubing rollers—occlude the pump tubing segment to move fluid through the extracorporeal circuit. (E) Flow-rate chart—provides the approximate relationship between revolutions per minute and liters per minute for several common tubing sizes. This can be used for rough calibration of the liter per minute display. (F) Tubing roller guide—helps keep the tubing centered in the pump raceway. There are four upper and four lower tubing roller guides in the pump head. (G) Hand-crank hole—allows the hand crank to be inserted into the pump head for manual rotation of the pump should a power loss occur. (H) Universal tubing clamp adjustment knobs (two)—sets retention force on the pump tubing. These knobs control position of the universal tubing clamps and can be adjusted to allow the clamp to accommodate a wide range of tubing sizes. (I) Pump cover—shields the moving parts of the pump when it is running. The pump head will not rotate with the cover open.

sive phase. Thus, the tubing is always compressed by one of the two rollers. The flow produced is relatively nonpulsatile.

Multiple-Roller Pump

The multiple-roller pump has been proposed for extracorporeal blood handling.[21] Using three or more rollers, the curvature of the backing plate can be reduced to 120° or less. However, since it has been shown that an increase in the number of rollers increases hemolysis, this design has never gained acceptance in clinical settings.

Reciprocating Pumps

The reciprocating pump is a second type of positive displacement pump in which a fluid chamber is alternately filled and emptied, creating pulsatile flow (Figure 11.9).[25] This type of pump incorporates some type of actuator to expel blood from the pump chamber. The actuator may be in direct contact with the blood or separated from it by a diaphragm. Reciprocating pumps require valves to force the proper direction of blood flow.

Two advanced types of reciprocating pumps are *diaphragm* and *ventricle* pumps.[25] Diaphragm pumps, commonly used for long-term ventricular assistance, propel blood from the holding chamber when acted upon by a hydraulic, pneumatic, or mechanical force. Ventricle pumps have a flexible ventricular chamber encased in a rigid housing. The chamber is compressed by infusion of fluid or air into the housing, causing the ejection of blood. Unidirectional blood flow is achieved with valves at both the inlet and the outlet ports. This design has been used recently to create a successful ventricular assist device, the BVS System 5000 (Abiomed, Danvers, MA) (Figure 11.10). This external blood pump is the first device to be approved by the Food and Drug Administration for ventricular assistance for postcardiotomy cardiogenic shock. The BVS System 5000 consists of two flexible sacks. The

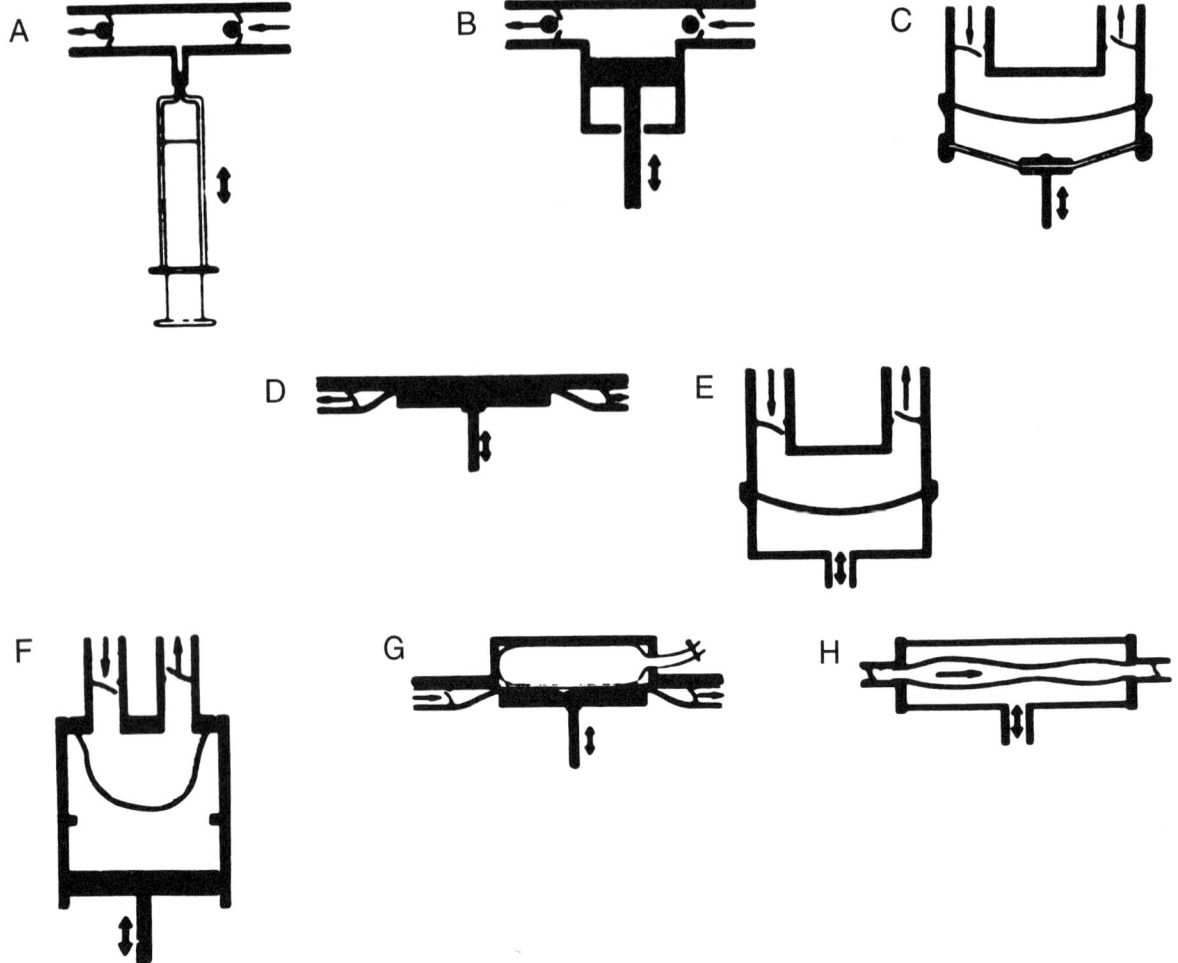

FIGURE 11.9. Reciprocating pumps. These types of pumps incorporate some type of actuator to expel blood from the fluid chamber. Diagrams of the early-stage piston, bellow, and bar compression pumps, as well as the more advanced diaphragm and ventricular pumps, are seen in this figure. Piston pumps: (A) syringe type; (B) plunger type. Diaphragm: (E) hydraulic-driven; (C) gas-driven. Bar compression: (G) solid plate; (D) resilient plate. Ventricle: (H) hydraulic-driven; (F) gas-driven.

upper chamber collects atrial blood by gravity drainage while the lower chamber is emptied by pneumatic pressure. Two tri-leaflet polyurethane valves provide unidirectional blood flow. This pump is also described in Chapter 27.

Blood Pumps Used Primarily for Partial CPB Support

Archimedean Screw Pumps

The Archimedean screw pump is a positive displacement pump consisting of two helical components, a rotor and a stator (Figure 11.11).[21] The rotor is spun within the stator, which is made of a resilient material. Since the stator has a double internal, helical thread, its pitch is twice the pitch of the rotor. When the rotor is inserted into the stator, fluid cavities are formed. As the rotor spins, these fluid cavities, trapped between the rotor and the stator, progress forward toward the outlet of the pump, providing a continuous flow. Throughout this process, spiral seals between the rotor and the stator are intermittently formed, preventing possible backflow. Blood handling is gentle with this type of pump. The blood itself, which is contained in the fluid cavities formed between the rotor and the stator, is practically motionless, resulting in minimal turbulence. An Archimedean screw pump was utilized for clinical CPB in the early 1960s.

A left ventricular assist device, the Nimbus Hemopump (Rancho Cordova, CA) (Figure 11.11), is somewhat similar to the Archimedean screw pump, in that both a stator and a rotor are used. Because there are no occlusive seals between the rotor and the stator, this pump might also be compared to a jet turbine in its mechanism. The device is attached to a cannula that goes across the aortic valve into the left ventricle. The stator-and-rotor portion of the Hemopump is positioned in the descending aorta just distal to the subclavian artery. By means of a flexible shaft, the rotor and stator are attached to an external motor, so that the rotor is spun by a rotating electromagnetic field. This spinning motion can lead to speeds up to 25,000 rpm which will yield an output of 3 to 3.5 L/min. The pump thereby withdraws oxygenated blood from the left ventricle and deposits it into the aorta.

Other pumps designed for short-term, intermediate-term, and long-term ventricular assistance are more fully described in Chapter 27.

References

1. Bahnson HT. Characteristics of an ideal pump for extracorporeal circulation. In: Allen JG, ed. *Extracorporeal Circulation*. Springfield, Ill: Charles C Thomas; 1958:9.
2. Melrose DG. Pumping and oxygenating systems. *Br J Anaesth* 1959;31:393–400.
3. Kolff WJ. Mock circulation to test pumps designed for permanent replacement of damaged hearts. *Cleveland Clin Q* 1959;26:223–226.
4. Pumping of liquids and gases. In: *Chem Eng Handbook*. 5th ed. New York: McGraw-Hill; 1973:3.
5. Stepanoff AJ. *Centrifugal and Axial Flow Pumps: Theory, Design and Application*. New York: John Wiley and Sons Inc; 1957:121–127.
6. *The Bio-Medicus Training Manual*. Education and Technical Support Dept., Eden Prairie, MN: Medtronic Biomedicus Inc, 1987.
7. Landis GH, Mandl JP, Holt D. Pump flow dynamics of the roller pump and constrained vortex pump. *J Extracorp Tech* 1979;6:210–213.
8. Kay PH. *Techniques in Extracorporeal Circulation*. 3rd ed. Oxford: Butterworth-Heinemann Ltd; 1992:36–37.
9. Iatridis E, Chan T. An evaluation of vortex, centrifugal and roller pump systems. Presented at the International Workshop on Rotary Blood Pumps, Vienna, 1991.
10. Edelman W, Levendusky J, Lichtenstein I. Alternate views of hydraulics for an impeller centrifugal pump. *Perfusion* 1992;13:70–72.
11. Akers T, Bolen G, Gomez J, et al. In vitro comparison of ECC blood flow measurement techniques. Presented at the Annual Meeting of the American Society of Extracorporeal Technology, Dallas, Texas, 1990.
12. Wagoner PA. The effect of hematocrit, amplifier input impedance and magnetic excitation frequency on the accuracy of electromagnetic flowmeter. *J Extracorp Tech* 1985;17:56–64.
13. Stoney WS, Alford WC Jr, Burrus GR, et al. Air embolism and other accidents using pump oxygenators. *Ann Thorac Surg* 1980;29:336–340.
14. Wheeldon D, Bethune D, Gill R. Vortex pumping for routine cardiac surgery. A comparative study. *Perfusion* 1990;5:135–143.

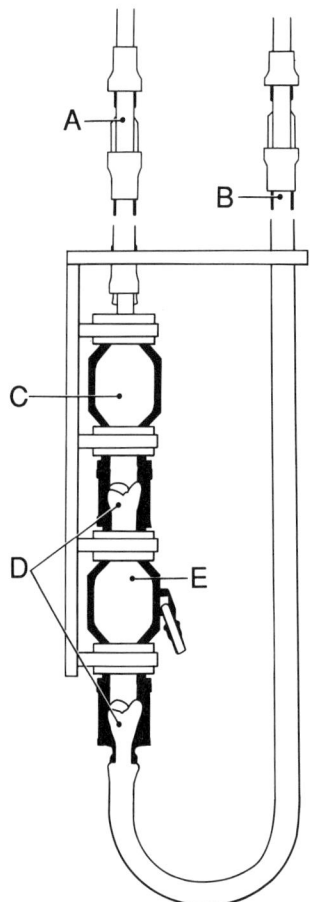

FIGURE 11.10. The Abiomed BVS System 5000. (A) Inflow to the assist device, which occurs via gravity. (B) Outflow from the Abiomed system. (C) Atrial chamber, which collects blood from either the left or right atrium. (D) Two tri-leaflet polyurethane valves, which provide unidirectional blood flow. (E) Ventricular chamber, which, when acted upon by pneumatic pressure, expels blood through the second valve.

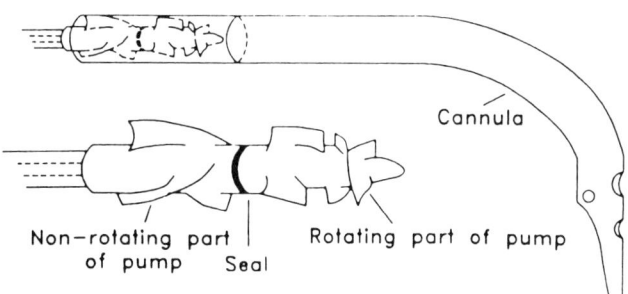

FIGURE 11.11. Pumps/cannula assembly of the Nimbus Hemopump. The Nimbus Hemopump utilizes the Archimedean screw flow principle to trap and raise blood continuously by means of spiral vanes rotating inside a closely fitted tube.

15. Riley JB, Kirven D, Stammers A. Similarity in gaseous microemboli separation characteristics of the commercially available centrifugal blood pumps. Presented at the Annual Meeting of the American Society of Extracorporeal Technology, San Francisco, 1991.
16. Reed CC, Kurusz M, Lawrence A Jr. *Safety and Techniques in Perfusion*. Stafford, Tex: Quali-Med Inc; 1988:79–91.
17. Vertrees R, Brownstein L. Centrifugal pump induced alterations in red cell morphology. Presented at Pathophysiology and Techniques in Cardiopulmonary Bypass, San Diego, 1992.
18. Hoerr H, Kraemer M, Williams J, et al. In vitro comparison of the blood handling by the constrained vortex and twin roller blood pumps. *J Extracorp Tech* 1987;19:316–321.
19. Horton A, Butt W. Pump induced hemolysis: is the constrained vortex pump better or worse than the roller pump? *Perfusion* 1992;7:103–108.
20. Bolles RE. Centrifugal pumps for routine cardiopulmonary bypass. St. Jude Lifestream centrifugal pump system. Presented at Pathophysiology and Techniques in Cardiopulmonary Bypass, San Diego, 1993.
21. Galletti PM, Brecher GA. *Heart-Lung Bypass: Principles and Techniques of Extracorporeal Circulation*. New York: Grune & Stratton; 1962:141–153.
22. Cooley DA. Development of the roller pump for use in the cardiopulmonary bypass circuit. *Texas Heart Inst J* 1987;14:113–118.
23. Reed CC, Stafford TB. *Cardiopulmonary Bypass*. Houston: Texas Med Press Inc; 1985:376–379.
24. James SD, Peters J, Maresca L, et al. The roller pump does produce pulsatile flow. *J Extracorp Tech* 1987;19:376–383.
25. Galletti PM, Brecher GA. *Heart-Lung Bypass: Principles and Techniques of Extracorporeal Circulation*. New York: Grune & Stratton; 1962:131–140.

12
Conduits and Filters for Extracorporeal Circulation

Kathy K. Spitzer and Charles T. Walker

Introduction

This chapter discusses the conduits used for conducting blood through the extracorporeal circuit. These conduits must be large enough to offer a low resistance to flow, yet small enough to minimize priming volume. To avoid trauma to formed blood elements, they should have smooth, nonwettable inside surfaces. Filters are incorporated into the circuit to remove air, debris, and aggregated blood elements. Each of these three circuitry components—tubing, cannulas, and filters—is considered separately.

Tubing

The function of the tubing is to provide a safe and effective route between the cannulas and the venous reservoir, to function as a pumping chamber within the arterial pump head or suction pumps, and to return blood to the patient. Tubing should be transparent to allow inspection for oxygenation and air. It should be resilient, allowing it to reexpand after repeated compression by clamps and roller pumps, and it must withstand high hydrostatic pressures (pressures as high as 500–700 mm Hg on the arterial side). It should be flexible and kink-resistant. To prevent microscopic air leakage on the venous side through negative pressure air entrainment, it must be crack-proof and rupture-proof. It should be nontoxic and should minimize the body's inflammatory responses to foreign surface exposure. There should be minimal leaching into the bloodstream of chemicals used in its manufacture. Spallation (release of pieces of the tubing material related to trauma from roller pumps or the sheer stress of blood flow) also should be minimized. The tubing ideally should tolerate heat sterilization as well as extremes of cold (which might occur during shipping).

The majority of medical-grade tubing currently in use is a clear, flexible variety of polyvinyl chloride. This polyvinyl chloride tubing needs to have both flexibility and resilience, or "memory." Flexibility allows turning and looping during packaging and use, with resistance to kinking. Resilience permits the tubing to resume its original shape after compression or occlusion. These properties are achieved by blending polyvinyl chloride resin with organic oils, called *plasticizers*, and organo-metal soaps, called *stabilizers*.[1] As much as 40% of the tubing may be plasticizer oil.[2]

Another important property of the tubing is its hardness, or *durometer*. The higher the durometer number, the harder the tubing. The flexible polyvinyl chloride tubing ordinarily used in extracorporeal circuits is generally between 65 and 72 durometer. Intravenous tubing is 80 durometer.[1] Silicone rubber tubing is softer and therefore has a lower durometer than polyvinyl chloride tubing. This softness gives silicone rubber a truer stroke volume in an arterial pump head and an increased fatigue life at low temperatures, but the softness also increases the incidence of spallation.[2-5] Increasing durometer increases both the strength of the tubing and the fatigue life. The fatigue life is the maximum period of time the tubing can be compressed by rollers, within a pump raceway, before it ruptures. Super Tygon is a variation of Tygon, with higher durometer, that is used for long-term support within a roller pump.

Vinyl tubing is susceptible to wear, which not only damages the internal surface but also erodes tubing and can lead to spallation. The most common site of spallation is tiny cracks that occur in the tubing near the line of flexion in a roller pump. The bulk of particle release occurs in the first 2 to 4 hours of cardiopulmonary bypass (CPB). The primary determinant of the extent of spallation is the revolutions per minute of the pump head. The durometer and age of the tubing also influence the degree of spallation.[2,3,6]

For most cardiovascular applications, polyvinyl chloride tubing can be considered thermally stable. It does, however, become softer at higher temperatures and

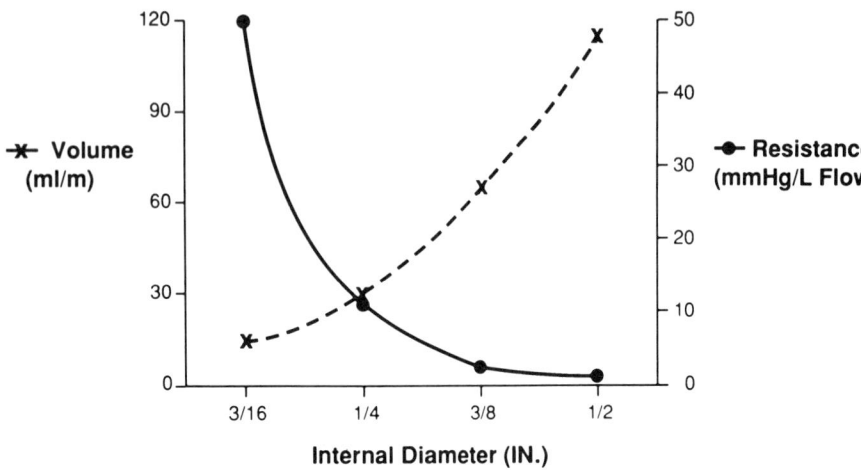

FIGURE 12.1. Relationship of internal tubing diameter, volume, and resistance. As tubing internal diameter increases, tubing volume increases and resistance decreases.

harder at lower temperatures. For this reason, the stroke volume increases exponentially as the perfusate temperature increases. The degree of flow change with temperature change is greater with higher-durometer tubing.[7]

In the past, silicone rubber tubing was often used in roller-pump heads. The softer silicone rubber tubing exhibits truer stroke volume characteristics at lower temperatures and has increased fatigue life, but it has a higher incidence of spallation than polyvinyl chloride tubing. Polyvinyl chloride tubing also appears to cause less hemolysis than other tubing. This is perhaps related to the stiffness of the vinyl and less displacement of the internal wall with rotation of the roller.[8]

The size of tubing used is a compromise between the need for a low priming volume and the low resistance offered by larger tubing, and the fact that larger tubing can deliver the desired flow with lower pump speed (and, thus, cause less hemolysis). Figure 12.1 illustrates the rapid rise in priming volume as tubing diameter is increased and shows the falling resistance that occurs with increasing tubing size.

Improvement in the biocompatibility of tubing and the blood-contacting surfaces of oxygenators is a continuing research effort. When blood comes in contact with the internal surface of the tubing, the inflammatory system is activated, resulting in complement and platelet activation, cellular adhesion, and protein deposition.[9,10] (These phenomena are discussed in Chapters 5 and 8.) The clotting cascade is also initiated. All of these reactions have been used as indices of biocompatibility. Albumin coating of the circuit is beneficial as a surface passivating film. The contact surfaces of polyvinyl chloride and silicone are negatively charged, since they contain chloromethyl and ether groups. This causes positively charted proteins to become bound upon initiation of CPB. Precoating the circuit with albumin by recirculating for at least 30 minutes inhibits this reaction and reduces postoperative platelet depletion.[11]

TABLE 12.1. Advantages and disadvantages of various types of extracorporeal circuit tubing.

Tubing type	Advantages	Disadvantages
Polyvinyl chloride (PVC)	Thermal stability Clear Resilience (memory) Biocompatibility	Stiffness Cannot be used for long-term support within a roller pump
Silicone silastic	Truer stroke volume Biocompatibility	Spallation Lack of thermal stability Fatigue
Heparin-bonded	Thermal stability Clear Resilience (memory) Higher level of biocompatibility Use in long-term support Decreased thrombin production	Stiffness

One useful and commercially available technique recently has been developed for coating the internal surfaces of equipment in the extracorporeal circuit. This technique covalently bonds partially degraded heparin to the internal surface (Carmeda Bioactive Surface, CARMEDA AB, Stockholm, Sweden).[12] The result is a highly thromboresistant coating that is compatible with platelets and effectively inhibits thrombin and complement activation.[13,14] Ionic bonding of heparin to the polymer surface also has been described.[15] The Carmeda system, however, has a higher thrombin-inhibiting capacity than ionic-bonded heparin surfaces.[16] Furthermore, ionic heparin complexes are not stable and may wash off in contact with blood.[17] In both animal and human studies, the Carmeda surface has been associated with decreased complement activation, decreased neutrophil activation, and a reduction in protamine use.[18-20] In most clinical settings, systemic heparinization is used in conjunction with the Carmeda surface, although full heparinization may not be necessary.[21] The types of tubing currently available for extracorporeal circuits are listed in Table 12.1.

Boonstra and colleagues[22] assessed the effects on postoperative hemostasis of employing heparin-bonded extracorporeal circulation circuits. The use of a Duraflo II (Bentley/Baxter Inc., Uden, The Netherlands) heparin-coated extracorporeal circuit in elective coronary revascularization procedures resulted in higher plasma heparin levels and decreased thrombin activity when compared to the use of nonheparinized circuits (Figure 12.2). How-

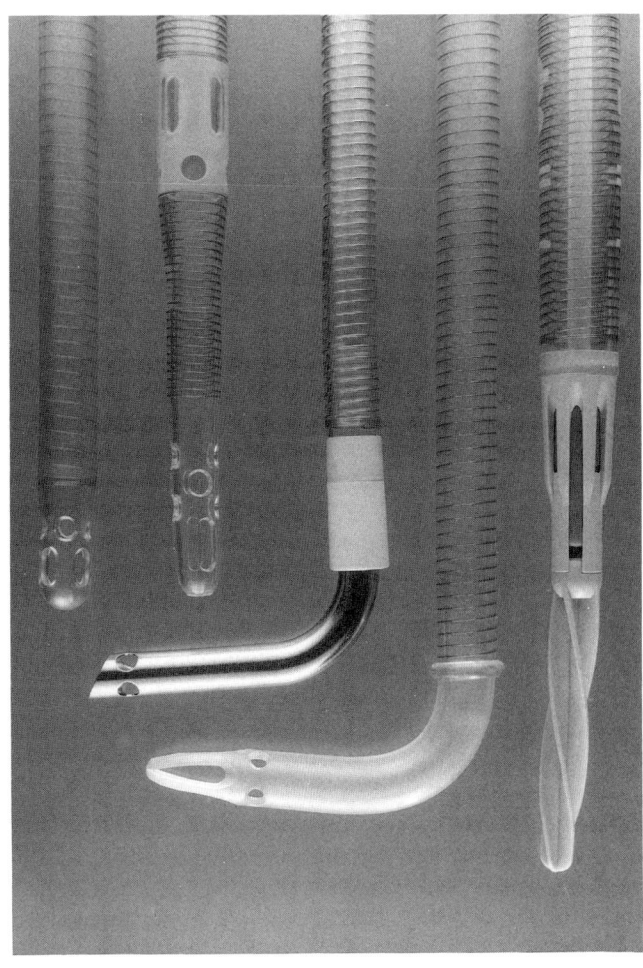

FIGURE 12.3. Various types of venous wire-wound cannulas. Left to right: closed-end dual caval (basket type); open-end single atrial cannula (two stage); open-end, right-angle, dual caval; closed-end, right-angle, dual caval (basket type); and a variation of open-end flexible type.

ever, postoperative bleeding time, blood loss, and donor blood transfusions were similar in both groups. The authors suggested that postoperative hemostasis was similar in both groups because the heparinized circuit did not prevent fibrinolysis and platelet activation.

The best connector used in extracorporeal circuits appears to be a disposable polycarbonate one with a smooth inner surface. A connector is used with a fluted external surface that has an outside diameter slightly larger than the inside diameter of the plastic tubing or cannulas into which it is inserted.

Cannulas

Venous drainage from the patient to the extracorporeal circuit is generally accomplished by gravity. Because the cannula usually needs to go upward to exit the chest, a si-

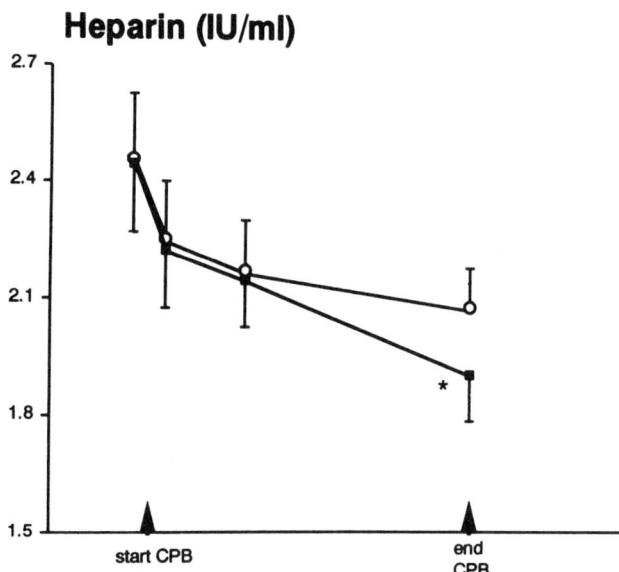

FIGURE 12.2. Plasma heparin concentrations measured with heparin-bonded (○) and non-heparin-bonded (■) extracorporeal circuits. Heparin concentration, measured by factor Xa inhibition in plasma, was significantly higher in the heparin-bonded group. (From Boonstra et al,[22] by permission of *J Thorac Cardiovasc Surg.*)

teristics of a particular cannula configuration usually are provided by the manufacturer and should be readily available in the operating room.

Single atrial caval cannulation is accomplished by inserting a single cannula into the right atrium, which extends down into the inferior vena cava. Drainage holes are designed so that a basket tip is positioned in the inferior vena cava and side holes are positioned in the cannula in the right atrium. Cannulas are usually made of a flexible plastic, with or without a wire reinforcement. It should be noted that the sizes of venous cannulas are ordinarily designated by the external circumference (using French sizes). The resistance to flow is determined by the internal diameter. Since various cannulas have varying wall thicknesses, various venous cannulas of the same external size may have greatly different flow characteristics.

Arterial cannulas should provide adequate flow (2.5 to 3 $L/m^2/min$) without an excessive pressure gradient across the cannula. Various cannulas for arterial cannulation are depicted in Figure 12.4. The portion of the can-

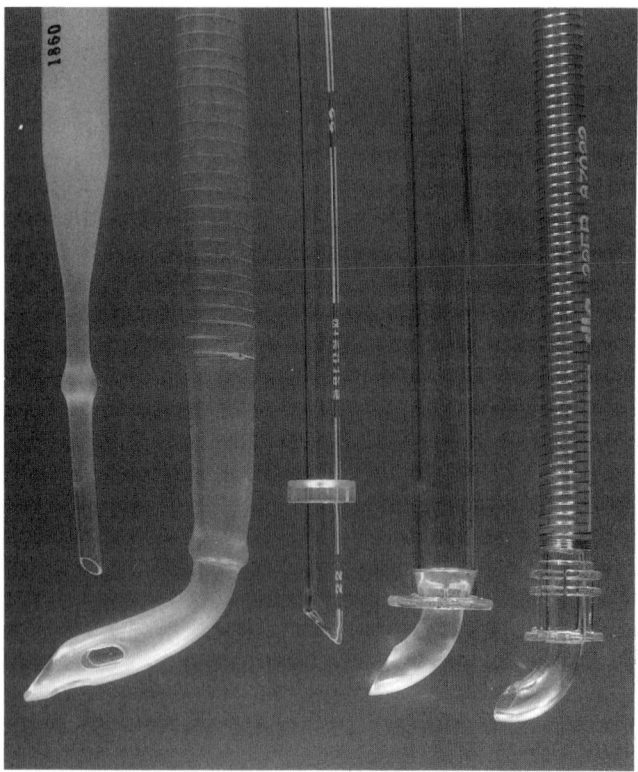

FIGURE 12.4. Types of arterial cannulas. The cannula depicted at the far left is for femoral artery access. The other four pictured cannulas are for aortic cannulation. Left to right: wire-wound, side-hole, right-angle; straight tip with support ring; curved semiridged tip with support ring; wire-wound, curved, ridged tip with support ring.

phon system usually exists. The theoretical limit to venous return is the amount of blood returning to the heart from the body. If the siphonage is too great, negative pressure may be created in the collapsible cavae or atrium, leading to intermittent collapse of the vessel walls around the ends of the venous cannulas, causing "chattering," which can actually decrease venous drainage. Various types of basket and fluted tips are used on the end of venous cannulas to prevent this occlusion by the vascular walls (Figure 12.3).

The venous cannulas are designed for either dual caval cannulation or atriocaval cannulation. The cannula used for dual caval cannulation is straight, with a basket tip designed for insertion through a purse string in the right atrium, into the superior vena cava or the inferior vena cava (Figure 12.3). Alternatively, right-angle plastic cannulas or, occasionally, cannulas with right-angle metal tips are designed for direct insertion into the superior vena cava and inferior vena cava (Figure 12.3). Generally, about two thirds of the venous return comes back to the inferior vena cava, and one third to the superior vena cava. For this reason, the cannula inserted into the inferior vena cava should generally be slightly larger than the cannula used in the superior vena cava. The flow charac-

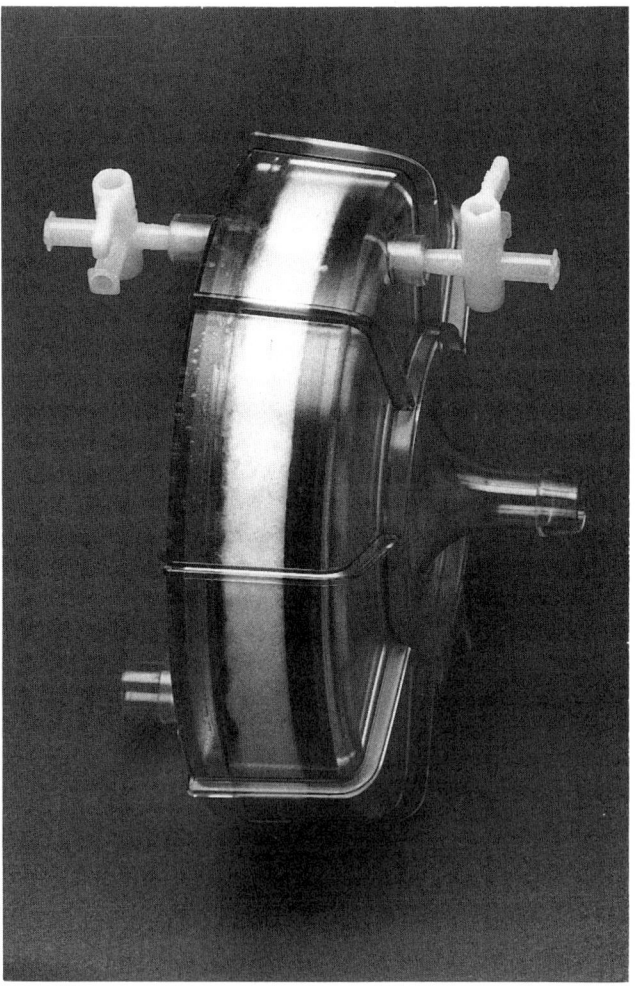

FIGURE 12.5. Swank depth filter.

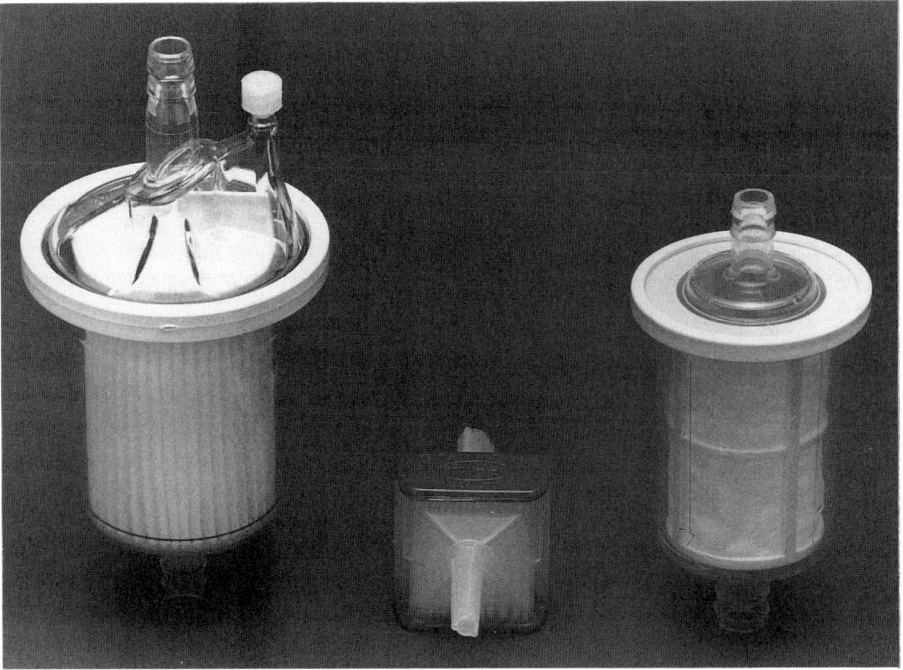

FIGURE 12.6. Various types of screen filters. *Left:* heparin-bonded arterial line blood filter. *Center:* blood transfusion line filter. *Right:* crystalloid prime prebypass filter.

nula that inserts into the aorta is the narrowest part of the extracorporeal circuit. This narrow portion of the cannula should be as short as possible to decrease the pressure gradient. Hard, thin-walled plastic or metal tips provide the best inside-to-outside diameter ratios, but these cannulas are often difficult to insert without excessive damage to the aorta. The expected pressure gradient across a specific cannula should be known to the perfusionist. Pressure gradients greater than 100 mm Hg are not acceptable because of excessive hemolysis and protein denaturation. For pediatric use, the choice of the arterial cannula is particularly important, since varying flows are necessary and arterial access may be very limited. For this purpose, the perfusionist should have at hand a table of acceptable cannulas for various anticipated flows. Venous and arterial cannulas for extracorporeal circulation are also discussed in Chapter 15.

Filters

Filters are used in numerous locations in extracorporeal circuits. As blood is suctioned from the patient through the cardiotomy suction line, a filter may be used prior to returning this blood to the oxygenator or venous reservoir. Stored blood and autotransfused blood may be filtered through a transfusion line filter. The arterial line blood may be filtered prior to infusion into the patient, but only after oxygenation, heat exchange, and pumping have occurred, as a final trap for macroemboli and microemboli. Crystalloid filtration may be used during recirculation of prebypass priming fluids and during infusion of crystalloid cardioplegia solutions, to remove small particulate matter. Finally, gas line filtration may be used for removal of bacteria from medical gases.

Arterial Line Filters

During the early years of extracorporeal circulation, filters offered considerable resistance to flow, were difficult to debubble, and frequently produced more emboli than were strained out. Fortunately, improvement in filter technology has eliminated many of these problems, and blood filtration is commonly used today. Studies by Swank and Porter[23] in 1963 demonstrated more macroemboli in the arterial blood than in the venous blood of clinical CPB circuits, implying that these macroemboli were being filtered out in the patient's vasculature. Later studies by Jenevien and Weiss[24] showed platelet emboli in the myocardium and renal glomeruli of patients who died within 4 days after operation. In 1969, Patterson and Kessler[25] evaluated the tendency toward formation of gaseous emboli in CPB circuits. They found that temperature increases in blood increased the number of gaseous emboli, due to deceasing gas solubility with increasing temperature.

Because emboli are both particulate and gaseous, the arterial line filter must be effective in both bubble-trapping and particulate-filtering, yet have a large enough pore size to minimize flow resistance. The ease with which a bubble will pass through a certain pore in a filter is described by the equation:

$$BPP = \frac{4Y\cos\emptyset}{D}$$

where BPP = bubble point pressure, Y = surface tension (dependent on the liquid used), $\cos \oslash$ = wetting angle (dependent on the filter material), and D = diameter of the filter pore. If BPP is exceeded by the pressure gradient across the filter, the bubble will pass through the medium.[26] As can be seen, the smaller the pore size, the more effective the filter is in trapping gaseous emboli, but the small pore size also contributes to the damage to formed blood elements and to increased resistance to flow.

Two types of arterial line filters in use are depth filters and screen filters. Depth filters consist of packed fibers or porous foam. An example of this is the Swank Dacron wool filter (Figure 12.5), which has no defined pore size, and removes particles by impaction filtration. These filters often lose their bubble-retaining capabilities due to channeling in the medium. They also tend to trap platelets and cause more hemolysis than screen filters.

Screen filters are usually made of pleated polyester strands which are lock woven with a defined pore size (Figure 12.6). Polyester has a low reactivity with blood. The appropriate pore size for screen filters requires a balance between microemboli and gaseous emboli removal, and damage to formed blood elements. The most desirable arterial filter is one with an intermediate pore size (approximately 30 μm).[27]

The most recent advancement in arterial line filters is the use of heparin-bonded surfaces.[28] Heparin is bonded to benzalkonium chloride and this complex is then applied to the arterial line filter media. This filter is easier to prime and debubble, but the heparin benzalkonium coating may leach off during fluid flow.[29]

The surface area of an arterial line filter must be large enough to assure low blood velocities through the mesh, with negligible blood trauma and a low pressure gradient at both high and low flow rates.[30] The pressure drop across the filter is a function of the fluid viscosity, fluid flow, and filter design. As hematocrit and temperature change, the viscosity can change.[31] An increase, however, in pressure gradient at a constant temperature and hematocrit indicates occlusion of the arterial filter with particulate matter.[31] In this instance, it is important that the arterial line have a bypass line or loop past the filter, so that the occluded filter can be excluded from the circuit.

Ease of priming is another important consideration in choosing an arterial line filter. The vent site on the filter should be positioned close to the inlet port, creating a short escape route for entrained air. The filter element should be easily wettable to facilitate bubble release. A baffle should be positioned to direct air towards the vent site. Finally, the filter should be made of a clear polycarbonate housing to facilitate visualization of air. Table 12.2 outlines desirable characteristics of an arterial line filter.

TABLE 12.2. Desirable characteristics of arterial line filters.

Very low resistance
Easy to debubble
Not a source of emboli
Removes both particulate and gaseous emboli
Produces minimal blood trauma
Easily purged of trapped air
Wettable table
Clear housing
Minimal hold-up volume

Cardiotomy Filters

Cardiotomy suction contains microemboli—related to blood trauma and platelet activation in the pericardium—fat particles, and bone wax. These microaggregates and particles are best removed by a cardiotomy line filter (Figure 12.7). Since flow is smaller, screen filters with a 20-μm filter pore size are often used in this circuit.[32-34]

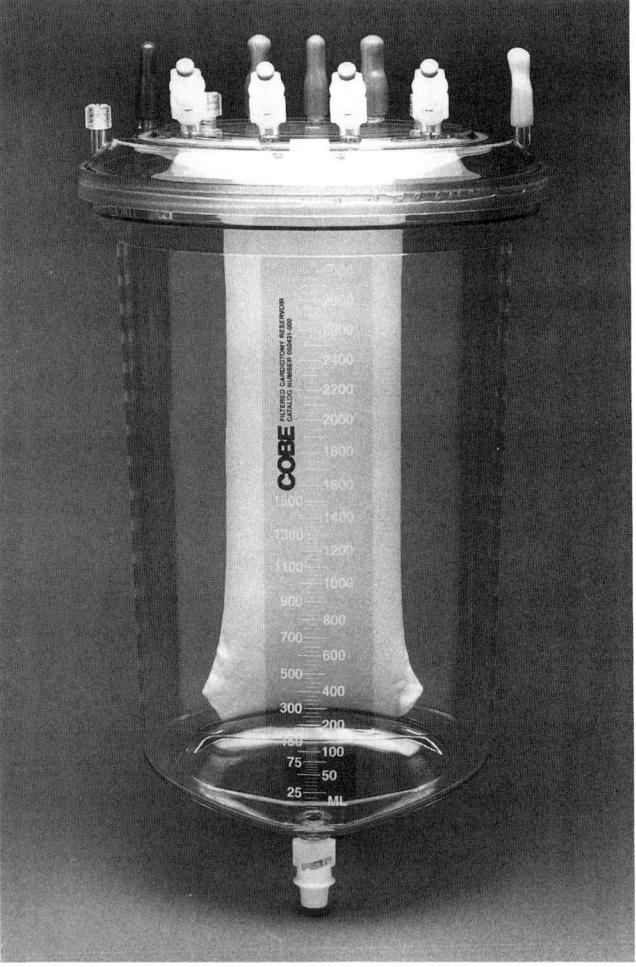

FIGURE 12.7. Cardiotomy reservoir with both gross and fine particulate filter.

FIGURE 12.8. Gas line sterilizing filter (*center*) and a crystalloid filter (*periphery*).

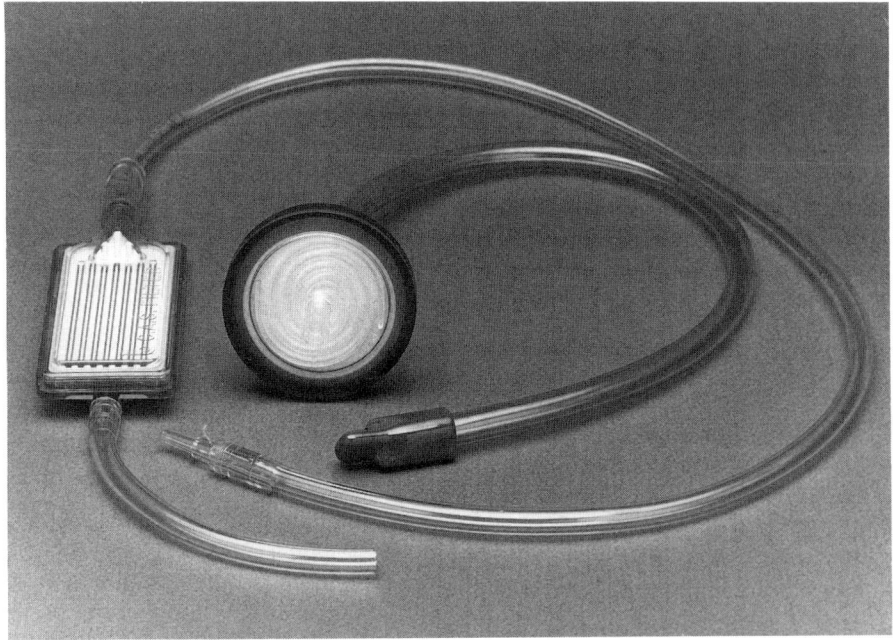

Prebypass Filters

Extracorporeal circuits invariably contain particles of all forms and sizes, including glass, plasticizers, bits of tubing from spallation, and even endotoxins.[35,36] A prebypass filter with a pore size of 0.2 to 5 μm can be used during recirculation prior to filling the circuit with blood to remove these particles from the circuit (Figure 12.8).

Transfusion Filters

Despite improvements in methods of collecting and storing blood, filtration of stored blood or autotransfused blood is very important, particularly when large volumes of blood products are being used. Transfusion filters, because of lower flows than arterial and cardiotomy line filters, are smaller and more compact (Figure 12.6).[37] Screen filters, depth filters, and combinations of the two have been used. Most screen filters have a pore size of about 40 μm and are effective in handling up to 1 L of stored blood.

Gas Filters

In most oxygenators, with the exception of true membrane oxygenators, there is direct contact between gas and blood. Viable bacteria do exist in medical oxygen as a result of nonsterile production and storage procedures.[38] The introduction of a filtering device into the oxygen line before it is attached to the oxygenator will reliably and effectively remove bacteria and trap debris that may be present in the medical gases. These filters usually have a pore size of 0.2 μm and can handle flow rates up to 40 L/min (Figure 12.8).[39,40]

Cardioplegic Solution Filters

Particulate contaminants have been demonstrated in crystalloid cardioplegic solutions. By filtration of this crystalloid solution, using a screen filter with a pore size of 0.2 to 5 μm, particulate matter may be removed from the crystalloid solution as it is infused into the patient. If blood cardioplegia is being utilized, the crystalloid portion of the cardioplegic solution should be filtered prior to mixing with blood from the oxygenator.

Summary of Filtration

In summary, the problem of embolization during CPB and its attendant morbidity has been well documented over the last 40 years. The importance of using filters in multiple extracorporeal circulation locations is accepted by perfusionists and those caring for patients during CPB. Kurusz and colleagues[41] reported that 81% of perfusionists use an arterial line filter, 94% an oxygen line filter, 50% a prebypass filter, and 91% a cardiotomy filter.

References

1. Direct communication with Lawrence E. Czyz, Vice President and General Manager, Plastron. 19555 E. Arenth Ave., City of Industry, CA 91748.
2. Hoenich NA, Thompson J, Varini E, et al. Particle Spall-

ation Plasticizer (DEHP) release from extracorporeal circuit tubing materials. *Int J Artif Organs* 1990;13:55-62.
3. Hodge R, Leverett B, Akers WW. *Abrasion of Pump Sets in Roller Pumps.* Report No. 6503, Bio-Medical Engineering Laboratory, Rice University, Houston, TX, 1965.
4. Boretos JW. *Silicone Polymers in Medicine and Surgery.* New York: Plenum Press; 1975:87-98.
5. Kurusz M, Christman E, Williams E, et al. Roller-pump induced tubing wear: another argument in favor of arterial line filtration. *J Extracorp Tech* 1980;12:49-59.
6. Bretz G, Schermeyer T, Donnelly T. Long term tubing fatigue characteristics. *J Extracorp Tech* 1979;11:151-156.
7. Pfaender LM, Riley JB, Whitehead JB, et al. An in vitro comparison of the effects of temperature on the stroke volume and occlusion setting of various tubing types in a roller pump. *J Extracorp Tech* 1979;11:78-88.
8. Wesolowski SA, Martinez A, McMahon JD. Use of artificial materials in surgery. *Curr Prob Surg* 1966;12:1-86.
9. Nilsson L, Nilsson U, Venge P, et al. Inflammatory system activation during cardiopulmonary bypass as an indicator of biocompatibility: a randomized comparison of bubble and membrane oxygenators. *Scand J Thorac Cardiovasc Surg* 1990;24:53-58.
10. van Oeveren W, Wildevuur CR. Blood compatibility of cardiopulmonary bypass circuits. *Perfusion* 1987;2:237-244.
11. Gurjar Y, Bowman JM. Prevention of platelet adhesion to extracorporeal surfaces. *J Extracorp Tech* 1984;16:104-107.
12. Larm O, Larsson R, Olsson P. A new non-thrombogenic surface prepared by selective covalent binding of heparin via a modified reducing terminal residue. *Biomat Med Devices Artif Organs* 1983;2:161-173.
13. Pasche B, Kodama K, Larm O, et al. Thrombin inactivation of surfaces with covalently bonded heparin. *Thromb Res* 1986;44:739-748.
14. Videm V, Mollnes T, Garred P, et al. Biocompatibility of extracorporeal circulation. *J Thorac Cardiovasc Surg* 1991;101:654-660.
15. Barbucci R, Magnani A, Albanese A, et al. Heparinized polyurethane surface through ionic bonding of heparin. *Int J Artif Organs* 1991;14:499-507.
16. Shumway R, Lowe N, Wirth L, et al. Functional characteristic determination of an immobilized bioactive heparin surface, a direct biological assay. Presented at the American Academy of Cardiac Perfusionists; September 1990; Chicago.
17. Medtronic/Carmeda Bioactive Surface, An Overview. Anaheim, CA: Medtronic, Compendium of Scientific Information; 1990.
18. Nilsson L, Storm K, Thelin S, et al. Heparin-coated equipment reduces complement activation during cardiopulmonary bypass in the pig. *Artif Organs* 1990;14:46-48.
19. Thelin S, Bylock A, Bagge L, et al. Heparin coated cardiopulmonary bypass sets during surgery-clinical study. Presented at the American Society of Extracorporeal Technologists Annual Meeting; April 1990; Dallas.
20. Videm V, Svennevig J, Fosse E, et al. Complement activation with a heparin coated cardiopulmonary bypass device. Presented at American Heart Association, Dallas, November, 1990.
21. Bindslev L, Bohm C, Jolin A, et al. Extracorporeal carbon dioxide removal performed with surface-heparinized equipment in patients with ARDS. *Acta Anaesth Scand Supplementum.* 1991;95:125-130.
22. Boonstra PW, Gu YJ, Akkerman C, et al. Heparin coating of an extracorporeal circuit partly improves hemostasis after cardiopulmonary bypass. *J Thorac Cardiovasc Surg* 1994;107:289-292.
23. Swank RL, Port GA. Disappearance of microemboli transfused into patients during cardiopulmonary bypass. *Transfusion* 1963;3:192-197.
24. Jenevein EP, Weiss DL. Platelet microemboli associated with massive blood transfusion. *Am J Pathol* 1964;45:313-325.
25. Patterson RH, Kessler J. Microemboli during cardiopulmonary bypass detected by ultrasound. *Surgery* 1969;129:505-510.
26. Berman L, Marin F. Micropore filtration during cardiopulmonary bypass. In: Taylor M, ed., *Cardiopulmonary Bypass: principles and management.* Cambridge: University Press, 1986:355-374.
27. Bailey R, Lumley J. Some observations on blood microfilters. *Ann R Coll Surg* 1975;43:578-581.
28. Hill AG, Groom RG, Kurusz M, et al. Arterial filtration: heparin bonded or unbonded: a comparison. *Proc Am Acad Cardiovasc Perf* 1985;6:132-139.
29. Palanzo DA, Kurusz M, Butler BD. Surface tension effects of heparin coating on arterial line filters. *Perfusion* 1990;5:277-284.
30. Rand PW, Lancombe E, Hunt HE, et al. Viscosity of normal human blood under normo-thermic and hypothermic conditions. *J Appl Physiol* 1964;19:119-122.
31. Pfaender LM, Riley JB. Viscosity-induced resistance changes during bypass with hemodilution and hypothermia. Presented at the American Society of Extracorporeal Technology, Boca Raton, FL, 1984.
32. Kemma GD, Doeherty JP. Why filter the cardiopulmonary circuit pre-bypass? *J Extracorp Tech* 1979;11:121-124.
33. Ream AK, Fogdall RR. *Acute Cardiovascular Management.* Philadelphia: JB Lippincott;1982:444.
34. Reed CC, Stafford TB. *Cardiopulmonary Bypass.* Houston: Texas Medical Press;1985:344.
35. Lin ELC, Goldstein R, Syvannen M. *Bacteria, Plasmids, and Phages: An Introduction to Molecular Biology.* Cambridge, Mass: Harvard University Press;1984:25.
36. Jenkins BS. The clinical manifestation of endotoxin shock arising from high level contamination. In: *Microbiological Hazards of Infusion Therapy.* Proceedings of an international symposium held at the University of Sussex, England, March 1976. Littleton, Mass: Publishing Sciences Group; 1976:93-97.
37. Lowe GD. Filtration in IV therapy—Review of the clinical and technical aspects of intravenous fluid and blood filtration in four parts—IV: Blood filters. *Br J Intraven Ther* 1981;2:24-38.
38. Mortensen JD, Smith SM, Hill G. Bacterial contamination of oxygen used in cardiopulmonary bypass. *J Thorac Cardiovasc Surg* 1961;41:675-679.
39. Mortenson JD, Hurd G, Hill G. Bacterial contamination of oxygen used clinically—importance and one method of control. *Dis Chest* 1962;42:567-572.

40. Mortenson JD, Hill G. Clinical and bacteriologic evaluation of a new filter designed specifically for bacteriologic decontamination of oxygen used clinically. *Dis Chest* 1964;45:508-514.

41. Kurusz M. Perfusion accidents in the 1970s and 1980s: comparison of two surveys. Presented at the Second World Congress on Open Heart Technology; October 7-11, 1986; Tampa.

13
Assembling and Monitoring the Extracorporeal Circuit

Richard B. Davis, Jeffrey N. Kauffman, Terry L. Cobbs, and Sharon L. Mick

Introduction

Cardiopulmonary bypass (CPB) began as a groundbreaking but unpredictable adjunct to cardiac surgery that often resulted in additional trauma to already debilitated patients. Over the last 40 years, it has evolved into an indispensable and efficient process with a reliability that often exceeds 99.9%. This remarkable evolution is evidenced by the fact that hundreds of patients can now undergo operations without major mishaps caused by CPB. In the early 1980s, at Emory University, coronary artery bypass patients with single- and double-vessel disease were reviewed, using three of the criteria from the Coronary Artery Surgery Study (CASS): age ≤65, ejection fraction >35%, and no history of congestive heart failure. Over 1300 such patients were identified who had undergone operations in the previous 5 years. In this series of routine coronary bypass patients, only one death had occurred, a 0.07% mortality.[1] This is a remarkable accomplishment for perfusion technology.

CPB has become dependable, reliable, and safe through improvements in methods and materials, as discussed in the preceding chapters. Fail-safe systems also have been developed for the use of CPB. This includes fail-safe systems for setup of perfusion circuitry, redundant systems to accommodate potential equipment failure, and monitoring systems to detect equipment malfunction before it can affect the patient.

Preparation for Extracorporeal Circuit Assembly

Choice of Equipment

In assembling the bypass circuit, the perfusionist must consider the patient's condition, his or her pathophysiology (both cardiac and other organ systems), the planned conduct of the operation by the surgeon, and the planned anesthetic management. These factors will determine the needed priming volume of the system (attempting to maintain the hemodiluted hematocrit greater than 20%), the choice of cardioplegic solutions and techniques, the use of hemoconcentrators or diuretics, the need for a large venous reservoir or no reservoir, and the use or nonuse of optional monitoring equipment. In general, one seeks to have a standardized system of CPB which can be modified to suit the individual patient, the specific anesthetic, and the surgical requirements. The standard system is frequently custom-designed and packaged with preconnected tubing, filters, purge lines, connectors, and oxygenator/heat exchanger combinations. If a large amount of cardiotomy suction is anticipated, a separate cardiotomy reservoir may be added to the circuit. If the patient is in congestive heart failure preoperatively, the addition of a hemoconcentrator is frequently appropriate.

Historically, fresh blood was used to prime the heart-lung machine. Today, crystalloid solutions are the major component of the prime for the CPB machine. This intentional hemodilution aids perfusion of the microcirculation, especially when hypothermia is used. A physiologic solution, an analog of the body's extracellular fluid, such as Normosal R or Plasmalyte A, is used to prime the pump. Normally, a colloid, such as hetastarch or albumin, is added to the prime as well as an osmotic diuretic such as mannitol. Mannitol is useful not only as an osmotic diuretic but also in reducing intracellular edema.

Great emphasis is placed upon avoiding blood transfusion during cardiac surgery, due to the ever-present danger of blood-transmitted diseases, such as AIDS and hepatitis. The blood conservation device most widely used during cardiac cases is the cell salvage machine (see Figure 31.3). This unit is used to salvage blood suctioned from the operative field before and after the interval of complete heparinization. This blood is then spun down into packed red blood cells, which are washed with normal saline and then returned to the patient. This unit can also retrieve blood remaining in the CPB circuit after disconnection of the circuit from the body.

A hemoconcentrator may be attached within the CPB circuit to remove relatively large volumes of crystalloid from the circulating blood volume. The hemoconcentrator has a large number of semipermeable hollow fibers in a cylindrical configuration placed on the arterial side of the circuit (see Figure 31.4). The hydrostatic pressure across the hollow fibers forces crystalloid out of the blood, retaining the large-molecular-weight blood components. Thus, cellular and protein blood components are retained (molecules smaller than 20,000 daltons are removed). Both cell salvage devices and hemoconcentrators are discussed in Chapter 31.

Assembling the Extracorporeal Circuit

The components of a complete extracorporeal circuit are diagrammed in Figure 13.1. Ordinarily, two separate sterile packs of polyvinyl chloride (PVC) tubing are used in setting up the extracorporeal circuit: the "pump pack" and the "table pack." This enables the perfusionist to set up the pump oxygenator, prime and debubble it, and then receive, from the scrub nurse or surgeon, the ends of the arteriovenous (A-V) loop from the table pack.

Initially, the oxygenator is placed in its holder, and water connection is made to the heat exchanger. The water is then recirculated, and the integrity of the heater/cooler circuit is checked. Next, tubing from the pump pack is aseptically connected to the appropriate ports of the oxygenator. The isolated arterial filter is then flushed with carbon dioxide gas at a flow of 100 to 200 mL/min for 5 minutes. Priming of the tubing then proceeds.

An asanguinous prime is used to prime the system. Components used in our institution include a pH-balanced physiologic saline solution (Normosal R or Plasmalyte A), a volume expander (500 mL of Hespan or hetastarch), and 22.5 g of mannitol. A prebypass checklist is used to minimize errors in pump setup (Table 13.1).[2]

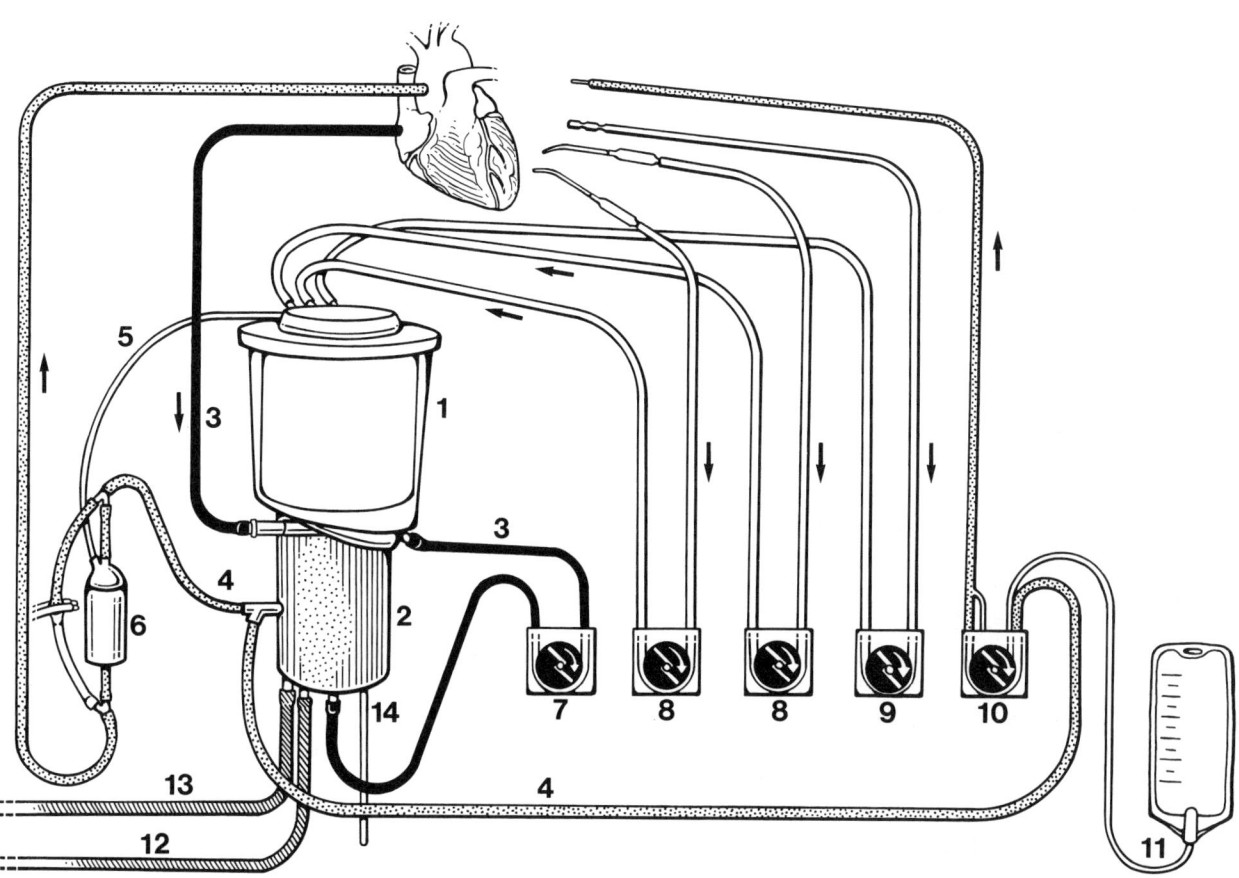

FIGURE 13.1. Components of the extracorporeal circuit: (1) integral cardiotomy reservoir; (2) membrane oxygenator bundle; (3) venous blood line; (4) arterial blood line; (5) arterial filter purge line; (6) arterial line filter; (7) venous blood pump (also called the "arterial" pump head; this pump forces venous blood through the membrane oxygenator and "arterialized" blood to the patient's aortic root); (8) cardiotomy suction pump; (9) ventricular vent pump; (10) cardioplegia pump; (11) crystalloid cardioplegia; (12) water inlet line; (13) water outlet line; and (14) gas inlet line.

TABLE 13.1. Perfusionist's prebypass checklist.

1. Equipment inspection. List each device and include physical inspection of each and verification of major control operation and displays.
2. Verification of utilities. List each required utility, including electrical outlets, primary gas sources and backup, suction, and vaporizer, including verification of availability and function.
3. Circuit inspection. Circuit paths, circuit connections, pump head/flow direction; occlusions, pressure/flow/air detector/temperature/level detector probes, and gas flow including verification of correct setup and integrity. Mounting brackets for major components should be verified as secure. Check for bubbles or leaks.
4. Check of supplies. Spare perfusion components, spare fuses, drugs, handcranks, flashlight(s), and extra tubing clamps should be verified.

It is helpful if two people can perform the prebypass check together, with the person who set up the system going through the list, and the other doing the checks.

Monitoring and Safety Devices

Monitoring devices provide information to the perfusionist about the conduct of CPB so that the perfusionist can correct any problem that might arise. Safety devices not only monitor the conduct of CPB, but automatically prevent an unforeseen event from affecting patient safety. An example of a *monitoring* device is a pressure transducer in the arterial line connected to an alarm that will alert the perfusionist if arterial line pressure becomes too high. An example of a *safety* device is a level detector in the oxygenator that will shut off or greatly reduce pump flow if the blood level in the oxygenator becomes dangerously low, thus preventing catastrophic air embolization. The locations of commonly employed monitoring and safety devices on the extracorporeal circuit are diagrammed on Figure 13.2.

Monitoring devices are being used with increasing frequency. A 1990 study focused on the use of monitoring and safety devices in pediatric perfusion in 127 different programs.[3] Level detectors were used by 63%, air bubble detectors by 71%, gas supply oxygen analyzers by 27%, and continuous blood gas monitoring by 62% of the respondents.

Continuous monitoring devices are now available at pump-side for many of the parameters previously measured on an intermittent basis from a remotely located laboratory. These pump-side devices must be accurate. This usually requires calibration of the device by adjusting the offset or zero at one point and the gain or slope at a second point (two-point calibration) if there is linearity between the patient parameter and the device reading (Figure 13.3). Another important consideration is the response time of the monitoring device. This can be expressed as a time constant, the time required for the device to indicate 63% of an instantaneous change in its input (Figure 13.4). After three time constants have passed, the device reflects 95% of the full change. Similarly, the rise time, the time required for a 90% change to a new value, is a measure of response time. If the patient variable changes significantly faster than the response time of the device, the monitoring device is not useful.

Temperature Monitoring

Certain ceramic semiconductors respond to temperature changes with changes in electrical resistance.[4] These devices, thermistors, work very well within the physiologic temperature range. Change in electrical resistance is nonlinear, so that linearizing circuits or scales are required in the monitoring device. The thermistor is part of a temperature probe which is precalibrated, usually by the manufacturer. Actual calibration of the temperature probes by the user is seldom done. The small mass required for the thermistor results in a fast response time (although the mass of the supporting probe structure may increase the response time slightly).

Another type of electronic temperature probe is the thermocouple, which is formed by the junction of two dissimilar metals placed at the temperature monitoring site.[5] A reference junction is formed by another pair of metals at a known temperature, bonded together and connected in series with the first. A voltage proportional to the temperature difference between the reference junction and the monitoring thermocouple is generated by the circuitry. Thermocouples have relatively small output signals, with temperature changes in the physiologic range. They can, however, be made exceptionally small (as small as 0.1 mm), allowing them to be made into very small sensors with time constants as short as 1 millisecond.

There are several points in the perfusion circuit at which temperature must be monitored. The water temperature in the fluid entering the heat exchanger directly affects the temperature of the arterial blood and must be monitored. In addition to the temperature display, an audible alarm is desirable for high temperatures in order to call attention to failures. If the water is provided by a heater/cooler, the heater/cooler should also have a monitor to detect excessive heating and a backup thermostat which can act as a second safety device to limit the upper temperature that can be reached.

Blood temperatures proximal and distal to the heat exchanger, the venous and arterial blood temperatures, respectively, are also needed. These temperatures are typically measured with permanent nonsterile temperature probes that insert into a well on the combined oxygenator/heat exchanger (Figure 13.5). The well is lined with a material that conducts heat efficiently from the arterial or venous blood and isolates the probe from direct contact with the blood.

Patient temperature monitoring, using thermistors as

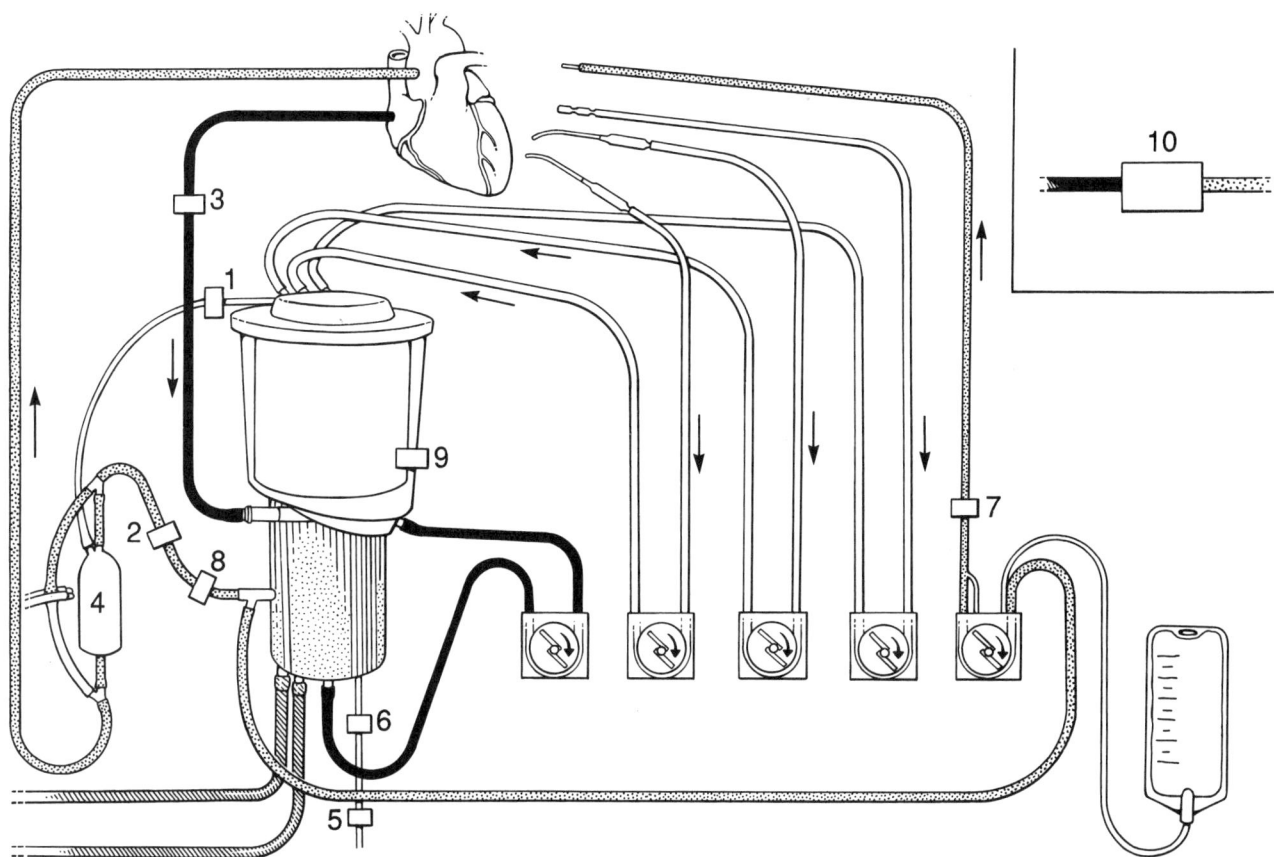

FIGURE 13.2. Type and location of commonly employed extracorporeal circuit safety and monitoring devices: (1) purge line unidirectional valve; (2) air emboli detector/pressure alarm; (3) venous blood saturation and hematocrit, and temperature monitor; (4) arterial line filter; (5) oxygen/air differential alarm; (6) gas line filter; (7) cardioplegia line filter and temperature and pressure monitors; (8) arterial blood gas and temperature monitor; (9) blood level sensor; and (10) prebypass filter.

temperature probes, is accomplished ordinarily by probes measuring rectal, esophageal, and/or bladder temperatures. Each of these sites has unique problems. The rectal temperature is subject to long time constants when poor tissue contact is caused by feces. The bladder temperature similarly can have a slow time constant if urine output is low. Esophageal temperature may not reflect core body temperature if the pericardium or the pleural cavity is filled with cold (or warm) irrigating solution. Tympanic and nasopharyngeal monitoring sites are used to reflect cerebral temperatures.

Cardioplegic solutions are ordinarily cooled prior to myocardial delivery. An in line thermistor distal to the heat exchanger validates the temperature of the cardioplegic solution during its administration (Figure 13.6). The effectiveness of the solution in cooling the myocardium is best monitored through the use of myocardial temperature probes. Typically, thermocouple probes are used, as they are easily fabricated into needlelike configurations. In addition to validating initial cooling by cardioplegic solutions, myocardial temperature probes alert the operating team to rewarming and identify the need for additional cardioplegic cooling.

Blood Pressure Monitoring

Pressure monitoring of the perfusion circuit is distinct from hemodynamic monitoring of the patient. Often referred to as "line pressures," these pressures provide information about the function of the components in the perfusion circuit.[6] Generally, the pulsatile pressure in these areas is not needed, and these devices can monitor and display mean pressure only. These pressure monitoring devices are sterilely isolated from the blood pathway and should have an operating range of 0 to 500 mm Hg. There are three locations for line pressure monitoring: proximal to the membrane oxygenator, proximal to the arterial filter, and proximal to the arterial cannula. These pressures, along with the patient's mean arterial pressure, allow calculation of the pressure gradient for each of the perfusion circuit components listed above. Typical pressure gradients are about 200, 30, and 50 mm Hg for the membrane

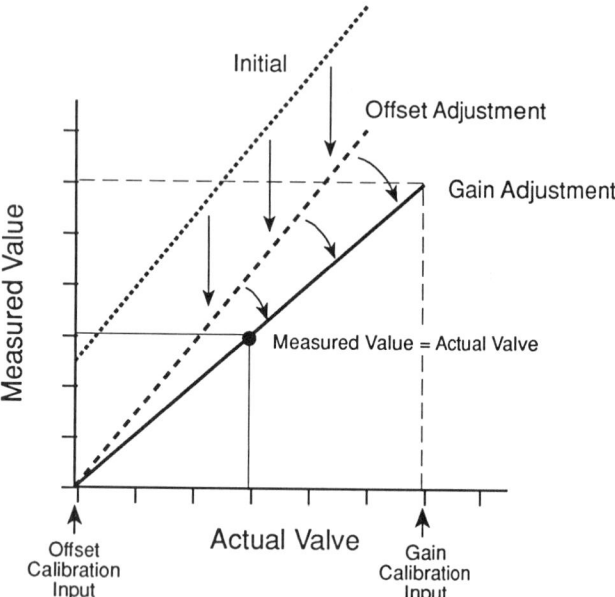

FIGURE 13.3. A two-point calibration adjusts for offset errors by using a known low value to position the calibration line and gain errors, and by using a known high value to adjust the slope of the calibration line. Measured values then accurately represent actual values for linear measurement devices.

pressure is typically monitored directly from a second lumen on the cannula. Pressure is more critical with a recommended limit of approximately 40 mm Hg.

Flow Monitoring

Measurement of blood flow from the arterial pump head is a requirement for centrifugal pumps, because they are pressure dependent in their flow output (see Chapter 11). With proper setting of the occlusion of a roller pump, blood flow measurement is not necessary. Blood flow in tubing is typically measured using one of two techniques, electromagnetic or ultrasonic (Doppler) flow measurements.

Clinical electromagnetic blood flow meters use electromagnets to generate a magnetic field and small electrodes in direct contact with the blood to measure the induced voltage. Permanent extracorporeal electromagnetic flow probes have integral fluid paths that can be inserted in line with standard tubing sizes. A probe with a disposable fluid path has been developed utilizing a permanent component (housing the electromagnet) that clamps around a special tubing connector containing electrodes molded into the connector to contact the blood.

Ultrasonic techniques use mechanical vibrations generated by a piezoelectric crystal that vibrates at the desired frequency. The ultrasound is detected by a receiving crystal that, when deformed by the mechanical vibrations originating from the first crystal, induces a voltage pro-

oxygenator, the filter, and the cannula, respectively.[7-9] If the pressure gradient across the oxygenator or arterial filter increases, the probable cause is occlusion due to inadequate anticoagulation. Excessive pressure gradients across the aortic cannula may be due to undersizing for the required flow, a kink in the arterial tubing, or malposition of the tip of the cannula (with the tip possibly against the aortic wall or possibly occluded because of dissection of the aorta).

Administration pressures for cardioplegic solution can be similarly monitored. This is more critical for cardioplegia administered by roller pump than that given by pressure bag, since the pressure bag inherently limits pressure.[10] It is important to know the pressure gradient across the cardioplegia cannula and filter for typical flow rates in order to compute the pressure at the administration site. For antegrade administration, the pressure at the administration site should approximate normal mean arterial pressure. High pressure in the cardioplegia line during antegrade cardioplegia flow could indicate poor cannula position or inadequate capacity to carry the selected flow (down a vein graft with a severely diseased distal coronary artery). In the aortic root, a very low pressure may indicate an incompetent aortic valve causing poor delivery of cardioplegic solution. For retrograde infusion, the

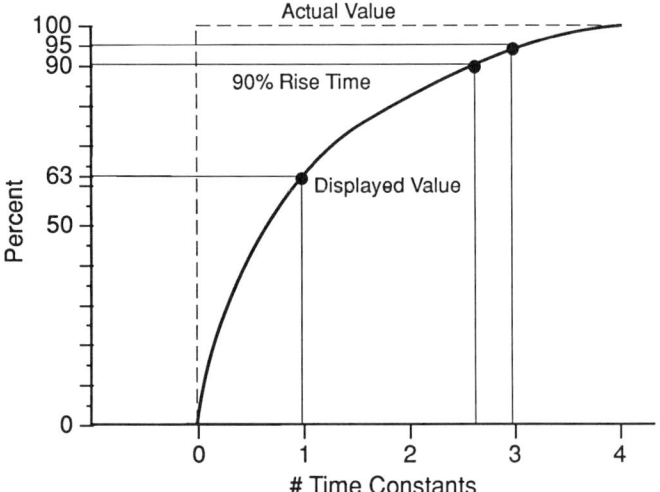

FIGURE 13.4. Device response times to instantaneous input changes are typically specified as a value for the time constant. For example, a device with a 10-second time constant would require 30 seconds (3 time constants) to reach 95% of the input change. Alternately, the rise time specifies the time to rise to the denoted percentage of change, often 90%.

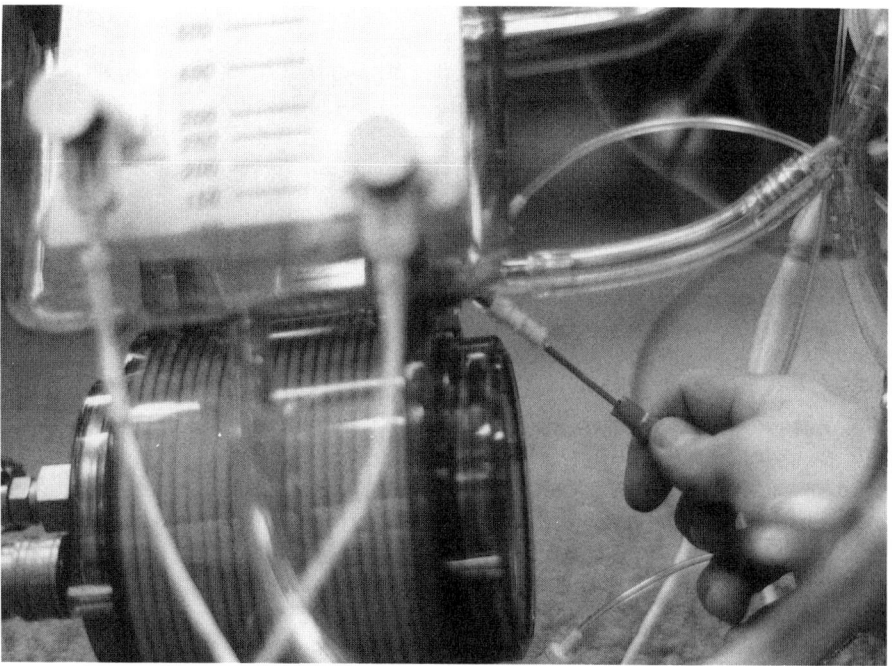

FIGURE 13.5 The oxygenator reservoir temperature is measured by inserting a temperature probe into an integral well on the oxygenator which is designed to accept it. The temperature is then monitored on the heart-lung machine display.

portional to the deformation. Two different ultrasonic methods are used to measure flow. The Doppler principle states that the frequency of sound coming from a source will shift in proportion to the velocity of that source relative to the receiver. With Doppler flow probes, a transmitting crystal is used to generate an ultrasonic signal. This signal reflects off the particulate matter and is then received by a second signal. The particulate matter, in reflecting the ultrasonic signal, acts as the source, and the frequency shift detected by the receiving crystal can be used to determine the velocity of the blood particles. This velocity, in combination with the diameter of the flow path, can be used to calculate the actual blood flow. A second technique is a transit time flow meter which uses a transmitting crystal to direct an ultrasound pulse either upstream or downstream towards a receiving crystal. The time for the pulse to reach the receiving crystal is shifted by the speed of the fluid between the two crystals. This change in the time can then be used to detect fluid velocity (and, in combination with tubing diameter, flow). The transmit time flow meters can be used for all types of fluid, while the Doppler flow meter requires fluid-containing particles.

Monitoring Blood Variables

One of the earliest parameters of the blood to be monitored continuously was oxygen saturation. Reduced hemoglobin has a different light absorbance spectrum than oxyhemoglobin. The absorbencies are maximally different for red light, with a wave length near 660 nm, whereas the absorbance characteristics are virtually the same for both forms of hemoglobin at certain points in the infrared range. By detecting the ratio of absorbance of red light to the infrared absorbance, the fraction of hemoglobin that is oxygenated can be calculated.[11] The accuracy of units

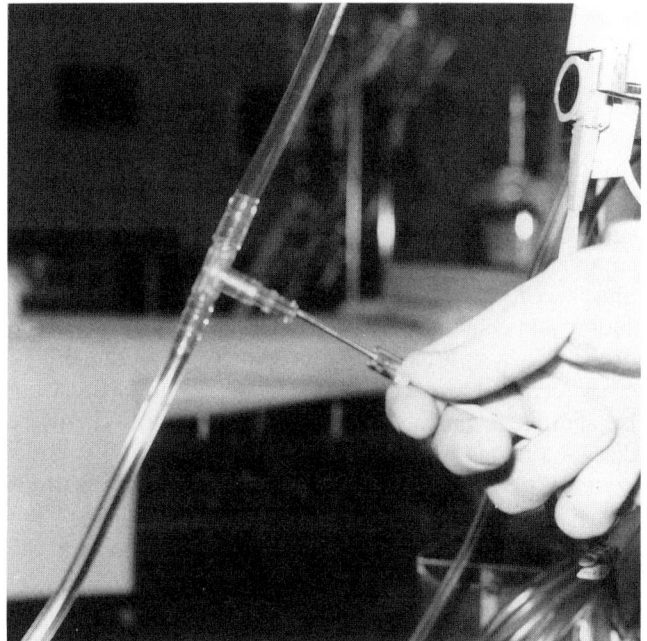

FIGURE 13.6. Cardioplegic solution temperature is measured as it passes through an in line housing that accepts a temperature probe.

on the market for in line saturation monitoring compare very favorably to more sophisticated benchtop analyzers. Response time is limited only by electronic filtering to stabilize the display, and is typically several seconds. More recently, a number of different technologies have evolved for continual monitoring of blood gases: Po_2, Pco_2, and pH. The first, Mallinckrodt Sensor Systems (Ann Arbor, MI), uses conventional blood-gas machine technology, with automatic calibration and direct sampling from the extracorporeal circuit. The accuracy of this system is comparable to that of benchtop analyzers, but it is not a fully continuous measurement device, since the results are available approximately 90 seconds after sampling.

An in line continuous system for the measurement of blood gases has been developed (CDI, 3M Healthcare, Irvine, CA). This single-use sensor uses dyes that fluoresce at intensities that vary with the concentration of oxygen, carbon dioxide, and hydrogen ion.[12] The accuracy of this device is less reliable, and periodic conventional blood-gas measurements are ordinarily used to confirm absolute values. The 90% response time to changes in Po_2, Pco_2, and pH have been reported at 210, 238, and 217 seconds, respectively.[12]

Another in line continuous blood-gas system uses optical measurement techniques based on light from a fiberoptic bundle passed through a pH-sensitive dye and returned, via fiberoptic bundle, to the instrument (Biomedical Sensor Ltd. Bucks, UK). This technology is limited in accuracy and response time, similar to the unit mentioned above.[13]

Continuous blood-gas monitoring is a relatively new addition to CPB monitoring systems. Because of its cost (it adds approximately 10% to the direct cost of the CPB circuit), much attention has been directed to its application and accuracy. It is not yet fully cost effective, but if improvements in accuracy and response time allow near elimination of the need for additional samples processed in the blood-gas laboratory (now necessary to validate periodically the continuously monitored results), the technique will certainly become more widely adopted.

A closely related parameter that is primarily for safety is a measurement of the percentage of oxygen that is provided to the oxygenator from the blender (the FiO_2). This is a relatively inexpensive device that is used to validate blender performance. It is common to have an audible alarm, so that low levels of oxygen can be detected.

Electrolytes are among the parameters that can now be monitored in the operating room (Mallinckrodt Sensor Systems, Ann Arbor, MI). Sodium, potassium, and calcium ions are measured by the same disposable sensor system described above for blood gases.[14] Accuracy is consistent with benchtop analyzers, and the delay before the reading is available is about 90 seconds. This system also provides a measure of hematocrit, using the electrical conductivity of the blood.

Perfusion Circuit Safety Devices

A comprehensive survey of over 1000 perfusionists was performed in 1985.[15,16] The authors reported the following incidence for common accidents: air embolism, 1 per 8316; oxygenator failure, 1 per 13,662; disseminated intravascular coagulopathy, 1 per 19,786; reversed left ventricular vent, 1 per 22,069; mechanical failure, 1 per 170,446. Since massive gas embolism is by far the most common fatal perfusion accident, much attention has been directed toward safety devices for its prevention. The worst scenario is sudden occlusion of the venous line when the pump is pumping at full arterial flow. When this occurs, the time before a massive air embolism occurs is equal to the total volume of the reservoir and oxygenator divided by the arterial flow. For an arterial flow of 5 L/min and a total volume of 1 L, this time is 12 seconds. This demonstrates the need to maintain oxygenator volume at a reasonable level, to allow the perfusionist time to react to sudden changes. One of the first safety devices used on CPB circuits was an oxygenator reservoir level detector (Figure 13.7). A light source and a photodetector are used to monitor the level in the perfusion circuit, with an alarm to alert the perfusionist to stop the arterial pump head immediately and correct the cause of reduced volume. Alternatively, the detection device can be connected to the arterial pump head to stop the pump automatically.

Newer models use ultrasonic level detectors that will work on all types of fluids (photodetectors generally require opaque fluids). An alternative detector that has been used is based on the weight of the oxygenator and its volume.

Air detectors are based on principles similar to those of the level detectors. They are placed distal to the arterial pump head but as far away from the patient as practical, to maximize the time between the detection of bubbles and the introduction of these bubbles into the patient. The simplest system is based on a light source-photodetector combination.[17] If a bubble large enough to change the opacity of blood passes through the tubing, the light source and detector trigger an alarm. Bubbles that can be detected are approximately proportional to the tubing cross-sectional area (about 1 mL in ⅜" tubing) and are harder to detect in high-flow situations. Arterial filters are designed to remove both particulate matter and gaseous emboli. By gravity, the gas collects in the top of the filter, where a constantly flowing purge line can be connected to bleed off accumulated gas to a low pressure point in the extracorporeal circuit.

Ball valves can also be used in line with the arterial or cardioplegia tubing to prevent delivery of air to the patient (Figure 13.8). The principle is straightforward, in that the ball floats on the liquid in a position out of the mainstream of flow. The device is positioned so that the flow

FIGURE 13.7. Oxygenator level detectors (indicated by *arrowheads*) are positioned on the oxygenator at the lowest desirable blood volume, to prevent undetected emptying of the reservoir, and at the highest desirable volume, to prevent overfilling.

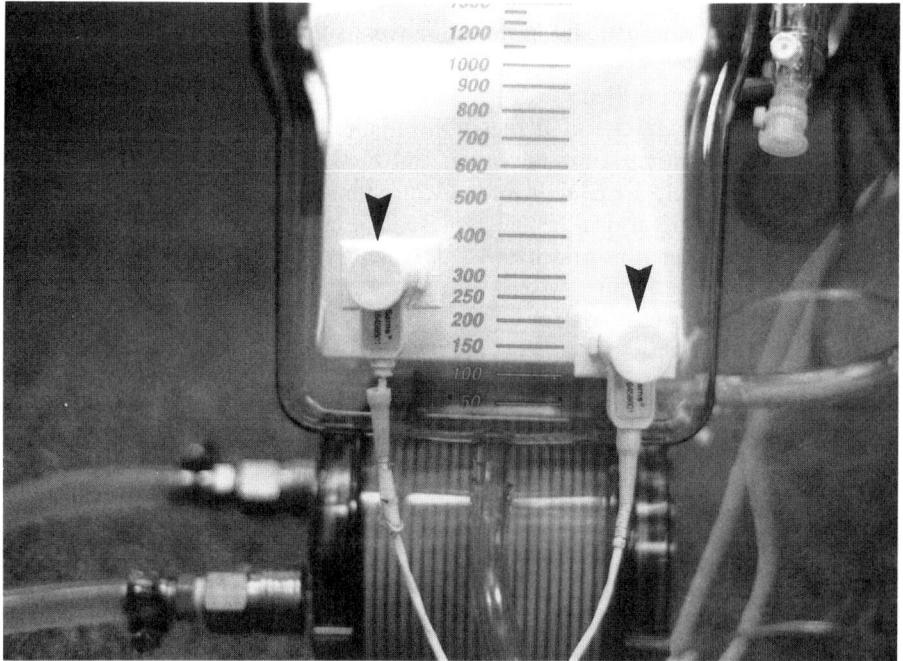

is from top to bottom. If the float chamber is emptied by advancing air, the ball no longer floats and it sinks to the bottom, where it seats in a seal and blocks further flow. These valves should be used proximal to the respective pump head, since the negative pressure generated, once the ball seats, collapses the tubing and prevents further pumping. If placed distal to the pump head, particularly if some liquid flow is restored, very large positive pressures can be generated against the seated ball, and the circuit may separate.

Pressure relief valves are used on suction lines, particularly the left ventricular vent, to prevent excessive negative pressures from developing if the proximal end becomes occluded or the ventricle is emptied.[18] The valve allows room air to be aspirated at a determined point or adjusted negative pressure. The air mixes with the blood that is still being suctioned, to make a total flow equal to the set pump flow rate. In order to minimize hemolysis, it is desirable to minimize air flow rate by reducing pump flow rate to nearly the blood flow rate.

Summary

The final common pathway for all monitoring and safety devices is a careful, vigilant perfusionist. Circuitry setup should be accomplished with verification by a checklist.

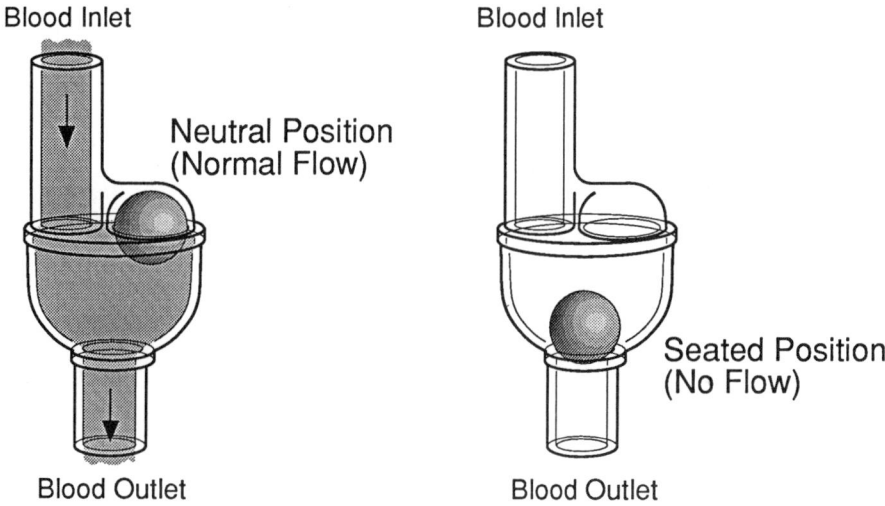

FIGURE 13.8. Ball valves are inserted into the arterial circuit between the oxygenator reservoir and the arterial pump head to prevent infusion of air. If the circuit remains filled with liquid, the ball floats out of the flow path (*left*). If the liquid level drops, the ball falls and seats to prevent air flow to the pump head and patient (*right*).

Appropriately designed documentation sheets, used during the perfusion run, also aid in detecting trends in patient and circuitry parameters that might alert the perfusionist to upcoming problems.

The extracorporeal circuit depicted in Figure 13.1, when used by attentive, knowledgeable, and meticulous perfusion personnel, with appropriate communication with anesthesia and surgical teams, represents a current compromise between the priorities of complete system monitoring and redundant system features versus the present emphasis on cost control.

References

1. Arcidi JM Jr, Powelson SW, King SB, et al. Trends in invasive treatment of single-vessel and double-vessel coronary disease. *J Thorac Cardiovasc Surg* 1988;95:773–781.
2. Crane TN, Keen WR Jr, Spiller CE, et al. A prebypass checklist—Why aren't you using one? *Proc Am Acad Cardiovasc Perf* 1986;7:98–100.
3. Hill AG, Groom RC, Akl BF, et al. 1990 pediatric perfusion survey II: expanded multivariate data analysis. *Proc Am Acad Cardiovasc Perf* 1991;12:96–102.
4. Webster JG, ed. *Medical Instrumentation Application and Design*. New York: Houghton-Mifflin Co; 1978:73–79.
5. Webster JG, ed. *Medical Instrumentation Application and Design*. New York: Houghton-Mifflin Co; 1978:70–73.
6. Vinansky RP, Hill AG, Groom RC, et al. Pressure measurement and safety with a self-contained device. *Proc Am Acad Cardiovasc Perf* 1986;7:101–104.
7. American Bentley. In-vitro, ex-vivo and in-vivo performance characteristics of the Bentley® BOS-CM40 and BOS-CM50 capillary fiber membrane oxygenators. Irvine, Calif: American Bentley; 1984 (PN Q83280-184-3PG).
8. Justison GA, Lewis HD, Hamilton DG, et al. A comparison of a heparin-coated and a non-coated ECC arterial line blood filter. *J Extracorp Tech* 1986;18:55–60.
9. Pfaender LM. Hemodynamics in the extracorporeal aortic cannula: review of factors affecting choice of the appropriate size. *J Extracorp Tech* 1981;13:224–232.
10. Grover FL, Fewel JG, Ghidoni JJ, et al. Comparison of roller pump versus pressurized bag administration of potassium cardioplegia solution. *Ann Thorac Surg* 1982;34:278–287.
11. Webster JG, ed. *Medical Instrumentation Application and Design*. New York: Houghton-Mifflin Co; 1978:86,93–94.
12. Lautier A, Gaillard D, Juvin AM, et al. Monitoring of blood gases during extracorporeal circulation with an artificial lung. *Int J Artif Organs* 1990;13:117–124.
13. Meyerhoff ME. New in vitro analytical approaches for clinical chemistry measurements in critical care. *Clin Chem* 1990;36:1557–1572.
14. Mansouri S, Mitsuhashi A. A new blood gas and electrolyte analyzer for point-of-care use. Presented at the 13th International Symposium on Methodology and Clinical Applications of Blood Gases, pH, Electrolytes and Sensor Technology; October 6–9, 1991; Hakone, Japan.
15. Kurusz M, Conti VR, Arens JF, et al. Perfusion accident survey. *Proc Am Acad Cardiovasc Perf* 1986;7:57–65.
16. Kurusz M, Faulkner SC. Follow-up comments from the 1985 perfusion accident survey. *Proc Am Acad Cardiovasc Perf* 1987;8:210–212.
17. Vivian WA, Stander KH, Smith RG. An air embolism detection device for use with a non-occlusive arterial pump head. *J Extracorp Tech* 1987;19:406–407.
18. Lewis GS, Czaplicka C. In vitro comparison tests of three LV vent valves. *J Extracorp Tech* 1990;22:125–131.

14
Heat Exchange in Extracorporeal Systems

Richard L. Rigatti and Roger Stewart

Introduction

In the early years of clinical heart-lung bypass, blood-warming devices were used to maintain the patient's normal (37°C) temperature during cardiopulmonary bypass (CPB). The development of hypothermic CPB techniques led to the development of heat-exchange devices for the extracorporeal circuit that are capable of rapidly warming or cooling blood.

The principal requirement of a heat-exchange unit is the capacity for a large caloric exchange. The temperature of the surface in contact with moving blood can safely be as low as 1°C or as high as 42°C without significant damage to formed blood elements. While cooling, a large temperature gradient may exist between the patient's blood and the heat-exchange unit; therefore, cooling is generally quickly and efficiently accomplished. With warming, the permissible temperature gradients are smaller (usually 10°–12°C to avoid formation of microbubbles[1]) and the maximum tolerable blood temperature is only a few degrees above normothermia (37°C). Therefore, warming occurs much more slowly. This chapter outlines the physical principles governing heat transfer, describes heat exchange device design, and discusses the clinical use of heat exchangers in extracorporeal circulation.

Modes of Heat Transfer

Heat transfer occurs by conduction, convection, and radiation (Table 14.1). Heat *conduction* is the term applied to energy exchange by direct contact from one mass to another or from one part of a mass to another part. This exchange is in the form of kinetic energy of motion of molecules in direct communication, or by the drift of free electrons in the case of heat conduction in metals. The distinguishing feature of conduction is that it takes place within the boundaries of a mass, or across the boundary of a mass into another mass placed in contact with the first, without appreciable displacement of the matter comprising the mass.

Convection is the term applied to heat transfer that occurs within a fluid by mixing of one portion of the fluid with another portion due to gross movements of the mass of fluid. On the molecular level, the actual process of energy transfer from one fluid particle or molecule to another is still one of conduction, but the energy is transported from one point to another by displacement of the fluid itself. If the fluid motion is caused by an external mechanical means (eg, by a pump), it is termed *forced* convection. If the fluid motion is caused by density differences that are created by the temperature differences in the fluid, the process is termed *free* or *natural* convection.

The third basic mode of heat transfer is *radiation*. This term is used to describe the electromagnetic radiation that is emitted from the surface of a body that has been thermally excited. This electromagnetic radiation is emitted in all directions, and when it strikes another body, the radiation may be reflected, transmitted, or absorbed.

Heat exchange occurs in extracorporeal circuits by all three modes of heat transfer—conduction, convection, and radiation—but the primary modes are conduction and convection.

Heat Transfer Theory

An assessment of the performance characteristics of heat-exchange devices in extracorporeal circuits (which generally utilize hot or cold water to control blood temperature) includes analyses of the processes of both conduction and convection. Forced convection occurs on

TABLE 14.1. Modes of heat transfer.

Conduction
Convection
Radiation

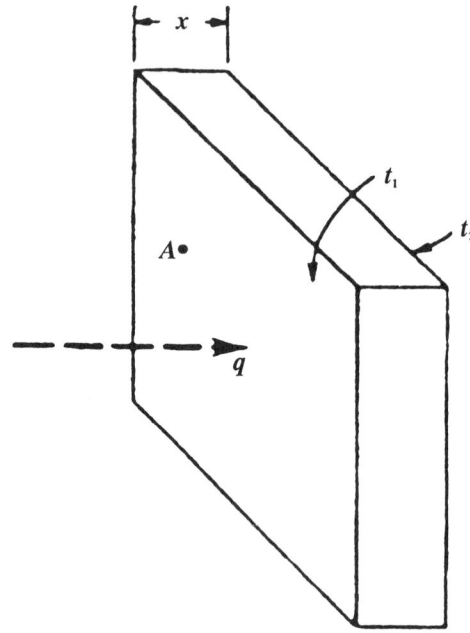

FIGURE 14.1. Variables used in the calculation of the thermal conductivity (k) of a hypothetical material with thickness x, cross-sectional area A, temperatures t_1 and t_2 on either side of the material, and rate of heat flow q.

both the water and blood sides of the heat-exchange barrier. Conduction occurs through the material barrier used to separate the two fluids.

The principles of thermal conduction can be examined in an idealized example of a material of thickness X and cross-sectional area A, with a temperature equal to t_1 on one side and t_2 on the other side (Figure 14.1).[2] If q is the rate of heat flow (ie, ∆ energy per unit time) through the plate, then q is described by the relationship:

$$q = kA \frac{(t_1 - t_2)}{x}$$

where k is the constant of proportionality called the *thermal conductivity of the material*. Thermal conductivity is a property dependent only upon the composition of the material, not on its geometric configuration. The term *unit thermal conductance* (C) is used to express the heat-conducting capacity per unit of surface area of a given physical configuration. Thus, if C represents the unit thermal conductance, then the rate of heat flow through the material is described by this equation:

$$\frac{q}{A} = C(t_1 - t_2)$$

where q equals the rate of heat flow; A equals the cross-sectional area of the material, and t_1 and t_2 equal the temperature on either side of the material. The term C is not a physical property of the material but depends on the geometric configuration of the heat-exchange system.

The forced convection that occurs in the fluid regions of the heat-exchange device is dependent upon fluid motion. It is therefore necessary to consider some of the principles of fluid dynamics in order to understand these processes of convection. The flow in the region can be either laminar or turbulent, depending in large part upon the viscosity of the fluid, the degree to which the surface is covered by fluid (wettability), and the velocity of flow. Figure 14.2 shows the difference in the velocity profile of a laminar and a turbulent boundary layer.

To understand how these conditions affect convective heat transfer, one can examine the case of a solid material surface maintained at temperature t_S with a fluid of temperature t_F flowing over it (Figure 14.3). This concept of the thermal boundary layer is similar to that of the velocity boundary layer described in Figure 14.2. The thermal

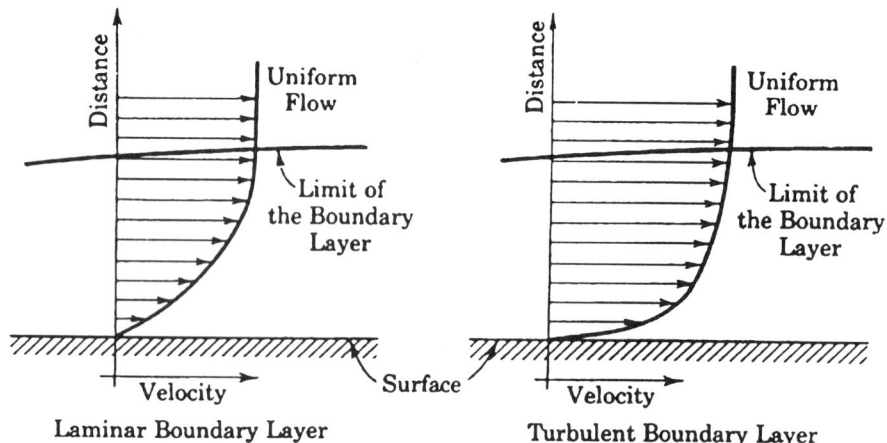

FIGURE 14.2. Diagrammatic representation of the difference in the velocity profile of laminar and turbulent boundary layers. When a fluid moves past a solid surface, the fluid velocity varies from 0 at the surface to a finite value at some distance away from the surface. The region between the surface and the point at which the fluid velocity is equal to the bulk flow velocity is referred to as the *velocity boundary layer*.

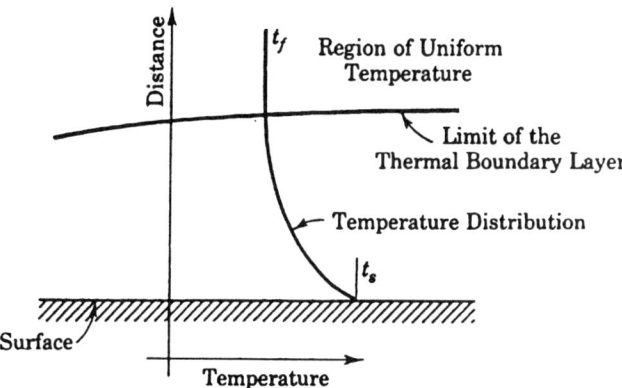

FIGURE 14.3. Diagrammatic representation of convective heat transfer in a solid material at temperature t_s with fluid of temperature t_F flowing over it. The temperature of the fluid flowing past the surface will vary. Most of the temperature variation occurs close to the surface and within the thermal boundary layer.

boundary layer is generally not precisely coincident with the velocity boundary layer. The complexities of this analysis are summarized in a formula similar to that describing the process of conduction:

$$\frac{q}{A} = h(t_S - t_F)$$

where q equals the rate of heat flow; A equals the cross-sectional area of the material; t_S and t_F are the temperatures of the solid material surface and the fluid flowing over it, respectively; and h is the film coefficient, a unit of conductance (the same as C) that is dependent upon the composition of the fluid and the nature of the fluid motion over the surface. The film coefficient, h, represents the overall effect of convection and does not explain the actual mechanism of heat transfer. In very simple cases, the film coefficient may be calculated, but in most cases, the geometry and fluid flows are sufficiently complex that the film coefficients are best determined experimentally.

To understand the interrelationship of variables that affect the performance of an extracorporeal blood heat exchanger, consider the problem depicted in Figure 14.4. This is a model of a modern heat-exchange device in which a biocompatible material coats the blood side of the heat exchanger. Water at a temperature t_1 flows over a plain surface, forming a boundary layer with film coefficient h_{12}. The material separating the two fluids is made up of two layers with thermal conductivities k_{23} and k_{34}. The material separating the two fluids is separated into two layers. The biocompatible coating is usually very thin but typically has very poor thermal conductivity, and therefore can reduce the overall efficiency of heat transfer significantly. Blood at a temperature t_5 flows over the other surface in the opposite direction, forming a boundary layer with film coefficient h_{45}. The series of resistances to heat flux are shown schematically at the bottom of Figure 14.4 (using an analogy with electrical circuitry) in which the *total thermal resistance* (R) is the inverse of conductance (C) or:

$$R = \frac{1}{C} = \frac{1}{h}$$

where h equals the film coefficient. Using these definitions and the electrical resistance analogy, the overall heat flux from water to blood can be summarized as:

$$\frac{q}{A} = \frac{t_1 - t_5}{\frac{1}{h_{12}} + \frac{\Delta x_{23}}{k_{23}} + \frac{\Delta x_{34}}{k_{34}} + \frac{1}{h_{45}}}$$

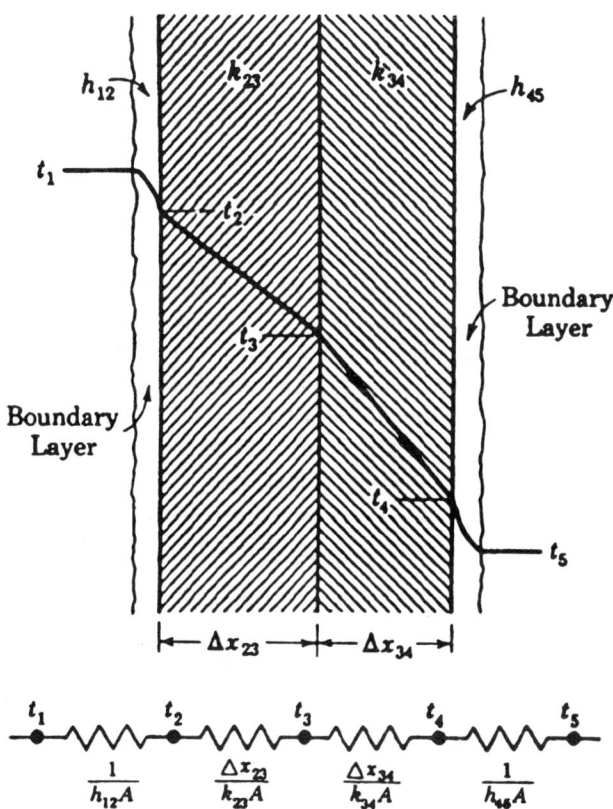

FIGURE 14.4. Diagrammatic representation of the heat-exchange device composed of two materials with thermal conductivity values of k_{23} and k_{24} and widths x_{23} and x_{24}. Water at temperature t_1 flows over one surface and forms a boundary layer with film coefficient h_{12}. Another fluid (eg, blood) with temperature t_5 flows in the opposite direction over the other surface, forming a boundary layer with a film coefficient of h_{45}. The sum of the multiple resistance ($1/h_{12}A$, $\Delta x_{23}/k_{23}A$, $\Delta x_{34}/k_{34}A$, $1/h_{45}A$) to heat flux in the system is the total thermal resistance.

where q equals the rate of heat flow; A equals the cross-sectional area of the system; t_1 and t_5 equal the temperatures of the two fluids (eg, water and blood), respectively; Δx_{23} and Δx_{34} equal the thickness of the materials separating the two fluids; k_{23} and k_{34} are the thermal conductivity values of the two materials; and h_{12} and h_{45} are the film coefficients in the water and blood pathways. The total heat flux per unit of heat transfer surface area is therefore a function of the temperature differences between the two fluids, the film coefficients (h) in the water and blood pathways, the thickness (x) of the materials separating the two fluids, and the conductivity (k) of the materials. A common misconception is that the blood-film coefficient is the primary performance-determining factor. As can be seen from the above equation, the water side of the film coefficient can be equally important. Generally speaking, it is desirable to have high flow (low resistance) and turbulent flow on the water side to achieve a high film coefficient. On the blood side, it is important to maintain laminar flow to minimize damage to formed blood elements and to keep the total blood pathway thickness as small as possible to improve thermal energy transfer.

Materials in Heat-Exchange Devices

The material to be selected for the separation of blood and water flows should be as thin as possible so that it will provide efficient hear transfer and still have sufficient integrity to withstand the expected water and blood pressures without failure. It is also important to have a material that has a high thermal conductivity (k).

Unfortunately, the most biocompatible materials (plastics and stainless steel, etc.) used in extracorporeal blood handling have relatively poor thermal conductivities. Table 14.2 lists the thermal conductivities of materials and coatings typically used in blood-heat exchangers. Some devices use materials with higher thermal conductivities (such as aluminum) and coat them with a very thin layer of biocompatible material (using plastic coating or anodizing). This technique has not gained wide acceptance, however, because traces of aluminum have been detected in extracorporeal circulating blood, and aluminum emboli have been found at autopsy in infants undergoing extracorporeal membrane oxygenation (ECMO) with circuits utilizing coated aluminum heat exchangers.[3-5] Stainless steel appears to be the best all around heat-exchanger material when considering biocompatibility, thermal conductivity, and structural integrity.

Heat Exchanger Performance Evaluation

An evaluation of the performance capability of a given heat-exchange device design is easily carried out in an in vitro laboratory model. Although the results obtained may not directly correlate with the performance achieved in a clinical setting, precise steady-state conditions and temperature measurements allow a reliable comparison of one heat exchanger with another.

The in vitro test circuit is characterized by a relatively large (15 L) reservoir of blood (or saline as a substitute) that is maintained at a constant temperature of 30°C. The "blood flow" is controlled by a roller pump similar to the pumps used in clinical application. The water side flow of the heat exchanger is controlled at 40°C, and the flow is typically varied to simulate various clinical water sources.

Analysis of the performance of a specific heat-exchanger design is expressed in terms of *effectiveness, efficiency*, or *performance factor* (P_f). The thermal potential (mc_p) of a fluid is the product of the mass flow rate of the fluid times the specific heat of the fluid. The specific heat of a fluid is the quantity of heat transferred per unit temperature difference. Thus, the mc_p of a fluid takes into consideration the flow rate, density, and thermal capacity of the fluid. The equation for determining P_f on the blood side of the heat exchanger for all water flows is[1]:

$$P_f = \frac{(mc_p)_{\text{blood}} (t_{\text{bo}} - t_{\text{bi}})}{(mc_p)_{\text{min}} (t_{\text{wi}} - t_{\text{bi}})}$$

where $(mc_p)_{\text{blood}}$ and $(mc_p)_{\text{min}}$ are the thermal potentials for blood and water, respectively; t_{bo} (temperature of blood out) is the temperature of the blood exiting the heat exchanger; t_{bi} (temperature of blood in) is the temperature of the blood entering the heat exchanger; and t_{wi} (temperature of water in) is the temperature of the water entering the heat exchanger. The numerator of the performance factor represents the total amount of heat flux to the blood as it passes through the heat exchanger. The denominator is the maximum amount of heat that can be transferred. This maximum amount of heat that can be transferred is limited to the maximum temperature difference (the difference between the inflow temperatures of the two fluids) available in the heat exchanger multiplied by the smaller of the two (mc_p) values of the two fluids.

TABLE 14.2. Thermal conductivity values (k) of different materials and coatings used in heat-exchange devices.

Material	k (10^4 cal cm/s cm² °F)
Aluminum	5374
Stainless steel	311
Polyurethane	5
Silicone	5
Polycarbonate	4.7
Epoxy	4.5

The performance factor is simply the ratio of the heat transferred to (or from) the blood to the maximum amount of heat transfer that theoretically could occur. The performance factor varies between 0 and 1 with an efficiency of 1 being impossible to achieve. Since the typical clinical water flow rate (6–20 L/min) through an extracorporeal heat-exchange device is most often higher than the typical blood flow (1–6 L/min), and the specific heat of blood is very close to that for water, the term $(mc_P)_{blood}$ is usually equal to $(mc_P)_{min}$ and cancels out of the equation. Thus, the most commonly used form of the performance factor is:

$$P_f = \frac{t_{bo} - t_{bi}}{t_{wi} - t_{bi}}$$

It should be remembered, however, that if the water flow is less than the blood flow, the more general form of the performance factor must be used.

Heat-Exchange Devices in Extracorporeal Circulation

Heat-Exchange Device Designs

Figure 14.5 is a schematic of the fundamental components of an extracorporeal bypass circuit utilizing a membrane oxygenator. Although the flow through the various components of the perfusion circuit is most often as shown in this diagram, there are several notable exceptions, including the COBE CML, Terumo Capiox E, and Bentley Univox oxygenators.

The COBE CML integrates the heat exchanger into the venous reservoir, so that gravity flow from the patient drives the blood through both the venous reservoir and the heat exchanger before the pump pushes the blood through the membrane lung and back to the patient. The Terumo Capiox E utilizes gravity pressure to push blood first through the heat exchanger, then the membrane lung, and then into the arterial reservoir before the pump returns blood to the patient. In both of these designs, the only driving force for blood through the heat exchanger is the head of pressure afforded by the height of the patient above the oxygenator. For this reason, it is very important in these designs that the heat exchanger have a very low resistance to flow.

The Bentley Univox is similar to many other membrane oxygenator systems in that the heat exchanger is distal to the arterial pump. However, in the Univox design, the heat exchanger is integrated into the membrane lung, so that heat exchange and gas exchange occur at the same time. This simultaneous process allows a very low priming volume of the heat exchanger-oxygenator combination.

With these exceptions in mind, the majority of heat-exchanger designs integrated with membrane oxygenator systems today utilize the flow path shown in Figure 14.5. Table 14.3 lists the construction and performance characteristics of many of the oxygenators clinically used today.

The performance factors, determined in vitro, of various heat exchangers listed in Table 14.3 are outlined in Figure 14.6. The primary reason for a difference between in vitro laboratory evaluation and clinical application of heat exchangers is a variability imposed by the water source used for water temperature control in the operating room[6] (Table 14.4).

There is significant variation in the performance capability of the various heater/cooler units used for heat exchange during extracorporeal circulation. Table 14.4 lists the performance specifications of some of the most commonly utilized units. The maximum flow and maximum pressure vary greatly with the heater/cooler unit evaluated. The heat-exchange performance test results shown in Figure 14.6 were determined with the water side flow rate set with either 12 psi inlet pressure of 20 L/min maximum flow, reflecting some of the limitations in water supply capability outlined in Table 14.4. If the wall water supply is used, the pressures and flows achievable through the heat exchanger can be substantially higher, depending upon the hospital plumbing system.

The usual procedure for safe setup and priming of a heat exchanger requires that the water source be connected to the heat exchanger and water circulated for a minimum of 5 to 10 minutes to detect a possible leak prior to priming the blood side of the extracorporeal circuit. Like the arterial filters, some heat-exchange devices are

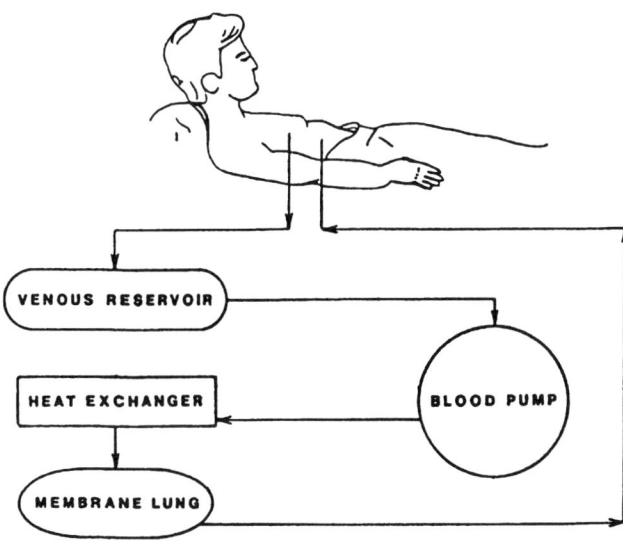

FIGURE 14.5. Blood flow path in an extracorporeal circuit that includes a heat-exchanger/membrane lung. Blood flows from the patient, by gravity, to the venous reservoir. Blood is pumped from the venous reservoir through the heat exchanger and membrane lung and ultimately returned to the patient.

TABLE 14.3. Comparison of type, heat-exchanger materials, and surface area and volume of available heat-exchange devices.

Heat exchanger/ oxygenator Manufacturer/ model	Type	Material	Approximate surface area (cm^2)	Approximate volume (mL)
BARD/HF5000	Shell and tube	Polyurethane	9000	250
Bentley/Univox	Bellows	Stainless steel	3260	0
COBE/CML 30	Convoluted coil	Stainless steel	1290	150
Dideco/COMPACTFLO	Textured folded sheets	Stainless steel	2200	90
Medtronics/Maxima	Shell and tube	Epoxy-coated aluminum	1160	100
SARNS/SMO	Bellows	Stainless steel	1580	60
SORIN/Monolyth	Textured folded sheet	Stainless steel	1700	65
Terumo/Capiox 350	Shell and tube	Stainless steel	1630	150

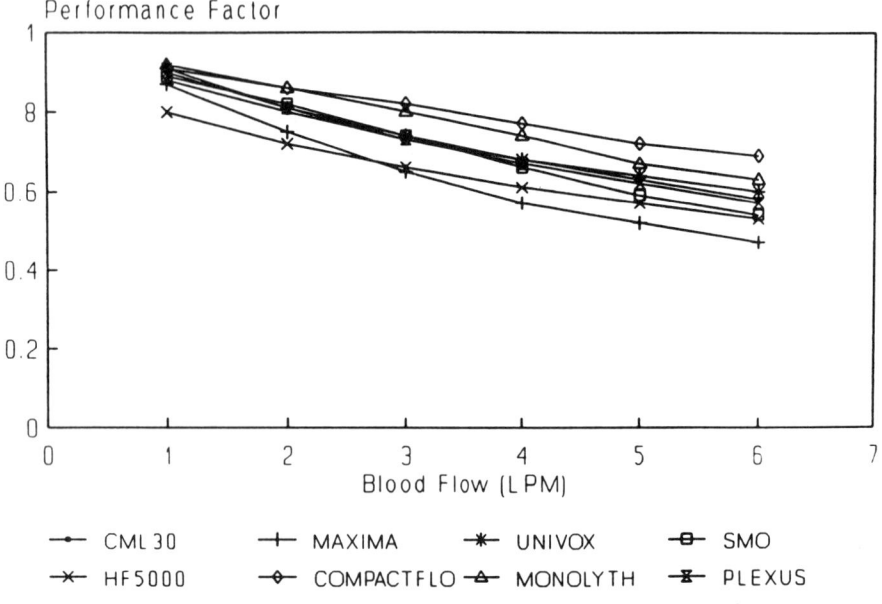

FIGURE 14.6. A comparison of performance factors in available heat exchangers at blood flows of 1 to 6 liters per minute (LPM).

TABLE 14.4. Comparison of method of cooling and performance specifications (maximum heating, flow, and pressure outputs) of available heater/cooler units.

Manufacturer	Model	Method of cooling	Maximum heating capability (watts@volts)	Maximum water flow (L/min)	Maximum output pressure (psi)
Biomedicus	Bio-cal 370	Ice	1500W@115V	20	10
Cincinnati Sub Zero	Hemotherm 400M	½ HP compressor	1200W@115V 1200W@240V 1000W@100V	19	15
Sarns	Dual cooler/ heater	Ice maker	1500W@115V	40	11
Sarns	TCMII	Ice	1550W@115V	21	9.3

difficult to fully debubble. The air must be swept through the heat exchanger by the circulation of water through the circuit (unlike the microporous membrane oxygenation compartment, where much of the air can pass across the membrane material). Because of this difficulty, many perfusionists flush the entire extracorporeal circuit with carbon dioxide, as flooding the blood path with this highly soluble gas allows simple removal of all highly insoluble air.

Patient Cooling and Rewarming Times

When normothermic bypass is employed, the performance of the heat exchanger usually is not challenged, since very little caloric transfer is necessary to maintain blood and patient temperature at 37°C. The performance of the heat exchanger comes under much more intense scrutiny when hypothermic temperatures (less than 28°C patient core temperatures) are employed. The clinically relevant performance features are the speed with which the patient can be cooled and the speed with which the patient can be subsequently rewarmed with a given extracorporeal circuit.

Because of temperature gradients between various parts of the patient's body, several different monitoring sites, or combinations of sites, are used for clinical patient temperature monitoring. Among the most commonly used sites are esophageal,[7] nasopharyngeal, tympanic,[7-10] pulmonary arterial, rectal, urinary bladder, subcutaneous (or muscle), and skin. The nasopharyngeal and tympanic membrane temperatures are the most accurate monitors of brain temperature. Often the esophageal, rectal, or bladder temperatures are used as indicators of patient core temperatures. Each of these sites has its own particular problem. Concerns about typmpanic membrane perforation limit the usefulness of this type of temperature monitoring probe. The esophageal probe can be influenced by ice or cold saline solution around the heart in the thoracic cavity. The rectal probe can be insulated by feces. Bladder temperatures can be affected by the rate of urine production. The measurement of patient core temperature in an accurate manner is important during warming, since patient temperature "afterdrop"[11] can occur after bypass. This postbypass drop in patient temperature occurs when warming has not continued long enough, and contributes to shivering, excessive oxygen demand, coagulopathies, and increased myocardial stress during the recovery interval after bypass.[12]

Blood "overheating" is also a potential problem. Blood temperature may be greater than 37°C as it exits the heart-lung machine. This overheated blood usually is infused into the aortic root and quickly reaches the brain. It has been shown that even small increases in brain temperature can exacerbate ischemic brain injury.[12] The problem of temperature and cerebral injury is discussed further in Chapter 6.

Clinical rewarming times are dependent on more than just the performance of the heat exchanger. There are differences seen in the rewarming times of the top-rated heat exchangers in Figure 14.6 compared to the lower-performing units in the clinical environments. However, the actual differences are not as extreme as the in vitro performance factor comparisons would imply. Heat exchange must occur not only between the water and the blood in the heat exchanger but also between the blood and the tissues in the body. If the patient has a high systemic vascular resistance, resulting in shunting of blood away from body tissues, or has been hypothermic for a prolonged period of time, rewarming time will be significantly prolonged.[13]

An obvious method for improving thermal transfer to blood with a given heat-exchange design is to increase the temperature difference between the blood and the water. Early experimental work demonstrated the dangers of excessive water-to-blood thermal gradients.[1] Temperature differences of 17°C were shown to cause continuous generation of gaseous microemboli due to the deceased solubility of oxygen as a function of rising temperature. In clinical practice, during the warming phase, a 10° to 12°C water-to-blood temperature gradient is not exceeded because of this potential problem.

Future Directions of Heat-Exchange Systems

The development of new heat-exchange systems is being influenced by emphasis upon cost-effectiveness and blood conservation. Integrated membrane oxygenators and heat exchanges are likely to be developed with low priming volumes. Cooling might be accomplished by a refrigerant rather than water, and heating might be accomplished by electrical warming of the material in contact with blood. Thus, the bulky heater/cooler with attached water hoses may be eliminated as computer circuitry becomes sufficiently reliable to allow safe application of other cooling and heating systems.

References

1. Donald DE, Fellows JL. Relation of temperature, gas tension and hydrostatic pressure to the formation of gas bubbles in extracorporeally oxygenated blood. *Surg Forum* 1960;10:589–592.
2. Chapman AJ. *Heat Transfer*. New York: Macmillan Publishing Co Inc; 1974:11–63.
3. Braun PR, Hommedieu BD, Klinedinst WJ, et al. Aluminum contamination by heat-exchangers during cardiopulmonary bypass. Presented at the American Academy of

Cardiovascular Perfusion; September 1988:69–72; New Orleans.
4. Vogler C, Sotelo-Avila C, Lagunoff D, et al. Aluminum-containing emboli in infants treated with extracorporeal membrane oxygenation. *N Engl J Med* 1988;319:75–79.
5. Berglin E, Hanson HA, William-Olsson G. Polytetrafluoroethylene and anodized aluminum surfaces in an extracorporeal circuit: scanning electron microscopic study. *Artif Organs* 1982;6:54–57.
6. Haveland SM. Blood heat-exchange: myths and reality. *Scanmag* 1990;2:19–23.
7. Webb GE. Comparison of esophageal and tympanic temperature monitoring during cardiopulmonary bypass. *Anesth Analg* 1973;52:729–733.
8. Benzinger TH, Taylor GW. Cranial measurements of internal temperature in man. In: *Temperature—Its Measurement and Control in Science and Industry*. New York: Reinhold Publishing Corp; 1963:1111–1120.
9. Dickey WT, Ahlgren EW, Stephen CR. Body temperature monitoring via the tympanic membrane. *Surgery* 1967;67:981–984.
10. Wilson RD, Knapp C, Traber DL, et al. Tympanic thermography: a clinical and research evaluation of a new technique. *South Med J* 1971;64:1452–1455.
11. Jani K, Carli FM, Bidstrup BP, et al. Prevention of body temperature reduction (afterdrop) following hypothermic perfusion. *Perfusion* 1988;3:301–306.
12. Ralley FE, et al. The effects of shivering on oxygen consumption and carbon dioxide production in patients rewarming from hypothermic cardiopulmonary bypass. *Can J Anaesth* 1988;35:332–337.
13. Dietrich WD, Busto R, Valdes I, et al. Effects of normothermic venous mild hyperthermic forebrain ischemia in rats. *Stroke* 1990;21:1318–1325.

Part IV
Conduct of Cardiopulmonary Bypass for Cardiac Surgery

15
Aortoatriocaval Cannulation for Cardiopulmonary Bypass

Mark W. Connolly

In the more than 300,000 operations requiring cardiopulmonary bypass (CPB) performed yearly in the United States, aortoatriocaval cannulation is the most frequently used standard method for venous drainage and arterial perfusion. Following the landmark contributions to extracorporeal circulation and oxygenators by Gibbon,[1] Dennis,[2] Lillehei,[3] and Kirklin[4] in the 1940s and 1950s, arteriovenous cannulation progressed from femorovenous to aortoatriocaval cannulation in the mid-1960s. In 1968, Gerbode[5] reported on a new technique of arterial perfusion that involved cannulating the ascending aorta, and in 1970, Taylor and Effler[6] reported their experience with this technique in 9000 cases with only one lethal complication.

Although ascending aortoatriocaval cannulation is now the most widely used method, it should not be considered routine. The patient population undergoing CPB today is older and has a higher incidence of diabetes mellitus, peripheral vascular disease, hypertension, and hypercholesterolemia than did the patients of the 1960s and 1970s. These risk factors are associated with an increased incidence of aortic atherosclerosis, aortic aneurysmal formation, and friable, more severely calcified aortic and atrial tissue, which can lead to such drastic complications as aortic dissections, atrial tears, cerebrovascular accidents, and hemorrhage. Therefore, each cannulation should be planned and performed as carefully as a distal coronary anastomosis; otherwise, life-threatening complications may occur.

Preoperative Evaluation of the Aorta

Every patient about to undergo CPB should provide a complete medical history, undergo a thorough physical examination, and have a chest x-ray. The history should be directed towards risk factors for aortic atherosclerotic diseases, such as diabetes mellitus, hypertension, hyperlipidemia, peripheral vascular disease, carotid artery disease, and previous cerebrovascular accidents (Table 15.1). Examination of all peripheral pulses (specifically noting the presence of carotid bruits) and screening for abdominal aortic aneurysm and peripheral emboli, suggested by the "blue toe" syndrome and/or visual field defects, should be a part of every preoperative physical examination. The PA and lateral chest x-ray may demonstrate dilatation or calcification of the ascending aorta. Further evaluation by computed axial tomography scan, magnetic resonance imaging, and transthoracic and/or transesophageal echocardiography may be indicated preoperatively to evaluate further the extent of aortic disease.

Technique of Aortoatriocaval Cannulation

After hemodynamic monitoring lines have been placed and anesthesia induced, the patient is prepped with betadine solution and draped. A standard midline sternotomy is performed, the thymus divided, and pericardial traction sutures are placed. The pericardial attachments to the superior ascending aorta and innominate artery are incised to provide maximal aortic length for cannulation and proximal vein graft anastomosis. The pericardial attachments to the right side of the diaphragm are incised laterally and inferiorly to increase exposure for atrial cannulation. Heparin (3 mg/kg) is given intravenously before cannulation to achieve clotting time greater than 300 sec-

TABLE 15.1. Risk factors for ascending aortic disease.

Diabetes mellitus
Hypertension
Hyperlipidemia
Peripheral vascular disease
Carotid artery disease
Cerebral vascular accident

onds. Anticoagulation for CPB is discussed further in Chapter 5.

Ascending Aortic Cannulation

The site of aortic cannulation (Figure 15.1) is approximately 1 to 2 cm proximal to the origin of the innominate artery, and left lateral to the midline aorta. This area usually has stronger adventitial and medial aortic tissue, in contrast to the weaker aortic tissue near the innominate artery takeoff area, which is more easily injured and more difficult to repair. The aorta is palpated for the presence of atherosclerotic disease and calcification or ectatic thinning. If any question of intraluminal disease exists, direct epiaortic ultrasonography can accurately display its presence. The adventitial fat is then cleaned from the cannulation site with electrocautery coagulation. Nonabsorbable 2-0 braided suture is used to form a double, four-sided, box purse string; pledgets may be used as additional reinforcement (Figure 15.1). The suture should not be full thickness, penetrating only the adventitial and medial layers. Full-thickness intimal aortic suture bites cause hematoma formation and possible local dissection, increasing the risks of cannulation.

The systolic arterial blood pressure should be lowered with short-acting vasodilators to between 90 and 105 mm Hg. Intravenous nitroglycerin, 2–3 µg/kg, sodium nitroprusside, 0.1–0.8 µg/kg, sodium thiopental, 0.1–1.0 µg/kg, propofol 50–100 µg/kg, or just elevating the head of the table to decrease preload are some of the methods that may be used to actively lower blood pressure. Cannulation at higher pressures would require a more forceful insertion, possibly producing intimal tears and aortic dissection. Next, a 1-cm aortic incision, within the box purse string, is made with a No. 15 scalpel. Bleeding from this site may be controlled with finger pressure or by pulling the adventitia distal to the purse string downward with forceps. An 8-mm, plastic, curved-tip arterial cannula (Sarnes, Inc. Ann Arbor, Michigan) is gently slipped through the aortic incision and then rotated 180° to direct distal arterial perfusion. (Other arterial cannulas for aortic cannulation are further described and illustrated in Chapter 12.) The purse-string sutures are tightened with rubber tourniquets which are secured to the cannula with a heavy cloth-tape ligature (Figure 15.2). At Emory, an aortic side-biting "J" clamp is not used to control the aorta during cannulation, since an increased incidence of air embolism has been reported with this method.[7] The cannula is de-aired, hooked to the arterial line, and secured with a plastic band. The cannula and arterial line are secured to the drapes with towel clips to prevent any disruption of the cannulation site during the procedure. Finally, the perfusionist checks the arterial line for flow and pressure. Methods used by the perfusionist to assess proper placement of the aortic cannula and arterial line are discussed in Chapters 13 and 16.

Right Atriocaval Cannulation

Single Venous Cannula

For coronary artery bypass, aortic valve replacement, ascending and transverse aortic repair, and other operations not requiring opening of the right atrium, single cannulation of the right atrium provides adequate venous return and decompression of the right and left ventricles. A 2-0 nonabsorbable suture is placed in a circular, purse-string fashion around the right atrial appendage. The tip of the appendage and the trabecular tissue are incised with Metzenbaum scissors. A single, 51F, double-stage venous cannula is placed through the appendage opening, positioning the tip into the inferior vena cava and the proximal basket holes in the mid-right atrium. This large, double-

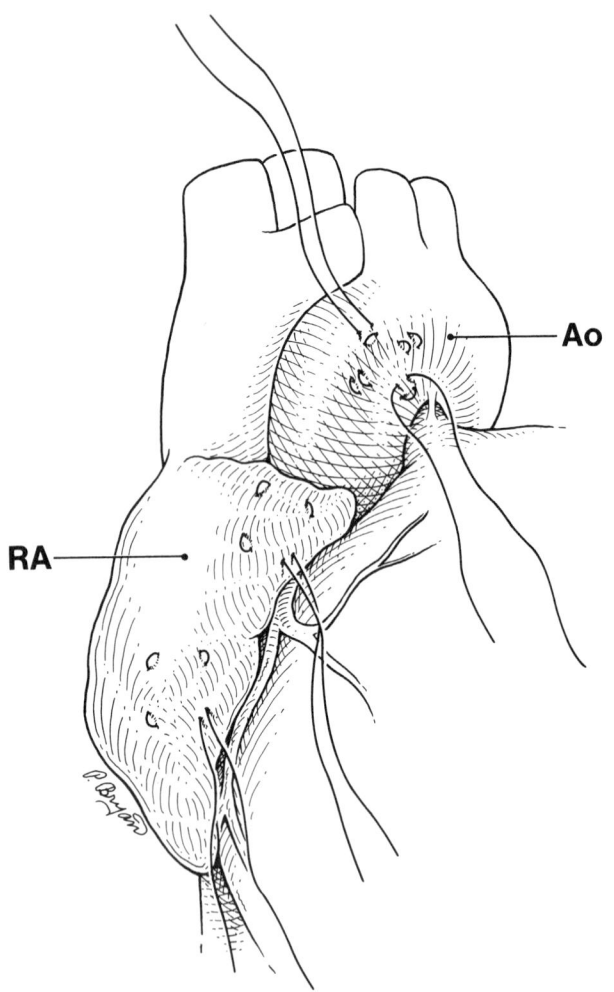

FIGURE 15.1. Position of aortic (Ao) and right atrial (RA) cannulation sites demonstrated by placement of purse-string sutures.

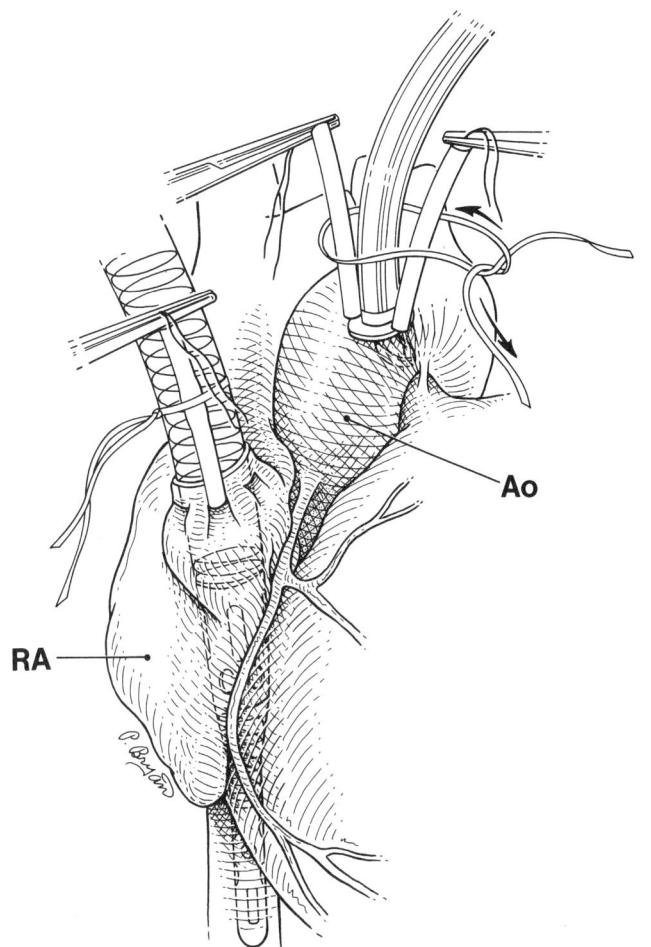

FIGURE 15.2 Aortic (Ao) and single, double-staged, right atrial (RA) cannulation. Note drainage holes of venous cannula in right atrium and inferior vena cava.

stage venous cannula is used exclusively at Emory for single, right atrial drainage. (Other venous cannulas are further discussed in Chapter 12.) The purse-string suture is tightened with a rubber tourniquet that is secured to the cannula with a cloth ligature. Finally, the cannula is connected to the venous return line, and bypass is ready to be instituted (Figure 15.2).

Double Right Atrial Cannulas

For operations requiring isolation of the right atrium (tricuspid valve or atrial septal defect), two venous cannulas are placed through the right atrium into the superior and inferior vena cava. A 34F, wire-bound venous cannula is placed through the right atrial appendage, and its drainage holes are positioned in the superior vena cava. The inferior, 38F, wire-bound cannula is positioned through a box purse-string suture placed 2 to 3 cm superior and anterolateral to the inferior vena cava. The drainage holes are positioned in the subdiaphragmatic vena cava. This inferior cannula should not be pushed too far into the hepatic veins, as decreased venous return and hepatic congestion from hepatic venous obstruction may occur. The correct position is assured by placing the proximal drainage holes of the cannula just inferior to the diaphragm. The cannulas are hooked to a Y-connector and then to the venous return line. Cloth tapes are passed around each vena cava, and each is snared to produce complete isolation of venous blood flow from the right atrium (Figure 15.3).

Comparing the single and double atriocaval cannula techniques, Louaqie et al[8] showed no difference in postoperative supraventricular tachyarrhythmias, right and left ventricular hemodynamic performance, hemodilution, or postoperative respiratory dysfunction. Bennett[9] proved that venous return and atrioventricular decompression were just as efficient when using the single 51F double-stage cannula as when using double caval cannula-

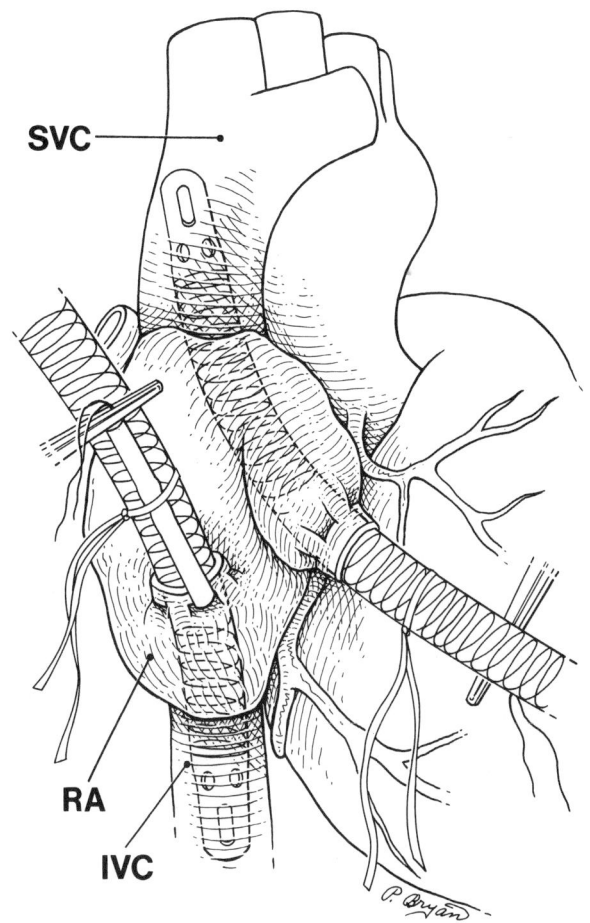

FIGURE 15.3. Position of two-venous cannulation of right atrium (RA) with placement of drainage holes into superior vena cava (SVC) and inferior vena cava (IVC). Aortic cannula not shown.

tion. The two-venous-cannula technique is necessary only when the right atrium or right ventricle has to be isolated from the bypass circuit, although many surgeons prefer this method for left atrial operations also.

Special Operative Considerations

Alternative Incisions

Although the preferred incision for the majority of cardiac procedures is the median sternotomy, special circumstances may require other incisions to obtain maximal exposure. Table 15.2 lists these alternative incisions and the clinical situations where they may provide better operative exposure during cardiothoracic surgery.

Femoral Arteriovenous Cannulation

When cannulation of the ascending aorta and/or the right atrium is not technically possible or carries a prohibitive complication risk, cannulation of the femoral vessels is necessary. Table 15.3 lists clinical operative situations where standard aortoatrial cannulation may not be technically possible. Advantages of femoral arteriovenous cannulation include increased exposure to the operative field (cannulas separate from the main operative site), technically simple procedure (femoral vessels are superficial and accessible), and decreased complication rate in high-risk patients. Furthermore, femoral cannulation may be the only arteriovenous access available to the cardiac surgeon, as in the case of surgery on the descending thoracic aorta through a left posterolateral thoracotomy, where access to the right-sided venous system is difficult.

The groin incision extends from the inguinal crease, two finger breadths from the lateral edge of the pubic symphysis, for approximately 6 cm vertically downward. If the femoral artery can be palpated, the incision is begun over this area. Dissection continues through Scarpa's fascia, through the femoral sheath, to the common femoral artery.

The artery is dissected free and proximal; distal and side branch vascular control is obtained with cloth tapes. Similar proximal and distal control of the femoral vein is ob-

TABLE 15.2. Alternative thoracic incisions for cardiovascular operations.

Operative approach	Indication
Right thoracotomy	Previous sternotomy and mitral valve procedures and/or atrial septal defect
Left thoracotomy	Descending thoracic aorta surgery Redo coronary artery surgery Left atrial-to-femoral artery bypass Left ventricular apical-aortic conduit

TABLE 15.3. Absolute and relative indications for femoral arteriovenous cannulation.

Substituted vessel	Indication
Ascending aorta	Severe atherosclerotic disease (risk emboli) Severe calcification ("porcine" aorta) Ascending and transverse aortic arch surgery Acute dissection repair Acute rupture repair Chronic aneurysm repair Traumatic injury Redo sternotomy
Descending thoracic aorta	Acute rupture repair Traumatic transection repair Chronic aneurysm repair
Right atrium and vena cava	Redo sternotomy Fibrosing mediastinitis Invasive renal tumors Right atrial myxomas Traumatic injury Constrictive pericarditis
Other	Preoperative cardiac arrest with cardiopulmonary resuscitation Damage to great vessels and heart during reoperation

tained. Frequently, dissection extends under the inguinal ligament to gain adequate vessel length for cannulation, particularly in calcified, diseased arteries. The external iliac or the other femoral artery may serve as alternative access sites.

Again, the patient must be heparinized prior to arterial cannulation. Proximal and distal femoral artery clamps are applied and side branches are snared. A transverse arteriotomy is performed with a No. 11 blade and enlarged with a Potts scissors. A straight arterial cannula is gently slipped into the lumen as the proximal clamp is released. A proximal snare is tightened around the artery and cannula. The size of the cannula is predetermined by the patient's body surface area and calculated flow rates, ranging from 16F to 24F in adults. The arterial line and cannula are connected after all the air is removed. Finally, the arterial line is tested by the perfusionist.

Femoral vein cannulation is performed in a similarly controlled fashion, except that a longitudinal venotomy is performed. Long femoral vein cannulas of 26F to 34F diameter are used. To ensure good venous return, the cannula must be positioned past the junction of the inferior vena cava and the iliac vein, well into the abdominal vena cava and/or the right atrium.

After CPB is completed, the cannulas are carefully removed and the vessels are repaired with 5-0 nylon suture.

As with aortoatrial cannulation, complications can occur. Femoral artery stenosis, injury, distal atheroemboli, dissection, aneurysm formation, and femoral vein injury, as well as constriction and thrombosis, all can cause significant patient morbidity. Infrequently, chronic lymphatic drainage from the wound can be a difficult postoperative management problem.

Cannulation for Reoperation Procedures

When the aorta and right atrium have been cannulated during a previous operation, there are several additional considerations. After adequate dissection of adhesions, and mobilization of the aorta and right atrium, the sites of cannulation are carefully chosen. The innominate vein is carefully identified and dissected off the aorta. Usually, the old cannulation site is adhered to the undersurface of the innominate vein. Entering the previous aortic cannulation site may be difficult due to previously used Teflon pledgets and scar tissue, and manipulation of this area may increase the risk of embolization of intraluminal debris. The new site is usually lateral, or just distal, to the old site. If the new cannulation site does not provide sufficient room to apply an aortic crossclamp distal to previously placed proximal vein grafts, or leave enough room to place new vein grafts, femoral cannulation should be considered. Right atrial cannulation can be difficult because the atrial tissue is usually thinned and friable after dissection of the pericardial adhesions. Teflon or pericardial-pledgeted suture can be used to reinforce a thinned-out atrial cannulation site. The techniques of aortic and venous cannulation then proceed as previously outlined. Femoral vessel cannulation should always be considered if aortoatrial cannulation for reoperation becomes difficult.

Left Ventricular Decompression

Removal of blood from the left side of the heart provides many advantages for the cardiac surgeon. Adequate drainage of the right heart is accomplished by a single double-staged right atrial venous cannula and, if necessary, by vena caval cannulation and caval snaring. During CPB, noncoronary blood enters the left heart through mediastinal collaterals. Left ventricular venting evacuates this systemic blood to provide a bloodless operative field when performing operations on the left heart (aortic valve replacement, mitral valve replacement, etc), to prevent myocardial rewarming during cold cardioplegia, and to prevent potentially damaging ventricular distension.

Left ventricular decompression is most commonly achieved by placing a suction or drainage catheter through the right superior pulmonary vein directly into the left ventricle or into the main pulmonary artery obtaining retrograde drainage through the left atrium and pulmonary veins. Drainage catheters can also be placed through the left atrium or directly through a stab wound in the left ventricular apex. The venting catheter is connected to roller-pump suction tubing that drains into the venous reservoir.

Importantly, all of the venting techniques introduce air into the left side of the heart, increasing the risk of cerebral air embolism. After the operative repair, careful de-airing maneuvers are necessary to prevent this drastic complication.

For many cardiac procedures, such as coronary artery bypass, left ventricular venting is not necessary, since adequate right heart venous drainage provides good left heart decompression. Patients with severe preoperative left ventricular dysfunction usually require left heart venting.

Complications of Aortoatrial Cannulation

Complications of aortic and atrial cannulation can be life-threatening and are associated with a high postoperative morbidity. These specific complications are outlined in Table 15.4. Chapter 18 further discusses this group of CPB complications.

Complications of Aortic Cannulation

Air Embolism

Significant air embolism during aortic cannulation rarely occurs, particularly now that the partial occluding aortic clamp is no longer used for standard cannulation. Care must be taken to de-air the arterial line and cannula meticulously when cannula hookup takes place.

Not infrequently, air may be seen in the arterial cannula after cessation of bypass, particularly when the aorta or left ventricle has been opened (aortic valve replacement, ventricular septal defect repair) during the operation. When air in the aortic cannula is noticed, infusion of volume through the pump should be immediately stopped, the cannula clamped and disconnected from the arterial line, and de-airing maneuvers performed. The arterial can-

TABLE 15.4. Complications of aortoatriocaval cannulation.

Aortic
    Air embolism
    Atheroembolism
    Fat embolism
    Acute dissection
    Late dissection
Venous
    Decreased blood return
    Air lock
    Venous obstruction
    Vena caval tear

nula should be closely watched for the presence of air bubbles. Massive air embolism during CPB and treatment following this untoward event are discussed in Chapter 18.

Atheroembolism

The risk of dislodging atherosclerotic plaque is always present during aortic cannulation. Preoperative evaluation of the extent of aortic atherosclerosis and thorough, gentle palpation before cannulation may decrease the incidence of this drastic complication.

Intraluminal disease can be more adequately assessed with transesophageal and direct epiaortic ultrasonography than with palpation. Wareing et al[10] used direct epiaortic ultrasonic scanning in 500 patients undergoing cardiac operations and modified their operative technique in 68 patients who demonstrated atherosclerotic aortic disease. Palpation of the aorta did not identify intraluminal disease. No perioperative strokes occurred in these 68 high-risk patients. Intraoperative techniques, such as ultrasonography, are becoming increasingly necessary as our patient population ages. Alternative cannulation sites, such as the femoral artery, should be used if an increased risk of cerebrovascular emboli is suspected. Gentle insertion of the cannula during well-controlled arterial pressure is equally important.

Fat Embolism

The cannulation site should be thoroughly cleansed of adventitial adipose tissue to prevent the introduction of debris into the aorta during cannula insertion.

Dissection

Acute aortic dissection may be local at the cannulation site or extensive, propagating from the aortic annulus to the descending aorta. Gott and Jones[11] reviewed the Emory experience of 11,145 consecutive cardiac operations from 1982 to 1988 and reported a 0.24% incidence (27 patients) with intraoperative ascending aortic dissection. Ten of the 27 patients had dissection originating at the aortic cannulation site. Hospital mortality in these 27 patients was 14.8%. Thus, although the incidence of acute aortic dissection is low, morbidity can be significant.

Local dissection presents as an adventitial hematoma around the cannulation site that bleeds briskly when the adventitia is incised. If the patient is still on CPB, arterial perfusion should be switched to the femoral artery. The cannula should be removed, the injured site excluded with a curved aortic clamp, and local repair with large Teflon-pledgeted prolene suture performed. The entire dissection site should be oversewn to preclude any intimal tears and subsequent dissection.

Extensive dissection may extend from the cannulation site to the aortic valve, encompassing proximal vein graft sites. In this situation, femoral arterial perfusion should be quickly established, and repair performed with an albumin-coated Dacron aortic conduit. Vein grafts are then anastomosed to a pericardial patch sutured to the Dacron graft repair. If an aortic crossclamp cannot be placed distal to the intimal injury site, circulatory arrest may be necessary for the distal aortic anastomosis. If dissection tracks down into the aortic valve annulus, valve replacement or resuspension may be necessary.

Postoperative cannulation complications, such as late dissection and late aneurysm formation, have also been reported,[9] occurring years after operations.

Complications of Venous Cannulation

Decreased Venous Return

The perfusionist quickly notices decreased venous return when the venous reservoir volume lowers, requiring a reduction in perfusion flow rates to prevent the introduction of air into the bypass system. The causes of decreased return are numerous. Malpositioned venous cannulas, air lock in the venous return line, obstruction of the cannula drainage holes caused by manipulation of the heart, kinking of the cannula or return line, and low patient blood volume from preoperative dehydration or third-space fluid sequestration all can contribute to inadequate venous drainage to the reservoir. After the perfusionist has indicated decreased venous return, attention should be directed toward recognizing and correcting the causes. If the above-stated causes are not present, raising the height of the table usually improves gravity drainage.

Air Lock

Significant amounts of air in the venous line can block blood returns, and in this case, bypass flow must be decreased by the perfusionist to prevent emptying of the venous reservoir. When an air pocket is detected, the line should be manipulated to move the air pocket toward the reservoir so adequate flow can be resumed. If this maneuver is not successful, the venous cannula should be clamped, disconnected from the venous line, and quickly filled with saline solution. The cannula and line are reconnected, and bypass is resumed. Backward slippage of the venous cannula exposing the drainage holes to the atmosphere, a tear in the right atrium, a nonocclusive purse-string suture around the cannula site, or, rarely, the presence of an atrial septal defect after opening of the left side of the heart or aorta (aortic valve replacement), all can introduce air into the system. Usually, readjustment of the cannula is all that is necessary to prevent further air entry.

Venous Obstruction

Malpositioned or inappropriately large venous cannulas placed in the vena cava may produce venous obstruction. A superior vena cava-like syndrome, with swelling of the head and upper extremity or hepatic congestion, can occur, particularly in patients with small body surface areas, such as infants or children. Decreased venous return is always present during venous obstruction. Repositioning or replacing the large cannulas with smaller ones is necessary to provide adequate drainage.

Vena Caval Injury

In reoperations where the venae cavae are relatively fixed by pericardial adhesions and thinned from reentry dissection, caval injury can occur. Gross manipulation of the venous cannula(s), particularly during double atriocaval cannulation, can tear the superior vena cava at the innominate vein or the inferior vena cava at the diaphragm. Care should be used when manipulating the cannulas, as vena caval injury can be very difficult to repair.

Summary

Aortoatriocaval cannulation is the preferred method of arteriovenous cannulation for CPB. The advantages of this method, compared to femoral vessel cannulation, are the relative ease of insertion, decreased operative time, presence of cannulas in the operative field for observation, and improved venous drainage with equally adequate arterial perfusion. Careful individual preoperative and intraoperative patient evaluation is necessary to decrease the incidence of cannulation complications. Although these complications occur infrequently, they may result in significant morbidity leading to permanent neurologic injury or death.

References

1. Gibbon JH Jr. Application of a mechanical heart and lung apparatus to cardiac surgery. In: *Recent Advances in Cardiovascular Physiology and Surgery*. Minneapolis: University of Minnesota; 1953:47-62.
2. Dennis C, Spreng DS Jr, Nelson GE, et al. Development of a pump oxygenator to replace the heart and lungs: an apparatus applicable to human patients and application to one case. *Ann Surg* 1951;134:709-713.
3. Worden HE, Cohen M, Read RC, et al. Controlled cross circulation for open intracardiac surgery. *J Thorac Surg* 1955;28:331-339.
4. Kirklin JW, Dushane JW, Patrick RT, et al. Intracardiac surgery with the aid of a mechanical pump oxygenator system (Gibbon type): report of eight cases. *Proc Staff Meet Mayo Clin* 1955;30:201-211.
5. Gerbode F, Kerth WJ, Kovacs G, et al. Cannulation of the ascending aorta for perfusion during cardiopulmonary bypass. A new technique and analysis of results. *J Cardiovasc Surg* 1968;9:293-296.
6. Taylor PC, Effler DB. Management of cannulation for cardiopulmonary bypass in patients with adult-acquired heart disease. *Surg Clin North Am* 1975;55:1205-1215.
7. Beckman CB, Hurley F, Mammana R, et al. Risk factors for air embolization during cannulation of the ascending aorta. *J Thorac Cardiovasc Surg* 1980;80:302-307.
8. Louagie Y, Gonzales M, Collard E, et al. Assessment of two venous drainage techniques in coronary artery bypass graft surgery. *J Thorac Cardiovasc Surg* 1989;37:169-173.
9. Bennett EV Jr, Fewel JH, Ybarra J, et al. Comparison of flow differences among venous cannulas. *Ann Thorac Surg* 1983;36:59-65.
10. Wareing TN, Davila-Roman VG, Barzilai B, et al. Management of the severely atherosclerotic ascending aorta during cardiac operations: a strategy for detection and treatment. *J Thorac Cardiovasc Surg* 1992;103:453-462.
11. Gott JP, Cohen CL, Jones EL. Management of ascending aortic dissections and aneurysms early and late following cardiac operations. *J Cardiac Surg* 1990;5:2-13.

16
Initiation and Maintenance of Cardiopulmonary Bypass

James R. Zaidan

Cardiopulmonary bypass (CPB) creates many acute physiologic and pharmacologic changes and gives rise to countless questions related to clinical management. Many specialized areas of concern are examined in other chapters. This chapter focuses attention on the clinical context of some of these concerns and controversies by examining patient monitoring, initiation of bypass, maintenance of bypass, and adequacy of perfusion.

Patient Monitoring

Monitoring provides important data for a well-controlled induction of anesthesia and a smooth initiation and termination of CPB. Thus, the majority of monitors are placed prior to anesthesia induction. Patient variables that should be continuously assessed during cardiac surgery are listed on Table 16.1. In the first part of this chapter, the importance of monitoring these variables and the monitors employed will be discussed. The perfusionist additionally monitors bypass circuit flow rates, oxygen flow rates, and venous oxygen saturation. Methods to monitor these variables are discussed in Chapter 13.

TABLE 16.1. Patient variables and monitors for cardiopulmonary bypass.

Variable	Monitor

Cardiac electrical activity	ECG
	    Surface
	    Endocardial
	    Esophageal

Blood pressure	Intraarterial catheter and transducer system
Ventricular filling pressures	Pulmonary arterial (PA) catheter
Cardiac output	Thermodilution pulmonary arterial catheter, transesophageal echocardiography probe
Temperature	Bladder, esophageal, and PA catheter probes
Renal function	Urinary output
Muscle activity	Blockade monitor Mixed venous oxygenation
Cerebral electrical activity	Electroencephalography (EEG)

Electrocardiogram (ECG)

Electrocardiographic monitoring ascertains data concerning heart rate, myocardial ischemic patterns, and cardiac rhythm. It is important to assure that the digital readout is correctly sensing each R wave before determining the heart rate. For example, the digital readout could doubly count the heart rate in the presence of atrial and ventricular pacing and in the presence of hyperkalemia associated with a small R wave and a tall T wave. As shown in Figures 16.1 to 16.3, the ECG can be distorted by electrical and mechanical problems and lead to an incorrect diagnosis. One electrical problem shown in Figure 16.4 is that of a "pump artifact." When the motor of the bypass circuit turns within the column of blood located in the pump head, an electrical artifact occurs that looks very much like ventricular tachycardia. This artifact, which could be due to a piezoelectrical or static electrical effect, is most bothersome when the ECG should reveal electrical silence after the cardioplegic solution has been infused.[1] The pump artifact looks like cardiac electrical activity that should be treated by administering subsequent doses of cardioplegic solution. It is occasionally necessary to slow the pump flow for a few seconds to determine if the activity on the ECG is, in fact, real or artifactual. To eliminate the problem, ground the metal connector in the aortic cannula to the ground on the CPB machine. Increasing the room temperature above 20°C and the humidity above 50% and spraying the bypass circuit tubing with water sometimes helps to eliminate this problem.[1]

Nonartifactual myocardial electrical activity occurring on the surface ECG is an important clinical finding that implies an unprotected and ischemic myocardium.[2-5] It is

16. Initiation and Maintenance of Cardiopulmonary Bypass

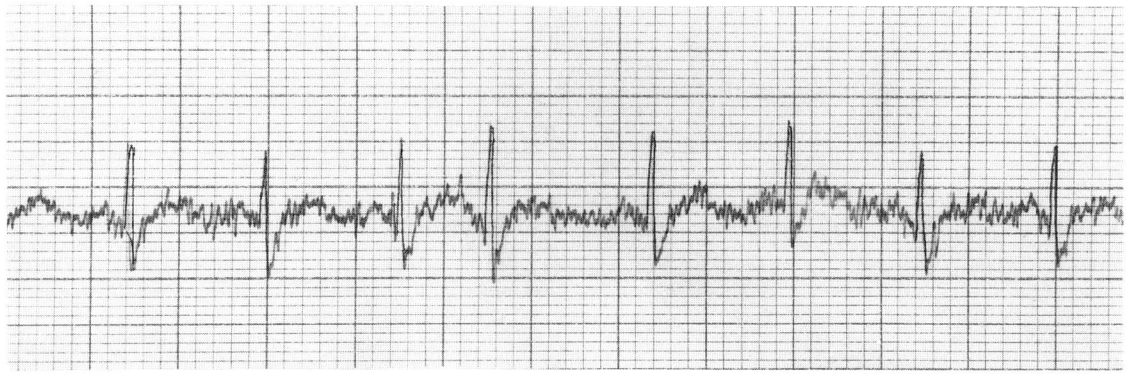

FIGURE 16.1. Muscle artifact distorts the baseline, making it difficult to interpret subtle ST segment changes. (By permission of Zaidan JR: Electrocardiography, in Barash PG, Cullen, BF, Stoelting RK (eds), *Clinical Anesthesia*, 1989, p 589. Philadelphia, J.B. Lippincott Company.)

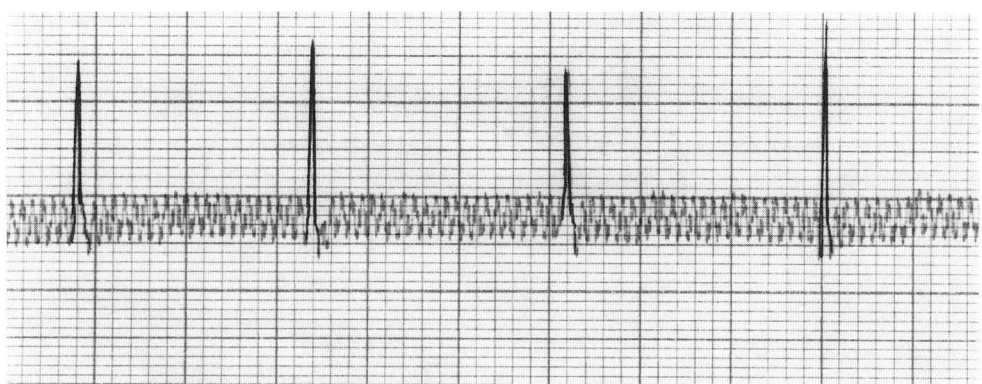

FIGURE 16.2. 60-cycle electrical interference obliterates the ST segment. (By permission of Zaidan JR: Electrocardiography, in Barash PG, Cullen BF, Stoelting RK (eds), *Clinical Anesthesia*, 1989, p 589. Philadelphia, J.B. Lippincott Company.)

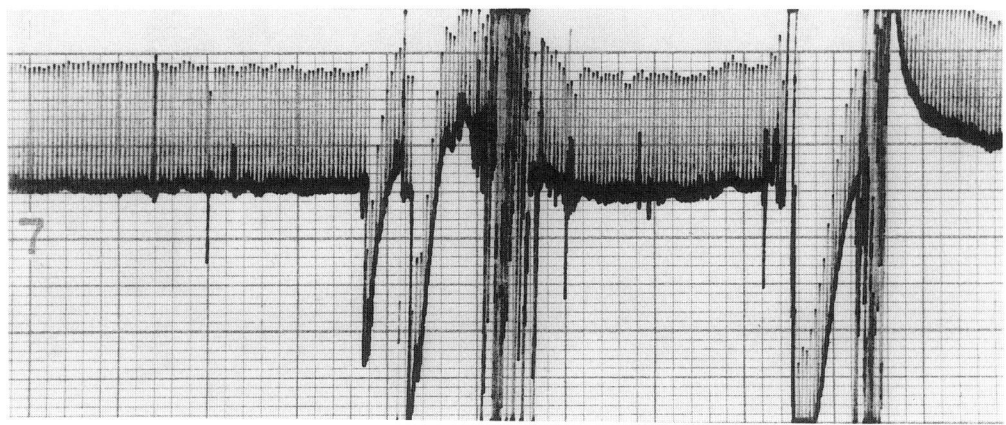

FIGURE 16.3. Effect of the electrocautery on the ECG.

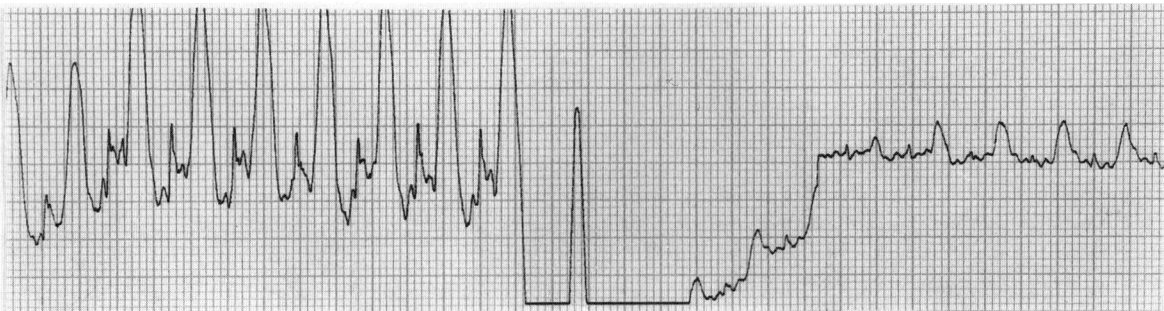

FIGURE 16.4. The large "pump artifact" in the left portion of the V_5 ECG tracing was reduced in size by grounding the CPB machine to the ground in the electrical outlet.

also possible for the surface ECG to be silent while the ventricular electrogram derived from the pacing pulmonary arterial catheter reveals electrical activity.[6] Figure 16.5 demonstrates this kind of problem. Any electrical activity, whether it is visible on the surface ECG or only on the right ventricular electrogram, should be treated by administering additional doses of cardioplegic solution to avoid depressed myocardial contractility when separating from bypass.

Ischemia detection, an important aspect of ECG monitoring, is modified by electrical filtering.[7] Figure 16.6 shows the effects of different filters on the configuration of the surface electrocardiogram. High-pass filtering of 0.05 Hz yields correct ST segment analysis and ischemia detection but results in a wandering baseline. High-pass filtering of 0.5 Hz stabilizes the baseline so that the ECG will remain visible on the monitor but distorts the ST segment. On a monitor with "diagnosis" and "monitor" selections, as was used in Figure 16.7, use the "diagnosis" mode with 0.05 Hz high-pass filtering to interpret ST segments and the "monitoring" mode with 0.5 Hz high-pass filtering to monitor rhythm and maintain a stable baseline.

Lead placement is just as important as electrical filtering in terms of detecting ischemia. The exploring ECG electrode that monitors one area of the myocardium can be used to localize the ischemic area.[8] These correlations are listed in Table 16.2. Intraoperatively, it is impossible to monitor the entire myocardium, and ischemia can be present without ECG manifestation. It is currently recommended that the leads V5 and II be continuously moni-

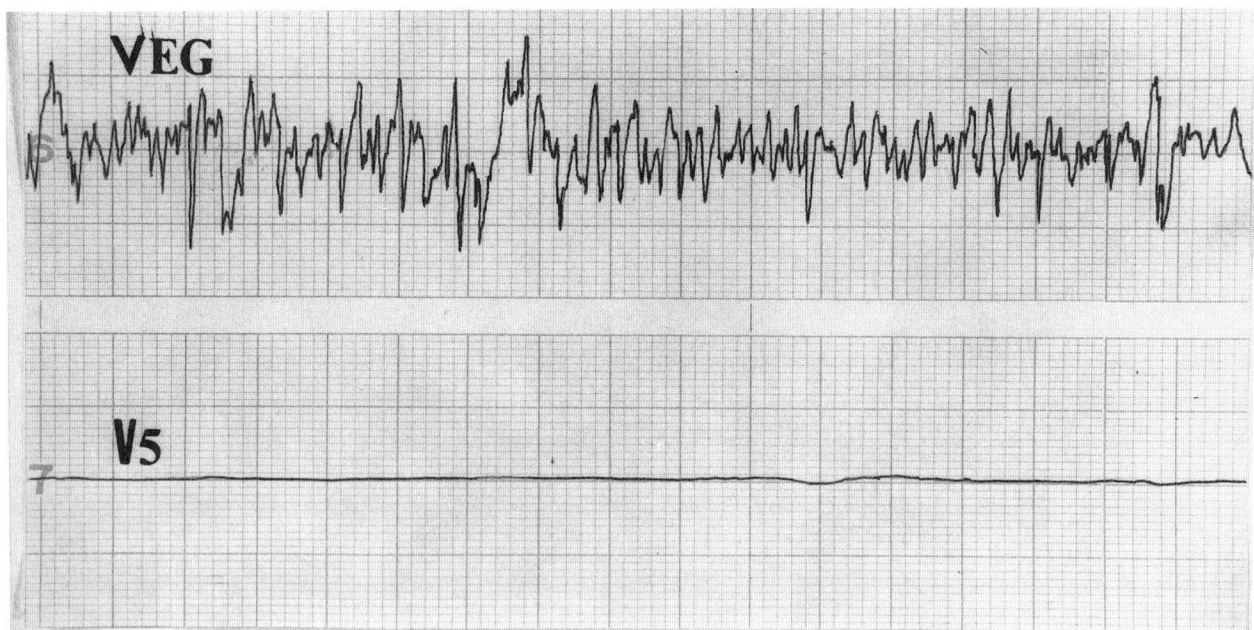

FIGURE 16.5. Electrical activity in the heart can exist even when the surface ECG is silent. In this figure, electrical activity is recorded from the right ventricular endocardium through a pacing pulmonary arterial catheter while concurrent surface ECG monitoring reveals a flat line. (From Roth JV, Zaidan JR,[6] by permission of *Journal of Clinical Monitoring*.)

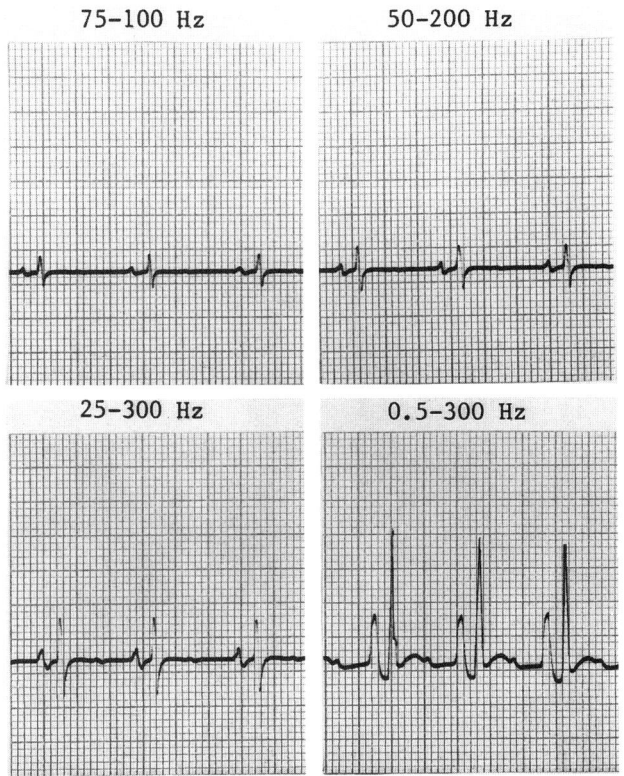

FIGURE 16.6. Electrical filtering changes the contour of the ECG tracing. Notice that the T wave does not "appear" until high-pass filtering reaches 0.5 Hz.

tored during surgery.[9] Even with V5 monitoring, changes in lead position during chest opening and closure could acutely discover ongoing myocardial ischemia. For this reason, it is important to observe not only for changes in the ECG, but also for hemodynamic changes and alterations in venous waveform.[10]

Blood Pressure Monitoring

Arterial cannulation is necessary to evaluate beat-to-beat blood pressure pre- and post-bypass, to measure mean arterial blood pressure during bypass, and to draw blood samples for arterial gas analysis and coagulation status. Most practitioners monitor blood pressure by placing a 20-gauge catheter in the radial artery; however, the axillary, femoral, and brachial arteries are other choices.[11-13] Problems with radial arterial cannulas and direct arterial pressure measurements include temporary and permanent arterial clotting and effects of damping and frequency response. Bedford found a 34% incidence of temporary occlusion of the radial artery after cannulation with an 18-gauge catheter and an 8% incidence after using a 20-gauge catheter.[14] In another study, Bedford[15] also determined that small wrist size (less than 18 cm circumference) led to a 25% incidence of radial arterial occlusion when an 18-gauge catheter was used. Conversely, Slogoff et al[16] could not find a correlation between the size or composition of the arterial catheter and thrombogenicity.[16]

One other difficulty with direct arterial pressure measurement is the damping and frequency response.[17] The most obvious frequency-related problem arises during systole when high-frequency components of the waveform occur. The resulting overshoot falsely elevates the systolic pressure. It is impossible to eliminate this problem; however, one can diminish the effect by reducing the length of the tubing to less than 1.3 m, including no more than one stopcock in the system, using low-compliance tubing, and eliminating air bubbles in the transducer and tubing. Management of blood pressure during bypass is discussed in the second part of this chapter. (See Maintenance of Bypass, Blood Pressure.)

Central Venous Pressure Monitoring

Controversy surrounds the use and meaning of filling pressures and cardiac output during cardiac surgical procedures. Filling pressure is defined by the pressure inside the atrium minus the pressure outside the atrium. When the chest is open, the pressure outside the atrium is zero (atmospheric), so that the filling pressure is the value that is on the recorder or digital readout. When the chest is closed, the filling pressure is the recorded pressure minus the mean airway pressure. It is possible for the filling pressure, and therefore the cardiac output and blood pressure, to decrease when closing the sternum even when the digital readout displays a higher number.

The pulmonary arterial catheter commonly used to monitor intracardiac pressures is associated with problems such as arrhythmias, conduction blocks, damage to the tricuspid and pulmonary valves, pulmonary infarction, pulmonary arterial rupture, and infection. The usually self-limiting atrial and ventricular arrhythmias that occur during insertion of the catheter occasionally require treatment.[18-21] Right bundle branch block can occur as the catheter passes through the right ventricular outflow track.[22,23] If the patient already has complete left bundle branch block, third-degree heart block might occur. One may avoid the consequences of third-degree block by applying transcutaneous pacing electrodes, by first inserting a temporary ventricular pacing electrode, or by using a pacing pulmonary arterial catheter. Some clinicians will wait until the mediastinum is open to insert the catheter from the central venous pressure to the wedge position. In this way, ventricular pacing can be rapidly established if a third-degree block does occur.

Pulmonary arterial rupture and infarction rarely occur, but they present devastating results when they do arise.[24,25] The incidence of these complications can be reduced by withdrawing the catheter into the proximal pulmonary artery before initiating bypass, or by inserting the catheter

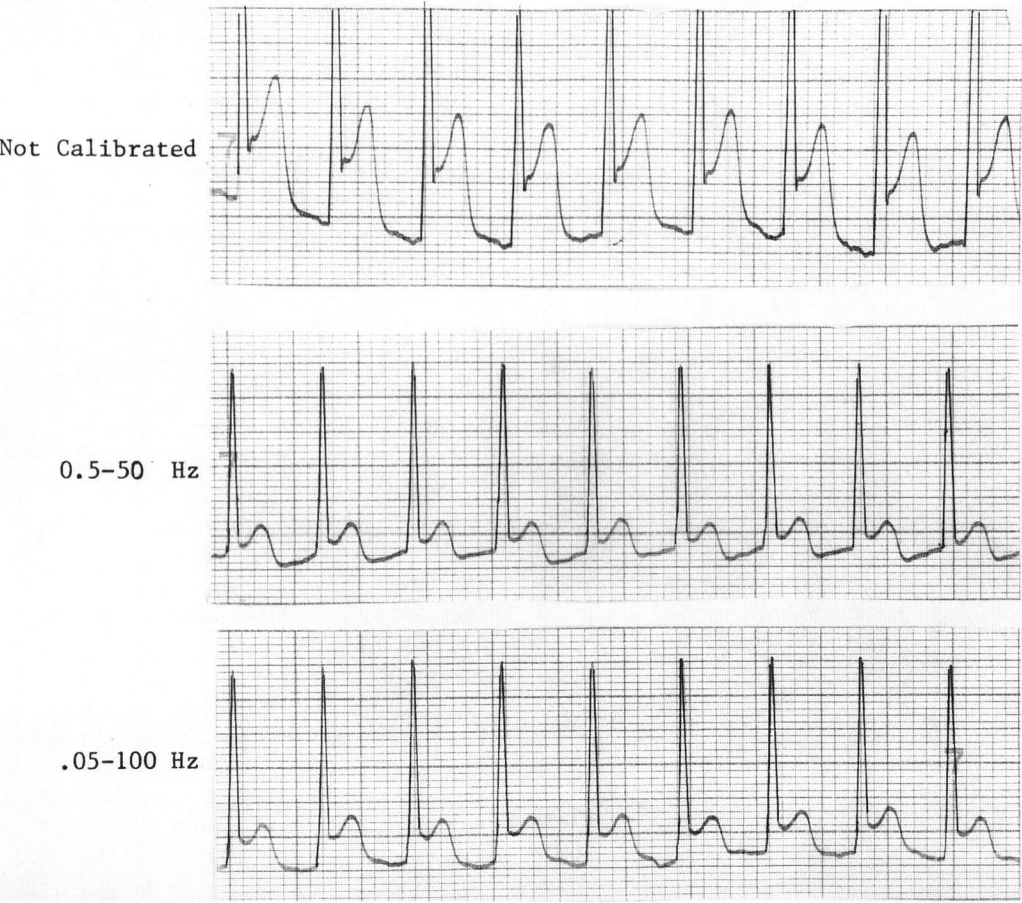

FIGURE 16.7. This figure shows the effect both of filtering and of not calibrating on the ST segment. The top tracing is not calibrated to 1 cm = 1 mV. The middle tracing, which is calibrated and filtered at 0.5–50 Hz, is the standard for monitoring heart rate. ST segment analysis of the ECG should occur in the presence of 0.05–100 Hz filtering. This patient was experiencing 4 mm elevation of the ST segment. (By permission of Zaidan JR: Electrocardiography, in Barash PG, Cullen BF, Stoelting RK (eds), *Clinical Anesthesia*, 1989, p 590. Philadelphia, J.B. Lippincott Company.)

(in centimeters) no farther than 60% of the patient's height (in inches). As an example, a patient who is 70 inches tall should have the catheter inserted approximately 42 centimeters as measured from the skin entry site

TABLE 16.2. ECG lead placement.

Area monitored	ECG lead location
I, aV_L, V_3, V_4	Anterior
II, III, aV_F	Inferior
I, aV_L, V_5, V_6	Lateral
Reciprocal changes in V_1, V_2	Posterior
V_{1-6}	Anterolateral
V_{1-4}	Anteroseptal
Inferior + V_5, V_6	Inferolateral
V_{4R}-V_{6R}	Right ventricle

(By permission of Zaidan JR. Electrocardiography. In: Barash PG, Cullen BF, Stoelting RK (eds). *Clinical Anesthesia*. Philadelphia, J.B. Lippincott, 1989.)

in the right neck. It is important not to develop a wedge tracing at the instant that the pulmonary arterial catheter balloon is inflated. The pressure inside the balloon, which can approach 500 mm Hg, could be transmitted to and, therefore, rupture the pulmonary artery.[26]

To assure that the clinician will not inflate the balloon if the catheter is permanently wedged, it is important to distinguish a large V wave from a pulmonary arterial trace (Figure 16.8). The upstroke of the V wave will lag behind that of the pulmonary and radial arterial tracings, and the V wave will have its peak approximately at the dicrotic notch of the radial arterial tracing. The V wave as described here is actually a regurgitant wave, signifying that blood is being ejected from the left ventricle to the left atrium through an incompetent mitral valve. The valve could have a primary disease process or the valve ring could have an enlarged diameter because of fluid overload. In these situations, the patient should receive vasodilators to increase forward flow through the aortic valve

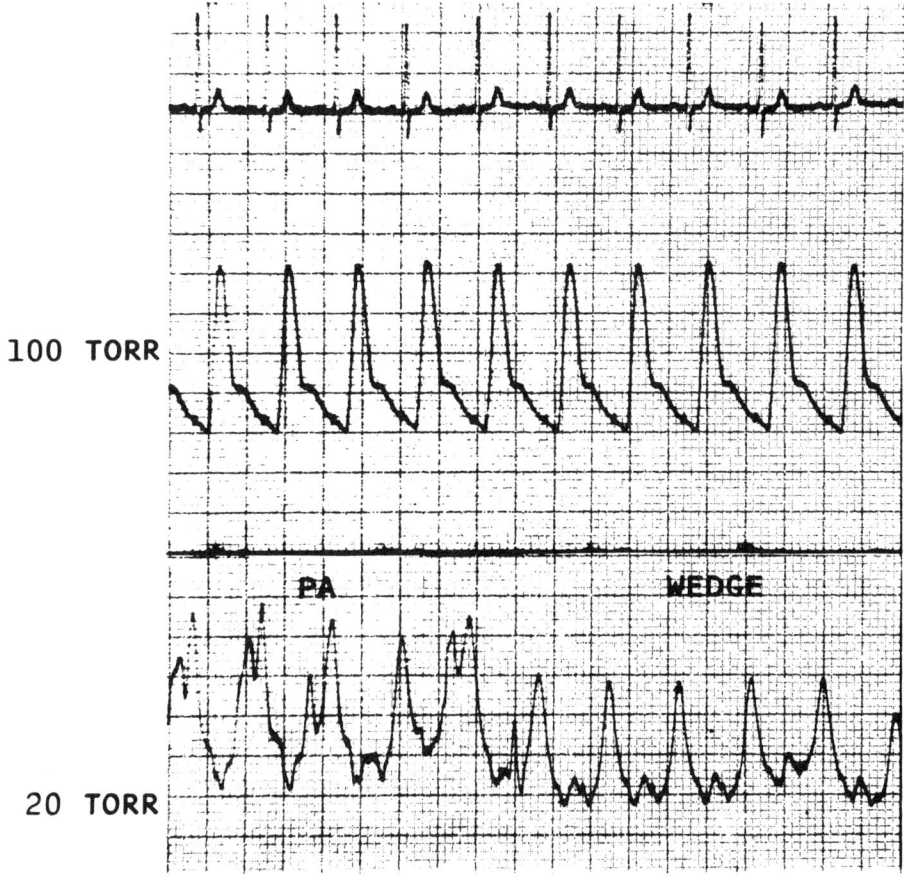

FIGURE 16.8. The wedge tracing (*lower tracing*) reveals V waves whose upstrokes begin approximately at the dicrotic notch of the arterial trace (*middle tracing*). V waves with this absolute pressure and contour could be confused with pulmonary arterial tracings and lure the anesthesiologist to advance the catheter through the wall of the pulmonary artery.

and reduce retrograde flow through the incompetent mitral valve. A-V wave in the classical sense occurs during atrial filling and is not due to mitral insufficiency.

Pulmonary arterial catheters are used to determine intraventricular pressures during bypass. Increases in pulmonary artery pressure, which are most obvious when the patient has aortic insufficiency and fibrillates during the initial phase of bypass, also occur in patients undergoing coronary artery bypass surgery. In contrast to the sudden increase in pressure associated with lifting the heart to observe the posterior wall, blood entering the heart results in a slow increase in the pulmonary arterial pressure. Figure 16.9 shows a sustained, elevated pulmonary arterial pressure that was relieved by venting the left ventricle through the right pulmonary vein and mitral valve. It is necessary to communicate to the surgeon that this pressure is increasing so that the heart can be vented. Elevated intraventricular pressures occurring during bypass result in reduced subendocardial coronary perfusion and unsatisfactory distribution of cardioplegic solution. Application of data derived from the pulmonary arterial catheter to terminate bypass is discussed in Chapter 17.

The pulmonary arterial diastolic pressure does not always reflect the occlusion pressure or left atrial pressure. Failure to occasionally determine the occlusion pressure could lead to an overestimation of the filling pressure if the patient has pulmonary arterial hypertension and an associated diastolic-to-occlusion pressure gradient. One can expect to see this gradient, like the example shown in Figure 16.10, in the presence of chronic obstructive pulmonary disease, long-standing mitral valvular disease, or long-standing coronary arterial disease.

Cardiac Output

Cardiac output during bypass is determined solely by the bypass flow rate. Before and after bypass, however, thermodilution is the commonly used technique to determine cardiac output. Thermodilution cardiac output correlates very closely with dye dilution techniques.[27,28] Room temperature or iced injectate can be used without noticing clinical differences in cardiac output.[29] The underlying principle suggests that the warmer the bolus of cold injectate reaching the thermistor, the higher the cardiac output. Warming the injectate requires thorough mixing with the blood in the atrium and the ventricle. Any condition that permits greater than normal mixing of the injectate with blood will falsely raise the cardiac output. Examples of such conditions are intracardiac lesions, such as an atrial or ventricular septal defect or tricuspid insufficiency. Injecting less than 10 mL of cold saline could lead to a falsely elevated cardiac output if the calibration factor has been adjusted for 10 mL.[30] Conversely, injecting more than 10 mL will result in a falsely low cardiac output. The cardiac output determined in a patient who has received a heterotopic heart transplant is not indicative of the output from either heart, but might estimate an "overall" output from the combination of the two hearts.

Temperature

The ideal location for measuring temperature during bypass remains undefined, because temperature gradients constantly change during bypass. Most clinicians measure either rectal or bladder temperature in addition to esophageal temperature. The esophageal temperature probe cannot measure central temperature during bypass if the surgeon has used local, pericardial cooling of the heart. The pulmonary arterial catheter temperature also cannot be reliably used until pulmonary blood flow is re-established.

The body responds to hypothalamic temperature change by shivering when the hypothalamus is hypothermic and sweating when it is hyperthermic. These changes are unrelated to bladder or rectal temperature, so that a patient could have a low bladder temperature and still sweat if the hypothalamic temperature was greater than the patient's set point.[31] To have a full understanding of these relationships during surgery, it is necessary to use nasopharyngeal or tympanic membrane temperatures. Potential complications of these temperature probes include nasopharyngeal bleeding and tympanic membrane perforation.

Electroencephalogram (EEG)

Anesthesiologists use EEG monitoring in several clinical settings that include determining the depth of anesthesia, detecting ischemia, and monitoring adequacy of barbiturate coma. Intraoperative cerebral ischemia followed by a residual neurologic deficit is a devastating complication of cardiac surgical procedures. Although multiple-channel EEG monitoring helps to detect cortical ischemia, the clinician has few, if any, treatment modalities. Regional ischemia during cardiac surgical procedures may be related to microemboli that probably cannot be stopped.[32] If the microemboli are due to air from an open ventricular procedure, then barbiturate coma might improve long-term neurologic outcome.[33] However, infusing thiopental to 30- to 45-second burst suppression does not lower the incidence of strokes following coronary artery surgery.[34] Global ischemia from insufficient oxygen delivery possibly can be treated by increasing the bypass flow rate and increasing the perfusion pressure.

Because it derives its electrical signals mostly from the cortex, the EEG is potentially useful to monitor cerebral ischemia. Despite the fact that it will not necessarily monitor for ischemia of the brain stem or the nuclei, clinicians have used the EEG to determine when the patient is experiencing generalized ischemia. The unprocessed EEG signal includes an overwhelming amount of information. For this reason, engineers have developed a processed EEG that conveys data concerning the frequency and amplitude of the EEG waveform. Sensitivity, linearity, frequency response, and bandwidth are several of the factors that influence the processed EEG.

The sensitivity of the EEG monitor is the magnitude of the input voltage required to obtain a standard output voltage. The ratio of output to input voltage, called the gain, is generally over one hundred thousand.

Linearity indicates that the output signal is always proportional to the input signal. Generally, linearity is given as a range. A dynamic range of 5 to 100 μV indicates that an input of 5 to 100 μV will result in a proportional voltage output. A system that is not linear over the operational input voltage could lead to errors in interpretation of the output data.

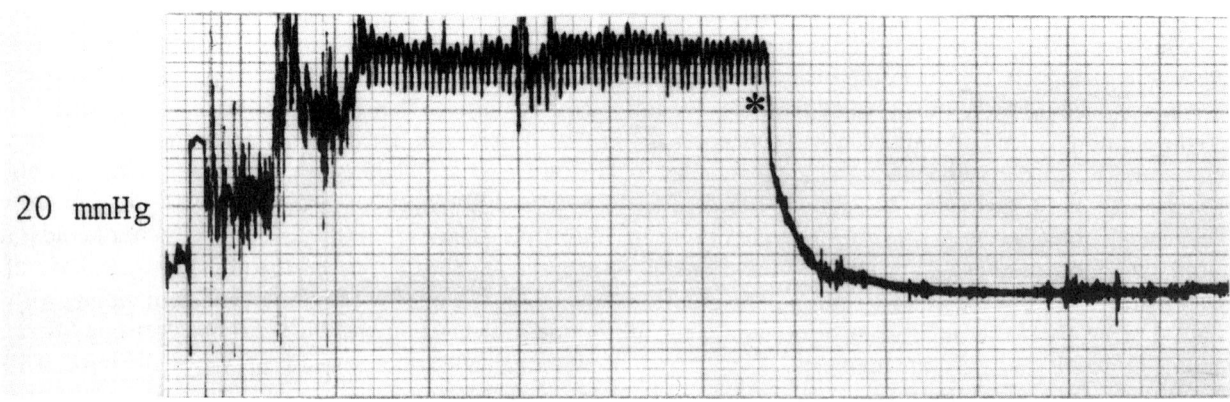

FIGURE 16.9. This figure reveals a slow increase in the pulmonary arterial pressure in a fibrillating heart during CPB associated with a full ventricle as described by the surgeon. At the asterisk, the left ventricle was vented by way of the pulmonary vein.

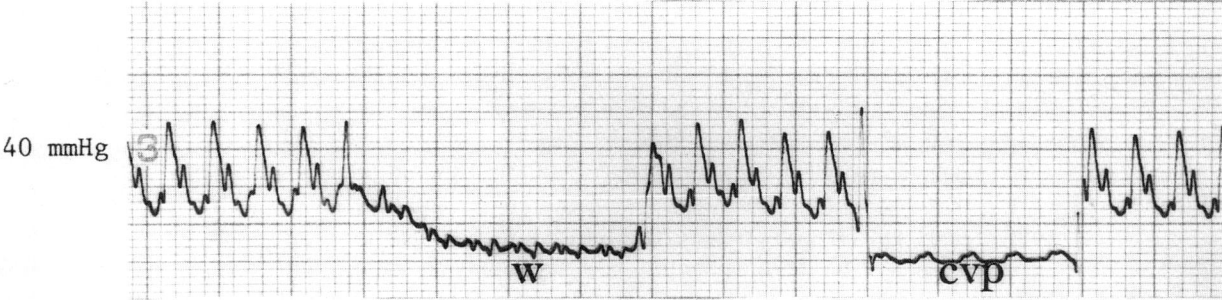

FIGURE 16.10. The pulmonary arterial diastolic pressure does not always correlate with the wedge pressure. In this case, the pulmonary arterial pressure was 45/28 mm Hg, while the wedge pressure and CVP were 12 mm Hg. CVP = central venous pressure tracing; W = wedge tracing.

An EEG should be able to amplify the input signal over a wide range of frequencies without distorting the signal. The frequency response is the range of frequencies in hertz over which the output signal is not distorted. The sensitivity will be zero at low and high frequencies and horizontal at some range of intermediate frequencies. This range of frequencies over which the sensitivity is stable is called the bandwidth. To eliminate distortion, the bandwidth is created by using low- and high-pass filters.

Noise is the inherent ability of the electrical system to develop an output signal when there is no input signal. Specific filters are used to eliminate the noise and simultaneously maintain the desired signal.

Several clinically important artifacts distort the processed EEG and result in the false persistence of electrical activity. These artifacts are well summarized by Edmonds and Wauquier.[35] Many of these artifacts can be diagnosed simply by simultaneously observing the unprocessed and the processed EEG. One of the best known of these artifacts is the R wave of the ECG. Impulses from cardiac pacemakers also lead to noncerebral artifacts on the EEG. These artifacts are easily diagnosed by observing the unprocessed EEG and occasionally eliminated by changing the location of the scalp leads.

Electrical activity occurring in the frontalis muscle can increase the amplitude of the beta waves (13-30 Hz) and distort the processed EEG. It is for this reason that an electromyelogram (EMG) of the frontalis muscle can be important in interpreting the EEG. Muscle activity from the tongue also can result in false EEG activity. Asking the awake patient to swallow will allow one to assess the frequency band of this artifact. Another artifact that leads to false EEG activity derives from ocular voltage potentials across the iris and cornea and also from movement of the eye. These artifacts will be most commonly located in the frontal EEG. There are no solutions to these problems, but it is important to know that they exist.

The electrode-skin interface gives rise to a potentially large voltage depending on skin temperature, sweating, and cutaneous blood flow. If the impedance of one pair of electrodes increases, then that pair of electrodes might show ischemic changes. For this reason, it is important to measure the impedance of the electrodes and to replace the electrodes if the impedance increases.

Electrode placement remains a difficult issue. Visualizing regional areas of cerebral ischemia requires multiple sets of bipolar electrodes. Since placing multiple electrodes is impractical in emergency situations, it would be advantageous to place only two sets of electrodes in such a way that they will diagnose ischemic events in most patients. It has been suggested that parietooccipital EEG monitoring might detect ischemic changes.[36]

Neuromuscular Blockade

Neuromuscular blocking agents react with the nicotinic receptor at the neuromuscular junction and block acetylcholine, the endogenous transmitter, from gaining access to the receptor. Blocking agents have various cardiovascular side effects, durations of actions, metabolic pathways, and routes of elimination that must be carefully considered before administration of the drug. In fact, the drugs can be chosen for their side effects. For example, if fentanyl slows the patient's heart rate enough that ventricular escape beats develop or cardiac output decreases, then pancuronium could be used to establish a more physiologic heart rate. Another possibility is to use d-tubocurarine to lower blood pressure in a hypertensive patient through histamine release and ganglionic blockade.

The side effects of this class of drug are only one consideration. Timing of drug administration is another important factor. Although some clinicians administer blocking agents without monitoring, the nerve stimulator provides valuable clinical information. The nerve stimulator emits a supramaximal impulse over the ulnar nerve. Generally, the stimulating electrode is applied over the ulnar nerve at the elbow and the ground electrode is applied at the wrist. Monitoring can be performed by observing the muscle twitch from a single stimulus, a tetanus, or four impulses delivered over a 2-second duration. This last type of monitoring is the train-of-four. The initial response in the train-of-four will be larger than the last and indicates that a nondepolarizing neuromuscular blocking agent is taking effect. All four twitches are abolished when the patient receives larger amounts of the drug. Surgical relaxation occurs when one reduced response twitch occurs with the train-of-four.

In the absence of muscle relaxants, hypothermia reversibly increases the height of the EMG action potentials while decreasing twitch height associated with ulnar nerve stimulation.[37] Clinically, these changes can increase muscle tone and total body metabolic rate enough to reduce venous and then arterial oxygen tension during hypothermic bypass. Since the bypass circuit has a finite ability to oxygenate the blood, some clinicians administer relaxants to abolish muscle tone. If arterial blood-gas analysis reveals that mixed venous oxygen tension is decreasing, then it is reasonable to administer a muscle relaxant during bypass to decrease muscle tone and increase oxygen tension. Pancuronium and d-tubocurarine abolish twitch height and increase EMG activity, whereas vecuronium decreases twitch height and EMG activity.[38] Clinically, all of these neuromuscular blocking agents increase mixed venous oxygen tension and secondarily increase arterial oxygen tension.

Total blockade of the neuromuscular junction should be balanced against the need to have a responsive patient after surgery. The ability to observe spontaneous movement and central nervous system function is especially important in patients who have undergone open-chamber cardiac procedures and in patients who have heavily calcified aortas.

Initiation of Cardiopulmonary Bypass

Clinical Observations

Before initiating bypass, the anesthesiologist should ensure that the patient is anticoagulated after administering heparin, 300 to 400 units per kilogram. The activated clotting time (ACT), the standard test, should increase to 450 to 500 seconds before proceeding with aortic cannulation; however, exceptions to this guideline can occur. The reader is referred to Chapter 5 for standards of heparinization.

Before the aorta is cannulated, the bypass circuit should be de-aired by priming through a micropore filter, and then the anesthesiologist and the surgeon should observe for air in the aortic and venous cannulas. Air in the aortic cannula must be immediately removed, whereas small amounts of air in the venous cannulas travel to the bypass reservoir without difficulty. Additionally, it is necessary to ensure that the connections are complete and banded on the arterial cannula and that the blood flow will proceed in the correct direction.

Ventilation should be maintained throughout the initiation period, and the ventilator stopped only when the heart has stopped ejecting blood into the aorta. The anesthesiologist should observe the patient's face as the pump begins to control cardiac output. It is common for the patient's face to become white since the pump is initially flowing only crystalloid. The face very quickly should return to normal color. Any persistence of this problem of more than 10 to 15 seconds implies that the aortic cannula is flowing in the wrong direction or that the aorta is dissecting into the ipsilateral carotid artery. Observing the patient's forehead for venous engorgement will indicate when the superior vena cava cannula is not properly functioning or if the cannula has been inserted past the junction of the jugular and innominate veins.

Once the patient's blood pressure and venous saturations are stable, the anesthesiologist should discontinue the ventilator, turn off the anesthetic vaporizers, decrease the intravenous flow rate to "keep-open," and discontinue any vasoactive drugs that were used in the prebypass period. Some clinicians will also decrease the oxygen flow rate on the anesthesia machine. From this point on, it is important to make continuous checks of the surgical procedure and of the patient's hemodynamic status, anticoagulation, and arterial blood gases. A brief checklist is presented in Table 16.3.

Acute Complications

Aortic and venous cannulas give rise to complications such as aortic dissection, air in the aortic cannula, misdirection of the aortic cannula, and failure of venous return that must receive immediate attention. Although these problems are discussed in Chapter 18, they are also briefly reviewed here.

Aortic dissection requires a high degree of suspicion to make the diagnosis and then instant correction. Suspect this problem if the patient has a heavily calcified or thin, dilated aorta, if the surgeon does not insert the cannula at right angles to the ascending aorta, or if the aorta is clamped and unclamped multiple times. Clinical signs in-

TABLE 16.3. Checklist for initiation of cardiopulmonary bypass.

Aortic and venous cannulas correctly connected.
Cannulae de-aired
ACT adequately elevated
Drugs prepared to maintain blood pressure
Transducers recalibrated
Observe face and neck for color and venous engorgement
Ventilation continued until CPB flow stable
Turn off vaporizers and intravenous infusions

clude a dilating ascending aorta with a bluish discoloration, high pressure measured in the aortic line, and sudden systemic hypotension. A kink in the aortic cannula can mimic these pressure changes. If the dissection proceeds to the innominate or left carotid artery, then the ipsilateral face should turn white and the pupil could dilate. Depending on the course of the dissection, the arterial tracing could disappear. Since the blood cannot return to the patient, the venous reservoir fills. The best treatment is prevention by eliminating hypertension, especially if the aorta is heavily calcified, and by avoiding calcified areas for the cannulation site. Treatment is centered around relocating the aortic cannula and repairing the dissection. If the patient is still ejecting blood from the heart, decrease the blood pressure by infusing vasodilators and lower the dP/dT by administering β-blockade. If the patient is no longer ejecting blood, then the perfusionist should decrease bypass flow to minimize the extent of the dissection.

Air in the aortic cannula is easy to locate as the surgeon is connecting the pump tubing to the cannula. Even the smallest air bubble must be cleared from the tubing before initiating bypass. If air enters the aortic cannula during bypass, stop the pump and place the patient in a head-down position. Once the surgeon has removed the air from the tubing, return to bypass. A more difficult management issue occurs at the end of bypass if air enters the aortic cannula. If the patient is ejecting blood, then it might be possible to stop the pump and simply leave the patient off bypass. Be aware, however, that air entering the coronary arteries acutely causes myocardial ischemia that might require returning to bypass. In this case, do not withdraw the aortic cannula. De-air the cannula and be prepared to initiate bypass for acute ventricular failure.

Although it is typical for the patient's face to turn white for a few seconds during the initiation phase of bypass, persistence of this situation should alert the anesthesiologist to the rare problem of a misdirected or a distally placed aortic cannula. Neither the surgeon nor the perfusionist will have access to this information. It is easily remedied by informing the surgeon who can redirect the cannula.

Failure of venous return can occur for various reasons. Since it is measured in the right atrium, the central venous pressure does not necessarily increase when venous return decreases. One must, instead, rely on the appearance of the face and heart to determine when venous return is inadequate. Venous air lock is one of the obvious and easily corrected problems. Occasionally, an excessive amount of air will remain in the venous tubing while the patient is being cannulated. As the pump flow starts, blood will not flow past the trapped air. It is important immediately to stop pump flow to avoid getting air into the aortic cannula. Raise the pump tubing so that the air follows the highest point in the tubing back to the venous reservoir, and then resume pump flow. An air lock can develop more insidiously if the purse-string suture around the superior vena cava cannula begins to tear the atrium. In this case, the air is entrained in ever-increasing quantities, and, eventually, the venous tubing is filled with foam. The perfusionist will be able to detect this problem by noticing a decreasing level of blood in the venous reservoir. The problem is created by placing traction on the venous cannula and is alleviated by maneuvering the venous tubing (as described above) to clear the air while the surgeon is placing another suture around the superior vena cava cannula.

Another cause of failure of venous return is incorrect placement of the cannulas. A superior vena cava cannula that is inserted past the origin of the innominate vein could cause decreased return and clinically result in a distended left external jugular vein. If the inferior vena cava cannula is inserted past the hepatic vein, the venous return could be slower; however, there is no clinical method of determining why the return is slow unless the pressure is being measured below the diaphragm. Suspect a problem if the diaphragm begins to rise into the surgical field. This change is likely caused by hepatic engorgement. These problems are easily corrected by repositioning the cannulas.

Maintenance of Bypass

Blood-Gas Analysis

Blood-gas temperature correction remains a clinical question. The question is not whether or not to correct, but rather what set of "normal" values to accept, regardless of whether temperature is corrected.[39,40] As temperature decreases, more carbon dioxide is dissolved in the blood, decreasing the Pa_{CO_2} and increasing the pH. One method of interpreting the results of the analysis is called the "pH-stat" method. With this method, one corrects the arterial blood gas to the patient's temperature, but adds carbon dioxide to the bypass to artificially decrease the pH to 7.4 and increase the Pa_{CO_2} to 40 mm Hg. If the analysis is not corrected to the patient's temperature, then the pH-stat method would result in a Pa_{CO_2} that might be as high as 70 mm Hg. The second method of interpreting blood gases, the "alpha-stat" method, implies that one should not add carbon dioxide to the bypass but rather should accept the values that would be found at the patient's temperature during hypothermia. For example, at 28°C, the pH should be 7.52 and the Pa_{CO_2} should be 28 mm Hg. If the results were not temperature corrected, then the alpha-stat method would result in the familiar pH = 7.4 and Pa_{CO_2} = 40 mm Hg.

The theory behind the use of alpha-stat blood-gas analysis suggests that it is best to maintain not the pH per se, but, instead, the neutrality of the cell. It has long been known that the pH at which neutrality occurs increases as temperature decreases. When neutrality is maintained, the proper charge remains on intracellular proteins and intermediary metabolites to carry on normal cellular function.[41] Adding carbon dioxide to the bypass to correct the pH to 7.40 at 28°C will render the patient acidotic.

Several investigators have studied the effect of blood-gas management on cerebral blood flow (CBF).[42,43] CBF autoregulation implies that flow remains stable over a wide range of pressures. The pH-stat method of blood-gas analysis results in cerebral vasodilatation, a concomitant increase in CBF, and a loss of autoregulation during hypothermia. Alpha-stat maintains the autoregulated pressure-flow relationship. One of the clinical implications of pH-stat analysis is that an increased number of microemboli could flow to the dilated cerebral vasculature.[42] Another implication is that CBF is dependent on pump flow, so that if pump flow decreases, CBF could decrease below that which is required to supply the oxygen requirements. Alpha-stat analysis, however, allows for an increase in the fraction of the pump flow that supplies the brain when the pump flow decreases. It also theoretically affords some protection from microemboli, because the cerebral vasculature is constricted as the patient cools.[43]

Oxygenation

Arterial oxygenation during bypass should be easily maintained at 250 mm Hg with a mixed venous Po_2 (Pvo_2) of 40 mm Hg. One of the causes of hypoxemia during bypass is a decreased Pvo_2. The membrane in the bypass circuit has a finite ability to add oxygen to the blood. If the Pvo_2 is low, the membrane cannot add enough oxygen to the blood and the patient becomes progressively hypoxemic and acidotic. The underlying cause is a metabolic demand that outstrips the oxygen supply. Large patient size, light levels of anesthesia, and increased muscle tone are three possible causes of a low mixed venous Po_2 leading to a low Pao_2. Light levels of anesthesia, occurring especially when the patient is warm, can be treated by adding enflurane or isoflurane to the bypass circuit or by administering intravenous anesthetic agents. Increased muscle tone is easily remedied by administering one of the neuromuscular blocking agents.

The Pvo_2 can rise without affecting the base deficit if the patient's metabolic rate markedly decreases. However, when the Pvo_2 begins to rise in the presence of a worsening base deficit, then shunting at the precapillary level becomes a theoretical possibility. Treat this change first by infusing a vasodilator, then by administering bicarbonate. The vasodilator will eliminate the underlying problem; however, the base deficit could worsen as the capillaries open and the blood flow washes out the metabolic acids. A reasonable dose of bicarbonate is 20% of the patient's weight in kilograms times the base deficit. For example, a 70-kg adult with a base deficit of minus 8 could receive approximately 100 mEq bicarbonate. This method obviously requires serial evaluations of arterial and venous blood gases.

The present standard of care is to draw arterial blood and send the sample to the laboratory for analysis approximately every 30 minutes. Future development dictates on-line analysis of arterial blood gas tensions that would help to eliminate problems associated with sampling techniques and long transport time. Electrodes that serve as optical sensors can be placed in arterial catheters for up to 72 hours to monitor Pao_2, $Paco_2$, and pH.[44-47] Monitoring can be continuous or on demand by withdrawing blood into a sampling chamber and waiting for the analysis for approximately 90 seconds.

Blood Pressure

It is typical for blood pressure to decrease during the early phase of bypass. Consistent with early studies, most clinicians will maintain a mean pressure range of 50 to 100 mm Hg.[48,49] Later studies reveal that there is no evidence of neurologic, hepatic, or renal failure associated with short periods of decreased perfusion pressure.[50-52] Initially, the patient receives only crystalloid from the pump. Crystalloid contains neither endogenous catecholamines nor the appropriate viscosity to maintain blood pressure. These problems can be overcome by slowly starting bypass and maintaining pulsatile perfusion until the patient begins to receive the returned blood through the aortic cannula. At this point, the bypass flow can be increased to empty the patient's heart and prepare for administration of the cardioplegic solution. Hypotension occurring after the initial phase of bypass can be treated by administering an α-adrenergic agent. Therapeutic suggestions include infusions of phenylephrine or norepinephrine at a rate sufficient to maintain a reasonable mean arterial blood pressure.

Hypertension occurring during bypass theoretically has undesirable side effects. It is possible to overcome cerebral autoregulation and cause cerebral edema if hypertension becomes severe. Also, high perfusion pressure increases noncoronary collateral flow that washes out the cardioplegic solution and warms the heart. Hypertension can be treated by administering commonly used vasodilators such as nitroglycerin or nitroprusside or by adding enflurane or isoflurane to the bypass circuit.

It is common to follow the blood pressure during the early phase of bypass without treating hypotension. Unclamping the aorta and warming the patient can lead to progressive hypotension during a time when the metabolic rates of the brain and heart are increasing. It is important to maintain a physiologic, but unfortunately not yet defined, blood pressure at this time during bypass to ensure that the coronary and cerebral circulations are receiving adequate blood flow. Clinically, a blood pressure of approximately 80 mm Hg will permit reasonable perfusion and oxygen delivery before terminating bypass.

Above all, it is most important to ensure that the blood pressure recorded by the monitor is, in fact, correct.[53] Recalibrate and relevel the transducers several times during bypass. The arterial catheter might require only a flush if the systolic pressure decreases simultaneously with an increase in diastolic pressure (Figure 16.11). If the systolic and diastolic pressures concurrently decrease (Figure 16.12), then the problem is not with the transducer or with the catheter, but rather with the patient. When in doubt about the systemic pressure measured in the radial artery, the surgeon should insert a small-gauge needle into the ascending aorta or into the femoral artery and measure a central pressure. The needle should not be inserted into the aortic cannula, because entrainment of air into the patient is possible should there be a need to recannulate to return to bypass. Commonly, the radial and central aortic pressures will reveal a significant pressure gradient, causing the radial arterial pressure to read up to 25 to 30 mm Hg lower.[54,55] When this problem occurs, the anesthesiologist should continue using the central aortic pressure and the surgeon should insert a femoral arterial catheter whenever it is convenient. The pressure gradient should resolve spontaneously.

Anticoagulation

Anticoagulation is a complex subject that is discussed in Chapter 5. The anesthesiologist remains the final common pathway to ensure that the patient has received heparin and that the heparin is actually functioning. Clinicians have many different protocols for the dose and route of administration of heparin. Three hundred to 400 units of heparin per kilogram given through a central venous catheter is a reasonable protocol. Full anticoagulation can require up to 30 minutes. Determine the ACT 5 to 10 minutes after administering the heparin, and if the ACT is low, draw another sample and run the test again. More time may be needed for heparin to become fully effective. If the ACT remains low, then perform a protamine titration test to determine if the patient received heparin. An adequate protamine titration coupled with a low ACT indicates that the heparin is present but not effective. The therapeutic options consist of administering subsequent doses of heparin in 10,000-unit increments and infusing fresh frozen plasma to increase antithrombin III activity.[56] Patients with inadequate responses to heparin include those who have congenitally decreased levels of antithrombin and those who have been receiving heparin infusions for several days.

The upper and lower limits for the ACT test remain undefined. Lower limits are important, because insufficient anticoagulation could initiate disseminated intravascular coagulation during bypass and excessive postbypass bleeding.[57] Values as low as 300 seconds and as high as 400 seconds have been reported for the lower limits of the ACT.[58,59] The ACT becomes nonlinear with respect to heparin dose once the ACT is above 500 seconds. It is assumed, therefore, that an ACT greater than 500 seconds indicates not only that anticoagulation is adequate for bypass but also that a more prolonged ACT is unnecessary.[60]

Once the patient is decannulated and the bleeding from the aorta is controlled, it is appropriate to administer protamine. A reasonable dose can be calculated based on the half-life of heparin.[61,62] When the protamine infusion is complete, observe the ACT. An elevated ACT indicates that a protamine titration should be performed to determine the heparin concentration. If the protamine titration test reveals heparin, then administer protamine. If the heparin concentration is zero, then the administration of clotting factors could be the correct choice.

Patients who have successfully separated from bypass will occasionally require a second emergency bypass after they have received protamine. It is reasonable practice to administer a second dose of 400 units of heparin per kilo-

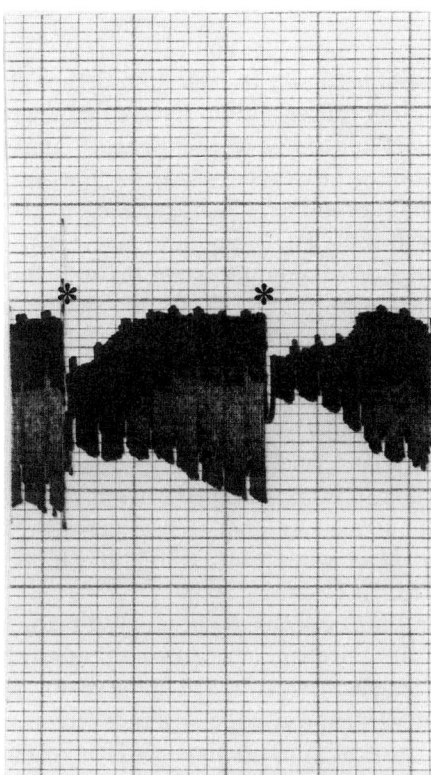

FIGURE 16.11. At each asterisk, the arterial catheter was flushed with heparinized saline and revealed that the decrease in the systolic blood pressure was artifactual. This fact could be predicted by noting the simultaneous increase in diastolic blood pressure. The recorder speed was 25 mm/min.

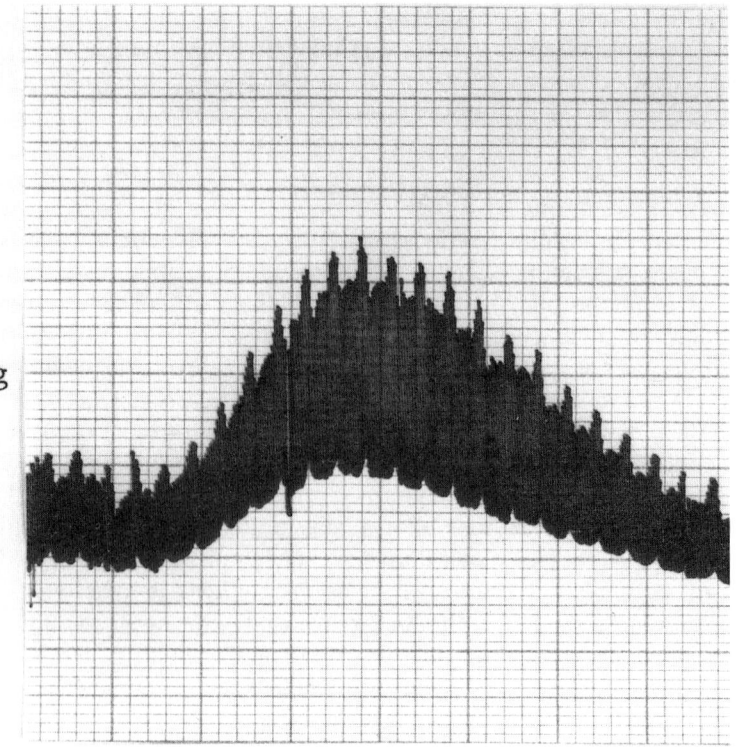

FIGURE 16.12. In contrast to Figure 16.11, the changes in systolic pressure are tracked by the changes in diastolic blood pressure. The systolic hypotension, therefore, is related to changes in the patient and not in the transducer system. The recorder speed was 25 mm/min.

gram through a central venous catheter and to request that, if the patient does not have adequate perfusion, the perfusionist place 20,000 units of heparin into the venous reservoir. In an emergent situation, administer the heparin, proceed with bypass, and draw a blood sample for the ACT as soon as possible.

Potassium

Serum potassium constantly changes during bypass. Cardioplegic solution used to protect the myocardium contains up to 20 mEq potassium per liter. This source of potassium, along with other extraneous sources and acidosis, can lead to serum concentrations greater than 6 mEq/L that are balanced by the patient's urine output, intracellular shifting, and protein concentration.

Although there are no specific guidelines for the management of potassium during bypass, it is reasonable to maintain the serum concentration between 4.5 and 6.5 mEq/L. To accomplish this requires frequent blood analysis, and it is, therefore, common practice to obtain serum electrolytes with each arterial blood gas sample. Observe the ECG before treating the serum concentration, because the ECG will offer evidence of the myocardial concentration. It is possible for the serum concentration to be normal in the presence of an elevated myocardial concentration determined by ECG changes. As suggested in Table 16.4, if the ECG does not have evidence of heart block, arrhythmias such as premature atrial contractions (PACs) and premature ventricular contractions (PVCs), or tall T waves, it is unnecessary to treat a borderline elevated serum potassium concentration. Ensure that the patient has a normal pH and is not receiving, apart from the cardioplegic solution, an external source of potassium. Administration of furosemide, glucose and insulin, or calcium chloride will acutely attenuate the myocardial effects of potassium. Furosemide decreases the total body potassium by increasing its renal clearance. Glucose and insulin shifts potassium into the cell and acutely lowers serum concentration. The potassium remaining in the body, however, can increase the serum level again within several hours. Calcium reverses the effect of potassium on conduction without otherwise lowering the serum concentration. The duration of action of calcium is only approximately 30 minutes. Another clinical maneuver is to start pacing the heart while waiting for the ECG changes to clear. All that is necessary is time.

Hypokalemia occasionally occurs just before terminating bypass if the patient has had an excessively high urine output. Potassium can be added to the venous reservoir in a dose sufficient to raise the serum concentration to 4.5 mEq/L. The dose is approximately 20% of the patient's ideal body weight multiplied by the calculated serum deficit. For example, a 70-kg patient has a potassium serum concentration of 3.5 mEq/L. If the desired serum concentration is 4.5, then the deficit is 1 mEq/L. The patient has 14 L of extracellular fluid and should receive 14 × 1 mEq/L or 14 mEq of potassium administered over 15

16. Initiation and Maintenance of Cardiopulmonary Bypass

TABLE 16.4. Treatment of hyperkalemia.

No ECG changes	Terminate CPB as usual
	Determine serial [K$^+$] until normal
Typical ECG changes	Ca^{+2} and pacing
	Furosemide
	Glucose + insulin or insulin alone if hyperglycemia

minutes. This dose will not replace the total body potassium, but will acutely raise the concentration to the calculated level. Within a few minutes, potassium will be redistributed and the serum concentration will decrease.

Glucose

It is important to control glucose concentrations in the perioperative period, because hyperglycemia leads to volume and electrolyte disturbances from osmotic diuresis, ketosis and acidosis, impaired wound healing and leukocyte phagocytosis, and, possibly, exacerbation of CNS damage if cerebral hypoxia occurs.[63-67] Several studies suggest that diabetic patients have a higher mortality rate.[68-70]

Glucose concentrations increase secondary to the stress response associated with surgery. Catecholamines, adrenocorticotropic hormone (ACTH), cortisol, and growth hormone increase and counteract the action of insulin.[71-74] Also, insulin resistance occurs.[75,76] It is impossible to control this response during cardiopulmonary bypass, and many clinicians simply allow the glucose to follow its usual course of increasing with initiation of hypothermic bypass and decreasing after bypass. Although not specifically studied, warm bypass during which the core body temperature is maintained at 37°C appears to be associated with higher glucose concentrations that are not amenable to correction by insulin therapy. In clinical practice, glucose concentrations as high as 600 mg/dL rapidly occur early in the bypass period and require control with insulin boluses to 50 U and infusions to 20 U/h. Short bypass periods complicate the problem, because the long

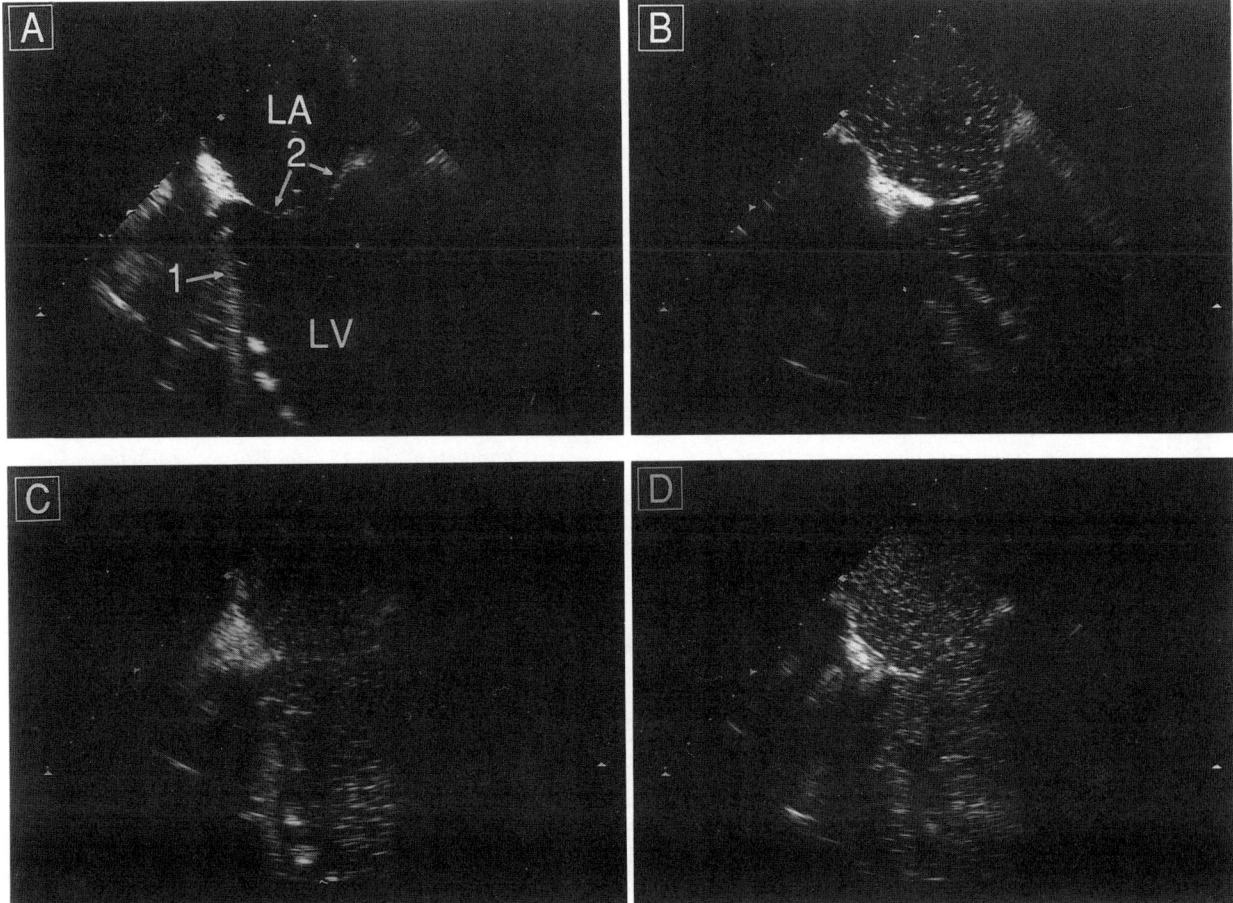

FIGURE 16.13. This series of transesophageal echocardiographic images shows air entering the heart from the pulmonary veins. (A) Before the first breath after the atrium was closed. (B-C) Air filling the left atrium (LA) and left ventricle (LV) during de-airing maneuvers. (Courtesy of Dr. Jack Shanewise, Emory University.)

onset of insulin will not acutely decrease glucose during bypass. Hirsh et al[67] suggest evaluating glucose concentrations at least every 30 minutes, limiting the quantity of infused glucose, and titrating the insulin infusion as required.

De-Airing Procedures

Before beginning the procedure of terminating bypass, it is important to eliminate the air that enters the heart during aortic or mitral valve replacement. If an esophageal echocardiogram is in place, use it to judge the adequacy of de-airing maneuvers. Figure 16.13 shows the appearance of air in the left atrium and ventricle after the patient was placed on the ventilator. This air cannot clear the heart if the aortic valve remains closed, and therefore de-airing cannot commence before the heart has enough volume to open the mitral and aortic valves. It is impossible to clear 100% of the air, but sinus rhythm, a to-and-fro movement of the electric operating room table, and ventilating with large tidal volumes help to move air from the pulmonary veins and through the heart to the ascending aorta. The aorta should be vented before starting the de-airing maneuvers. Discontinuation of cardiopulmonary bypass is discussed further in Chapter 17.

If the patient has undergone coronary artery surgery, ensure that air has been removed from the vein grafts and from the ascending aorta. Even a small air embolus through the vein grafts will severely compromise blood flow. Treatment of ventricular failure secondary to a coronary air embolus might include only maintenance of a high diastolic blood pressure, but it might also include reheparinization, a second bypass period, and intraaortic balloon support.

Summary

This book contains state-of-the-art knowledge concerning CPB. Just as important as the knowledge itself is the ability to use the scientific information to improve patient outcome. Therefore, this chapter draws from science to formulate clinical concepts related to monitoring, initiation, and maintenance of bypass, and adequacy of perfusion. The vital concept is that the approach to patient management is through a team effort, with communication and vigilance among the anesthesiologist, perfusionist, and surgeon the essential ingredients.

References

1. Khambatta HJ, Stone JG, Wald A, Mongero LB. Electrocardiographic artifacts during cardiopulmonary bypass. *Anesth Analg* 1990;71:88–91.
2. Landymore RW, Marble AR, Trillo A, et al. Effect of small-amplitude electrical activity on myocardial preservation in the cold potassium-arrested heart. *J Thorac Cardiovasc Surg* 1986;91:684–689.
3. Brandt B, Richardson JV, O'Bryan P, Ehrenhaft JL. Intramyocardial electrical and metabolic activity during hypothermia and potassium cardioplegia. *Ann Thorac Surg* 1981;31:117–120.
4. Ferguson TB, Smith PK, Buhrman WC, et al. Monitoring of the electrical status of the ventricle during cardioplegic arrest. *Circulation* 1983;68(suppl II):27–33.
5. Ferguson TB, Smith PK, Lofland GK, et al. The effects of cardioplegic potassium concentration and myocardial temperature on electrical activity in the heart during elective cardioplegic arrest. *J Thorac Cardiovasc Surg* 1986;92:755–765.
6. Roth JV, Zaidan JR. Use of the pacing pulmonary arterial catheter to detect endocardial electrical activity during hypothermic cardioplegic arrest. *J Clin Monit* 1988;4:178–180.
7. Clements FM, De Bruijn NP. Electrocardiography: Monitoring for Ischemia. In: Lake CL, ed. *Clinical Monitoring*. Philadelphia: WB Saunders Company; 1990:27–52.
8. Robertson D, Kostok WJ, Ahuja SP. The localization of coronary artery stenosis by 12-lead ECG response to graded exercise test. *Am Heart J* 1976;91:437–444.
9. Kaplan JA, King SB III. The precordial electrocardiographic lead (V_5) in patients who have coronary-artery disease. *Anesthesiology* 1976;45:570–574.
10. Kaplan JA, Wells PH. Early diagnosis of myocardial ischemia using the pulmonary artery catheter. *Anesth Analg* 1981;60:789–793.
11. Gordon LH, Brown M, Brown OW, Brown EM. Alternative sites for continuous arterial monitoring. *South Med J* 1984;77:1498–1500.
12. Barnes RW, Foster EJ, Janssen GA, Boutros AR. Safety of brachial arterial catheters as monitors in the intensive care unit: prospective evaluation with Doppler ultrasonic velocity detector. *Anesthesiology* 1976;44:260–264.
13. Adler DC, Bryan-Brown CW. Use of the axillary artery for intravascular monitoring. *Crit Care Med* 1973;1:148–150.
14. Bedford RF. Radial arterial function following percutaneous cannulation with 18- and 20-gauge catheters. *Anesthesiology* 1977;47:37–39.
15. Bedford RF. Wrist circumference predicts the risk of arterial occlusion after cannulation. *Anesthesiology* 1978;48:377–378.
16. Slogoff S, Keats AS, Arlund C. On the safety of radial artery cannulation. *Anesthesiology* 1983;59:42–47.
17. Hunziker P. Accuracy and dynamic response of disposable pressure transducer tubing systems. *Can J Anesth* 1987;34:409–414.
18. Shaw TJI. The Swan-Ganz pulmonary artery catheter. Incidence of complications, with particular reference to ventricular dysrhythmias and their prevention. *Anaesthesia* 1979;34:651–656.
19. Sprung CL, Jacobs LJ, Caralis PV, et al. Ventricular arrhythmias during Swan-Ganz catheterization of the critically ill. *Chest* 1981;79:413–415.
20. Geha DG, Davis NJ, Lappas DG. Persistent atrial arrhythmias associated with placement of a Swan-Ganz catheter. *Anesthesiology* 1973;39:651–653.

21. Salmenpera M, Peltola K, Rosenberg P. Does prophylactic lidocaine control cardiac arrhythmias associated with pulmonary artery catheterization? *Anesthesiology* 1982;56:210-212.
22. Luck JC, Engel TR. Transient right bundle branch block with "Swan-Ganz" catherization. *Am Heart J* 1976;92:263-264.
23. Thomson IR, Dalton BC, Lappas DG, Lowenstein E. Right bundle branch block and complete heart block caused by the Swan-Ganz catheter. *Anesthesiology* 1979;51:359-362.
24. Barash PG, Nardi D, Hammond G, et al. Catheter-induced pulmonary artery perforation. Mechanisms, management, and modifications. *J Thorac Cardiovasc Surg* 1981;82:5-12.
25. Hart U, Ward DR, Gillilian R, Brawley RK. Fatal pulmonary hemorrhage complicating Swan-Ganz catheterization. *Surgery* 1982;91:24-27.
26. McDonald D, Zaidan JR. Hemodynamic effects of pancuronium and pancuronium plus metocurine in patients taking propranolol. *Anesthesiology* 1984;60:359-361.
27. Fischer AP, Benis AM, Jurado RA, et al. Analysis of errors in measurement of cardiac output by simultaneous dye and thermal dilution in cardiothoracic surgical patients. *Cardiovasc Res* 1978;12:190-199.
28. Hillis LD, Firth BG, Winniford MD. Comparison of thermodilution and indocyanine green dye in low cardiac output or left-sided regurgitation. *Am J Cardiol* 1986;57:1201-1202.
29. Shellock FG, Riedinger MS, Bateman TM, Gray RJ. Thermodilution cardiac output determination in hypothermic postcardiac surgery patients: room vs ice temperature injectate. *Crit Care Med* 1983;11:668-670.
30. Reininger EJ, Troy BL. Error in thermodilution cardiac output measurement caused by variation in syringe volume. *Cathet Cardiovasc Diag* 1976;2:415-417.
31. Benzinger TH. Heat regulation: homeostasis of central temperature in man. *Physiol Rev* 1969;49:671-759.
32. McKibbin DW, Bulkley BH, Green WR, Gott VL, Hutchins GM. Fatal cerebral atheromatous embolization after cardiopulmonary bypass. *J Thorac Cardiovasc Surg* 1976;71:741-745.
33. Nussmeier NA, Arlund C, Slogoff S. Neuropsychiatric complications after cardiopulmonary bypass: cerebral protection by a barbiturate. *Anesthesiology* 1986;64:165-170.
34. Zaidan JR, Klochany A, Martin WA, Ziegler JS, Harless DM, Andrews RB. Effect of thiopental on neurologic outcome following coronary artery bypass grafting. *Anesthesiology* 1991;74:406-411.
35. Edmonds HL, Wauquier A. *Computerized EEG Monitoring in Anesthesia and Critical Care*. Helsinki, Finland: Instrumentarium Science Foundation.
36. Sotaniein KA, Seilg IA, Hokkanen TE. Quantitative EEG as a measure of cerebral dysfunction before and after open heart surgery. *Electroenceph Clin Neurophysiol* 1980;50:81.
37. Buzello W, Pollmaecher R, Schluermann D, Urbanyi B. The influence of hypothermic cardiopulmonary bypass on neuromuscular transmission in the absence of muscle relaxants. *Anesthesiology* 1986;64:279-281.
38. Buzello W, Schluermann D, Pollmaecher T, Spillner G. Unequal effects of cardiopulmonary bypass-induced hypothermia on neuromuscular blockade from constant infusion of alcuronium, d-tubocurarine, pancuronium, and vecuronium. *Anesthesiology* 1987;66:842-846.
39. Ream AK, Reitz BA, Silverberg G. Temperature correction of P_{CO_2} and pH in estimating acid-base status: an example of the emperor's new clothes? *Anesthesiology* 1982;56:41-44.
40. Marshall BE, Williams JJ. A fresh look at an old question. *Anesthesiology* 1982;56:1-2.
41. Hickey PR, Hansen DD. Temperature and blood gases: the clinical dilemma of acid-base management for hypothermic cardiopulmonary bypass. In: Tinker J, ed. *Cardiopulmonary Bypass: Current Concepts and Controversies*. Philadelphia: WB Saunders Company; 1989:1-20.
42. Govier AV, Reves JG, McKay RD, et al. Factors and their influence on regional cerebral blood flow during nonpulsatile cardiopulmonary bypass. *Ann Thorac Surg* 1984;38:592-600.
43. Henriksen L, Hjelms E, Lindeburgh T. Brain hyperperfusion during cardiac operations. *J Thorac Cardiovasc Surg* 1983;86:202-208.
44. Shapiro B. In-Vivo monitoring of arterial blood gases and pH. *Resp Care* 1992;92:165-169.
45. Saari LA, Seitz WR. pH sensor based on immobilized fluoresceinamine. *Ann Chem* 1982;54:821-825.
46. Gehrich HL, Lubbers DW, Opitz N, Hansmann DR, Miller WW, Tusa JK, et al. Optical fluorescence and its application to an intravascular blood gas monitoring system. *IEEE Trans Biomed Eng* 1986;33:117-132.
47. Miller WW, Gehrich JL, Hansmann DR. Continuous in vivo monitoring of blood gases. *Lab Med* 1988;19:629-632.
48. Murkin JM, Farrar JK, Tweed WA, et al. Cerebral autoregulation and flow/metabolism coupling during cardiopulmonary bypass: The influence of Pa_{CO_2}. *Anesth Analg* 1987;66:825-832.
49. Stockard JJ, Bickford RG, Myers RR, et al. Hypotension-induced changes in cerebral function during cardiac surgery. *Stroke* 1974;5:730-746.
50. Tufo HM, Ostfeld AM, Shekelle R. Central nervous system dysfunction following open heart surgery. *JAMA* 1970;212:1333-1340.
51. Slogoff ST, Girgis KZ, Keats AS. Etiologic factors in neuropsychiatric complications associated with cardiopulmonary bypass. *Anesth Analg* 1982;61:903-911.
52. Heikkinen L. Clinically significant neurologic disorders following open heart surgery. *J Thorac Cardiovasc Surg* 1985;33:201-206.
53. Kolkka R, Hilberman M. Neurologic dysfunction following cardiac operation with low-flow, low-pressure cardiopulmonary bypass. *J Thorac Cardiovasc Surg* 1980;79:432-437.
54. Barbierei LT, Kaplan JA. Artifactual hypotension secondary to intraoperative transducer failure. *Anesth Analg* 1983;62:112-114.
55. Stern DH, Gerson JI, Allen FB, Parker FB. Can we trust the direct radial artery pressure immediately following cardiopulmonary bypass? *Anesthesia* 1985;62:557-561.
56. Mohr R, Lavee J, Goor DA. Inaccuracy of radial artery pressure measurement after cardiac operations. *J Thorac Cardiovasc Surg* 1987;94:286-290.
57. Sabbagh AH, Chung GKT, Shuttleworth P, et al. Fresh frozen plasma: a solution to heparin resistance during cardiopulmonary bypass. *Ann Thorac Surg* 1984;37:466-468.

58. Ellison N, Jobes DR, Swartz AJ. Heparin therapy during cardiac surgery. In: Ellison N, Jobes DR, eds. *Effective Hemostasis in Cardiac Surgery*. Philadelphia: WB Saunders Company; 1988:1-14.
59. Young JA, Kisker CT, Doty DB. Adequate anticoagulation during cardiopulmonary bypass determined by activated clotting time and the appearance of fibrin monomer. *Ann Thorac Surg* 1978;26:231-240.
60. Jobes DR, Schwartz AJ, Ellison N, et al. Monitoring heparin anticoagulation and its neutralization. *Ann Thorac Surg* 1981;31:161-166.
61. Cohen JA. Activated coagulation time method for control of heparin is reliable during cardiopulmonary bypass. *Anesthesiology* 1984;60:121-124.
62. Guffin AV, Dunbar RW, Kaplan JA, et al. Successful use of a reduced dose of protamine after cardiopulmonary bypass. *Anesth Analg* 1976;55:110-113.
63. McMurray JF. Wound healing with diabetes mellitus: better glucose control for better healing in diabetes. *Surg Clin North Am* 1984;64:769-778.
64. Goodson WH, Hunt TK. Status of wound healing in experimental diabetes. *J Surg Res* 1977;22:221-227.
65. Rosen RB, Enquist IF. The healing wound in experimental diabetes. *Surgery* 1961;50:525-528.
66. Yue DK, McLennan S, Marsh M, Mai YW, Spaliviero J, Delbridge L, Reeve T, Turtle JR. Effects of experimental diabetes, uremia, and malnutrition on wound healing in diabetes. *Diabetes* 1987;36:295-299.
67. Hirsch IB, McGill JB, Cryer PE, White PF. Perioperative management of surgical patients with diabetes mellitus. *Anesthesiology* 1991;74:346-359.
68. Fowkes FGR, Lunn JH, Farrow SC, Robertson IB, Samuel P. Epidemiology in anesthesia: III. Mortality risk in patients with coexisting physical disease. *Br J Anaesth* 1982;54:819-824.
69. Hjortrup A, Sorensen C, Dyremose E, Hjortso NC, Kehlet H. Influence of diabetes mellitus on operative risk. *Br J Surg* 1985;72:785-787.
70. Farrow SC, Fowkes FGR. Epidemiology in anesthesia: a method for predicting hospital mortality. *Eur J Anesthesiol* 1983;1:77-84.
71. Zaloya GP. Catecholamines in anesthetic and surgical stress. *Int Anesthesiol Clin* 1988;26:187-198.
72. Yao M, Matsuke A, Fukushi S, Kudo T, Dudo M, Oyama T. Episodic secretions of ACTH during halothane anesthesia and surgery. *Jpn J Anesth* 1984;33:525-531.
73. Wagner RL, White PF. Etomidate inhibits adrenocortical function in surgical patients. *Anesthesiology* 1984;61:647-651.
74. Goldberg NJ, Wingert TD, Levin SR, Wilson SE, Biljoen JF. Insulin therapy in the diabetic surgical patient: metabolic and hormonal response to low dose insulin infusion. *Diabetes Care* 1981;4:279-284.
75. DeFronzo RA, Ferrannini E, Kovisto V. New concepts in the pathogenesis and treatment of non-insulin-dependent diabetes mellitus. *Am J Med* 1983;74(suppl 1A):52-81.
76. Reaven GM. Role of insulin resistance in human disease. *Diabetes* 1988;37:1595-1606.

17
Discontinuation of Cardiopulmonary Bypass

Luis G. Michelsen and Jack S. Shanewise

Discontinuation of cardiopulmonary bypass (CPB) is an obvious, necessary part of every operative procedure that includes extracorporeal circulation. This process removes the functions of blood flow and respiration from the heart-lung machine and returns them to the patient's heart and lungs. To avoid mishap, it should be approached in a systematic, thorough manner. In this chapter, we will discuss the preparations for discontinuing bypass support and the mechanics of weaning a patient from CPB. We will then review cardiovascular pharmacologic support in the peri-CPB period, and management of the patient who cannot be readily weaned from CPB support.

As in most important endeavors, proper preparation is critical to successful CPB weaning. Scrambling in the immediate postbypass period to complete tasks that could have been completed while the patient was supported on CPB is unnecessary and can be dangerous. The preparations for taking a patient off CPB may be divided into three parts: (1) preparing the heart, (2) preparing the lungs, and (3) preparing the rest of the patient. These steps are discussed in detail below and are outlined in Tables 17.1 to 17.3.

Preparing the Heart for CPB Weaning

Preparing the heart to resume its pump function means optimizing four of the five hemodynamic factors we can readily manipulate: rhythm, rate, afterload, and myocardial contractility. Preload is the fifth controllable hemodynamic variable, and is manipulated during the process of weaning.

An organized cardiac rhythm is a necessary prerequisite to discontinuing CPB. Ideally, this occurs spontaneously, but often the heart resumes electrical activity with ventricular fibrillation after aortic crossclamp removal. When the blood temperature reaches 30°C, the heart may be defibrillated using 10 to 20 J with internal paddles. Attempting to defibrillate at lower temperatures may be unsuccessful, because hypothermia may precipitate ventricular fibrillation.[1-3] The ideal rhythm for coming off bypass is normal sinus rhythm (NSR), which provides an atrial contribution to ventricular filling and a normal contraction sequence to systole.[4,5]

Atrial flutter or fibrillation often can be successfully converted to NSR with synchronized cardioversion, even if present before CPB. Ventricular arrhythmias should be treated by correcting underlying causes, such as potassium or magnesium deficits,[6] and, if necessary, with antiarrhythmic drugs such as lidocaine. External pacing may be needed to provide an organized rhythm. Atrial pacing is functionally close to NSR and is a good rhythm for discontinuing bypass, but atrial-ventricular (A-V) sequential pacing may be necessary when there is 3°, or complete, heart block. Occasionally, if no organized atrial rhythm is present, and A-V pacing cannot be achieved, simple ventricular pacing is the only option. However, ventricular pacing results in the loss of the often important contribution of atrial contraction to ventricular filling.[4,5]

A moderately elevated heart rate (75–95 bpm) helps maximize cardiac output in the immediate post-CPB period. In general, the heart rate should be 75 to 95 bpm before discontinuing CPB support. Even higher rates may be needed in hearts with a limited stroke volume (eg, hearts undergoing ventricular aneurysmectomy), and lower rates may be desirable in hearts with residual ischemia or incomplete revascularization. Slower rates are most easily controlled by pacing, but atropine and β-adrenergic drugs may also be used. Tachycardia before coming off CPB is more worrisome and difficult to manage; causes—including hypercarbia, inadequate anesthesia, and ischemia—should be identified and treated. Sinus tachycardia often improves as the heart is filled during the weaning process. Cardioversion is the preferred treatment of supraventricular tachycardias, but digoxin and/or calcium channel blockers may be needed to control the ventricular rate. Systemic vascular resistance (SVR)—the most controllable component of afterload—is a major determinant of myocardial work and oxygen consumption.[7] Thus, interventions to decrease SVR during the CPB-weaning process will improve the heart's ability to resume its function, which has been temporarily provided by the heart-lung machine. Therefore, in preparation for discontinuing bypass support, a high SVR should be treated by deepening anesthesia or by administering direct arterial vasodilators, such as sodium nitroprusside. Alternatively, a low SVR (as manifested by a low mean arterial pressure with high pump flow) should be treated with α-agonists (such as phenylephrine or norepinephrine) to ensure an adequate coronary artery perfusion pressure.

Finally, myocardial contractility should be optimized before discontinuing CPB support. The likelihood of diminished myocardial contractility after bypass is increased with pre-existing ventricular impairment (low ejection fraction [EF], high left ventricular end-diastolic pressure [LVEDP]), advanced age of patient, prolonged bypass and aortic crossclamp times, and problems with myocardial preservation.[8] A heart with poor contractility often has visibly weak contractions while on bypass, in contrast to the more vigorous snap of a normally contracting heart. If significant depression of myocardial contractility is suspected, inotropic support should be started before attempting to wean from CPB.

Some thought should be given to cardiac preload while preparing to discontinue bypass. The ventricular filling pressures prior to initiation of CPB may indicate what the value should be after bypass; a heart with elevated filling pressures prior to bypass often requires high filling pressures after CPB. Additionally, the modality by which the left ventricular preload will be assessed in the post-CPB period should be determined prior to discontinuing bypass support. Pulmonary hypertension, severe ventricular dysfunction, or the inability to obtain a pulmonary artery occlusion pressure (PAOP) are reasons to consider placing a left atrial pressure (LAP) cannula while the patient is on CPB.[9] Transesophageal echocardiography (TEE) is a useful monitor for weaning from CPB, since it provides visualization of the volume status, and of contractility of the left ventricle.[10,11] The surgeon must evacuate any intracardiac air before taking the patient off bypass, and TEE is helpful in this regard.

Finally, in preparing the heart to come off bypass, major sites of bleeding should be controlled; the cardiac vent suction should be turned off; all clamps on the heart and great vessels should be removed; bypass grafts should be checked for kinks; and tourniquets around the caval cannulas should be loosened. Table 17.1 summarizes recommendations for optimizing cardiac rate, rhythm, contractility, and preload, and manipulating SVR prior to discontinuing CPB.

TABLE 17.1. Discontinuation of CPB: preparing the heart.

Rhythm
  Sinus rhythm, the ideal rhythm (atrial pacing functionally close to sinus rhythm)
  A-V sequential pacing for 3° block
  Ventricular pacing needed if organized atrial rhythm absent
  Ventricular fibrillation: defibrillate when T > 30°C
  Ventricular arrhythmias
    Correct K^+, Mg^{2+} deficits
    Lidocaine, procainamide, bretylium
    Attempt cardioversion for atrial fibrillation, flutter, and supraventricular tachycardia (SVT)
Rate
  75–95 bpm desirable
    Faster with limited stroke volume
    Slower with residual ischemia
  Bradycardia
    Increase rate with pacing, atropine, β-adrenergic drugs
  Tachycardia
    Identify and treat causes
      Hypercarbia
      Inadequate anesthesia
      Ischemia
    Sinus tachycardia often improves as heart fills
    SVTs: atrial fibrillation, flutter
      Attempt synchronized cardioversion
      Control rate with digoxin, Ca^{2+} channel blockers, β-blockers
Afterload
  ↑ SVR: ↑ myocardial work and O_2 consumption
    Deepen anesthesia
    Direct vasodilators: nitroprusside
  ↓ SVR: inadequate coronary artery perfusion pressure
    α-Agonist: phenylephrine and norepinephrine
Contractility
  Risk factors for low contractility after CPB
    Pre-existing ventricular impairment
    Advanced age
    Prolonged CPB and aortic crossclamp times
    Problems with myocardial preservation
  Consider inotropic support if low contractility is suspected
    Catecholamines (see Figures 17.2 and 17.3)
      Epinephrine, norepinephrine, dopamine, dobutamine
    Phosphodiesterase inhibitors
      Amrinone, milrinone
Preload
  Manipulated when weaning from CPB
  Modalities to assess preload
    CVP, PAP, PAOP, LAP
    Appearance of heart
    TEE
Miscellaneous
  Evacuate intracardic air
  Control bleeding
  Cardiac vent suction off
  Clamps off heart and great vessels
  Coronary artery bypass grafts inspected for kinks
  Caval tourniquets loosened

Preparing the Lungs for CPB Weaning

As CPB is discontinued, and the patient's heart provides the impulse supporting circulation, the lungs once again become the site of gas exchange, delivering oxygen and eliminating carbon dioxide. Before weaning from bypass, suction the trachea and, if necessary, lavage the lungs with saline to clear any secretions. Suction the stomach to ensure gastric distension does not impair ventilation after bypass. Reinflate the lungs by hand with large respiratory sighs using 30 to 40 cm H_2O pressure, and then mechanically ventilate with 100% oxygen. If an in situ internal mammary artery (IMA) bypass graft is present, visually monitor the lungs as they are inflated to prevent tearing of the IMA-coronary artery anastomosis. Both lungs should be rising and falling with each breath, and should be inspected for residual atelectasis. Lung compliance can be judged with hand ventilation (the cardiac anesthesiologist should have a very "educated" hand). Stiff or noncompliant lungs suggest there may be oxygenation and/or ventilation problems after bypass. Activate the ventilation alarms and monitors. The surgeon should check both sides of the chest for fluid and a tension pneumothorax. Auscultate for wheezing and give bronchodilators if necessary. In its worst form, pulmonary dysfunction after bypass may require treatment with positive end-expiratory pressure (PEEP) or even a more sophisticated ventilator; the time to obtain this equipment and have it ready is *before* attempting to wean the patient from CPB. Methods to ensure and optimize pulmonary function post-CPB are listed in Table 17.2.

Preparing the Patient for CPB Weaning

Patient systems, and variables other than heart and lung function, must be assessed and corrected prior to discontinuing bypass. The patient should be warm (37°C bladder or rectal) before attempting to wean from CPB. Normal patient temperature optimizes cell biochemical function. Incomplete rewarming jeopardizes the patient's ability to maintain a physiologic temperature and may re-

TABLE 17.2. Discontinuation of CPB: preparing the lungs.

Lavage and suction trachea
Suction gastric tube
Reinflate lungs by hand under direct vision
Mechanically ventilate with 100% O_2
Inspect lungs for residual atelectasis
Estimate compliance of lungs by "feel"
Activate respiratory monitors and alarms
Check pleural spaces for fluid and pneumothorax
Auscultate for wheezing, give bronchodilators if necessary
Consider the need for PEEP and/or sophisticated ventilator

TABLE 17.3. Discontinuation of CPB: final preparations.

Patient temperature
   Rewarm to 37°C before weaning
   Fluid warmer, circuit heater, and warming pad functioning
   Warm room temperature if necessary
Metabolic balance
   Correct acidosis
   Correct K^+
      KCl in pump resevoir if too low
      Diuresis, $NaHCO_3$, CaCl, and/or glucose-insulin if too high
   Correct Ca^{2+} deficit
Hematocrit 20-25%
Consider adequacy of anesthesia
Final preparations
   Level table and re-zero transducers
   Resuscitation drugs and volume fluids available
   Monitors activated and functioning properly
   Lungs ventilated with 100% O_2
   Vaporizers off 20-30 minutes before weaning
   Check drug infusions for rate and content

sult in cellular dysfunction and bleeding. Once off bypass, the patient will steadily lose heat, and measures to keep the patient warm, including fluid warmers, a breathing-circuit heater-humidifier, and a warming pad, should be set up and employed before CPB weaning. The operating room temperature may need to be increased as well.

Check the acid-base status of the patient and correct any abnormalities. Severe metabolic acidosis depresses myocardium[12,13] and should be treated with $NaHCO_3$ or tromethamine (THAM).[14,15] Potassium and calcium levels should be normalized and the hematocrit maintained in the 20% to 25% range before taking the patient off bypass. Consider the adequacy of anesthesia at this time.

The final preparations for taking the patient off bypass include leveling the operating table, re-zeroing the transducers, checking on the availability of resuscitation drugs and appropriate volume fluids, ensuring the proper function of all monitoring devices, and, once again, determining that the lungs are being ventilated with 100% oxygen. Be sure that the anesthetic agent vaporizers have been off for 20 to 30 minutes before taking the patient off bypass,[16] and that only those drugs you intend to administer are being infused. Table 17.3 lists final preparations for terminating CPB.

Termination of CPB Support

Weaning a patient from CPB involves occluding the venous drainage to the heart-lung machine (thus diverting blood back into the heart), and then decreasing the heart-lung machine's arterial flow as the heart's contribution to systemic flow increases. This can be done most abruptly by clamping the venous cannulas and transfusing with the pump until the heart fills and the preload appears optimal. Some patients can tolerate this method of coming off bypass, but many cannot; therefore, a more gradual transfer of the systemic flow from the pump to the heart is usually desirable. The poorer the anticipated cardiac function, the slower the weaning from bypass should be. *Close and clear communication among the perfusionist, the surgeon, and the anesthesiologist is imperative while weaning from bypass*, and one of these individuals should be clearly in charge of the process.

When ready to wean a patient from bypass, ask the perfusionist for three values: (1) the volume in the pump reservoir, (2) the oxygen saturation of the blood returning to the pump from the patient, and (3) the flow rate of the pump. The volume indicates how much blood is available for transfusion to fill the heart and lungs as bypass is discontinued. If this number is low—less than 400 to 500 mL (8 mL/kg in children)—more fluid (or blood if the hematocrit is low) may be added to the pump before weaning. The oxygen saturation of the venous return (Svo_2) helps estimate the adequacy of peripheral perfusion on CPB. If the Svo_2 is greater than 60%, oxygen delivery during bypass is adequate: if it is less than 50%, oxygen delivery is inadequate, and measures to improve oxygen delivery (increase flow, hematocrit) and/or decrease consumption (deepening anesthesia, muscle paralysis) should be instituted before taking the patient off bypass. An Svo_2 between 50% and 60% is marginally acceptable and must be followed closely. As the patient is weaned from CPB, a rising Svo_2 suggests that the heart and lungs will support the circulation off CPB; a falling Svo_2 indicates that the contribution of the patient's cardiac output to total blood flow is inadequate and that further intervention is needed before weaning from bypass.

Weaning from CPB is initiated by partially occluding the venous return cannula. This may be done on the field by the surgeon, or at the pump by the perfusionist. As the heart fills with blood, the left ventricle will begin to eject, and the arterial waveform will become pulsatile. Next, the perfusionist *gradually* decreases the pump flow rate. This is necessary to avoid emptying the pump reservoir—and thus possibly pumping air into the arterial circulation—as more of the venous return goes through the heart. It is best to bring the filling pressure being monitored (eg, central venous pressure [CVP], PAOP, LAP) to a specific, predetermined level—which should be somewhat lower than what may be ultimately necessary—and then assess cardiovascular performance. Further filling of the heart should proceed in small increments, guided by the ventricular filling pressures, and continued until satisfactory hemodynamics are achieved, as judged by the arterial pressure, the appearance of the heart, and the Svo_2 trend. Overfilling and distension of the heart will lead to myocardial fibril disruption and should be avoided at all costs. If the patient has two venous cannulas, the smaller of the two may be removed when the pump flow is reduced by half the full flow rate. This will facilitate the movement of blood from the great veins into the right atrium. When the pump flow has been decreased to 1 L/min or less (in an adult) and the hemodynamics are satisfactory, the venous cannula is completely clamped and the pump flow turned off. The patient is now off bypass.

At this critical point in the operation, pause and review/reassess important patient care factors: confirm that (1) the lungs are being ventilated with oxygen; (2) the hemodynamic status of the patient is acceptable and stable; (3) the heart does not appear to be distending; (4) only prescribed drugs and infusions are being administered; and (5) the ECG and/or TEE do not demonstrate new signs of ischemia. Further "fine-tuning" of the preload can be accomplished by transfusing 50- to 100-mL aliquots through the arterial cannula and noting the effect on patient hemodynamics. When it is clear that the patient has successfully resumed cardiorespiratory function, the venous cannula may be removed from the heart. If there is acute failure of the circulation, as evidenced by unstable rhythm, falling arterial and rising filling pressures, or visible distension of the heart, put the patient back on CPB and begin the process of assessment and intervention again.

Before removing the arterial cannula, transfuse as much as possible of the pump reservoir blood into the patient. It is usually easier and quicker to give this volume through the arterial cannula than through intravenous lines after decannulation. Venous capacitance can be increased by tipping the patient's head up and/or giving nitroglycerin, but be more cautious with these maneuvers in patients with impaired cardiac function. Filling the vascular space while the patient is on nitroglycerin, with the head up, increases your ability to manage volume loss after aorta decannulation, by enabling you to augment central vascular volume quickly by simply tipping the head back or decreasing the nitroglycerin rate. (This is much like storing extra volume in an easily accessible space.) The venous cannula and tubing may be drained into the reservoir and transfused, if the patient is stable and not likely to be put back on bypass.

When this transfusion is completed, carefully assess the patient's condition before deciding to remove the arterial cannula, since, once this is done, returning to bypass becomes much more difficult and time-consuming. The patient should be hemodynamically stable, with an adequate cardiac output (greater than 2.3 L/min/m^2) and arterial pressure (mean arterial pressure [MAP] $\geq$ 65-70 mm Hg). Adequate oxygenation and ventilation should be confirmed by arterial blood gas or pulse oximetry and capnography. Patient bleeding should not be allowed to exceed that manageable through the vascular access available after aorta decannulation. (Be sure the perfusionist is not transfusing significant amounts of blood through the arterial cannula before removing it; you may not be able to keep up with the blood loss through IV infusions.) Also, bleeding from behind the heart may have to be repaired on bypass if the patient cannot tolerate lifting of the heart to expose the problem area. Keep the systolic arterial pressure between 95 and 105 mm Hg for decannulation, to avoid dissection or tearing of the aorta.[17] Tip the patient's head up or give small boluses of sodium nitroprusside to bring the pressure down, if necessary. Once the arterial cannula has been removed, and control of the bleeding from the cannulation site ensured, protamine may be started. Alternatively, if the patient is at risk for a protamine reaction (see Chapter 5), the aortic cannula may be left in place until half of the protamine has been administered. This will facilitate return to CPB if the patient has an untoward reaction to protamine. Suction that returns blood to the bypass circuit should be stopped before the administration of protamine. Protamine should be given slowly over 7 to 15 minutes, watching for systemic hypotension and pulmonary hypertension, which may indicate that a reaction to protamine is occurring.[18-20] Technically flawed coronary bypass grafts may thrombose with protamine administration, causing acute ischemia and left ventricular failure mimicking a protamine reaction. When protamine has been given and the patient remains hemodynamically stable, the process of discontinuing CPB is complete.

Discontinuation of CPB: Pharmacologic Considerations

Although cardiac surgery is intended to improve myocardial function, improvement may not be apparent at the end of CPB, when the effects of cardioplegia, ischemic injury, and reperfusion can cause significant myocardial depression. Therefore, patients having cardiac surgery will often need pharmacologic support to be weaned from CPB, particularly those with preoperative ventricular dysfunction, advanced age, poor intraoperative myocardial protection, inadequate revascularization, and/or persistent mechanical problems.[8,21]

Pharmacologic support at the end of CPB may also be needed in "healthier" patients. Cardiac surgery and CPB frequently cause a deterioration of ventricular function that extends into the early postoperative period, even in patients who have undergone uneventful surgery.[22-27]

Deciding to Initiate Pharmacologic Support

We believe that the need for perioperative pharmacologic support does not represent a failure of surgery in any way, and we recommend its use early, rather than late, in the peri-CPB period. Attempting to wean from CPB or to maintain a patient with a failing heart off CPB risks distending the ventricles, causing subendocardial ischemia, and worsening the situation. Pharmacologic support may be initiated during one of the distinct peri-CPB periods: (1) *prior* to initiating weaning from CPB, (2) *during* the CPB weaning process, and (3) *after* discontinuing CPB support. The characteristics of each of these periods are discussed below.

Initiating Pharmacologic Support Prior to CPB Weaning

The decision to start inotropic support before attempting to wean the patient from CPB may be based on the patient's previous cardiac function, length of ischemic arrest time, adequacy of myocardial protection, and general appearance of the heart.

For example, patients with chronic congestive heart failure (CHF) have been shown to have a decrease in the density of myocardial β-receptors and a decreased response to catecholamines.[28] These patients require high levels of endogenous catecholamines to maintain even marginal cardiac output. CHF patients undergoing cardiac surgery are likely to require exogenous catecholamines for successful weaning from CPB. In addition, CPB is associated with a large surge in endogenous catecholamines,[29] which can acutely cause further down-regulation of the β-receptors.[30,31]

Some indicators of the heart's function may be seen at the end of CPB. One encouraging sign is the ejection of blood from the left ventricle (noted in the arterial line tracing as a pulsatile waveform) when the beating heart is allowed to fill. The appearance of the exposed surface of the heart may also be an indicator of ventricular function, even though most of the visible surface is the right ventricle. However, although global dysfunction may be visible, regional defects in contractility may not be. Blood ejection related to filling pressures (CVP, LAP, pulmonary artery [PA], or PAOP) and the arterial waveform upstroke slope are other clues to myocardial contractility. Global and regional myocardial contractility can be evaluated with intraoperative echocardiography.[32] A blood-filled heart that has little or no ejection is an ominous finding.

When inotropes are started during CPB, it is important to do so *after* the heart is warm and adequately reperfused. Starting the inotropes 5 to 10 minutes before weaning allows enough time to achieve adequate effect on the heart, and avoids increasing myocardial oxygen consumption early after the cardiac arrest, when myocardial energy stores are depleted.

Importantly, before any pharmacologic treatment decisions are made, be sure that the pressures and readings obtained are accurate, and not the result of a dampened tracing, malfunctioning transducer, inappropriate reference level, etc. Serious mistakes can occur when critical decisions are based on faulty information. Constantly compare and correlate the data obtained with that from all other sources (ie, palpate the pulses, look at and touch the skin to assess temperature and perfusion).

Initiating Pharmacologic Support During Weaning from CPB

During the process of CPB weaning, a persistently low blood pressure with a narrow pulse range (despite increasing filling pressures) suggests ventricular dysfunction. In the failing heart, the systemic pressure will decline as the filling pressures rise and the heart distends. The heart must be unloaded and supported with rapid return to full CPB. This will prevent further myocardial distension and worsening ischemia. Cardiovascular parameters should be reassessed and appropriate therapy started before attempting to wean again from CPB support.

Initiating Pharmacologic Therapy After Discontinuing CPB

In a third group of patients, the weaning process is completed with normal (or even high) systemic arterial pressures but low cardiac output (less than 2 L/min/m^2). This reflects the fact that an adequate systemic blood pressure is not equivalent to an adequate cardiac output, and that blood pressure and physical examination may not correlate well with actual cardiac output determinations after cardiac surgery.[33] In this circumstance, inotropic drugs may improve cardiac output by improving myocardial contractility. However, as noted above, preload should be optimized, and vasodilators may be necessary to decrease SVR.

In many circumstances, a single dose of ephedrine (5–10 mg) or epinephrine (2–8 μg) will provide the necessary pharmacologic support to wean the patient from CPB. Calcium chloride (5–10 mg/kg) is also frequently given in this setting, but the potential for worsening reperfusion injury,[34-36] causing vasoconstriction[37] and coronary spasm,[38] has made its use controversial. However, calcium remains a useful therapy in the presence of hypocalcemia, the persistence of hyperkalemia, or the occurrence of hypotension after rapid infusion of citrated blood.

Choosing Inotropic/Vasodilator Drug Therapies

Once the decision to use an inotrope is made, one must consider the multiple actions of each drug. The Appendix of this chapter briefly outlines the action of commonly used inotropic and vasodilator drugs. A discussion of the rationale for selecting a specific inotrope or vasodilator is given below. Figure 17.1 outlines drug treatment strategies to facilitate CPB weaning.

Inotropic Drugs and CPB Weaning

Although there are multiple studies comparing different inotropic medications used after cardiac surgery, few of them address the use of inotropic support while weaning from CPB, probably because this is a period of hemodynamic instability in which few variables can be controlled. Achieving the goal of restoring blood flow to tissues may require not only intervention to increase myocardial contractility, but also pharmacologic therapy to alter vascular tone. In most circumstances, a single drug cannot effect optimal hemodynamics, but combinations of inotropic and vasoactive medications favorably modify the body's response. Figure 17.2 lists commonly used inotropes.

In many medical centers, dopamine (or dobutamine) is the first-line drug when inotropic support is needed.[39,40] Dopamine has the advantage of acting on renal dopaminergic receptors when used at low doses.[41] However, as higher doses are used, the α-adrenergic effects predominate, leading to vasoconstriction; tachycardia also occurs due to chronotropic stimulation.[42] The actions of dopamine are also partially dependent on the release of endogenous norepinephrine,[43] and this makes its effects unreliable in conditions such as CHF, in which endogenous stores are depleted. Dobutamine's β-adrenergic effects in the peripheral vasculature can cause mild vasodilation.[44,45] Although this effect is favorable in patients with an increased SVR, it may cause hypotension in patients who are already vasodilated.[46]

We favor the use of epinephrine as a first-line inotropic agent for weaning patients from CPB. It is a potent drug with direct action and is effective in a wide dose range. At lower doses, the β-adrenergic effects predominate, while at the higher range the α-adrenergic effects are more marked.[47,48] α-Adrenergic effects can be controlled by a variable infusion of sodium nitroprusside or nitroglycerin, allowing for potent inotropic action without increases in the filling pressures or SVR.[49] Epinephrine increases cardiac output more consistently than dopamine or dobutamine in patients being weaned from CPB.[50] The potential for tachycardia is one of its primary limitations, but adjusting for potency, epinephrine causes less tachycardia than dopamine or dobutamine.[47,51] Arrhythmias occur mainly when high doses are given, and we recommend that these not exceed 0.15 μg/kg/min.

In patients with marked vasodilation and low systemic blood pressures, norepinephrine is probably the drug of choice, since its β-adrenergic action is equipotent to that of epinephrine, while its α-adrenergic action leads to an increase in blood pressure,[52] which is important for maintaining coronary perfusion, particularly in hypertrophied ventricles.[53] Some advocate the use of norepinephrine mixed with a fixed dose of a vasodilator, such as phentolamine;[54] this mixture has pharmacodynamic effects similar to those of epinephrine. Norepinephrine can also be

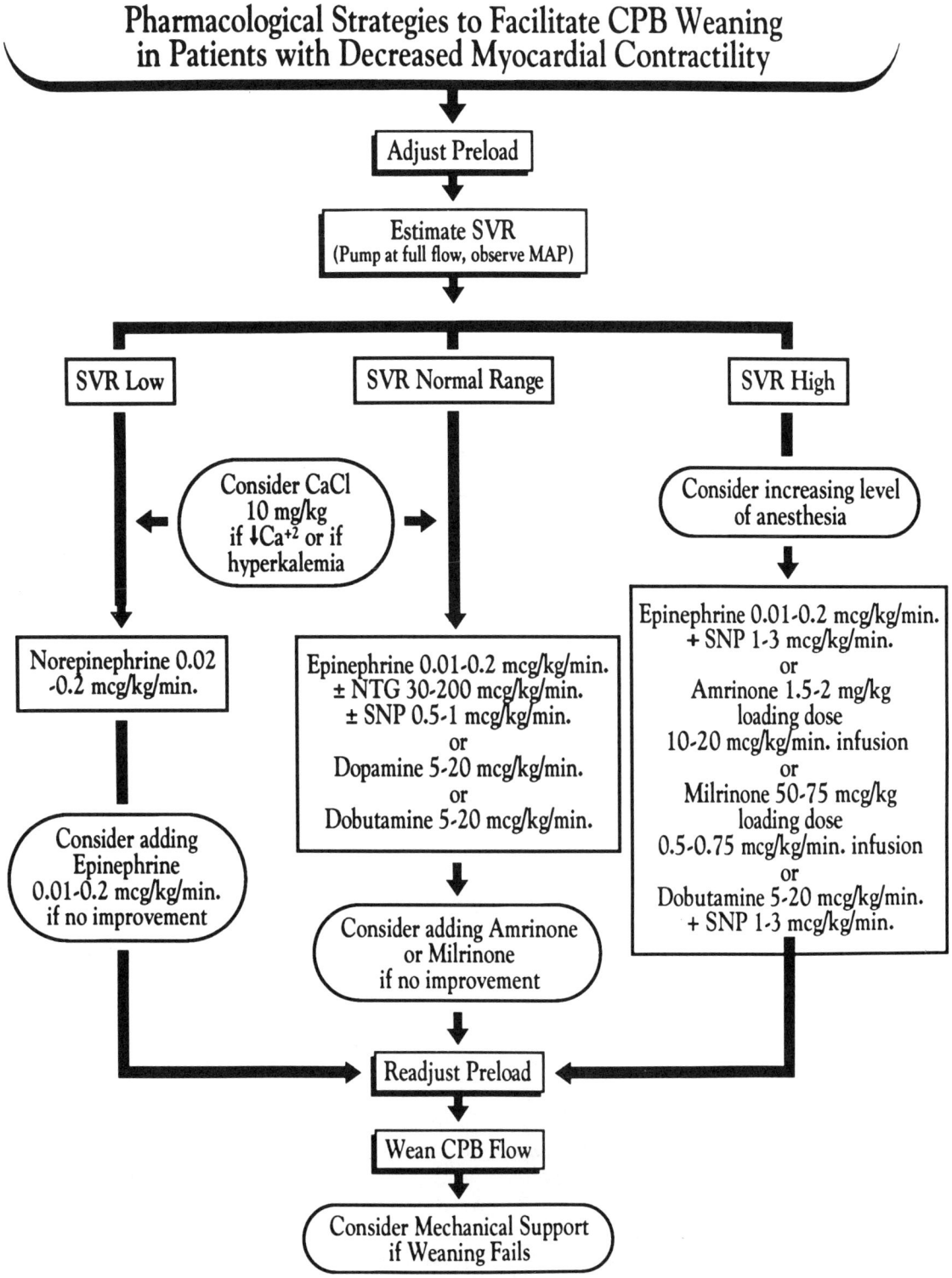

FIGURE 17.1. Pharmacologic strategies to facilitate CPB weaning in patients with decreased myocardial contractility. SVR, systemic vascular resistance; MAP, mean arterial pressure; SNP, sodium nitroprusside; NTG, nitroglycerin.

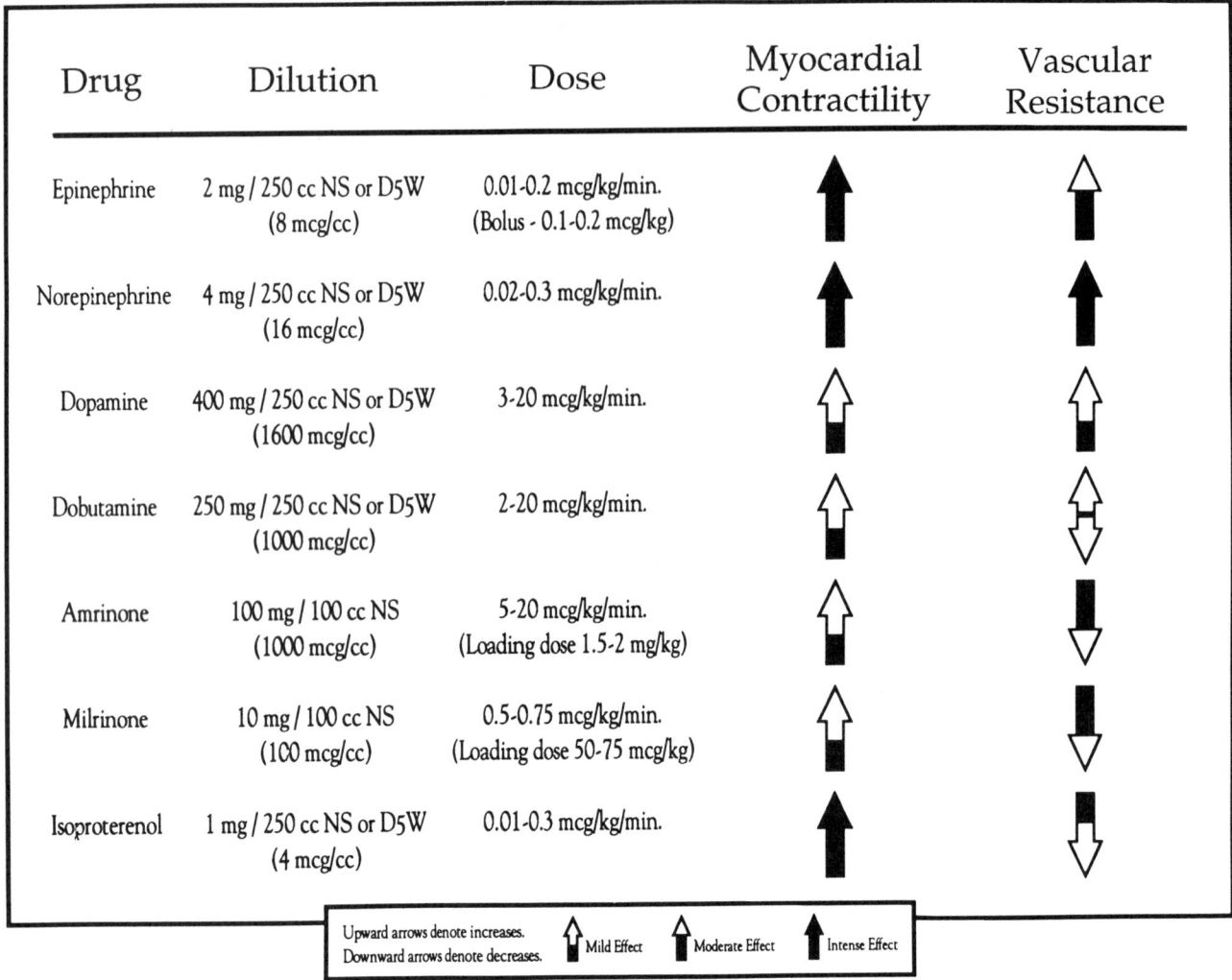

FIGURE 17.2. Dosages, methods of preparation, and effects on myocardial contractility and vascular resistance of commonly used inotropic drugs. NS, normal saline; D_5W, 5% dextrose in water.

combined with low-dose dopamine to maintain renal blood flow,[55] and, in fact, it may be better than dopamine for this effect in severely vasodilated patients.[56] Norepinephrine is useful in counteracting excessive hypotension that may be caused by fraction III phosphodiesterase (PDE III) inhibitors, while adding to the inotropic effect of these agents.[57,58]

PDE III inhibitors (amrinone, milrinone) are frequently used in patients who require a second inotrope, but they also have been advocated as first-line drugs.[59,60] These drugs increase intracellular calcium (enhancing myocardial contractility) by inhibiting intracellular phosphodiesterase activity. Unlike catecholamines, the effectiveness of amrinone is not dependent on adrenergic membrane receptor populations. Therefore, this type of drug can provide inotropic action when a ceiling effect has been reached with the cathecholamines.[61,62] Although clinical experience in weaning from CPB with amrinone is more abundant, milrinone is now taking a predominant role, due to its lower cost and decreased incidence of thrombocytopenia. PDE III inhibitors are also useful in right ventricular failure, as they increase contractility without elevating pulmonary vascular resistance.[63,64] However, efforts must be made in this setting to avoid systemic hypotension, which will reduce right ventricular coronary perfusion.

Isoproterenol, a potent catecholamine with marked β_1-adrenergic action, has a limited role in myocardial revascularization surgery, due to its chronotropic effects, which may increase myocardial oxygen demand beyond the supply, resulting in myocardial ischemia or infarction.[65] It has an important role, however, in those cases in which an increased heart rate and vasodilation are desirable (eg, pediatric cardiac surgery or after heart transplantation). The drug's action on the bronchial tree and pulmonary vasculature favors its use in patients with bronchospasm or pulmonary hypertension.

Vasodilators and CPB Weaning

As noted earlier, vasodilators can be combined with inotropic drugs to optimize hemodynamics by reducing vascular resistance and facilitating forward flow, or they can be used alone when a patient has acceptable ventricular function but requires reduction in afterload and/or preload. The most commonly used vasodilators in this setting are sodium nitroprusside and nitroglycerin, since they can be given by intravenous infusion and have a rapid onset of action and response to titration.

Sodium nitroprusside is a potent vasodilator that relaxes the smooth muscle in the precapillary arterioles, decreasing afterload. It also lowers the preload, but to a smaller degree. In the setting of decreased preload, sodium nitroprusside can cause marked hypotension, and to avoid this, intravascular volume should be optimized before and during the infusion of sodium nitroprusside. It is a nonspecific vasodilator, and as such it also decreases pulmonary vascular resistance. This is useful in patients with pulmonary hypertension, but this same vasodilation may cause increased intrapulmonary shunting and lower arterial Po_2. Sodium nitroprusside can also cause coronary steal (shunting of blood from ischemic to adequately perfused areas of the myocardium) and worsen ischemia.[66,67] Sodium nitroprusside is given mainly by infusion (see Appendix). It can also be used topically to relieve spasm of the internal mammary artery,[68] or in small boluses (1–3 μg/kg) when a brief episode of hypotension is desired, such as for removal of the aortic cannula.

Nitroglycerin is a vasodilator with more pronounced effects on the venous side, lowering preload and myocardial oxygen consumption. In fact, this action appears to be more important than coronary vasodilation in the drug's ability to relieve angina.[69] At higher doses, its effect on afterload becomes more apparent, and hypotension may occur. Nitroglycerin is a useful vasodilator during weaning from CPB, because it mildly decreases the afterload and moderately lowers the preload, so that the blood volume left in the pump can be transfused back to the patient and the cannulas can be removed. Under these circumstances, the patient becomes his own venous reservoir, with decreases in the dose of nitroglycerin and tilting of the operating room table to the Trendelenburg position resulting in blood transfer to the central compartment, compensating, as needed, for simultaneous blood loss.

In patients with severe reactive pulmonary hypertension, a useful combination that facilitates CPB weaning is prostaglandin E_1, a potent pulmonary vasodilator, and norepinephrine, a potent inotrope and vasoconstrictor. Prostaglandin E_1 should be administered through a central vein or pulmonary artery catheter, with norepinephrine given through a left atrial line to counteract the systemic hypotension that would occur if the prostaglandin E_1 were given alone.[70,71] Since norepinephrine is rapidly metabolized before reaching the lungs, it will exert most of its effects on the heart and systemic vasculature when given through a left atrial line, while the vasodilatory effects of prostaglandin E_1 will predominate in the lungs.

Although not clinically available yet, a very promising alternative for the management of patients with pulmonary hypertension is inhaled nitric oxide. Nitric oxide, known also as endothelial-derived relaxing factor (EDRF), is a powerful vasodilator produced by vascular endothelial cells.[72] Nitric oxide can be given as an inhalant to produce pulmonary vasodilation.[73] However, unlike other vasodilators, the effect of nitric oxide is apparently restricted to the pulmonary circulation, because as soon as it diffuses into the bloodstream, it reacts with hemoglobin and becomes inactivated.[74] Several reports have shown the beneficial effects of inhaled nitric oxide in patients with pulmonary hypertension in a variety of settings,[75-78] but further studies will be necessary before inhaled nitric oxide is approved by the US Food and Drug Administration.

Before finishing this section, we would like to emphasize some important points concerning the use of both inotropic and vasodilator drugs. These are potent agents that can have severe side effects if extravasated or bolused inadvertently. Inotropic drugs should be given through a central line in controlled doses, preferably through an infusion pump, while the hemodynamic effects are closely monitored. Care must be taken to be sure that boluses of other medications are not given through the same line, to avoid combining inotropes with other infusions that cause inactivation, and to prevent accidental disconnections. Finally, when giving medications through a left atrial line, air must be meticulously removed from the tubing to avoid systemic air embolism.

Failure to Wean from CPB

When a patient cannot be weaned from CPB, several important points must be considered. First, the safety of extracorporeal support must be maintained. It is easy to forget that heparin is being metabolized and that continuous assessment of anticoagulation is imperative. Second, during *each* attempt at weaning from CPB, the sequence outlined at the beginning of this chapter should be meticulously followed. If an organized sequence is not followed, critical steps, such as re-establishing lung ventilation, can be forgotten, turning a difficult-to-wean case into an impossible one. Third, one must reassess the accuracy of the information being used to facilitate the discontinuation of bypass. As an example, in some patients, the pressure readings from the radial artery may be much lower than the central aortic pressure. This demonstrates how easy it is to be misled by information that, earlier in the case, was dependable.[79-81]

Next, re-evaluate the patient and attempt to establish the cause(s) of failure to wean. Even when the cause(s) seem evident, other contributing factors should be sought and treated. We recommend a systematic approach to assessing failure to wean a patient from CPB.

The following discussion may facilitate recognition of causative factors in failure to wean. Figure 17.3 summarizes these factors.

1. Is the Myocardium Contracting?

If myocardial dysfunction is present, is it global or regional? Global dysfunction suggests inadequate protection of the heart during arrest, but other simple causes, such as hyperkalemia and inadvertent administration of negative inotropes (an open anesthetic vaporizer), must be eliminated as possible causes. In our experience, it is not unusual for the heart to recover significantly from global injury with the passage of time, as long as it is supported; a period of "rest" on CPB, at normothermia, with inotropic drugs off and adequate coronary perfusion pressures for 30 minutes to 1 hour, may be warranted. Replenishing myocardial energy stores with an infusion of glucose-insulin-potassium may also be helpful.[82,83] If the myocardial dysfunction is regional, the considerations noted above are still valid, but it is necessary to evaluate the possibility of acute obstruction or spasm of the grafts on native coronary arteries.[68,84] TEE echocardiography is a very useful tool in determining the affected area, but in its absence, the heart may be lifted while on CPB and the grafts inspected. Coronary air embolism is a common cause of transient myocardial dysfunction. It is characterized by abrupt onset and, usually, resolution after several minutes, provided that coronary perfusion pressure is maintained and 100% oxygen administered.[85,86] In some patients, especially children, the air bubbles can be seen in the coronary arteries.

2. Are the Rate and Rhythm Appropriate?

The contribution of the atrial contraction to the total cardiac output is very significant in patients with reduced ventricular compliance, and every effort should be made

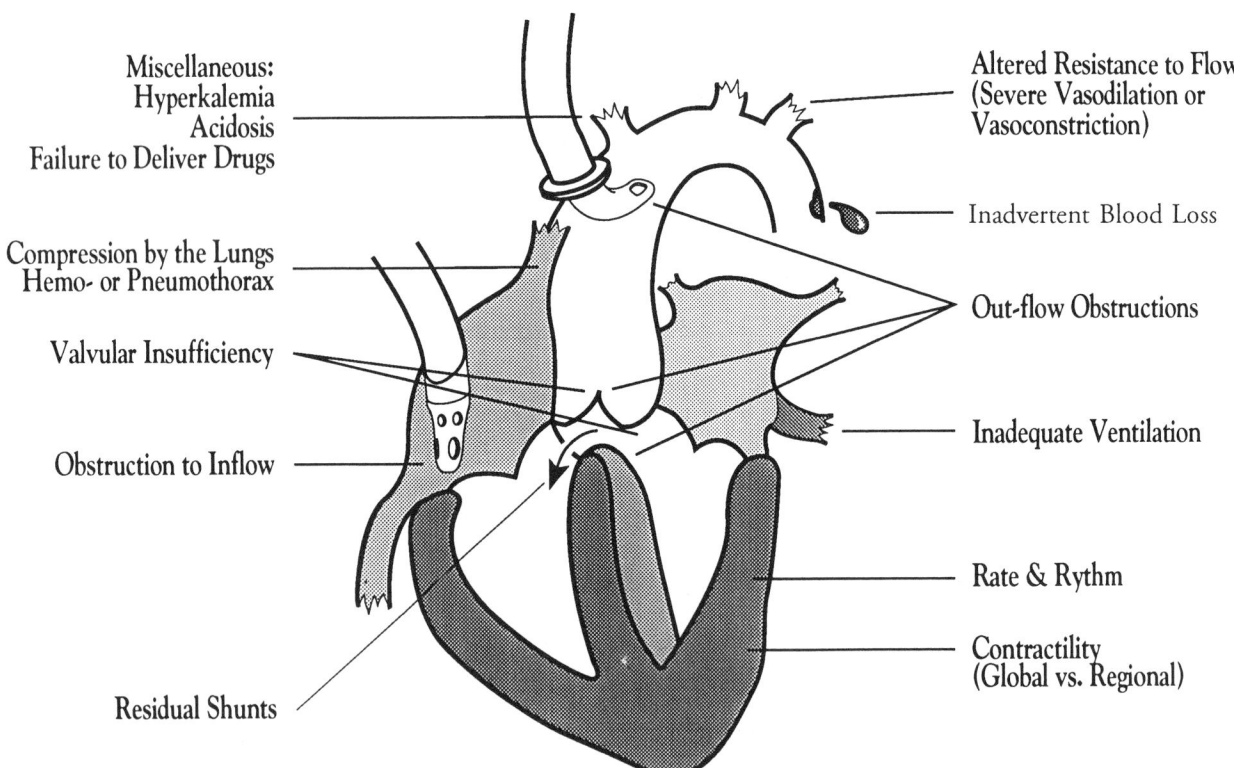

FIGURE 17.3. Factors that can impede successful weaning from CPB.

to have synchronous atrial-ventricular contraction. For most adult patients, a heart rate of 80 to 90 beats per minute maximizes cardiac output, without markedly impairing diastolic filling and coronary perfusion. However, this may vary with the individual patient, depending on the pre-existing lesion and compensatory mechanisms (ie, at the end of CPB, the ventricle remains dilated despite replacement of an insufficient aortic valve), persistence of the original lesion (eg, incomplete revascularization in coronary artery bypass surgery), or presence of new problems (ie, global myocardial dysfunction after a prolonged aortic crossclamp time).

3. Are There Any Obstructions to Flow?

Flow obstruction may be caused by a previously undiagnosed stenotic valve, after placement of a mitral ring, a malfunctioning prosthetic valve, a large aortic cannula, or acute aortic dissection (fixed obstructions); or by subaortic infundibular stenosis (dynamic obstruction). Obstructions to flow should be suspected when the heart appears to contract vigorously but the blood pressure and cardiac output are low. Using a sterile extension tubing and a needle, the surgeon can measure the pressures above and below the suspected obstruction to confirm the diagnosis. Dynamic obstruction can also be diagnosed by intraoperative echocardiography,[32] with the additional advantage that the effectiveness of therapy can be assessed throughout the case.[87] The underlying cause of obstruction should be treated.

4. Are Any of the Valves Insufficient?

Significant problems are usually related to aortic or mitral valve insufficiency and may be caused by inadvertent injury to the valve during surgery, a malfunctioning prosthetic valve, large perivalvular leaks, or, in the case of the mitral valve, by papillary muscle dysfunction due to ischemia.[88] Failure of the pulmonary or tricuspid valves is usually not as critical, unless associated with pulmonary hypertension, in which case the right ventricle can fail and cause significant hemodynamic compromise. Intraoperative echocardiography is useful in making this diagnosis,[89] but in its absence, the diagnosis may be suspected from the pressure waveforms and hemodynamic measurements. Once the diagnosis is made, the underlying cause should be treated.

5. Is the Preload Adequate?

Difficulty in filling the heart should lead to the suspicion of obstruction to venous inflow or rapid inadvertent blood loss. Obstructions to venous inflow can be caused by failure to remove the tourniquets around the venous cannulas, by the cannulas themselves, or by reduction in the size of the cava due to a large purse-string suture.[90,91] The heart will appear empty, and the veins will be distended up to the place of obstruction. Rapid, inadvertent blood loss can be the result of suctioning through a vent; inadequate clamping of the venous or aortic cannula, allowing blood to be drained to the pump circuit; disconnected arterial line; or bleeding into the thorax or abdomen (especially bleeding from the aorta due to spontaneous dissection, or from injury to the aortic wall during a recent heart catherization or placement of an intraaortic balloon pump). Checking the pump return, and looking at the patient should indicate where the blood is being lost, and action should be taken to prevent further loss.

Preload can be compromised by overdistending lungs. The heart can be compressed even though the chest is open. The most common cause is overdistended lungs that do not deflate on exhalation due to bronchospasm and secretions. Other causes of compression are pneumothorax, hemothorax, or, rarely, a lap sponge left behind the heart. The diagnosis may be obvious in some cases, such as those in which the lungs meet over the heart and will not deflate ("kissing lungs"). Or it may be less obvious in other cases, in which a localized compression impedes adequate filling of the heart.

In evaluating the preload, a more difficult situation arises when the filling pressures are high and the heart appears to have adequate volume, but the actual volume in the ventricles is low. This occurs particularly in patients with reduced ventricular compliance, in whom the operative procedure may have eliminated the main pathologic condition, but not other dysfunctions, such as ventricular hypertrophy secondary to aortic stenosis. Even in patients with good ventricular function, the myocardial changes induced by CPB, cardioplegic arrest, and cardiac surgery may alter significantly the correlation between filling pressures and ventricular end-diastolic volume.[92] TEE can be very useful in this setting, guiding the magnitude of volume replacement far beyond what conventional wisdom would indicate if filling pressures were to be followed.[93] In the absence of echocardiography, it is reasonable to try to determine the patient's position on the Frank-Starling curve by increasing the preload until there are no further increases in the cardiac output and blood pressure.

6. Is There Marked Vasodilation or Vasoconstriction?

Marked hypotension may be the result of anaphylactic shock, anaphylactoid reactions, severe anemia, hyperthermia, inadvertent administration of vasodilators, or release of toxins.[94] Hypertension may be caused by inadequate anesthesia, inadvertent administration of vasoconstrictors, or low levels of oral antihypertensives in patients with a history of hypertension. Since the extracorporeal pump can provide a constant cardiac output, the blood pressure at full flow gives an idea of the systemic vascular resistance, so that changes can be made before attempting to wean the patient again.

7. Are the Patient's Metabolic Demands Excessive?

In a patient with limited cardiac reserve, increased metabolic demands can quickly lead to acidosis and further decreases in cardiac output. Increased metabolic demands can result from hyperthermia (excessive rewarming, spontaneous fever), inadequate anesthesia, or shivering. The patient should be adequately anesthetized, paralyzed, and normothermic before weaning is attempted again.

8. Miscellaneous

Residual shunts, severe hyperkalemia, profound acidosis, and malignant arrhythmias are other causes of failure to wean from CPB, and they should be treated specifically. Another important pitfall is failure to deliver the inotropic drugs because of a disconnected line, empty carrier fluid, or extravasation, and this can be suspected when marked changes in the dose of drugs have little or no effect on the patient. Connections should be checked and intravascular delivery confirmed, and if doubt remains, the drugs should be given by a different line.

Following a methodological approach to weaning patients from CPB, and in selecting inotropic drugs and addressing difficulties, maximizes the likelihood of a successful outcome. If the patient cannot be weaned from CPB, even after all the potential causes have been addressed, mechanical support should be used. The different modalities and indications for mechanical support are discussed in Chapter 27.

APPENDIX
Inotropic and Vasodilating Drugs Commonly Used in Cardiac Surgery

Inotropes

Epinephrine

Epinephrine is an endogenous catecholamine with significant effects on the cardiovascular system. At low doses (0.01–0.03 µg/kg/min) it acts on vascular smooth muscle β_2-receptors, leading to vasodilation.[95,96] As the dose increases, the effect at β_1-receptors causes increase in contractility, stroke volume, and heart rate, whereas the effect on α-receptors causes vasoconstriction and elevation of the systemic blood pressure. Except for brief periods, doses above 0.15 to 0.2 µg/kg/min are not recommended, as high doses produce marked vasoconstriction, tachycardia, and arrhythmias.[48] Epinephrine also has favorable effects on the lungs, causing bronchodilation through stimulation of β_2-receptors.[97]

An infusion of epinephrine can be prepared by mixing 2 milligrams in a 250-mL bag of normal saline (final concentration = 8 µg/mL) and giving it in a central vein, preferably through an infusion pump. Small boluses of epinephrine (8–32 µg) can be used when a very rapid effect is needed.

Norepinephrine

Norepinephrine affects β-receptors (potency equivalent to that of epinephrine) and it is also a potent α-agonist that causes peripheral vasoconstriction and increases the systemic vascular resistance.[52] Therefore, this drug is particularly useful in patients with marked vasodilation and marginal or low cardiac output.

An infusion is prepared by mixing 4 mg in 250 mL of normal saline, giving a final concentration of 16 µg/mL. The dose required usually varies from 0.02 to 0.3 µg/kg/min.

Dopamine

An endogenous catecholamine and precursor of norepinephrine, dopamine is unique in its action on dopaminergic receptors. The stimulation of this type of receptor causes vasodilation in the renal and splanchnic vasculatures.[41] Dopamine also is a direct β_1-agonist and releases endogenous norepinephrine.[43] The effect of dopamine on the cardiovascular system is dose dependent, with low doses (1–4 µg/kg/min) increasing renal blood flow, moderate doses (5–10 µg/kg/min) increasing cardiac output and myocardial contractility, and high doses (>10 µg/kg/min) primarily increasing heart rate and systemic vascular resistance.[42] Dopamine also increases preload through vasoconstriction.[98]

An infusion is prepared by mixing dopamine, 200 to 400 mg, in a 250-mL bag of normal saline or 5% dextrose in water; the final concentration will be 800 or 1600 µg/mL.

Dobutamine

Dobutamine stimulates β_1-receptors, increasing contractility,[44] and has balanced effects on β_2- and α-receptors, causing little change in vascular tone.[45] Dobutamine's primary advantage is its ability to increase cardiac output without increasing afterload. Clinical doses range from 2 to 20 µg/kg/min. At the higher dose range, dobutamine can cause tachycardia, arrhythmias, and myocardial ischemia by increasing myocardial oxygen demand in excess of supply.[46,99]

Dobutamine is prepared by mixing 250 mg in 250 mL of normal saline of 5% dextrose in water (D_5W), giving a final concentration of 1 mg/mL.

Isoproterenol

Isoproterenol is a synthetic catecholamine with marked β-adrenergic receptor effects and little or no α-adrenergic receptor interactions. It increases contractility and is a potent chronotropic agent, but can cause excessive tachycardia, arrhythmias, and myocardial ischemia. In healthy subjects, isoproterenol enhances the elastic recoil of the myocardium and improves ventricular filling.[100] It is a bronchodilator and also reduces pulmonary vascular resistance. The clinical isoproterenol dose varies from 0.01 to 0.3 µg/kg/min.

Isoproterenol is prepared by diluting 1 mg in 250 mL of normal saline or D_5W, giving a concentration of 4 µg/mL.

Amrinone

Amrinone is a bypiridine derivative that exerts its effects through inhibition of PDE III, resulting in an increase in intracellular cyclic AMP and calcium concentration.[101] Since its action is independent of β-adrenergic receptors, it is frequently used in patients with a persistent low cardiac output despite large doses of catecholamines. Amrinone causes marked venous and arterial vasodilation, reducing both preload and afterload.[102-104] Although there is some dispute concerning amrinone's positive inotropic action at clinically useful doses,[105] pressure-volume analysis, separating ventricular from vascular changes, demonstrates that amrinone increases myocardial contractility independent of afterload reduction.[106,107] When used to wean a patient from CPB, a loading dose of 1.5 to 2 mg/kg should be used, followed by an infusion at 10 to 20 µg/kg/min.[103] Since amrinone has a long half-life ($t_{1/2} \approx$ 5h), changes in the infusion rate do not result in immediate hemodynamic changes, as with catecholamine-type inotropes.

An infusion is prepared by diluting 1 ampule of 100 mg (20 mL) into 80 mL of normal saline, giving a final concentration of 1 mg/mL.

Milrinone

Milrinone, a PDE III inhibitor 10 to 30 times more potent than amrinone, is available for clinical use in the United States. Initial studies suggest it is as effective as amrinone and does not interfere with platelet number and function.[108] Milrinone, 50 to 75 µg/kg IV over 10 minutes, followed by an infusion of 0.5 to 0.75 µg/kg/min, will result in therapeutic plasma levels.

An infusion is prepared by diluting one or two 10-mg ampules in normal saline for a total volume of 100 mL, giving a final concentration of 100 or 200 µg/mL.

Calcium

Calcium is necessary for myocardial cell function, and the effect of most inotropes is ultimately to increase intracellular calcium levels.[109] Since calcium administration increases contractility and blood pressure, calcium salts (calcium chloride, calcium gluconate) are frequently administered at the end of CPB to facilitate weaning.[110] However, calcium has been implicated in myocardial cell injury during ischemia and reperfusion,[34] and its use at the end of CPB is controversial.[110-115] Although it is probably best to avoid giving calcium just before, or in the first 15 minutes after, removing the aortic crossclamp, or when there is evidence of ongoing ischemia, it can be useful for weaning patients with low ionized calcium levels or with persistent hyperkalemia. In adults, calcium is usually given as calcium chloride in boluses of 5 to 10 mg/kg. For children, some prefer calcium gluconate (15–30 mg/kg), since it can be given peripherally, while others recommend calcium chloride, because it provides greater bioavailability of free calcium.[116]

Other Drugs

Enoximone, an imidazole rather than a bypiridine derivative, is also a PDE III inhibitor with similar actions to other drugs in this group.[117] Its role in cardiac surgery is being established, but it appears to have favorable hemodynamic effects, lowering afterload and increasing myocardial contractility.[118] Dopexamine, another synthetic catecholamine, has $β_2$-adrenergic receptors and dopaminergic (DA_1 receptors) activity with no α-adrenergic effects and minimal $β_1$-receptor stimulation.[119,120] Although the combination of vasodilation, increased contractility, and reduction of renal vascular resistance[121] appears favorable, further studies are needed to define its use in cardiac surgery.

Vasodilators

Sodium Nitroprusside

Sodium nitroprusside is a potent nonselective vasodilator that acts mainly on arterioles and to a smaller degree on venules. In the presence of heart failure, it improves hemodynamics by decreasing the afterload, slightly reducing the preload and allowing for increases in the cardiac output. Due to its potency and short effect, sodium nitroprusside is usually given by infusion, but small (1–3 µg/kg) boluses can be given when very rapid control of elevated blood pressure is needed. It is decomposed by light, so the infusion bag should be covered. An infusion is made by diluting 50 mg in 250 mL of normal saline or D_5W, giving a concentration of 200 µg/mL. The dose range varies from 0.5 to 5 µg/kg/min. Due to the drug's metabolism, infusion rates over 3 µg/kg/min can lead to thiocyanate and cyanide toxicity.[122]

Nitroglycerin

Nitroglycerin is an organic nitrate that relaxes smooth muscle in the vein walls, and, to a lesser degree, in the arteries. It decreases coronary resistance and improves collateral blood flow in the coronary bed.[123] The vasodilatory action appears to be mediated by the formation of nitric oxide and increases in the cyclic AMP in smooth muscle.[124] Nitroglycerin is rapidly taken up and metabolized both by vascular tissue and by the liver, and its metabolites, although less potent, may accumulate over time.[125] An infusion is made by mixing 50 mg in 250 mL of D_5W, giving a concentration of 200 µg/mL. The infusion dose usually varies from 30 to 200 µg/kg/min, depending on the effect sought. Nitroglycerin can bind to certain types of plastic,[126] so the infusion should be contained in a glass bottle, and low-absorption, nonpolyvinyl chloride (PVC) tubing is preferred to deliver it. Patients develop tolerance to the effects of nitroglycerin when it is given continuously for more than 24 hours,[127] so it may be better to administer it when needed rather than running continuous "prophylactic" infusions.

Prostaglandin E_1 (PGE_1)

PGE_1, or alprostadil, is an eicosanoid derivative normally produced in the body. It is a powerful vasodilator that also decreases platelet aggregation. It is used to treat episodes of pulmonary hypertension that fail to respond to more conventional vasodilators. When administered intravenously, a large portion of the drug is cleared on the first pass through the lungs by the pulmonary endothelium,[128] but, despite this, it may cause significant systemic hypotension necessitating a simultaneous infusion of norepinephrine through a left atrial line. In neonates, PGE_1 relaxes the smooth muscle surrounding the ductus arteriosus, and because of this, the drug is primarily used to keep the ductus open in newborns with ductus-dependent congenital heart disease. An infusion is made by diluting 0.5 mg in 250 mL of normal saline or D_5W, giving a concentration of 2 µg/mL. The starting dose is 0.01 µg/kg/min and the drug is titrated for clinical effect up to 0.1 µg/kg/min.

References

1. Tofler OB. Electrocardiographic changes during profound hypothermia. *Br Heart J* 1962;24:265-268.
2. Schwab RH, Lewis DW, Killough JH, Templeton JY. Electrocardiographic changes occurring in rapidly induced deep hypothermia. *Am J Med Sci* 1964;248:290-303.
3. Trevino A, Razi B, Beller BM. The characteristic electrocardiogram of accidental hypothermia. *Arch Intern Med* 1971;127:470-473.
4. Braunwald E. The hemodynamic significance of atrial systole. *Am J Med* 1964;37:665-669.
5. Konstadt SN, Reich DL, Thys DM, et al. Importance of atrial systole to ventricular filling predicted by transesophageal echocardiography. *Anesthesiology* 1990;72:971-976.
6. England MR, Gordon G, Salem M, Chernow B. Magnesium administration and dysrhythmias after cardiac surgery. *JAMA* 1992;268:2395-2402.
7. Evans GL, Smulyan H, Eich RH. Role of peripheral resistance in the control of cardiac output. *Am J Cardiol* 1967;20:216-221.
8. Royster RL, Butterworth JF, Prough DS, et al. Preoperative and intraoperative predictors of inotropic support and long-term outcome in patients having coronary artery bypass grafting. *Anesth Analg* 1991;72:729-736.
9. Entress JJ, Dhamee S, Olund T, et al. Pulmonary artery occlusion pressure is not accurate immediately after cardiopulmonary bypass. *J Cardiothorac Anesth* 1990;4:558-563.
10. Konstadt SN, Thys D, Mindich BP, et al. Validation of quantitative intraoperative transesophageal echocardiography. *Anesthesiology* 1986;65:418-421.
11. Abel MD, Nishimura RA, Callahan MJ, et al. Evaluation of intraoperative transesophageal echocardiography. *Anesthesiology* 1987;66:64-68.
12. Cingolani HE, Mattiazzi AR, Blesa ES, Gonzalez NC. Contractility in isolated mammalian heart muscle after acid-base changes. *Circ Res* 1970;26:269-278.
13. Gerst PH, Fleming WH, Malm JR. Increased susceptibility of the heart to ventricular fibrillation during metabolic acidosis. *Circ Res* 1966;19:63-70.
14. Kassirer JP. Serious acid-base disorders. *N Engl J Med* 1974;291:773-776.
15. Bleich HL, Schwartz WB. TRIS buffer (THAM). *N Engl J Med* 1966;274:782-786.
16. Nussmeier NA, Moskowitz GJ, Weiskopf RB, et al. In vitro anesthetic wash-in and wash-out via bubble oxygenators. *Anesth Analg* 1988;67:982-987.
17. Murphy DA, Craver JM, Jones EL, et al. Recognition and management of ascending aortic dissection complicating cardiac surgical operations. *J Thorac Cardiovasc Surg* 1983;85:247-256.
18. Moorthy SS, Pond W, Rowland RG. Severe circulatory shock following protamine (an anaphylactic reaction). *Anesth Analg* 1980;59:77-78.
19. Lowenstein E, Johnston WE, Lappas DG, et al. Catastrophic pulmonary vasoconstriction associated with protamine reversal of heparin. *Anesthesiology* 1983;59:470-473.
20. Horrow JC. Protamine: a review of its toxicity. *Anesth Analg* 1985;64:348-361.
21. Cohn LH. Dobutamine in the postcardiac surgery patient. In: Chatterjee K, ed. *Dobutamine—A Ten-Year Review*. New York: NCM Publishers Inc;1989:123-138.
22. Breisblatt WM, Stein KL, Wolfe CJ, et al. Acute myocardial dysfunction and recovery: a common occurrence after cardiopulmonary bypass surgery. *J Am Coll Cardiol* 1990;15:1261-1269.
23. Mangano DT. Biventricular function after myocardial revascularization in humans: deterioration and recovery patterns during the first 24 hours. *Anesthesiology* 1985;62:571-577.
24. Gray R, Maddahi J, Berman D, et al. Scintigraphic and hemodynamic demonstration of transient left ventricular dysfunction immediately after uncomplicated coronary artery bypass grafting. *J Thorac Cardiovasc Surg* 1979;77:504-510.
25. Khuri SF, Warner KG, Josa M, et al. The superiority of continuous cold blood cardioplegia in the metabolic protec-

tion of the hypertrophied human heart. *J Thorac Cardiovasc Surg* 1988;95:442-454.
26. Sell TL, Purut CM, Silva R, et al. Recovery of myocardial function during coronary artery bypass grafting. Intraoperative assessment by pressure-volume loops. *J Thorac Cardiovasc Surg* 1991;101:681-687.
27. Fowler MB, Laser JA, Hopkins GL, et al. Assessment of the beta adrenergic receptor pathway in the intact failing human heart: progressive receptor down-regulation and subsensitivity to agonist response. *Circulation* 1986;74: 1290-1302.
28. Bristow MR, Ginsburg R, Minobe W, et al. Decreased catecholamine sensitivity and β-adrenergic receptor density in failing human hearts. *N Engl J Med* 1982;307:205-211,
29. Reves JG, Karp RB, Buttner EE, et al. Neuronal and adrenomedullary catecholamine release in response to cardiopulmonary bypass in man. *Circulation* 1982;66:49-55.
30. Spahn DR, Frasco P, Smith LR, et al. Cardiopulmonary bypass induces physiologic β-adrenergic receptor desensitization. Abstracts of the 14th Annual Meeting of the Society of Cardiovascular Anesthesiology. 1992;178.
31. Mantz J, Marty J, Pansard Y, et al. β-Adrenergic receptor changes during coronary artery bypass grafting. *J Thorac Cardiovasc Surg* 1990;99:75-81.
32. Sharvan K. Transesophageal echocardiography; how valuable is it for heart monitoring during cardiac surgery? *Curr Opin Anesth* 1992;5:94-103.
33. Bailey JM, Levy JH, Kopel MA, et al. Relationship between clinical evaluation of peripheral perfusion and global hemodynamics in adults after cardiac surgery. *Crit Care Med* 1990;18:1353-1356.
34. Barry WH. Mechanisms of myocardial cell injury during ischemia and reperfusion. *J Card Surg* 1987;2:375-383.
35. Borgers M. The role of calcium in the toxicity of the myocardium. *Histochem J* 1986;13:839-848.
36. Nayler WG. Calcium and cell death. *Eur Heart J* 1983; 4(suppl C):33-41.
37. Scheidegger D, Dropp LJ, Schellenberg JC. Role of the systemic vasculature in the hemodynamic response to changes in plasma ionized calcium. *Arch Surg* 1980;115:206-211.
38. Engleman RM, Harji-Rousou S, Bres RH, et al. Rebound vasospasm after coronary revascularization in association with calcium antagonist withdrawal. *Ann Thorac Surg* 1984;37:469-472.
39. Sethna DH, Gray RJ, Moffit EA, et al. Dobutamine and cardiac oxygen balance in patients following myocardial revascularization. *Anesth Analg* 1982;61:917-920.
40. Van Trigt P, Spray TL, Pasque MK, et al. The comparative effects of dopamine and dobutamine on ventricular mechanics after coronary artery bypass grafting: a pressure-dimension analysis. *Circulation* 1984;(suppl I):112-117.
41. Goldberg LI, Hsuh Y, Resnekov L. Newer catecholamines for treatment of heart failure and shock: an update on dopamine and a first look at dobutamine. *Prog Cardiovasc Dis* 1977;19:327-340.
42. Lawless CE, Loeb HS. Pharmacokinetics and pharmacodynamics of dobutamine. In: Chatterjee K, ed. *Dobutamine: A Ten Year Review.* New York: NCM Publishers;1989: 33-47.
43. Leier CV, Heran PT, Huss P, et al. Comparative systemic and regional hemodynamic effects of dopamine and dobutamine in patients with cardiomyopathic heart failure. *Circulation* 1978;58:466-475.
44. Tuttle RR, Mills J. Development of a new catecholamine to selectively increase cardiac contractility. *Circ Res* 1975; 36:185-196.
45. Ruffolo RR Jr, Spradlin TA, Pollock GD, et al. Alpha and beta adrenergic effects of the stereoisomers of dobutamine. *J Pharmacol Exp Ther* 1981;219:447-452.
46. Leier CV, Unverferth DV. Dobutamine. *Ann Intern Med* 1983;99:490-496.
47. Stephenson LW, Blackstone EH, Korchoukos NT. Dopamine vs epinephrine in patients following cardiac surgery: randomized study. *Surg Forum* 1976;27:272-275.
48. Sung BH, Aubison C, Thadani U, et al. Effects of L-epinephrine on hemodynamics and cardiac function in coronary disease: dose response studies. *Clin Pharmacol Ther* 1988;43:308-316.
49. Tinker J. Pro: strong inotropes (ie, epinephrine) should be drugs of first choice during emergence from cardiopulmonary bypass. *J Cardiothorac Anesth* 1987;1:256-258.
50. Stenn PA, Tinker JH, Pluth JR, et al. Efficacy of dopamine, dobutamine and epinephrine during emergence from cardiopulmonary bypass in man. *Circulation* 1978;57:378-384.
51. Butterworth JF IV, Prielipp RC, Royster RL, et al. Dobutamine increases heart rate more than epinephrine in patients recovering from aortocoronary bypass surgery. *J Cardiothorac Vasc Anesth* 1992;6:535-545.
52. Zaritsky AL, Chernow B. Catecholamines, sympathomimetics. In: Chernow B, ed. *The Pharmacologic Approach to the Critically Ill Patient.* Baltimore: Williams & Wilkins; 1983:481-509.
53. Dole WP. Autoregulation of the coronary circulation. *Prog Cardiovasc Dis* 1987;29:293-323.
54. Lemmer JH, Bothma MJ, McKenney P, et al. Norepinephrine plus phentolamine improves regional blood flow during experimental low cardiac output syndrome. *Ann Thorac Surg* 1984;38:108-116.
55. Schaer GL, Fink MP, Parrillo JF. Norepinephrine alone versus norepinephrine plus low-dose dopamine: enhanced renal blood flow with combination pressor therapy. *Crit Care Med* 1985;13:492-496.
56. Lucas CE. A new look at dopamine and norepinephrine for hyperdynamic septic shock. *Chest* 1994;105:7-8.
57. Lathi KS, Shulman MS, Diehl JT, et al. The use of amrinone and norepinephrine for inotropic support during emergence from cardiopulmonary bypass. *J Cardiothorac Vasc Anesth* 1991;5:250-254.
58. Robinson RJS, Tchervenkov C. Treatment of low cardiac output after aortocoronary artery bypass surgery using a combination of norepinephrine and amrinone. *J Cardiothorac Anesth* 1987;1:229-233.
59. Dupuis J, Bondy R, Cattran C, et al. Amrinone and dobutamine as primary treatment of low cardiac output syndrome following coronary artery surgery: a comparison of their effects on hemodynamics and outcome. *J Cardiothorac Vasc Anesth* 1992;6:542-553.
60. Royster RL, Whiteley JW, Butterworth JF IV. Amrinone

therapy during emergence from cardiopulmonary bypass. *J Thorac Cardiovasc Surg* 1991;101:942-943.
61. Colucci WS, Wright RF, Braunwald E. New positive inotropic agents in the treatment of congestive heart failure: mechanisms of action and recent clinical developments. (Second of two parts) *N Engl J Med* 1986;314:349-358.
62. Gage J, Rutman H, Lucido D, et al. Additive effects of dobutamine and amrinone on myocardial contractility and ventricular performance in patients with severe heart failure. *Circulation* 1986;74:367-373.
63. Bondy R, Ramsay JG. Reversal of refractory right ventricular failure with amrinone. *J Cardiothorac Vasc Anesth* 1991;5:255-257.
64. Hines R. Use of amrinone in perioperative states. *Pract Cardiol* 1987;9(suppl):33-37.
65. Udelson JE, Cannon RU III, Bacharack SL, et al. Beta-adrenergic stimulation with isoproterenol enhances left ventricular diastolic performance in hypertrophic cardiomyopathy despite potentiation of myocardial ischemia. *Circulation* 1989;79:371-382.
66. Chiarello M, Gold HK, Leibach RC, et al. Comparison between the effects of nitroprusside and nitroglycerin on ischemic injury during acute myocardial infarction. *Circulation* 1976;54:766-733.
67. Kaplan JA, Jones EL. Vasodilator therapy during coronary artery surgery: comparison of nitroglycerin and nitroprusside. *J Thorac Cardiovasc Surg* 1979;77:301-309.
68. Cooper GJ, Wilkinson GA, Angelini GD. Overcoming perioperative spasm of the internal mammary artery: which is the best vasodilator? *J Thorac Cardiovasc Surg* 1992;104:465-468.
69. Ganz W, Marcus HS. Failure of intracoronary nitroglycerin to alleviate pacing-induced angina. *Circulation* 1972;46:880-889.
70. D'Ambra M, La Raia P, Philbin D, et al. Prostaglandin E_1 — a new therapy for refractory right heart failure and pulmonary hypertension after mitral valve replacement. *J Thorac Cardiovasc Surg* 1985;89:567-572.
71. Vincent JL, Carlier E, Pinsky MR, et al. Prostaglandin E_1 infusion for right ventricular failure after cardiac transplantation. *J Thorac Cardiovasc Surg* 1992;103:33-39.
72. Palmer RMJ, Ashton DS, Mocada S. Vascular endothelial cells synthesize nitric oxide from L-arginine. *Nature* 1988;333:664-666.
73. Frostell CG, Blomqvist H, Hedenstierna G, et al. Inhaled nitric oxide selectively reverses human hypoxic pulmonary vasoconstriction without causing systemic vasodilation. *Anesthesiology* 1993;78:427-435.
74. Pearl RG. Inhaled nitric oxide. The past, the present, and the future. *Anesthesiology* 1993;78:413-416.
75. Girard C, Lehot JJ, Pannetier JC, et al. Inhaled nitric oxide after mitral valve replacement in patients with chronic pulmonary artery hypertension. *Anesthesiology* 1992;77:880-883.
76. Sellden H, Winberg P, Gustafsson LE, et al. Inhalation of nitric oxide reduced pulmonary hypertension after cardiac surgery in a 3.2-kg infant. *Anesthesiology* 1993;78:577-580.
77. Roberts JD, Polaner DM, Lang P, et al. Inhaled nitric oxide in persistent pulmonary hypertension of the newborn. *Lancet* 1992;340:818-819.
78. Rossaint R, Falke KJ, Lopez F, et al. Inhaled nitric oxide for the adult respiratory distress syndrome. *N Engl J Med* 1993;328:399-405.
79. Stern DH, Gershon JI, Allen FB, et al. Can we trust the direct radial artery pressure immediately following cardiopulmonary bypass? *Anesthesiology* 1985;62:557-561.
80. Pauca AL, Hudspeth AS, Wallenhaupt SL, et al. Radial artery-to-aorta pressure difference after discontinuation of cardiopulmonary bypass. *Anesthesiology* 1989;70:935-941.
81. Pauca AL, Wallenhaput SL, Kon ND. Reliability of the radial arterial pressure during anesthesia. Is wrist compression a possible diagnostic test? *Chest* 1994;105:69-75.
82. Gradinac S, Coleman GM, Taegtmeyer H, et al. Improved cardiac function with glucose-insulin-potassium after aortocoronary bypass grafting. *Ann Thorac Surg* 1989;48:484-489.
83. Coleman GM, Cradinac S, Taegtmeyer H, et al. Efficacy of metabolic support with glucose-insulin-potassium for left ventricular pump failure after aortocoronary bypass surgery. *Circulation* 1989;80(suppl I):91-96.
84. Jain U, Sullivan HJ, Pifarre R, et al. Graft atheroembolism as the probable cause of failure to wean from cardiopulmonary bypass. *J Cardiothorac Anesth* 1990;4:476-480.
85. Justice C, Leach J, Edwards WS. The harmful effects and treatment of coronary air embolism during open heart surgery. *Ann Thorac Surg* 1972;14:47-53.
86. Profeta J, Silvay G. Perioperative right ventricular failure due to air in the coronary vein graft. In: Reves JG, Hall KD, eds. *Common Problems in Cardiac Anesthesia*. Chicago: Year Book Medical Publishers Inc;1987:304-309.
87. van Herwerden LA, Fraser AG, Bos E. Left ventricular outflow tract obstruction after mitral valve repair assessed with intraoperative echocardiography. *J Thorac Cardiovasc Surg* 1991;102:461-463.
88. Doty DB. The surgeon's response to a low-output state after cardiopulmonary bypass: etiologies and remedies. *J Card Surg* 1990;5(suppl):256-258.
89. Reichert SLA, Visser CA, Moulijn AC, et al. Intraoperative transesophageal color-coded doppler echocardiography for evaluation of residual regurgitation after mitral valve repair. *J Thorac Cardiovasc Surg* 1990;100:756-761.
90. Hill RF. Increased central venous pressure during cardiopulmonary bypass. In: Reves JG, Hall KD, eds. *Common Problems in Cardiac Anesthesia*. Chicago: Year Book Medical Publishers Inc;1987:27-30.
91. Kirklin JK, Kirklin JW, Pacifico AD. Cardiopulmonary bypass. In: Arciniegas E, ed. *Pediatric Cardiac Surgery*. Chicago: Year Book Medical Publishers;1985:67-77.
92. Hansen RM, Viquerat CE, Matthay MA, et al. Poor correlation between pulmonary arterial wedge pressure and left ventricular end-diastolic volume after coronary artery bypass surgery. *Anesthesiology* 1986;64:764-770.
93. Reichert CLA, Visser CA, Koulen JJ, et al. Transesophageal echocardiography in hypotensive patients after cardiac operations. Comparison with hemodynamic parameters. *J Thorac Cardiovasc Surg* 1992;104:321-326.
94. Andersen LW, Baek L, Degn H, et al. Presence of circulating endotoxins during cardiac operations. *J Thorac Cardiovasc Surg* 1987;93:115-119.
95. Freyschuss U, Hjemdahl P, Juhlin-Dannfelt A, et al. Car-

diovascular and metabolic responses to low-dose adrenaline infusion: an invasive study in humans. *Clin Sci* 1986; 70:199-206.
96. Stratton JR, Pfeifer MA, Ritchie JL, et al. Hemodynamic effects of epinephrine: concentration-effect study in humans. *J Appl Physiol* 1985;58:1199-1206.
97. Jaimovich D, Kecshes SA. Management of reactive airway disease. In: Viayasagar D, Carlson R, Geheb MA, eds. *Critical Care Clinics*. Philadelphia: WB Saunders Co; 1992;8:147-162.
98. Loeb HS, Ostrenga JP, Gaul W, et al. Beneficial effects of dopamine combined with intravenous nitroglycerin on hemodynamics in patients with severe left ventricular failure. *Circulation* 1983;68:813-820.
99. Monrad ES, Baim DS, Smith HS, et al. Milrinone, dobutamine and nitroprusside: comparative effects on hemodynamics and myocardial energetics in patients with severe congestive heart failure. *Circulation* 1986;73(III):168-174.
100. Udelson JE, Bacharach SL, Canon RO III, et al. Minimum left ventricular pressure during β-adrenergic stimulation in human subjects. *Circulation* 1990;82:1174-1182.
101. Honerjager P, Schafer-Korting M, Reiter M. Involvement of cyclic AMP in the direct inotropic action of amrinone: biochemical and functional evidence. *Naunyn-Schmiedeberg's Arch Pharmacol* 1981;318:112-120.
102. Firth BG, Ratner AV, Grassman ED, et al. Assessment of the inotropic and vasodilator effects of amrinone versus isoproterenol. *Am J Cardiol* 1984;54:1331-1336.
103. Levy JH, Ramsay J, Bailey JM. Pharmacokinetics and pharmacodynamics of phosphodiesterase III inhibitors. *J Cardiothorac Anesth* 1990;4(suppl 5):7-11.
104. Levy JH, Bailey JM. Amrinone: its effect on vascular resistance and capacitance in human subjects. *Chest* 1994;105: 62-64.
105. Wilmshurst PT, Thompson DS, Juul SM, et al. Effects of intracoronary and intravenous amrinone infusions in patients with cardiac failure and patients with near normal cardiac function. *Br Heart J* 1985;53:493-506.
106. Kass DA, Grayson R, Marino R. Pressure-volume analysis as a method for quantifying simultaneous drug (amrinone) effects on arterial load and contractile state in vivo. *J Am Coll Cardiol* 1990;16:726-732.
107. Konstram MA, Cohen SR, Weiland DS, et al. Relative contribution of inotropic and vasodilator effects to amrinone-induced hemodynamic improvement in congestive heart failure. *Am J Cardiol* 1986;57:242-248.
108. Anderson JL, Baim DS, Fein SA, et al. Efficacy and safety of sustained (47 hours) intravenous infusions of milrinone in patients with severe congestive heart failure: a multicenter study. *J Am Coll Cardiol* 1987;9:711-722.
109. Rutman HI, LeJemtel TH, Sonneblick EH. Newer cardiotonic agents: implications for patients with heart failure and ischemic heart disease. *J Cardiothorac Anesth* 1987;1: 59-70.
110. DiSesa V. The rational selection of inotropic drugs in cardiac surgery. *J Card Surg* 1987;2:385-406.
111. Vitex TS. Pro: Calcium salts are contraindicated in the weaning of patients from cardiopulmonary bypass. *J Cardiothorac Anesth* 1988;2:567-569.
112. Koski G. Con: Calcium salts are contraindicated in weaning patients from cardiopulmonary bypass coronary artery surgery. *J Cardiothorac Anesth* 1988;2:570-575.
113. Johnston WE, Robertie PG, Butterworth JF IV, et al. Is calcium or ephedrine superior to placebo for emergence from cardiopulmonary bypass. *J Cardiothorac Vasc Anesth* 1992;6:528-534.
114. Royster RL, Butterworth JF IV, Prielipp RE, et al. A randomized, blinded, placebo-controlled evaluation of calcium chloride and epinephrine for inotropic support after emergence from cardiopulmonary bypass. *Anesth Analg* 1992;74:3-13.
115. Urban MK, Hines R. The effect of calcium on pulmonary vascular resistance and right ventricular function. *J Thorac Cardiovasc Surg* 1992;104:327-332.
116. Broner CW, Stidham GL, Westen-Kirchner DF, et al. A prospective, randomized, double-blind comparison of calcium chloride and calcium gluconate therapies for hypocalcemia in critically ill children. *J Pediatr* 1990;117:986-989.
117. Dage RL, Kariya T, Hsieh CP, et al. Pharmacology of enoximone. *Am J Cardiol* 1987;60:10c-14c.
118. Boldt J, Kling D, Moosdorf R, Hempelmann G. Enoximone treatment of impaired myocardial function during cardiac surgery: combined effects with epinephrine. *J Cardiothorac Anesth* 1990;4:462-468.
119. Brown RA, Dixon J, Farmer JB, et al. Dopexamine: a noval agonist at peripheral dopamine receptors and β₂-adrenoreceptors. *Br J Pharmacol* 1985;85:599-608.
120. Smith GN, Hall JC, Farmer JB, et al. The cardiovascular actions of dopexamine hydrochloride, an agonist at dopamine receptors and β₂-adrenoreceptors in the dog. *J Pharm Pharmacol* 1987;39:636-641.
121. Ghosh S, Gray B, Odura A, et al. Dopexamine hydrochloride: pharmacology and use in low cardiac output states. *J Cardiothorac Vasc Anesth* 1991;4:382-389.
122. Parrillo JE. Vasodilator therapy. In: Chernow B, ed. *The Pharmacological Approach to the Critically Ill Patient*. Baltimore: Williams & Wilkins;1983:283-302.
123. Cohen MV, Downey JM, Sonnenblick EH, et al. The effects of nitroglycerin on coronary collateral and myocardial contractility. *J Clin Invest* 1973;52:2836-2847.
124. Moncada S, Radomski MW, Palmer RM. Endothelium-derived relaxing factor: identification as nitric oxide and role in the control of vascular tone and platelet function. *Biochem Pharmacol* 1988;37:2495-2501.
125. Haefeli WE, Bumbleton M, Zenet L, et al. Comparison of vasodilatory responses to nitroglycerin and its dinitrate metabolites in human veins. *Clin Pharmacol Ther* 1992;52: 590-596.
126. Cossum PA, Galbraith AJ, Roberts MS, et al. Loss of nitroglycerin from intravenous infusion sets. *Lancet* 1978;2: 349-350.
127. Dupuis J, Lalonde G, Lemieux R, et al. Tolerance to intravenous nitroglycerin in patients with congestive heart failure: role of increased intravascular volume, neurohumoral activation and lack of prevention with *n*-acetylcystine. *J Am Coll Cardiol* 1990;16:923-931.
128. Said SI. Pulmonary metabolism of prostaglandin and vasoactive peptides. *Annu Rev Physiol* 1982;44:257-268.

18
Safety and Management of Perturbations During Cardiopulmonary Bypass

Scott M. Sadel

Introduction

Since its first clinical use in the 1950s, cardiopulmonary bypass (CPB) has evolved and expanded each year to change the lives of thousands of people who have congenital or acquired cardiac disease. Although CPB now saves lives routinely, its use does result in an abnormal physiologic state. Drs. Kirklin and Barratt-Boyer have remarked, "The patient whose arterial blood flow is temporarily provided by means of a pump oxygenator is in an abnormal state that affects most, if not all, of the body's physiologic processes."[1]

Beginning in the 1980s, the issue of safety during this temporary, but abnormal, physiologic state has been addressed extensively. There have been, to date, three large retrospective studies conducted by questionnaire, asking physicians or perfusionists about common accidents that occur during CPB.[2-4] Even though the incidence of perfusion accidents is quite small, ranging from 0.3% to 1% (Table 18.1), in an effort to decrease the risk of CPB there has been much discussion about prevention strategies by the authors of these outcome studies and others. In addition, every perfusionist should be prepared to deal quickly and efficiently with any potential accident or error.

In this chapter, we discuss why extracorporeal circulation (ECC) involves substantial risk. The previously mentioned surveys will be discussed, focusing on some of the more frequent complications. Methods of prevention and, lastly, management of some of the more serious complications will be considered.

System Analysis

As with any complex, highly technical system, CPB is vulnerable to accidents. At the time that safety in perfusion was beginning to become an important issue, several articles appeared in the anesthesia literature evaluating similar concepts.[5-10] Gaba et al[5] described characteristics that predispose a system to accidents. They extrapolated these characteristics to anesthesia, but these can be just as true for the complexities of CPB.

Gaba describes *complexity of interactions* and *tightness of coupling* as two key elements that make a system vulnerable to accidents. Complex interactions can be divided into those having *intrinsic* complexity, *proliferation* complexity, and *uncertainty* complexity. Coupling can be either *tight* or *loose*.

Intrinsic complexity is a property of highly technical systems that require extraordinary effort and close coordination among their various components in order to function properly. Proliferation complexity is a property of a system that requires multiple simple components that interface in a complex fashion. Uncertainty complexity occurs when a process, although relatively straightforward, is not well understood and contains a degree of unpredictability.

The other element described that renders a system susceptible to accidents is *tight coupling*. This element exists when different components of the system affect each other intimately, leaving no room for error. In contrast, *loose coupling* describes the property of a system in which interaction between different components allows some margin for error, so that a mistake in one component will not cause the whole system to fail. This type of system is therefore less predisposed to mishaps.

TABLE 18.1. Summary of survey data on the incidence of perfusion accidents.

Investigator	Incidence/accidents	Incidence of permanent injury or death
Stoney[2]	1/300	1/1000
Wheeldon[3]	1/300	1/1500
Kurusz[4]	1/100	1/1000

TABLE 18.2. Causes of CPB accidents.

	Device	vs.	User
CPB[4]	19.5%		72.3%
Anesthesia[7,8]	14%		82%
	4%		96%

It is easy to apply this type of system analysis to CPB. Multiple complex interactions must be carefully integrated for successful ECC. Health professionals from varying backgrounds (perfusionists, surgeons, nurses, and anesthesiologists) must communicate effectively. Of equal complexity is the coordination required of the mechanical aspects of CPB. The perfusionist's multiple responsibilities and activities during bypass contribute to the proliferative complexity of bypass. Finally, the problem of uncertainty persists in CPB, since it is difficult to judge the adequacy of organ perfusion.

Gaba's analysis implies that a system becomes complex and prone to mishap due to the interfacing of multiple, interdependent components. In today's technological world, this interfacing requires human involvement and quick reaction to different possible outcomes, resulting in the potential for human error. This idea is supported by several studies that looked at anesthetic accidents in a retrospective manner to evaluate their causes and develop possible preventive measures. Keenan and colleagues[6] looked at cardiac arrests during anesthesia over a 15-year period, and determined that errors in judgment accounted for 75% of the 27 anesthetic-related arrests that occurred during those years.

Cooper et al[7] interviewed anesthesiologists to obtain histories of preventable incidents that had occurred in the operating room. They found that 82% of the incidents involved human error. Similarly, the vast majority of perfusion accidents are related to human error rather than machine malfunction (Table 18.2).[4] In Cooper's study, factors found to be associated with errors were equipment design that promoted errors, inadequate experience, unfamiliarity with equipment, inadequate communication, haste, and distraction. They also noted that almost half of the incidents occurred during the maintenance portion of the anesthetic, which may indicate a lack of vigilance.[7]

In a later study, Cooper and colleagues[8] developed a larger database by interviewing and observing a larger number of anesthetists, and they also identified incidents that resulted in a "substantive negative outcome." These incidents were then categorized into judgmental errors, technical errors, and monitoring or vigilance errors. From the data obtained, Cooper was able to describe several strategies to decrease the incidence of mishaps. These included changing training procedures and supervising inexperienced anesthetists, more complete preoperative assessment and equipment inspection, additional monitoring, and improved communication among operating room personnel.

The technical sophistication and know-how required to administer an anesthetic can be compared to that required to maintain a patient on CPB, since many of the properties that make a system prone to mishaps are present in CPB. Also, the errors noted by Cooper can just as easily be made by a perfusionist while maintaining a patient on bypass, as was shown in the studies investigating CPB mishaps.

CPB Complication Surveys

As noted, there has been much interest in perfusion accidents in the last decade. Of the three most commonly cited surveys, the first was performed by Stoney et al[2] who submitted questionnaires to cardiac surgeons in the United States and Canada asking about accidents that occurred between the years 1972 and 1977 (including approximately 374,819 pump cases). The short (26-question) survey[11] focused on the problems of arterial line air embolism, mechanical pump failure, electrical pump failure, disseminated intravascular coagulation (DIC), oxygena-

TABLE 18.3. Perfusion accidents: Stoney survey.

Type of accident	Incidents	Permanent injuries	Deaths
Arterial line air embolism	429	61	92
Disseminated intravascular coagulation	472	28	163
Electrical failure	253	1	3
Mechanical failure	141	4	4
Oxygenator failure	124	6	2
Total	1419	100	264

The number of accidents that were specifically inquired about and the number of resulting permanent injuries and deaths in 374,819 patients from 1972 to 1977 ([Reprinted with permission from the Society of Thoracic Surgeons (*The Annals of Thoracic Surgery*, 1980, 29:336–340).]

TABLE 18.4. Perfusion accidents: UK survey.

Type of accident	Incidents	Permanent injuries	Deaths
Arterial line embolism	26	4	2
Vent air embolism	4	1	2
Electrical failure	33	1	1
Mechanical failure	9	0	0
Oxygenator failure	16	0	0
Inadequate perfusion	10	2	4
Donor blood	3	0	2
Disseminated intravascular coagulation	9	0	3

The number of accidents that occurred and the number of resulting permanent injuries or deaths in approximately 33,000 patients from 1974 to 1979 (Data from Wheeldon DR.[3])

tor failure, and the occurrence of permanent injury or death.

The study showed that accidents with the pump oxygenator occurred once in every 300 procedures, with death or permanent injury occurring once in every 1000 procedures. The most common accidents, from most to least prominent, included DIC, arterial line air embolism, electrical failure, mechanical failure, and oxygenator failure (Table 18.3). Ruptured arterial line connector and air pumped into the left ventricle via a left ventricular vent by reversing the tubing were also listed occasionally.

Stoney concluded that most occurrences of air embolism are due to human error and may be decreased with the use of electronic warning devices. He also concluded that the incidence of DIC may be decreased by following the activated coagulation time (ACT), and he recommended that the perfusionist should be aware of "the multitude of other problems that can arise," to help in preventing these problems.

A survey performed in the United Kingdom, from the years 1974 to 1979, including information on approximately 33,000 perfusion cases, was reported by Wheeldon.[3] This study elicited reports of similar accidents to those of the Stoney study (Table 18.4), with inadequate perfusion, air embolism, DIC, problems with donor blood, and electrical failure being the most severe, life-threatening problems.

The last and most recent survey was performed by Kurusz et al[4] who evaluated accidents that occurred from 1982 to 1985 in the United States and Canada. This survey included data from approximately 573,785 perfusion cases. Table 18.5 lists 15 accidents reported in the Kurusz study, ranked by their relative frequencies and by patient outcomes. The most common accidents reported were protamine reaction, hypoperfusion, inadequate oxygenation, electrical failure, drug errors, and gas embolism (from most to least common). The accidents most likely to result in permanent injury or death included (from most to least common): protamine reaction, hypoperfusion, gas embolism, drug errors, and inadequate oxygenation.

The five most common accidents noted by each study, in incidence per 1000, as well as the incidence per 1000 of permanent injury or death, are listed in Table 18.6. Each incident is also ranked in frequency. As can be seen from the chart, the most common reported complication in the earliest study, coagulopathy, decreased significantly in incidence in both later studies. This is most likely due to better understanding of the variability of patient response to heparin, the phenomenon known as *heparin resistance*,[12-14] and the need to monitor carefully the response to heparin as initially described by Bull.[15] In addition, heparin-protamine titrations are now easily accessible as an aid to

TABLE 18.5. Perfusion accidents: Kurusz survey.

Type of accident	No. cases	Morbidity/mortality
"Protamine reaction"	1 (1606)	1 (21/133)
Hypoperfusion	2 (548)	2 (24/63)
Inadequate oxygenation	3 (506)	5 (10/32)
Electrical failure	4 (482)	13 (0/2)
Drug errors	5 (469)	4 (14/34)
Gas embolism	6 (458)	3 (26/43)
Blood clotting	7 (388)	7 (4/27)
Transfusion reaction	8 (319)	6 (5/33)
Line separation	9 (281)	11 (0/5)
Blood leaks	10 (242)	13 (2/0)
Gross contamination	11 (176)	9 (1/8)
Mechanical failure	12 (166)	12 (3/1)
Consumption coagulopathy	13 (119)	8 (2/27)
Flow meter/blender failure	14 (64)	14 (1/0)
Wrong unit blood	15 (54)	10 (3/5)

The 15 most common perfusion complications from 1982 to 1985 involving 573,785 patients. The complications are ranked from most common to least common in number of accidents and associated morbidity and mortality. The numbers in parentheses are the actual number of each accident and its associated morbidity and mortality (By permission of Kurusz M, Conti VR Arens JF, et al. *Proceed Am Acad Cardiovasc Perf* 1986;7:57–65)

TABLE 18.6. Comparison of the five most common accidents from the three perfusion surveys.[2-4]

	Stoney[2] 1972–1977		Wheeldon[3] 1974–1979		Kurusz[4] 1982–1985	
	Incidents	PI/D	Incidents	PI/D	Incidents	PI/D
Air embolism	(2) 1.14	0.41	(2) 0.79	0.18	(6) 0.80	0.12
Coagulopathy	(1) 1.26	0.51	(6) 0.26	0.09	(8) 0.21	0.05
Electrical failure	(3) 0.67	0.01	(1) 1.00	0.06	(4) 0.84	0.003
Mechanical failure	(4) 0.38	0.02	(5) 0.27	0	(7) 0.30	0.007
Inadequate oxygenation	(5) 0.33	0.02	(3) 0.59	0	(3) 0.88	0.07
Hypoperfusion	–	–	(4) 0.30	0.18	(2) 0.96	0.15
Protamine reaction	–	–	–	–	(1) 2.80	0.22
Drug error	–	–	–	–	(5) 0.82	0.08

PI/D, Permanent injury or death.
The five most common complications for each study are listed as incidence per 1000 perfusions and the number of permanent injuries and mortalities as incidence per 1000 perfusions. The numbers in parentheses are the rank of each complication from most to least.

determining heparin levels before and during CPB (especially during long pump runs).

The problem of air embolism during CPB is cited prominently in all perfusion safety surveys. There are several mechanisms by which air can enter the arterial circulation (Table 18.7). This complication can occur by allowing a previously opened heart to eject air into the ascending aorta. Air can also enter the heart during a closed heart procedure if the left ventricular vent tubing is reversed at the pump head, or air is entrained at the left ventricular vent or aortotomy entry sites. The most devastating and feared cause of air embolism is the pumping of air directly from the aortic cannula. This may occur when (1) the aortic cannula is not properly "de-aired" prior to bypass; (2) there is a rupture in the arterial pump head or arterial line; or (3) rotation of the arterial pumphead occurs unnoticed. Inattention to the reservoir level or a mechanical failure called "runaway pumphead" (uncontrolled acceleration of the pump) may result in the pumping of air from the reservoir into the arterial cannula.[16] In Kurusz's study, more than half of the occurrences of gas embolism resulted from inattention to the reservoir level. Interestingly, although the incidence had decreased from the first to the later two studies, it is very similar in these two studies and resulted in similar incidences of personal injury and death.

The decrease in the incidence of air embolism in the Wheeldon and Kurusz surveys is most likely due to the increased use of alarms, such as level detectors on the reservoir, air detectors on the proximal arterial line, and especially arterial filters that allow some margin of error if air is pumped into the arterial line. This is because the filter will allow accumulation of air and removal of air from the circuit. Most importantly, increasing awareness in the literature provides a constant reminder that this type of accident, which can be avoided by vigilance, can happen to anyone.

Both electrical failure and mechanical failure were noted in all three studies, but both were associated with a low incidence of permanent injury or death. Electrical failure occurred secondary to loss of hospital power, master breaker burnout, fire, faulty plug or power cord, wall circuit-breaker activation, or a pump accidentally unplugged by operating room personnel. Types of mechanical failure included roller pump cessation, runaway roller

TABLE 18.7. Circumstances and events that may result in entrapment of air into the arterial circulation.

Events at the bypass machine
  Inattention to the reservoir level
  Ruptured arterial pump-head tubing
  Arterial line separation
  Unnoticed rotation of the arterial pump head
  Runaway pump head
  Reversal of pump-head rotation
  Reversal of tubing connected to the ventricular vent
  Inadvertent detachment of oxygenator during CPB
  Air transmitted through the membrane oxygenator by an occluded scavenger line
  Clotted oxygenator
  Pressurized cardiotomy reservoir
Events on the operative field
  Unexpected resumption of heartbeat
  Opening of beating heart
  Aortic root air during cardioplegic solution administration
  Aortic root air accumulation secondary to suction for returning retrograde cardioplegic solution
  Inadequate de-airing after cardiotomy
  High flow suction deep in pulmonary artery
  Use of an intraaortic blood pump while aorta is open
  Rupture of pulsatile assist device
  Difficult insertion of a vent line

pump head, or loss of revolutions per minute (rpm) indicator.[11]

The incidence of oxygenator failure is noted to increase with later studies. In comparing the Stoney study and the Kurusz study, Kurusz writes, "The apparent increase in the number of reported oxygenator failures can be explained in two ways. First, there was a difference in wording of the question on the two surveys. Stoney asked about 'failure of delivery of oxygen to the pump,' while Kurusz asked about 'inadequate oxygenation' during CPB. Secondly, surgeon respondents versus perfusionist respondents may have accounted for an increased number of observations (124 v 506, respectively) by perfusionists for this particular complication."[9]

Oxygenator failure can occur secondary to clot formation within the oxygenator. The outer shell can be mechanically injured by collision with some object or person in the operating room or by contact with a solvent, such as spilled inhalational agent from a nearby anesthetic vaporizer. A pressurized bubble oxygenator can burst or have a reduction in its defoaming capacity.

Inadequate oxygenation can occur without an oxygenator problem, if the supply of oxygen to the oxygenator is too low, as can occur with an oxygen/air blender malfunction or a failure in the oxygen supply. If a patient is not paralyzed and is shivering, oxygen use will increase, possibly resulting in inadequate oxygenation. Also, using a membrane oxygenator inappropriate for a patient's size may result in inadequate oxygenation, since these oxygenators have fixed gas transfer rates.

Hypoperfusion occurs when an inadequate amount of flow is produced by the pump. Adequacy of flow is mostly determined indirectly, by following venous saturation and acid-base status. Some possible reasons for decreased perfusion include inadequate blood volume in the bypass machine reservoir, aortic dissection, problems with cannulation, malposition of the aortic cannula,[17-19] and poor venous return. Accidental line separation, especially in the high-pressure arterial side, may also interrupt perfusion.

Protamine reaction, which was only noted in the Kurusz study, was the most common complication in that study. Kurusz and Wheeldon[11] speculate that, since it is not uncommon for hemodynamic instability to occur soon after discontinuation of bypass, some of the hemodynamic perturbations noted may not be due to protamine reactions, but may be interpreted as such because of the temporal relationship. Actually, adverse reactions to administration of protamine are quite common and can be divided into three categories. In Type I reactions, hypotension, related to rapid administration of protamine, occurs. This type of reaction is fairly common but is usually self-limited, and can be treated with vasopressors or volume. The second category (Type II) includes anaphylactic or anaphylactoid reactions. These types of reactions are less common but more severe, and result in a decrease in systemic vascular resistance, bronchospasm, and edema. Type III reactions can be very severe and are associated with pulmonary vasoconstriction, right ventricular distension, pulmonary artery hypertension, decreased left ventricular filling, and systemic hypotension.[20]

The etiologies of Type I and III protamine reactions are not clear. There have been many animal and human studies and case reports looking at effects on specific hemodynamic variables—histamine release, antibody reactions, platelet interactions, and complement activation—without elucidating a common cause. Hypotensive reactions cannot be predicted, although some data do show a significant correlation with patients who are diabetic, those who take NPH insulin, and those who have a previous exposure to protamine.[21] At present, there are no laboratory evaluations that reliably predict risk of protamine reaction. The problem of adverse reactions to protamine administration is also discussed in Chapter 5.

The problem of drug errors, which was only noted in the Kurusz study, refers to drugs accidentally administered to the patient by any member of the cardiac team. The reported problems were mostly due to overdoses of vasodilators or vasoconstrictors, or were problems with coagulation, resulting from heparin overdoses or administration of protamine while on bypass.[4]

Prevention of Perfusion Accidents

Prevention of untoward events during CPB begins with the perfusionist's experience and knowledge of all the possible errors that may occur. This knowledge fosters the anticipation of problems and promotes vigilance. Many of the accident prevention strategies described by Cooper, including communication, better monitoring devices, thorough equipment inspection, and supervision of inexperienced operators, apply to the use of ECC.

Preventing Air Embolism

The prevention of air embolism has been discussed extensively in the literature, and many safety devices have been introduced to help the perfusionist prevent the introduction of air into the arterial line and the heart.[22] Safety devices commonly used today include level detectors that warn the perfusionist of a low blood level in the CPB machine reservoir (see Figure 13.7). These devices can set off an auditory alarm, and some are servoregulated to the pump, turning down the flow or stopping the pump automatically. Air sensors located on the proximal arterial line are also utilized as alarms.[23] Another safety device used is an artrial line filter that traps any air entering the arterial line and allows aspiration of that air. This filter gives the perfusionist added time to identify the problem and take the appropriate steps before air is pumped into the patient (loosening the coupling as per Gaba's model). Other devices used include an arterial line ball valve that stops all flow through the arterial line when air enters the device, and one-way pressure relief valves in the left ventricular vent line to avoid sucking air into a collapsed left ventricle[24] (see Figure 13.8). These devices are described in more detail in Chapter 13. The Kurusz survey addressed the use of these devices and showed that 81% of perfusionists who answered the survey used arterial line filters, 70% used low-level alarms, 48% used bubble detectors, and 35% used one-way pressure relief valves in the left ventricular vent line.[4]

It should be noted that the above devices are aids to preventing air embolism and are not substitutes for vigilance, experience, and communication. Some of these devices have potential hidden hazards, such as residual air trapped in the arterial line filter that cannot be seen after bleeding a bubble out, ball-check valves that will not reopen after air is cleared, and level detectors set too low on the reservoir that may allow a vortex to form at that level, drawing air bubbles into the perfusate.[25]

Other practices recommended to help prevent possible air embolism include clearly marking the direction of flow on the pump heads and their controls to prevent reversal of flow in a left ventricular vent line.[2] Clamping the arterial line on the field before and after bypass will prevent accidental initiation of flow before the line can be inspected for bubbles[11] (sometimes air from a previously opened heart can be trapped in the aortic root and can passively travel into the aortic cannula after CPB). Purging the bypass circuit with carbon dioxide before priming with crystalloid causes the circuit to be filled with more soluble carbon dioxide, so that, if there is a gas bubble left in the circuit, it should dissolve into the prime fluid. If an intraaortic balloon (IABP) pump is in use, it should be stopped during placement or removal of the aortic cannula, since massive air embolism to the aorta has occurred during IABP deflation in combination with arteriotomy.[11] If a procedure requires opening the heart, or if air in the heart is suspected during a closed-heart procedure, the heart should be aggressively de-aired by allowing it to eject with a de-airing vent in the proximal aorta before attempting to separate from bypass. The lungs should be ventilated at this time to remove air trapped in the pulmonary veins. Transesophageal echocardiography (TEE) can be useful as an aid to identifying intracardiac air and determining when the heart is devoid of air.[26,27]

Preventing Coagulopathies

The incidence of coagulopathy decreased from the Stoney study to the subsequent studies. This is most likely due to the increased use of an activated coagulation time (ACT) monitor to assess the adequacy of anticoagulation prior to initiating CPB. The use of a heparin-protamine titration during long pump runs can also be helpful, to be sure that appropriate blood heparin levels are maintained. Since the speed of heparin metabolism varies among patients and changes depending on the patient's body temperature and distribution of blood flow, monitoring the heparin level as well as the ACT can be very important, because the ACT is very nonspecific and will continue to rise despite low levels of heparin as DIC develops.

Preventing Mechanical and Electrical Failures

To help prevent mechanical and electrical failures, scheduled preventive maintenance should be done on all CPB equipment, and should consist of routine safety and performance testing, lubrication, cleaning, and component replacement. Instruments should be periodically calibrated and realigned. After a certain amount of use, pump components should be overhauled to assure longevity of function.[28] Some feel that a prebypass checklist is very important to be sure that all components of the CPB system have been installed correctly and are functioning properly prior to initiating bypass[29] (see Table 13.1). Lastly, backup equipment, such as a hand crank, a battery power supply, additional pump heads or a backup pump, and a backup oxygen source, should be checked and made easily available prior to the initiation of bypass.

Avoiding Inadequate Oxygenation

Inadequate oxygenation can be avoided by frequent blood-gas analysis while the patient is on bypass. In-line blood-gas analyzers can be used but should be verified periodically with arterial blood gases (see Chapter 13). Monitoring of continuous venous oxygen saturation is a common practice during CPB. A slowly decreasing saturation in a patient who is receiving adequate flow may be an early warning of a decrease in oxygen delivery, but it may also signify an increase in oxygen use, as in the case of a lightly anesthetized patient who is shivering or moving.

If a membrane oxygenator is in use, it should be properly sized to the patient (see Chapter 10). The oxygenator (any type) should be positioned in a place where it is not likely to be knocked over or kicked. A spare oxygenator should always be readily available in case of oxygenator failure or physical damage. If an oxygen-air blender is in use, an oxygen analyzer with an audible alarm should be placed in the gas line to the oxygenator, to ensure that the blender is functioning properly. As mentioned above, an auxiliary oxygen source should be readily available in case of oxygen wall-supply failure.

Preventing Inadequate Perfusion

Hypoperfusion is mostly due to other causes, as listed in the previous section (CPB Complications Surveys). The perfusionist should always be prepared to add volume (including packed red blood cells) to the CPB machine reser-

TABLE 18.8. Signs associated with aortic cannulation site problems.

	Arterial line pressure	Blood pressure		Face		Late findings	Metabolic	Misc.
		RRA	LRA	Right	Left			
Cannula toward innominate artery	↑	↑	↓	Plethoric	Pale	Right facial edema, otorrhea, rhinorrhea	↓ U/O ↓ pH	—
Cannula toward left common carotid artery	↑	↓	↑	Pale	Plethoric	Left facial edema, otorrhea, rhinorrhea	↓ U/O ↓ pH	—
Cannula toward aortic valve	↑	—	—	—	—	—	—	Severe AI Left ventricular distention
Aortic dissection	↑	↓	↓	Variable		—	↓ U/O ↓ pH	Decreasing venous reservoir level

RRA, right radial artery; LRA, left radial artery; U/O, urine output; AI, aortic insufficiency

voir in case of low volume. A manometer located in the arterial line will warn the perfusionist of abnormally high resistance and will warn of impending arterial line rupture in the event of sudden kinking or occlusion of that line. Elevated arterial line pressures should make the perfusionist think of all the critical possibilities, such as aortic dissection (especially if elevated pressure is associated with decreasing reservoir volume and hypotension) and malposition of the aortic cannula. Any suspicion or concern should be communicated to the surgeon and the anesthesiologist immediately, so that possible problems can be further investigated (Table 18.8). Lastly, all tubing connections should be banded to decrease the chance of line separation.

Preventing Protamine and Incorrect Drug Administration

A protamine reaction cannot be predicted, and the entire cardiac team must be aware that an untoward life-threatening response to protamine may occur in any patient. When protamine is started, cardiotomy suction should be stopped so that no protamine interacts with the heparinized blood in the pump. Thus, the pump will be ready to go, in the event that the patient becomes extremely hemodynamically compromised and needs to go back on bypass. Protamine should always be given slowly to decrease the possibility of developing hypotension.

All drugs that are administered to the patient should be in clearly labeled syringes with the concentration plainly marked. The perfusionist or anesthesiologist who administers the drug should double-check its name and concentration prior to injecting it. Positioning the label so that it lies along the long axis of the syringe, just below the gradations, ensures that the person who is injecting the drug sees the label, since that person has to look at the gradations to see the volume to be injected.

Management of Perfusion Complications

Air Embolism

Even though the incidence of massive air embolism is very low (0.08–0.2%),[2–4,30] these occurrences are well represented in the literature.[30–35] Numerous case reports and articles document the severity of this problem once it occurs and also offer interventions, hopefully to decrease its associated morbidity (Table 18.9).

If an air embolism occurs, the bypass pump must be stopped immediately. Some recommend reversing the pump temporarily to aspirate as much air as possible from the aorta.[32] The patient should be placed in a steep Trendelenburg position to allow air in the ascending aorta to

TABLE 18.9. Management of massive air embolism during CPB.

Intraoperative interventions
   Immediately discontinue bypass
   Institute Trendelenburg position
   Remove aortic cannula
   Reprime CPB circuit
   Initiate retrograde perfusion of superior vena cava
   Reinstitute CPB with hypothermia, increased perfusion pressure, and 100% oxygen
   Bleed air from coronary arteries
   Consider pharmacologic interventions:
      Barbiturates
      Steroids
      Mannitol
Postoperative interventions
   Institute hyperbaric oxygen treatment
   Place patient in reverse Trendelenburg position
   Institute slight hyperventilation
   Avoid hyperglycemia and hyponatremia

accumulate at the aortic root. The aortic cannula should be removed to allow escape of air to the atmosphere through the cannulation site. If the source of embolization is the pump, the entire circuit must be reprimed and cleared of air.

In many reported cases, retrograde perfusion of the cerebral circuit via the superior vena cava was used to flush air from the cerebral vessels back to the aortic arch and allow air to escape through the cannulation site in the ascending aorta.[30,36-38] This is performed by attaching the aortic cannula (after the circuit has been de-aired) to a cannula in the superior vena cava and initiating flow of 1 to 2 L/min[30,36,38] or keeping a pressure of 40 mm Hg[37] for 1 to 10 minutes or until no more air can be detected escaping from the hole in the ascending aorta. Temporary pressure on the carotids during this maneuver will promote retrograde purging of air from the vertebral system.[30] Hendriks et al[39] evaluated the effectiveness of venoarterial perfusion by injecting a known quantity of nitrogen into the arterial line of pigs on CPB, and measuring the amount of gas that returned to the aortic root during retrograde perfusion. They found that only 47% of the gas could be retrieved after 15 minutes. This study shows that this technique is effective in removing *some* of the embolized gas, but a large portion is still left behind, with the potential to cause ischemia.

Next, the patient should be placed back on CPB with hypothermia (18°-30°C), the systemic pressures should be increased, and 100% oxygen should be administered. Decreasing the temperature of the blood will increase the solubility of the gas in the bubbles, hopefully decreasing their size. Increasing the perfusion pressure will drive the smaller bubbles more distally, or possibly even to the venous side, to allow perfusion of more of the microvasculature. Some recommend pulsatile perfusion to increase further cerebral blood flow.[31] The use of 100% oxygen will increase the partial pressure gradient for nitrogen, promoting faster absorption of air bubbles. In addition, hypothermia will decrease cerebral metabolism, so that cerebral parenchyma that is temporarily ischemic, as bubbles decrease in size or move distally, is less likely to undergo permanent damage.

One group has recommended placing small puncture holes in the distal coronary arteries with a 25-gauge needle while massaging these arteries, to remove air from the coronary circuit before attempting separation from CPB.[30]

Pharmacologic treatment of air embolism includes high-dose barbiturates, high-dose steroids, and mannitol. Sodium pentothal has been used in some cases, with doses ranging from 2 g to 10 mg/kg.[30,32] Dexamethasone, 1 to 10 mg/kg,[30,31,34] methylprednisolone, 2 g,[32] and 20% mannitol[31] have also been used to attenuate the ischemic morbidities associated with air embolism.

Hyperbaric oxygen has also been used for the treatment of air in the arterial circulation. Since the late 1800s, it has been known that increasing atmospheric pressure can be used to treat a decompression sickness that is secondary to nitrogen bubbles in the blood. There are many case reports of hyperbaric oxygen treatments producing a probable improvement in neurologic outcome in patients with air emboli.[33,38,40-42] Increasing atmospheric pressure will decrease the volume (and size) of gas bubbles in the blood. Hyperbaric oxygen significantly increases the partial pressure of oxygen in the blood, increasing the diffusion gradient for nitrogen, which promotes air bubble absorption. Also, the increased oxygen tension in the blood will increase the blood-to-tissue gradient and promote better oxygen delivery to tissues with already compromised blood flow.[41] Since, after all the intraoperative measures are taken, there will probably still be a large amount of air remaining in the cerebral vasculature, as demonstrated by Hendriks et al,[39] it is best to initiate this treatment as early as possible to decrease the amount of irreversible ischemic injury. Some recommend starting treatment even before the patient awakens from the anesthesia, if it is known that a large air embolus has occurred. Even after a delay in treatment, however, there have been reports of postoperative improvement.[41,42]

Other postoperative measures that can be taken include decreasing intracranial pressure by tilting the head of the bed up, keeping the head in neutral position to decease jugular vein distension, slight hyperventilation, and avoiding hyponatremia to keep cerebral edema to a minimum. In addition, since hyperglycemia likely is associated with increased neurologic injury, maintaining a normal glucose may be important.

Electrical and Mechanical Failures

The problems associated with electrical or mechanical failures can be minimized by having (1) well-developed and well-rehearsed backup plans that can be followed quickly and efficiently, even under stressful conditions, and (2) readily available equipment. In the event of an electrical failure, the perfusionist should be able to maintain perfusion with minimal delay, using a hand crank and then a well-charged backup battery power source until wall power can be restored by hospital maintenance personnel. In the event of a mechanical failure, the perfusionist should have at hand a backup pump head and should be able to switch heads quickly. Additional perfusion personnel can be very helpful in this situation, and a backup, complete CPB machine should always be available.

Inadequate Oxygenation and Hypoperfusion

A decrease in the venous saturation while flow is at an adequate cardiac index may be an early warning of a decrease in oxygen delivery secondary to a decrease in the fraction of oxygen in the inlet gas (FiO_2), a decrease in hematocrit, or a failing oxygenator. It also may be due to increased oxygen use. An arterial blood-gas analysis should be requested immediately, but in the meantime, the problem should be communicated to the cardiac team. If the anesthesiologist determines that the patient is not paralyzed, additional muscle relaxant and anesthetic can be administered to decrease shivering and the concomitant increase in oxygen use. If the blood-gas analysis shows adequate PaO_2 but there is a metabolic acidosis and a low hematocrit, administration of packed red blood cells can be considered. If the PaO_2 is low, a failing oxygenator or a decrease in the FiO_2 should be considered. The oxygen pressure and the oxygen monitor should be checked, and the oxygen-air blender should be turned to 100%. If the wall oxygen supply has failed, an oxygen cylinder should be connected to the oxygen input. The perfusionist should bypass the blender if it is suspected to be malfunctioning. If the oxygen source and the blender appear to be working, failure of the oxygenator should be considered. All perfusionists should be well versed in emergency oxygenator changes and should periodically rehearse this procedure. Of course, as mentioned previously, a spare oxygenator should be readily available.

Many of the causes of hypoperfusion are not in the control of the perfusionist. If the perfusionist must decrease the pump flow because of inadequate volume, this fact should be communicated to the rest of the cardiac team so that the surgeon can check the venous line for obstruction (air lock or mechanical obstruction) and look for lost volume in the pleural space or undetected blood loss. The anesthesiologist should decrease any venodilating drugs that might be in use. An increase in aortic line pressure should be immediately announced so that the surgeon can check for kinks in the line or evidence of malposition of the aortic cannula or dissection.

Extracorporeal Circuit Line Separation

A line separation is in the control of the perfusionist, who should have on hand replacement connectors and tubing (in case of contamination of the separated line), and should be able to repair and de-air the separated line expeditiously.

Protamine Reactions

The management of a protamine reaction depends on the specific type of the reaction. If the reaction is just mild hypotension, the treatment can consist of adding volume, or a small dose of vasoconstrictor, such as phenylephrine or norepinephrine. These reactions are usually self-limited and may not require any treatment at all. If the reaction is anaphylactic or anaphylactoid, the treatment consists of 100% oxygen, intravenous fluids, antihistamines, steroids, and early aggressive use of epinephrine and vasoconstrictors, to maintain adequate perfusion pressure.[20] Aminophylline and possibly isoproterenol can be used to treat bronchospasm. With a Type III reaction that involves severe pulmonary vasoconstriction and systemic hypotension, aggressive administration of epinephrine and isoproterenol is indicated. The CPB machine should be still available and uncontaminated with protamine, so that CPB can be initiated in the event of inadequate perfusion due to the critical transpulmonary gradient and right ventricular failure. If vasoconstrictors are deemed necessary, they should be administered through a left atrial line to avoid the pulmonary circuit and decrease the chance of exacerbating the pulmonary hypertension.

Drug Errors

Treatment of drug errors depends, of course, on the particular drug that was given incorrectly. If an overdose of a vasoconstrictor is given and the resultant hypertension is significant, it can be treated with a titrated dose of a vasodilator, such as sodium nitroprusside. If the patient is off bypass, the reverse Trendelenburg position decreases preload to the heart and decreases blood pressure. If an overdose of a vasodilator is given, significant hypotension can be treated with a vasoconstrictor or the Trendelenburg position (if the patient is not on bypass). Accidental administration of protamine while the patient is on CPB is a life-threatening error which should be treated immediately with an additional dose of heparin while a second oxygenator is made ready in the event the oxygenator becomes clotted. Blood products, such as fresh frozen plasma, platelets, and cryoprecipitate, should be made ready in the blood bank to treat the consumptive coagulopathy that will most likely be present after separation from CPB.

The treatment of post-CPB coagulopathy is a complicated issue that will not be discussed in this section. It is addressed extensively in Chapter 9.

Conclusion

Due to the complex nature of cardiac surgery and perfusion practice, there always exists the possibility of error and resultant patient morbidity or death. We have seen that systems such as CPB are vulnerable to accidents. Three studies that evaluated accidents with CPB, however, demonstrated only a small incidence of various mishaps, with even fewer resulting in permanent injury or death. It must be remembered that these studies were all retrospective, by survey, and prone to all of the biases that these types of studies exhibit. The true value of the studies is that they delineate the vast majority of possible perfusion mishaps, so that the cardiac team can anticipate, attempt to prevent, and be prepared to deal, quickly and efficiently, with any perturbation that occurs. This calls for keen awareness of the possible accidents, constant vigilance, good communication among team members, and mental preparedness.

References

1. Kirklin JW, Barratt-Boyer BG. Hypothermia, circulatory arrest, and cardiopulmonary bypass. In: Kirklin JW, Barratt-Boyer BG, eds. *Cardiac Surgery* 2nd ed. New York: Churchill Livingstone; 1993;75.
2. Stoney WS, Alford WC Jr, Burrus GR, et al. Air embolism and other accidents using pump oxygenators. *Ann Thorac Surg* 1980;29:336-340.
3. Wheeldon DR. Can cardiopulmonary bypass be a safe procedure? In: Longmore DB, ed. *Towards Safer Cardiac Surgery*. Lancaster, London: MTP; 1981:427-446.
4. Kurusz M, Conti VR, Arens JF, et al. Perfusion accident survey. *Proc Am Acad Cardiovasc Perf* 1986;7:57-65.
5. Gaba DM, Maxwell M, Deanda A. Anesthetic mishaps: breaking the chain of accident evolution. *Anesthesiology* 1987;66:670-676.
6. Keenan RL, Boyan CP. Cardiac arrest due to anesthesia—a study of incidence and causes. *JAMA* 1985;253:2373-2377.
7. Cooper JB, Newbower RS, Long CD, et al. Preventable anesthesia mishaps: a study of human factors. *Anesthesiology* 1978;49:399-406.
8. Cooper JB, Newbower RS, Kitz RJ. An analysis of major errors and equipment failures in anesthesia management: considerations for prevention and detection. *Anesthesiology* 1984;60:34-42.
9. Utting JE, Gray TC, Shelley FC. Human misadventure in anaesthesia. *Can Anaesth Soc J* 1979;26:472-478.
10. Lunn JN, Hunter AR, Scott DB. Anaesthesia-related surgical mortality. *Anaesthesia* 1983;38:1090-1096.
11. Kurusz M, Wheeldon DR. Risk containment during cardiopulmonary bypass. *Semin Thorac Cardiovasc Surg* 1990;2:400-409.
12. Chung F, David TE, Watt J. Excessive requirement for heparin during cardiac surgery. *Can Anaesth Soc J* 1981;28:280-282.
13. Anderson EF. Heparin resistance prior to cardiopulmonary bypass. *Anesthesiology* 1986;64:504-507.
14. Esposito RA, Culliford AT, Colvin SB, et al. Heparin resistance during cardiopulmonary bypass—the role of heparin pretreatment. *J Thorac Cardiovasc Surg* 1983;85:346-353.
15. Bull BS, Korpman RA, Huse WM, et al. Heparin therapy during extracorporeal circulation—I. Problems inherent in existing heparin protocols. *J Thorac Cardiovasc Surg* 1975;69:674-684.
16. Kurusz M, Shaffer CW, Christman EW, et al. Runaway pump head: new cause of gas embolism during cardiopulmonary bypass. *J Thorac Cardiovasc Surg* 1979;77:792-795.
17. Taylor PC, Groves LK, Loop FD, et al. Cannulation of the ascending aorta for cardiopulmonary bypass: experience with 9,000 cases. *J Thorac Cardiovasc Surg* 1976;71:255-258.
18. Ross WT, Lake CL, Wellons HA. Cardiopulmonary bypass complicated by inadvertent carotid cannulation. *Anesthesiology* 1981;54:85-86.
19. McLeskey CH, Cheney FW. A correctable complication of cardiopulmonary bypass. *Anesthesiology* 1982;56:214-216.
20. Horrow JC. Protamine: a review of its toxicity. *Anesth Analg* 1985;64:348-361.
21. Weiler JM, Gellhaus MA, Carter JG, et al. A prospective study of the risk of an immediate adverse reaction to protamine sulfate during cardiopulmonary bypass surgery. *J Allergy Clin Immunol* 1990;85:713-719.
22. Hill AG, Lefrak EA. Cardiopulmonary bypass safety devices and techniques. *Proc Am Acad Cardiovasc Perf* 1985;6:38-42.
23. Vivian WA, Stander KH, Smith GR. An air embolism detection device for use with a non-occlusive arterial pumphead. *J Extracorp Technol* 1987;19:406-407.
24. Blanche C, MacKay D, Lee ME. A new overpressure safety valve for use in the venting line during cardiopulmonary bypass. *Mt Sinai J Med* 1986;53:239-240.
25. Stofer RC, Reed CC. The hidden hazards of perfusion. *Proc Am Acad Cardiovasc Perf* 1982;3:46-48.
26. Oka Y, Inoue T, Hong Y, et al. Retained intracardiac air—transesophageal echocardiography for definition of incidence and monitoring removal by improved techniques. *J Thorac Cardiovasc Surg* 1986;91:329-338.
27. Orihashi K, Matsuura Y, Hamanaka Y, et al. Retained intracardiac air in open heart operations examined by transesophageal echocardiography. *Ann Thorac Surg* 1993;55:1467-1471.
28. Kurusz M, Crane TN, Speer D. Preventive maintenance of heart-lung machines. *Proc Am Acad Cardiovasc Perf* 1985;6:34-37.
29. Crane TN, Keen WR, Spiller CE, et al. A prebypass checklist—why aren't you using one? *Proc Am Acad Cardiovasc Perf* 1986;7:98-100.
30. Mills NL, Ochsner JL. Massive air embolism during cardiopulmonary bypass—causes, prevention, and management. *J Thorac Cardiovasc Surg* 1980;80:708-717.
31. Bayindir O, Paker T, Akpinar B, et al. Case 6 1991—A 58-year-old man had a massive air embolism during cardiopulmonary bypass. *J Cardiothorac Vasc Anesth* 1991;5:627-634.
32. Spampinato N, Stassano P, Gagliardi C, et al. Massive air embolism during cardiopulmonary bypass: successful treatment with immediate hypothermia and circulatory support. *Ann Thorac Surg* 1981;32:602-603.
33. Peirce EC. Specific therapy for arterial air embolism. *Ann Thorac Surg* 1980;29:300-303.
34. Kumar AS, Jayalakshmi TS, Kale SC, et al. Management of massive air embolism during open heart surgery. *Int J Cardiol* 1985;9:413-416.
35. Ghosh PK, Kaplan O, Barak J, et al. Massive arterial air embolism during cardiopulmonary bypass. *J Cardiovasc Surg* 1985;26:248-250.
36. Stark J, Hough J. Air in the aorta: treatment by reversed perfusion. *Ann Thorac Surg* 1986;41:337-338.
37. Brown JW, Dierdorf SF, Moorthy SS, et al. Venoarterial cerebral perfusion for treatment of massive arterial air embolism. *Anesth Analg* 1987;66:673-674.
38. Toscano M, Chiavarelli R, Ruvolo G, et al. Management of

massive air embolism during open-heart surgery with retrograde perfusion of the cerebral vessels and hyperbaric oxygenation. *Thorac Cardiovasc Surg* 1983;31:183–184.

39. Hendriks FFA, Bogers AJJC, de la Riviere AB, et al. The effectiveness of venoarterial perfusion in treatment of arterial air embolism during cardiopulmonary bypass. *Ann Thorac Surg* 1983;36:433–436.

40. Kol S, Ammar R, Weisz G, et al. Hyperbaric oxygenation for arterial air embolism during cardiopulmonary bypass. *Ann Thorac Surg* 1993;55:401–403.

41. Armon C, Deschamps C, Adkinson C, et al. Hyperbaric treatment of cerebral air embolism sustained during an open-heart surgical procedure. *Mayo Clin Proc* 1991;66:565–571.

42. Bitterman H, Melamed Y. Delayed hyperbaric treatment of cerebral air embolism. *Israel J Med Sci* 1993;29:22–26.

Part V(a)
Cardiopulmonary Bypass in Special Patient Populations
Complete Cardiopulmonary Bypass

19
Pediatric Cardiopulmonary Bypass

James M. Bailey and William L. Daly

Introduction

Advances in the treatment of congenital heart disease have resulted in an increase in the number of children, infants, and neonates undergoing surgical procedures that require cardiopulmonary bypass (CPB). In a 1990 survey of 127 North American pediatric programs, Groom et al[1] reported 11,721 pediatric surgical procedures with CPB in 1988, 12,826 in 1989, and an estimated 14,473 in 1990. Innovative procedures have been developed for the correction of complex lesions.[2-4] Implementation of extracorporeal circulation for these procedures is complicated by the technical difficulties associated with patient size and the multiple types and complexity of congenital heart abnormalities (Table 19.1). What are usually routine procedures for establishing and conducting CPB in adults with normal cardiac anatomy are more complicated in the patient with congenital heart disease. These difficulties are compounded by the fact that, according to Groom et al,[1] 81% of pediatric cases are done in institutions that do fewer than 150 cases annually.

In this chapter, we will focus on aspects of CPB which are unique to pediatric patients, particularly neonates and infants. Additionally, details of anesthetic management and patient monitoring will be discussed. Long-term support for respiratory distress or extracorporeal membrane oxygenation (ECMO) is not discussed in this chapter, but rather in Chapter 29. We have tried to avoid duplicating discussions found elsewhere in this volume, but this is difficult, since many techniques and practices in pediatric perfusion are extrapolations from experience with adults. This is illustrated by the fact that a standard, computerized literature search, cross-indexed to the search terms "cardiopulmonary bypass" and "pediatrics," yielded only 168 articles for the period from 1966 to 1991. Because many aspects of pediatric CPB have not been rigorously investigated, our discussion inevitably draws heavily on our own experience. We hope we have sufficiently emphasized that established fact (or near-fact) and local custom are not always synonymous.

The fundamental problems in conducting pediatric extracorporeal circulation are (1) small circulating volumes and (2) high oxygen consumption.[5,6] Additionally, difficulties in thermoregulation, due to ratios of body surface area to weight, the use of profound hypothermia (with and without total circulatory arrest), and a reduced tolerance of microemboli are characteristic of pediatric perfusion.[7,8] The wide range of patient sizes and blood flow requirements precludes the standardization of pediatric perfusion circuitry. Other complicating factors are congenital cardiac anomalies that result in collateral blood flow, intra- and extracardiac shunts, and lesions that usually require open cardiac chambers during the repair.

Preparation for CPB: Equipment

Oxygenators

A complete discussion of both membrane and bubble oxygenators is found in Chapter 10. This section focuses on issues unique to pediatric oxygenators. Modern pediatric oxygenators and circuitry are increasingly adaptable, and may be integrated in multiple configurations for specific patient and institutional requirements. Both integrated and component system membrane lungs, as well as bubble oxygenators, have reduced priming volumes and enhanced gas transfer characteristics; for the above-noted reasons, these features are important in the diverse pediatric patient population. In the 1990 survey by Groom et al,[1] 102 of 126 responding institutions performing pediatric CPB used membrane oxygenators exclusively. Unfortunately, the minimum dynamic volume requirement of these oxygenators commonly equals or exceeds the patient's entire circulating volume.[9] Therefore, the specific

TABLE 19.1. Diagnostic frequencies of congenital cardiac lesions requiring CPB for repair.

Ventricular septal defect	15.7%
D-transposition of the great arteries	9.9%
Tetralogy of Fallot	8.9%
Hypoplastic left ventricle	7.4%
Endocardial cushion defect	5.0%
Pulmonary stenosis	3.3%
Pulmonary atresia (intact ventricular septum)	3.1%
Atrial septal defect, secundum	2.9%
Total anomalous pulmonary venous return	2.6%
Tricuspid atresia	2.6%
Single ventricle	2.4%
Aortic stenosis	1.9%
Double outlet right ventricle	1.5%
Truncus arteriosus	1.4%

Data from Fyler DC. Report of the New England Regional Infant Cardiac Program. *Pediatrics* 1980; 65 (suppl): 375–461.

metabolic requirements of the patient and the length and complexity of the particular procedure must be considered when selecting a device for a patient. The oxygenator's prime should be as small as possible to minimize hemodilution and heterologous blood requirements, but large enough to adequately transfer sufficient oxygen and carbon dioxide for the duration of the CPB perfusion. The smallest membrane lungs have membrane surface areas between 0.4 and 0.6 m^2, with static priming volumes between 135 and 290 mL, and are suitable for flows up to 1.5 L/min. Component membrane systems and bubble oxygenators have smaller static priming volumes, but very similar dynamic volume requirements during operation. Different oxygenators have specific advantages and disadvantages, and this is especially true of pediatric devices. Many suitable bubble and membrane artificial lungs require several discrete devices dictated by patient size, necessitating device-matching decisions and increased inventory. Bubble oxygenators offer no independent oxygen and carbon dioxide control, the latter being important in cerebral autoregulation of flows and metabolism.[10,11] There is evidence that bubble oxygenators cause greater blood trauma, especially in very long procedures.[12,13] Some closed-membrane systems require complex setup and debubbling procedures. Additional disadvantages of these systems include poor venous reservoir resolution and venous air handling capabilities due to nonvented soft-bag reservoirs. In addition to the oxygenator's capacity to provide consistent long-term support, accurate volume resolution and venous air handling characteristics are critical aspects of pediatric perfusion that distinguish it from adult perfusion. In our institution, the Cobe Variable Prime Membrane Lung is utilized because it is an open, integrated system with a compartmentalized membrane surface area, suitable for most patients under approximately 50 kg (Figure 19.1). The SciMed Membrane Oxygenator is currently being used for long-term support (ECMO), and hollow-fiber membrane oxygenators with heparin-bonded and bioactive coatings are being investigated. These coatings are now widely available on artificial lungs and tubing, and, although they are more expensive, they may increase the life expectancy of the devices

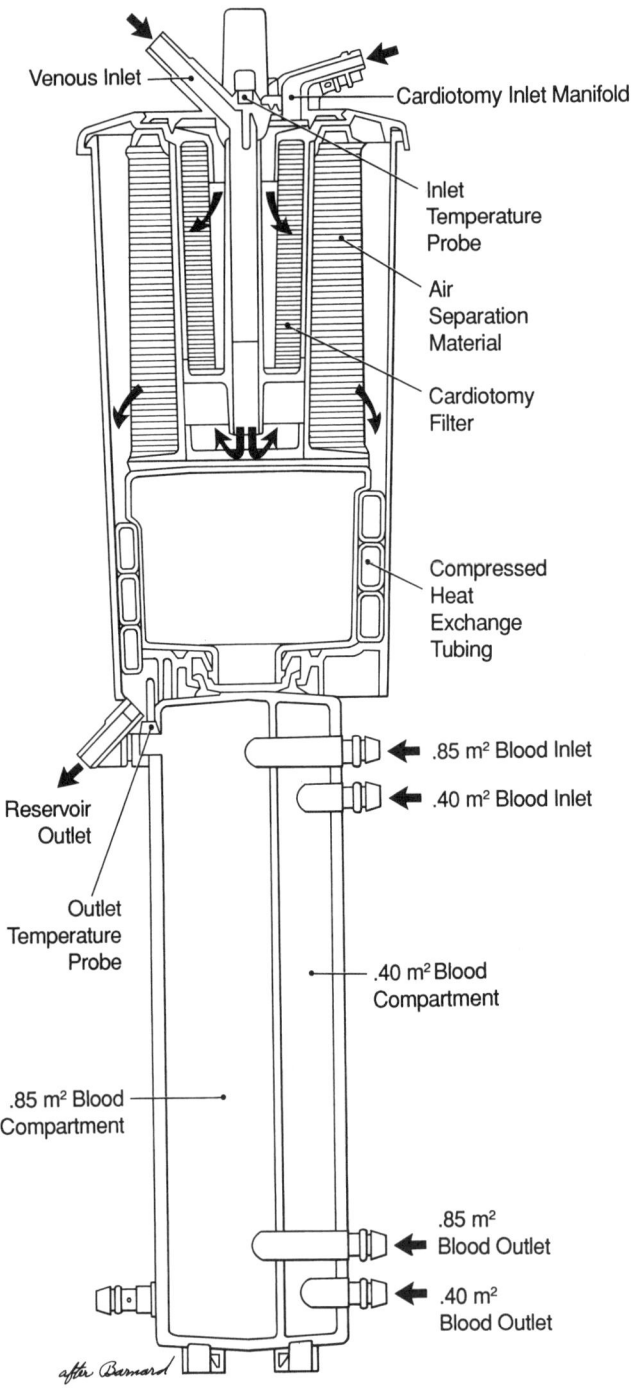

FIGURE 19.1. Diagram of a typical membrane oxygenator.

TABLE 19.2. Tubing prime volume.

¼-inch tubing	9.6 mL/foot
⅜-inch tubing	21.7 mL/foot
½-inch tubing	38.6 mL/foot

and promise to diminish certain coagulation and inflammatory response problems.[14-16]

Tubing

After the oxygenator, the extracorporeal tubing constitutes the largest reservoir of circuit volume. The tubing type and size, the dynamic holdup, and the performance characteristics must be considered when constructing the extracorporeal circuit and calculating the total priming volume. The length of the tubing should be minimized to decrease resistance to flow and lessen hemodilution and blood product usage. Conversely, the tubing must be of adequate size and tube wall thickness to ensure satisfactory flow and line pressure characteristics and to ensure durability and flexibility. Priming volumes are dependent on internal diameter of the tubing and are generalized in Table 19.2.

Flows of 2 L/min or less are necessary for ¼-inch arterial lines and pump headers, as a higher flow necessitates an increase in the head rotations per minute (rpm); this results in excessive arterial line pressures and an increased rate of tubing fatigue that can threaten circuit integrity. These problems can be eliminated by using ⅜-inch tubing when flows greater than 2 L are required. The use of ⅜-inch venous line tubing minimizes resistance, maximizes venous return to the oxygenator, and enhances the perfusionist's control of venous volumes in the majority of pediatric patients. However, in the smallest neonates, many perfusionists prefer to use ¼-inch venous lines. Although this size tubing is adequate for low pump flows, it can be very difficult to reprime manually in the event of an air lock or to partially occlude the tubing when weaning from bypass or performing other maneuvers. One-half-inch venous line tubing, commonly used for adults, is used in very large adolescents who require higher pump flows because of higher metabolic rates and larger body surface areas. Improvements in tubing durability and the availability of heparin-impregnated and bioactive, bonded tubing may also result in decreased anticoagulation requirements and an attenuated inflammatory response associated with CPB.[17-19]

Filters

Arterial line filters are widely used in adult extracorporeal circuits[20] and, as reported by Groom et al,[1] over 81% of pediatric CPB procedures include arterial line filtration. CPB circuit filters, as used in adult perfusion, are discussed in detail in Chapter 12. In pediatric perfusion, arterial line filters should have small priming volumes, low resistances, and acceptable low- and high-flow characteristics in order to minimize hemodilution, excessive line pressures, and damage or aggregation of formed blood elements. Membrane oxygenators are thought to produce fewer microemboli than bubble oxygenators; therefore, arterial line filters are particularly important in the latter system.[21] We utilize all types of filtration, including pre-bypass circuit, arterial line, cardiotomy reservoir, blood transfusion, leukocyte removal, and gas line filters. We use the Pall Pre-Bypass Plus Filter, which has the smallest pore size available (0.2 μm) for filtration of the noncellular components of the perfusate. These are effective in eliminating particulate debris or bacterial contamination of the extracorporeal circuit.[22] We also include Pall Ultipor 40-μm extracorporeal blood filters in our arterial lines with either ¼-inch ports and 35-mL priming volume for pump flows of 2 L or less, or ⅜-inch ports and 190-mL priming volume for higher flows. The arterial line filter is an important safety device, as it acts as the final "trap" for air or particulate emboli.[23] Although greater line resistance, hemodilution, and blood trauma may be potentially undesirable features of CPB circuit filters, there is evidence that neonates and infants are especially vulnerable to the untoward effects of particulate microembolization,[24,25] and, in general, there are few reasons to exclude filters on any CPB circuit. Filters on both the arterial and venous sides of the extracorporeal circuit are important safety devices, and the prophylactic benefits far outweigh any potential problems associated with their use, especially in pediatric CPB.

Prime/Hemodilution

Both the volume and the composition of the circuit prime may have an impact on the outcome of extracorporeal perfusion of the pediatric patient, especially the neonate.[26-28] A common pediatric pump circuit has a total prime volume of between 500 and 1200 mL. The constituents of a typical circuit prime are listed in Table 19.3. The primary component is a balanced electrolyte solution. In addition, albumin is often added to the prime to precoat the circuit, particularly the membrane, and as a volume expander, because of its osmotic and colloidal properties.[29] Addition of albumin to the prime may also enhance platelet function after CPB.[30] Mannitol is included in the prime because it may enhance renal function on CPB.[31,32] These additives lower the crystalloid and/or heterologous blood requirement of the prime and possibly decrease fluid requirements during perfusion, although this is still a debated issue.[32-35]

In most pediatric cases, some degree of hemodilution is well tolerated and even beneficial, if only temporarily,

TABLE 19.3. Constituents of prime for pediatric extracorporeal circuit.

Constituent	Volume/amount
Plasma-lyte-A or Normosol-R (pH 7.40)	400–1200 mL
Red packed cells or fresh whole blood	0–600 mL
Mannitol 15%	1 g/kg
Albumin 25%	50 mL
NaHCO$_3$	25 mEq/L
CaCl$_2$	30 mg/kg
Heparin	2 U/mL prime
Total volume	700–1200 mL

during hypothermia.[36,37] Hemodilution improves peripheral circulation by decreasing sludging in the capillaries and prevents damage to formed elements, while decreasing heterologous blood requirements.[38,39] However, the extent of hemodilution should reflect the diagnosis, degree of functional impairment, and planned surgical procedure of the specific patient. Palliative procedures such as systemic-pulmonary shunts, atrial septectomy, or relief of critical valvular stenosis in the newborn often necessitate normal physiologic hematocrits, since the patient may remain cyanotic after the procedure or because normothermic CPB is employed.[40,41] In order to calculate the degree of hemodilution, one must consider circuit prime volume, patient blood volume, and hematocrit.[42] A formula to determine the volume of blood that must be added to the prime to achieve a given hematocrit after the initiation of CPB is given in Figure 19.2. (Note that this formula does not take into account hemodilution secondary to cardioplegia.) Blood conservation should be undertaken during all phases of the surgical procedure.[43,44] In our institution, we use autologous blood collection and hemofiltration in every case; use of a hemoconcentrator during CPB, in particular, seems to have decreased use of bank blood. The size of the patient and the type or extent of the repair will largely determine the blood requirements of a specific case.[45,46] When blood products are required in the prime, we prefer fresh (<48 hours), cytomegalovirus-negative, leukocyte-depleted packed cells. Fresh whole blood, when available, is preferred for neonates during CPB or in the postbypass period.[47] Heterologous blood should not be necessary for surgical repair of isolated, less complex cardiac lesions, such as atrial septal defects. These may require aggressive blood salvaging while on CPB, with immediate rinsing and use of all volume left in the pump circuit.[44–46,48] However, even simple repairs on smaller patients may require heterologous blood, and it is often not possible to manage complex procedures using CPB without blood.

$$V = [H_d \times (BV + CV) - H_p \times BV]/H_b$$

V = volume of blood needed in prime
H$_d$ = desired hematocrit on CPB
H$_p$ = patient hematocrit prior to CPB
H$_b$ = hematocrit of blood to be added to prime
BV = patient's circulating blood volume
CV = extracorporeal circuit volume

FIGURE 19.2. Formula for the calculation of the volume of blood needed in the extracorporeal circuit prime.

Preparation for CPB: The Patient

Anesthesia

There is increasing evidence that anesthetic technique affects the neurohumoral response to CPB; thus, any discussion of CPB must include the topic of anesthetic management for the pediatric cardiac surgical patient. Details of the "stress response" to bypass are discussed in Chapter 9, where there are also references to the extensive literature describing hormonal and inflammatory changes during CPB. This response appears to be much more pronounced in the pediatric patient.[49] While the stress response has an obvious adaptive value to an organism, some believe that excessive neurohormonal and inflammatory responsivity may be harmful. Anand et al[50] have found that the magnitude of the hormonal response to noncardiac thoracic surgery in preterm infants correlates with outcome. In this study, nitrous oxide anesthesia for patent ductus arteriosus ligation was compared to nitrous oxide supplemented with fentanyl (10 mg/kg). Patients receiving fentanyl had a blunted stress response and fewer perioperative complications. More recently, Anand and Hickey[51] have compared two groups of neonates undergoing cardiac surgery. One group received halothane/morphine as the primary anesthetic/postoperative analgesic while the other group was given high-dose sufentanil. Both the hormonal response and mortality were higher in the patients receiving halothane/morphine. These studies suggest that overly "light" anesthesia may be as deleterious as excessively "deep" anesthesia. Importantly, the observation that neonates have neurohormonal responses to what would be regarded as a painful stimulus by adults has discredited (as has other evidence) the notion that neonates are insensitive to noxious stimuli and do not require anesthesia.

Anesthesia for adult cardiac surgery that requires CPB is discussed elsewhere in this book; therefore, this chapter will be confined to anesthetic management considerations specific to the pediatric patient. Since infants and children are seldom as cooperative as adult patients, anesthetic induction is made more pleasant for the patient, and for the operating room staff, if the patient receives appropriate premedication. Premedication appears to be generally safe, even for the cyanotic patient.[52] Because children fear needles, oral premedication is preferred. Pentobarbital, 1 to 4 mg/kg, is effective and can be given with an elixir of meperidine and atropine in children who are older or more active.[53] As an alternative, oral midazolam can provide excellent sedation with a relatively rapid onset.[54] We routinely include oral atropine in our premedication to attenuate cardiovascular depression during induction of anesthesia with halothane.[55] In general, we do not administer any sedative-hypnotic as premedication to infants under 6 months of age, and use only pentobarbital for children who are 6 months to 1 year old. Obviously, the selection of premedication must be individualized. It should be noted that there has been a great deal of recent interest in the pediatric anesthesia literature on alternative routes of delivering premedicants. Fentanyl "lollipops," nasal midazolam, and rectal barbiturates are among the "preinduction" sedative techniques that have been investigated. The role of these techniques in pediatric cardiac anesthesia has not been established.

Induction is often a stressful period for the patient and the pediatric cardiac anesthesiologist. If the patient arrives in the operating room with a venous catheter in place, or if venous access can be readily established, anesthesia induction can proceed as it would for an adult using any of several intravenous agents. We prefer intravenous opioid induction anesthesia in high-risk patients. Even neonates tolerate a fentanyl or sufentanil induction if bradycardia is averted by the appropriate use of pancuronium or atropine.[56,57]

Inhalation or intramuscular induction of anesthesia is indicated in children who do not have, or who resist placement of, an intravenous catheter. This is the major difference in anesthetic management for pediatric and adult patients.

The safety of inhalation induction is attested to by years of clinical experience, but myocardial depression does occur, with halothane causing more depression than isoflurane.[58] Halothane is our preferred inhalational induction agent, however, as it is less irritating to the airway and is less likely to result in increases in pulmonary artery pressure due to coughing, laryngospasm, and/or hypercarbia.[59] Even in cyanotic patients, halothane and nitrous oxide, administered with attention to airway maintenance, heart rate, blood pressure, and peripheral perfusion, induce general anesthesia safely and effectively.[60–62]

As an alternative to inhalation agents, anesthesia can be induced by intramuscular injection of ketamine, 2 to 5 mg/kg.[63] Although ketamine has a long history of use in congenital heart disease patients, there have been concerns that it might increase pulmonary vascular resistance. However, Morray et al[64] and Hickey et al[65] demonstrated insignificant hemodynamic changes after ketamine administration, as long as the airway and ventilation were maintained. The hemodynamic stability after ketamine administration would suggest that it is well suited for the induction of anesthesia in critically ill neonates. The safety of this agent in cyanotic patients has been confirmed in recent studies.[60,61]

Table 19.4 outlines the advantages and disadvantages of different induction techniques for children undergoing cardiac surgery.

After induction, anesthesia may be maintained with opioids or inhalation agents. In patients undergoing less complex operations, in which hemodynamic stability and possible early extubation are anticipated, inhalation agents (supplemented with opioids for analgesic effects) are appropriate. This necessitates that the extracorporeal circuit be equipped with a vaporizer. Conversely, in more complex cases, opioids are used as the primary maintenance anesthetics, as the myocardial depressant effects of inhalation agents may not be tolerated. There is also evidence that the stress response is more pronounced with inhalation agents.[51] Opioid anesthetic requirements are not well defined for pediatric patients. Yaster[66] has demonstrated that fentanyl, 10 to 12.5 mg/kg, is an adequate dose for the first 30 minutes of thoracic surgery (patent ductus arteriosus ligation) in neonates, when hemodynamic responses are used as the indicators of inadequate anesthetic level. For cardiac surgery involving CPB (and procedures lengthier than patent ductus arteriosus ligation), a variety of doses have been reported, most ranging from 50 to 100 mg/kg of fentanyl (with comparable doses of other opioids). Dosage is usually based on hemodynamic responses to noxious stimuli, although it is important to remember that critically ill patients may not be capable of mounting a hemodynamic response, and paralysis will mask the movement that would be a sign of inadequate anesthesia. This is an important issue which deserves further study in light of Anand and Hickey's[50] data suggesting that suppression of the stress response improves outcome. In this study, the patients in the sufentanil group (who had a lower mortality rate) received a minimum 20 mg/kg in the operating room, with additional sufentanil for sedation during the first 24 hours in the intensive care unit. Their results imply that optimal opioid doses may be higher than previously thought, although confirmation of this requires further study. Addition of a benzodiazepine should lower opioid requirements, although this has not been systematically studied in the pediatric cardiac surgical patient.

Monitoring

Noninvasive monitoring of the pediatric patient is very similar to that of the adult patient and includes (1) an electrocardiogram with multiple lead capabilities, (2) noninvasive blood pressure measurement, (3) tempera-

TABLE 19.4. Pediatric cardiac anesthetic induction techniques.

Technique	Advantages	Disadvantages
Inhalation	Control of anesthetic depth	Airway irritation myocardial depression
Intramuscular	Ease of administration	Poorly controlled plasma levels
Intravenous	Ease of administration More predictable plasma levels (vs IM)	Need for access prior to induction

ture measurement from multiple sites (nasopharyngeal, esophageal, or tympanic and a core temperature such as bladder or rectal), and (4) pulse oximetry (Table 19.5). We view pulse oximetry as one of our most important monitors, since the majority of patients with congenital heart disease have some sort of communication between the systemic and pulmonary circulations, with the possibility of left-to-right or right-to-left shunting. Pulse oximetry often allows quick detection of changes in the magnitude and direction of shunt flow. We also view the pulse oximeter as a useful indirect indicator of the adequacy of cardiac output. A decrease in peripheral perfusion will result in a loss of the pulse oximeter signal.[67] It is our clinical impression that in the normothermic patient, the inability of the pulse oximeter to detect a pulse indicates poor peripheral perfusion and probably low cardiac output. This is often a harbinger of metabolic acidosis and decreased urine output. Since pulse oximetry is one of our most important monitors, we often employ multiple probes, including one on the tongue or buccal mucosa, which often can be used to monitor oxygenation when the signal is lost on a distal extremity due to hypothermia or poor perfusion.[68]

Invasive monitoring in infants and children is best initiated after induction of general anesthesia and establishment of venous access. This will include bladder catheterization, placement of an arterial catheter for monitoring of blood pressure and collection of samples for blood-gas analysis, and, in many institutions, placement of a central venous catheter. Invasive monitoring catheters can be placed either percutaneously or by surgical "cutdown." We believe that surgical cutdown should be used only after percutaneous cannulation has been attempted, as it is well documented that the incidence of catheter-associated infection is significantly reduced by percutaneous insertion.[69]

Appropriate sites for arterial catheter placement include the radial, axillary, and femoral arteries. The radial artery has been commonly employed because the consequences of ischemia due to arterial occlusion are presumably less. However, it has been demonstrated that blood pressure measured in the radial artery is often falsely low (relative to a central aortic pressure) after CPB.[70] Furthermore, the more distal, smaller radial artery is often more difficult to cannulate than larger, more central, axillary or femoral arteries, and we often employ an axillary or femoral artery catheter in small infants and neonates. The safety of axillary or femoral arterial catheters has been documented in recent reports.[71,72] In general, we expect the femoral or axillary pressure to more accurately reflect central aortic pressure, although we have observed significant pressure gradients between the femoral artery and the aorta in a few patients (Figure 19.3).

At our institution, we routinely place central venous catheters via the internal jugular vein (although we may cannulate the subclavian, femoral, or external jugular veins). Central venous catheters are not essential to the conduct of surgery or CPB, since intracardiac catheters can be placed by the surgeon.[73] However, we find them helpful, providing the anesthesiologist with an index of preload and a secure route for the administration of vasoactive drugs into the central circulation. This is especially important for patients presenting for "redo" surgery, when opening the sternum is often time-consuming and is sometimes complicated by profuse hemorrhage and dysrhythmias. In the past 5 years, we have had no complication of central venous catheter insertion more significant than minor hematomas. The primary consequence of the procedure is an increase in the time required for preparation of the patient for surgery. Our experience is consistent with a recently published study.[74]

Pulmonary artery catheters, which are often used for

TABLE 19.5. Pediatric patient monitors for cardiac surgery and CPB.

Noninvasive
  Precordial and esophageal stethoscope
  Pulse oximeter
  ECG
  Blood pressure
  End-tidal CO_2
  Temperature (multiple sites)
  Echocardiography
  EEG
Invasive
  Blood pressure
  Bladder catheter
  Central venous pressure (optional)
  Right atrial pressure (optional)
  Left atrial pressure (optional)
  Pulmonary artery pressure (optional)
  Cardiac output thermistor (optional)

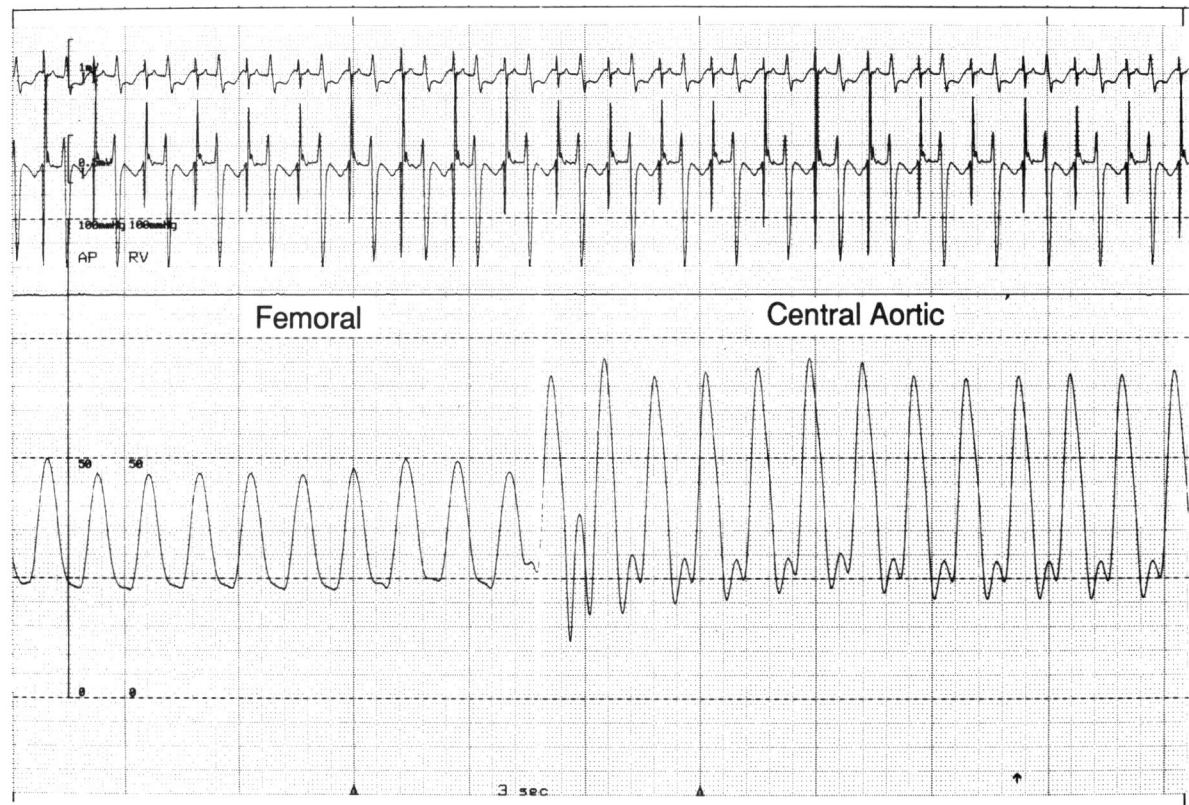

FIGURE 19.3. An illustration of the discrepancy between central aortic and femoral arterial blood pressure which may be found after CPB.

monitoring of adult cardiac surgical patients, are seldom used in pediatric patients. The size of the catheters, relative to the size of the patients, and the difficulty of floating the tip into the pulmonary artery in patients with intracardiac lesions, have greatly limited the use of percutaneous, balloon-tipped catheters. Recently, Introna et al[75] reported on the use of a new generation of smaller pulmonary artery catheters in pediatric patients. The report was interesting, although it was apparent that flotation into the pulmonary artery was difficult and sometimes required fluoroscopy. In general, if measurement of pulmonary artery pressures is desired, a transthoracic pulmonary artery catheter is more expeditiously placed by the surgeon. Similarly, if measurement of cardiac output by thermodilution is essential to postoperative management, a thermistor can be placed directly in the pulmonary artery.[76] However, the need for additional intracardiac catheters is the reason that measurement of pulmonary artery pressure and thermodilution cardiac output is not routine in pediatric patients. The alternative for direct monitoring of cardiac output is dye dilution, which is more time-consuming and not suited to frequent repetitive measurements.

Table 19.5 summarizes monitoring techniques for pediatric cardiac surgery.

Anticoagulation

Management of anticoagulation for the pediatric patient is very similar to that in adult practice, which is extensively reviewed in Chapter 5. Young et al[77] demonstrated that fibrinolysis could not be detected in five pediatric patients (as indicated by fibrin monomer formation) if the activated clotting time (ACT) was 450 seconds or higher. Although other studies suggest that even lower ACT values are safe,[78] an ACT > 450 seconds provides a margin of safety against the risks of fibrinolysis and precipitation of disseminated intravascular coagulation during CPB. There is some institutional variation in the initial doses of heparin used to achieve this ACT value, and doses as low as 200 U/kg have been reported.[49] Excessive heparin doses require higher protamine for neutralization, with a greater risk of protamine neutralization-related complications. We employ an initial dose of heparin of 400 U/kg, which is somewhat higher but consistent with the usual length of operation at our institution. We monitor the level of anticoagulation with frequent ACT measurement. It is common for the ACT to be quite prolonged during profound hypothermia, and then to drop precipitously during rewarming. Accordingly, we continuously monitor the ACT during rewarming, drawing a new sample for measure-

TABLE 19.6. Arterial cannula guide: flow requirement vs cannula size.

Flow (L/min)	Cannula size (French)
0–0.5	8
0.5–1.0	10
1.0–1.75	12
1.75–2.75	14
2.75–3.5	16
3.5–4.5	18

ment as soon as the previous one exceeds 600 seconds. We have not found direct measurement of heparin levels (by automated protamine titration) to be of value, since heparin concentrations inhibiting fibrinolysis have not been defined. However, this opinion must be tempered by the realization that very few studies of the management of anticoagulation for CPB have specifically addressed the pediatric patient.

Cannulation

Arterial and venous cannulation in the pediatric patient, and especially the neonate, can be difficult. Small hearts and hypoplastic vessels make the size and type of cannula used critical in minimizing the morbidity associated with extracorporeal perfusion. In general, an 8F aortic cannula can be used for flows up to 500 mL/min and should be increased 2 French sizes for every additional 500 to 700 mL/min flow. The actual internal diameter and pressure drop across the cannula, the circuit configuration, the size of the aorta, and the existence of shunts or collaterals will influence the size actually used and the difficulty of insertion. A guide to approximate aortic cannula sizes is presented in Table 19.6.

Arterial line pressures should always be monitored in order to diagnose misplaced or improperly sized cannulas. An arterial cannula that is malpositioned may result in nonuniform perfusion or coronary ischemia. Furthermore, an overly large or malpositioned aortic cannula may obstruct normal ejection and greatly complicate separation from CPB by masking the true hemodynamics of the patient (Figure 19.4). Modifications of aortic cannulation are often necessary for specific cases, such as the repair of hypoplastic left heart syndrome or interrupted aortic arch. Discontinuity, or near-discontinuity, of the ascending and descending aorta makes it necessary to "Y" the arterial line into two cannulas (Figure 19.5), allowing separate perfusion of upper and lower systemic circulations. Insertion of a "T" connector between the arterial line and the cannula in the hypoplastic aorta allows cardioplegic solution to be delivered via the aortic arterial cannula once the ascending aorta has been clamped distal to the cannula and the aortic line is clamped proximal to the "T" connector after circulatory arrest. Venous cannulation can be equally troublesome. Choosing the proper size cannula is more difficult and more subjective than the typical one-size-fits-all approach used for many adults. General guidelines are presented in Table 19.7. The manner of venous cannulation will obviously depend on the planned procedure. For cases to be performed under circulatory arrest, a single venous cannula in the systemic venous atrium will often suffice. Otherwise, total bypass with

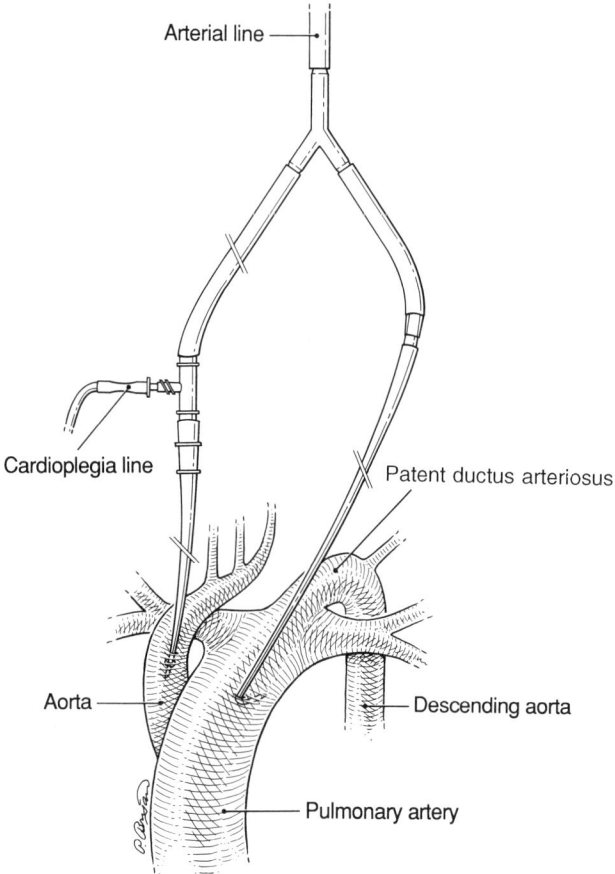

FIGURE 19.5. Double cannulation of the ascending aorta and the pulmonary artery used for severe aortic atresia or interrupted aortic arch via a Y-connector. Note that the left and right branch pulmonary arteries must be occluded distal to the cannula during CPB to prevent runoff into the pulmonary circulation.

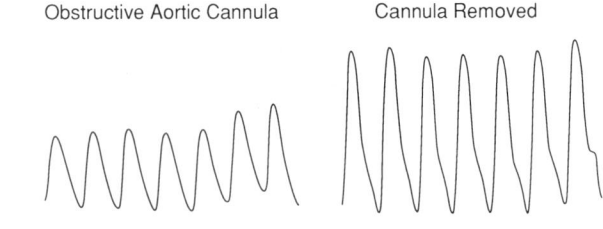

FIGURE 19.4. An illustration of the effects of an obstructive aortic cannula on systemic blood pressure.

TABLE 19.7. Venous cannula guide: flow vs size in double and single cannula.

Flow (L/min)	Size (French)	
	Double venous	Single venous
0–0.5	16	18
0.5–1.0	18	20
1.0–1.25	20	24
1.25–1.6	22	26
1.6–1.8	24	28
1.8–2.2	26	30
2.2–2.8	28	32
2.8–3.2	30	32
3.2–3.6	32	34
3.6–4.0	34	36

cannulas extending up and down the venae cavae with caval tapes may be necessary to maintain a clear surgical field. In some procedures that involve intraatrial manipulation, the venae cavae may be directly cannulated using right-angle catheters for improved access and visibility of the heart. The presence of a persistent left superior vena cava may also necessitate its separate cannulation.

Conduct of CPB

Initiation of CPB

The initiation of CPB should provoke careful assessment of the adequacy of perfusion, by the perfusionist and surgeon and by the anesthesiologist. This is facilitated by monitoring of systemic blood pressure, filling pressures, the electrocardiogram, and temperature gradients, and by constant visual inspection of the patient and the surgical field. In-line monitors of the extracorporeal circuit are listed in Table 19.8. A suggested "checklist" that may be used to assess the adequacy of perfusion on initiation of CPB is provided in Table 19.9.

Hypotension is common at the onset of CPB. This is often ameliorated by a slow initiation of CPB, maintaining some cardiac ejection on the part of the patient. If the hypotension does not resolve after a few minutes, the monitoring system should be recalibrated and blood pres-

TABLE 19.8. Extracorporeal circuit monitors.

Arterial line pressure
Venous hemoglobin oxygen saturation
Cardioplegia line pressure
In-line arterial blood gas analysis
Arterial blood temperature
Venous blood pressure
Myocardial temperature
Cardioplegia temperature

TABLE 19.9. Initiation of CPB checklist: assessing adequacy of perfusion.

Evaluate the adequacy of flow
  Blood pressure
  Arterial line pressure
  Mixed venous hemoglobin oxygen saturation
  Uniformity of peripheral perfusion (color, capillary refill)
  Temperature gradients
Evaluate the adequacy of venous return
  Appearance of the heart
  Filling pressures
  Inspection of the face (superior vena cava syndrome)
  Palpation of the anterior fontanel
  Inspection of the abdomen (distension)
  Net circuit volume balance
Evaluate metabolic status
  In-line acid/base monitor
  In-line hematocrit measurement
  Arterial blood gas

sure also measured in the aortic root to ensure that the hypotension is real, and then consideration should be given to the various possible causes. The most common cause is decreased systemic vascular resistance secondary to hemodilution. However, mechanical factors must be considered. There is always the risk of a malpositioned aortic cannula in neonates or infants, causing apparent hypotension (depending on the site of blood pressure measurement). It is imperative that this possibility be considered and, if confirmed, corrected. Another possible cause of hypotension is the presence of open systemic-pulmonary vascular shunts. Because of the low impedance of the pulmonary vasculature, a "steal" phenomenon will occur, with hypoperfusion of the systemic circulation and hyperperfusion of the pulmonary circulation, both of which are undesirable. Systemic-to-pulmonary shunts such as a patent ductus arteriosus, pre-existing palliative shunts, or even naturally occurring collateral vessels should be closed, whenever possible, prior to or at the initiation of CPB.

The majority of pediatric cases require some degree of hypothermia, and passive surface cooling can be started prior to CPB, simply by not taking measures to maintain normothermia. This can be quite effective in small infants, and there may be theoretical advantages to surface cooling (while there is pulsatile flow),[79] although one must be prepared for the hemodynamic consequences, bradycardia and hypotension.[80] In general, however, cooling is most efficiently accomplished on bypass. Optimal flows during cooling and rewarming have not been strictly determined. Several studies have demonstrated that, as flow rate is decreased, tissue oxygenation is initially maintained by increasing oxygen extraction, with a resultant lowering of the mixed venous oxygen content. However, as perfusion is further decreased, oxygen extraction becomes limited and both total oxygen consumption and tissue oxygenation decrease. This is associated with lactic acidosis.[81,82] It seems logical to assume that this may be a clear indication of inadequate flow, with impending tissue damage. It also suggests that mixed venous oxygenation saturation can be used as a global indicator of the adequacy of flow rates. By using an in-line monitor of venous oxygen saturation (SvO_2), continuous assessment of perfusion is readily available.[83]

We usually employ flow rates of 120 to 150 mL/kg during normothermia, cooling, and rewarming. This maintains tissue oxygenation, as evaluated by mixed venous oxygen saturation, and provides for efficient cooling and rewarming. Excessively high flow rates should be avoided, since they may result in greater edema and may exacerbate the inflammatory response to CPB.[84]

The most common limiting factor to flow rates is venous return, and all members of the team should be vigilant for signs that it is inadequate. At various times, the venous return can come not only from venous cannulas, but also from pump "suckers" and intracardiac vents. Even in the smallest circuits, the dynamic holdup of the tubing alone can be significant and complicate patient management, especially when on "sucker" bypass. Additional fluids added to maintain circuit integrity, or irrigation scavenged from the field, must be identified and carefully considered when evaluating venous return. The perfusionist should keep a careful record of fluid balance, and the surgeon and anesthesiologist should frequently evaluate the volume of the heart, inspect the abdomen for signs of ascites, and inspect the face and head (especially the anterior fontanelle in the infant) for a superior vena cava syndrome (Figure 19.6). This is especially important after caval tapes are tightened to produce total bypass. In some situations, venous return can be improved simply by raising the height of the operating room table. The venous cannulas may need to be repositioned, or a different size cannula used, if venous return remains inadequate. Inadequate venous drainage also can result from cannulas being inserted too far into either the superior or the inferior vena cava, obstructing the innominate vein or the hepatic vein respectively, and causing either cerebral edema or liver and mesenteric distension. Inadequate venous return, with a persistently flooded surgical field after caval tape tightening, should suggest the possibility of a persistent left superior vena cava.

There is evidence that neurologic injury after hypothermic arrest, or low-flow bypass, may be exacerbated by hyperglycemia and may be diminished by alkalosis.[85,86]

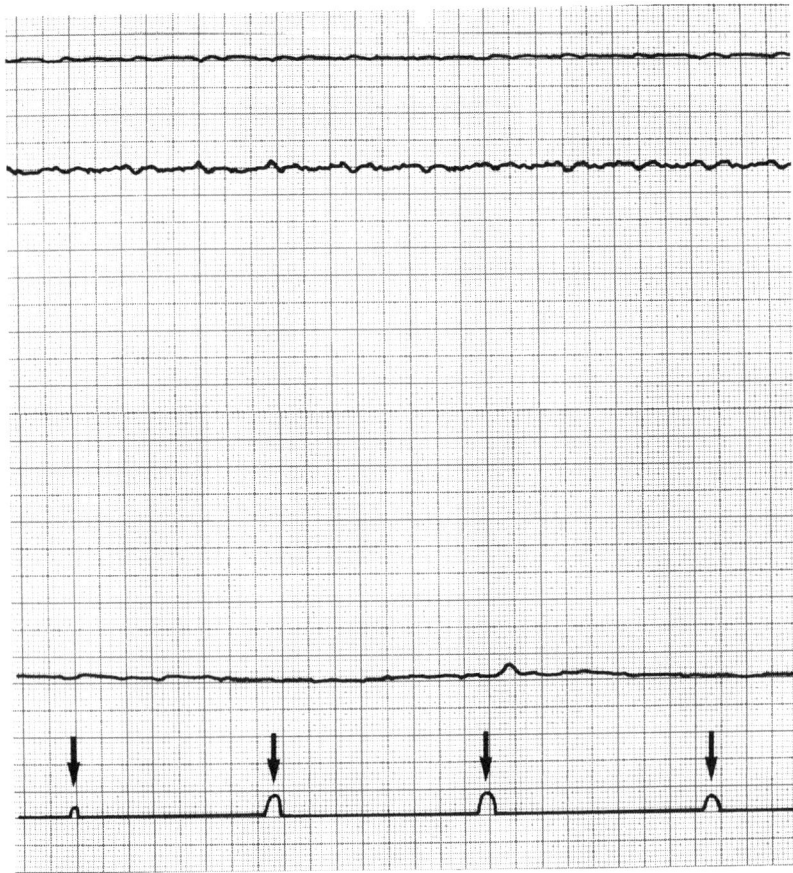

FIGURE 19.6. Impaired venous return on CPB results in increased anterior fontanel pressure as manifested by the increases in central venous pressure (*arrows*, lower trace) associated with palpation of the fontanel.

Therefore, after the initiation of CPB, the patient's metabolism must be monitored with frequent measurement of arterial blood gases, electrolytes, and glucose.

Maintenance of CPB

General Considerations

To be a surgically useful tool, CPB must be not only safe but also flexible. Arterial flow is one variable that can be manipulated, with reduction in flow rates resulting in better operating conditions. Surgical field requirements can, to a large extent, determine flow rates. In order for lower flow rates to be tolerated, some degree of hypothermia is necessary, and it is logical to classify pediatric perfusion in terms of the degree of hypothermia (Table 19.10).

Normothermic perfusion is primarily employed for older children and straightforward cases, such as the repair of an atrial septal defect, although it is occasionally used for infants having very simple operations (such as an atrial septectomy) or for larger children having more complicated procedures. Because hypothermia is not employed, higher flow rates are required. It should also be noted that normothermia may necessitate higher hematocrits while the patient is on CPB.

Moderate hypothermic perfusion (25°–30°C) is also frequently employed for larger children undergoing straightforward repairs. The repair of a ventricular septal defect or subaortic membrane in children who are out of infancy are examples of procedures in this category. Flow rates may be lowered and titrated to global tissue oxygenation on the basis of mixed venous hemoglobin oxygen saturation.[81-83] However, since most congenital heart surgery includes intracardiac repair, bicaval cannulation and total bypass may be required. Inadequate venous return may limit flow rates and result in fluid losses and unnecessary patient edema.

Profound hypothermic perfusion (18°C or lower) is used when the complexity of the repair and/or the small size of the heart, necessitates the superior operating conditions provided by low flows. Limits to safe flow rates are discussed below. Venous blood returns via atrial cannulas extending up and down the cavae or by direct caval cannulation, and is often supplemented by suction from the surgical field and intracardiac vents. Even with low CPB flows, net loss of fluid from the pump to the patient may occur.

The final category of pediatric perfusion is circulatory arrest. As discussed in detail in Chapter 3, circulatory arrest offers superb operating conditions and appears to be safe when limited in duration. When circulatory arrest is anticipated, only a single venous cannula is necessary. Prior to arrest, the patient is exsanguinated by keeping the venous line open until the administration of cardioplegia is complete, and by inflating the lungs to force blood from the pulmonary veins. During the arrest period, gas flow is stopped or significantly reduced, and the perfusate is recirculated through the oxygenator. Resumption of perfusion requires meticulous attention to the prevention of air embolism, including aspiration of air from the ascending aorta, often via the same catheter used to administer cardioplegia.

As we have noted above, decreased oxygen consumption with hypothermia allows bypass flow rates to be lowered without compromising global tissue oxygenation (as assessed by acid-base balance and mixed-venous hemoglobin oxygen saturation). However, although mixed venous hemoglobin oxygen saturation content may remain within normal physiologic limits during hypothermia, specific tissue damage may occur, since an indicator of *total* body tissue oxygenation does not guarantee that specific organs are not hypoperfused. Very little is known about regional perfusion regulation during hypothermic low flow. Although both renal failure and hepatic dysfunction are relatively common in the pediatric patient after CPB, it is generally agreed that the organ most sensitive to hypoperfusion is the brain. Greely et al[87] have demonstrated that the cerebral metabolic rate is an exponential function of temperature, thus documenting what has been an article of faith in pediatric cardiac surgery. The reduction in metabolic rate at 18°C, and the coupling of cerebral blood flow and metabolism, would suggest that very low flows should prevent cerebral ischemia at this temperature.

The question of whether deep hypothermic total circulatory arrest (DHTCA) is preferable to low-flow bypass is still a topic of intense debate.[88,89] The advantages of DHTCA include a bloodless surgical field and less trauma

TABLE 19.10. Classification of pediatric CPB cases by intraoperative temperature requirements.

Normothermia
    Atrial septal defect repair
    Aortic or pulmonary valvotomy
    Atrial septectomy
    Systemic-pulmonary shunts (requiring CPB)
Moderate hypothermia
    Ventricular septal defect repair
    Subaortic membrane resection
    Repair of pulmonary stenosis
    Bidirectional Glenn shunt
Profound hypothermia
    Ventricular setpal defect repair (infant)
    Atrioventricular canal defect repair
    Tetralogy of Fallot repair (infant)
    Arterial switch
Circulatory arrest
    Hypoplastic left heart syndrome palliation (Norwood stage I)
    Procedures cited for profound hypothermia when completion requires < 1 h

to blood elements, presumably with a less pronounced inflammatory response to CPB. If continuous-flow CPB is employed rather than DHTCA, it is logical that the lowest safe flows should be employed. Fox et al[90] have shown that cerebral oxygen consumption is maintained in monkeys with flows as low as 0.5 L/min/m^2 during profound hypothermia. Watanabe et al[91] found that canine brain tissue oxygen tension was maintained with flows of 25 mL/kg/min during profound hypothermia. Rebeyka et al[92] noted that somatosensory neural transmission was maintained in dogs at flows as low as 0.25 L/min/m^2. Miyamoto et al[93] found that cerebral oxygen consumption in dogs did not decrease with flows as low as 30 mL/kg/min, a value for the threshold of maintenance of cerebral oxygen consumption identical to that reported for infants and children by Kern et al.[94]

It would appear from these studies that flows as low as 30 mL/kg/min or 0.5 L/min/m^2 will preserve neurologic function. However, there are contradictory data. Rossi et al[86] have found equally high elevations in a marker of cerebral ischemia, creatinine kinase BB, after low-flow bypass and hypothermic arrest. Also Taylor et al[95] have observed immediate loss of middle cerebral artery flow (using transcranial Doppler measurements of blood velocity) upon reduction of pump flow to 0.6 L/min in neonates during profound hypothermia. This group has suggested that these disparities may be explained by postulating a critical opening pressure for the cerebral circulation, and noted that studies of cerebral blood flow at low systemic flow have not controlled cerebral perfusion pressure. This assumption is consistent with the observations of Greely et al[96] that cerebral flow becomes pressure dependent with profound hypothermia (loss of autoregulation). In a subsequent study, Taylor et al[97] demonstrated that there is no cerebral blood flow during profound hypothermia in neonates and infants if the cerebral perfusion pressure is less than 10 torr. Conversely, these studies suggest that flows as low as 30 mL/kg/min during profound hypothermia are neurologically tolerated if cerebral perfusion pressure exceeds 10 torr. More recently, Newburger et al[98] have prospectively compared neurologic outcome in the perioperative period for neonates randomly assigned to repair of transposition of the great arteries (via the arterial suited procedure) with circulatory arrest or continuous low-flow perfusion. The low-flow group had perfusion maintained at 50 mL/kg/min (roughly 0.7 L/min/m^2) during the primary repair. Patients in the circulatory arrest group had a high risk of perioperative surgeries, as well as more pronounced electroencephalographic and laboratory (creatinine kinase BB) evidence of neurologic dysfunction.

An interesting clinical question is whether raising the blood pressure pharmacologically, while maintaining a constant systemic flow rate, offers any benefit to the patient. This question has not yet been addressed in any systematic study. We do not attempt to control blood pressure independently of flow rate during low-flow bypass and profound hypothermia, because this issue is unresolved and because it is our clinical impression that pediatric patients are very unresponsive to α-agonists during profound hypothermia. However, during normothermic bypass, we do attempt to maintain mean systemic blood pressures above 40 torr in neonates and infants, since Kurth et al[99] have shown, using near infrared reflectance spectroscopy, that brain oxyhemoglobin levels decrease below this pressure threshold.

Although there are numerous studies of cerebral blood flow and metabolism during bypass, virtually nothing is known about the relationship between systemic perfusion and pressure, the flow to other organs (liver, mesentery, kidney), the extent to which organ function is impaired by low-flow bypass, and whether blood pressure is an independent determinant of function. Hopefully, a better understanding of these questions will evolve in the near future.

Acid-Base Management During CPB

Since acid-base management (alpha-stat versus pH-stat) is discussed elsewhere in this book (see Chapters 3 and 6), we will only note that alpha-stat management preserves coupling of cerebral flow and metabolism and pressure-flow autoregulation at temperatures above 22°C and has been advocated, for this reason, in adults. However, it is not clear which is the optimal acid-base management for the pediatric patient. Kern et al[100] have shown that the response of the cerebral circulation to carbon dioxide is preserved during hypothermia in infants and children, although the magnitude of this response is diminished by deep hypothermia and also when it is employed in children under 1 year. Thus, pH-stat management could be deleterious because of hyperperfusion of the brain with increased cerebral edema. Conversely, during very low flows (an uncommon situation in adult surgery), basal cerebral flow may be inadequate and pH-stat management could be protective. Presently, it is impossible to judge which is the optimal approach. We currently utilize alpha-stat management, primarily because autoregulation is preserved during moderate hypothermia with this approach, and also because of evidence that neurologic injury may be diminished if the patient is alkalotic.[85,86] However, as we have tried to emphasize, further studies may show this approach to be inappropriate.

Separation from CPB

Preparation for separation from CPB begins during rewarming. Blood and blood products should be ordered, if needed. Vasoactive drug requirements for separation from CPB should be anticipated and infusions prepared (with appropriate pumps) prior to their expected use. Blood samples should be drawn frequently for analysis and correction of metabolic abnormalities and adjustment of the hematocrit. Recommendations for preparation for separation from CPB are listed in Table 19.11.

Efficient rewarming requires higher flows than are needed during the primary surgical repair. When flow rate is increased, vasoconstriction will often become apparent with an elevated blood pressure. There is evidence that administration of a vasodilator will not only control hypertension, but will promote more uniform rewarming and result in less extreme thermal fluctuations in the postoperative period.[101] Phentolamine has frequently been employed, with 0.1 mg/kg given at the start of rewarming.[49] However, we prefer to use sodium nitroprusside, because its pharmacokinetic properties facilitate rapid titration to effect control of blood pressure. If hypertension cannot be readily controlled by doses of sodium nitroprusside of 4 to 5 mg/kg/min, then phentolamine can also be administered, or isoflurane can be added via a vaporizer incorporated into the circuit. Usually, as rewarming progresses, patients become less constricted and vasodilators are not tolerated. Excessive rewarming can result in significant vasodilation and is not only associated with sinus tachycardia but also with other, more malignant, atrial dysrhythmias.[102] There is considerable institutional variation in the temperatures accepted for separation from CPB. We strive for an esophageal temperature of 37°C, but no more than 38°C, with a bladder temperature of 35.5°C or greater.

When the primary surgical repair is completed and an organized rhythm is established, caval tapes can be released, cannulas withdrawn into the atrium, and vents removed, resulting in partial bypass. The next step in preparation for separation from CPB is re-establishment of ventilation. The mediastinum and pleural spaces should be inspected while the lungs are gently inflated. Bilateral lung expansion should be confirmed and atelectatic areas reexpanded. We find it useful to irrigate and suction the endotracheal tube to ensure patency and to clear secretions. The pleural spaces, if open, should be drained of fluid. The importance of these simple procedures cannot be overstated, since a major cause of hemodynamic instability in the pediatric patient is pulmonary hypertension. This can be greatly exacerbated by hypoxia and hypercarbia, so it is vital that pulmonary function be optimized.[103]

Separation from CPB should not be attempted until the hematocrit and metabolic status are appropriate for the patient. The optimal hematocrit may vary markedly from patient to patient. Anemia is often well tolerated, because it is compensated for by a decrease in afterload, due to lower blood viscosity, and an increase in contractility, due to increased endogenous sympathetic tone.[104] However, this is not the case if myocardial function or hemoglobin oxygenation is impaired. Administration of blood should be done on a case-by-case basis. For example, patients undergoing palliative procedures, who will depend on a shunt for pulmonary blood flow, will be relatively hypoxic after the repair. The normal response to this hypoxia is polycythemia, and it would seem rational to adjust the hematocrit accordingly prior to separation from CPB. However, a healthy 4-year-old having a simple procedure, such as correction of an atrial septal defect, will tolerate a very low hematocrit.

In general, acid-base status and electrolytes should be within normal limits. We would, in particular, emphasize the importance of normocalcemia. Recent studies have demonstrated that the inotropic state of the immature myocardium is very dependent on plasma ionized calcium, presumably due to a poorly developed sarcoplasmic reticulum.[105] Ionized calcium levels decrease with the initiation of CPB.[106] Although calcium levels tend to normalize after this initial decline, this is not a consistent finding. Furthermore, the administration of blood at the end of bypass exacerbates this hypocalcemia. We routinely administer 45 mg/kg of calcium chloride (in divided doses of 30 and 15 mg/kg) prior to separation from CPB. Frequently, in small infants, even these doses do not fully correct the hypocalcemia caused by CPB and by the administration of heterologous blood.

Once the patient is adequately rewarmed, ventilation re-established, and hematocrit, acid-base balance, and electrolytes adjusted as appropriate to the specific patient, separation from bypass can be attempted. Decision-making during this procedure is facilitated by considering the determinants of cardiac output. Table 19.12 lists strategies to maximize cardiac output on separation from CPB. Cardiac output is equal to the product of heart rate and stroke volume. Thus, before attempting to wean from CPB, an appropriate heart rate and rhythm must be established. Heart block is a major risk of congenital heart surgery, and when it occurs, pacing may be necessary. Atrial

TABLE 19.11. Preparation for separation from CPB.

Airway
   Evacuation of pleural spaces/chest tube insertion, if indicated
   Irrigation and suction of endotracheal tube
   Bilateral lung expansion with appropriate airway pressures
   Treatment of bronchospasm, if indicated
Balance of physiologic parameters
   Temperature control (room, warming blanket)
   Continuous monitoring of anticoagulation
   Availability of blood and/or blood products
   Correction of hematocrit
   Correction of acid-base and electrolyte status
Circulation
   Pacemaker availability (preferably with DDD mode)
   Treatment of vasoconstriction or vasodilation on CPB
   Preparation of inotrope infusions

TABLE 19.12. Strategies for optimizing cardiac output after CPB.

Rate and rhythm
  Bradycardia
    May be corrected with atropine, catecholamines, or pacing. Atrial pacing is generally preferable to ventricular pacing. If bradycardia is due to conduction block, atrial-ventricular pacing is employed. If there is a rapid supraventricular rate, use of temporary DDD pacing is recommended.
  Tachycardia
    Cardioversion for atrial fibrillation, atrial flutter, supraventricular tachycardias, and, obviously, ventricular tachydysrhythmias. Treat possible underlying causes of sinus or nodal tachycardia, such as light anesthesia, hypovolemia, or hyperthermia. Otherwise, exercise caution, as the tachycardia may be the patient's only means of maintaining cardiac output.
Stroke volume
  Optimize preload.
  When preload is optimized, add inotropic support.
  Consider afterload reduction when systemic and/or filling pressures are stable.
Assess the repair (PRIMARY IMPORTANCE)
  Pressure measurements in relevant chambers of the heart and great vessels.
  Hemoglobin oxygen saturations in relevant chambers and great vessels.
  Intraoperative echocardiography.

pacing is preferred, but when atrial pacing is not possible, atrial-ventricular pacing is preferred over ventricular (if the intrinsic atrial rate is slow enough), as the atrial "kick" augments stroke volume. We usually pace at a rate near the normal value for the patient's age, but there is considerable room for empirical adjustment of the rate to maximize cardiac output. Unfortunately, it is not uncommon for the intrinsic atrial rate in a patient with heart block to be too high to allow efficient atrial-ventricular (A-V) pacing using commonly employed demand A-V sequential (DVI) pacing units. However universal, fully automatic (DDD) pacing units are now available for temporary use in the operating room, and they promise to enhance our pacing capabilities.

After establishment of an acceptable heart rate and rhythm, one can focus on the generation of an adequate stroke volume. Stroke volume is determined by preload, contractility, and afterload. Preload can sometimes be assessed by monitoring of central venous pressure, or right atrial pressure, but often it is vital to monitor both right atrial (or central venous) and left atrial pressure. We begin separation from bypass by having the perfusionist lower the flow by 25% while gently filling the heart. The response to this maneuver can be used to assess the contractile state of the heart. If the pulse pressure remains low, despite a significant increase in filling pressure, inotropic agents may be started. Our first-line inotrope is dopamine, primarily because of its mixed dopaminergic, α-agonist, β-agonist activity.[107-109] Once the inotrope is started (and sufficient time has elapsed for the dead space of the line of administration to be cleared), the flow is lowered by another 25% increment. The response to this maneuver is evaluated by consideration of the pulse pressure and the filling pressures. Since dopamine's inotropic property is in part mediated indirectly via the release of norepinephrine stores, it may be relatively ineffective in patients with depleted catecholamine stores and additional inotropic support may be needed. The β_1 and β_2 properties of isoproterenol may be beneficial for patients in heart block or with pulmonary hypertension, especially since dopamine may raise pulmonary pressure,[110] although this is not a consistent finding at usual doses.[108,109] Dobutamine is an alternative which has been touted as causing less tachycardia than isoproterenol, although this is not a consistent finding.[111] Epinephrine is used to treat frank hypotension in the presence of adequate filling of the heart, when dopamine is ineffective.

It should be remembered that if cardiac performance is significantly impaired, afterload reduction may be beneficial. Both sodium nitroprusside and amrinone have been shown to improve cardiac output in the pediatric patient after cardiac surgery,[112-114] and they can be particularly beneficial when α-agonists (epinephrine or high-dose dopamine) are required for separation from CPB. A not uncommon cause of hemodynamic instability in the pediatric patient is pulmonary hypertension and right heart failure. A variety of vasodilators (sodium nitroprusside, nitroglycerin, prostaglandin E_1) can be used in this instance, although the mainstay of therapy is adequate depth of anesthesia and appropriate ventilation.[103,109,115,116] We recommend using a vasodilator during separation from bypass only when some pressure, either systemic, atrial, or pulmonary, is excessively high.

Once decisions about the use of inotropes and/or vasodilators have been made and therapy has been instituted, separation from bypass can be completed in a controlled manner. When the patient is completely separated from bypass, it is important to conduct diagnostic studies. It is uncommon for primary myocardial failure to be the cause of hemodynamic instability after congenital heart surgery. We wish to emphasize that a significant inotropic requirement often indicates an inadequate repair. Thus, after or during separation from CPB, an "operating room catheterization" should be done, with measurement of pressures in all the chambers of the heart and in the pulmonary artery. Residual ventricular defects can be detected by measurement of hemoglobin oxygen saturation in samples drawn from the superior vena cava, inferior vena cava, right atrium, right ventricle, and pulmonary artery, or by dye-dilution curves. Intraoperative echocardiography has a documented role in the evaluation of the surgical repair,[117] and even if not used routinely, as advocated by some centers, it should be available.

Summary

CPB for infants and children presents challenges which are distinct from those encountered during extracorporeal circulation in adult patients. The "one size fits all" approach often used for adults obviously must be modified for a patient population that includes 70-kg adolescents and 3-kg neonates. Furthermore, the conduct of CPB will be determined by the specific anatomic features of each patient and by the need to optimize surgical operating conditions.

The obvious unique characteristics of pediatric perfusion are the size of the patients and the broad spectrum of congenital heart disease. Although it has been possible to downsize equipment, in general, miniaturization has not been proportional to the size of the patients. For many cases, the equipment is "larger than the patient," and this leads to a number of difficulties. Mechanical factors can be a major cause of morbidity associated with CPB, and each member of the operating room team should be aware of this. Both arterial and venous cannulas may be obstructive and easily malpositioned. Venous return is often not sufficient during total CPB to support a normal flow rate without resulting in an obscured surgical field and a markedly positive fluid balance.

The complexity of congenital heart disease and the surgeon's need for a clear, bloodless field will typically necessitate the use of low flows and profound hypothermia. Currently, evidence suggests that very low flows are tolerated by the central nervous system during profound hypothermia. Further investigation will be needed to confirm this and to define more sharply the limits of safe perfusion. Hopefully, future research will also focus on the effects of low flows and deep hypothermia on the function of other organ systems, and on the inflammatory and neuroendocrine response to CPB and how it might be managed.

References

1. Groom RC, Hill A, Kurusz M, et al. Pediatric perfusion survey. *Proc Am Acad Cardiovas Perf* 1990;11:78-84.
2. Laks H. Advances in the repair of complex congenital heart disease. *Pediatr Ann* 1982;11:926-931.
3. Castaneda AR, Mayer JE Jr, Jonas RA, Lock JE, Wessel DL, Hickey PR. The neonate with critical congenital heart disease: a surgical challenge. *J Thorac Cardiovasc Surg* 1989;98:869-875.
4. Esposito G, Keeton BB, Sutherland GR, Monro JL, Manners JM. Open heart surgery in the first 24 hours of life. *Pediatr Cardiol* 1989;10:33-36.
5. Sugimura S, Starr A. Cardiopulmonary bypass in infants under four months of age. *J Thorac Cardiovasc Surg* 1977;73:894-899.
6. Hartley-Winkler M, Lambert JJ, Rohre C. Perfusion considerations for infants weighing ten kilograms or less. *J Extracorp Tech* 1985;17:31-36.
7. Stammers AH, Bove EL. The neonatal heart: developmental differences, response to ischemia and protection during cardiopulmonary bypass. *J Extracorp Tech* 1986;18:210-220.
8. Ferry PC, Neurological sequelae of open-heart surgery in children. *AJDC* 1990;144:309-312.
9. Conley JC, Zografos CA. Bloodless prime in pediatric cardiopulmonary bypass circuits. *J Extracorp Tech* 1991;23:80-82.
10. Murkin JM, Farrar JK, Tweed WA, McKenzie FN, Guiraudon G. Cerebral autoregulation and flow/metabolism coupling during cardiopulmonary bypass: the influence of $Paco_2$. *Anesth Analg* 1987;66:825-832.
11. Bashein AL, Townes BD, Nessly ML. A randomized study of carbon dioxide management during hypothermic cardiopulmonary bypass. *Anesthesiology* 1990;72:7-15.
12. Belboul A, Khaja NA, Hirayama T, Dahlin A, Karlson H, Roberts D. Comparison of Terumo fiber membrane and Harvey 1500 bubble oxygenators using red cell microrheology analysis during cardiopulmonary bypass. *J Extracorp Tech* 1987;19:209-215.
13. Wright JS, Fisk GC, Torda TA, Stacey RB, Hicks RG. Some advantages of the membrane oxygenator for open heart surgery. *J Thorac Cardiovasc Surg* 1975;69:884-890.
14. Von Segesser LK, Lachat M, Leskosek B, Turina M. Cardiopulmonary bypass with low systemic heparinization: an experimental study. *Perfusion* 1990;5:267-276.
15. Olsson P. Non-thrombogenic systems for extra-corporeal gas exchange. *Int J Artif Organs* 1990;13:594.
16. Nilson L. Heparin-coated equipment reduces complement activation during cardiopulmonary bypass in the pig. *Int J Artif Organs* 1990;14:46-48.
17. Andrade JD, Coleman DL, Didisheim P. Blood materials interactions, 20 years of frustration. Synopsis of panel conference. *Trans Am Soc Artif Intern Organs* 1981;27:659.
18. Mottaghy K, Oedekoven B, Poppel K, et al. Heparin free long-term extracorporeal circulation using bioactive surfaces. *ASAIO Trans* 1989;35:635-637.
19. Barry YA, Labow RS, Keon WJ, Tocchi M, Rock G. Perioperative exposure to plasticizers in patients undergoing cardiopulmonary bypass. *J Thorac Cardiovasc Surg* 1989;97:900-905.
20. Hill JD. Blood filtration during extracorporeal circulation. *Ann Thorac Surg* 1973;15:313-316.
21. Demierre D, Maass E, Garcia E, Turina M. ECC Sources of gaseous microemboli. *J Extracorp Tech* 1985;17:20-26.
22. Ueda M, Kondo Y, Makuuchi H, Konishi T. Removal of particle contamination in the extracorporeal circuit detected by an in-line particle counter. *J Extracorp Tech* 1989;21:24-28.
23. Mollison DR, Streczyn MV. In depth evaluation of arterial line filtration of air emboli in bubbler and membrane oxygenators. *AMSECT Proc* 1976:99-102.
24. Orenstein JM, Sato N, Aaron B, Buchholz B, Bloom S. Microemboli observed in deaths following cardiopulmonary bypass surgery. *Hum Pathol* 1982;13:1082-1090.
25. Muraoka R, Yokota M, Aoshima M, Kyoku I, Nomoto S, Kobayashi A, Nakano H, Ueda K, Saito A, Hojo H. Sub-

clinical changes in brain morphology following cardiac operations as reflected by computed tomographic scans of the brain. *J Thorac Cardiovasc Surg* 1981;81:364–369.
26. Ratcliffe JM, Wyse RK, Hunter S, Albert KG, Elliot MJ. The role of priming fluid in the metabolic response to cardiopulmonary bypass in children less than 15 kg body weight undergoing open-heart surgery. *J Thorac Cardiovasc Surg* 1988;36:65–74.
27. Hosking MP, Beynen FM, Raimundo HS, Oliver WC, Williamson KR. A comparison of washed red cells versus packed red blood cells (AS-1) for cardiopulmonary bypass prime and their effects on blood glucose concentration in children. *Anesthesiology* 1990;72:987–990.
28. Ridley PD, Ratcliffe JM, Alberti MM, Elliot MJ. The metabolic consequences of a "washed" cardiopulmonary bypass pump-priming fluid in children undergoing cardiac operations. *J Thorac Cardiovasc Surg* 1990;100:528–537.
29. Hallowell P, Bland JHL, Dalton BC, Eardmann AJ, Lappas DG, Laver MB, Philbin D, Thomas S, Lowenstein E. The effect of hemodilution with albumin or Ringer's lactate on water balance and blood use in open-heart surgery. *Ann Thorac Surg* 1978;25:22–29.
30. Boldt J, Zickman B, Ballesteros BM, Stertmann F, Hempelmann G. Influence of five different priming solutions on platelet function in patients undergoing cardiac surgery. *Anesth Analg* 1992;74:219–225.
31. Rigden SP, Dillon MJ, Kind PR, deLeval M, Stark J, Barratt TM. The beneficial effect of mannitol on postoperative renal function in children undergoing cardiopulmonary bypass surgery. *Clin Nephrol* 1984;21:148–151.
32. Utley JR, Stephens DB, Wachtel C. Effect of albumin and mannitol on organ blood flow, oxygen delivery, water content, and renal function during hypothermic hemodilution cardiopulmonary bypass. *Ann Thorac Cardiovasc Surg* 1982;33:250–257.
33. Marelli D, Paul A, Samson R, Edgell D, Angood P, Chiu RC. Does the addition of albumin to the prime solution in cardiopulmonary bypass affect clinical outcome? *J Thorac Cardiovasc Surg* 1989;98:751–756.
34. D'Ambra MN, Philbin DM. Con: colloids should not be added to the pump prime. *J Cardiothorac Anesth* 1990;4:406–408.
35. London MJ. Pro: colloids should be added to the pump prime. *J Cardiothorac Anesth* 1990;4:401–405.
36. Hirsch DM Jr, Hadidan C, Neville WE. Oxygen consumption during cardiopulmonary bypass with large volume hemodilution. *J Thorac Cardiovasc Surg* 1968;56:197–202.
37. Milam JD, Austin SF, Nihill MR, Keats AS, Cooley DA. Use of sufficient hemodilution to prevent coagulopathies following surgical correction of cyanotic heart disease. *J Thorac Cardiovasc Surg* 1985;89:623–629.
38. Lilleaasen P, Stokke O. Moderate and extreme haemodilution in open-heart surgery. Evaluation of haemolysis, cell damage and protein changes. *Scand J Clin Lab Invest* 1979;39:133–141.
39. Utley JR, Wachtel C, Cain RB, Spaw EA, Collins JC, Stephens DB. Effects of hypothermia, hemodilution, and pump oxygenation on organ water content, blood flow and oxygen delivery, and renal function. *Ann Thorac Surg* 1981;31:121–133.
40. Kawamura M, Minamikawa O, Yokochi H, Maki S, Yasuda T, Mizukawa Y. Safe limit of hemodilution in cardiopulmonary bypass—comparative analysis between cyanotic and acyanotic congenital heart disease. *Jpn J Surg* 1980;10:206–211.
41. Burch M, Redington AN, Carvalho JS, Rusconi P, Shinedourne EA, Rigby ML, Paneth M, Lincoln C. Open valvotomy for critical aortic stenosis in infancy. *Br Heart J* 1990;63:37–40.
42. Newland PE, Pasoriza PJ, McMillan J, Smith BF, Stirling GR. Maximal conservation and minimal usage of blood products in open-heart surgery. *Anesth Intens Care* 1980;8:178–182.
43. Kawaguchi A, Bergsland J, Subramanian S. Total bloodless open heart surgery in the pediatric age group. *Circulation* (suppl) 1984;70:I30–I37.
44. Cosgrove DM, Loop FD, Lytle BW. Blood conservation in cardiac surgery. *Cardiovasc Ther* 1981;12:165–175.
45. Henling CE, Carmichael MJ, Keats AS, Cooley DA. Cardiac operation for congenital heart disease in children of Jehovah's Witnesses. *J Thorac Cardiovasc Surg* 1985;89:914–920.
46. Stein JI, Gombotz H, Rigler B, Metzler H, Suppan C, Beitzke A. Open heart surgery in children of Jehovah's Witnesses. *Pediatr Cardiol* 1991;12:170–174.
47. Manno CS, Hedberg KW, Kim HC, Bunin GR, Nicolson S, Jobes D, Schwartz E, Norwood WI. Comparison of the hemostatic effects of fresh whole blood, and components after open heart surgery in children. *Blood* 1991;77:930–936.
48. Zobel G, Stein JI, Kuttnig M, Beitzke A, Metzler H, Rigler B. Continuous extracorporeal fluid removal in children with low cardiac output after cardiac operations. *J Thorac Cardiovasc Surg* 1991;101:593–597.
49. Anand KJS, Hansen DD, Hickey PR. Hormonal-metabolic stress response in neonates undergoing cardiac surgery. *Anesthesiology* 1990;73:661–670.
50. Anand KJS, Sippell WG, Aynsley-Green A. Randomized trial of fentanyl anaesthesia in preterm neonates undergoing surgery: effects on the stress response. *Lancet* 1987;1:62–66.
51. Anand KJS, Hickey PR. Halothane-morphine compared with high-dose sufentanil for anesthesia and postoperative analgesia in neonatal cardiac surgery. *N Engl J Med* 1992;326:1–9.
52. DeBock TL, Davis PJ, Tome J, Petrilli R, Siewers RD, Motoyama EK. Effect of premedication on arterial oxygen in children with congenital heart disease. *J Cardiothorac Anesth* 1990;4:425–429.
53. Nicolson SC, Betts EK, Jobes DR, Christiansan LA, Walters JK, Mayes KR, Korevaar W. Comparison of oral and intramuscular preanesthetic medication for pediatric inpatient surgery. *Anesthesiology* 1989;71:8–10.
54. Fields LH, Negus JB, White PF. Oral midazolam preanesthetic medication in pediatric patients. *Anesthesiology* 1990;73:831–834.
55. Miller BR, Friesen RH. Oral atropine premedication in infants attenuates cardiovascular depression during halothane anesthesia. *Anesth Analg* 1988;67:180–185.
56. Hickey PR, Hansen DD. Fentanyl- and sufentanil-oxygen-

pancuronium anesthesia for cardiac surgery in infants. *Anesth Analg* 1984;63:117-124.
57. Moore RA, Yang SS, McNicholas KW, Gallagher JD, Clark DL. Hemodynamic and anesthetic effects of sufentanil as the sole anesthetic for pediatric cardiovascular surgery. *Anesthesiology* 1985;62:725-731.
58. Wolf WJ, Neal MB, Peterson MD. The hemodynamic and cardiovascular effects of isoflurane and halothane in children. *Anesthesiology* 1986;64:328-333.
59. Fisher DM, Robinson S, Brett CM, Perin G, Gregory GA. Comparison of enflurane, halothane, isoflurane for diagnostic and therapeutic procedures in children with malignancies. *Anesthesiology* 1985;63:647-650.
60. Greeley WJ, Bushman GA, Davis DP, Reves JG. Comparative effects of halothane and ketamine on systemic arterial oxygen saturation in children with cyanotic heart disease. *Anesthesiology* 1986;65:666-668.
61. Laishley RS, Burrows FA, Lerman J, Roy WL. Effect of anesthetic induction regimens on oxygen saturation in cyanotic congenital heart disease. *Anesthesiology* 1986;65:673-677.
62. Hensley FA, Larach DR, Martin DE, Stauffer RA, Waldhausen JA. The effect of halothane/nitrous oxide/oxygen mask induction on arterial hemoglobin saturation in cyanotic heart disease. *J Cardiothorac Anesth* 1987;11:289-296.
63. Bland JW, Williams WH. Anesthesia for treatment of congenital heart defects. In: Kaplan JA, ed. *Cardiac Anesthesia*. New York: Grune and Stratton; 1979:281-346.
64. Morray JP, Lynn AM, Stamm SJ, Herndon PS, Kawabori I, Stevenson JG. Hemodynamic effects of ketamine in children with congenital heart disease. *Anesth Analg* 1984;63:895-899.
65. Hickey PR, Hansen DD, Cramolini GM, Vincent RN, Lang P. Pulmonary and systemic responses to ketamine in infants with normal and elevated pulmonary vascular resistances. *Anesthesiology* 1985;62:287-293.
66. Yaster M. The dose response of fentanyl in neonatal anesthesia. *Anesthesiology* 1987;66:433-435.
67. Lawson D, Norley I, Korban G, Loeb R, Ellis J. Blood flow limits and pulse oximeter signal detection. *Anesthesiology* 1987;67:599-603.
68. Jobes DR, Nicolson SC. Monitoring of arterial hemoglobin saturation using a tongue sensor. *Anesth Analg* 1988;67:186-188.
69. Band J, Maki D. Infections caused by arterial catheters used for hemodynamic monitoring. *Am J Med* 1979;67:735-741.
70. Gallagher JD, Moore RA, McNicholas KW, Jose AB. Comparison of radial and femoral arterial blood pressure in children after cardiopulmonary bypass. *J Clin Monit* 1985;1:168-171.
71. Glenski JA, Beynen FM, Brady J. A prospective evaluation of femoral artery monitoring in pediatric patients. *Anesthesiology* 1987;66:227-229.
72. Lawless S, Orr R. Axillary arterial monitoring of pediatric patients. *Pediatrics* 1989;84:273-275.
73. Gold JP, Jonas RA, Lang P, Elixson EM, Mayer JE, Castenada AR. Transthoracic intracardiac monitoring lines in pediatric patients: a ten-year experience. *Ann Thorac Surg* 1986;42:185-191.
74. Hayashi Y, Uchida O, Tataki O, Ohnishi Y, Nakajima T, Kataoka H, Kuro M. Internal jugular vein catheterization in infants undergoing cardiovascular surgery: an analysis of the factors influencing successful catheterization. *Anesth Analg* 1992;74:688-693.
75. Introna RPS, Martin DC, Pruett JK, Philpot TE, Johnston JF. Percutaneous pulmonary artery catheterization in pediatric cardiovascular anesthesia: insertion technique and use. *Anesth Analg* 1990;70:562-566.
76. Colgan FJ, Stewart S. An assessment of cardiac output by thermodilution in infants and children following cardiac surgery. *Crit Care Med* 1977;5:220-225.
77. Young JA, Kisker CT, Doty DB. Adequate anticoagulation during cardiopulmonary bypass determined by activated clotting time and the appearance of fibrin monomer. *Ann Thorac Surg* 1978;26:231-240.
78. Metz S, Keats AS. Low activated coagulation time during cardiopulmonary bypass does not increase postoperative bleeding. *Ann Thorac Surg* 1990;49:40-44.
79. Williams GD, Seifer AB, Lawson NM, Norton JB, Readinger RI, Dungen TW, Callaway JK. Pulsatile perfusion versus conventional high flow nonpulsatile perfusion for rapid core cooling and rewarming of infants for circulatory arrest in cardiac operation. *J Thorac Cardiovasc Surg* 1979;78:667-677.
80. Mohri H, Dillard DH, Crawford EW, Martin WE, Merendino KA. Method of surface-induced deep hypothermia for open-heart surgery in infants. *J Thorac Cardiovasc Surg* 1969;58:262-270.
81. Clowes GHA, Neville WE. The relationship of oxygen consumption, perfusion rates, and temperature to the acidosis associated with cardiopulmonary bypass. *Surgery* 1958;44:220.
82. Kirklin JK, Kirklin JW, Pacifico AD. Cardiopulmonary bypass. In: Arciniegas E, ed. *Pediatric Cardiac Surgery*. Chicago: Year Book Medical Publishers; 1985:67-77.
83. Swan H, Sanchez M, Tyndall M, Koch C. Quality control of perfusion: monitoring venous blood oxygen tension to prevent hypoxic acidosis. *J Thorac Cardiovasc Surg* 1990;99:868-872.
84. Kirklin JK, Westaby S, Blackstone EH, Kirklin JW. Complement and the damaging effects of cardiopulmonary bypass. *J Thorac Cardiovasc Surg* 1983;86:845-857.
85. Ekroth R, Thompson RJ, Lincoln C, Scallen M, Rossi R, Tsang V. Elective deep hypothermia with total circulatory arrest: changes in plasma creatinine BB, blood glucose, and clinical variables. *J Thorac Cardiovasc Surg* 1989;97:30-35.
86. Rossi R, Ekroth R, Thompson RJ. No flow or low flow? A study of the ischemic marker creatine BB after deep hypothermic procedures. *J Thorac Cardiovasc Surg* 1989;98:193-199.
87. Greeley WJ, Kern FH, Ungerleider RM, Boyd JL, Quill T, Smith LR, Baldwin B, Reves JG. The effect of hypothermic cardiopulmonary bypass and total circulatory arrest on cerebral metabolism in neonates, infants, and children. *J Thorac Cardiovasc Surg* 1991;101:783-794.
88. Hickey PR. Use of hypothermic circulatory arrest rather than low-flow bypass for repair of complex cardiac defects in infants. Pro: Deep hypothermic circulatory arrest is pref-

erable to low-flow bypass. *J Cardiothorac Vasc Anesth* 1991;5:635-637.
89. Greeley WJ. Use of hypothermic circulatory arrest rather than low-flow bypass for repair of complex cardiac defects in infants. Con: Deep hypothermic arrest must be used selectively and discreetly. *J Cardiothorac Vasc Anesth* 1991; 5:638-640.
90. Fox LS, Blackstone E, Kirklin JW, Bishop S, Bergdahl LAL, Bradley EL. Relationship of brain blood flow and oxygen consumption to perfusion flow rate during profoundly hypothermic cardiopulmonary bypass. *J Thorac Cardiovasc Surg* 1984;87:658-664.
91. Watanabe T, Orita H, Kobayashi M, Washio M. Brain tissue pH, oxygen tension, and carbon dioxide tension in profoundly hypothermic cardiopulmonary bypass. *J Thorac Cardiovasc Surg* 1989;97:396-401.
92. Rebeyka IM, Coles JG, Wilson GJ, Watanabe T, Taylor MJ, Adler SF, Mickle DAG, Romaschin AD, Ujc H, Burrows FA, Williams WG, Trusler GA, Kielmanowics S. The effect of low-flow cardiopulmonary bypass on cerebral function: an experimental and clinical study. *Ann Thorac Surg* 1987;43:391-396.
93. Miyamoto K, Kawashima Y, Matsuda H, Okuda A, Maeda S, Hirose H. Optimal perfusion flow rate for the brain during deep hypothermic cardiopulmonary bypass at 20°C. *J Thorac Cardiovasc Surg* 1986;92:1065-1070.
94. Kern FH, Greeley WJ, Ungerleider RM, Quill TJ, Baldwin B, Smith LR, Reves JG. Cerebral blood flow and metabolism are independent of pump flow rate during hypothermic cardiopulmonary bypass in children. *Anesthesiology* 1990;73:A1107.
95. Taylor RH, Burrows FA, Bissonnette B. No flow during low-flow cardiopulmonary bypass. *J Thorac Cardiovasc Surg* 1991;101:362-364.
96. Greeley WJ, Ungerleider RM, Kern FH, Brusinof G, Smith LR, Reves JG. Effects of cardiopulmonary bypass on cerebral blood flow in neonates, infants, and children. *Circulation* 1989;80:1209-1215.
97. Taylor RH, Burrows FA, Bissonnette B. Cerebral pressure-flow velocity relationships during hypothermic cardiopulmonary bypass in neonates and infants. *Anesth Analg* 1992;74:636-642.
98. Newburger JW, Jonas RA, Wesnovsky G, et al. A comparison of the perioperative neurological effects of hypothermic circulatory arrest versus low-flow cardiopulmonary bypass in infant heart surgery. *N Engl J Med* 1993;329:1057-1064.
99. Kurth CD, Steven JM, Nicolson SC, Chance B. Arterial pressure (BP) thresholds for cerebral oxygenation in neonates with congenital heart disease. *Anesthesiology* 1989; 71:A1034.
100. Kern FH, Ungerleider RM, Quill TJ, Baldwin B, White WD, Reves JG, Greeley WJ. Cerebral blood flow response to changes in arterial carbon dioxide tension during hypothermic cardiopulmonary bypass in children. *J Thorac Cardiovasc Surg* 1991;101:618-622.
101. Noback CR, Tinker JH. Hypothermia after cardiopulmonary bypass in man. *Anesthesiology* 1980;53:277-280.
102. Gillette PC. Diagnosis and management of post-operative junctional ectopic tachycardia. *Am Heart J* 1989;118:192-194.
103. Graves ED, Redmond CR, Arensman RM. Persistent pulmonary hypertension in the neonate. *Chest* 1988;93:638-641.
104. Priebe HJ. Hemodilution and oxygenation. In: Brodsky JB, ed. *International Anesthesiology Clinics*. Boston: Little, Brown; 1981:237-255.
105. Klitzner TS. Maturational changes in excitation-contraction coupling in mammalian myocardium. *J Am Coll Cardiol* 1991;17:218-225.
106. Das JB, Eraklis AJ, Adams JG Jr, Gross RE. Changes in serum ionic calcium during cardiopulmonary bypass with hemodilution. *J Thorac Cardiovasc Surg* 1971;62:449-453.
107. Lang P, Williams RG, Norwood WI, Castenada AR. The hemodynamic effects of dopamine in infants after corrective cardiac surgery. *J Pediatr* 1980;96:630-634.
108. Williams DB, Kiernan PD, Schaff HV, Marsh HM, Danielson GK. The hemodynamic response to dopamine and nitroprusside following right atrium-pulmonary artery bypass (Fontan procedure). *Ann Thorac Surg* 1982;34:51-57.
109. Drummond WH, Gregory GA, Heymann MA. The independent effects of hyperventilation, tolazine, and dopamine on infants with persistent pulmonary hypertension. *J Pediatr* 1981;98:603-611.
110. Mentzer RM, Alegre CA, Nolan SP. The effects of dopamine and isoproterenol on the pulmonary circulation. *J Thorac Cardiovasc Surg* 1976;71:807-814.
111. Bohn DJ, Poirier CS, Edmonds JF. The hemodynamic effects of dobutamine after cardiopulmonary bypass in children. *Crit Care Med* 1980;8:367-371.
112. Benzing G, Helmsworth JA, Schreiber JT, Kaplan S. Nitroprusside and epinephrine for treatment of low output in children after open-heart surgery. *Ann Thorac Surg* 1978; 27:523-528.
113. Applebaum A, Blackstone E, Kouchoukos NT, Kirklin JW. Afterload reduction and cardiac output in infants after intracardiac surgery. *Am J Cardiol* 1977;39:445-451.
114. Taylor RH, Skippen PW, Bohn D. Amrinone versus dopamine following cardiac surgery in children. *Anesth Analg* 1990;70:S405.
115. Rubis LJ, Stephenson LW, Johnston MR. Comparison of effects of prostaglandin E_1 and nitroprusside on pulmonary vascular resistance in children after open-heart surgery. *Ann Thorac Surg* 1981;32:563-570.
116. Rasch DK, Lancaster L. Successful use of nitroglycerin to treat post-operative pulmonary hypertension. *Crit Care Med* 1987;15:616-617.
117. Ungerleider RM, Greeley WJ, Sheikh KH, Philips J, Pearce F, Kern FH, Kisslo JA. Routine use of intraoperative epicardial echocardiography and Doppler color flow imaging to guide and evaluate repair of congenital heart lesions. *J Thorac Cardiovasc Surg* 1990;100:297-309.

20
Thoracic Aortic Surgery and Cardiopulmonary Bypass

Tomas D. Martin

Diseases of the aorta are common and most are surgically correctable.[1-4] Aneurysmal disease alone is said to account for 1% to 2% of all deaths in industrialized countries.[5] Unfortunately, no adequate medical therapy is currently available. It is not within the scope of this chapter to cover each of these diseases in detail. The goal is, however, to review the intraoperative surgical techniques used to approach the thoracic aorta, focusing on cardiopulmonary bypass (CPB) and its variations. The surgical, anesthetic, and bypass and perfusion techniques are dictated by the segment or segments of the aorta that need to be replaced or repaired (ie, ascending aorta, aortic arch, and/or descending/thoracoabdominal aorta; Figure 20.1). The institution and management of CPB will be reviewed for each type of aortic vascular disease.

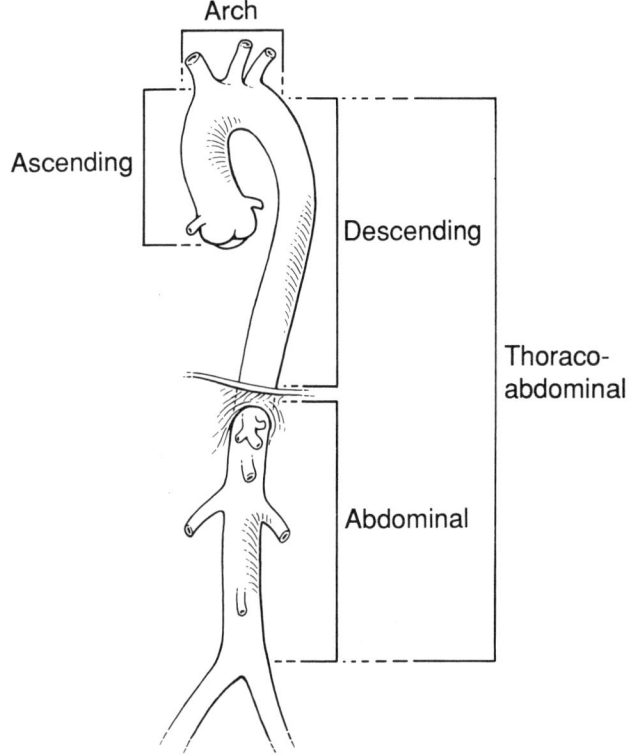

FIGURE 20.1. Various segments of the thoracoabdominal aorta.

Ascending Aorta

The ascending aorta begins at the aortic annulus and extends to the base of the innominate artery as seen in Figure 20.1. The two most common surgically treatable abnormalities are degenerative aneurysmal disease and dissection, with the etiology being variable.[5,6] The surgical treatment is resection and graft replacement, and may or may not include aortic valve repair or replacement or coronary ostia reimplantation.

Cannulation

Cannulation techniques vary according to the location and extent of pathology. This is particularly true for arterial cannulation. With aneurysmal disease, the site of arterial cannulation is most commonly the distal ascending aorta or the common femoral artery. Cannulating the distal ascending aorta is preferable, since it avoids a groin incision, which has its own potential complications. If, however, the aneurysm extends into the distal ascending aorta, or if there is evidence of thrombus or debris in the distal ascending aorta, then an alternate cannulation site is chosen, most frequently the common femoral artery. Direct cannulation of an aneurysmal segment (ascending or arch) is possible with the assistance of transesophageal and epiaortic ultrasound to evaluate the luminal contents of the aorta.[7] Other cannulation options include the aortic arch, the innominate artery, or even the left ventricular apex.[8]

Direct cannulation of the common femoral artery is a commonly used and safe technique; however, it is not without potential complications. These include retrograde femoral/iliac dissection and prolonged arterial occlusion leading to lower extremity ischemic complications. In order to avoid these problems, we have recently used a technique in which an 8-mm knitted collagen-impregnated Dacron graft is sutured onto the common femoral artery, using a transverse arteriotomy (Figure 20.2). A 22F or 24F femoral cannula will easily fit into the 8-mm graft, thereby preventing the possibility of intimal elevation and dissection when directly cannulated. This technique also allows perfusion of the distal extremity, as well as the entire body, preventing prolonged lower extremity ischemia.

In patients with acute or chronic dissections, the common femoral artery is the cannulation site of choice. Cannulation of the ascending aorta in dissections is fraught with difficulty and should be avoided. In patients with acute DeBakey type I dissections, the dissection may or may not extend into the iliac and femoral vessels. If it does, the majority will extend into the left side. Therefore, in most cases, cannulation is safer via the right femoral artery.

In most patients, venous cannulation is possible via the right atrium, utilizing a single two-stage cannula. There are cases, however, in which the ascending aorta has reached such a large size that the right atrium is so displaced inferiorly and posteriorly that cannulation is extremely difficult and potentially hazardous. In this case, femoral venous cannulation is warranted. Femoral cannulation should also be considered in those cases in which the aorta has reached such a large size that sternotomy alone poses a risk of entering the aorta. This is particularly true with large aneurysms in patients who have had previous sternotomies.[9]

Cannulation of the femoral vein alone often leads to poor venous return due to its small size. Therefore, most surgeons attempt to pass the venous cannula cephalad into the inferior vena cava. In many patients, this is impossible secondary to the tortuosity of the venous system and the large caliber of cannulas used. Recently, wire-guided cannulas (28F or 32F), which can easily be placed into the inferior vena cava or even the right atrium, have become available. In most cases, adequate venous return is easily obtained using these cannulas.[10]

CPB Management

When dealing with a pathologic process of the ascending aorta, not involving the aortic arch, anesthetic and perfusion management are no different than that for coronary revascularization or valve replacement. In most, moderate to high pump flows (≥ 2.25 L/m^2/min), moderate systemic hypothermia ($\leq 28\,°C$), and intermittent cold oxygenated cardioplegia are employed. One liter of cold cardioplegic solution is delivered in an antegrade fashion (directly into the root if there is no significant aortic insufficiency or directly into the coronary ostia). This is followed by an initial 300 mL in a retrograde fashion via the coronary sinus and then 300 mL every 20 minutes also via the retrograde system (see Chapter 2). This easily maintains myocardial diastolic arrest and hypothermia. Retrograde cardioplegia allows the surgeon to continue working without having to stop periodically to deliver antegrade cardioplegia. If, however, retrograde delivery is not possible, then delivery directly into the coronary ostia should be accomplished at least every 30 minutes. Myocardial protection is the key to a good outcome.

Continuous retrograde warm blood cardioplegia is an alternative myocardial protection technique that has been associated with good results.[11] However, difficulty with visualization of the coronary ostia and aortic valve may occur, as blood is continuously streaming out of the coronary ostia. Continuous antegrade warm blood cardioplegia has also been described.[12] Cannulas placed directly into the coronary ostia for antegrade delivery of cardioplegia may be cumbersome and often leak, potentially exacerbating visualization problems. This technique, however, is used by some with excellent success.[12]

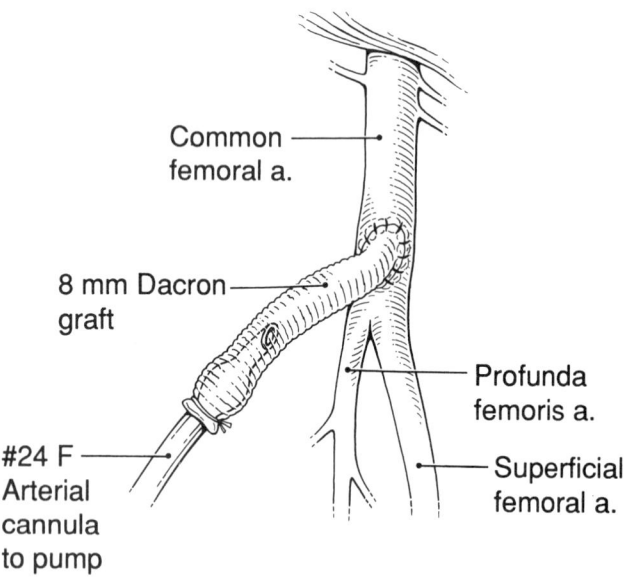

FIGURE 20.2. Technique to limit complications associated with femoral artery cannulation. An 8-mm, knitted, collagen-impregnated, Dacron graft is sutured to the common femoral artery. A 22F or 24F femoral cannula will fit into the 8-mm graft. Both the distal extremity and the entire body can be perfused.

The Aortic Arch

The true aortic arch begins at the anterior border of the base of the innominate artery and extends to the posterior border of the left subclavian artery (Figure 20.1). Again,

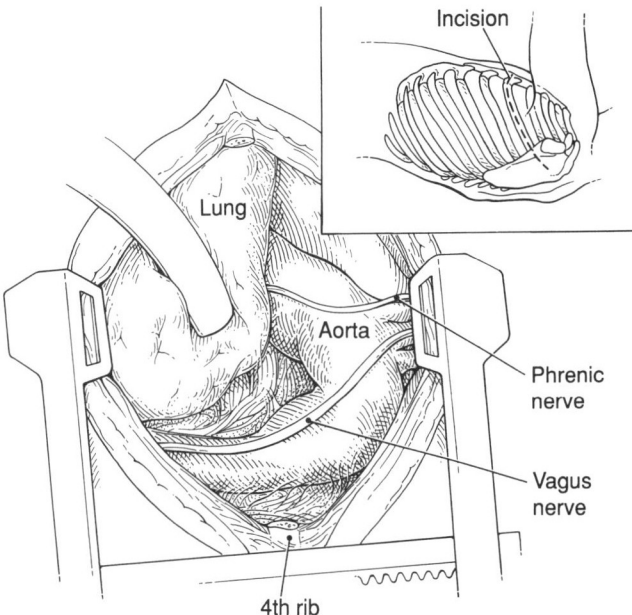

FIGURE 20.3. High left thoracotomy incision for operative procedures limited to the arch of the descending aorta. The incision is made between the 3rd and 4th interspace.

the two most common surgical problems affecting the aortic arch are dissection and aneurysmal disease.[5,6] In most cases, the same pathologic process that affects the arch also affects the ascending aorta, the descending thoracic aorta, or both. The proximal arch is the most common portion involved; therefore, the surgical approach is usually via a median sternotomy. However, in patients who have lesions isolated to the arch of the descending aorta, a high left thoracotomy (3rd or 4th interspace) provides excellent exposure (Figure 20.3).[13]

Cannulation sites will vary depending on the type and extent of the pathology. If the ascending aorta is normal, the arterial cannula can easily be placed here. As the proximal arch and ascending aorta are often simultaneously affected, femoral arterial cannulation is usually required (as described previously). Alternate cannulation sites are available and include the ascending aorta (even when diseased), the innominate, carotid, and subclavian arteries, or even the descending thoracic aorta.[11] Venous cannulation, as previously described for the ascending aorta, is via the right atrium or femoral vein.

CPB Management

Anesthetic and perfusion management strategies for arch surgery are varied and distinctly different from other routine bypass cases. In contrast to most cardiovascular procedures, repair of such lesions requires interruption of cerebral circulation, selective arch vessel perfusion, or retrograde cerebral perfusion. Cerebral protection is as important as myocardial protection. Most arch procedures are performed under profound hypothermia (core temperature <21°C) (see Chapter 3) and circulatory arrest. This technique has proven easy, safe, and effective,[9,14-21] with Crawford reporting the largest series (>650 patients). In this series, in-hospital mortality was 10% and the stroke rate was 3%.[20]

After arterial and venous cannulation, cooling is initiated. In children, it appears that the rate of cooling may affect the incidence of postoperative cerebral dysfunction. In an experimental canine model by Almond et al,[22] brain cell necrosis and death correlated with large gradients between perfusate and body temperatures while cooling. In adults, there is no conclusive evidence that the rate of cooling leads to cerebral dysfunction; however, at the present time, many institutions limit the gradient between the blood and the water bath temperatures to 10°C for both cooling and rewarming.

The purpose of cooling is to reduce the metabolic activity of all tissues, but especially the brain, since it is *the* organ most susceptible to ischemia. The exact temperature at which a prolonged "safe" circulatory arrest period can be tolerated without obvious neurologic injury is controversial.[19-26] Clinically, the only practical method of evaluating cerebral activity is with electroencephalography (EEG). Burst suppression of EEG activity and complete electrocerebral silence both suggest marked decrease in cerebral metabolism.[27] Several studies have shown that detectable EEG activity ceases at a brain temperature of 20° to 21°C.[28] This level of inactivity may reflect a 50% reduction in cerebral metabolism (see Chapter 6). Determining exact brain temperature is not practical, and in most cases "core" temperature is used. There is, however, no clear definition of "core" temperature. Is it rectal, bladder, esophageal, nasopharyngeal, or tympanic? In order to establish a consistent and reliable method of determining the appropriate level of hypothermia prior to circulatory arrest, Coselli and Crawford[29] prospectively studied 56 patients requiring circulatory arrest during aortic surgery. Nasopharyngeal, esophageal, and rectal temperatures were continuously recorded during cooling, and correlated with EEG activity. Their results showed a wide variation in temperature among the body sites when electrocerebral silence occurred: nasopharyngeal, 10.1° to 24.1°C; esophageal, 7.2° to 23.1°C; and rectal, 12.8° to 28.6°C. None of these sites, or combinations of sites, consistently predicted electrocerebral silence.[29] Tympanic membrane temperature most likely correlates best with brain temperature; however, most anesthesiologists are reluctant to place tympanic probes due to the risk of tympanic perforation and the cost of the infrared probes. At the present time, bladder and rectal temperatures are most commonly used. The topic of temperature monitoring is also discussed in Chapters 13 and 14.

In our own experience, a bladder or rectal temperature

of 17° to 20°C, combined with pharmacologic cerebral suppression and EEG monitoring, has allowed cerebral ischemic times of up to 45 minutes without detectable gross neurologic deficits. In the study by Cosseli and Crawford,[29] the use of a 10-lead EEG to determine the presence of electrocerebral silence (regardless of the "core" temperature) proved extremely effective. Thirty-day survival in the 56 patients in whom circulatory arrest was used for aortic arch procedures was 91%. Only three (5.9%) of the survivors had neurologic deficits. Four died of cardiac causes, and one secondary to multiple brain emboli from atherosclerotic intimal debris. Circulatory arrest time ranged from 14 to 109 minutes (mean 39 minutes).[29] The use of a 10-lead EEG is not practical in most circumstances. Some type of cerebral monitoring is recommended, since there are many good, smaller EEG units available.

Several anesthetics and other types of drugs suppress EEG activity and therefore presumably decrease cerebral metabolism. These include inhalational anesthetic drugs (halothane, isoflurane), barbiturates (thiopental, methoxital, pentobarbital), corticosteroids, calcium channel blockers (nimodipine), and, potentially, propofol.[30-34] The subject of cerebral metabolism and protection during cardiac surgery is discussed in detail in Chapter 6. Our preferred technique for cerebral monitoring and protection during aortic arch surgery in adult patients is outlined in Table 20.1.

Management of pH during hypothermia is also controversial. Hypothermia in itself affects pH, since there is an inverse relationship between temperature and gas solubility leading to an apparent metabolic alkalosis by making carbon dioxide more soluble.[35] Some have used a process termed *pH-stat management* in which exogenous carbon dioxide is added to the circuit to maintain a temperature-corrected pH 7.40. It has been reported, however, that this is unphysiologic.[30] It has been demonstrated that pH-stat management produces cerebral hyperemia as a result of a pressure-passive flow phenomenon that uncouples the normally tight relationship between cerebral blood flow and metabolism. Therefore, cerebral blood flow during hypothermic CPB varies with perfusion pressure and may lead to excessive flow, which may unnecessarily place the brain at risk for damage from excessive emboli or high intracranial pressure.[30] Most surgeons and anesthesiologists prefer *alpha-stat management*, in which a more normal transmembrane gradient (0.6 pH units) is sought. This is achieved by not correcting pH values for temperature. This method better preserves cerebral autoregulation, leading to lower and perhaps metabolically more appropriate cerebral blood flow.[30]

Cerebral circulatory arrest of up to 45 minutes is usually well tolerated. As stated before, the exact "safe" cerebral ischemic time is unknown and most likely varies from patient to patient depending on a number of factors (age, cerebral vascular disease). Children are obviously different from adults and it may be that the younger the patient, the longer the "safe" ischemic time. In both children and adults, however, there seems to be a demonstrable adverse effect on intellectual capacity and development when arrest time exceeds 60 minutes.[36-38] We have noted in our own adult experience that when arrest time exceeds 45-60 minutes, a much higher incidence of postoperative confusion, hallucinations, and personality changes are seen.

Other methods to provide cerebral protection during aortic arch surgery include retrograde cerebral perfusion via the SVC (superior vena cava) and antegrade perfusion with selective cannulation of the arch vessels.[18,39-48]

Two of the earliest reports on the use of retrograde cerebral perfusion (RCP) were by Stoney[49] in 1980 and Valk[43] in 1982 when it was recommended for the treatment of massive air embolism during CPB. More recently, this technique has been advocated for use during surgery of the aortic arch, in hopes of extending the safe period of circulatory arrest and preventing cerebral air embolism and thromboembolism (Figure 20.4).[40,51,52] Safi[51] in 1993 reported on 11 patients undergoing arch replacement in whom retrograde cerebral perfusion was utilized in an attempt to minimize cerebral ischemia. Systemic hypothermia (15° to 24°C) was combined with retrograde cerebral perfusion (15° to 24°C) administered via the superior vena cava with mean cerebral ischemic and retrograde perfusion times of 36 minutes (9-71 minutes). Throughout the retrograde perfusion period, blood samples were drawn from the innominate and left carotid arteries for analysis of oxygen content, total creatine kinase level, and creatine kinase BB fraction.[51]

In this series, there were no deaths and only one major stroke. The stroke occurred in a patient with a large thoracoabdominal aortic aneurysm, in whom femoral-femoral bypass was necessary. The stroke was felt to be secondary to emboli from the thoracoabdominal aneurysm. In a comparison of the intraoperative EEGs with a historical control, there was no difference, and the creatinine kinase BB band was not identified as a reliable marker of brain injury. It was felt, however, that retrograde cerebral perfusion was a valuable adjunct to brain protection.[51]

Several experimental studies have been reported to evaluate retrograde cerebral perfusion, with most using a ca-

TABLE 20.1. Monitoring and protection during circulatory arrest.

"Core" temperature <18°C
EEG silent or burst suppression pattern
Barbiturate 10-15 mg/kg thiopental[a]
Steroid 10 mg/kg methylprednisolone
Alpha-stat pH blood-gas management

[a]Administered at least 3-5 minutes prior to circulatory arrest.

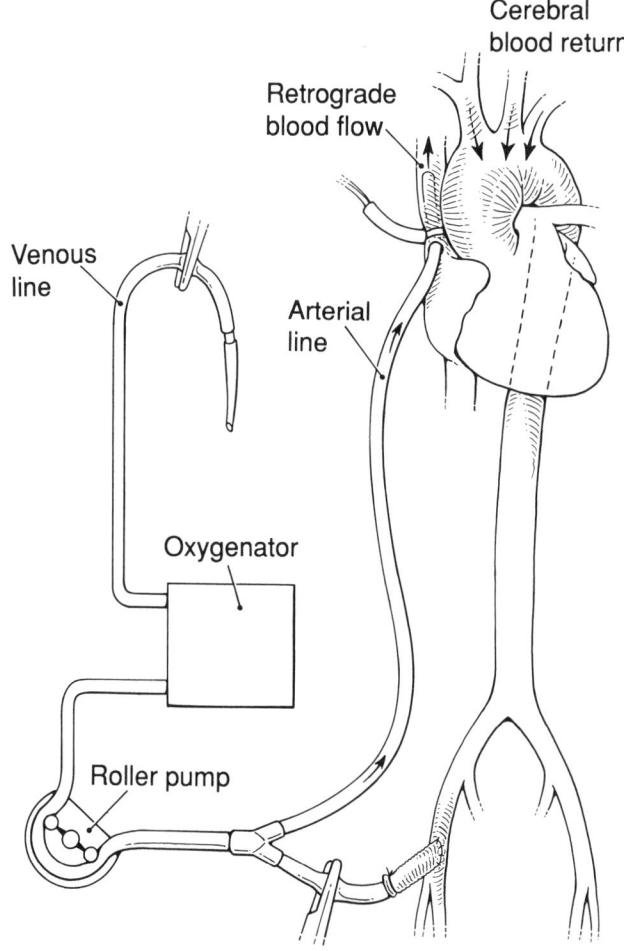

FIGURE 20.4. Diagram of technique for providing retrograde cerebral perfusion. Using a bypass circuit that includes an oxygenator and roller pump, oxygenated blood is infused into the superior vena cava. In humans, valves in the cerebral venous circulation are mostly absent. Cerebral blood return is to the aortic arch vessels.

nine model.[40-42] It appears from these studies that RCP may be beneficial, providing half the cerebral tissue blood flow and one third of the oxygen normally delivered during CPB, while allowing 20% discharge of the carbon dioxide.[40] There is also some evidence that pulsatile flow provides more cerebroprotective effects than nonpulsatile flow[42] and that perfusion pressure, when too high (>25 mm Hg), causes cerebral edema, while low pressures (<20 mm Hg) provide significantly lower cerebral tissue blood flow,[42,43] potentially leading to ischemic problems. One major problem with laboratory investigation in this area is the development of a reliable animal model. The major cerebral venous drainage in the dog is the external jugular vein, which contains many functioning valves that obstruct retrograde perfusion in many animals. This certainly places the reliability of these studies in question.

Other animals (sheep and baboon) have been used and may provide a better model. In an unpublished National Institutes of Health study by Crittenden, retrograde cerebral perfusion in sheep resulted in very poor protection with virtual brain death in all animals.

Several other points must be considered. To date, all experimental and clinical studies of RCP have included systemic hypothermia (17°–24°C). It is therefore difficult to adequately ascertain the benefits of RCP, when hypothermia and circulatory arrest would, in most patients and animals, yield similar results. It also must be recognized that most humans have some component of venous valves in the internal jugular system. The majority of these valves are incompetent, but in some cases they may interrupt RCP.[40]

Selective perfusion of the arch vessels was the initial method used for successful arch surgery and was reported by DeBakey in 1957.[52] In this and other reports, fairly complex methods of perfusion were used relying on multiple pump heads and separate cannulation of each arch vessel.[45,53-55] Results with these techniques were extremely variable. The techniques were simplified and results improved, although morbidity and mortality were still high.[46,47,56]

With the evolution of profound hypothermia and circulatory arrest, with their simple techniques and improved results, antegrade cerebral perfusion fell out of favor in the late 1970s. Due to the often long perfusion times necessary for cooling and rewarming and multiple hematologic and organ abnormalities that can occur with prolonged CPB, antegrade cerebral perfusion using moderate hypothermia (28°C) and simplified cerebral perfusion techniques (Figure 20.5) has recently seen a revival.[57-59] It has also been recognized that some of the cerebral complications seen with antegrade perfusion in the 1960s and 1970s were due, in part, to high cerebral pressures and blood flow.[57] The most recent reports utilizing antegrade perfusion have paid special attention to these parameters, with flow ranging from 500 to 1000 mL/min and pressures of 40 to 60 mm Hg. Kazui[58] has specifically recommended using a roller pump for cerebral perfusion separate from the systemic circulation, and perfusing at 10 mL/kg/min with a pressure (arterial) of 50 to 70 mm Hg.

From June 1990 to December 1993, the author performed 80 aortic arch procedures employing profound hypothermia and using the methods outlined (Table 20.1) without retrograde or selective antegrade perfusion. In this group, two patients had cerebral ischemia times greater than 70 minutes (75 and 78 minutes). Both had extremely complicated problems. One had a previous coronary bypass complicated by a chronic type II dissection, ascending and arch aneurysms, and acute dissection of the aortic arch. The other had an infected ascending and arch graft with pseudoaneurysms of the proximal ascending anastomosis and great vessel anastomosis. Neither had a

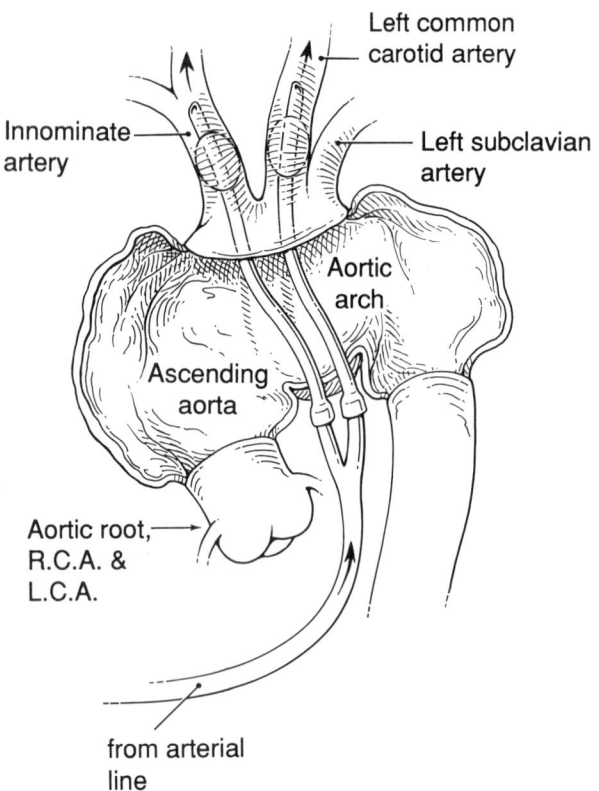

FIGURE 20.5. Diagram of technique for providing antegrade cerebral perfusion during total CPB. Separate cannulas are introduced into the innominate artery and the left common carotid artery. A separate arterial pump head can be used to provide cerebral perfusion.

and dissections are the most common surgical problems.[5,6] Diffuse atheromatous disease, often referred to as "shaggy" aorta, which causes repetitive distal emboli, is a less common problem but is receiving increased surgical interest.

The surgical approach to these areas varies, depending on the extent of aortic involvement. A standard posterolateral thoracotomy is the approach of choice for lesions confined to the descending thoracic aorta. However, once the pathology traverses the diaphragm, a thoracotomy must be combined with a transcostal extension into the abdomen (Figure 20.6). A retroperitoneal approach via a paramedian incision is preferable to transperitoneal laparotomy, since it keeps the intestines inside the peritoneum, limits intraoperative fluid loss and intestinal edema, and may decrease postoperative intestinal dysfunction. In most cases, the aorta is replaced with a prosthetic graft. Surgically, this can be accomplished by several methods, including simple clamping of the descending thoracic aorta without any provision for distal flow; shunting with various shunts from the ascending aorta, aortic arch, descending aorta, or even the left ventricle; or some type of bypass.

Clamping of the descending thoracic aorta causes profound hemodynamic and multiple neurohumoral changes,[45,56,57,60] including a sudden and severe increase in peripheral resistance, leading to proximal hypertension, increased ventricular afterload, and increased stroke work. Significant plasma elevations of epinephrine, norepinephrine, and renin also occur. Depending on the site of clamping, as much as two thirds of the body becomes acutely ischemic, leading to significant acidosis and multiple electrolyte changes (primarily a marked increase in serum potassium). Massive bleeding, combined with multifactorial coagulopathies, is not uncommon, and release of the clamp after the grafting procedure has been completed again produces profound hemodynamic changes. All of the above, combined with single-lung anesthesia and its attendant problems, presents the anesthesiology and surgical teams one of their greatest challenges.[61,62] Saleh[61] in 1980 outlined in detail the anesthetic management necessary for success when clamping without distal perfusion.[64] The basics, modified and updated from Saleh, include:

1. A thorough preoperative evaluation, including cardiac, pulmonary, renal, and neurologic status;
2. Preoperative review of current medications;
3. Invasive monitoring intraoperatively, including an oximetry pulmonary artery catheter, central venous pressure, and arterial lines;
4. Close monitoring of arterial blood gases, electrolytes, and coagulation;
5. Spinal fluid drainage, maintaining a spinal pressure ≥ 10 mm Hg;

discrete stroke, and both fully recovered, but both had prolonged periods of recovery with profound confusion and neuropsychiatric disorders (hallucinations, paranoia, loss of short-term memory, and disorientation). At the present time, it is difficult to recommend retrograde or antegrade cerebral perfusion in all patients requiring aortic arch reconstruction. In complicated cases, such as those described, however, where prolonged (more than 45 to 60 minutes) arch reconstruction is required, some type of adjunctive technique of cerebral perfusion is most likely beneficial.

Descending and Thoracoabdominal Aorta

The descending thoracic aorta begins at the distal base of the left subclavian artery and extends to the diaphragmatic aortic hiatus (Figure 20.1). The thoracoabdominal aorta is that part which traverses the diaphragmatic aortic hiatus. As with the other portions of the aorta, aneurysms

FIGURE 20.6. Surgical incision and exposure for vascular disease that includes both the thoracic and abdominal segments of the aorta.

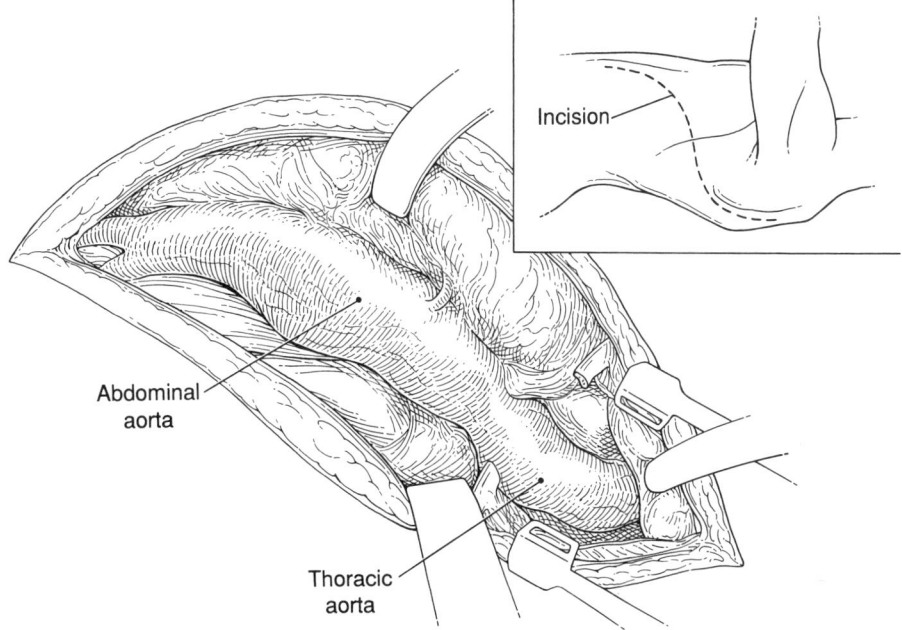

6. A double-lumen endobronchial tube or bronchial blocker tube placed and bronchoscopic confirmation of the tube position;
7. Adequate venous access (at least two 14-gauge peripheral IVs and an 8F intravenous catheter in a large vein);
8. A rapid infusion device with blood warmers (see Figure 26.2);
9. Two separate cell-salvage lines, and, occasionally, two machines (Figure 31.4);
10. Transesophageal echocardiography (TEE) for continuous cardiac evaluation;
11. Intravenous nitroglycerin with increasing doses to volume load prior to clamping;
12. During the "clamp" period (absence of distal perfusion), a continuous infusion of sodium bicarbonate at 3 mEq/kg/h;
13. Blood pressure maintained at or slightly above preoperative values.

CPB Management

At the present time, management of CPB for descending and thoracoabdominal aortic procedures is varied (Table 20.2). The use of perfusion is in itself controversial and is tailored to treat, prevent, or attenuate the above-described morbidities.[63-69]

If distal perfusion is used, partial CPB support can be initiated and managed in a variety of ways. The most common method is left atrial to left femoral artery bypass, using a centrifugal force pump and no oxygenator (Figure 20.7).[65-68,70-72] The advantages of this method include its relative ease of institution, since it does not require heparin anticoagulation, and it has few complications. It is important when using this technique to realize that drainage to the pump comes from the preload chamber of the left ventricle, and that increasing pump flow decreases ventricular filling, cardiac output, and systemic pressure. It is therefore imperative to monitor upper-body and lower-body pressures simultaneously. Improper drainage of the left atrium can result in upper-body hypotension leading to cerebral and cardiac ischemia.

There are reports in the literature that advocate distal perfusion to decrease the incidence of perioperative spinal cord ischemia.[65,69,71-75] However, other reports contradict this theory.[65] In fact, most recent studies, which report a marked reduction in postoperative spinal cord problems, utilize no distal perfusion.[76,77] These reports utilize a variety of surgical hemodynamic and pharmacologic manipulations combined with spinal fluid drainage, and have reduced their spinal cord injury rate to less than 10% in all groups. At the present time, distal perfusion is not recom-

TABLE 20.2. Surgical approaches to repair descending and thoracoabdominal aortic disease.

Simple crossclamp
Left atrium to left femoral artery bypass
Left ventricle to left femoral artery shunt
Passive shunt (Gott shunt) (proximal to distal aortic)
Partial CPB (femoral a. to femoral v.)
Total CPB with hypothermia (femoral a. to femoral v.)

mended for routine use. However, it may be advantageous in patients with poor myocardial function, since mechanical loading and unloading of the heart is in many cases more readily accomplished and more reliable than pharmacologic manipulations.[65-68] Distal perfusion is also recommended in patients with decreased renal function (serum creatine > 2.5), since it will either limit or eliminate renal ischemia and, hopefully, postoperative renal dysfunction.[66-68]

Other methods to provide lower-body perfusion include a proximal-to-distal aortic shunt such as that proposed by Gott[73,74] and even direct left ventricle-femoral artery shunts.[75] The Gott shunt, along with other "simple" shunts, utilizes plastic tubing placed into the aorta proximal to the proximal clamp and distal to the distal clamp (Figure 20.8). Flows with these types of shunts are quite variable and very difficult to assess intraoperatively.

Finally, femoral-femoral bypass, using CPB with an oxygenator and full anticoagulation (heparin 3–4 mg/kg), may be used. This method, combined with profound

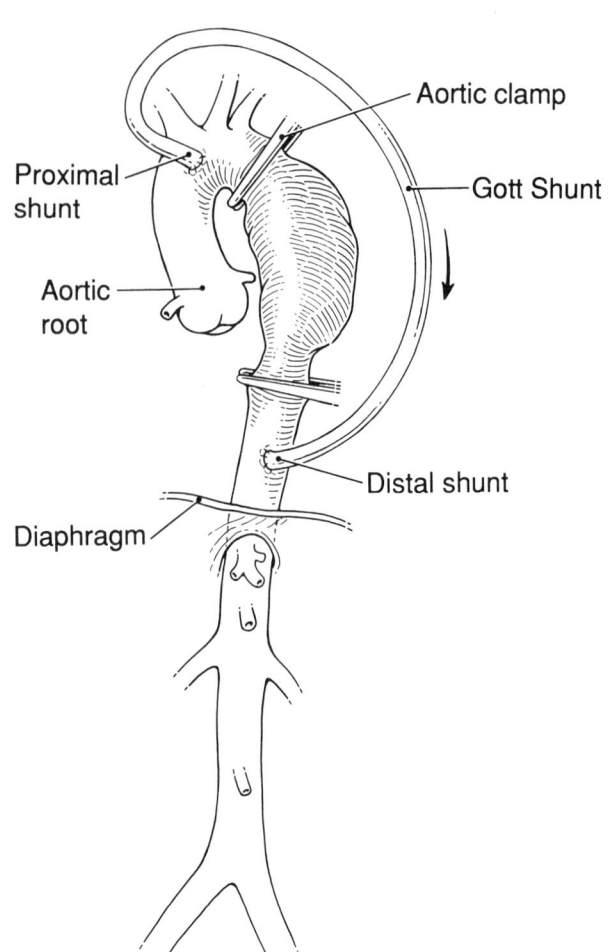

FIGURE 20.8. The Gott shunt. A piece of plastic tubing is placed proximal and distal to the clamps isolating the diseased aortic segment.

hypothermia and circulatory arrest, has recently been recommended by Kouchoukos and others[78-80] for extensive thoracoabdominal aneurysms. This allows prolonged visceral and intercostal ischemia with little risk of postoperative problems. In the author's experience with these techniques, the drawbacks include a much longer operative time, increased perioperative bleeding and coagulation problems, and an increased incidence of postoperative pulmonary morbidity. Reported results with this technique, however, are good.[78]

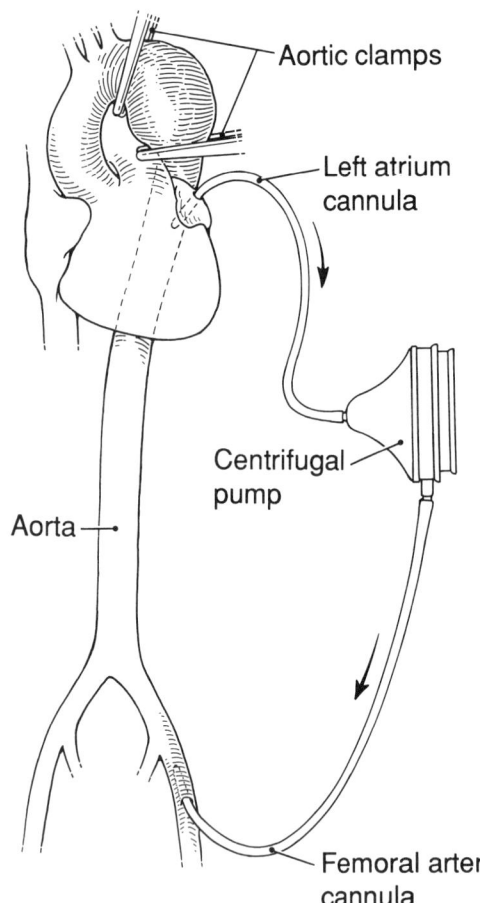

FIGURE 20.7. Technique for perfusing the distal thoracic aorta through proximal cannulation of the left atrium and distal cannulation of the femoral artery with an intervening centrifugal pump head.

References

1. Fradet G, Jamieson WRE, Janusz MT, et al. Aortic dissection: a six-year experience with 117 patients. *Am J Surg* 1988;155:697-670.
2. Svensson LG, Crawford ES, Hess KR, et al. Dissection of the aorta and dissection of aortic aneurysms: improving early and long-term surgical results. *Circulation* 1990; 82(suppl IV):24-38.

3. Stanson AW, Kazmier FJ, Hollier LH, et al. Penetrating atherosclerotic ulcers of the thoracic aorta: natural history and clinicopathologic correlations. *Ann Vasc Surg* 1986;1:15-23.
4. Cohen M, Fuster V, Steele PM, et al. Coarctation of the aorta: long-term follow up and prediction of outcome after surgical correction. *Circulation* 1989;80:840-845.
5. Kuivaniemi H, Tromp G, Prockop DJ. Genetic causes of aortic aneurysms. *J Clin Invest* 1991;88:1441-1444.
6. McNamara JJ, Pressler JM. Natural history of arteriosclerotic thoracic aortic aneurysms. *Ann Thorac Surg* 1978;25:468-473.
7. Martin TD, Accola KA. Megaaorta and aortoiliac obstruction: alternate method of cannulation. *Ann Thorac Surg* 1992;53:889-891.
8. Robicsek F. Apical aortic cannulation: application of an old method with new paraphernalia. *Ann Thorac Surg* 1991;51:330-332.
9. Crawford ES, Crawford JL, Safi HJ, et al. Redo operations for recurrent aneurysmal disease of the ascending aorta and transverse aortic arch. *Ann Thorac Surg* 1985;40:439-455.
10. Rosenbloom M, Muskett AD. Simplified method for femoral venous cannulation. *Ann Thorac Surg* 1991;51:846-847.
11. Martin TD, Craver JM, Gott JP, et al. A prospective randomized trial of retrograde warm blood cardioplegia: myocardial benefit and neurologic threat. *Ann Thorac Surg* 1994;57:288-304.
12. Lichtenstein SV, Able JG, Salerno TA. Warm heart surgery and results of operation for recent myocardial infarction. *Ann Thorac Surg* 1991;52:455-460.
13. Crawford ES, Coselli JS, Safi HJ. Partial cardiopulmonary bypass, hypothermic circulatory arrest, and posterolateral exposure for thoracic aortic aneurysm operations. *J Thorac Cardiovasc Surg* 1987;94:824-827.
14. Massimo Carlo G, Presenti LF, Marranci P, et al. Extended and total aortic resection in the surgical treatment of acute type A aortic dissection: experience with 54 patients. *Ann Thorac Surg* 1988;46:420-424.
15. Wareing TH, Davila-Roman VG, Barzilai B, et al. Management of the severely atherosclerotic ascending aorta during cardiac operations. *J Thorac Cardiovasc Surg* 1992;103:453-462.
16. DeBakey ME, Lawrie GM, Crawford ES, et al. Surgical treatment of dissecting aortic aneurysms: 28 years experience with 527 cases. *Contemp Surg* 1984;9:25.
17. Caramutti VM, Dantur JR, Favaloro MR, et al. Deep hypothermia and circulatory arrest as an elective technique in the treatment of type B dissection aneurysm of the aorta. *J Card Surg* 1989;4:206-215.
18. Bachet J, Teodori G, Goudot B, et al. Replacement of the transverse aortic arch during emergency operations for type A acute aortic dissection. *J Thorac Cardiovasc Surg* 1988;96:878-886.
19. Graham JM, Stinnett DM. Operative management of acute aortic dissection using profound hypothermia and circulatory arrest. *Ann Thorac Surg* 1987;44:192-198.
20. Crawford ES, Svensson LG, Coselli JS, et al. Surgical treatment of aneurysm and/or dissection of the ascending aorta transverse aortic arch. *J Thorac Cardiovasc Surg* 1989;98:659-674.
21. Greeley WJ, Kern FH, Meliones JN, et al. Effect of deep hypothermia and circulatory arrest on cerebral blood flow and metabolism. *Ann Thorac Surg* 1993;56:1464-1466.
22. Almond CH, Jones JC, Snyder HM, et al. Cooling gradients and brain damage with deep hypothermia. *J Thorac Cardiovasc Surg* 1964;48:890-897.
23. Griepp RB, Ergin MA, Lansman SL, et al. The physiology of hypothermic circulatory arrest. *Semin Thorac Cardiovasc Surg* 1991;3:188-193.
24. Hollier LH. Protecting the brain and spinal cord. *J Vasc Surg* 1987;5:524-528.
25. Vanderlinden J, Astudillo R, Ekroth R, et al. Cerebral lactate release after circulatory arrest but not after low flow in pediatric heart operations. *Ann Thorac Surg* 1993;56:1485-1489.
26. Mohri H, Sadahiro M, Akimoto H, et al. Protection of the brain during hypothermic perfusion. *Ann Thorac Surg* 1993;56:1493-1496.
27. Williams MD, Rainer G, Fieger HG, et al. Cardiopulmonary bypass, profound hypothermia and circulatory arrest for neurosurgery. *Ann Thorac Surg* 1991;52:1069-1075.
28. Woodhall B, Sealy WC, Hall KD, et al. Craniotomy under conditions of guinidine protected cardioplegia and profound hypothermia. *Ann Surg* 1960;152:37-44.
29. Coselli JS, Crawford ES, Beall AC Jr, et al. Determination of brain temperatures for safe circulatory arrest during cardiovascular operations. *Ann Thorac Surg* 1988;45:638-642.
30. Murkin JM. Anesthesia, the brain and cardiopulmonary bypass. *Ann Thorac Surg* 1993;56:1461-1463.
31. Nussmeier NA, Arlund C, Slogoff S. Neuropsychiatric complications after cardiopulmonary bypass: cerebral protection by a barbiturate. *Anesthesiology* 1986;64:165-170.
32. Zaidan JR, Klochany A, Martin W, et al. Effect of thiopental on neurologic outcome following coronary artery bypass grafting. *Anesthesiology* 1991;74:406-411.
33. Woodcock TE, Murkin JM, Farrar JK, et al. Pharmacologic EEG suppression during cardiopulmonary bypass: cerebral hemodynamic and metabolic effects of thiopental or isoflurane during hypothermia and normothermia. *Anesthesiology* 1987;67:218-224.
34. Forsman M, Olsnes BT, Semb G, et al. Effects of nimodipine on cerebral blood flow and neuropsychological outcome after cardiac surgery. *Br J Anesth* 1990;65:514-520.
35. Reeves RB. An imidazate alpha state hypothesis for vertebrate acid-base regulation: tissue carbon dioxide content and body temperature in bullfrogs. *Respir Physiol* 1972;14:219-236.
36. Dickinson DF, Sambrooks JE. Intellectual performance in children after circulatory arrest with profound hypothermia in infancy. *Arch Dis Child* 1979;54:1-6.
37. Charleson PM, MacArthur BA, Barret-Boyes BG, et al. Developmental progress after cardiac surgery in infancy using hypothermia and circulatory arrest. *Circulation* 1980;62:855-861.
38. Messmer BJ, Schallberger U, Garriker R, et al. Psychomotor and intellectual development after deep hypothermia and circulatory arrest in early infancy. *J Thorac Cardiovasc Surg* 1976;72:495-502.
39. Veda Y, Miki S, Husuhara K, et al. Surgical treatment of aneurysm of dissection involving the ascending aorta and

40. aortic arch, utilizing circulatory arrest and retrograde cerebral perfusion. *J Cardiovasc Surg* 1990;31:553-558.
40. Usui A, Hotta T, Hiroura M, et al. Retrograde cerebral perfusion through a superior vena caval cannula protects the brain. *Ann Thorac Surg* 1992;53:47-53.
41. Usui A, Oohara K, Liu T, et al. Determination of optimum retrograde cerebral perfusion conditions. *J Thorac Cardiovasc Surg* 1994;107:300-308.
42. Mori A. Retrograde cerebral perfusion using pulsatile flow under conditions of profound hypothermia. *Ann Thorac Surg* 1993;56:1497-1498.
43. Valk A, Kanten RA, Oosterheert M. Treating massive air embolism. *J Extracorp Technol* 1982;14:325-327.
44. DeBakey ME, Beall AC, Cooley DA, et al. Resection and graft replacement of aneurysms involving the transverse arch of the aorta. *Surg Clin North Am* 1966;46:1057-1071.
45. Bloodwell RD, Hallman GL, Cooley DA. Total replacement of the aortic arch and the "subclavian steal" phenomenon. *Ann Thorac Surg* 1968;5:236-245.
46. Pearce CW, Weichert RF III, del Real RE. Aneurysms of the aortic arch. Simplified technique for excision and prosthetic replacement. *J Thorac Cardiovasc Surg* 1969;58:886-890.
47. Crawford ES, Saleh SA, Schuessler JS. Treatment of aneurysms of the transverse aortic arch. *J Thorac Cardiovasc Surg* 1979;78:383-393.
48. Cooley DA, Oh DA, Frazier OH, et al. Surgical treatment of aneurysms of the transverse aortic arch: experience with 25 patients using hypothermic technique. *Ann Thorac Surg* 1981;32:260-272.
49. Stoney WS, Alford WC, Burrus GR, et al. Air embolism and other accidents using pump oxygenators. *Ann Thorac Surg* 1980;29:336-340.
50. Yamashita C, Nakamura H, Nishikawa Y, et al. Retrograde cerebral perfusion with circulatory arrest in aortic arch aneurysms. *Ann Thorac Surg* 1992;54:566-568.
51. Safi HJ, Brien HW, Winter JN, et al. Brain protection via cerebral retrograde perfusion during aortic arch aneurysm repair. *Ann Thorac Surg* 1993;56:270-276.
52. DeBakey ME, Cooley DA, Crawford ES, et al. Successful resection of fusiform aneurysm of the aortic arch with replacement by homograft. *Surgery* 1957;105:657-664.
53. DeBakey ME, Cooley DA, Crawford ES, et al. Aneurysms of the thoracic aorta. *J Thorac Surg* 1953;36:393-420.
54. Muller WH, Warren WD, Blanton FS Jr. A method for resection of aortic arch aneurysms. *Ann Surg* 1960;151:225-230.
55. Bjork VO. Successful replacement of the total aortic arch for aneurysm. *J Thorac Cardiovasc Surg* 1963;45:817-823.
56. Dubost CH, Blondeau PH, Piunica A, et al. Treatment chirurgical des aneurysms de l'aorte thoracique à propos de 25 cas explores chirurgicalement. *J Chir* 1962;83:331-359.
57. First WH, Baldwin JC, Vaughn AS, et al. A reconsideration of cerebral perfusion in aortic arch replacement. *Ann Thorac Surg* 1986;42:273-281.
58. Kazui T, Inoue N, Yama O, et al. Selective cerebral perfusion during operation for aneurysms of the aortic arch: a reassessment. *Ann Thorac Surg* 1992;53:109-114.
59. Tabayashi K, Niibori K, Iguchi A, et al. Replacement of the transverse aortic arch for type A acute aortic dissection. *Ann Thorac Surg* 1993;55:864-867.
60. Symbas PN, Pfaender LM, Drucker MH, et al. Cross-clamping of the descending aorta: hemodynamic and neurohumoral effects. *J Thorac Cardiovasc Surg* 1983;85:300-305.
61. Saleh SA. Anesthesia and monitoring for aortic aneurysm surgery. *World J Surg* 1980;4:689-692.
62. Spargo P, Crosse MM. Anesthetic problems in cross clamping of the aorta. *Ann R Coll Surg Eng* 1988;70:64-68.
63. Svensson LG, Crawford ES, Hess KR, et al. Thoracoabdominal aortic aneurysms associated with celiac, superior mesenteric, and renal artery occlusive disease: methods and analysis of results in 27 patients. *J Vasc Surg* 1992;16:378-389.
64. Schepens MA, Defauw JJ, Hamerlijnck RP, et al. Surgical treatment of thoracoabdominal aortic aneurysms by simple cross clamping: risk factors and late results. *J Thorac Cardiovasc Surg* 1994;107:134-142.
65. Borst HG, Jurmann M, Buhner B, et al. Risk of replacement of descending aorta with a standardized left heart bypass technique. *J Thorac Cardiovasc Surg* 1994;107:125-133.
66. VonSegesser LK, Kilher I, Jenni R, et al. Improved distal circulatory support for repair of descending thoracic aortic aneurysms. *Ann Thorac Surg* 1993;56:1373-1380.
67. Svensson LG, Coselli JS, Safi HJ, et al. Appraisal of adjuncts to prevent acute renal failure after surgery on the thoracic or thoracoabdominal aorta. *J Vasc Surg* 1989;10:230-239.
68. Carlson DE, Karp RB, Kouchoukos NT. Surgical treatment of aneurysms of the descending thoracic aorta: an analysis of 85 patients. *Ann Thorac Surg* 1983;35:58-69.
69. Najafi H. 1993 Update: descending aortic aneurysmectomy without adjuncts to avoid ischemia. *Ann Thorac Surg* 1993;55:1042-1045.
70. Crawford ES, Mizrahi EM, Hess KR, et al. The impact of distal aortic perfusion and somatosensory evoked potential monitoring on prevention of paraplegia after aortic aneurysm operation. *J Thorac Cardiovasc Surg* 1988;95:357-367.
71. deMol B, Hamerlijnck RP, Boezeman E, et al. Prevention of spinal cord ischemia in surgery of thoracoabdominal aneurysms: the biomedicus pump, the recording of somatosensory evoked potentials and the impact on surgical strategy. *Eur J Cardiothorac Surg* 1990;4:658-664.
72. Walls JT, Curtis JJ, Boley T. Sarns centrifugal pump for repair of thoracic aortic injury: case reports. *J Trauma* 1989;29:1283-1285.
73. Gott VL, Whippen JD, Dutton RC. Heparin bonding on colloidal graphite surfaces. *Science* 1963;142:1297-1298.
74. Verdant A, Page A, Cossette R, et al. Surgery of the descending thoracic aorta. Spinal cord protection with the Gott Shunt. *Ann Thorac Surg* 1988;46:147-154.
75. Murray GF, Young WG. Thoracic aneurysmectomy utilizing direct left ventriculo femoral shunt (TDMAC-heparin) bypass. *Ann Thorac Surg* 1976;21:26-29.
76. Acher CW, Wynn MM, Archibald J. Naloxene and spinal fluid drainage as adjuncts in the surgical treatment of thoracoabdominal and thoracic aneurysms. *Surgery* 1990;108:755-762.
77. Wisselink W, Becker MD, Nguyen JH, et al. Protecting the

ischemic spinal cord during aortic clamping: the influence of selective hypothermia and spinal cord perfusion pressure. *J Vasc Surg* 1994;19:788–795.
78. Kouchoukos NT, Wareing TH, Izumoto H, et al. Elective hypothermia and cardiopulmonary bypass and circulatory arrest for spinal cord protection during operations on the thoracoabdominal aorta. *J Thorac Cardiovasc Surg* 1990;99:659–664.
79. Dumanian AV, Hoeksema TD, Santschi DR, et al. Profound hypothermia and circulatory arrest in the surgical treatment of traumatic aneurysm of the thoracic aorta. *J Thorac Cardiovasc Surg* 1970;59:541–545.
80. Berguer R, Porto J, Fedoronko B, et al. Selective deep hypothermia of the spinal cord prevents paraplegia after aortic cross clamping in the dog model. *J Vasc Surg* 1992;15:62–72.

21
Intracranial Surgery with Cardiopulmonary Bypass

Brian L. Thomas

Background

The introduction of profound hypothermia and circulatory arrest into complex neurosurgical procedures coincided with the refinement of this technique in patients undergoing congenital cardiac and aortic arch repairs.[1-3] The use of deep hypothermia and total circulatory arrest (DHTCA) for a neurosurgical operation was initially described in 1960 by Woodhall.[4] A circulatory arrest of 10 minutes at 4°C was employed to facilitate drainage of a large subcortical tumor cyst in a 39-year-old man with metastatic carcinoma of the lung. Cannulation for pulmonary bypass (CPB) was via the femoral artery and jugular vein. The patient recovered uneventfully from this procedure yet succumbed to his pulmonary disease some 3 months later.

Over the next several years, a number of studies evaluating DHTCA for intracranial aneurysm surgery were published. Patterson and Ray[5] reported a series of seven patients in 1962, five of whom survived their operation with complete neurologic recovery. Circulatory arrest times averaged 24 minutes (range 9 to 42.5 minutes) at an esophageal temperature of 5°C. In 1964, Michenfelder[6] reported 15 patients from the Mayo Clinic undergoing aneurysm surgery using closed-chest DHTCA as described initially by Drew.[2] Bilateral femoral venous cannulas were employed to facilitate drainage into the reservoir, and patients were cooled to a nasopharyngeal temperature of 13° to 16°C prior to circulatory arrest. Only three operative deaths were reported in this series.

Despite these early successes, the technique of DHTCA for neurosurgery fell from favor in the late 1960s, in large part due to problems with coagulopathy encountered following hypothermic CPB. Drake[7] found that complications resulting from hypothermic CPB were responsible for three deaths in a series of 10 patients after surgery for intracranial aneurysm. Uihlein[8] reported a mortality rate of 22% for 66 patients undergoing intracranial surgery with DHTCA in 1968. Although the feasibility of closed-chest bypass was supported by this paper, coagulation defects were responsible for over half of the perioperative deaths in this study.

Improvements in neurosurgical management, particularly the arrival of microsurgical techniques, allowed successful operation on a greater number of complex neurovascular cases without circulatory arrest in the 1970s. Surgical options for patients with "giant" (>2.5 cm in greatest dimension) aneurysms, however, were frequently limited to parent vessel ligation, wrapping of the aneurysm, or exploration alone. Adjuncts including "controlled" systemic hypotension without hypothermia were employed to reduce turgor in large intracranial aneurysms at craniotomy, yet many centers abandoned this technique due to an unacceptable rate of systemic and neurologic complications.[9] Temporary aneurysm clips have proven quite effective for control of giant aneurysms where collateral flow is reasonably well developed and exposure is excellent, such as the carotid circulation. Transient occlusion of a brain stem vessel, however, may portend disastrous neurologic consequences. Exposure in the posterior fossa also limits the feasibility of temporary feeder vessel clipping. Even in the best of hands, direct occlusion of giant aneurysms without DHTCA (including temporary occlusion of their parent vessels), carries a significant risk. Symon and Vajda[10] operated on 35 patients with giant aneurysms, reporting poor neurologic outcomes in 20% and an 8% mortality. Patients with posterior circulation (basilar artery) aneurysms frequently experience poor outcomes when excision or clipping is attempted.[11,12] In 1979, Drake[13] reported a mortality rate of 25% and an overall complication rate exceeding 50% in a large series of patients with posterior circulation lesions. Fortunately, advances in neuroanesthesia and perioperative monitoring, combined with an enhanced understanding of the pathophysiology of CPB, have revitalized interest in the use of

DHTCA for patients with giant aneurysms that, without this technique, would frequently be deemed inoperable.

Rationale

The rationale for employing hypothermia in intracranial surgery is based upon the premise that lowering the cerebral metabolic rate for oxygen ($CMRO_2$) of neuronal tissue by decreasing body temperature confers a measure of protection against cerebral ischemia. $CMRO_2$ in humans is reduced to 50% of normal at 30°C, 15% of normal at 20°C, and less than 10% of normal at 15°C.[14] Several studies have demonstrated the protective effect of profound hypothermia in the face of cerebral ischemia.[5] The allowable period of cerebral ischemia may be extended by deep hypothermia, both in experimental animal models and in humans.[15] Several clinical series have also shown that cooling humans to core temperatures of 13° to 15°C may be undertaken without significant adverse effects.[16] The maximum allowable duration of circulatory arrest is unknown, although several investigators have suggested "safe" periods on the basis of laboratory and clinical experience. Lundar[17] has suggested a "safe period" of 50 minutes based on neurologic morbidity in adults undergoing open cardiac procedures. Taylor[18] has shown a slight increase in neurologic sequelae as circulatory arrest times approach 60 minutes. Longer circulatory arrest times have been successfully employed in pediatric patients undergoing cardiac repair, with satisfactory neurologic outcome seen in infants following arrest times of up to 90 minutes.[19] In the majority of studies involving intracranial aneurysm surgery, the duration of arrest was less than 1 hour, averaging just under 15 minutes.[20]

Barbiturates are employed by most centers along with DHTCA to augment cerebral protection. Barbiturates reduce metabolic requirements of neuronal tissue at normothermia, though it is unclear whether further reductions occur under conditions of deep hypothermia (Figure 21.1). There is convincing evidence for the protective effect of barbiturates when administered before the onset of focal ischemia.[21] The efficacy of barbiturates for global cerebral protection is controversial, however. Although Zaidan[22] found no neurologic benefit from prophylactic administration of thiopental in patients undergoing CPB, many neurosurgeons feel that the administration of pentothal in giant aneurysm cases is not deleterious, and indeed may be helpful.[20]

The technical advantages afforded by DHTCA allow performance of the neurosurgical procedure in cases where it might otherwise be impossible. The anatomy of a giant aneurysm, especially the parent vessels at the base of the lesion, may be clearly defined when the sac is collapsed under conditions of circulatory arrest with venous drainage.[23] Rupture of the sac (and its attendant consequences) is thus avoided, and clipping or endaneurysmorrhaphy may be safely carried out.[24]

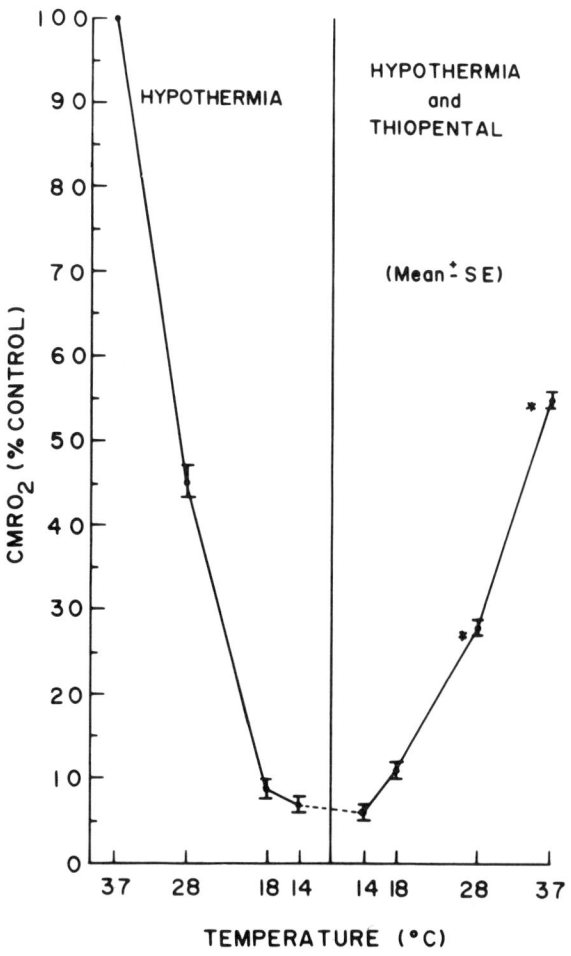

FIGURE 21.1. Canine $CMRO_2$ during cooling with spinal anesthesia (*left*) and during rewarming with the addition of deep barbiturate anesthesia (*right*). $CMRO_2$ is plotted as a percentage of control vs temperature in degrees centigrade. Asterisks indicate $CMRO_2$ values significantly different from those measured at the same temperature without thiopental ($p < 0.05$). Although barbiturates reduce metabolic requirements of neuronal tissue at normothermia, it is unclear whether thiopental affords additional reductions in $CMRO_2$ under conditions of deep hypothermia.

Technique

Employing DHTCA for intracranial aneurysm surgery requires extraordinary coordination (Table 21.1). Teams of anesthesiologists, perfusionists, operating room nurses,

TABLE 21.1. Typical anesthetic and operative sequence for intracranial surgery employing DHTCA.

Preoperative medication
Peripheral IV access, arterial line placement in holding area
To operating room
Induction of anesthesia, endotracheal intubation
Central venous pressure on pulmonary artery catheter, 2nd IV or arterial line to remove autologous blood
Place TEE probe, EEG monitors
Final positioning, external defibrillator pads
Head holder on
Prep and drape
Normovolemic hemodilution
Craniotomy, initial dissection, surface cooling, IV mannitol
Heparinization, cannulation
Burst suppression with thiopental
On CPB—cool to 15°–18° C
Circulatory arrest
Restart pump at low flow once lesion controlled
Rewarm if repair acceptable (with nitroprusside), defibrillate if needed
Separate from CPB at 36° C
Protamine after decannulation
Platelets; fresh frozen plasma or cryoprecipitate if needed
Wound closure
To intensive care unit

---

avoided, especially in those patients with elevated intracranial pressure. Anesthesia is induced with a combination of barbiturates and narcotics (eg, fentanyl). A neuromuscular blocking agent such as vecuronium is routinely administered. Tracheal intubation is accomplished after the patient is deeply anesthetized to prevent any hypertensive response or "bucking" during direct laryngoscopy. Anesthesia may be maintained with an infusion of narcotic in combination with inhaled isoflurane. Invasive monitoring lines are best placed after induction of anesthesia, and before insertion of the TEE probe. A dedicated large-bore intravenous line or second arterial line should be placed for drainage of autologous blood before initiation of CPB. Cortical electroencephalographic (EEG) tracings, somatosensory evoked potentials, brain stem auditory evoked responses, and cerebral artery blood flow[26] may be monitored according to the preferences of the attending neurosurgeon and neuroanesthesiologist. External defibrillator pads should be placed before final positioning of the patient. Positioning of the patient must allow free access to both groins as well as the sternum.

electroencephalographers, cardiac surgeons, and neurosurgeons are routinely involved to ensure optimum efficiency and patient safety. Only the largest operating rooms can accommodate the equipment and people (including observers) requisite to these procedures (Figure 21.2). The requirement for electrical outlets and power is likewise prodigious, and special engineering considerations may need to be addressed.

Appropriate patient selection requires communication between the neurosurgeon, the cardiac surgeon, and the anesthesiologist well in advance of the planned procedure. Patients typically present with a giant posterior circulation lesion amenable to surgical correction only with the exposure afforded by circulatory arrest. The patient should be evaluated by the cardiac surgeon to assess the feasibility of cannulation by way of the femoral vessels. Intraoperative transesophageal echocardiography (TEE) is routinely performed at many centers to verify satisfactory placement of femoral venous cannulas and assess distension of the cardiac chambers while CPB is underway.[25] The preanesthetic evaluation must identify contraindications to TEE, as well as coexisting cardiovascular disease. Preoperative transthoracic echocardiography can detect valvular lesions, including aortic insufficiency, which, if sufficiently severe, may be a contraindication to closed-chest CPB. The patient should be informed that median sternotomy may be necessary if femoral cannulation proves unsuccessful or should intractable cardiac distension occur during bypass.

Premedication must be sufficient to blunt any hemodynamic response to intravenous and radial arterial cannulation. Myocardial and ventilatory depression must be

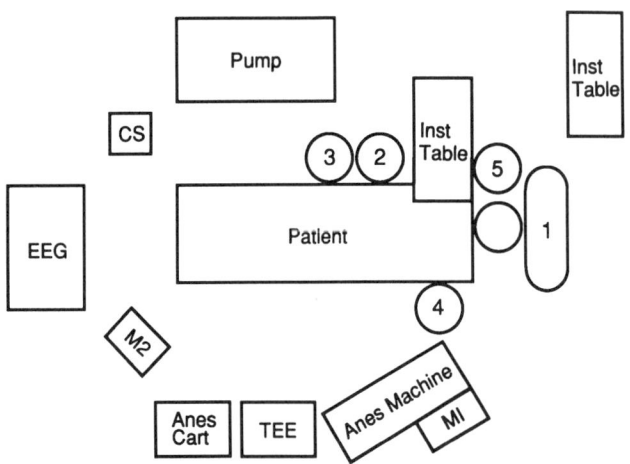

FIGURE 21.2. Schematic of an operating room setup for clipping of a basilar artery aneurysm using DHTCA. M1 represents the primary monitor screen, M2 the secondary or "slave" monitor. CS represents the cell saver apparatus. TEE represents the TEE console. The probe must course along the left axilla toward the patient's head, and is draped out of the field. [1] represents the area occupied by the neurosurgeon, the microscope chair, and the neurosurgical assistants. [2] represents the primary cardiothoracic surgeon. [3] and [4] represent cardiothoracic assistants. The assistant will most commonly be at position [3] for a right groin cannulation, position [4] for sternotomy. [4] may also be a neurosurgical assistant. There is often very little room on the side of the patient closest to the anesthesiologist. [5] represents the scrub nurse assisting either the cardiac or neurosurgeon. The patient is supine with the right shoulder slightly elevated. Access to the head, chest, and both groins is maintained. The two surgical instrument tables may rotate into the field depending on which team is operating. Only the largest operating rooms can accommodate this type of procedure.

Control of blood pressure is of paramount importance, especially in cases where there has been a recent aneurysm rupture. Anesthetic depth must be appropriate to the varying levels of stimulation encountered during the procedure. β-Blockade or nitroprusside may be required during episodes of maximal stimulation, such as application of the head fixator.

During the initial phases of the craniotomy, several units of autologous blood are removed for reinfusion after discontinuation of CPB. Volume may be replaced with isotonic crystalloid or 5% albumin to achieve a target hematocrit of 20% upon initiation of bypass. Typically, 3 to 5 L of cold perfusate are required for hemodilution in the average patient. Surface cooling is augmented by lowering the ambient temperature and applying cooling blankets beneath the exposed patient. Mannitol (0.5–1.0 g/kg) is administered during the initial dissection, and barbiturate loading is begun prior to CPB. A set amount of thiopental (25 mg/kg) may be administered, or the dose may be titrated to achieve EEG burst suppression using an infusion technique. The pump is primed with 25 g mannitol, 500 mL 6% hetastarch, with the balance as Plasma-Lyte® based on the patient's body surface area.

Dissection of the aneurysm proceeds while surface cooling is under way. When no further intracranial operation is feasible under conditions of spontaneous circulation, heparin sulfate (300–400 U/kg) is administered. Femoral cannulation is accomplished using a long 28F to 36F venous catheter placed through the saphenous bulb, and an 18F to 22F femoral artery cannula appropriate to the patient's body surface area. If a second femoral vein cannula is required for adequate drainage, the ipsilateral femoral artery should be clamped upon initiation of CPB. The long venous cannula is advanced under TEE guidance to the level of the right atrium. Should femoral cannulation prove unsuitable, cannulation of the ascending aorta and right atrium via median sternotomy is performed. Venting of the cardiac chambers may be necessary if distension should occur on bypass, particularly in patients with aortic insufficiency. Partial bypass is initiated with flow rates of 40 mL/kg/min, and cooling at a rate of 0.2°C/min is begun. Ventricular fibrillation will occur when the core temperature is between 23° and 27°C.[27] Potassium chloride may be given in 20-mEq boluses to achieve cardiac standstill. P_{CO_2} is adjusted to maintain a pH of 7.42 or greater when blood gases are measured at 37°C.[28] When brain temperature reaches 16° to 18°C, the pump is stopped. The head may be elevated and the venous lines drained to improve exposure, though overaggressive drainage may predispose to air emboli or tearing of small vascular structures.[20] If feasible, a slight head-down tilt may prevent this negative pressure gradient, reducing the likelihood of air embolus through the intracranial vasculature.

During circulatory arrest, mobilization of the aneurysm is completed, and ligation, clipping, or aneurysmectomy is performed. When this portion of the procedure is finished, perfusion is reinitiated at 16°C to test the competency of the repair. If control and hemostasis are deemed adequate, warming of the perfusate may begin. Warming may be augmented by administration of sodium nitroprusside,[29] with phenylephrine as needed to maintain an adequate perfusion pressure.

Return of spontaneous cardiac activity occurs between 23° and 28°C. External defibrillation (300 W/s) was required in 9 of 15 patients in one recent series.[30] Bypass is terminated when spontaneous cardiac function is adequate to maintain perfusion and the core temperature is ≥36°C. Protamine sulfate (10 mg/1000 U heparin) is administered after decannulation, and the patient's warm blood is returned to the circulation. Heparin reversal is optimally guided using a heparin titration method, such as the HepCon® system.

Hemostasis and Coagulation

The effects of hypothermia and CPB on the coagulation system are myriad and are only now beginning to be understood. Defects in platelet function and membrane receptor expression following bypass[31] have led many centers to "routinely" administer platelets along with the patient's warm, autologous blood after separation from the (frequently prolonged) pump run. The propensity toward using blood products in these patients stems from the fact that a small amount of postoperative hemorrhage within the cranial vault is much more problematic than the same amount in the mediastinum. Empiric administration of other procoagulants has likewise been advocated in the majority of recent series. Platelets (8–16 U), fresh frozen plasma (2–4 U), calcium chloride (1–2 g), and/or factor IX complex (1–2 U) may be administered following satisfactory heparin neutralization. The use of antifibrinolytics such as aprotinin or ε-aminocaproic acid may prove valuable in the future. Use of the thromboelastogram to guide blood product administration may be prudent in this age of viral blood-borne diseases. (Coagulation defects following CPB are further addressed in Chapter 5.)

Recent Clinical Series (Since 1981)

Advances in the anesthetic management of neurosurgical patients combined with refinements in extracorporeal circulation techniques encouraged several centers to re-evaluate the use of DHTCA for selected complex intracranial lesions in the last decade (Table 21.2). Gonski[32] reviewed 40 patients with intracranial aneurysms treated between 1974 and 1984. Thirty of these patients survived the perioperative period. The majority of complications were related to sternotomy and cardiopulmonary bypass; indeed, 4 of the 10 deaths resulted from intractable postoperative

TABLE 21.2. Recent studies of intracranial aneurysm surgery employing CPB.

Author	Year	Pts (n)	Deaths (n)	Living independently postop	Circulatory arrest time (min)	Arrest temp (°C)
Silverberg[24]	1981	9	0	9	9–51	18–22
Baumgartner[30]	1983	15	0	15	5–51	16–20
Richards[33]	1987	11	3	7	5–39	14–22
Spetzler[20]	1988	7	1	6	7–53	18–22
Williams[34]	1991	10	1	8	1–60	8–14
Solomon[35]	1991	14	0	13	8–51	15–18

hemorrhage. Morbidity and mortality decreased through later years of the study, however, perhaps because of improved patient selection. There was no correlation between duration of bypass or circulatory arrest and their perioperative mortality.

Silverberg[24] managed 8 patients undergoing 9 operations (8 giant aneurysms and 1 hemangioblastoma) with DHTCA. There were no perioperative deaths. Circulatory arrest times ranged from 9 to 51 minutes, averaging 15 minutes. Minimum core temperatures achieved were between 18° and 22°C. CPB times averaged 142 minutes (range 66–282 minutes). There was no correlation between length of bypass or circulatory arrest and postoperative course; indeed, all patients enjoyed a good or excellent outcome. One patient suffered a small stroke presenting as homonymous hemianopsia 6 months after surgery, resulting from thrombosis of the residual aneurysm sac. Angiography showed this patient's aneurysm clip had slipped, and the sac was no longer excluded from the circulation. Two patients suffered small pulmonary emboli without clinical sequelae. Both of these patients received preoperative antifibrinolytic therapy and were at bed rest following their presenting subarachnoid hemorrhages. Two patients suffered temporary ipsilateral third nerve palsies with contralateral hemiparesis, which subsequently cleared completely. One patient sustained a small frontal lobe hematoma near the site of a retractor, which resolved without further intervention.

Baumgartner[30] reported 14 patients undergoing 15 neurosurgical procedures using DHTCA. Two of these patients (three procedures) were also reported in Silverberg's series above. Two patients suffered from medullary hemangioblastoma, while the remainder presented with intracranial aneurysms. Femoral cannulation was employed, and circulatory arrest times averaged 21 minutes (range 5–51 minutes). Core temperatures at the time of arrest ranged from 16° to 20°C. Bypass time averaged 146 minutes (range 66–282 minutes). Cardiac distension on CPB was not encountered, and no perioperative deaths were reported. Four patients suffered transient thromboembolic complications, each having received antifibrinolytic therapy before surgery. Three patients suffered permanent neurologic sequelae, but all were able to leave the hospital and function independently. Three patients developed temporary neurologic palsies that resolved.

Richards[33] treated 11 patients with giant anterior or basilar circulation aneurysms who were considered inoperable without the use of DHTCA. The duration of circulatory arrest averaged 19.8 minutes, with a range of 5 to 39 minutes. Seven patients had an excellent outcome and returned to a normal life. A 46-year-old man succumbed to a left middle cerebral artery infarct. Again, postmortem examination revealed that an aneurysm clip had slipped, partially occluding the main trunk of the parent artery. One patient died from a late myocardial infarction, and another died from persistent intracranial hemorrhage. One patient underwent uneventful clipping of a basilar artery aneurysm but awoke in a persistent vegetative state. No correlation could be found between outcome and duration of circulatory arrest.

Spetzler[20] treated 7 patients with giant posterior circulation aneurysms using DHTCA. Femoral cannulation was utilized in all patients, and circulatory arrest times averaged 11 minutes (range 7–53 minutes) at 18° to 22°C. No complications related to CPB were reported. Four of these patients enjoyed excellent neurologic outcomes. One patient suffered a massive brain stem infarction and died 8 weeks later. Another patient left the hospital after ventricular shunting for a third nerve palsy with a minimal residual hemiparesis, but succumbed to a myocardial infarction 7 months postoperatively. The last patient was discharged with an improving third nerve palsy and mild contralateral hemiparesis.

Two encouraging series were published in 1991. Williams[34] treated 10 patients with complex intracranial pathology, including aneurysms, arteriovenous malformations (AVM), glomus jugulare tumors, and a cerebellar hemangioblastoma judged inoperable by conventional techniques. These patients were cooled to core temperatures of 8.4° to 13.7°C. Bypass times averaged 174 minutes, and circulatory arrest ranged in length from 1.25 to 60 minutes (average 24.5 minutes). One patient did not require circulatory arrest. Average operating room time was just over 13 hours. Eight of 10 patients enjoyed an excellent outcome. One patient with an AVM suffered from postoperative brain swelling and hemorrhage and endured a prolonged, albeit successful, recovery. The other patient in this study with an AVM died from increased intracerebral pressure after an intraventricular bleed. One patient with a vertebral artery aneurysm sustained severe postoperative neurologic deficits, including blindness and dysarthria, and required prolonged rehabilitation.

Solomon[35] reviewed 14 patients operated on for giant anterior and posterior circulation aneurysms at Columbia-Presbyterian Medical Center, including 3 who had undergone previous surgery in an attempt to control their lesion. There were no operative deaths in this series. Mean core temperature at the time of circulatory arrest was 18.3°C. Bypass time averaged 119 minutes, and circulatory arrest times averaged 22 minutes (range 8-51 minutes). Twelve patients enjoyed good neurologic outcomes. One patient suffered an intraoperative thalamic infarction and continues with a moderate right hemiparesis and aphasia after 6 months of rehabilitation. One patient sustained a subcortical infarction during the perioperative period yet was living independently one year later. Minor complications included three temporary third nerve palsies, two superficial groin infections, and one lower extremity deep venous thrombosis. Five of these patients presented after subarachnoid hemorrhage with moderate to severe preoperative deficits. These patients as a group did well postoperatively; indeed, three were living independently at the time of the report.

Conclusion

No randomized prospective trials comparing DHTCA to conventional surgical techniques have been attempted to this date, nor would they be likely, given the potential morbidity and rarity of these intracranial lesions. Comparing currently available data against historical "controls," it may be concluded that the use of DHTCA in selected high-risk patients may allow safe treatment of complex intracranial lesions that could not otherwise be successfully addressed. The frequent, life-threatening complications related to the use of CPB in the late 1960s are not apparent in more recent series. Although the results with intracranial aneurysms have been encouraging, the treatment of large AVMs remains problematic, however approached. Further refinements in surgical techniques and a clearer understanding of the hemostatic defects resulting from CPB may yield superior results for these difficult cases in the years ahead.

References

1. Brown IW, Smith WW, Emmons WO, et al. An efficient blood heat exchanger for use with extracorporeal circulation. *Surgery* 1958;44:372-377.
2. Drew CE, Anderson IM. Profound hypothermia in cardiac surgery: report of three cases. *Lancet* 1959;1:748-750.
3. Horicuchi T. Radical operations for ventricular septal defect in infancy. *J Thorac Cardiovasc Surg* 1963;46:180-190.
4. Woodhall B, Sealy WC, Hall KD, et al. Craniotomy under conditions of quinidine-protected cardioplegia and profound hypothermia. *Ann Surg* 1960;152:37-44.
5. Patterson RH, Ray BS. Profound hypothermia for intracranial surgery: laboratory and clinical experiences with extracorporeal circulation by peripheral cannulation. *Ann Surg* 1962;156:377-393.
6. Michenfelder JD, Kirklin JW, Uihlein A, et al. Clinical experience with a closed-chest technique of profound hypothermia and total circulatory arrest in neurosurgery. *Ann Surg* 1964;159:125-130.
7. Drake CG, Barr HWK, Coles JC, et al. The use of extracorporeal circulation and profound hypothermia in the treatment of ruptured intracranial aneurysm. *J Neurosurg* 1964;21:575-581.
8. Uihlein A, MacCarty CS, Michenfelder JD, et al. Deep hypothermia and surgical treatment of intracranial aneurysms: a five-year survey. *JAMA* 1966;195:639-641.
9. Heros RC, Nelson PB, Ojemann RG, et al. Large and giant paraclinoid aneurysms: surgical techniques, complications and results. *Neurosurgery* 1983;12:153-163.
10. Symon L, Vajda J. Surgical experiences with giant intracranial aneurysms. *J Neurosurg* 1984;61:1009-1028.
11. Sundt, Jr, TM, Piepgras DG. Surgical approach to giant intracranial aneurysms. Operative experience with 80 cases. *J Neurosurg* 1979;51:731-742.
12. Onuma T, Suzuki J. Surgical treatment of giant intracranial aneurysms. *J Neurosurg* 1979;51:33-36.
13. Drake CG. Giant intracranial aneurysms: experience with surgical treatment in 174 patients. *Clin Neurosurg* 1979;26:12-95.
14. Cucchiara RF, Black S, Steinkeler JA. Anesthesia for intracranial procedures. In: Barash PG, Cullen BF, Stoelting RK, eds. *Clinical Anesthesia*. Philadelphia: JB Lippincott; 1989:867-868.
15. Haneda K, Sands MP, Thomas R, et al. Prolongation of the safe interval of hypothermic circulatory arrest: 90 minutes. *J Cardiovasc Surg* 1983;24:15-21.
16. Rittenhouse EA, Mohri H, Dillard DH, et al. Deep hypothermia in cardiovascular surgery. *Ann Thorac Surg* 1974;17:63-98.
17. Lundar T, Frøysaker T, Noornes H. Cerebral damage following open-heart surgery in deep hypothermia and circulatory arrest. *Scand J Thorac Cardiovasc Surg* 1983;17:237-242.
18. Taylor C. Surgical hypothermia. *Pharmacol Ther* 1988;38:169-200.
19. Bland JW Jr, Dunbar RW, Kaplan JA, et al. Anesthetic technic using profound hypothermia for correction of congenital heart defects in infants and small children. *South Med J* 1976;69:831-833.
20. Spetzler RF, Hadley MN, Rigamonti D, et al. Aneurysms of the basilar artery treated with circulatory arrest, hypothermia, and barbiturate cerebral protection. *J Neurosurg* 1988;68:868-879.
21. Todd MM, Hehls DG, Drummond JC, et al. A comparison

of the protective effects of isoflurane and thiopental in a primate model of temporary focal cerebral ischemia. *Anesthesiology* 1985;63:A412.
22. Zaidan JR, Klochany A, Martin WM, et al. Effect of thiopental on neurologic outcome following coronary artery bypass surgery. *Anesthesiology* 1991;74:406-411.
23. McMurtry JG III, Housepian EM, Bowman FO Jr, et al. Surgical treatment of basilar artery aneurysms. Elective circulatory arrest with thoracotomy in 12 cases. *J Neurosurg* 1974;40:486-494.
24. Silverberg GD, Reitz BA, Ream AK. Hypothermia and cardiac arrest in the treatment of giant aneurysms of the cerebral circulation and hemangioblastoma of the medulla. *J Neurosurg* 1981;55:337-346.
25. Young WL. Hypothermic cardiac arrest for giant intracranial aneurysm clipping: anesthetic considerations. In: Mora CT, ed. *Cardiopulmonary Bypass in the 90's*. Atlanta: Emory University; 1991:87-92.
26. Young WL, Solomon RA, Pedley TA, et al. Direct cortical EEG monitoring during temporary vascular occlusion for cerebral aneurysm surgery. *Anesthesiology* 1989;71:794-799.
27. Griepp RB, Stinson EB, Hollingsworth JF, et al. Prosthetic replacement of the aortic arch. *J Thorac Cardiovasc Surg* 1975;70:1051-1063.
28. Rahn H, Eeves RB, Howell BJ. Hydrogen ion regulation, temperature, and evolution. *Am Rev Respir Dis* 1975;112:165-172.
29. Michenfelder JM. *Anesthesia and the Brain*. New York: Churchill Livingstone;1988:155-159.
30. Baumgartner WA, Silverberg GD, Ream AK, et al. Reappraisal of cardiopulmonary bypass with deep hypothermia and circulatory arrest for complex neurosurgical operations. *Surgery* 1983;242:242-248.
31. George GN, Pickett EB, Saucerman S, et al. Platelet surface glycoproteins; studies on resting and activated platelets and platelet membrane microparticles in normal subjects, and observations in patients during adult respiratory distress syndrome and cardiac surgery. *J Clin Invest* 1986;78:340-348.
32. Gonski A, Acedillo AT, Stacey RB. Profound hypothermia in the treatment of intracranial aneurysms. *Aust NZ J Neurosurg* 1986;9:639-643.
33. Richards PG, Marath A, Rice-Edwards JM, et al. Management of difficult intracranial aneurysms by deep hypothermia and elective cardiac arrest using cardiopulmonary bypass. *Br J Neurosurg* 1987;1:261-269.
34. Williams MD, Rainer WG, Fieger HG, et al. Cardiopulmonary bypass, profound hypothermia, and circulatory arrest for neurosurgery. *Ann Thorac Surg* 1991;52:1069-1075.
35. Solomon RA, Smith CR, Raps EC, et al. Deep hypothermic circulatory arrest for the management of complex anterior and posterior circulation aneurysms. *Neurosurgery* 1991;29:732-738.

22
Emergency Coronary Artery Bypass and Cardiopulmonary Bypass

Joseph M. Craver

Introduction

During the past 12 years, percutaneous transluminal coronary angioplasty (PTCA) has undergone remarkable growth as a revascularization modality in the care of patients with coronary artery obstructive disease.[1] With the increasing number of institutions offering coronary angioplasty services, an increasing number of cardiac surgical services will be involved in the surgical support of angioplasty patients. Since 4% to 7% of coronary angioplasty procedures result in acute ischemic complications necessitating emergency coronary artery revascularization, the cardiac surgery team must be familiar with the medical and surgical problems associated with this group of patients in their often difficult and urgent clinical circumstances.[2] To be successful in managing these failed angioplasty patients, it is essential to establish and maintain cooperative teamwork among the caregivers: the physician who performs the angioplasty, the cardiac anesthesiologist, the cardiac surgeon, the perfusionist, and the operating room nurses.

In this chapter, we will discuss the Emory experience of the last 12 years and outline our developed patient management strategies for failed angioplasty patients, including the role of intraaortic balloon pump support and emergency cardiopulmonary bypass (CPB). Our practice continues to evolve as both angioplasty procedures and the angioplasty patient change. Patients in the early years typically had arteriosclerotic heart disease requiring single-vessel angioplasty; however, the majority of patients now being considered for angioplasty have multivessel disease. The efforts to salvage these patients, who may have had previous coronary artery bypass grafting and poor ventricular function, require more sophisticated coordination and management. We are pleased that the operative mortality has remained under 3% for this difficult group of patients, and that their long-term course following angioplasty has been excellent.[3]

Spectrum and Onset of Clinical Symptoms

Most of the acute coronary injuries associated with angioplasty are manifested immediately in the cardiac catheterization laboratory. However, these lesions also may appear later, following delayed sudden closure of the coronary artery, long after the patient has left the cardiac catheterization laboratory.[4] When heparin infusion is utilized following difficult or complicated angioplasty, delayed coronary occlusion can occur after the heparin infusion has been stopped. The signs and symptoms of acute myocardial ischemia following complicated angioplasty range from acute chest pain without electrocardiographic changes, to chest pain with electrocardiographic changes, and cardiogenic shock.

The potential for delayed coronary artery occlusion requires the availability of the operating room team for a period of 24 hours following any coronary angioplasty procedure. That these ischemic events can occur within a time frame far removed from the actual angioplasty procedures necessitates that the hospital with angioplasty services have surgical and perfusion support available at all times.

Angioplasty Suite Patient Management and Treatment Strategies

Successful management of failed angioplasty patients with acute myocardial ischemia depends on well-coordinated and cooperative efforts between the angioplasty team and the surgical and perfusion teams. Management strategies are intended to (1) identify and document acute coronary occlusion, (2) moderate the effects of the myocardial ischemia, and (3) minimize the length of time during which the patient is subject to acute ischemia. If acute coronary occlusion is suspected, an immediate diagnostic arteriogram should be obtained to determine the cause of ischemia and to assess the extent to which the myocardium has been jeopardized.[5] If angiography demonstrates coronary occlusion in a previously dilated artery, then the angioplasty team will attempt to reverse the ischemia, using nonsurgical methods to minimize its severity and treat any hemodynamic deterioration. Ischemia is further treated by increasing the fraction of oxygen in the inspired air, correcting arrhythmias, adding afterload-reducing agents to reduce the work of the myocardium, and allaying patient anxiety with verbal reassurance and sedative-hypnotics. Table 22.1 outlines treatment strategies for the patient with suspected coronary artery occlusion following failed angioplasty.

If myocardial ischemia persists in the angioplasty suite, more invasive therapies to improve myocardial oxygen supply-demand ratios should be considered. If hemodynamic function is severely depressed by the acute ischemic event, additional measures may be needed to support the patient. These measures should be instituted while diagnostic and therapeutic strategies are formulated for the acutely compromised patient.

Patient oxygenation and myocardial oxygen delivery can be improved with endotracheal intubation and positive pressure ventilation. Vasoactive and inotropic drugs may increase cardiac index and diastolic blood pressure. Percutaneous intraaortic balloon pumping may be used both to increase diastolic blood pressure and coronary artery perfusion and decrease afterload.[5,6] Strategies for management of the hemodynamically unstable, failed angioplasty patient are outlined in Table 22.2. Uses of intraluminal perfusion devices, coronary stents, and intraaortic balloon pumps in the failed coronary angioplasty patient are discussed in detail below. A more detailed discussion of the pharmacologic support of the failing heart is in Chapter 17.

TABLE 22.1. Management of hemodynamically stable patients with suspected coronary artery occlusion following angioplasty.

1. Repeat coronary angiography in angioplasty suite
2. Identify occluded vessel and jeopardized myocardium
3. Treat myocardial ischemia to improve myocardial oxygen supply-demand ratio:

↑ O_2 supply	↓ O_2 demand
↑ FiO_2	↓ Anxiety
Nitroglycerin (50–200 μg/min)	Verbal assurance
	Sedation (morphine sulfate midazolam)
	Rx tachycardia or dysrhythmia
	β-Blockers
	Antiarrhythmics
	↓ Preload
	Nitroglycerin (50–200 μg/min)
	↓ Afterload
	Nitroglycerin
	ACE inhibitors

4. Monitor patient for resolving or accelerating signs and symptoms of ischemia

FiO_2, Fraction of oxygen in the inlet gas; ACE, angiotensin-converting enzyme

TABLE 22.2. Management of hemodynamically *unstable* patients following failed angioplasty.

1. Alert surgeon, anesthesiologist, perfusionist, and operating room
2,3. Same as for stable patient
4. Administer inotropic drugs to increase cardiac index and perfusion to vital organs
   Dopamine, 3–10 μg/kg/min, IV
   Epinephrine, 1–8 μg/min, IV
   Amrinone, 1–3 mg/kg, IV (loading dose)
              5–10 μg/kg/min, IV (maintenance)
5. Aggressive therapy to improve myocardial oxygen supply-demand ratio:

↑ O_2 supply	↓ O_2 demand
↑ FiO_2 (intubation, controlled ventilation if cardiogenic shock[a])	Controlled ventilation[a]
↑ Coronary perfusion pressure IABP	↓ Afterload IABP or Sedation or paralysis[a]
↑ Diastolic blood pressure (phenylephrine, 50–200 μg/min)	
Coronary artery perfusion catheter	
Intraluminal coronary artery stents	

6. If ischemia persists, prepare patient to be transported to operating room

[a]Anesthesiologist should be present for sedation, paralysis, and initiation of controlled ventilation
FiO_2, Fraction of oxygen in the inlet gas; IABP, intraaortic balloon pump

Perfusion Catheters and Intraluminal Devices

In an effort to reduce acute myocardial ischemia by restoring some degree of distal perfusion, several intraluminal devices have been developed for use while the patient is still in the catheterization laboratory.[7] Stack autoperfusion catheters (Advanced Cardiovascular Systems, Inc., Santa Clara, California) have multiple luminal ports whereby blood can enter the catheter lumen above the injured arterial zone, pass through the catheter spanning the injury zone, and exit through ports in the catheter distal to the injury. Perfusion of the coronary vessels and capillary beds distal to acutely occluded zones by these "bail-out" catheters may reduce the severity of ischemia, improve hemodynamic stability, reduce the need for intraaortic balloon support, and often allow for a more normal induction of anesthesia for emergency surgical revascularization. The Stack catheter and other autoperfusion catheters provide only passive perfusion; therefore, catheter blood flow depends on, and is directly related to, the patient's mean arterial pressure. Thus, catheter effectiveness is severely limited if the patient is hypotensive. The Emory experience with the Stack "bail-out" catheter has been favorable; however, results in other centers have been inconsistent and associated with arterial perforation and other complications.

Intraluminal stents are being studied and developed in several centers. At Emory, our early experience has been gained with a balloon expandable wire coil stent (Cook Inc., Bloomington, Indiana).[7] The stent was developed to address problems of acute closure as well as long-term restenosis. The clinical utility of the stent is still evolving, as there may be difficulty with proper insertion and positioning, an increased incidence of hemorrhage and false aneurysm at the femoral artery insertion site, mandatory permanent anticoagulation, and early restenosis in spite of the stent's apparent successful placement. In the management of coronary artery acute closure requiring surgery, most surgeons would prefer that the patient's arterial injury be splinted with the guide wire alone, or treated with a "bail-out" catheter with hemodynamic support provided by balloon pumping. The patient could be sent more quickly for emergency revascularization without the usual considerable delay necessary for proper stent placement.

Intraaortic Balloon Pump

The use of the intraaortic balloon pump in patients who develop acute myocardial ischemia as a complication of coronary angioplasty has several theoretical advantages.[5,6] Counterpulsation with an intraaortic balloon may reduce myocardial oxygen demand during systole and enhance the coronary flow to the ischemic myocardial zone during diastole by augmentation of diastolic pressure. In patients who develop acute ischemia during angioplasty, the electrocardiographic signs of myocardial ischemia improve with initiation of intraaortic balloon pumping. Furthermore, intraaortic balloon counterpulsation may provide the added benefit of raising mean arterial pressure and cardiac output in patients with hemodynamic deterioration due to acute myocardial ischemia. Stabilization and improvement of hemodynamic parameters in patients with acute myocardial ischemia may prevent extension of the ischemic zone, thus avoiding cardiac arrest and end-organ injury, and allowing an orderly transfer of the patient to the operating room. When a complication occurs during an angioplasty, and acute myocardial ischemia becomes refractory to medical management, the intraaortic balloon pump should be inserted while the patient is still in the cardiac catheterization laboratory.[5] If a patient develops myocardial ischemia on the ward after leaving the cardiac catheterization laboratory, balloon counterpulsation should be seriously considered, especially if the surgical standby has been disbanded and a delay in prompt surgical revascularization is anticipated. Intraaortic balloon pumping should also be considered when the patient has had previous cardiac surgery, with resultant mediastinal and epicardial scarring, which will require prolonged dissection before bypass grafting can be achieved.

Rapid implementation of counterpulsation in patients who develop acute injury during angioplasty can be facilitated by a number of preparations: (1) stationing of a balloon pump console and intraaortic balloon catheters in the angioplasty suite, (2) ensuring immediate availability of skilled balloon pump technicians, and (3) preparing both groin areas prior to the angioplasty procedure. Intraaortic balloon insertion can be achieved very rapidly using a percutaneous puncture and guide wire technique.[6] The potential complications arising from the use of an intraaortic balloon pump can be minimized by allowing only experienced personnel to insert the balloon catheter, using fluoroscopy, and removing the balloon catheter during the postoperative period as soon as the patient's hemodynamic condition permits.

Deciding on Coronary Artery Bypass Graft (CABG) Surgery Following Failed Angioplasty

It is our policy to carry out emergency bypass surgery following angioplasty on patients who have preinfarction myocardial ischemia that is refractory to nonsurgical treatments. The decision to proceed with emergency bypass surgery is reserved for those patients who are in a preinfarction state and for whom medical and interventional techniques have failed to reverse the ischemic process. However, the decision to perform emergency bypass surgery is also made for those additional patients without continuing ischemic chest pain after acute arterial closure when there is a significant amount of myocardium in jeopardy as determined by diagnostic angiography, regardless of whether ischemic changes are present on the electrocardiogram.

At Emory University Hospital, the angioplasty service notifies the surgical, anesthesia, perfusion, and nursing teams immediately when there are any signs of impending complications. Coordination of the emergency support and revascularization effort is provided by the staff cardiac anesthesiologist in charge at the time. Early notification ensures that members of the cardiac surgery and anesthesia teams will be dispatched to the angioplasty suite where they will participate in further decisions regarding patient management. When it seems likely that the patient will go to the operating room for emergency coronary revascularization, the surgical, anesthesia, perfusion, and nursing teams rapidly prepare to receive the patient.

In summary, early identification and intervention following failed angioplasty are critical to the preservation of jeopardized myocardium and, therefore, patient survival. Treatment is initiated in the angioplasty suite to reestablish coronary artery blood flow (via angioplasty or intracoronary perfusion catheters and stents) and to minimize myocardial oxygen demand while maximizing myocardial oxygen delivery. The cardiac surgeon, anesthesiologist, nurse, and perfusionist should be alerted early to the status of failed angioplasty patients who may require CABG surgery.

Coordination of Surgical Support

As noted above, when the decision is made to proceed with emergency bypass surgery, time is of the essence. During the initial 2 months at Emory University Hospital, surgical support for any angioplasty procedure involved having a cardiac surgical operating room standing ready with a full complement of personnel and a cardiopulmonary perfusion unit available. In the third and fourth months, angioplasty procedures were performed at those times when a cardiac operating room was not in use, ie, between elective operations or at the end of the day. From that time forward, there has been no formal coordination between angioplasty procedures and the cardiac surgical schedule. Patients who require emergency myocardial revascularization are accommodated in the first operating room available. There are four cardiac surgical operating rooms at Emory University Hospital and two at Crawford Long Hospital. When angioplasty procedures are scheduled during nonworking hours for the surgery team, such as after hours or on weekends, the nursing personnel and at least one member of the perfusion team will be present in the hospital along with the cardiothoracic resident on duty. The angioplasty attending physician must notify the attending surgeon and cardiac anesthesiologist to secure their availability. In smaller institutions, stricter coordination of the angioplasty and elective cardiac surgical schedules may be necessary to allow for immediate availability of cardiac surgical personnel and facilities.

Intraoperative Patient Management Following Failed Angioplasty

Once the patient has arrived in the operating room, the strategies for intraoperative care will vary according to the local experience. It has been our practice to tailor the procedure to the stability of the patient. Obviously, if the patient is in cardiogenic shock, anesthesia preparation and monitoring must be kept at a minimum to expedite CPB and myocardial reperfusion. Fortunately, most patients arriving in the operating room, even with ongoing ischemia, are hemodynamically stable because the therapeutic measures described above were instituted early in the course of the acute closure. In our experience, insertion of comprehensive monitoring catheters prior to anesthesia induction has not significantly delayed surgery. Pulmonary artery catheters were placed in over 95% of our patients prior to anesthesia induction.[5,8] The pulmonary artery catheter permits the rational selection of vasoactive and cardiotonic drugs on the basis of objective hemodynamic data, and facilitates the salvage of these acutely ischemic patients. Frequently, we employ the catheters placed by cardiology for venous access and for monitoring the arterial blood pressure during anesthesia induction. Supplementary venous access is virtually always needed. In those few cases in which it is not possible to place a pulmonary artery catheter prior to induction, the catheters are placed during the procedure prior to discontinuation of CPB support so that hemodynamic data can be available for post-CPB management. In addition, radial or femoral artery catheters, temperature probes, and indwelling bladder catheters are always utilized. Failed angioplasty emergency surgery patients can be hemodynamically tenuous, necessitating a careful selection of anesthetic induction and maintenance drugs. High-dose synthetic opioids, benzodiazepines, ketamine, and etomidate, or a combination of these drugs, may facilitate hemodynamic stability during anesthesia.

Surgical Technique

Surgical management is focused on placing the patient on CPB support as quickly as possible. This unloads the heart, thereby decreasing the oxygen demand in the jeopardized area and providing a measure of salvage for that zone. This is the first step in rescuing the injured myocardium. Further steps include reducing the workload of the area by implementing cardioplegia (which provides substrates and oxygenation to the injured zone) and restoring the blood supply to the area by revascularization.

As soon as the induction of anesthesia is achieved, a median sternotomy is performed. Intraoperative findings frequently include discoloration and dysfunction of the left ventricle in the distribution of the injured coronary artery.[4,5] Less commonly, there may be areas of periarterial hemorrhage proximally or distally along the course of the injured artery. Cannulation of the heart is rapidly carried out, and CPB is instituted as quickly as possible. In the case of patients with previous cardiac surgery who are hemodynamically unstable despite intraaortic balloon pumping, CPB is instituted via the femoral arteries while the heart is exposed. Following institution of CPB, no time should be wasted for systemic cooling prior to aortic cross-clamping and administration of cardioplegia. Persistent ST-segment elevation is frequently seen on the electrocardiogram in this group of patients, despite an empty, beating, perfused heart supported on CPB. During the first decade of caring for failed angioplasty patients, myocardial preservation was achieved by the institution of cold oxygenated crystalloid cardioplegia or cold blood cardioplegia, with solutions infused antegradely via the aorta and retrogradely via the coronary sinus. If more than one vein graft was planned, the injured artery or arteries were bypassed first, and cardioplegia was induced by 200 mL of cardioplegic cold blood administered immediately through the completed vein graft perfusing the area of ischemic myocardium. Cardioplegic solutions administered via the aorta often cannot reach the ischemic area, due to acute arterial occlusion and lack of collateral vessels. Therefore, prior to and during the time when the proximal anastomoses were being constructed, we administered continuous cardioplegic cold blood by retrograde coronary sinus infusion and via the completed grafts when multiple distal grafts are employed. We have also used the internal mammary artery (IMA) for the bypass conduit when the patient was stable preoperatively. However, the additional time required to harvest and prepare the IMA, and the inability to infuse cardioplegic solutions through this artery, limit its desirability in ischemic, hemodynamically unstable patients. The use of cardioplegia instituted with warm blood administered both antegradely and retrogradely via a coronary sinus catheter was begun in 1990. This is a promising technique, and perhaps is superior for patients with acute closure syndrome who require emergency surgical bypass.[9]

Following completion of bypass graft anastomoses, and re-establishment of flow into the distribution of the injured artery, we "rest" the heart on CPB in a warm, empty, beating state for 30 minutes. During this period of reperfusion, improvement in color and function of the previously ischemic muscle is frequently observed.[4,10] In severely ischemic ventricles, a "hot shot" of warm, hyperkalemic blood cardioplegia, administered just before aortic crossclamp removal, has been used to induce myocardial arrest.

In patients who have had prior bypass surgery, special technical considerations may be necessary in cases of acute myocardial ischemia resulting from the balloon dilation of an old aortocoronary vein graft. In this particular setting, angioplasty of atherosclerotic vein grafts may have resulted in embolization of atherosclerotic debris into the distal coronary artery. If this complication is recognized before or during the operation, embolectomy of the distal involved coronary artery can be performed, but frequently with only limited success. Usually, a new saphenous vein graft, placed beyond the site of embolic debris, results in better myocardial reperfusion.

Fortunately, only rarely do we perform emergency coronary bypass on angioplasty patients who have had previous CABG surgery. When this occurs, and the patient's hemodynamic condition is quite poor or unstable, it may be necessary to place the patient on femoral-to-femoral bypass. It also may be advisable to consider doing this if a difficult mediastinal dissection is anticipated. Placing the patient on femoral bypass, however, does not guarantee safety, since arrhythmias or other problems may arise, which can only be managed by having direct access to the myocardium. Opening the chest quickly is paramount and should proceed while the designated member of the team establishes the femoral perfusion route. We have had little experience in our hospital with percutaneous femoral CPB, a modality that may be beneficial in this situation in the future.

In our experience, approximately 30% of patients will require inotropic drug support to be successfully separated from the CPB.[8] We have also observed that by applying intraaortic balloon pumping to all patients with chest pain and persistent ST-segment elevation preoperatively, it was rarely necessary to employ balloon pumping in any additional patients after emergency surgery.[5,10]

Probability of Myocardial Infarction

Among our patients undergoing emergency bypass surgery for angioplasty-induced acute ischemia, slightly more than half manifested some degree of myocardial necrosis by the criterion of serum creatinine phosphokinase elevation. Twenty percent of these patients had signs of transmural myocardial infarction by the criterion of new Q-wave(s) on the electrocardiogram.[3,5]

Our experience also indicates that there is a strong correlation between the severity of preoperative ischemia and evidence of postoperative transmural myocardial infarction.[3,5] We have also observed that there is a connection between the extent of myocardial damage and the length of time from onset of ischemia to surgical intervention, although we have not been able to demonstrate a statistically significant correlation between the two factors.[4,10,11] It seems likely, however, that the duration of ischemia is an important determinant of the degree of myocardial necrosis in these patients. This belief is based on experimental studies in canines and clinical studies of intracoronary streptokinase infusion in humans with acute coronary thrombosis, which demonstrate a significant reduction in myocardial necrosis when myocardial reperfusion is achieved in less than 3 hours.[12,13] Our inability to prove a correlation between the duration of ischemia and the extent of myocardial necrosis may be related to the fact that those patients at high risk for myocardial infarction—the patients with persistent ST elevation—were more expeditiously processed to surgery.[4,5,10]

Procrastination After Angioplasty Complications

A disturbing trend in angioplasty practice is the willingness of angioplasty physicians to accept complications or unsuccessful results occurring at angioplasty as long as there is no associated severe hemodynamic compromise.

Failure to send patients for emergency surgery after complicated angioplasty, when large areas of myocardium are potentially jeopardized, is inexcusable. Whether motivated by a desire to hold down a team's emergency surgery rate, or to avoid interrupting a surgical colleague's elective schedule, this lack of effort shows an inability to recognize impending injury to the patient; it will certainly deny the patient an optimal revascularization result.

Conclusion

Despite careful patient selection and meticulous attention to technique, a small percentage of patients undergoing PTCA will develop acute myocardial ischemia distal to the instrumented artery. Immediate diagnostic coronary arteriography allows for recognition of the cause of the ischemic process and assessment of the mass of myocardium jeopardized by the obstructed artery. When myocardial infarction appears imminent, or when the area of jeopardized myocardium is large, emergency surgical revascularization is the therapy of choice. The ability, at this juncture, to mobilize quickly the operating team of surgeon, cardiac anesthesiologist, nurse, and cardiopulmonary perfusionist is essential if the patient's life is to be saved and myocardial injury minimized. Without question, the infarction process starts the moment the angioplasty instrumentation produces closure of a vessel on which myocardium is still dependent. Minimizing the length of time the myocardium must work in an ischemic state prior to its revascularization minimizes the amount of muscle mass that will ultimately be lost, and the resultant degree of future disability for the patient. Prompt notification of potential complications and early employment of pharmacologic support or intraaortic balloon counterpulsation may serve to preserve ischemic myocardium and prevent hemodynamic deterioration. Prompt bypass revascularization and the use of preoperative intraaortic balloon pumping has been associated with a 20% incidence of transmural infarction and very low mortality in this difficult group of patients.

References

1. Gruentzig A. Results from coronary angioplasty and implications for the future. *Am Heart J* 1982;103:779–783.
2. Dorros G, Crowley MJ, Simpson J, et al. Percutaneous transluminal coronary angioplasty: report of complications from the National Heart, Lung, and Blood Institute PTCA Registry. *Circulation* 1983;67:723–730.
3. Talley JD, Weintraub WS, Roubin, GS, et al. Dailey elective percutaneous transluminal coronary angioplasty requiring coronary artery bypass surgery. *Circulation* 1990;82:1203–1213.
4. Murphy DA, Craver JM, Jones EL, et al. Surgical revascularization following unsuccessful percutaneous transluminal coronary angioplasty. *J Thorac Cardiovasc Surg* 1982;84:342–348.
5. Murphy DA, Craver JM, Jones EL, et al. Surgical management of acute myocardial ischemia following PTCA: role of the intraaortic balloon pump. *J Thorac Cardiovasc Surg* 1984;87:332–339.
6. Margolis JR. The role of the percutaneous intraaortic balloon in emergency situations following percutaneous transluminal coronary angioplasty. In Kaltenback M, Gruentzig A, Rentrop K, Bussman WD, eds. *Transluminal Coronary Angioplasty and Intracoronary Thrombolysis*, New York: Springer-Verlag; 1982:144–150.
7. Roubin GS, Douglas JS, Lembo NJ, et al. Intracoronary stents for acute closure following percutaneous transluminal coronary angioplasty (PTCA). *Circulation* 1988;78(suppl):1621.
8. Curling PE, Waller JL, Murphy DA, Craver JM, Jones EL, Freniere S. Resuscitation, monitoring, and anesthesia for failed percutaneous transluminal coronary angioplasty. Abstracts of the 6th Annual Meeting of the Society of Cardiovascular Anesthesiologists, Boston, MA. May 1984:227–228.
9. Salerno TA, Houck JP, Barrozo CA, et al. Retrograde continuous warm blood cardioplegia: a new concept in myocardial protection. *Ann Thorac Surg* 1991;51:245–247.
10. Jones EL, Craver JM, Gruentzig AR, et al. Percutaneous transluminal coronary angioplasty: role of the surgeon. *Ann Thorac Surg* 1982;34:493–503.
11. Kutcher MA, Gruentzig AR, Turina M, Craver JM, Jones EL, Douglas JS, King SB III. Can emergency coronary bypass surgery following acute failure of coronary angioplasty prevent myocardial infarction? *Am J Cardiol* 1982;49:956.
12. Riemer KA, Lower JE, Rasmussen MM, Jennings RB. The wave front phenomenon of ischemic cell death: myocardial infarct size vs duration of coronary occlusion in dogs. *Circulation* 1977;56:786–794.
13. Anderson JL, Marshall HW, Bray BE, et al. A randomized trial of intracoronary streptokinase in the treatment of acute myocardial infarction. *N Engl J Med* 1983;308:1312–1318.

23
Chest Trauma and Emergency Cardiopulmonary Bypass

Panagiotis N. Symbas

Trauma is the leading cause of absenteeism from work and the leading cause of death among young adults in the industrialized nations.[1,2] Injuries to the various intrathoracic structures play a major role in this morbidity and mortality.[3] Most injuries to the chest, including wounds to the heart, can be repaired without the aid of total or partial cardiopulmonary bypass (CPB) or any form of shunts. Only a few injuries to the heart, to the great vessels, and, occasionally, to the major airways call for some form of CPB support. The aim of this chapter is to describe the various traumatic lesions that require extracorporeal support for their repair.

Cardiac Wounds

Injury to the heart is usually caused by a penetrating wound or blunt trauma to the chest.[4] Less frequently, injury to the heart may be due to iatrogenic trauma, to ionizing radiation, or to electric current.

The vast majority of penetrating cardiac wounds, in civilian life, are gunshot or stab wounds. Injury to the heart is usually limited to the free cardiac wall, but occasionally the coronary arteries or the intracardiac structures may also be injured.[4,5] The vast majority of wounds of the free cardiac wall can be repaired without any form of extracorporeal support. In fact, during a 25-year period, of the 221 patients with penetrating wounds of the heart treated at Grady Memorial Hospital, only two required CPB for repair of the free cardiac wall.[4,6] One of these had a large, self-inflicted bullet wound to the anterolateral wall of the left ventricle. Because of the size of the wound and the adjacent contusion, primary repair of the myocardium could not be accomplished, and therefore the wound was repaired with a Dacron patch[7] (Figure 23.1A and B). The other patient sustained bullet wounds to the right and left ventricles and to the ventricular septum. The septal wound was repaired with a Teflon patch, and the right and left ventricular wounds with pericardial patches.

The repair of such wounds is accomplished under conventional CPB, following cannulation of the right atrium with single or bicaval cannulas and cannulation of the ascending aorta.

Injury to intracardiac structures may involve the aortic cusps, the mitral valve apparatus, leaflets, chordae tendineae, or papillary muscles, or the ventricular or atrial septa.[5] Wounds to these structures, which result in valvular regurgitation or intracardiac shunts, usually do not require repair at the same time the free cardiac wall is being repaired. Rather, these lesions are treated "semiurgently," or usually electively, after their hemodynamic significance is assessed by cardiac catheterization and/or echocardiography. The treatment of an injury to a valve consists of valvuloplasty or replacement, while treatment of the atrial or ventricular septum is primary closure or closure with a patch, which is similar to the treatment of other acquired lesions of these structures. Conventional CPB is used for these nonemergent repairs.

Coronary artery trauma must be repaired emergently. The type of repair is dependent upon the myocardium at risk. Wounds to a small coronary artery are treated by ligation of the injured artery without the aid of extracorporeal circulation, whereas injury of larger coronary arteries is either primarily repaired or bypassed, as are other acquired coronary artery lesions. Again, conventional CPB is employed if coronary artery repair or bypass is required.

Other rare residual or delayed lesions or penetrating wounds to the heart that may require total CPB include retained missiles in the heart and traumatic aneurysm of the heart (Figure 23.2A and B). The treatment of intracardiac retained missiles is dependent upon the site, size, and shape of the missile, and upon the presence or absence of symptoms.[8,9] Symptomatic missiles, missiles in a left cardiac chamber or partially protruding into it, and those located next to any artery, should be removed. The extraction of these missiles, as well as repair of a traumatic aneurysm of the heart, is accomplished under conventional total CPB.

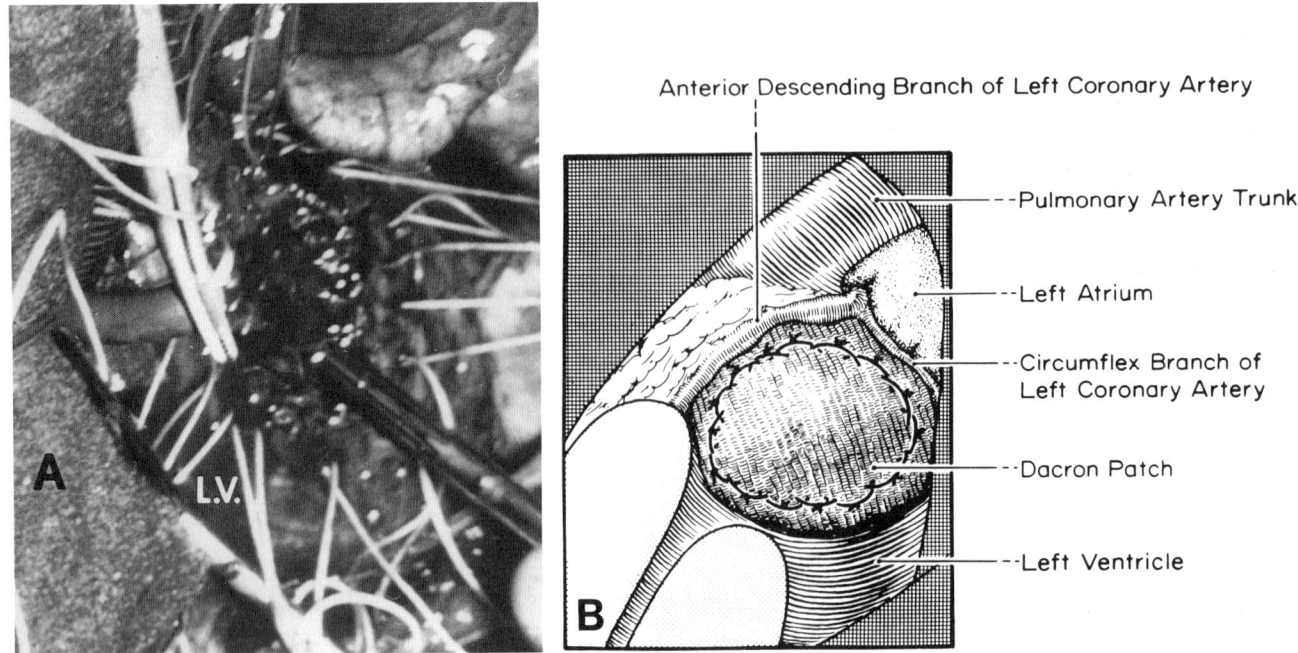

FIGURE 23.1. (A) Photograph of a large wound of the left ventricle. (B) Diagrammatic illustration of the wound repaired (From Symbas PN, Tyras DA, McGraw DB,[7] by permission of *J Thorac Cardiovasc Surg*.)

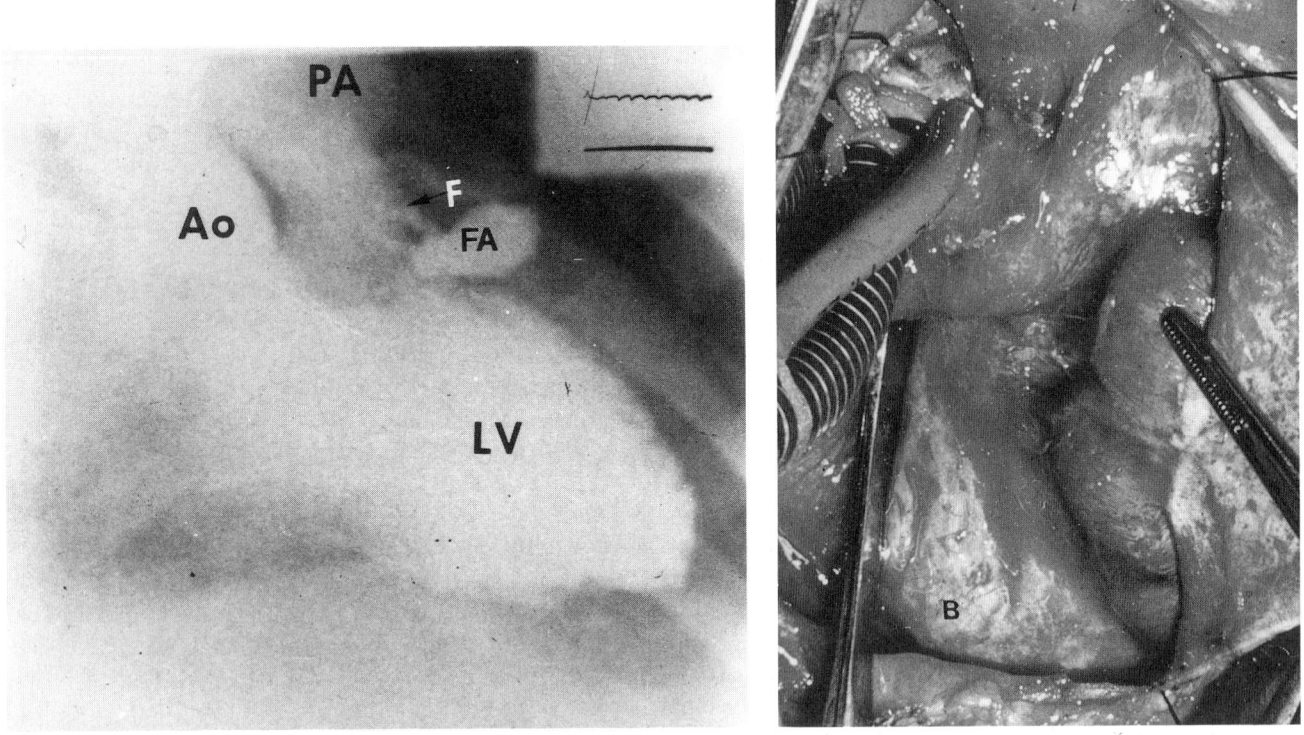

FIGURE 23.2. (A) Left cineventriculogram showing simultaneous opacification of the right ventricle, pulmonary artery (PA), aorta (Ao), and left ventricle (LV), and a false aneurysm (FA). (B) Photograph of the pseudoaneurysms of the left and right ventricles (By permission of Symbas PN, Ware RE, Belenki I et al, *J Thorac Cardiovasc Surg* 1972;64,648.)

Although, as was mentioned earlier, the current number of patients requiring CPB for the repair of lesions from penetrating wounds to the heart is limited, this number may increase in the future. The increase may be caused by an increase in the number of penetrating cardiac injuries, if the current trend toward violence continues, and to possible expansion of the role of CPB in the management of acutely injured patients, such as temporary cardiac assist to patients who have sustained irreversible ventricular fibrillation.

Treatment of the vast majority of cardiac blunt injury cases is medical.[10] Only a few patients require surgical treatment, which is done with total CPB in almost all cases. Blunt trauma patients who need surgical treatment include those with rupture of the free cardiac wall, the ventricular septum, or the cardiac valves. Rupture of the free cardiac wall may involve the wall of any cardiac chamber, but most of the patients who survive long enough to be treated have a rupture of the atria.[11] Repair of these wounds is done as soon as the diagnosis is made, either by applying tangentially a vascular clamp at the site of the wound, for some ruptures of the atria, or under conventional total CPB for the rest of these cases. Repair of the ventricular septum and cardiac valves can be accomplished only under total CPB[3] (Figure 23.3).

Finally, intraaortic balloon counterpulsations[12] or, rarely, a biventricular support device may be the only treatment modalities for patients suffering a global cardiac contusion with refractory congestive heart failure. Intraaortic balloon counterpulsation is discussed in detail in Chapter 28.

Aortic Wounds

Injury to the aorta is usually due to penetrating or blunt trauma, and frequently results in death shortly after its occurrence.

The vast majority of penetrating aortic wounds can be repaired under the tip of the finger occluding the wound or after tangential partial occlusion of the aorta.[13] Occasionally, however, such wounds—particularly through-and-through or posterior wounds, and wounds associated with aorta-cardiac or aorta-pulmonary artery fistula—require the use of CPB for their repair. The repair of an aorta-cardiac or aorta-pulmonary artery fistula is done following crossclamping of the ascending aorta under conventional total CPB bypass and cardioplegia.[10] Through-and-through aortic or posterior aortic arch wounds are repaired with CPB bypass with profound hypothermia and circulatory arrest, as are other acquired aortic arch lesions. Through-and-through descending aortic wounds are repaired with the descending aorta crossclamped. If the repair of these wounds requires more than 25 minutes, aorta-to-aorta (or to femoral artery external shunt) or femoral vein-to-femoral artery partial CPB should be used.

The optimal method of repair of a rupture of the descending aorta is controversial.[14-20] This controversy stems from the significant incidence of paraplegia that accompanies the repair of this lesion. Several factors determine the incidence and magnitude of the ischemic spinal cord injury associated with the repair of aortic rupture. The length of the crossclamping period, the number of intercostal arteries ligated, the adequacy of perfusion to the spinal cord when a bypass device is used, and the degree and duration of spinal cord hypoperfusion prior to crossclamping of the aorta are factors that may contribute to spinal cord ischemia and resulting paraplegia. Numerous methods have been advocated for the repair of the rupture and protection of the spinal cord from ischemic injury during crossclamping, with varying success.[14-19] These methods include crossclamping of the aorta without any adjuvant, or with some form of bypass (femoral vein to femoral artery, left atrium to femoral artery or descending aorta, and aorta to femoral artery or to aorta temporary shunt); systemic administration of barbiturates or steroids; and drainage of the cerebrospinal fluid.[14-20] Unfortunately, none of these methods guarantees adequate protection of the spinal cord, nor do any of the bypass procedures guarantee its adequate perfusion. The size of the Gott shunt, or any kinking of its tubing, influences the adequacy of flow through the shunt. A small-sized or improperly placed outflow cannula in the left atrium or a femoral vein cannula not advanced into the inferior vena cava causes inadequate flow through the extracorporeal system and, thereby, hypoperfusion of the spinal cord. Since the cause of spinal cord ischemia is multifactorial, and since each of the available methods has advantages and disadvantages, the method of treatment of aortic rupture should be individualized according to the condition of the patient. Those with no central nervous system injury may undergo repair of the rupture with the use of the CPB unit and left-atrial-to-femoral-artery or femoral-vein-to-femoral-artery bypass. Patients in whom heparinization is contraindicated, including those with central nervous system injury, may undergo repair with the use of a temporary external shunt or with only crossclamping of the aorta and adjuvant pharmacologic (ie, barbiturates and/or steroids) support and drainage of the cerebrospinal fluid. As noted above, when the surgeon feels confident that the aortic repair can be accomplished within 25 minutes, the repair may be done with aortic crossclamping alone.[20] A complete discussion of the management of patients with thoracic aneurysms from nontraumatic causes is found in Chapter 20. Many of the same management strategies outlined in that chapter are applicable to patients with traumatic rupture of the thoracic aorta.

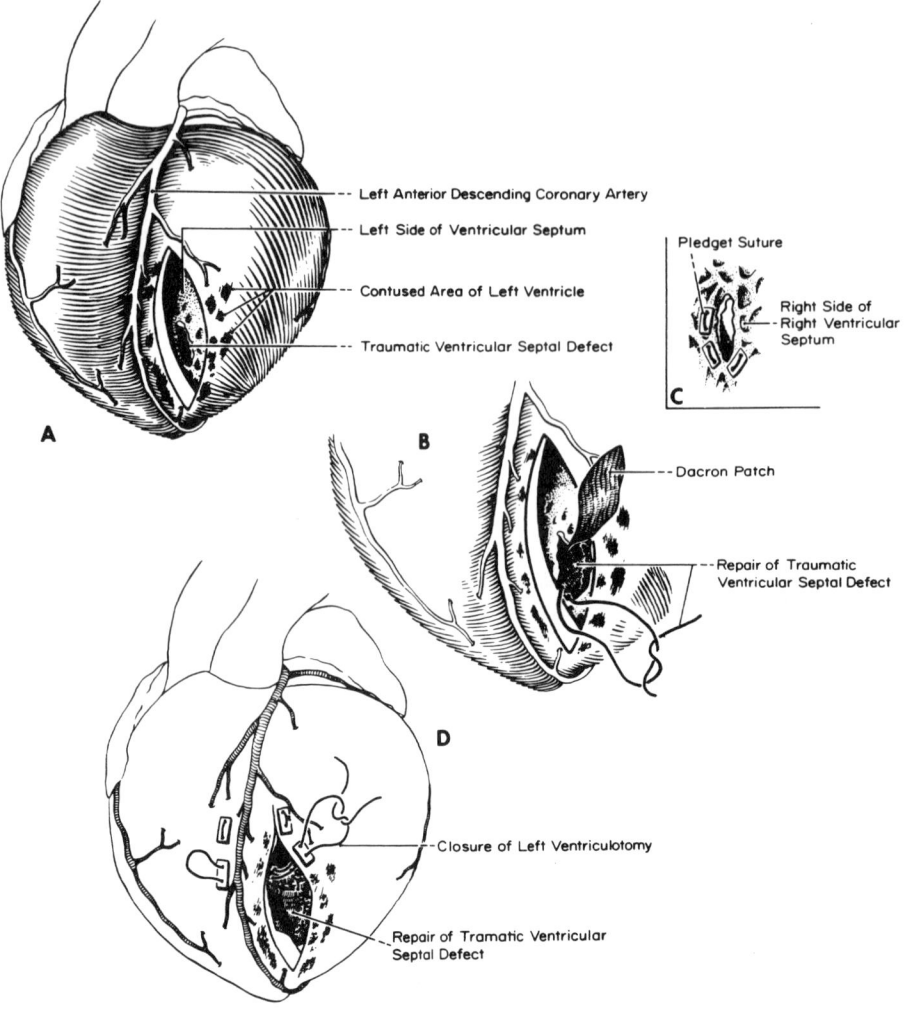

FIGURE 23.3. Diagrammatic illustration of the repair of ventricular septal rupture from blunt trauma. (By permission of Symbas PN: Trauma to the Heart and Great Vessels. Orlando, Grune & Stratton, pages 80–81, 1979.)

Major Airway Injuries

The tracheobronchial tree may be injured from penetrating or blunt trauma. The wound from blunt trauma may be a single transverse wound between the trachea rings, a longitudinal wound along the membranous segment of the airway, or a complex wound with a combination of transverse and longitudinal or multiple ruptures. The transverse rupture is the most common form, occurring in about 74% of cases; the longitudinal rupture accounts for 18%; and the complex rupture comprises the remaining 8%.[21]

Almost all major airway injuries can be repaired with conventional surgical techniques, using tissue flaps usually from parietal pleura, or occasionally from pericardium, intercostal muscle, or other tissues.[22,23] the few patients who require CPB are usually those who have suffered complex or extensive longitudinal rupture (Figure 23.4A and B) and for whom no other form of adequate ventilatory and/or circulatory support can be provided during the repair. Of the six patients with rupture of the airways who were treated at Grady Memorial Hospital during the last 20 years, only one patient, who had a longitudinal tear of both the anterior and posterior walls of the distal trachea extending into the carina, and transverse rupture of both main stem bronchi, required CPB bypass for the repair of these wounds[21] (Figure 23.4A and B). Among the 183 cases of rupture of the airway reported in the English literature during the same period, 14 had complex rupture, and only 4 of these were repaired with the use of CPB bypass. However, for the remaining 10 patients with complex rupture who were managed without CPB bypass, the treatment consisted of repair of the tracheal wound and resection of the lung, with ruptured bronchi in 5 patients, pneumonectomy in 3 patients, and lobectomy in 2.[21] Perhaps the use of CPB in the 5 patients with ruptured bronchi would have resulted in saving their resected lung. Therefore, when it is difficult to provide adequate ventilation or circulatory support in patients during the repair of airway injuries, CPB should be utilized. The judicious use of cardiopulmonary support in selected patients not only provides safety during the correction of

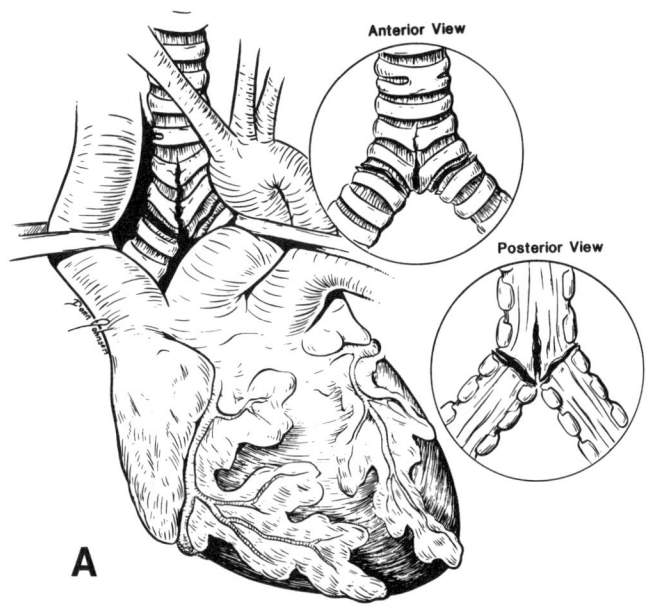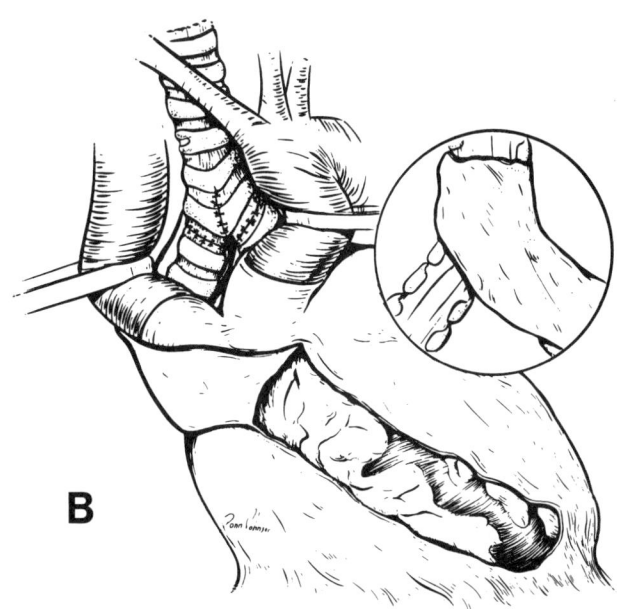

FIGURE 23.4. (A) Rupture of distal trachea and both main stem bronchi. (B) Diagram of primary repair of ruptured bronchi covered with a pericardial tissue flap. All ruptures repaired under total CPB. (Reprinted with permission from Symbas PN. *Cardiothoracic Trauma. Current Problems in Surgery*, page 788, 1991, and with permission from the Society of Thoracic Surgeons from Symbas PN, Justicz AG and Rickets RR. *Ann Thorac Surg*, July, 1992.)

the wounds, but may encourage repair of all ruptures rather than resection of the involved lung. However, the potential benefits of CPB must be weighed against the risks of heparinization of a patient with potential multiple injuries. Therefore, this technique should be reserved for those individuals in whom satisfactory ventilation and circulatory support cannot be provided by other means during the repair of the lesions. When CPB is used, the aorta or femoral artery is cannulated for the inflow and the right atrium, with double or single cannula, for the outflow.

In summary, the vast majority of traumatic injuries to the thoracic organs can be repaired without extracorporeal support. In a minority of patients, however, with penetrating wounds of the free cardiac wall or the aorta, or longitudinal or complex rupture of the major airways, and in almost al patients with rupture of the free cardiac wall and intracardiac structures, or with residual or delayed sequelae of traumatic injury, some form of extracorporeal support is required during correction of these injuries.

References

1. Unintentional and intentional injuries—United States. *MMWR* 1982;31:245–248.
2. Cost of injury—United States: a report to the congress, 1989. *JAMA* 1989;262:2803–2804.
3. Kemmerer WT. Patterns of thoracic injuries in fatal traffic accidents. *J Trauma* 1961;1:595–599.
4. Symbas PN, Harlaftis N, Waldo WJ. Penetrating cardiac wounds: a comparison of different therapeutic methods. *Ann Surg* 1976;183:377–381.
5. Symbas PN, Diorio DA, Tyras DH, et al. Penetrating cardiac wounds: significant residual and delayed sequelae. *J Thorac Cardiovasc Surg* 1973;66:526–532.
6. Symbas PN. Cardiothoracic trauma. *Curr Probl Surg* 1991; 16:741–797.
7. Symbas PN, Tyras DH, McCraw B. Repair of left ventricular traumatic defect with a dacron prosthesis. *J Thorac Cardiovasc Surg* 1972;63:608–612.
8. Symbas PN, Picone AL, Hatcher CR Jr, et al. Cardiac missiles: a review of the literature and personal experience. *Ann Surg* 1990;211:639–647.
9. Symbas PN, Harlaftis N. Bullet emboli in pulmonary and systemic arteries. *Ann Surg* 1977;185:318–320.
10. Symbas PN. *Cardiothoracic Trauma*. Philadelphia: WB Saunders Co; 1989:1–404.
11. Parmley LF, Manion WC, Mattingly TW. Nonpenetrating traumatic injury of the heart. *Circulation* 1958;18:371–396.
12. Snow N, Lucas AE, Richard JD. Intra-aortic balloon counterpulsation for cardiogenic shock from cardiac contusion. *J Trauma* 1982;22:426–429.
13. Symbas PN, Sehdeva JS. Penetrating wounds of the thoracic aorta. *Ann Surg* 1970;171:441–450.
14. Symbas PN, Tyras DH, Ware RE, et al. Traumatic rupture of the aorta. *Ann Surg* 1973;178:6–12.
15. Kirsh MM, Behrendt DM, Orringer MB, et al. The treatment of acute traumatic rupture of the aorta. A 10-year experience. *Ann Surg* 1976;184:308–316.
16. Pate JW. Traumatic rupture of the aorta: Emergency operation. *Ann Thorac Surg* 1985;329:531–537.

17. Laschinger JC, Cunningham JN, Cooper MM, et al. Prevention of ischemic spinal cord injury following aortic cross-clamping: use of corticosteroids. *Ann Thorac Surg* 1984;38:500–507.
18. Nylander WA Jr, Plunkett RJ, Hammon JW, et al. Thiopental modification of ischemic spinal cord injury in the dog. *Ann Thorac Surg* 1982;33:64–68.
19. Svensson LG, Von Ritter CM, Groneveld GT, et al. Cross-clamping of the thoracic aorta. *Ann Surg* 1986;24:38–47.
20. Vasko JS, Raess DH, Williams TE, et al. Non-penetrating trauma to the thoracic aorta. *Surgery* 1977;82:400–406.
21. Symbas PN, Justicz AG, Ricketts RR. Rupture of the airways from blunt trauma: treatment of complex injuries. *Ann Thorac Surg* 1992;54:177–183.
22. Symbas PN, Hatcher CR Jr, Boehm GA. Acute penetrating tracheal trauma. *Ann Thorac Surg* 1976;22:473–477.
23. Symbas PN, Hatcher CR Jr, Vlasis SE. Bullet wounds of the trachea. *J Thorac Cardiovasc Surg* 1982;83:235–238.

24
Pregnancy and Cardiopulmonary Bypass

Christina T. Mora

Background

Pregnancy, with its attendant stress on the cardiovascular system, is a significant cause of morbidity and mortality in the patient with heart disease. Cardiovascular pathology is present in 0.4% to 4.1% of all gravidae, and accounts for 30% of all maternal deaths.[1] Despite the overall decrease in deaths from cardiovascular disease among the general population in the last two decades, heart disease has become an increasingly likely cause of morbidity and mortality in the pregnant patient. But the prominence of heart disease is probably due to the decrease in other causes of maternal mortality. For example, Shearman[2] compared the causes of maternal death in Australia during two periods, 1970 to 1972 and 1982 to 1984, and found that heart disease had become the most likely cause of death in the latter period (Table 24.1).

Today, women with heart disease increasingly are encouraged to attempt pregnancy. (The exceptions are patients with pulmonary hypertension, coarctation of the aorta [complicated] or Marfan's syndrome with aortic involvement. These patients have a significant risk of death [25% to 50%] since they cannot tolerate the increase in cardiac output that occurs with pregnancy.[3]) Also, physicians caring for gravidae are now more likely to recommend heart surgery during pregnancy.[4] In 1982, Rush[5] opined, "Open heart surgery should be undertaken during pregnancy only in *exceptional* circumstances." By 1991, Clark[3] stated, "There are numerous reports of cardiovascular surgery during pregnancy. The reports are mostly favorable. . . ." Thus, clinicians should anticipate that gravid patients with heart disease will be referred increasingly for cardiac surgery and cardiopulmonary bypass (CPB).

As of this writing, no controlled studies have assessed the effects of cardiac surgery and extracorporeal circulation on obstetric physiology and/or fetal well-being and outcome. Although most authors advocate providing perioperative care that will ensure maternal well-being, appropriate investigation would enable clinicians to care optimally for *both* mother and fetus.

Although controlled studies are lacking, there are a few reviews[6-9] and many case reports that describe individual experience in caring for the gravid patient and fetus during cardiac surgery and extracorporeal circulation.[10-26] These surveys and anecdotal reports, along with an understanding of the well-studied physiology of pregnancy and the effects of cardiac therapeutics on fetal physiology, can serve as a basis for a rational approach to care of the pregnant patient and fetus during cardiac surgery and CPB.

This chapter summarizes the available survey data and case reports on pregnancy and cardiac surgery with CPB, and outlines the author's recommendations for perioperative management of the gravid patient requiring heart surgery. The basic principles for the perioperative management of the gravid patient undergoing cardiac surgery and

TABLE 24.1. Rank order of causes of maternal death in Australia from 1970 to 1972 and from 1982 to 1984[a].

Cause	Rank order 1970–1972	Rank order 1982–1984
Heart disease	4	1
Hemorrhage	3	2
Hypertension	5	3
Ectopic pregnancy	7	4[b]
Anesthesia	8	4[b]
Pulmonary embolism	2	4[b]
Infection	6	7
Abortion	1	8

[a]Data from ref. 2
[b]Ectopic pregnancy, anesthesia, and pulmonary embolism occurred in equal frequency

CPB are identical to those outlined by Levison and Shnider[27] for gravidae requiring *any* type of surgery: (1) maternal safety, (2) avoidance of teratogenic drugs, (3) avoidance of intrauterine asphyxia, and (4) prevention of preterm labor.

Survey Data on Maternal and Fetal Outcomes Following Cardiac Surgery and CPB

TABLE 24.2. Maternal and fetal mortality following cardiac surgery and CPB in gravida.

	Maternal death	Fetal death
Jacobs/Cooley[6] (1965)	0/3 (0%)	0/3 (0%)
Zitnik[7] (1968)	1/20 (5%)	7/20 (35%)
Becker[8] (1983)	1/68 (1.5%)	11/68 (16%)
Lapiedra[9] (1986)	0/23 (0%)	1/23 (4.3%)

In 1958, Dubourg and colleagues[28] were the first to report on the use of extracorporeal circulation in a gravida to correct a tetralogy of Fallot in a 10-weeks-pregnant patient. Although the patient recovered from her procedure, she aborted at 6 months. In 1961, Leyse[29] reported correcting an aortic valvular infundibular stenosis in a pregnant patient. This patient recovered and carried to term a fetus with multiple congenital abnormalities incompatible with life.

Four groups have published reports detailing either their individual experiences or survey data on maternal and fetal outcomes following cardiac surgery and CPB.[6-9] Cooley and colleagues[6] reported their experience with three gravid patients, at 8, 11, and 12 weeks, requiring cardiac surgery and extracorporeal circulation for repair of ventricular septal defects. All three gravidae recovered from their operative procedures and delivered normal term infants. It is noteworthy that the modal time of CPB in this series was 6½ minutes!

The first survey data on pregnancy and open-heart surgery were reported in 1969 by Zitnik and colleagues[7] from the Mayo Clinic. The authors randomly selected 20 of their cardiothoracic surgical colleagues in the United States and asked them to report on their experience in caring for the gravid patient undergoing cardiac surgery. A variety of lesions were corrected or repaired in gravid patients, including arterial and ventricular septal defects, aortic and mitral valve stenoses, tetralogy of Fallot, mitral valve insufficiency, and an aortic aneurysm. Total CPB time ranged from 6½ minutes to over 2 hours. There was only one maternal death, but seven fetuses died prior to term. The authors concluded that heart surgery does not increase the likelihood of death in the gravida with heart disease. (That is, a 5% mortality rate would be expected in this group of patients with these types of morbid diseases.) However, in this series there was a high incidence of fetal mortality, which could be related to the presence of congenital abnormalities, compromised fetal health prior to surgery (progeny of patients with uncorrected heart disease have an increased incidence of congenital abnormalities), or the adverse effects of CPB (Table 24.2). However, the authors believed the high fetal mortality associated with CPB was acceptable, because therapeutic abortion to save the mother's life would result in a fetal loss rate of 100%.

Lapiedra[9] and Becker[8] individually published reports in the 1980s on gravid patients undergoing heart surgery. Lapiedra and colleagues[9] reviewed their own experiences and found only one fetal death and no maternal mortality in their review of 23 cases. Becker surveyed members of the Society of Thoracic Surgeons on their experiences with cardiac surgery in pregnant patients. Of the 600 surgeons responding, 119 reported on a total of 169 gravid patients undergoing cardiac surgery, 68 of whom were managed with CPB (Table 24.3).

The most commonly reported procedure in this survey was mitral valve commissurotomy, most frequently performed for congestive heart failure in the second trimester of pregnancy. Both closed (without CPB) and open mitral commissurotomies were well tolerated by both mother and fetus. Open procedures may be preferable to closed procedures, since they provide more predictable short- and long-term results.[30,31] However, the avoidance of CPB has a theoretical advantage in gravid patients. The variety of other procedures reported in this survey included CPB (Table 24.3). Aortic and mitral valve replacements were associated with the highest rates of fetal loss. The authors speculated that the increased mortality may be related to the increased severity of illness and the longer duration of bypass in these two groups of patients. The maternal and fetal mortality rates (1.5% and 16%, respectively) reported in this 1983 study compared favorably with those reported by Zitnik et al[7] (Table 24.2). However, fetal mortality following cardiac surgery and CPB is a significant problem.

In conclusion, review of the reported experience on maternal and fetal outcomes following cardiac procedures with CPB suggests that cardiac surgery is well tolerated by the mother but poses a significant risk to the fetus. Extracorporeal circulation and the accompanying body temperature changes, nonpulsatile blood flow, and anticoagulation may adversely affect fetal well-being. The potential (though not well-studied) effects of CPB on fetal physiology and recommendations on the management of bypass in the gravida are outlined in Conduct of Perfusion in the Gravid Patient, below.

TABLE 24.3. Cardiac procedures performed during pregnancy: results of 1983 Society of Thoracic Surgeons survey.[a]

Procedure	Total patients	Maternal survivors	Fetal survivors[b]	Fetal deaths
Closed mitral commissurotomy[c]	101	101	98 (0)	3
Open mitral commissurotomy	23	23	22 (2)	1
MVR	19	18	15 (1)	4
AVR	10	10	6	4
Pulmonary embolectomy	3	3	2	1
ASD/VSD repair	8	8	7	1
CABG	3	3	3	0
Myxoma removal	2	2	2	0
Total CPB	68	67/68	57/68	11/68

[a]Data from ref. 7
[b]Numbers in parentheses represent premature deliveries
[c]Closed mitral commissurotomy done without CPB
MVR = mitral valve replacement; AVR = aortic valve replacement; ASD = atrial septal defect; VSD = ventricular septal defect; CABG = coronary artery bypass grafting

Preoperative Considerations

Premedication

Premedication should be appropriate for the specific cardiac lesion and physical status of the patient. Teratogenic drugs should be avoided, especially in the first trimester of pregnancy. After the 34th week of gestation, stomach emptying is delayed and patients are at increased risk for pulmonary aspiration. Although it is not possible to ensure gastric emptying prior to the induction of anesthesia, sodium citrate and an H_2-receptor antagonist may provide some protection against aspiration pneumonia.[32,33]

Patient Positioning

The gravid uterus obstructs both aortic flow and inferior vena cava blood return to the heart. Gravid patients should never be supine, and must be positioned with left uterine displacement during the perioperative period.

Monitors

The pregnant patient undergoing cardiac surgery requires the usual monitors employed during cardiac surgery, as well as monitors to assess fetal well-being. Monitors that help assess the adequacy of maternal cardiovascular performance and oxygen delivery to the fetus are of paramount importance. Table 24.4 lists appropriate maternal and fetal monitors for cardiac surgery and CPB in the gravid patient.

As discussed above, little is known about the actions of cardiovascular drugs and therapeutics in the pregnant cardiac patient. Appropriate monitors permit assessment of the effects of individual drugs and therapeutics on maternal and fetal oxygen delivery.

Maternal Monitors

Patient monitors for cardiac surgery and CPB are discussed in Chapters 16 and 17. These recommendations are summarized here. A two-lead (II, V_5) electrocardiogram (ECG), peripheral pulse oximeter, and blood pressure cuff should be placed first. These monitors provide information concerning cardiorespiratory function as other, more invasive monitors are placed.

TABLE 24.4. Maternal and fetal monitors for cardiac surgery and CPB. Monitors help assess the adequacy of oxygen delivery to both the mother and fetus.

Maternal
  "Routine"
    Blood pressure cuff
    Peripheral oximeter
    ECG
    Esophageal temperature probe
    End-tidal carbon dioxide monitor
    Neuromuscular blockade monitor
  Arterial catheter
  Pulmonary artery catheter (SvO_2)
  Transesophageal echocardiography probe
  Foley catheter with temperature transducer
  Tocodynamometer
  EEG
Fetal
  Fetal heart rate monitor (noninvasive)

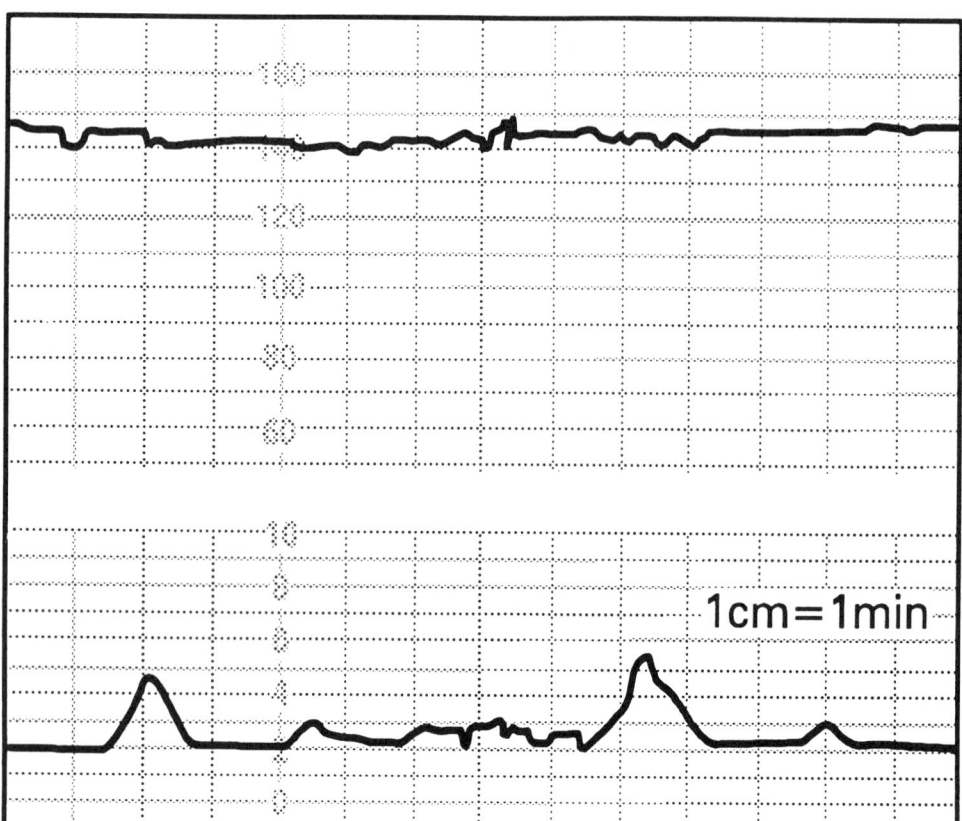

FIGURE 24.1. FHR (*upper tracing*) and uterine activity (*bottom tracing*) recorded at the end of a mitral valve replacement in a 23-year-old patient in her 32nd week of gestation. There are persistent uterine contractions and a loss of long-term FHR variability. (From Bahary, et al.[16] by permission of *Is J Med Sci*.)

Prior to the induction of anesthesia, radial artery and thermodilution pulmonary artery catheters should be introduced. These monitors provide beat-to-beat systemic and pulmonary artery blood pressure information and permit the measurement of cardiac output, as well as arterial and mixed-venous blood gases. A pulmonary artery catheter provides continuous information on venous oxygen saturation (Svo_2), an indirect, approximate measure of the adequacy of maternal tissue oxygen delivery.

Following anesthesia induction, a urinary bladder catheter with a temperature probe and a transesophageal echocardiography (TEE) probe should be placed. The former provides information on fluid balance and core temperature. TEE is especially important in the patient undergoing valvular or congenital heart surgery, since it can document pathology and help assess the adequacy of the repair. This author[18] reported a case of a gravid patient requiring replacement of both aortic and mitral porcine prosthetic valves. The patient was thought to have cardiac pathology limited to her aortic valve; however, after rewarming and an unsuccessful attempt to wean from CPB, mitral valve dysfunction was diagnosed, and a second period of CPB was required to replace the mitral valve. Pre-CPB TEE would have identified mitral valve dysfunction prior to extracorporeal circulation, and obviated the need for two separate periods of CPB.

Other maternal monitors include end-tidal expired gas concentrations, neuromuscular blockade, and electroencephalographic (EEG) monitors.

Uterine activity should be assessed continuously with a tocodynamometer applied to the maternal abdomen. This monitor transduces the tightening of the abdomen during uterine contractions.[34] As is the case with many other types of major surgery, the tocodynamometer should not interfere with the conduct of cardiac surgery[35]; if necessary, the monitor may be intermittently displaced by the operating surgeon. The use of an intra-amniotic catheter to monitor uterine activity and pressure may be inadvisable in a patient who will be fully anticoagulated.

Intraoperative uterine contractions may have a deleterious effect on fetal oxygen delivery (by causing an increase in uterine venous pressure and decrease in uterine blood flow [UBF]) and may signal the onset of preterm labor. Thus, utilization of the tocodynamometer is imperative, as it will provide important information about the state of the uterus and allow intervention if necessary.

Various case reports have documented the common occurrence of uterine contractions in association with cardiac surgery and CPB.[12,15-18] Uterine contractions may appear during any perioperative period, but occur most frequently intraoperatively following CPB, or in the postoperative time period (Figure 24.1). Therefore, it is important to leave the tocodynamometer in place after surgery is completed and the patient is transferred to the intensive care unit.

Perioperative uterine contractions occur frequently in the perioperative course, but they usually are treated effectively with magnesium sulfate, ritodrine, or ethanol infusions and do not result in preterm labor and fetal demise.[12,17,18,36,37]

Fetal Monitors

Fetal monitors should be employed in all gravidae after 16 weeks gestation, since one of the primary perioperative goals is to avoid fetal loss. The fetal heart rate (FHR) can be externally monitored at 16 to 20 week's gestation.[38] An FHR monitor records the FHR and FHR variability, as well as uterine contractions, and permits the recognition of fetal distress, allowing the clinician to institute measures to improve fetal oxygen delivery. A spinal electrode placed in the fetal scalp gives the most reliable fetal ECG and, hence, the best FHR information. However, this method may be undesirable because of maternal anticoagulation. External FHR monitoring, using ultrasound, phonocardiography, or external abdominal ECG, is less exact but is preferable in this clinical setting.

Interventions aimed at optimizing maternal blood oxygen content, correcting any acid-base imbalance, and replenishing fetal glycogen stores may alleviate signs of fetal hypoxia. Additionally, some clinicians recommend that the extracorporeal circuit pump flow be increased to improve fetal oxygen delivery (Figure 24.2).[8,11,12] (This is discussed further in Conduct of Perfusion in the Gravid Patient, below.)

The FHR may be normal, elevated, or slightly depressed prior to the initiation of CPB, but decreases precipitously with bypass, and remains below normal for the entire bypass period[11,14,16,17] (Figures 24.3 and 24.4). There are many potential causes of this observed decrease in FHR. Persistent fetal bradycardia is a classic sign of acute fetal hypoxia.[38] However, in the bypass setting, especially when hypothermia is employed, it is difficult to ascribe fetal bradycardia to hypoxia or to a decrease in fetal oxygen demand.

Fetal tachycardia typically occurs following the discontinuation of bypass support.[11-14,16,17] This tachycardia may represent a compensating mechanism for an oxygen debt incurred during CPB. The FHR usually returns to normal by the end of the operative period.

The cardiac surgeon and perfusionist may not be familiar with uterine and FHR monitors; the anesthesiologist is accustomed to caring for the gravida during labor and delivery and thus can assess uterine and FHR tracings. However, in some clinical circumstances, such as preoperative fetal distress or anticipated need for emergency cesarean section during cardiac surgery, the presence of a perinatologist and/or an obstetrician may be desirable.

Conduct of Perfusion in the Gravid Patient

The conduct of CPB can be characterized by the following variables: (1) machine blood flow, (2) absence or presence of blood flow pulsatility, (3) patient blood pressure, (4) maintenance of normothermia, or magnitude of hypothermia, (5) type of oxygenator (bubbler or membrane), (6) magnitude of patient hyperoxygenation, (7) patient hematocrit, (8) extracorporeal circuit prime, (9) type of cardioplegia, (10) anesthetic drugs and cardiovascular drugs and therapeutics, and (11) duration of perfusion. Perfusion techniques and the requisite condition of anticoagulation during CPB could theoretically impact fetal

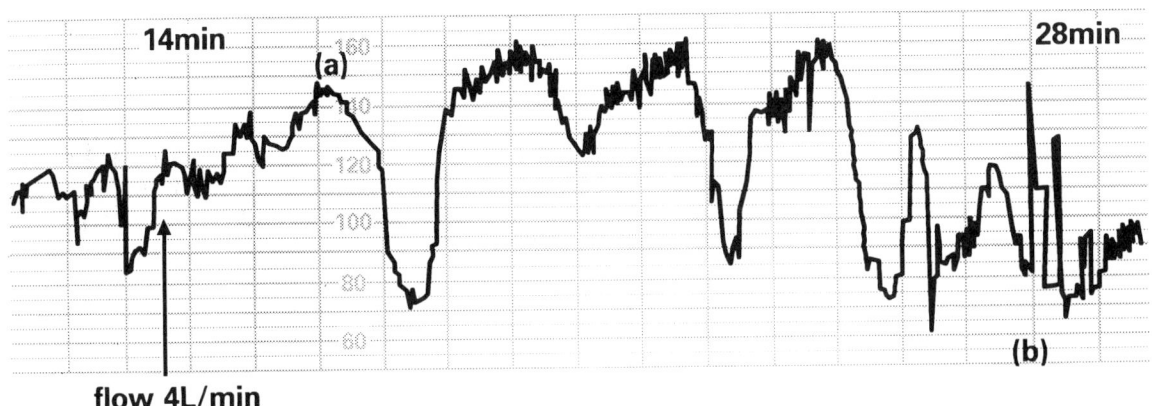

FIGURE 24.2. FHR tracing recorded between 14 and 28 minutes of bypass. Increasing blood flow from 3.1 to 4 L/min resulted in a transient improvement in FHR (a). A deep variable deceleration pattern then deteriorates to a persistent bradycardia (b) after 28 minutes of bypass. (From Lamb et al,[17] by permission of *B & J Obstet Gynecol.*)

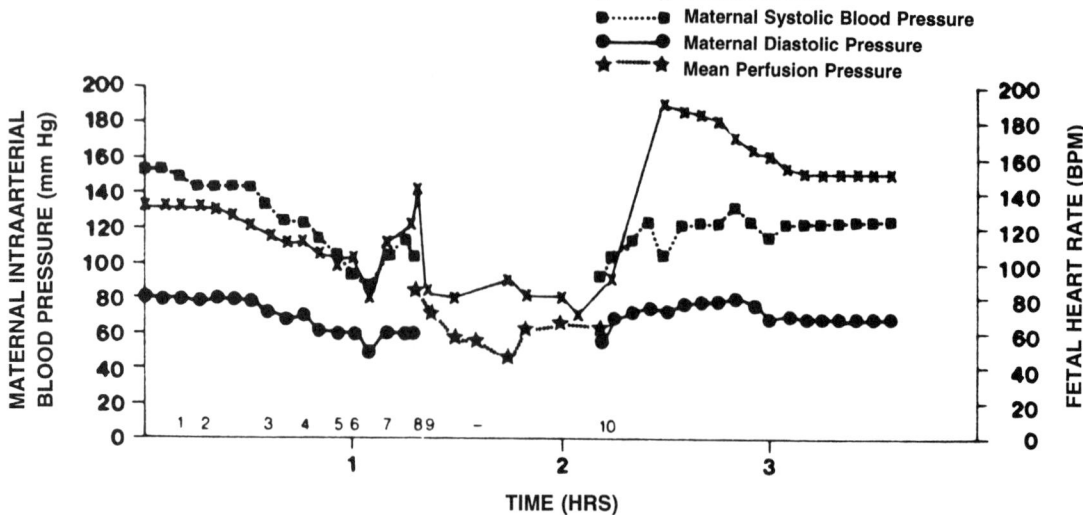

FIGURE 24.3. Maternal blood pressure and FHR changes during cardiac surgery and CPB: 1 = induction of anesthesia; 2 = ventilatory rate adjusted; 3 = median sternotomy; 4 = pericardiotomy; 5 = heparin given; 6 = aortic cannulation (with manipulation of the heart, there was a transient fall in maternal blood pressure and FHR); 7 = administration of scopolamine and pancuronium; 8 = start of CPB; 9 = fall in FHR with start of nonpulsatile flow and fall in maternal blood pressure; 10 = CPB discontinued. The increase in FHR after the discontinuation of bypass may reflect a fetal oxygen debt. (Reprinted with permission from The American College of Obstetricians & Gynecologists [*Obstet Gynecol* 1980,56:112–5].)

well-being during CPB. As noted above, there are no studies assessing the effect of any *one* of these variables on maternal and fetal outcomes. Summarized below are the author's recommendations for the management of some of these variables, based on the survey and anecdotal reports in the literature (Table 24.5). Recommendations and information on cardiovascular drugs and therapeutics for cardiac surgery and CPB in the gravid patient are summarized in the concluding section of this chapter (Rational Selection of Cardiovascular Drugs and Therapeutics in the Gravid Patient During Cardiac Surgery and CPB).

CPB Blood Flow

The optimal extracorporeal circuit blood flow in the *nongravid* patient is controversial. Some clinicians recommend that blood flow should be maintained at relatively normal values (ie, cardiac index ≥ 2.3 L/min/m^2). Others believe that lower blood flows, especially with hypo-

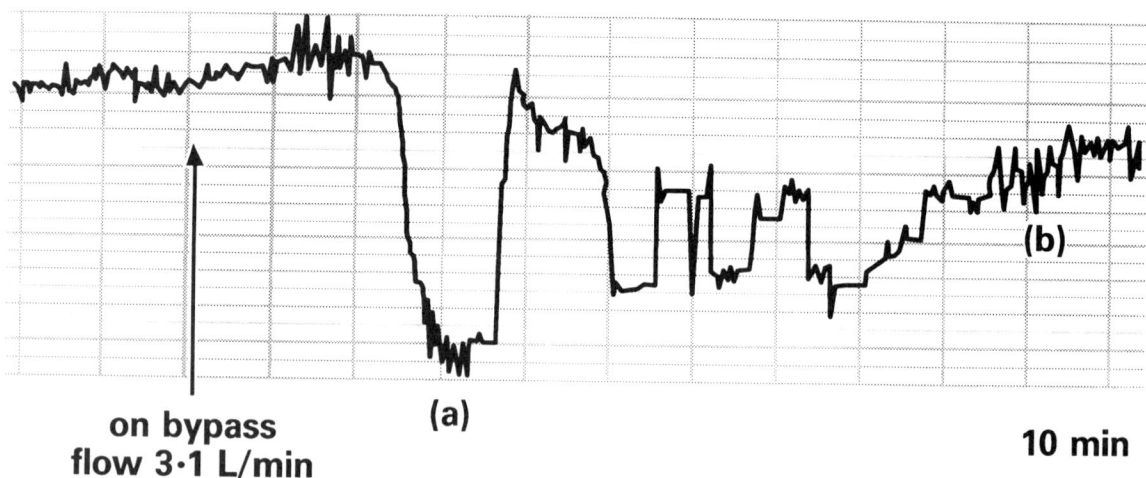

FIGURE 24.4. FHR tracing from the initiation of CPB at a perfusion flow rate of 3.1 L/min. A FHR deceleration occurs at (a) and there is increased FHR variability after 10 minutes of bypass (b). (From Lamb et al,[17] by permission of Br J Obstet Gynecol.)

TABLE 24.5. Recommendations for the conduct of extracorporeal circulation in the gravid patient.

Variable	Recommended value/ characteristic	Rationale
Blood flow	3.0 L/min/m^2	Cardiac index normally increased during pregnancy
Blood pressure (MAP)	60–70 mm Hg	UBF is dependent on maternal MAP
Temperature	28°–32° C	Hypothermia decreases fetal oxygen requirements
Oxygenator type	Membrane	Membrane oxygenators are associated with fewer embolic phenomena than bubblers
Hematocrit	25%–27%	The quantity of oxygen carried in maternal blood (and therefore the oxygen available to the fetus) is greatly dependent on hemoglobin concentration
Duration of perfusion	Minimized (?)	The duration of bypass is dictated by the complexity of the operative procedure
Cardioplegia	?	
Pulsatile perfusion	?	

thermia, are desirable, and may decrease the morbidity associated with bypass and the embolization of particulate matter.

Optimal CPB blood flow in the gravid patient is unknown. However, the increase in cardiac output associated with pregnancy is well defined, and one might argue that high blood flows during CPB are desirable in the gravid patient. Indeed, Becker and colleagues[8] suggested that flow during CPB in the pregnant patient be maintained at a minimum of 3.0 L/min/m^2. Additionally, there are a few reports demonstrating that increasing CPB circuit blood flow improves FHR, suggesting an improvement in fetal oxygen delivery.[11,12] In a report by Koh and colleagues,[11] FHR improved when pump blood flow was increased from 3100 to 3600 mL/min. Similarly, Werch and Lambert[12] reported an improvement in FHR when blood flow was increased from 2800 to 4600 mL/min. However, in other reported cases in which fetal monitors were used, increasing pump flow did not consistently improve FHR.[16,17] In one case, flow was increased from 3.1 to 4 L/min/m^2 resulting in a brief, unsustained apparent improvement in fetal oxygen delivery (Figure 24.2).[17]

Blood Pressure

Under normal conditions, UBF is determined solely by maternal blood pressure, as the placental vasculature is maximally dilated. However, it is not known what factors determine UBF during the very "abnormal" condition of CPB.[39] For example, we know that catecholamine levels increase many-fold during CPB[32]; therefore, uterine vascular resistance may increase during extracorporeal circulation in response to increased levels of norepinephrine and epinephrine. Regardless of the state of uterine vascular resistance during CPB, maternal blood pressure will be an important determinant of UBF and fetal oxygen delivery. Moderately high pressures (mean arterial pressure ≥ 65 mm Hg) should be employed during perfusion in the gravid patient.

There are no reports demonstrating that increasing blood pressure during CPB improves fetal oxygen delivery or FHR. Most reports on CPB in the gravid patient do not include information on maternal blood pressure during CPB. The few blood pressure values reported in gravid perfusion cases ranged from 55 to 95 mm Hg.[13,18,19,40] However, there are several reports documenting a decrease in FHR and loss of FHR variability during the initiation of CPB, a period in which blood pressure is acutely reduced (Figures 24.3 and 24.4).[11–17]

In theory, the use of short-acting vasodilators, such as nitroglycerin or sodium nitroprusside, may counteract the effects of CPB-induced increases in norepinephrine and epinephrine. If maternal blood pressure is maintained by increasing extracorporeal circuit pump flow, UBF and fetal oxygen delivery may be increased with the use of vasodilators. Again, controlled studies should be conducted to assess the effect of a given therapeutic on fetal oxygen delivery during CPB.

Temperature

Although hypothermic CPB has been the standard of care during the last 30 years, several groups have recently advocated the use of normothermic bypass and warm blood cardioplegia to improve myocardial protection.[41,42] However, the effects of warm compared to cold cardioplegia on myocardial function are controversial, and one group has reported an increase in adverse neurologic sequelae in patients treated with normothermic perfusion.[43] Thus, controversy exists regarding the optimal temperature management during CPB in the nongravid patient, although the vast majority of perfusions are conducted with hypothermia. There are few data, and no consensus exists, regarding temperature management in the gravid patient undergoing CPB.

There are theoretic advantages and disadvantages to the use of either normothermic or hypothermic CPB in the gravid patient. Hypothermia will cause fetal bradycardia and may lead to fetal ventricular dysrhythmias resulting in fetal loss. Also, rewarming following hypothermic bypass may precipitate uterine contractions and preterm labor.[8] This latter observation convinced Becker and colleagues[8] that CPB in the gravida should be conducted under normothermic conditions. However, others have noted the occurrence of uterine contractions at the time of discontinuation of bypass support, in spite of normothermic perfusion.[17] Moreover, uterine contractions occur at various times in the postbypass and postoperative period.[12,15-18] Therefore, the association of uterine contractions with rewarming following hypothermic bypass is unclear.

Hypothermic extracorporeal circulation may be protective to the fetus by decreasing fetal oxygen requirements. Asali and colleagues[44] demonstrated that induced hypothermia to 28°C in gravid dogs causes an increase in UVR but does not result in a decrease in UBF. Most importantly, in this study, hypothermia did not affect fetal survival, and the authors concluded that hypothermia is well tolerated by the fetus. There are several reports that discuss the effects of both deliberately induced and septicemia-associated hypothermia in gravid patients. In two reports, gravidae underwent neurologic vascular procedures at 30.5° and 26.5°C to decrease maternal cerebral oxygen demand.[10,45] In another report, a gravid patient suffered septicemia-induced hypothermia to 92°F.[46] The authors noted that FHR decreased with maternal hypothermia but improved with maternal rewarming (Figure 24.5).

Perfusion temperatures of 25° to 37°C have been used in gravidae undergoing CPB.[11,13,14,17-19] There is no apparent correlation between the temperature used during bypass and fetal loss. This author[18] reported a case in which hypothermic bypass at 25°C was required for 2 hours and 40 minutes, and in which the patient underwent two periods of rewarming. Uterine contractions noted in the early postoperative period were successfully treated with magnesium sulfate. Despite the magnitude and duration of hypothermia and the two periods of rewarming, a normal infant was delivered 10 days postoperatively.

In conclusion, we do not know the optimal temperature for the gravida and fetus during CPB. There are no data to suggest hypothermia is harmful to the mother or fetus undergoing bypass. Also, normothermic bypass may increase the likelihood of untoward neurologic sequelae in the mother.

Summary

We do not have definitive data to support the use of one perfusion technique over another in the gravid patient requiring cardiac surgery and CPB. Empirically, a perfusion technique that optimizes UBF (high machine blood flow, normal-to-elevated arterial pressure), decreases fetal oxygen requirements (moderate hypothermia), and minimizes the problem of air embolization (membrane oxygenators) would be most suitable in the gravid patient (Table 24.5). Appropriate maternal and fetal monitors provide continuous information on uterine activity, fetal oxygen delivery, and the effects of an intervention. Research focused on delineating the effects of CPB on maternal and fetal outcome is required to provide optimal care for the pregnant cardiac patient.

Rational Selection of Cardiovascular Drugs and Therapeutics in the Gravid Patient During Cardiac Surgery and CPB

The pregnant patient undergoing cardiac surgery and CPB may require vasoactive and inotropic drugs for perioperative cardiovascular support. Cardiovascular drug therapeutics are administered to the gravida to improve cell oxygen delivery to *both* mother and fetus. The incorrect choice may improve maternal hemodynamics but further compromise UBF and fetal oxygen delivery. Most clinicians select care for the gravida to ensure a satisfactory maternal outcome—even at the risk of fetal demise. A thorough understanding of the physiology of pregnancy and the actions of cardiovascular drugs on both maternal and fetal oxygen delivery allows the clinician to make rational therapeutic choices to optimize care for both mother and fetus.

Although there are a multitude of well-controlled studies documenting the effects of cardiac therapeutics on maternal hemodynamics and fetal oxygen delivery, there are few studies that assess the effects of a given pharmacologic intervention in the gravida with a specific cardiac lesion. For example, we know that in the healthy gravid ewe—without cardiac pathology—isoproterenol will increase cardiac output without increasing placental blood flow.[47] However, we can only speculate as to what happens to placental blood flow when isoproterenol is administered to a pregnant cardiac patient with 4+ mitral regurgitation. Theoretically, the effects of isoproterenol-increased heart rate and decreased systemic vascular resis-

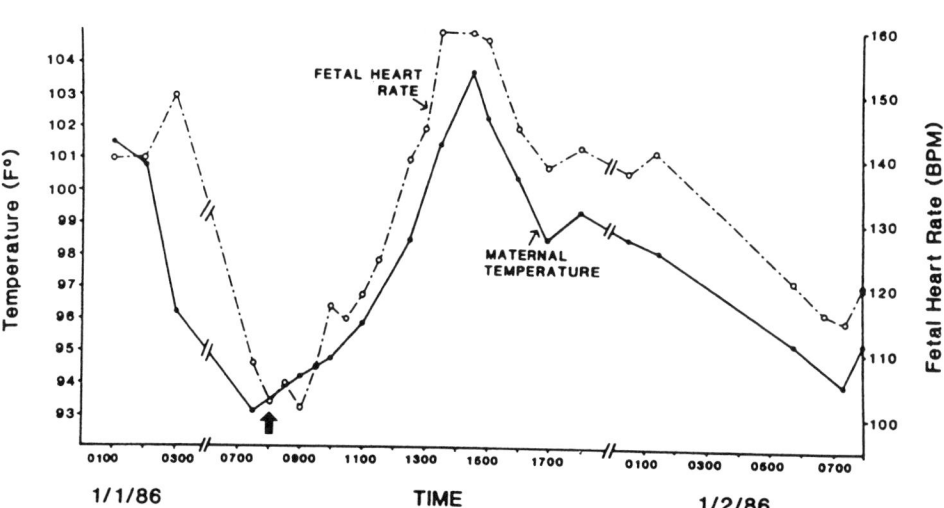

FIGURE 24.5. Maternal temperature and FHR in a pregnant patient with septicemia-induced hypothermia. FHR closely paralleled maternal temperature. Fetal brachycardia persisted until hypothermia was corrected. (Reprinted with permission from The American College of Obstetricians and Gynecologists [*Obstet Gynecol* 1988, 72:496-7].)

tance could significantly improve maternal cardiac output and blood pressure. These changes may improve UBF and fetal oxygen delivery.

Thus, although this section outlines the effects of commonly used cardiac therapeutics, it is intended only as a guide to treatment. Fortunately, appropriate patient monitoring during cardiac surgery in the gravida—namely, thermodilution pulmonary and radial artery catheters, uterine tocodynamometer, and continuous fetal ultrasound—can provide immediate information on the effects of a given therapy on maternal and fetal oxygen delivery.

Determinants of UBF

It is beyond the scope of this chapter to provide a full discussion of obstetric physiology; however, in order to care for the gravida requiring cardiac surgery, one must understand the determinants of UBF and fetal oxygen delivery to select appropriate cardiovascular therapeutics.

UBF normally represents approximately 10% of total maternal cardiac output. UBF is not autoregulated or affected by carbon dioxide or oxygen gas tensions, and it is directly proportional to maternal mean arterial blood pressure (MAP) and inversely related to uterine vascular resistance (UVR).[48] Any event or therapy that decreases maternal MAP increases UVR or uterine venous pressure (UVP) (ie, uterine contractions) will decrease fetal oxygen delivery. The factors determining UBF are summarized as follows:

$$UBF = \frac{MAP - UVP}{UVR}$$

Uterine muscle and vasculature contain both α- and β-adrenergic receptors, which respond to both endogenous and exogenous catecholamines.[48] Table 24.6 summarizes the effects of catecholamines on maternal blood pressure and UBF in the gravida. Since uterine vessels are maximally dilated under normal conditions, β-adrenergic drugs should not significantly decrease UVR or increase UBF. However, this class of drug may cause a slight decrease in uterine tonus and a concomitant decrease in UVP, thus slightly improving UBF. Stimulation of α-adrenergic receptors will have a deleterious effect on UBF by causing an increase in UVR. Table 24.7 summarizes the effects of α- and β-adrenergic receptor stimulation and blockade on maternal-fetal physiology.

There are a multitude of factors that may lead to a decrease in UBF (Table 24.8). However, in the gravida undergoing cardiac surgery, the most likely cause of decreased UBF is maternal hypotension resulting from inadequate cardiac performance. As noted above, appropriate selection of cardiac therapeutics and careful monitoring of the adequacy of maternal and fetal oxygen delivery may help ensure satisfactory maternal and fetal outcome.

TABLE 24.6. Effects of catecholamines on maternal blood pressure and UBF in the gravida.

	Maternal BP	UBF
Dobutamine	↑	↓
Dopamine	↑	↓↑
Ephedrine	↑	↑
Epinephrine	↑	↓
Isoproterenol	↑	↔
Norepinephrine	↑	↓

TABLE 24.7. Effects of α- and β-adrenergic receptor stimulation and blockade on maternal-fetal physiology.

	Stimulation		Blockade	
	α-Receptor	β-Receptor	α-Receptor	β-Receptor
Fetal heart rate	↔	↑	↔	↔↓
Maternal heart rate	↔	↑	↔	↓
Umbilical blood flow	↔	↑	↔	↓
Myometrial activity	↑	↓	↓	↑

Effects of Cardiovascular Drugs During Pregnancy and CPB

Inotropic and Vasoconstrictive Drugs

Amrinone

Amrinone is an intracellular phosphodiesterase inhibitor that causes an increase in intracellular cyclic AMP. Phosphodiesterase inhibitors have both positive inotropic and vasodilatory actions independent of β-receptors.[49]

In a study comparing amrinone and dopamine in anesthetized gravid baboons, amrinone in doses up to 40 μg/kg/min had no effect on MAP, heart rate, UBF, or UVR.[50] Dopamine at an intravenous dose of 40 μg/kg/min increased MAP and UVR (Figure 24.6.). Jelsema and colleagues[51] reported on the successful use of amrinone in an 18-week gravida with mitral regurgitation and pulmonary edema. Dopamine and dobutamine were ineffective in treating her heart failure, but amrinone, 2μg/kg/min, improved her condition.

Dobutamine

Fishburne and colleagues[52] compared the hemodynamic effects of dobutamine and dopamine in the gravid ewe. Dobutamine increased maternal heart rate and UVR but decreased UBF. Because dobutamine has less α-adrenergic activity than dopamine, it causes less uterine vasoconstriction and may be preferable in gravid patients (Figure 24.7).

Dopamine

Dopamine exerts its effects directly through dopaminergic receptors and indirectly through α- and β-adrenergic receptors. There are conflicting data describing the effects of dopamine on UBF. One group of investigators reported that dopamine, 2 to 10 μg/kg/min, administered to hypotensive patients undergoing cesarean section, improved maternal blood pressure but resulted in depressed umbilical arterial and venous oxygen tensions.[53] In a study of hypotensive gravid sheep, dopamine, 20 to 40 μg/kg/min, returned maternal blood pressure to control values but resulted in a 56% drop in UBF and a 50% increase in UVR.[54] The effects of lower doses of dopamine are also controversial. In one study, dopamine, 5 to 20 μg/kg/min, decreased UBF to 71% of control values[54]; Blanchard and colleagues[55] reported that UBF was maintained or increased with dopamine, 5 to 40 μg/kg/min.

Ephedrine

Ephedrine, and indirect- and direct-acting α- and β-adrenergic agonist (with β-adrenergic effects predominating), is effective in restoring maternal MAP through its chronotropic and inotropic effects. In a normotensive gravid ewe model, Ralston et al[56] demonstrated that ephedrine, administered at a dose sufficient to raise maternal MAP to 50% above control values, had no significant effect on UBF (Figure 24.8). In this same study, methoxamine and metaraminol (purely and predominantly α-adrenergic-agonist drugs, respectively), in doses sufficient to raise maternal MAP to 50% of control, resulted in decreases in UBF (Figure 24.8). In hypotensive pregnant ewes, ephedrine both restored maternal blood pressure and improved UBF to 85% of control values.[57]

Epinephrine

Epinephrine, like norepinephrine, is an α- and β-adrenergic agonist that also adversely affects UBF.[58,59] In a normotensive gravid ewe model, epinephrine, 0.29 μg/kg/min IV, had no effect on maternal blood pressure but caused a 38.5% decrease in UBF.[58] Importantly, the effect of any drug is influenced by a multitude of factors. Thus, although epinephrine will likely have a deleterious effect on UBF, in one case report, both maternal and fetal oxygen delivery may have improved with the administration of epinephrine following the discontinuation of extracorporeal support during cardiac surgery[17] (Figure 24.9).

TABLE 24.8. Conditions that will decrease uterine blood flow.

Uterine contractions
Hypotension
Hypertension
Vasoconstriction, catecholamines
    Endogenous
    Exogenous

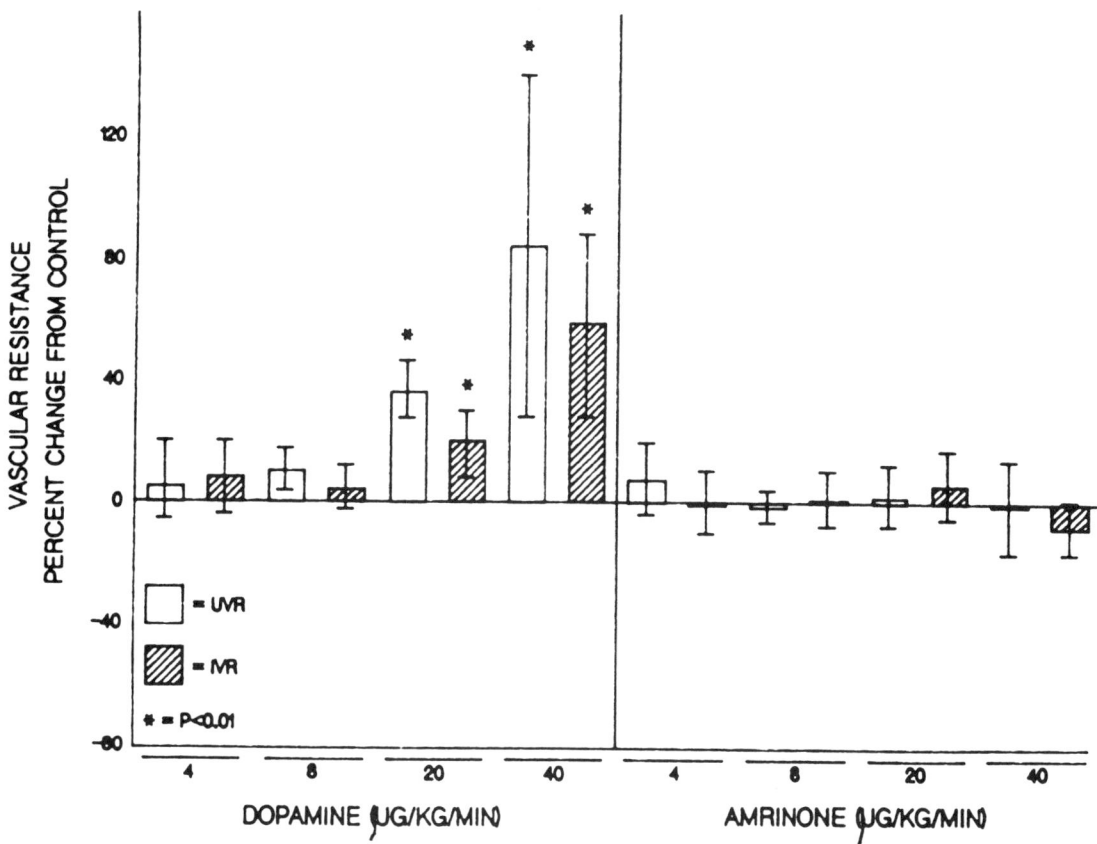

FIGURE 24.6. Effects of systemically infused dopamine and amrinone on uterine (UVR) and iliac (IVR) vascular resistance expressed as percent change from control. Dopamine at 20 and 40µg/kg/min significantly increased UVR. Amrinone had no effect on UVR at any dose. (From Fishburne et al,[50] by permission of *Am J Obstet Gynecol*.)

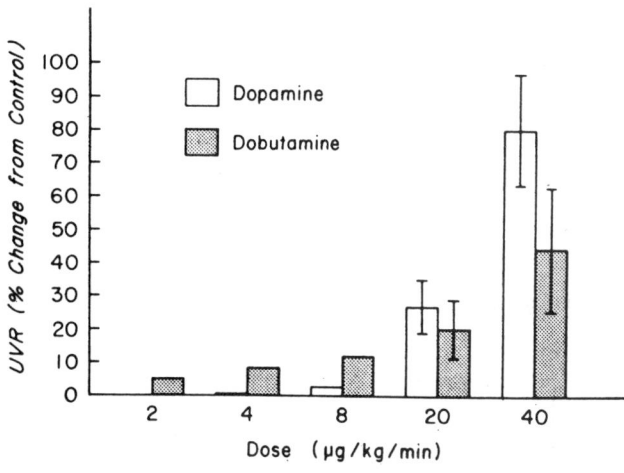

FIGURE 24.7. Comparison of average changes in calculated UVR at various rates of dopamine and dobutamine infusion in gravid ewes. Insignificant changes are noted at 2, 4, and 8 µg/kg/min. UVR increased with both drugs during high-dosage administration, but the rise was most pronounced with dopamine. The magnitude of UVR changes is greater for dopamine than for dobutamine ($p > 0.01$) at the 40 µg/kg/min infusion rate. (From Fishburne et al,[52] by permission of *Am J Obstet Gynecol*.)

Isoproterenol

This pure β-adrenergic agonist causes a 70% increase in cardiac output in gravid animals, but does not decrease UVR or increase blood flow to vessels supplying the placenta.[47] Because isoproterenol may decrease maternal blood pressure and vasodilate nonuterine vascular beds (causing a "steal" from uterine vessels), UBF may be adversely affected by this drug. There are no studies assessing the effect of isoproterenol in the gravida with cardiovascular compromise. However, in two separate case reports, isoproterenol, administered after CPB, improved maternal hemodynamics and, in one case, improved fetal oxygen delivery, as assessed by an FHR monitor.[14,18] Since isoproterenol may inhibit uterine contraction in doses of 2 to 8 µg/kg/min,[60] it may be considered a first-line drug of choice (in the absence of hypotension) to improve maternal cardiac output and increase UBF either by enhancing maternal cardiac output or, indirectly, by suppressing uterine contractions.

Mephentermine

This is a mixed α- and β-adrenergic drug with more α-adrenergic activity and, hence, more vasoconstrictive effects than ephedrine. When both drugs are administered

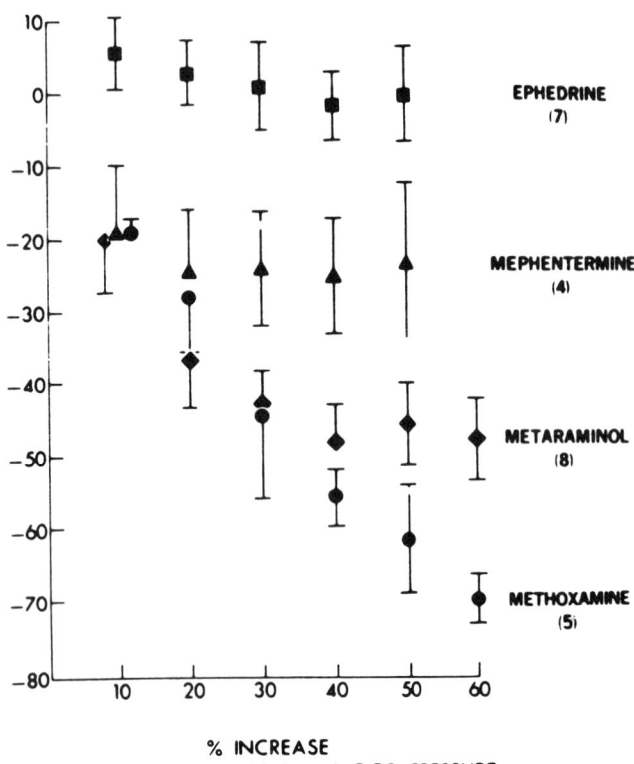

FIGURE 24.8. Mean changes in UBF at equal elevations of MAP after vasopressor administration. Metaraminol and methoxamine decrease UBF at all pressor levels. Ephedrine has negligible effects on UBF at doses that cause a 10% to 50% increase in maternal blood pressure. (From Ralston et al,[56] by permission of *Anesthesiology*.)

to increase maternal blood pressure, mephentermine causes a significant decrease in UBF compared to ephedrine (Figure 24.8).[56]

Metaraminol, Methoxamine

These drugs, potent adrenergic agonists, have undesirable effects on UBF, even when maternal arterial blood pressure increases 50% above control values (Figure 24.8).[56]

Milrinone

Milrinone is an analog of amrinone with similar, β-receptor-independent inotropic and vasodilatory effects.[61] In one report, milrinone caused an increase in maternal heart rate and UBF without affecting the fetus.[62] Further study will define the role of milrinone in pregnancy.

Norepinephrine

Norepinephrine is an α- and β-adrenergic agonist with undesirable effects in both the normotensive and the hypotensive gravid ewe. In a normotensive animal model, norepinephrine causes an increase in maternal blood pressure but decreases UBF.[63] Low-dose norepinephrine (0.1–0.2 µg/kg/min) causes no change in maternal blood pressure or UBF, but norepinephrine doses greater than 0.5 µg/kg/min result in decreased UBF, despite an increase in maternal blood pressure.[64] Importantly, high doses of norepinephrine may stimulate uterine contractions, resulting in further decreases in UBF and in preterm labor.[65]

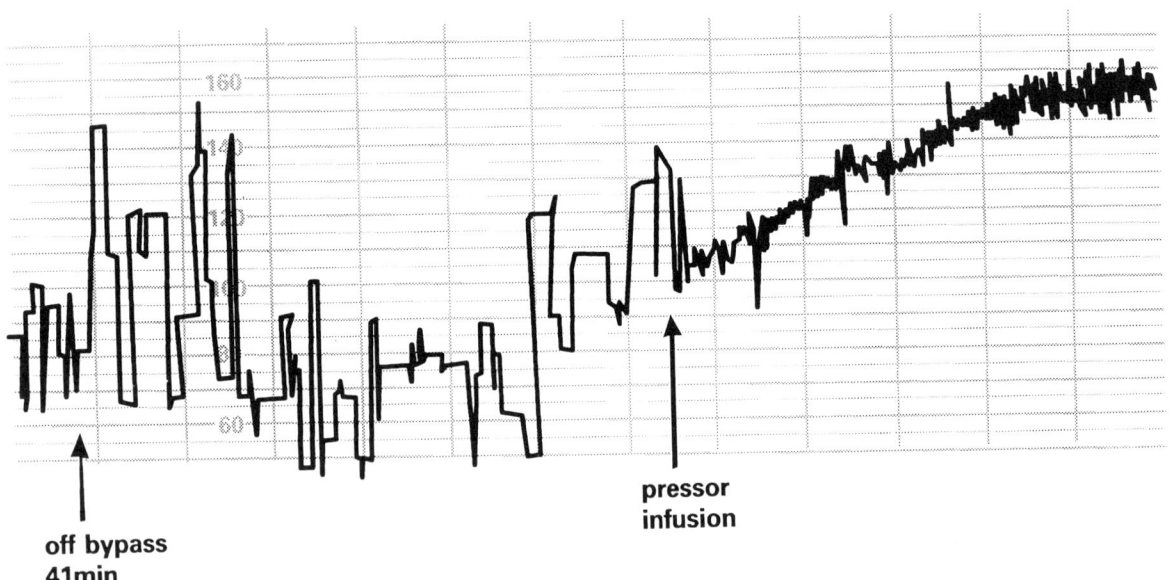

FIGURE 24.9. FHR after the discontinuation of bypass support. Maternal cardiac output and FHR were low, but both improved significantly with the administration of epinephrine (pressor). The improvement in FHR could be a direct effect of epinephrine or secondary to an improvement in fetal oxygen delivery. (From Lamb et al,[17] by permission of *Br J Obstet Gynecol*.)

Phenylephrine Hydrochloride

This pure α-adrenergic agonist will restore maternal MAP but increase UVR and decrease UBF; it is therefore of limited value in the hypotensive gravida.[66]

Vasodilators

Short-acting, titratable vasodilators are desirable in the gravid cardiac patient in the perioperative period. Although hydralazine (a direct-acting vasodilator with desirable effects on UBF and maternal hypertension) is commonly used in noncardiac obstetrical patients, it is not readily titratable, and it requires 10 to 20 minutes to achieve a therapeutic effect.[67] Additionally, this drug is no longer available for intravenous administration. In contrast, nitroglycerin and sodium nitroprusside are both short-acting, titratable drugs that may be used effectively in the gravid cardiac surgery patient. Most vasodilators cross the placenta, but fetal effects have not been well defined.

Nitroglycerin

Nitroglycerin dilates both arterial and venous capacitance vessels, with greater effect on the latter. When administered to normotensive gravid ewes, nitroglycerin causes a slight decrease in UBF.[68] Nitroglycerin will reverse norepinephrine-induced decreases in UBF, while effectively treating maternal hypertension. DeSimone and colleagues[69] demonstrated that nitroglycerin directly relaxes uterine muscles.

Nitroprusside

Sodium nitroprusside, like nitroglycerin, effectively treats maternal hypertension and improves UBF. It is a vasodilator, with its main effect on total peripheral vascular resistance. In the gravid ewe, with norepinephrine-induced hypertension, sodium nitroprusside reduces maternal blood pressure and restores UBF. Metabolism of sodium nitroprusside results in the release of cyanide; cyanide is converted by rhodanase to thiocyanate. Although sodium nitroprusside administered in the usual clinical doses, 0.1 to 1.0 μg/kg/min, does not cause maternal or fetal cyanide toxicity,[70] large doses may produce significant fetal cyanide levels.[71]

Anti-Arrhythmics

β-Blockers

All β-blockers cross the placenta and can reach clinically significant levels in the newborn.[72,73] Fears concerning β-blocker-induced intrauterine fetal growth retardation, fetal bradycardia and hypoglycemia, or premature labor have been tempered by the safe administration of this class of drugs to several generations of gravidae. Review of the literature suggests that β-blockers, given to treat hypertension associated with pregnancy, also improve fetal outcome.[74]

Esmolol

This short-acting, β-cardioselective receptor antagonist is metabolized rapidly in both the mother and the fetus. One group of investigators reported a transient and moderate decrease in maternal and fetal heart rate and MAP following administration of esmolol to the mother[75] (Figures 24.10 and 24.11). Maternal and fetal acid-base status were not affected.[75] However, others suggest that esmolol, administered as a continuous infusion for 60 to 90 minutes, may adversely affect the fetus by causing prolonged fetal bradycardia, hypoxemia, and acidosis.[76] In one report, esmolol was used safely in a pregnant patient undergoing intracranial surgery. FHR decreased somewhat, but heart-rate variability was maintained.[77]

Esmolol may be the first choice of drug for β-receptor blockade in the gravida undergoing cardiac surgery. This drug is titratable and has a short half-life ($t_{1/2}$ equals approximately 2 minutes). Thus, with esmolol one may assess the effect of β-blockade on maternal and fetal oxygen delivery without "committing" to prolonged β-adrenergic antagonism. However, fetal well-being should be monitored continuously if an esmolol infusion is prescribed.

Labetolol

Labetolol has a half-life similar to that of propranolol ($t_{1/2}$ equals 4 hours), but it is both an α- and a nonspecific β-adrenergic antagonist. Several studies report its safe use for the treatment of hypertension during pregnancy.[78-80] Labetolol pharmacokinetics do not differ between pregnant and nonpregnant patients.[81]

Metoprolol

Metoprolol is a $β_1$-cardioselective receptor antagonist with a half-life of 3 to 4 hours. In one study of 198 gravidae with hypertension resistant to diuretic therapy, all but 44 patients were successfully treated with the addition of metoprolol.[82]

Propranolol

As is the case with the vast majority of cardiac drugs, there are few prospective studies that have assessed the use of propranolol in gravid humans. However, propranolol given to treat the hypertension associated with pregnancy improves the likelihood of a satisfactory fetal outcome.[72,73]

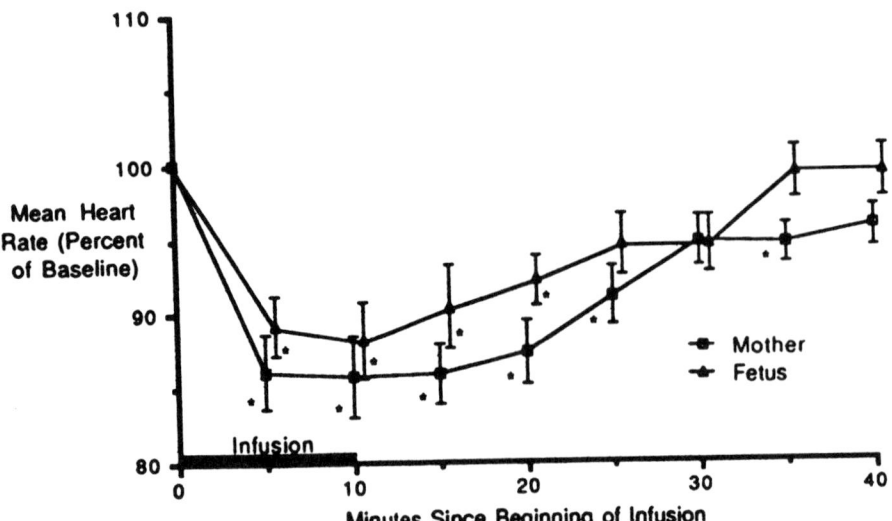

FIGURE 24.10. Maternal and fetal heart rate during and after esmolol infusion in chronically instrumented gravid ewes. The maximal decrease in maternal and fetal mean arterial pressure was 7 ± 2% (mean ± SEM) in both groups. All values are expressed as mean (± SEM) % of baseline. *$p < 0.05$ when compared to the baseline. (From Ostman et al,[75] by permission of *Anesthesiology*.)

Calcium Channel Blockers

Nifedipine, verapamil, and diltiazam cross the placental membranes but have not been shown to affect adversely fetal well-being.[83] However, these drugs may cause a decrease in UBF by causing a decrease in maternal blood pressure, especially in patients with cardiovascular disease.

Verapamil

Verapamil exerts its primary cardiovascular effects by prolonging atrioventricular nodal conduction and refractoriness. It has a pronounced effect on vascular and cardiac smooth muscle. It has been used effectively to treat both fetal and maternal supraventricular arrhythmias.[83,84]

Murad and colleagues[85] demonstrated that verapamil may decrease maternal blood pressure and adversely affect UBF. They administered verapamil, 0.2 mg/kg IV, over 3 minutes to awake, gravid ewes. Maternal cardiac output and systemic vascular resistance were unaffected, but systemic blood pressure and UBF decreased significantly. UBF fell to 75% at 2 minutes and 90% over the next 30 minutes following verapamil administration.

Nifedipine

Unlike verapamil, nifedipine primarily affects hemodynamics by causing peripheral vasodilation. Veille et al[86] studied gravid, awake pygmy goats and demonstrated that UBF was unaffected by a dose of nifedipine sufficient to reduce maternal blood pressure. Although nifedipine may inhibit uterine contractions late in pregnancy, normal therapeutic doses of verapamil do not.[87,88]

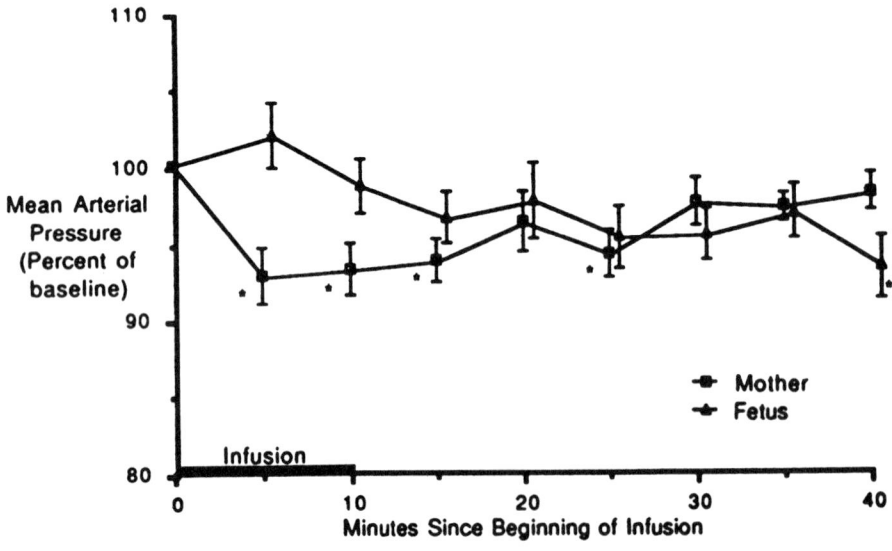

FIGURE 24.11. Maternal and fetal MAP during and after esmolol 500 μg/kg/min IV for 4 minutes and then 300 μg/kg/min for 6 minutes in chronically instrumented gravid ewes. All values are expressed as mean (± SEM) % of baseline. *$p < 0.05$ compared to the baseline. The maximal decrease of maternal and fetal heart rates was 7 ± 2% and 12 ± 3% (mean ± SEM) respectively. (From Ostman et al,[75] by permission of *Anesthesiology*.)

Other Commonly Used Anti-Arrhythmic Drugs

Lidocaine

Lidocaine effectively suppresses ventricular dysrhythmias at the usual therapeutic level (plasma lidocaine concentration equal to 2 to 5 µg/mL) in gravid patients. Lidocaine has no adverse effect on UBF or fetal blood gases at these therapeutic levels.[89,90] However, very high maternal blood levels (plasma lidocaine concentration greater than 200 µg/mL) cause a decrease in UBF.[91]

Procainamide

Procainamide may be used to treat both atrial and ventricular dysrhythmias in the gravid patient. Although procainamide crosses the placental membrane, it does not have apparent teratogenic effects.[83]

Bretylium

If lidocaine is ineffective in controlling dangerous arrhythmias, bretylium may be considered. There are no controlled studies on the use of bretylium in pregnancy, but there is a report of a gravid patient with prolonged QT interval syndrome who was successfully treated with bretylium and delivered a normal term infant.[92]

Digoxin

Digoxin has been administered to the gravid patient for the usual therapeutic indications. Although fetal levels are equal to maternal levels (digoxin readily crosses the placental membranes), digoxin has not been shown to be teratogenic.[93] Interestingly, digoxin may exert the same inotropic effect on the uterus as on the heart, thus shortening labor.[94]

References

1. McFaul PB, Dorman JC, Lamki H, et al. Pregnancy complicated by maternal heart disease. A review of 519 women. *Br J Obstet Gynaecol* 1988;95:861–867.
2. Shearman RP. Trends in maternal mortality in Australia: relevance in current practice. *Aust NZ J Obstet Gynaecol* 1990;30:15–17.
3. Clark SL. Cardiac disease in pregnancy. *Crit Care Clin* 1991;7:777–796.
4. In a conversation with John H. McNulty, Jr, MD (March, 1993).
5. Rush RW, Fraser RC, Commerford PJ. Management of heart disease in pregnancy. *S Afr Med J* 1982;61:192–195.
6. Jacobs WM, Cooley D, Goen GP. Cardiac surgery with extracorporeal circulation. Report of 3 cases. *Obstet Gynecol* 1965;25:167–169.
7. Zitnik RS, Brandenburg RO, Sheldon R, et al. Pregnancy and open heart surgery. *Circulation* 1969;39(suppl 39-40): I-257–I-262.
8. Becker RM. Intracardiac surgery in pregnant women. *Ann Thorac Surg* 1983;36:453–458.
9. Lapiedra OJ, Bernal JM, Ninot S, et al. Open heart surgery for thrombosis of a prosthetic mitral valve during pregnancy: fetal hydrocephalus. *J Cardiovasc Surg (Torino)* 1986;27:217–220.
10. Matsuki A, Oyama T. Operation under hypothermia in a pregnant woman with an intracranial arteriovenous malformation. *Can Anaesth Soc J* 1972;19:184–191.
11. Koh KS, Friesen RM, Livingston RA. Fetal monitoring during maternal cardiac surgery with cardiopulmonary bypass. *Can Med Assoc J* 1975;112:1102–1104.
12. Werch A, Lambert HM. Fetal monitoring and maternal open heart surgery. (Letter) *South Med J* 1977;70:1024.
13. Trimakas AP, Maxwell KD, Berkay S, et al. Fetal monitoring during cardiopulmonary bypass for removal of a left atrial myxoma during pregnancy. *Johns Hopkins Med J* 1979;144:156–160.
14. Levy DL, Warner RA, Burgess G. Fetal response to cardiopulmonary bypass. *Obstet Gynecol* 1980;56:112–115.
15. Eilen B, Kaiger IH, Buker R, et al. Aortic valve replacement in the third trimester of pregnancy: case report and review of the literature. *Obstet Gynecol* 1980;57:119–121.
16. Bahary CM, Ninio A, Gorodesky IG, et al. Tococardiography in pregnancy during extracorporeal bypass for mitral valve replacement. *Isr J Med Sci* 1980;16:395–397.
17. Lamb MP, Manners JM. Fetal heart monitoring during open heart surgery. *Br J Obstet Gynaecol* 1981;88:669–674.
18. Mora CT, Grunewald KE. Reoperative aortic and mitral prosthetic valve replacement in the third trimester of pregnancy. *J Cardiothorac Anesth* 1987;1:313–317.
19. Farmakides G, Schulman H, Mohtaschemi M, et al. Uterine-umbilical velocimetry in open heart surgery. *Am J Obstet Gynecol* 1987;156:1221–1222.
20. Katz JD, Hook R, Barash PG. Fetal heart rate monitoring in pregnant patients undergoing surgery. *Am J Obstet Gynecol* 1976;125:267–269.
21. Mooij PNM, deJong PA, Bavinck JH, et al. Aortic valve replacement in the second trimester of pregnancy: a case report. *Eur J Obstet Gynecol Reprod Biol* 1988;29:347–352.
22. Martin MC, Pernoll ML, Boruszak AN, et al. Cesarean section while on cardiac bypass: report of a case. *Obstet Gynecol* 1981;57:41S–44S.
23. Merin G, Bitran D, Donchin Y, et al. Traumatic rupture of the thoracic aorta during pregnancy. *Chest* 1981;79:99–100.
24. Salomon J, Yartner R, Levy M. Open heart surgery during pregnancy—case report. *Vasc Surg* 1975;9:257–259.
25. Meffert WG, Stansel HC Jr. Open heart surgery during pregnancy. *Am J Obstet Gynecol* 1968;102:1116–1120.
26. Korsten HHM, Van Zundert AAJ, Moois PNM, et al. Emergency aortic valve replacement in the 24th week of pregnancy. *Acta Anaesth Belg* 1989;40:201–205.
27. Levinson G, Shnider SM. Anesthesia for surgery during pregnancy. In: Shnider SM, Levinson G, eds. *Anesthesia for Obstetrics* 2nd ed. Baltimore: Williams and Wilkins; 1987:188–207.
28. Dubourg G, Broustet P, Bricand H. Complete correction of Fallot's triad with extracorporeal circulation. *Arch Mal Coeur* 1959;52:1389.
29. Leyse R, Ofstun M, Dillard DH, et al. Congenital aortic ste-

nosis in pregnancy corrected by extracorporeal circulation. Offering a viable male infant at term with anomalies eventuating in his death at four months of age—report of a case. *JAMA* 1961;176:1009-1012.
30. Halseth WL, Elliott DP, Walker EL, et al. Open mitral commissurotomy. *J Thorac Cardiovasc Surg* 1980;80:842-848.
31. Roe BB, Edmunds LH Jr, Fishman NH, et al. Open mitral valvulotomy. *Ann Thorac Surg* 1971;12:483-491.
32. Colman RD, Frank M, Longhnan BA, et al. Use of IM ranitidine for the prophylaxis of aspiration pneumonitis in obstetrics. *Br J Anaesth* 1988;61:720-729.
33. O'Sullivan G, Sear JW, Bullingham RES, et al. The effect of magnesium trisilicate mixture, metoclopramide and ranitidine on gastric pH, volume and serum gastrin. *Anaesthesia* 1985;40:246-253.
34. Miller AC, DeVore JS, Eisler EA. Effects of anesthesia on uterine activity and labor. In: Schnider SM, Levinson G, eds. *Anesthesia for Obstetrics*. 3rd ed. Baltimore: Williams and Wilkins; 1993:53.
35. Liu PL, Warren TM, Ostheimer GW, et al. Fetal monitoring in parturients undergoing surgery unrelated to pregnancy. *Can Anaesth Soc J* 1985;32:525-532.
36. Sheybany S, Murphy JF, Evans D, et al. Ritodrine in the management of fetal distress. *Br J Obstet Gynaecol* 1982;89:723-726.
37. Reece EA, Chervenak FA, Romero R, et al. Magnesium sulfate in the management of acute intrapartum fetal distress. *Am J Obstet Gynecol* 1984;148:104-106.
38. Schnider SM, Levison G, Parer JT. Diagnosis and management of fetal asphyxia. In: *Anesthesia for Obstetrics*. 3rd ed. Baltimore: Williams and Wilkins, 1993:657-670.
39. Reves JG, Karp RB, Butner EE, et al. Neuronal and adrenomedullary catecholamine release in response to cardiopulmonary bypass in man. *Circulation* 1982;66:49-55.
40. Estafanous FG, Buckley S. Management of anesthesia for open heart surgery during pregnancy. *Clev Clin Q* 1976;43:121-124.
41. Lichtenstein SV, Kassam AA, El-Dalati H, et al. Warm heart surgery. *J Thorac Cardiovasc Surg* 1991;52:1009-1013.
42. Salerno TA, Houck JP, Barrozo CAM, et al. Retrograde continuous warm blood cardioplegia: a new concept in myocardial protection. *Ann Thorac Surg* 1991;51:245-247.
43. Mora CT, Henson MB, Weintraub WS, et al. Neurologic events and neuropsychologic function after warm vs cold cardiopulmonary bypass: a prospective randomized trial in patients undergoing elective coronary bypass surgery. Presented at the 1993 American College of Cardiology Annual Meeting, Anaheim, CA.
44. Asali NS, Westin B. Effects of hypothermia on uterine circulation and on the fetus. *Proc Soc Exp Biol Med* 1962;109:485-488.
45. Boatman KK, Bradford VA. Excision of an internal carotid aneurysm during pregnancy employing hypothermia and a vascular shunt. *Ann Surg* 1958;148:271-275.
46. Jadhon ME, Main EK. Fetal bradycardia associated with maternal hypothermial. *Obstet Gynecol* 1988;72:496-497.
47. Van de Walle AFGM, Martin CB Jr. Effect of isoproterenol on uterine blood flow and cardiac output distribution in pregnant guinea pigs. *Am J Obstet Gynecol* 1985;152:1058-1062.
48. Shnider SM, Levinson G, Cosmi E. Obstetric anesthesia and uterine blood flow. In: Shnider SM, Levinson G, eds. *Anesthesia for Obstetrics*. 3rd ed. Baltimore: Williams and Wilkins; 1993:29-51.
49. Mancini D, LeJemtel TH, Sonnenblick EH. Intravenous use of amrinone for the treatment of the failing heart. *Am J Cardiol* 1985;56:8B.
50. Fishburne JI Jr, Dormer KJ, Payne GG. Effects of amrinone and dopamine on uterine blood flow and vascular responses in the gravid baboon. *Am J Obstet Gynecol* 1988;158:829-837.
51. Jelsema RD, Bhatia RK, Ganguly S. Use of intravenous amrinone in the short-term management of refractory heart failure in pregnancy. *Obstet Gynecol* 1991;78:935-936.
52. Fishburne JI, Meis PJ, Urban RB, et al. Vascular and uterine responses to dobutamine and dopamine in the gravid ewe. *Am J Obstet Gynecol* 1980;137:944-951.
53. Clark RB, Brunner JA. Dopamine as a vasopressor for the treatment of spinal hypotension during cesarean section. *Anesthesiology* 1980;53:514-517.
54. Rolbin SH, Levinson G, Shnider S, et al. Dopamine treatment of spinal hypotension decreases uterine blood flow in the pregnant ewe. *Anesthesiology* 1979;51:36-40.
55. Blanchard K, Dandavino A, Nuwayhid B, et al. Systemic and uterine hemodynamic responses to dopamine in pregnant and nonpregnant sheep. *Am J Obstet Gynecol* 1978;130:669-673.
56. Ralston DH, Schnider SM, deLorimier AA. Effects of equipotent ephedrine, metaraminol, mephentermine and methoxamine on uterine blood flow in the pregnant ewe. *Anesthesiology* 1974;40:354-370.
57. James FM III, Greis FC, Kemp RA. An evaluation of vasopressor therapy for maternal hypotension during spinal anesthesia. *Anesthesiology* 1970;33:25-34.
58. Rosenfeld CR, Barton MD, Meschia G. Effects of epinephrine on distribution of blood flow in the pregnant ewe. *Am J Obstet Gynecol* 1976;124:156-163.
59. Hood DD, Dewan DM, James FM III. Maternal and fetal effects of epinephrine in gravid ewes. *Anesthesiology* 1986;64:610-613.
60. Mahon WA, Reid DWJ, Day RA. The in vivo effects of beta adrenergic stimulation and blockade on the human uterus at term. *J Pharmacol Exp Ther* 1967;156:178-185.
61. Bailey JM, Levy JH, Kikura M, et al. Pharmacokinetics of milrinone in cardiac surgery patients. *Anesthesiology* 1994 (In press).
62. Baumann AL, Santos AC, Wlody D, et al. Maternal and fetal effects of milrindine and dopamine. *Anesthesiology* 1989;71:A855.
63. Greiss FC Jr, Pick JR. The uterine vascular bed: adrenergic receptors. *Obstet Gynecol* 1964;23:209-213.
64. Greiss FC Jr, Van Wilkes D. Effects of sympathomimetic drugs and angiotensin on the uterine vascular bed. *Obstet Gynecol* 1964;23:925-930.
65. Cibils LA, Pose SV, Zuspan FP. Effect of 1-norepinephine infusion of uterine contractibility and the cardiovascular system. *Am J Obstet Gynecol* 1962;84:307-317.

66. Greiss FC Jr, Gobble FL Jr. Effect of sympathetic nerve stimulation on the uterine vascular bed. *Am J Obstet Gynecol* 1967;97:962–967.
67. Ring G, Krames E, Shnider SM, et al. Comparison of nitroprusside and hydralazine in hypertensive gravid ewes. *Obstet Gynecol* 1977;50:598–602.
68. Wheeler AS, James FM III, Meis PJ, et al. Effects of nitroglycerin and nitroprusside on the uterine vasculature of gravid ewes. *Anesthesiology* 1980;52:390–394.
69. DeSimone CA, Norris MC, Leighton BL. Intravenous nitroglycerin aids manual extraction of a retained placenta. (Letter to the editor) *Anesthesiology* 1990;73:787.
70. Stempel JE, O'Grady JP, Morton MJ, et al. Use of sodium nitroprusside in complications of gestational hypertension. *Obstet Gynecol* 1982;60:533–538.
71. Naulty J, Cefalo RL, Lewis PE. Fetal toxicity of nitroprusside in the pregnant ewe. *Am J Obstet Gynecol* 1981;139:708–711.
72. Tcherdakoff PH, Colliard M, Berrard E, et al. Propranolol in hypertension during pregnancy. *Br Med J* 1978;2:670.
73. Bott-Kanner G, Schweitzer A, Reisner SH, et al. Propranolol and hydralazine in the management of essential hypertension in pregnancy. *Br J Obstet Gynaecol* 1980;87:110–114.
74. Rubin PC. β-Blockers in pregnancy. *N Engl J Med* 1981;305:1323–1326.
75. Ostman PL, Chestnut DH, Robillard JE, et al. Transplacental passage and hemodynamic effects of esmolol in the gravid ewe. *Anesthesiology* 1988;69:738–741.
76. Eisenach JC, Castro MI. Maternally administered esmolol produces fetal β-adrenergic blockade and hypoxemia in sheep. *Anesthesiology* 1989;71:718–722.
77. Losasso TJ, Muzzi DA, Cucchiara RF. Response of fetal heart rate to maternal administration of esmolol. *Anesthesiology* 1991;74:782–784.
78. Frishman WH, Chesner M. Beta-adrenergic blockers in pregnancy. *Am Heart J* 1988;115:147–152.
79. MacPherson M, Pipkin FB, Rutter N. The effect of maternal labetalol on the newborn infant. *Br J Obstet Gynaecol* 1986;93:539–542.
80. Michael CA. Intravenous labetalol and intravenous diazoxide in severe hypertension complicating pregnancy. *Aust NZ J Obstet Gynaecol* 1986;26:26–29.
81. Wood M, Wood AJJ. *Drugs and Anesthesia: Pharmacology for Anesthesiologists*. 2nd ed. Baltimore: Williams and Wilkins; 1990:428.
82. Sandstrom B. Antihypertensive treatment with the adrenergic beta-receptor blocker metoprolol during pregnancy. *Gynecol Obstet Invest* 1978;9:195–204.
83. Rotmensh HH, Elkayam U, Frishman W. Anti-arrhythmic drug therapy during pregnancy. *Ann Intern Med* 1983;98:487–497.
84. Kleinman CS, Copel JA, Weinstein EM, et al. In-utero diagnosis and treatment of fetal supraventricular tachycardia. *Semin Perinatol* 1985;9:113.
85. Murad SHN, Tabsh KMA, Conklin KA, et al. Verapamil: placental transfer and effects on maternal and fetal hemodynamics and atrioventricular condition in the pregnant ewe. *Anesthesiology* 1985;62:49–53.
86. Veille JC, Bissonnette JM, Hohimer AR. The effect of a calcium channel blocker (nifedipine) on uterine blood flow in the pregnant goat. *Am J Obstet Gynecol* 1986;154:1160–1163.
87. Kaul AF, Osathanondh R, Safon LE. The management of preterm labor with the calcium channel-blocking agent nifedipine combined with the β-mimetic terbutaline. *Drug Intell Clin Pharm* 1985;19:369–371.
88. Forman A, Gandrup P, Anderson KE, et al. Effects of nifedipine on oxytocin and prostaglandin $F_{2\alpha}$-induced activity in the post-partum uterus. *Am J Obstet Gynecol* 1982;144:665–670.
89. Biehl D, Shnider SM, Levinson G, Callender K. The direct effects of circulating lidocaine on uterine blood flow and foetal well being in the pregnant ewe. *Can Anaesth Soc J* 1977;24:445–451.
90. Biehl D, Shnider SM, Levinson G, et al. Placental transfer of lidocaine. *Anesthesiology* 1978;48:409–412.
91. Greiss FC Jr, Still JG, Anderson S. Effects of local anesthetic agents on the uterine vasculatures and myometrium. *Am J Obstet Gynecol* 1976;124:889–899.
92. Gutgesell M, Overholt E, Boyle R. Oral bretylium tosylate use during pregnancy and subsequent breast feeding: a case report. *Am J Perinatol* 1990;7:144–145.
93. Rogers MC, Willerson JT, Goldblatt A, et al. Serum digoxin concentrations in human fetus, neonate and infant. *N Engl J Med* 1972;298:1010–1013.
94. Weaver JB, Pearson JF. Influence of digitalis on time of onset and duration of labor in women with cardiac disease. *Br Med J* 1973;3:519–520.

Part V(b)
Cardiopulmonary Bypass in Special Patient Populations
Partial Cardiopulmonary Bypass

25
Cardiopulmonary Bypass–Supported Angioplasty

Steven K. Macheers

Introduction

Cardiopulmonary bypass (CPB), initiated percutaneously or via "cutdown," serves as an effective means of resuscitating patients suffering cardiac arrest in or out of the cardiac catheterization laboratory.[1-5] More recently, portable CPB units have been used to support patients undergoing "high-risk" angioplasty or valvuloplasty.[6-19] These portable bypass systems, available commercially as self-contained units, have been employed prophylactically during high-risk procedures for hemodynamic support, or have been employed in a standby fashion with either guide wires or femoral cannulas in place, with a perfusionist in attendance. This chapter will follow the evolution of supported percutaneous transluminal coronary angioplasty (S-PTCA) and delineate the role of this important treatment modality in the armamentarium of the cardiologist and cardiac surgeon.

Background

Since the introduction of percutaneous transluminal coronary angioplasty (PTCA) by Dr. Andreas Gruentzig in 1977,[14] the spectrum of problems addressed has steadily increased in complexity. The patients are older and sicker; the cardiac lesions are more complex and greater in number. Abrupt closure of vessels, or failed angioplasty, in patients with minimal reserve, can be catastrophic. Similarly, prolonged balloon inflation times in vessels serving critical masses of myocardium may result in hemodynamic compromise during angioplasty.

Portable CPB units (Figure 25.1A and B) have been employed successfully in the resuscitation of these patients as well as in other clinical settings—cardiogenic shock, hypothermia, allergic reactions, smoke inhalation, near-drowning, asthma attacks, pulmonary edema (Table 25.1)—for patients not responding to traditional therapy. Successful use of portable cardiopulmonary bypass (PCPB) in these settings, as well as in the cardiac catheterization lab, has led to the extrapolation of PCPB employed prophylactically to support high-risk patients undergoing PTCA (S-PTCA) or balloon valvuloplasty.[6]

Vogel et al[6] first reported the use of PCPB in a prophylactic setting in December 1987. Similar successful reports were soon to follow.[8-15] In 1988, a national registry was established to be used in a prospective study of the elective use of PCPB in this setting. A liberal set of criteria for entry into the study was established. Suggested indications for inclusion were (1) the presence of severe or unstable angina pectoris, (2) at least one likely dilatable coronary artery stenosis, and (3) left ventricular ejection fraction <25% or a target vessel supplying more than half of the viable myocardium, or both.[7] While the initial results from the 14 centers comprising the National Registry of Elective Cardiopulmonary-Bypass-Supported Coronary Angioplasty were touted as successful, complications associated with the prophylactic use of PCPB have tempered the indications for use of this modality.[16] The trend now is for the use of PCPB to be available in a standby setting, with either guide wires or cannula in place, with extracorporeal support reserved for hemodynamic compromise. Further controversy exists over whether this modality is physiologically beneficial when used prophylactically, and whether PCPB should be employed by physicians without formal training in extracorporeal circulatory support. Current use will determine future potential.

Equipment/Techniques

There are currently three systems commercially available for use as portable extracorporeal circulation units. They are:

1. Cardiopulmonary Bypass Support (CPS™) system (Bard, Tewksbury, MA);
2. Bio-Medicus™ Portable Bypass System (PBS™) (Medtronic, Inc., Minneapolis, MN);
3. Sarns™ Percart™ system (Ann Arbor, MI).

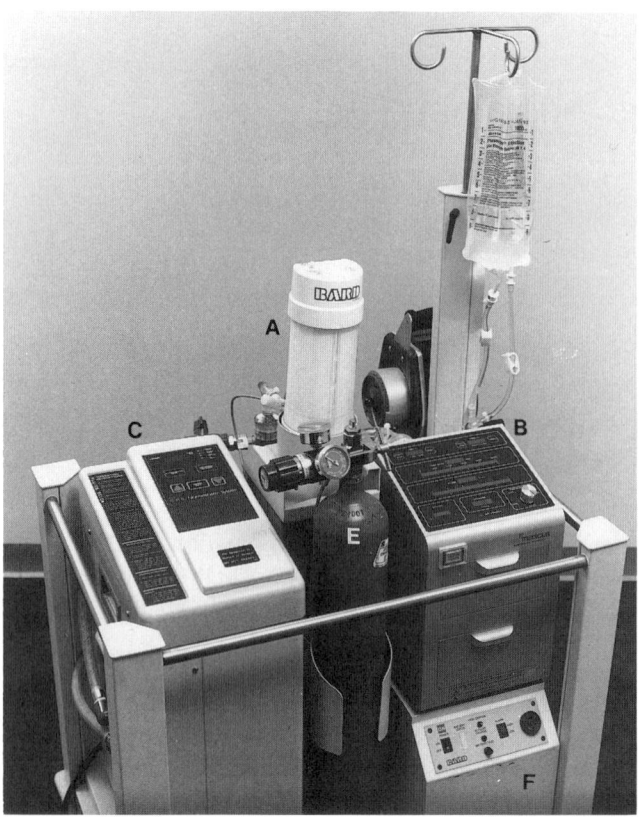
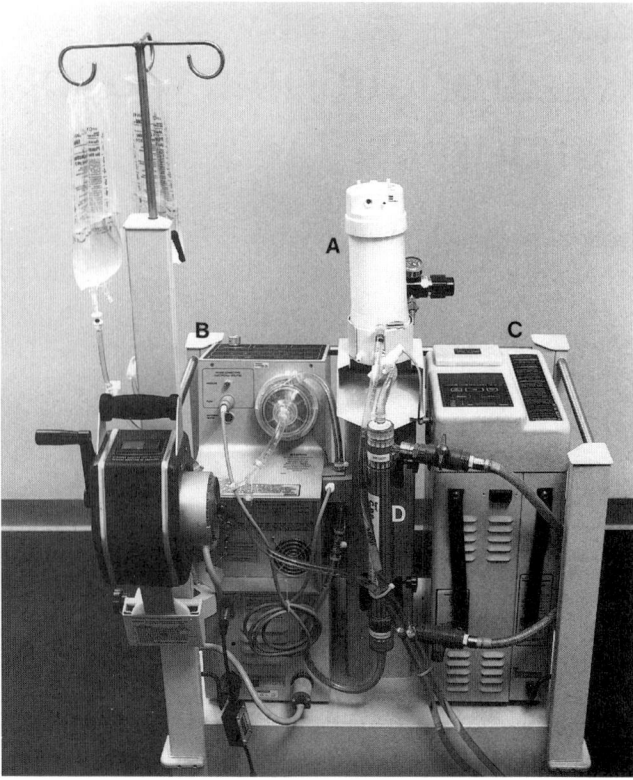

FIGURE 25.1 Front (A) and rear (B) views of self-contained portable CPB unit consisting of a membrane oxygenator (A), pump console with a centrifugal pump (B), warming unit (C), heat exchanger (D), oxygen source (E), and battery pack (F).

All three systems rely on three basic components:

1. Femoral artery and femoral vein percutaneous cannulation catheters (Figure 25.2A and B);
2. A portable, self-contained heart-lung machine (Figure 25.1A and B);
3. A preassembled perfusion circuit (Figure 25.3)

All systems employ a centrifugal pump rather than the more commonly used roller pump. These pumps work by creating a forced vortex in the blood generated by a smooth rotating cone which is then constrained and expelled. This type of pump is discussed further in Chapter 11. This system relies on active venous return rather than gravity return because it is necessary to overcome the increased resistance created by longer cannulas that are inserted distally via the femoral vessels.

The cannulas continue to undergo evolution as technology improves. Typically, large-bore, thin-walled Teflon™ cannulas measuring 18F or 20F are employed, and are inserted by cutdown, or percutaneously through the femoral vessels (Figures 25.2A, and B, 25.4).

The perfusion circuits employed are preassembled to assure sterility and ease of setup. Manufacturers suggest that equipment setup takes 5 to 10 minutes. The circuit includes a membrane oxygenator, capable of exchanging large volumes of respiratory gases, that also functions as a trap for air and gaseous emboli. An arterial line filter would be impossible to prime expeditiously in an emergency setting. Since the system utilizes active venous return, a reservoir is not included in the circuit. Thus, the circuit is isovolemic.

All available PCPB systems allow maximal flows of 5 to 6 L/min through single venous and arterial cannulas under optimal conditions. Unfortunately, flows of these magnitudes are not always obtained, due to resistance within the circuit and limited venous return. Volume must frequently be added to the patient-extracorporeal circuit to maintain adequate flows.

TABLE 25.1. Clinical uses of PCPB units.

Supported percutaneous transluminal coronary angioplasty
Cardiogenic shock
Cardiac arrest not responsive to advanced cardiac life support
Hypothermia
Severe allergic reactions not responding to medical treatment and causing cardiopulmonary collapse
Smoke inhalation
Near-drowning
Asthma not responding to medical therapy
Drug overdose
Pulmonary edema (reversible)
Short-term maintenance of cadaveric organs

25. Cardiopulmonary Bypass–Supported Angioplasty

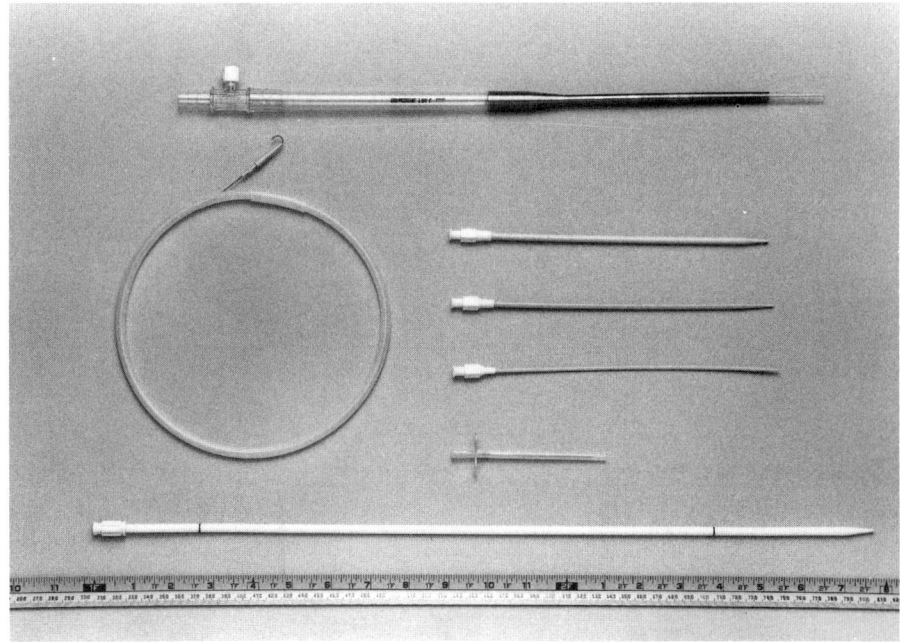

FIGURE 25.2. Femoral artery (A) and vein (B) cannulation catheters prepackaged in a sterilized kit for use with a portable CPB unit.

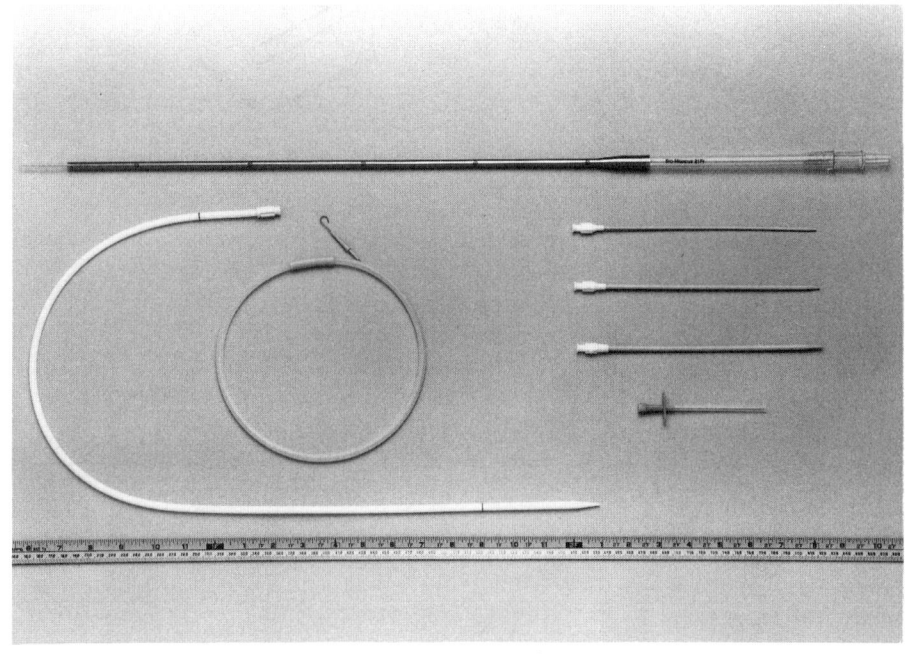

The primary limitation of PCPB systems is the inability of these devices to completely unload the heart. This deficit is magnified in the face of pathophysiologic conditions that leave the heart prone to distension, such as aortic insufficiency. Other limitations include the loss of circulating volume, red cells, and clotting factors which are left in the bypass circuit after successful patient resuscitation. Blood factor transfusion is frequently required when a PCPB unit is employed.

PCPB Unit: Placement of Cannulas

Initial experience required placement of the cannulas via femoral arterial and venous cutdown in the cardiac catheterization laboratory.[6] Subsequently, catheters have been placed percutaneously using a Seldinger technique—optimally, after the vessels have been visualized.[9] However, because of the size of the catheters required, placement in

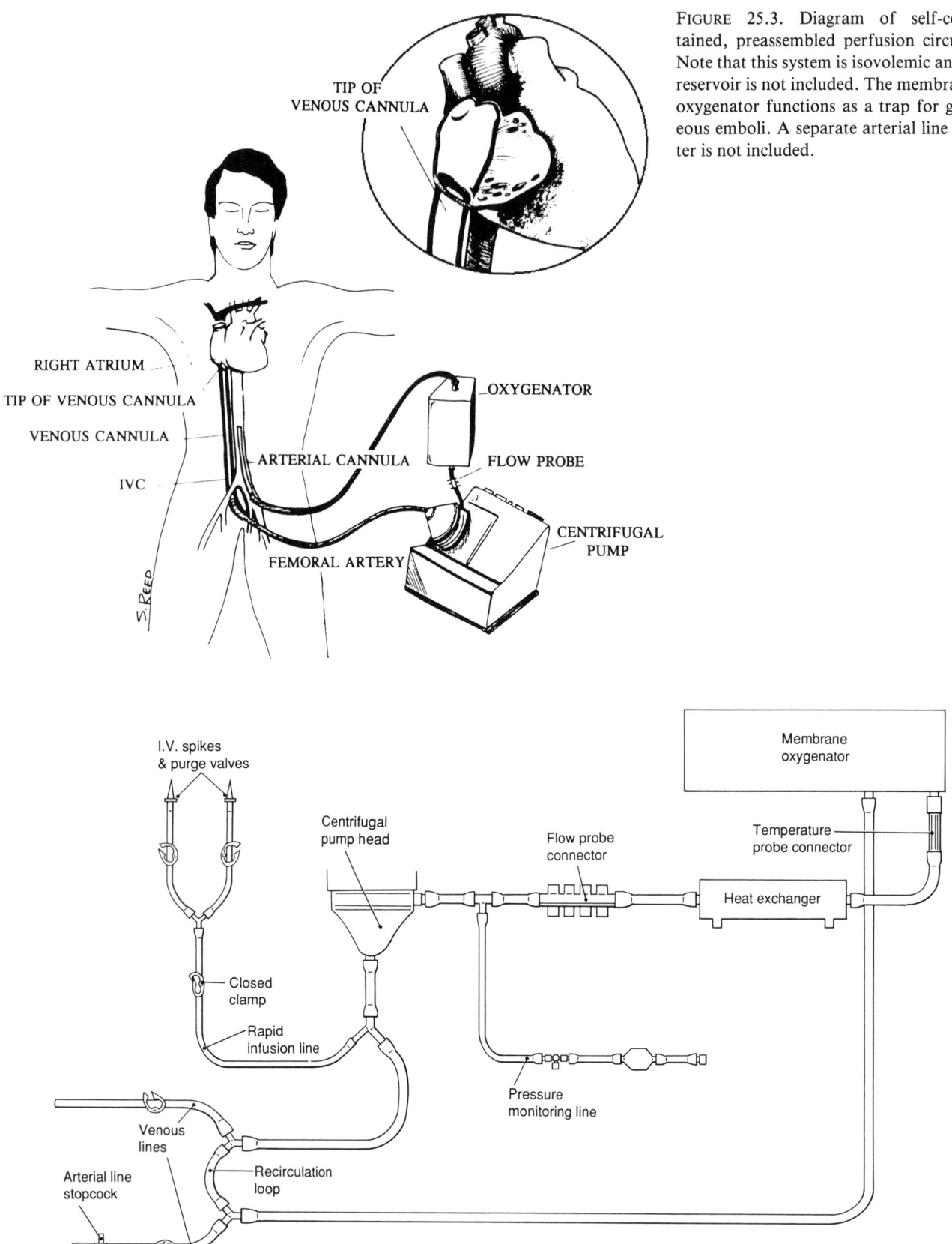

FIGURE 25.3. Diagram of self-contained, preassembled perfusion circuit. Note that this system is isovolemic and a reservoir is not included. The membrane oxygenator functions as a trap for gaseous emboli. A separate arterial line filter is not included.

FIGURE 25.4. Schematic representation of femoral vessel cannulation and the portable bypass circuit. The tip of the venous cannula should be advanced to the level of the right atrium to optimize venous return and cardiac decompression.

this fashion and subsequent removal have led to an unacceptable rate of morbidity in some series.[16,18] Therefore, the preferred method of cannula placement appears to be via cutdown if time permits. If the PCPB unit is to be used as a standby measure, the method of choice appears to be guide wires inserted in the femoral vessels, with cannula placement reserved for emergency situations. From a surgical standpoint, open cutdown and direct repair of the femoral vessels represents the most conservative and the only *certain* method of assuring long-term vessel patency.

Obviously, the use of PCPB units requires full heparinization, and is thus unacceptable in situations in which complete anticoagulation would be contraindicated.

Hemodynamic and Echocardiographic Changes During PCPB

Extracorporeal circulation via percutaneous portable bypass systems differs, in a number of fundamentally important ways, from CPB employed in the operating room: the patient remains awake, the heart continues to beat, and the protection provided by hypothermia is not employed. CPB utilized during open-heart procedures completely isolates the heart, allowing its complete unloading. When combined with hypothermia, myocardial oxygen demands are minimized. Typical flow rates necessary for full support of the patient during open-heart surgery are not achievable with these systems, due to limitations previously described. Although hemodynamic support and perfusion for systemic organs can be maintained, myocardial protection may not be optimal.

Typically, flow rates of 2 to 4.5 L/min are achievable with PCPB systems. Although this may provide a 50% reduction in pulmonary capillary wedge pressures, echocardiographically measured left ventricular internal diastolic dimension does not change significantly, nor does left ventricular shortening fraction.[20] Other hemodynamic changes include a significant drop in systolic arterial blood pressure with the initiation of CPB, when a large volume of venous return is shunted through the bypass circuit, causing a decrease in cardiac preload. This may result in a decreased coronary artery perfusion pressure, if not corrected pharmacologically or with volume replacement.

Pavlides et al,[20] in an echocardiographic study of 20 patients during S-PTCA, reported that myocardial regions supplied by a stenotic vessel deteriorated during bypass support, whereas regions supplied by a nonstenotic vessel did not. Regions supplied by a target vessel were shown to deteriorate further during balloon inflation. Thus, although PCPB in this setting results in decreased afterload, myocardial dysfunction in regions supplied by a stenotic vessel may generally worsen.[20,21]

Although PCPB has been touted as a way of supporting the high-risk patient, PCPB does not translate into myocardial protection. The cardiac changes characteristic of protracted angioplasty balloon inflation—chiefly, local decrease in myocardial wall function—are not lessened on PCPB.

Results

Early Results

Vogel[6] in 1988 reported his initial experience with 15 patients, 9 undergoing PTCA and 3 undergoing balloon valvuloplasty. Successful coronary artery dilation was performed in 11 of 12 attempts; success was defined as residual coronary artery stenosis less than 40% and residual gradient greater than 20 mm Hg. There were two deaths (2/15), resulting in a mortality rate of 13%. One patient died from a superior mesenteric artery thrombosis 8 hours after the procedure, and the other from ventricular fibrillation occurring 12 hours after balloon valvuloplasty. Transfusions of 3 to 8 units of blood were required in all patients.[6]

Similarly, Shawl et al[19] reported the use of PCPB-supported PTCA in 35 patients, successfully dilating 85 of 86 arteries. Although complications related to catheter insertion were reported, transfusions were required in only 43% of patients. Anecdotal experiences in smaller series and community settings have echoed the successful use of this technique.[5,8,10,11,15]

In 1989, Shawl and colleagues[18] reported a study of 51 high-risk patients undergoing elective S-PTCA. Angioplasty was successful in 115 of 117 attempted coronary artery dilations. There were three in-hospital deaths unrelated to bypass. Complications related to PCPB are listed in Table 25.2. Although morbidity was high, blood transfusions were necessary in only 38% of patients.[18]

Initial Report of the National Registry of Elective Cardiopulmonary Bypass Supported Coronary Angioplasty

The initial results of a multicenter trial involving 14 institutions were reported in January 1990.[7] Study entry criteria were ejection fraction less than 25%, a target vessel supplying more than half the myocardium, or both. One hundred five patients were entered into the Registry, with a mean age of 62 years. Twenty patients had vascular disease deemed too severe to permit bypass surgery and 30 patients had dilation of their only patent coronary vessel.

The S-PTCA success rate was 95% for 105 patients, with an in-hospital mortality of 7.6%. Forty-one patients suffered a complication, in most cases due to arterial, venous, or nerve injury associated with cannula insertion, removal, or both (Table 25.3). Symptomatic improve-

TABLE 25.2. Complications due to percutaneous cardiopulmonary bypass support in 51 patients.

	No.	Percent
Requiring surgical intervention		
Pseudoaneurysm of femoral artery[a]	3	6
Infection requiring debridement	2	4
Increasing hematoma	1	2
Embolus	1	2
Requiring nonsurgical intervention		
Femoral nerve weakness[b]	4	8
Superficial skin abrasion or necrosis[b]	4	8
Deep venous thrombosis[a]	1	2
Minor superficial infection[a]	1	2
Transient ischemic attack 48 hours after procedure[c]	1	2
Air embolus	1	2
Minor gastrointestinal bleeding	1	2

[a] Noted on follow up
[b] Due to clamp compression
[c] Patient also had bilateral carotid artery stenoses
(From Shawl, Domanski, Punja et al,[18] by permission of *Amer J Cardiol*.)

ment was seen in 91% of patients surviving hospitalization. Seventy-two percent of patients had residual Class I or II angina. Postangioplasty vessel closure occurred in 7 patients at 10 hours to 4 days following PTCA. Four patients died. An additional surgical procedure was required in 12 patients (11%). Indications for operation included coronary artery bypass graft (CABG) in 4 patients, repair of a femoral artery in 7 patients, and laparotomy for bowel infarction in 1 patient. Other causes of death in this series included abdominal hemorrhage, mesenteric artery thrombosis, and femoral artery occlusion (Table 25.3). Blood transfusions of 1 to 12 U (mean 3.7 U) were required in 45 patients (43%).[7]

Standby Versus Supported PTCA

In a series of patients reported by Tommaso et al,[16] standby PCPB-supported PTCA (equipment and personnel available for immediate initiation of PCPB) appeared to offer the advantages of S-PTCA without the associated morbidity. Although this study was nonrandomized, in the words of the authors, "When the significant morbidity associated with insertion of the cannulae was recognized, we switched to a strategy of standby supported-PTCA in the subsequent consecutive patients with similar indications."[16]

In this series, of the 12 patients undergoing PCPB-supported PTCA, 1 patient suffered a gastrointestinal bleed, 1 patient required re-exploration of the cannula insertion site for bleeding, and 8 patients required transfusions. There was one acute vessel closure 36 hours postprocedure, which was successfully managed with repeat PTCA. Among the 13 patients having standby PCPB-supported PTCA, 13 of 13 vessels were successfully dilated. There were no procedure-related complications or transfusions. One death occurred several days postprocedure, presumably due to late vessel closure.[16]

Further concerns over the morbidity associated with PCPB-supported PTCA were echoed by Feld et al[22] in 1991. In a series of 720 patients undergoing PTCA at Maimonides Medical Center in New York, 7.2% met the entry criteria suggested by the National Registry of Elective Supported Angioplasty. These records were then reviewed and compared to the results of the National Registry (Table 25.4). Although the Maimonides group patients may have been at higher risk than the Registry Group (14% of the Registry Group did not meet the entry criteria), there were no mortalities, despite an expected acute closure rate of 5% in the cardiology suite. The authors attribute this phenomenon to their use of the Stack perfusion catheter and intraaortic balloon pump (IABP). Morbidity and mortality were significantly less in this group than in the National Registry Group (Table 25.5).

Comparison of Alternative Strategies to PCPB-Supported Angioplasty

To date, no randomized studies have compared PCPB-supported angioplasty or valvuloplasty with unsupported PTCA or valvuloplasty. Although the procedure can be

TABLE 25.3. Initial report of the National Registry of Elective Cardiopulmonary Bypass Supported Angioplasty; morbidity in 105 coronary angioplasty patients treated with PCPB.

Vessel cannulation	
Femoral artery repair (required)	4
Femoral artery occlusion	1
Femoral artery pseudoaneurysm	3
Large hematoma	4
Thrombophlebitis	5
Cannula site infection or necrosis	8
Femoral nerve injury (transient)	2
Embolism	
Superior mesenteric artery embolus or thrombus	1
Cerebrovascular accident	1
Transient cerebral ischemia	1
Angioplasty	
Left ventricular dysfunction requiring IABP	1
Post-PTCA myocardial ischemia	5
Post-PTCA myocardial infarction	7
Cardiac arrest	1
Other	
Gastrointestinal bleeding	2
Diabetic ketoacidosis (bowel ischemia)	1
Acute renal failure	1

(Reprinted with permission from the American College of Cardiology [*Journal of the American College of Cardiology* 1990; 15(1):23–29].)

TABLE 25.4. Clinical and angiographic characteristics of high-risk coronary angioplasty patients managed with PCBP.

	Maimonides Medical Center high-risk study $n = 56$	National Registry of Elective Supported Angioplasty $n = 105$
Men	43 (76%)	84 (80%)
Age	66 (35–86)	62 (38–81)
Ejection Fraction (%)	37 (16–67)	32 (6–67)
Ejection Fraction (<25%)	20 (36%)	35 (33%)
Target vessel supplies		
All myocardium	5 (9%)	13 (12%)
>1/2 myocardium	14 (25%)	19 (18%)
<1/2 myocardium	6 (11%)	16 (15%)

(From Feld, Herz, Fred et al,[22] by permission of *Amer J Cardiol*.)

performed with the results detailed in the previous section, other alternatives are available.

Other strategies for the support or salvage of the high-risk patient undergoing PTCA have been studied extensively in animals and in humans. These strategies include (1) use of the IABP (see Chapters 17 and 28), (2) retrograde synchronized coronary artery retroperfusion, (3) use of the Hemopump™ (a temporary left ventricular assist device [LVAD] utilizing axial flow technology to draw blood out of the left ventricle and expel it into the aorta), (4) standard LVADs, and (5) use of autoperfusion catheters (catheters capable of providing flow beyond the point of acute occlusion or in situations where prolonged balloon inflation times are required). Although all of these strategies have merits and pitfalls, a full description and comparison is beyond the scope of this text. However, a brief overview is provided below.

LVADs are, unfortunately, reserved for postcardiotomy patients, thereby limiting their application. Synchronized coronary venous retroperfusion is a technique in which arterial blood is shunted from the femoral artery into the coronary sinus during the diastolic segment of the cardiac cycle. It has been shown to preserve regional and global myocardial function during abrupt coronary artery occlusion.[10] Although clinical studies are in progress, this technology has not been compared with other cardiac support systems. The Hemopump™, also a fledgling technology, shows promise in certain circumstances but cannot be compared with PCPB at this time. Two other strategies that are routine in many institutions are the use of autoperfusion catheters and the IABP.

Autoperfusion Catheters

The autoperfusion catheter, exemplified by the Stack Perfusion Dilation Catheter™ (Advanced Cardiovascular Systems, Mountain View, CA) has four potential roles: (1) for routine PTCA, (2) to salvage jeopardized myocardium following failed PTCA, (3) to perform PTCA in high-risk patients, and (4) as a bridge to definitive therapy, emergency CABG, in failed angioplasty procedures. Although no study has assessed the effect of autoperfusion catheters on outcome following emergency CABG surgery, their use as a bridge to the operating room is standard practice in many institutions.

IABP

Kahn and colleagues[23] reported on the use of the IABP in a series of 28 patients with high-risk characteristics. In this study, 90 of 94 vessels were successfully dilated. This included multivessel angioplasty in 75% of patients, and five left main coronary artery dilations. Decrease in systolic blood pressure to less than 70 mm Hg occurred in 11 patients, but augmented diastolic pressure was greater than 90 mm Hg at all times. There were no deaths or myo-

TABLE 25.5. Complications of PCPB in patients undergoing coronary angioplasty.

	Maimonides Medical Center high-risk study	National Registry of Elective Supported Angioplasty	*p* value
Death	0	8 (7.6%)	0.03
Emergent CABG	3 (5.4%)	4 (3.8%)	NS
Myocardial infarct	1 (1.8%)	7 (6.7%)	NS
Blood transfusion	2 (1.8%)	45 (4.3%)	0.0001
Vascular or nerve injury	1 (1.8%)	27 (26%)	0.0001
Other (gastrointestinal bleeding, diabetic ketoacidosis, acute renal failure, superior mesenteric artery embolus, cerebrovascular accident, transient ischemic attack)	0	(6.7%)	0.05

NS, not significant
(From Feld, Herz, Fred et al,[22] by permission of *Amer J Cardiol*.)

cardial infarctions. Vascular complications requiring surgery occurred in three patients, but all had good operative results and no need for transfusion.[23] Although this was not a randomized study, PCPB-supported PTCA must be compared with the results obtained with IABP support alone.

In a study using a porcine model, comparing the relative efficacy of PCPB and IABP in reducing infarct size after revascularization for acute coronary insufficiency, optimal recovery occurred in the IABP group. Although the PCPB group experienced less myocardial necrosis than did the unsupported control group, the IABP group had the highest ventricular wall-motion scores, the least change in tissue pH values from preischemia, and the least amount of myocardial necrosis.[24]

Do Circulatory Support Technologies (PCPB, IABP, Coronary Autoperfusion Catheters) Improve Patient Outcome Following PTCA?

Clearly, several strategies exist for the support of the high-risk patient undergoing PTCA. To date, there are no data demonstrating that the use of circulatory support technologies improves patient outcome following PTCA. Additionally, it is unclear whether the use of any one of these devices in *all* high-risk patients is superior to a strategy in which circulatory support technologies are reserved for patients with hemodynamic compromise or failed PTCA procedures. Time and prospective randomized trials are needed to determine the relative benefit and potential morbidities of these support technologies. Obviously, a comparison of morbidity and mortality in the unsupported versus the supported patient must be the gold standard.

To assess the frequency and outcome of emergency CABG for failed PTCA in patients with prior CABG, 2136 elective PTCA procedures, performed over a 10-year period, were reviewed by Kahn et al.[23] Emergency CABG was required in only 19 (0.9%) of the patients with prior CABG, compared with 130 of 6974 patients (1.9%) without prior CABG ($p = 0.001$). Three of these patients could not be weaned from CPB. The remaining 16 patients were discharged after a mean stay of 16 days. Of these patients, 15 of 16 were alive with no, or mild, angina at a mean follow-up of 52 months (range 3–99 months).[23] Their conclusion was that in patients without high-risk features, emergency repeat CABG can be accomplished with good results, both hospital and long-term.[23]

Personnel/Training

CPB and extracorporeal circulatory support represent a complex artificial intervention resulting in a unique and profound pathophysiology. When CPB is employed in the operating room by highly trained personnel, complications related to the procedure itself have been minimized. However, employment of this complex technology by those untrained in the unfamiliar with extracorporeal circulation may be fraught with significant difficulties. This problem is addressed in a policy statement issued by The Society of Thoracic Surgeons and Council of the American Association for Thoracic Surgery, here reproduced in its entirety[25]:

Extracorporeal circulation was introduced into clinical use by Dr. John Gibbon in 1953. Since then, the technology has undergone modification and is applied widely today for surgical treatment of diseases of the heart and great vessels.

The use of ECC traditionally has been under the direct supervision of the thoracic surgeon, the only medical specialist whose formal training and certification require theoretical knowledge and practical experience (case load requirements) with ECC including a thorough understanding of the scientific aspects, necessary apparatus, and complications associated with its use.

The distribution of blood flow during ECC, rheologic effects, impact on various organ systems (lungs, kidneys, immune system, clotting mechanism), and the effects of hemodilution, hypothermia, and non pulsatile flow are examples of the knowledge required of thoracic surgeons who are distinguished from other surgical specialists by their routine use of this technology in surgical applications.

Of great concern is the potential for patient injury with ECC. Vascular injury due to cannulation, aortic dissection, air embolism, thrombosis, hemolysis, with resultant renal injury, hemorrhage, protamine reactions, and failure to provide adequate perfusion are but a few of the potential hazards of ECC, many of which may be fatal. Less obvious is the cumulative, time-related cellular injury associated with ECC.

In addition to its use in operations on the heart and great vessels, ECC is applied in a limited way for other purposes such as treatment of hypothermia, limb perfusion for melanoma, hypothermia and circulatory arrest for certain neurosurgical procedures and for treatment of renal cell carcinoma with tumor extension into the IVC and atrium. These applications are undertaken in the operating room under the direct supervision of the thoracic surgeon.

Less commonly, ECC technology may be applied outside the operating room for other purposes, such as extracorporeal membrane oxygenation (ECMO) used in the ICU setting to treat reversible lung injury, or in the CCU or cardiac catheterization laboratory for patients in cardiogenic shock.

Medical specialists other than thoracic surgeons may be involved in the applications of ECC. Anesthesiologists who provide anesthesia for cardiac surgery are familiar with the administration of heparin, protamine reversal, and the effect of ECC on cardiopulmonary responses in the anesthetized patient. The vascular surgeon may become involved in treatment of vascular complications of ECC.

The perfusionist is knowledgeable in the physiology of ECC and has proficiency with the pump-oxygenator apparatus.

Recently, cannulas have been developed and marketed for percutaneous insertion. This has led to the use of ECC by the non-surgeon, who may insert cannulas percutaneously and connect them to portable pump-oxygenator systems for circulatory support during catheter interventions on the obstructed coronary artery. Experience with so-called "supported angioplasty" has been reported, including six abstracts (five recording clinical experience, and one an animal study) reported at the American College of Cardiology Meeting in Anaheim, California, April 1989.

It is of concern that ECC during "supported angioplasty" may be conducted without the participation and direct supervision of a physician who is both knowledgeable and experienced in the technique. There are a few non-surgeons who, because of professional commitment and long experience, are qualified, but these individuals are exceptional. In contrast, all American Board of Thoracic Surgery diplomates are qualified by virtue of education and examination, and most are currently experienced in the supervision of ECC. We therefore believe that, except under unusual circumstances, patient safety considerations require formal consultation with the thoracic surgeon whenever use of ECC is contemplated. If ECC is deemed appropriate, then the participation and supervision of a thoracic surgeon or an equally qualified physician are imperative.

We would emphasize the special relationship that exists between the thoracic surgeon and the perfusionist, in which the perfusionist functions under the supervision of the thoracic surgeon. In those instances in which the perfusionist is employed by the hospital, or functions as an independent contractor, and is asked to provide perfusion services under a physician not trained in ECC, serious liability questions may be raised for the hospital, perfusionist, physician, and manufacturer.*

Conclusions

Employment of PCPB units in emergency settings for salvage of failed angioplasty and valvotomy procedures, as well as for resuscitation of patients with cardiac arrest in, and out of, the cardiac catheterization laboratory, has been well established. When used by personnel trained in the use of the equipment and by physicians trained in the use of extracorporeal circulation, or by perfusionists under their direct supervision, the systems are safe and effective.

The desirability of the prophylactic use of PCPB units for support of the high-risk patient undergoing elective PTCA or valvuloplasty is less clear. High complication rates associated with the procedure itself—arterial injury, venous injury, nerve injury, limb loss, stroke—and a high rate of transfusion requirements make the prophylactic use of this technology less desirable.

Physiologic studies suggest that PCPB is ineffective in eliminating wall-motion abnormalities associated with vessel occlusion. In fact, regions supplied by a stenotic vessel may deteriorate during PCPB support. Myocardial regions supplied by a target vessel have been shown to deteriorate further during balloon inflation. Thus, PCPB employed in this setting does not protect the myocardium.

While PCPB is certainly capable of providing hemodynamic support in the case of failed procedures, acute vessel closure occurs in only 5% of cases. In reality, vessel closure and failed procedures are likely to be recognized as complications occurring hours after extracorporeal support has been discontinued.

Ultimately, PCPB-supported angioplasty must be compared to less invasive means of support of these patients, as well as to no support at all.

Conceptually, PCPB is more likely to be employed successfully in a standby setting. In this way, the efficacy of PCPB employed as a salvage procedure can be optimized and the complications associated with its routine use minimized.

References

1. Kanter KR, Pennington G, Vandormael M, et al. Emergency resuscitation with extracorporeal membrane oxygenation for failed angioplasty *J Am Coll Cardiol* 1988;11:149A. Abstract.
2. McDonnel BE, Napoli P, Bowman GA, et al. Evolving myocardial infarction during percutaneous transluminal coronary angioplasty: the use of portable percutaneous cardiopulmonary support. *Mil Med* 1990;155:565-567.
3. Phillips SJ, Zeff RH, Kongtahworn C, et al. Percutaneous cardiopulmonary bypass: application and indication for use. *Ann Thorac Surg* 1989;47:121-123.
4. Mattox KL, Beall AC. Resuscitation of the moribund patient using portable cardiopulmonary bypass. *Ann Thorac Surg* 1976;22:436-442.
5. Shawl FA, Domanski MJ, Wish MH, et al. Emergency cardiopulmonary bypass support in patients with cardiac arrest in the catheterization laboratory. *Cathet Cardiovasc Diagn* 1990;19:8-12.
6. Vogel RA. The Maryland experience: angioplasty and valvuloplasty using percutaneous cardiopulmonary support. *Am J Cardiol* 1986;62:11K-14K.
7. Vogel RA, Shawl F, Tommaso C, et al. Initial report of the National Registry of Elective Cardiopulmonary Bypass Supported Coronary Angioplasty. *J Am Coll Cardiol* 1990;15:23-29.
8. Wanner WR, Peterson SC, Blankenship WR, et al. Emergency portable cardiopulmonary bypass for abrupt left main occlusion during coronary angioplasty. Excellent long-term survival. *Chest* 1992;101:869-870.
9. Shawl FA, Domanski MJ, Wish MH, et al. Percutaneous cardiopulmonary bypass support in the catheterization laboratory: technique and complications. *Am Heart J* 1990;120:195-203.
10. Lincoff AM, Popma JJ, Ellis SG, et al. Percutaneous support devices for high-risk or complicated coronary angioplasty. *J Am Coll Cardiol* 1991;17:770-780.
11. Osamu U, Kyoji K, Nobuhiko K. Percutaneous transluminal coronary angioplasty with cardiopulmonary bypass for stenosis of the most proximal part of the left anterior descending coronary artery. *Br Heart J* 1990;63:178-179.
12. Vogel JH, Ruiz CE, Jahnke EJ, et al. Percutaneous (nonsurgical) supported angioplasty in unprotected left main disease and severe left ventricular dysfunction. *Clin Cardiol* 1989;12:297-300.
13. Gundry SR, Brinkley J, Wolk M, et al. Percutaneous cardio-

---

*Reprinted with permission from the Society of Thoracic Surgeons (*The Annals of Thoracic Surgery* 1990; 49:514).

pulmonary bypass to support angioplasty and valvuloplasty. Technical considerations ASAIO Trans 1989;35:725-727.
14. Shawl FA. Percutaneous cardiopulmonary support in high-risk angioplasty. *Cardiol Clin* 1989;7:865-875.
15. Freedman RJ Jr, Wrenn RC, Godley ML, et al. Complex multiple percutaneous transluminal coronary angioplasties with vortex oxygenator cardiopulmonary support in the community hospital setting. *Cathet Cardiovasc Diagn* 1989; 17:237-242.
16. Tommaso CL, Johnson RA, Stafford JL, et al. Supported coronary angioplasty and standby supported coronary angioplasty for high-risk coronary artery disease. *Am J Cardiol* 1990;66:1255-1257.
17. Vogel RA, Tommaso CL, Gundry SR. Initial experience with coronary angioplasty and aortic valvuloplasty using elective semipercutaneous cardiopulmonary support. *Am J Cardiol* 1988;62:811-813.
18. Shawl FA, Domanski MJ, Punja S, et al. Percutaneous cardiopulmonary bypass support in high-risk patients undergoing percutaneous transluminal coronary angioplasty. *Am J Cardiol* 1989;64:1258-1263.
19. Shawl FA, Domanski MJ, Punja S, et al. Percutaneous cardiopulmonary bypass to support high-risk electric coronary angioplasty. *J Am Coll Cardiol* 1989;13:160A. Abstract.
20. Pavlides GS, Hauser AM, Stack RK, et al. Effect of peripheral cardiopulmonary bypass on left ventricular size, afterload and myocardial function during elective supported coronary angioplasty. *J Am Coll Cardiol* 1991;16:499-505.
21. Axelrod HI, Galloway AC, Murphy MS, et al. A comparison of methods for limiting myocardial infarct expansion during acute reperfusion—primary role of unloading. *Circulation* 1987;76:v28-32.
22. Feld H, Herz I, Fred G, et al. Cardiopulmonary support increases morbidity and mortality in high-risk coronary angioplasty. *Am J Cardiol* 1991;68:790-792.
23. Kahn JK, Rutherford BD, McConahay DR, et al. Supported "high-risk" coronary angioplasty using intraaortic balloon pump counterpulsation. *J Am Coll Cardiol* 1990;15:1157-1165.
24. Lazar HL, Yang SM, Rivers S, et al. Role of percutaneous bypass in reducing infarct size after revascularization for acute coronary insufficiency. *Circulation* 1991;64(suppl 5): 416-421.
25. The Society of Thoracic Surgeons and Council of the American Association for Thoracic Surgery. The use of extracorporeal circulation for circulatory support during PTCA. *J Thorac Cardiovasc Surg* 1990;99:1011-1021.

26
Closed Chest Bypass for Liver Transplantation

Linda E. McLean, Scott M. Kreger, and Christina T. Mora

Historical Perspective

Preliminary investigation into the feasibility of organ replacement as a therapeutic modality for treatment of irreversible liver disease began in the early 1950s. Welch, in 1955, reported a technique of heterotopic liver transplantation by insertion of a donor graft into the pelvis of a dog, without removal of the native organ.[1] In 1956, the report of an experimental orthotopic liver transplantation (OLT) provided the first venture at whole organ replacement.[2] Individual groups at Boston (Moore) and Chicago (Starzl) began extensive research on liver transplantation in the canine model,[3,4] leading to the first attempt at human OLT in 1963. Relatively long-term success in human transplantation did not occur until 1967, however, when a recipient, one-and-a-half years old, survived for 13 months.[5]

The many medical disciplines that contribute to successful liver transplantation evolved most notably during the 20-year span from 1963 to 1983.[6] Improvements in surgical technique, immunosuppression therapies, and methods of homograft preservation, coupled with new techniques for rapid volume infusion, autologous blood recovery, and venous decompression of surgically obstructed vessels, reduced the number and severity of intraoperative and postoperative complications.[7-17]

In June 1983, the National Institutes of Health convened a consensus development conference on liver transplantation. The panel determined that transplantation was an accepted therapy for patients with end-stage liver disease.[18] Following this decision, many state and private insurance companies began paying for OLT and, as a result, transplant programs proliferated.[19] Starzl and colleagues[20] suggest that 4,000 to 50,000 liver transplantations a year may be needed. However, the insufficient number of donors limits the availability of this procedure.

Patient Selection

Evaluation of the transplant candidate remains a complex process of determining medical necessity, proper timing, technical feasibility, and absence of contraindicating factors.[21] Candidates for OLT must have irreversible liver disease not responsive to alternative methods of treatment.[12] In adults, the most common causative disease states are chronic active hepatitis, cryptogenic cirrhosis, alcoholic cirrhosis, primary biliary cirrhosis, various hepatic malignancies, primary sclerosing cholangitis, and acute hepatic necrosis.[54] Relative contraindications to OLT include active alcoholism or drug abuse, extrahepatic malignancies, pre-existing local or systemic infections, advanced pulmonary or cardiovascular disease, and other untreatable conditions.[21,54] The presence of hepatitis C or hepatitis B is not an absolute contraindication to liver transplantation, since the development of cirrhosis in the allograft is variable.[22,23] Tables 26.1 and 26.2 list the indications and relative contraindications to OLT.

Rationale for Venovenous Bypass During OLT

The phase of surgery during which mobilization and removal of the native liver occurs, and the anhepatic phase, remain the most crucial periods of the transplantation procedure. During these times, surgical obstruction of the inferior vena cava and portal vein is necessary. The subsequent interruption of venous return to the heart is often associated with an up to 50% reduction in cardiac output, and marked increase in systemic vascular resistance.[24] Engorgement of the subdiaphragmatic vessels occurs, increasing portal hypertension and bowel congestion. This congestion can lead to excessive hemorrhaging from high-

TABLE 26.1. Indications for liver transplantation.

Cirrhosis
    Primary biliary cirrhosis
    Chronic active hepatitis
    Cryptogenic cirrhosis
    Alcoholic cirrhosis
    Biliary atresia
    Autoimmune cirrhosis
    Primary sclerosing cholangitis
Fulminant hepatic failure
    Viral
    Drug-induced
    Toxin-induced
Metabolic disease
    Wilson's disease
    α_1-Antitrypsin deficiency
    Hemochromatosis
Isolated hepatic malignancy

pressure venous collaterals, third-space fluid sequestration, and possible peritoneal contamination with bowel flora.[21] Decreased renal function is commonly seen, possibly due to hypoperfusion of the kidneys secondary to increased pressure in the inferior vena cava.[25] Once reperfusion occurs, highly acidic and potassium-rich venous blood is suddenly reintroduced into the systemic circulation, further increasing the possibility of cardiac arrhythmias and hemodynamic instability.[24]

In an attempt to maintain more normal hemodynamics during the anhepatic phase, Calne and colleagues[26] first used a selective technique of partial cardiopulmonary support. Those high-risk patients who showed marked circulatory instability during trial clamping of the inferior vena cava were placed on venoarterial bypass, with an intervening oxygenator. Circulatory support was provided, but systemic heparinization was required. Severe hemorrhage often resulted from anticoagulation, limiting the procedure's usefulness.

The need for a successful method of venous decompression was addressed with the development of a closed bypass system that did not require heparinization. Dixon and Magovern[27] were the first to report long-term heparinless cardiac support, with the use of a constrained vortex pump. Employing this knowledge, Griffith and Shaw[28] designed a closed, venovenous bypass system for use during OLT. Their circuit was composed of heparin-bonded, Gott aneurysm-shunt tubing for drainage and return cannulas, a centrifugal blood pump, and connecting segments of ⅜-inch uncoated polyvinyl chloride tubing.

Similar heparinless closed circuits have been employed for femoral venoarterial bypass as an alternative method of circulatory support.[29] This technique provides venous decompression, but desaturated blood is delivered to the kidneys and lower extremities.[30] Due to this fact, some controversy exists as to the actual usefulness of this method. A direct comparison of the two types of bypass indicates a closer approximation of normal physiology with a venovenous bypass than with a venoarterial approach.[31] Since its introduction, heparinless venovenous bypass has become the predominant bypass technique employed during OLT.

Although definitive outcome studies are lacking, advocates for the use of venovenous bypass during OLT believe that this technique improves interoperative hemodynamic stability, reduces perioperative transfusion requirements, and decreases the likelihood of postoperative renal dysfunction.

The incorporation of venovenous bypass during OLT allows for maintenance of venous return and cardiac filling pressures during inferior vena cava occlusion. The degree to which an individual can tolerate the acute reduction in preload created by obstruction of venous return from the inferior vena cava and portal vein is variable. A relatively healthy patient may require very little support compared to a debilitated person in whom a rapid infusion of a large volume of fluid may be necessary to maintain an adequate cardiac output. Vigorous volume expansion at this point may cause volume overload once normal inferior vena cava flow is reinstated.[24] The ability to normalize hemodynamics may be especially beneficial in the patient with limited cardiac reserve.[32] Additionally, venovenous bypass may be especially useful in elderly patients with cholecystic disease and pulmonary hypertension, since this group is particularly prone to hemodynamic instability with caval inclusion.[33]

One group advocates the use of a hepatic occlusion test to determine which patients will require venovenous bypass to obviate the problem of hemodynamic instability.[34] If patients become hypotensive (>30% decrease in the mean arterial pressure) or have a greater than 50% reduction in their cardiac index during a 5-minute test period, in which the hepatic vessels are occluded, preparations for the institution of venovenous bypass are initiated. However, the technique of rapid volume infusion can be employed to minimize the hemodynamic alterations that occur during inferior vena cava and portal vein clamping.[35] Researchers at some institutions have found that the cirrhotic patient, who often presents with an elevated cardiac output and decreased systemic vascular resistance, can easily tolerate a 50% reduction in cardiac output during the anhepatic phase, and they therefore proceed without attempts at rectifying these alterations.[36]

Venovenous bypass may also reduce bleeding from

TABLE 26.2. Contraindications to liver transplantation.

Active alcohol or drug abuse
Extrahepatic malignancies
Sepsis
Advanced pulmonary, cardiac, or neurologic disease
Acquired immunodeficiency syndrome
Inability to continue immunosuppression and maintain medical follow-up care

TABLE 26.3. Potential theoretical advantages of venovenous bypass in liver transplant surgery.

Normalization of cardiac physiology
Improved renal perfusion/decreased renal failure
Decompression of the portal system/decreased transfusion requirements
Safe extension of the anhepatic phase

high-pressure venous collaterals, thereby reducing hemorrhage and the resulting amount of blood transfusion required. However, the effect of venovenous bypass on perioperative blood-product transfusion requirements is unclear.[24,34] One group, in a retrospective study of patients undergoing OLT, reported that 33 ± 25 units of packed red cells were transfused in patients who were not managed with venovenous bypass, compared with 19 ± 8 units transfused in the bypass group.[34] However, other researchers have not demonstrated that the use of bypass during OLT results in decreased transfusion requirements.[35]

Renal perfusion is compromised during the anhepatic phase of OLT. Caval occlusion results in a decrease in systemic arterial blood pressure and in elevation in renal venous pressure.[37] Because venovenous bypass improves renal blood flow by maintaining an adequate preload, cardiac output, and normal renal vein pressure, some believe that the use of bypass will reduce the incidence of postoperative renal dysfunction.[25] Again, controlled randomized clinical trials assessing the effect of venovenous bypass on renal outcome are not available. However, in a retrospective study, patients managed with venovenous bypass had a lower postoperative creatinine and were less likely to require postoperative hemodialysis than patients not exposed to bypass during OLT.[38] In contrast, others found no difference in postoperative creatinine levels.[34] Additionally, patients with normal preoperative renal function who were not exposed to venovenous bypass did not develop postoperative renal impairment.[34]

Further benefits of venovenous bypass include the safe extension of the venous occlusion period during more complicated cases and in training situations.[24] Potential benefits of venovenous bypass employed during OLT are listed in Table 26.3.

As noted above, there are those who deny the necessity of routine venovenous bypass in OLT. These clinicians agree that bypass may facilitate certain aspects of the surgery, but they challenge the idea that it is required to reduce blood loss or prevent renal failure.

Further research is required to determine the usefulness of venovenous bypass in OLT. While there are many potential benefits associated with the use of this technique, randomized clinical trials are required to assess the effect of venovenous bypass on specific outcome variables including allograft function, blood-product requirements, perioperative renal function, and overall patient morbidity and mortality.[39,40]

The Operative Procedure and Establishing Venovenous Bypass

The operation begins with the acquisition of appropriate peripheral venous, arterial, and central access. Anesthetic induction can either precede or follow line placement, depending on the relative stability of the patient.

When venovenous bypass will be used, saphenofemoral and axillary venous access should be established prior to incision, in case rapid cannulation becomes necessary. The abdomen is then opened, and the hepatic artery, portal vein, intrahepatic and suprahepatic inferior vena cava, and common bile duct are skeletonized.

Once the native liver is isolated, preparation for bypass (if used) is continued. Heparin-bonded No. 7 and No. 9 Gott Shunt tubing is utilized for axillary/femoral and portal vein cannulation, respectively. The portal cannula is advanced into the transected end of the portal vein, and the inferior vena cava cannula is placed through the saphenovenous junction at the origin of the iliac veins. Blood from the inferior vena cava and portal vein is drained to a centrifugal pump and returned to the axillary vein. Figure 26.1 diagrams a venovenous bypass circuit for OLT. Vascular clamps are placed on the hepatic artery, portal vein, and vena cava, above and below the native liver. These vessels are incised and the native organ is removed.

Questions concerning safe blood-flow rates during venovenous bypass remain incompletely answered. Early laboratory work demonstrated that platelet counts and fibrinogen levels decreased, while fibrin split-product accumulation increased when pump flow dropped below 800 mL/min. This phenomenon indicates that, when the rate at which blood passed through the circuit was reduced, activation of the coagulation cascade occurred. Consequently, the lower limit of bypass flow had been initially set at 1000 mL/min.[38] During bypass, malposition of the portal vein cannula or a decrease in the patient's circulating volume are the two most common causes of fluctuation in flow. If bypass is interrupted for more than a few minutes, the system should be changed, or bypass must be discontinued, even if heparin-bonded tubing has been employed.[33] To date, there are no data that define the blood-flow rate below which thrombus formation is a significant risk.

Graft insertion involves four vascular, and one biliary, anastomoses. The suprahepatic and infrahepatic caval anastomoses are usually made first. The portal vein anastomosis is then performed, and the portal vein cannula is clamped and removed. Portal venous blood flow is then reestablished by release of the portal and caval clamps. If the surgical team is satisfied with graft reperfusion, veno-

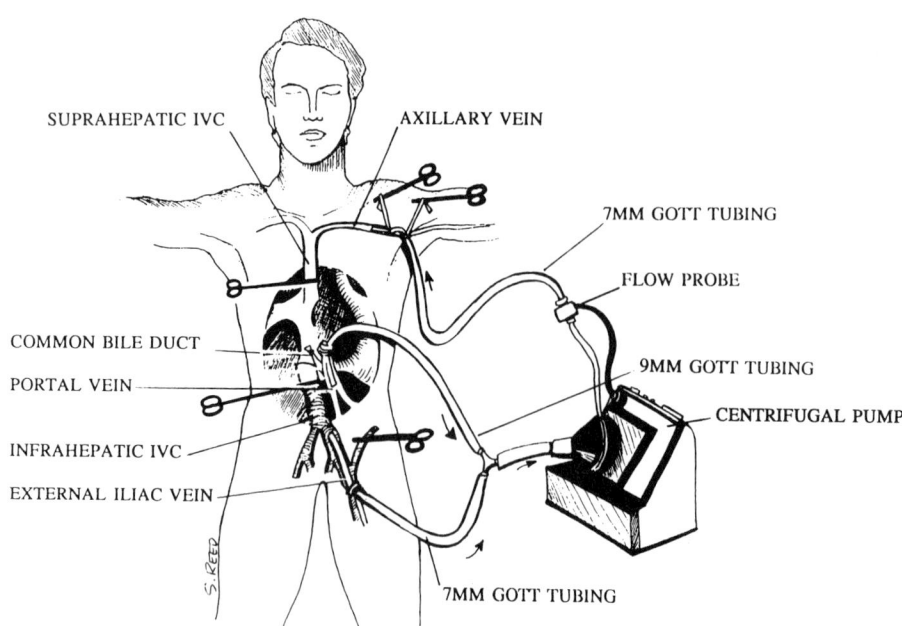

FIGURE 26.1. Venovenous bypass circuit for orthotopic liver transplantation. Venovenous bypass re-establishes blood return between the surgically obstructed vena cava and portal vein to the central venous circulation via the axillary vein. The circuit is composed of drainage cannulas in the obstructed vessels (blood drains by gravity) and a centrifugal pump that pumps blood into the axillary vein via the return cannula.

venous bypass is terminated and decannulation is completed.

The next step requires careful anastomosis of the hepatic artery. Due to the nature of the vessel, precise surgical skill is required to reduce the risk of arterial thrombosis, a potentially lethal complication.[55] Finally, the patient's biliary tract is reconstructed, the donor's gallbladder is removed, and the patient's abdomen is closed.

Complications of Venovenous Bypass

The risk-to-benefit ratio of venovenous bypass has been the center of great controversy. Complications, such as air and thrombus embolization, nerve injury, lymphocele formation, and wound infection, have been reported, but only rarely.[12,30,41,42] Documentation of thromboembolization of a pre-existing clot in patients with polycystic disease of the liver and acute Budd-Chiari syndrome suggests venovenous bypass is contraindicated in these groups of patients.[38] Air embolism with or without venovenous bypass is a potential problem during OLT.[43] Other potential problems associated with the use of venovenous bypass are listed in Table 26.4.

TABLE 26.4. Potential adverse effects of venovenous bypass.

Air or thrombus embolization
Brachial plexus injury
Lymphocele formation
Wound infection
Added cost in materials and personnel
Added surgical time

In vitro studies have shown that the centrifugal pump may generate embolic matter.[44] Examination of the pump, following in vivo use, indicates that thrombus formation is possible in areas of low shear rates, low flow rates, and temperature elevation.[45] Dixon and Magovern[27] hypothesized that, although platelet and coagulation factor activation does occur, a concurrent state of "controlled" fibrinolysis is present in the patient, preventing the accumulation of coagulation particles.

Thrombus formation should be a concern when the bypass circuit is assembled.[56] Exposure of blood to a smooth surface can reduce the risk of embolic formation; therefore, the fewer connectors used in the system, the better. The use of heparin-coated tubing may help to provide a less thrombogenic surface for blood contact. Although proponents of this product exist, others have found it provides little advantage over its noncoated counterpart.[46] The newer heparin-bonded tubing may offer the greatest advantage during low-flow states or complete bypass interruption.[38]

Autologous Blood Recovery and Rapid Transfusion Devices: Utility During OLT

Problems with hemostasis frequently occur during OLT. Hepatocellular failure is often associated with a decreased production in all the coagulation factors (except factor VIII), resulting in abnormal hemostasis.[47] Preoperative coagulopathics are exacerbated during OLT by the significant amount of intraoperative heat loss by the patient.

FIGURE 26.2. This schematic of a rapid infusion device depicts the unique features which allow for the delivery of up to 1500 mL/min of warm fluid. Fluid is contained in a 3-L reservoir and warmed to 30°C by a columnar countercurrent heat exchanger. Warmed fluids are infused into the patient by a nonocclusive roller pump. Interposed between the reservoir and the patient is a series of air detection monitors and pressure sensors that protect the patient from an air embolus.

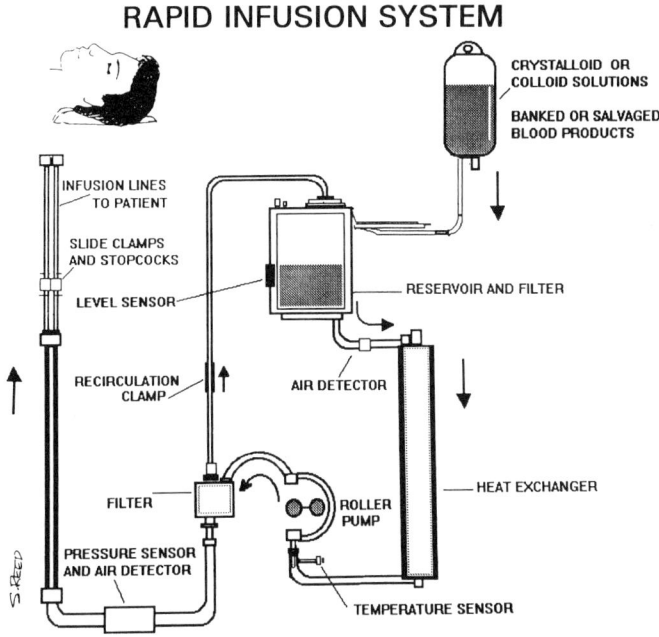

The extended period during which the abdominal contents are exposed to ambient temperatures, prolonged controlled ventilation, unwarmed intravenous fluids, extracorporeal circulation, and the grafting of a cold, preserved allograft all contribute to the development of hypothermia.[48] Additionally, damage incurred by the allograft may precipitate activation of both the coagulation and the fibrinolysis systems.[49] Finally, blood dilution, platelet aggregation in the extracorporeal system, and consumption of coagulation factors because of excessive hemorrhage all may contribute to coagulation abnormalities.

Both autologous blood recovery and rapid transfusion devices may attenuate the morbidity associated with massive blood loss. Although a rapid transfusion device may not be always required, it should be readily available for all cases. Autologous cell recovery reduces banked blood requirements without excessive blood cellular component damage.[50,51] The processed product is deficient in plasma content and platelets and is frequently supplemented by the administration of fresh frozen plasma and platelet concentrates.[12] Chapter 31 includes a detailed discussion of red blood cell salvaging techniques. The placement of 8.5F venous catheters permits the administration of large quantities of resuscitation fluids, and rapid transfusion devices can transfuse up to 1½ L of volume per minute if the viscosity of the infused fluids remains low. These devices include a roller pump, heat exchanger, reservoir filters, and temperature, pressure, and air-bubble monitors (Figure 26.2). The rapid transfusion device reservoir can be filled with crystalloid and/or colloid solutions, fresh frozen plasma, or red blood cells. As the microaggregate filter used with this device will remove most of the platelets, they should not be delivered with the rapid infuser.

Venovenous Bypass in Pediatric Patients Undergoing OLT

Every year, many children die as a consequence of liver failure. For some, liver transplantation is a viable and life-saving option.[52,53] The most common pediatric disease states requiring transplantation include biliary atresia, biliary hypoplasia, chronic hepatitis, and inborn errors of metabolism (ie, Wilson's disease, α_1-antitrypsin deficiency, tyrosinemia, glycogen storage disease, Crigler-Najjar syndrome, and protoporphyria).[57]

Venovenous bypass is used only occasionally in pediatric transplantation. Patient size limits cannulation capacity and attainable maximum pump flow.[38] Due to the nature of the heparinless system, and the danger of thrombus formation during low flow, patients below 30 to 40 kg are not typically candidates for venovenous bypass. Compensatory mechanisms in children make them more tolerant of the hemodynamic insult of venous occlusion, offsetting the need for venous decompression through venovenous bypass.[55] Bypass is more commonly indicated for a teenaged patient, or when profound portal hypertension exists.

Conclusion

Clinicians involved in liver transplant surgery are constantly searching for ways to reduce the operative risk of the procedure, a search that has led to the routine incorporation of a number of technological innovations. Paramount among those innovations is heparinless venovenous bypass. Although the routine use of this technique may be arguable, there is little doubt that, in select cases, venovenous bypass can significantly increase the margin of safety for this operation.

References

1. Welch CS. A note on transplantation of the whole liver of dogs. *Transplant Bull* 1955;2:54–55.
2. Cannon JA. Organs (communication). *Transplant Bull* 1956;3:7.
3. Starzl TE, Kaupp HA, Brock DR, et al. Reconstructive problems in canine liver homotransplantation with special reference to the postoperative role of the hepatic venous flow. *Surg Gynecol Obstet* 1960;11:733–743.
4. Moore FD. Experimental whole organ transplantation of the liver and the spleen. *Ann Surg* 1960;152:374–387.
5. Starzl TE, Iwatsuki S, VanThiel DH, et al. Evolution of liver transplantation. *Hepatology* 1982;2:614–636.
6. Smith SL. Liver transplantation. In: Smith SL, ed. *Tissue and Organ Transplantation: Implications for Professional Nursing Practice.* St Louis: Mosby Yearbook; 1990:273.
7. Starzl TE, Marchiaro TL, Vonkulla KN, et al. Homotransplantation of the liver in humans. *Surg Gynecol Obstet* 1963;117:659–676.
8. Vanthiel DG, Schade RR, Hakala TR, et al. Liver procurement for orthotopic transplantation: an analysis of the Pittsburgh experience. *Hepatology* 1984;4:66S–71S.
9. Stratta RJ, Wood RP, Langhas AN, et al. The impact of extended preservation on clinical liver transplantation. *Transplantation* 1990;50:438–443.
10. Starzl TE. *Liver Transplantation.* Chicago: Yearbook Med Pub Inc; 1990:14–18.
11. Kalayoglu M, Hoffmann RM, D'Alessandro AM, et al. Results of extended preservation of the liver for clinical transplantation. *Transplant Proc* 1989;21:3487–3488.
12. Lopez RR, Wright K, Donovan KL, et al. Overview of liver transplantation for the perfusionist. *J Extracorp Technol* 1992;24:26–32.
13. Mendez IB, Leddomado E. Orthotopic liver transplantation in children. *Mt Sinai J Med* 1989;56:71–75.
14. Hooks MA. Immunosuppressive agents used in transplantation. In: Smith SL, ed. *Tissue and Organ Transplantation: Implications for Professional Nursing Practice.* St Louis: Mosby Year Book; 1990:48–80.
15. Iwatsuki S, Starzl TE, Todo S, et al. Liver transplantation for treatment of bleeding esophageal varices. *Surgery* 1988;104:697–705.
16. Millis JM, Baquerizo A, Saleh S, et al. Preservation of renal function using OLT in liver transplant patients. *Transplant Proc* 1989;21:3551–3552.
17. Fabregat J, Fradera R, Jaurrieta E, et al. Clinical results of quadruple drug immunosuppression in liver transplantation. *Transplant Proc* 1992;24:148–149.
18. National Institutes of Health Consensus Development Conference Statement. *Liver Transplant Hepatol* 1984;4:107S–110S.
19. Roberts JP, Forsmark C, Lake JR, et al. Liver transplantation today. *Annu Rev Med* 1989;40:287–303.
20. Starzl TE, Demetris AJ, Van Thiel D. Liver transplantation. *N Engl J Med* 1989;321:1014–1022.
21. Smith SL. Liver transplantation. In: Smith SL, ed. *Tissue and Organ Transplantation: Implications for Professional Nursing Practice.* St Louis: Mosby Yearbook; 1990:276–283.
22. Samuel D, Bismuth A, Serres C, et al. HBV infection after liver transplantation in HBsAg positive patients: experience with long-term immunoprophylaxis. *Transplant Proc* 1991;23:1492–1494.
23. Shah G, Demetris AJ, Gravaler JS, et al. Incidence, prevalence, and clinical course of hepatitis C following liver transplantation. *Gastroenterology* 1992;103:323–329.
24. Shaw BW, Martin DJ, Marquez JM, et al. Venous bypass in clinical liver transplantation. *Ann Surg* 1984;200:524–534.
25. Brown M, Gunning T, Roberts C, et al. Biochemical markers of renal perfusion are preserved during liver transplantation with veno-venous bypass. *Transplant Proc* 1991;23:1980–1981.
26. Calne RY, McMaster P, Smith DP, et al. Use of partial cardiopulmonary bypass during the anhepatic phase of orthotopic liver grafting. *Lancet* 1979;2:612–614.
27. Dixon CM, Magovern GJ. Evaluation of the bio-pump for long-term cardiac support without heparinization. *J Extracorp Technol* 1982;14:331–336.
28. Griffith BP, Byers WS, Hardesty RL, et al. Venovenous bypass without systemic anticoagulation for transplantation of the human liver. *Surg Gynecol Obstet* 1985;160:270–272.
29. Calne RY, Williams R, Rolles K. Liver transplantation in the adult. *World J Surg* 1986;10:422–431.
30. Kang YG, Freeman JA, Aggarwal S, et al. Hemodynamic instability during liver transplantation. *Tranplant Proc* 1989;21:3489–3492.
31. Eason J, Tan K, Howard E, et al. Comparative hemodynamics of venovenous and venoarterial bypass during liver transplantation in the pig. *Transplant Proc* 1989;21:3525.
32. Taura P, Beltran J, Garcia-Valdecasas JC, et al. The need for venovenous bypass in orthotopic liver transplantation. *Transplantation* 1991;52:730–733.
33. Shaw BW. Some further notes on venous bypass for orthotopic transplantation of the liver. *Transplant Proc* 1987;19(suppl 3):13–16.
34. Veroli P, El Hage C, Ecoffey C. Does adult liver transplantation without venovenous bypass result in renal failure? *Anesth Analg* 1992;75:489–494.
35. Stock PG, Payne WD, Ascher NL, et al. Rapid infusion technique as a safe alternative to venovenous bypass in orthotopic liver transplantation. *Tranplant Proc* 1989;21:2322–2325.
36. Wall WJ, Grant DR, Duff JH. Liver transplantation without venovenous bypass. *Transplantation* 1987;43:56–61.
37. Merritt WT, Beattie C, Peck R, et al. Vena caval pressure gradients during liver transplantation. *Transplantation* 1990;50:336–338.
38. Shaw BW, Martin DJ, Marquez JM, et al. Advantages of venovenous bypass during orthotopic transplantation of the liver. *Semin Liver Disease* 1985;5:344–348.
39. Kelley SD. Venovenous bypass during liver transplantation. *Anesth Analg* 1992;75:481–483.

40. Carton EG, Plevak DJ, Kranner PW, et al. Perioperative care of the liver transplant patient: Part 2. *Anesth Analg* 1994;78:382-399.
41. Khoury GF, Mann ME, Porot MJ, et al. Air embolism associated with veno-venous bypass during orthotopic liver transplantation. *Anesthesiology* 1987;848-851.
42. Paulsen AW, Whitten CW, Ramsay MA, et al. Considerations for anesthetic management during veno-venous bypass in adult hepatic transplantation. *Anesth Analg* 1989;68:489-496.
43. Prager MC, Gregory GA, Ascher NL, et al. Massive venous air embolism during orthotopic liver transplantation. *Anesthesiology* 1990;72:198-200.
44. Martin BJ, Riley JB. Thrombus formation in centrifugal pumps. *J Extracorporp Technol* 1992;24:20-25.
45. Magovern GJ, Park SB, Maher TD. Use of a centrifugal pump without anticoagulants for postoperative left ventricular assist. *World J Surg* 1985;9:25-36.
46. van der Hulst VPM, Henny CP, Moulijn AC, et al. Veno-venous bypass without systemic heparinization using a centrifugal pump: A blind comparison of a heparin bonded circuit versus a non heparin bonded circuit. *J Cardiovasc Surg* 1989;30:118-123.
47. Morgan CH, Penner JA. Bleeding complications during surgery: Part II, Acquired hemorrhage disorders. *Lab Med* 1986;17:262-266.
48. Smith SL. Liver transplantation. In: Smith SL, ed. *Tissue and Organ Transplantation: Implications for Professional Nursing Practice*. St Louis: Mosby Yearbook; 1990:286-287.
49. Harper PL, Luddington RJ, Jennings I, et al. Coagulation changes following hepatic revascularization during liver transplantation. *Transplantation* 1989;48:603-607.
50. Calne R. *Liver Transplantation The Cambridge King's College Hospital Experience*. 2nd ed. Orlando: Grune and Stratton Ltd; 1987:193-197.
51. Kristiansson M, Lantz B, Gulliksson H, et al. Autotransfusion in liver transplantation. *Transplant Proc* 1989;21:35-38.
52. Gartner JC, Zitelli BJ, Malatack JJ, et al. Orthotopic liver transplantation in children: two year experience with 47 patients. *Pediatrics* 1984;74:140-145.
53. Vanthiel DH. Liver transplantation. *Pediatric Ann* 1985;14:474-480.
54. Starzl TE. *Liver Transplantation*. Chicago: Yearbook Med Pub Inc; 1990:119-130.
55. Shaw BW. Transplantation of the liver. In: Gitnick G, La Brecque DR, Moody FG, eds. *Diseases of the Liver and Biliary Tract*. St. Louis: Mosby Yearbook; 1989:635-638.
56. Musial J, Gluszko P, Edmunds H. Evaluation of surface-bound heparin and platelet inhibition in a centrifugal pump left ventricular assist system. *World J Surg* 1985; 9(1):72-77.
57. Mendez IB, Leddomado E. Orthotopic liver transplantation in children. *The Mount Sinai Journal of Medicine* 1989; 56(1):71-75.

Part VI
Mechanical Assist of the Failing Heart and Lung

27
Ventricular Assist Devices

Bradley L. Bufkin and Robert A. Guyton

Introduction

Extracardiac blood pumps may be used to allow temporary circulatory support in circumstances in which the pumping function of the heart is inadequate. Because of the complexity of these devices, the complications associated with their use, and cost considerations, all pharmacologic avenues of myocardial and circulatory support, as well as the intraaortic balloon pump (IABP) (see Chapter 28), are usually tried prior to resorting to ventricular assist devices. This chapter will consider the indications for the use of ventricular assistance, the devices that are appropriate for short-term assistance and those appropriate for longer-term assistance, and the complications associated with these devices.

Principles of Ventricular Assistance

Inadequate cardiac pumping function results in a hemodynamic situation characterized by high right atrial and/or left atrial pressures, low systemic blood pressures, and inadequate tissue perfusion. If volume loading, pharmacologic support, and IABP counterpulsation fail to rectify this situation, the patient will lapse into a state of cardiogenic shock with progressive end-organ damage from inadequate perfusion. If ventricular assistance is to be useful, it must be employed before significant end-organ damage has occurred. Ventricular assist devices are inserted parallel to the right ventricle and/or the left ventricle. Generally, these devices are capable of achieving cardiac outputs in the range of 3 to 10 L/min. They decrease preload by withdrawal of blood from the atrium (or, in some cases, from the ventricle itself) and infusion of blood into the pulmonary artery or into the aorta. In addition to restoring tissue perfusion by circulatory support, ventricular assist devices (VADs) allow the myocardium to rest by decreasing preload and thereby reducing end-diastolic and end-systolic ventricular size. Some VADs can also reduce afterload (when used in a manner synchronous with cardiac contraction) and thereby allow further systolic ventricular decompression. Preload reduction and reduction in cardiac size permit improvement in myocardial metabolism as less energy is required for each contraction, and the available energy can be used for repair of injured cardiac muscle.

Indications for Ventricular Assistance

The appropriate timing for initiation of ventricular assistance has been controversial. Many patients with poor ventricular function can be managed with volume loading, pharmacologic support, and intraaortic balloon counterpulsation, even though they might benefit from ventricular assistance. The establishment of guidelines for initiation of ventricular assistance has been necessary as experimental protocols have been developed (Table 27.1). Generally, the hemodynamic criteria for left ventricular assist device insertion are: (1) a cardiac index of less than 1.8 to 2 L/min/m^2, (2) a pulmonary capillary wedge pressure greater than 18 to 25 mm Hg, and (3) a mean arterial pressure less than 70 mm Hg despite maximal medical therapy including IABP counterpulsation. The indications for right ventricular assistance are a right atrial pressure greater than 18 to 25 mm Hg and a cardiac index less than 1.8 to 2 L/min/m^2. These criteria—particularly if filling pressures greater than 18 mm Hg and a cardiac in-

TABLE 27.1. Hemodynamic criteria for ventricular assistance.

Left ventricular failure	
Cardiac index	<1.8–2.0 L/m^2/min
Left ventricular filling pressure	>18–25 mm Hg
Mean arterial pressure	<70 mm Hg
Right ventricular failure	
Cardiac index	<1.8–2.0 L/m^2/min
Right ventricular filling pressure	>18–20 mm Hg
Mean arterial pressure	<70 mm Hg

dex of less than 2 L/min/m² are utilized—allow initiation of ventricular assistance prior to the development of profound and irreversible cardiogenic shock.

The most common indications for ventricular assistance are postcardiotomy cardiogenic shock (PCCS) and end-stage cardiomyopathy, as a bridge to transplantation (BTT). Ventricular assistance has been used less commonly for treatment of massive acute myocardial infarction, acute viral myocarditis, and rejection after transplantation. Short-term ventricular assistance, that is intended to permit myocardial recovery, is typically weaned within 2 to 7 days of device implantation. Long-term assistance is used for patients in whom there is only a very small possibility of myocardial recovery, and circulatory support is required until the patient undergoes heart transplantation.

Postcardiotomy Cardiogenic Shock

PCCS occurs in 2% to 6% of all patients undergoing coronary artery bypass grafting or valvular surgery.[1-3] Multiple factors can produce profound postoperative cardiac dysfunction, including prior myocardial infarction with depressed ventricular function, inadequate myocardial protection, and reperfusion injury. In general, ventricular assistance is not utilized if the patient has had a technically imperfect operation or an incomplete revascularization, as these hearts are not expected to recover. Additionally, a patient who suffers a large perioperative infarction has a very small chance of recovering even with ventricular assistance. In those centers in which VADs are used regularly, approximately 0.5% to 1% of patients undergoing cardiac surgery are managed with complete ventricular assistance to resuscitate postsurgical stunned myocardium and to maintain adequate systemic and pulmonary perfusion.[4,5] The original operative procedure (coronary bypass, valve operations, etc) does not predict the patient outcome following VAD implantation. If myocardial recovery is to occur, it generally happens within 1 week. Of the patients managed with a VAD for PCCS, 90% of those who survive require less than 1 week of assistance. A combined registry of experience in this group revealed that 45% of 965 patients requiring complete ventricular assistance were weaned from mechanical support and 25% of these patients achieved long-term survival.[6]

More liberal use of a VAD for treatment of PCCS may improve survival in this population.[7] Presently, most institutions reserve VAD support for patients unresponsive to IABP counterpulsation. But the survival of patients supported with an IABP for postcardiotomy low output is only 65%, indicating that a significant number of patients could benefit from complete ventricular assistance.[8]

The VAD as a Bridge to Transplantation

Cardiac transplantation is an effective therapy for end-stage cardiomyopathy of various etiologies. Of patients who are transplant candidates, 20% to 33% die while awaiting transplantation.[9,10] For a specific patient with inadequate cardiac pump function, ventricular assistance can provide interim circulatory support with hemodynamic stability and adequate end-organ perfusion, thereby extending the time for an appropriate donor organ to become available. Unfortunately, since there are other patients waiting for the same donor hearts who have not yet required ventricular assistance, an ethical dilemma arises. As there is an inadequate supply of donor hearts, should ventricular assistance be used to help specific patients compete for a heart that could be used in a less complex patient, perhaps with a better success rate and certainly with a lower cost?

The requirement for ventricular assistance for BTT is somewhat different than the requirement for the 1- to 2-week support necessary for PCCS. In the BTT population, cardiac dysfunction is considered to be permanent and myocardial recovery is not expected. The duration of circulatory support that will be required is unknown, and therefore safe, reliable assistance is necessary for extended time periods. Generally, patients requiring univentricular assistance have a slightly better outcome than those requiring biventricular assistance or total artificial heart implantation.[11,12] In a combined registry experience of 476 patients requiring a heart transplant and managed with a VAD, 69% were transplanted and 46% were long-term survivors.[12]

As in ventricular assistance for PCCS, early institution of VAD circulatory support before end-organ damage occurs is important in patients waiting for heart transplantation. If end-organ damage has occurred, it is important to continue ventricular assistance until complete end-organ recovery has occurred. These patients must recover from renal and/or respiratory failure, should be free of a coagulopathy, and should not be infected prior to transplantation. If these guidelines are followed, excellent long-term survival can be anticipated. Patients without other organ system failure who undergo univentricular support prior to heart transplantation have an 83% 2-year survival, a survival equivalent to that of isolated orthotopic cardiac transplantation patients without preceding ventricular assistance.[12] This success rate justifies the use of donor hearts in this population.

Appropriate Device Selection

An accurate diagnosis of the cause of ventricular failure is necessary for appropriate selection of the device for ventricular assistance. This permits an estimation of the expected duration of necessary circulatory support. Short-term support (4 days to 2 weeks) is used for patients with acute reversible processes. Examples of these patients and processes are (1) a patient with an acute myocardial infarction with early revascularization either by angioplasty or surgery with persistent stunned myocardium; (2) a patient with a technically successful cardiac operation with poor myocardial protection, in whom myocardial recovery is likely to occur with time; and (3) a transplanted heart with unexplained poor function immediately after transplantation, suggesting poor protection at the time of harvesting.

As noted above, long-term support (greater than 10 days) is utilized as interim therapy for permanent cardiac dysfunction as a BTT. Generally, the best candidates for this type of ventricular assistance are patients with cardiomyopathy (ischemic, viral, or other) who gradually deteriorate under medical observation. This type of assistance may also be utilized in a young patient with a massive myocardial infarction who is not revascularized quickly. VADs are generally classified as short-term or long-term devices (Table 27.2).

Short-Term VADs

Devices used for short-term circulatory support typically include extracorporeal circuits with free-standing pumps. An extracorporeal circuit is established by cannulation of the left atrium and ascending aorta for left ventricular assistance, and by cannulation of the right atrium and pulmonary artery for right ventricular assistance. These extracorporeal circuits generally do not permit patient mobility and require systemic anticoagulation. The devices differ, for the most part, in the type of pump employed. Either nonpulsatile roller pumps or centrifugal pumps, such as those used in standard cardiopulmonary bypass (CPB) circuits, may be employed. Additionally, a pneumatic pulsatile pump has been designed for short-term ventricular assistance. All of these devices are commercially available to all institutions for short-term circulatory support.

TABLE 27.2. Short- and long-term VADs.

Short-term VADs
  Nonpulsatile
    Roller pump systems
    Centrifugal pump systems—Biomedicus, Sarns, St Jude
  Pulsatile
    Abiomed BVS 5000
Long-term VADS
  Pneumatic
    Thoratec VAD system
    Thermo Cardiosystems HeartMate
    Symbion J-7 Total Artificial Heart
  Electric
    Novacor LVAS

Roller-Pump Devices as VADs

The system consists of standard CPB venous and arterial cannulas, silicone rubber, medical-grade pump tubing, and a portable roller pump. The roller pump includes two diametrically opposed rollers that rotate through an arch raceway (see Chapter 11). Maximal flow rates of 5 to 7 L/min can be achieved with this device. However, prolonged use of this device with flows in excess of 3 L/min has been associated with hemolysis and injury to blood components.[13]

The advantage of the roller pump is that it is readily accessible, since it is part of most CPB circuits, and it is reasonably successful. In a report of 72 patients undergoing left VAD (LVAD) support, 30 (42%) were weaned from the roller pump with 21 (29%) patients achieving long-term survival.[13] Several disadvantages of the roller pump are related to the mechanical trauma caused by the force applied to the tubing within the pump raceway. Spallation (breaking off of small particles of tubing which then enter the circulation) may occur. Tubing rotation helps prevent perforation and particulate embolization. Care must be taken to ensure unobstructed inflow and outflow, since roller pumps are not pressure limited. Constant attendance by a perfusionist is required when a roller pump is used as a ventricular assist device.

Centrifugal Pump Devices as VADs

Centrifugal pumps generate pressure by spinning blood as a solid body vortex, using impeller blades (see Chapter 11). This pump design allows pumping with decreased hemolysis and decreased damage to the blood elements.[14,15] The absence of tubing trauma prevents spallation of tubing and resultant embolic debris. Centrifugal pump systems have been widely employed for circulatory support for PCCS, and several centrifugal pump systems are commercially available. Despite the design advantages over roller pumps, these systems also require constant attention by an on-site perfusionist.

Results from the Combined Registry for the Clinical Use of Mechanical Ventricular Assist Devices demonstrate the effectiveness of centrifugal pumps in the treatment of PCCS.[12] Five hundred of the 965 patients in the registry were supported with centrifugal devices, with 45% of patients weaned from circulatory support and 26% surviving. When compared with pneumatic assist devices employed for PCCS support in this report, centrifugal pumps were associated with improved survival. A single institution report of 77 patients undergoing left, right, or biventricular mechanical assistance following cardiac surgery reflected the Combined Registry experience. Forty-three patients (56%) were weaned from support, with 27 (35%) long-term survivors.[16] In this series, survival rates increased from 25% to 45% during the last half of the decade reported, indicating progressive improve-

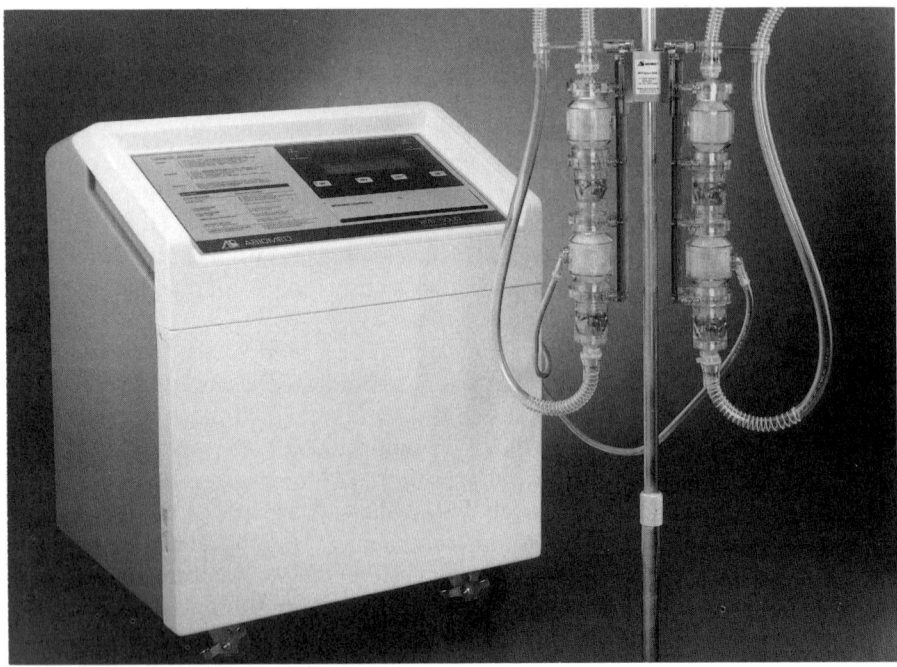

FIGURE 27.1. Abiomed BVS 5000 pump and console (Courtesy Abiomed, Inc., Danvers, MA).

ment based on experience, patient selection, and aggressive employment of circulatory support.

Abiomed BVS 5000

The Abiomed BVS 5000 (Abiomed Cardiovascular, Inc., Danvers, MA) is an extracorporeal pulsatile VAD composed of disposable blood pumps, transthoracic cannulas and a pneumatic drive console (Figures 11.10 and 27.1). The blood pump is a dual-chambered device with an atrial chamber that fills passively, and a ventricular chamber that collapses and fills in response to compressed air from the drive console. The blood pump is capable of delivering up to 4.8 L/min of pulsatile flow. Unidirectional flow is ensured by trileaflet polyurethane valves isolating the ventricular chamber. These trileaflet polyurethane valves are a particular advantage of the Abiomed BVS 5000, since they are much less expensive than the commercial disk or bioprosthetic valves used in other VADs.

The drive console initiates pulsatile flow that is asynchronous to the native cardiac rhythm. The control system monitors the air flow from the pumping chambers, and a microprocessor accurately adjusts blood pump function. Thereby, a pump stroke volume of near 80 mL is maintained, and the pulse rate of the ventricular assist pump is varied with venous return. This computer automation provides a system that is operator independent. A perfusionist is *not* necessary during operation of the BVS 5000. Attention to the patient's volume status and proper pump position for dependent drainage are necessary during operation. Weaning controls on the console allow independent pump-flow adjustments to a minimum of 0.5 L/min, although flows less than 1 L/min for an extended period of time are not recommended, as clotting may occur in the extracorporeal circuits. The drive console operates on alternating current or internal battery power, and a foot pump is also available for manual operation, if necessary.

A 1993 report from a multi-institutional clinical trial demonstrated the efficacy of the BVS 5000 for postcardiotomy cardiogenic shock.[17] BVS 5000 systems were implanted in 31 patients, with 17 (55%) weaned from support and 9 (29%) discharged. Adequate circulation was effectively restored by increasing the mean arterial pressure and the cardiac index, while left ventricular filling pressure decreased. These results compare favorably with the postcardiotomy experience reported by the Combined Registry for the Clinical Use of Mechanical Ventricular Assist Devices.[6]

The BVS 5000 is the first and only VAD to obtain U.S. Food and Drug Administration (FDA) approval for use as a cardiac assist device through the premarket approval process. In addition, Medicare recognizes the BVS 5000 as an approved therapy for postcardiotomy ventricular dysfunction and reimburses for application of the device in this setting. This device is a well-designed, functional system for short-term mechanical circulatory support providing pulsatile flow.

Summary

Each of these systems successfully provides short-term ventricular assistance, accomplishing the goals of adequate systemic perfusion and decompression of the heart to enhance recovery of stunned myocardium. Patient outcomes for short-term circulatory support are similar among these devices and reflect the experience of the Combined Registry for the Clinical Use of Mechanical Ventricular Assist Devices (Table 27.3). At present, there is significant experience with nonpulsatile ventricular assistance, and it is widely used for short-term circulatory support. Centrifugal pump systems have some design advantages over roller-pump systems, favoring their application for ventricular assistance. This type of device has been used for PCCS support in the majority of patients reported in the literature.

The recently introduced Abiomed BVS 5000 provides pulsatile circulatory support, which may be advantageous over nonpulsatile flow. The advantages and disadvantages of pulsatile and nonpulsatile blood flow are discussed below. Although no clinical benefit has been established for short-term circulatory support, pulsatile flow provides hemodynamic and metabolic benefits when compared with nonpulsatile perfusion.[18-20] The BVS 5000 represents a new generation of short-term VADs that are operator independent (an on-site perfusionist or technician is not necessary), unlike established centrifugal pump systems, and this cost advantage may offset the increased system cost.

Long-Term VADs

Several devices have been designed for long-term circulatory support. All of these devices employ pumps delivering pulsatile flow with pneumatic or electrical activation. These systems include paracorporeal devices and implantable pump devices with external console control. For the most part, long-term VADs are designed for left ventricular support, since right ventricular dysfunction generally improves with restored left ventricular output. Inotropic support of the right ventricle and afterload reduction with pulmonary vasodilators, usually allow right ventricular functional recovery after LVAD insertion.[21,22] With severe right ventricular dysfunction, temporary right-sided mechanical support may be necessary following implantation of an LVAD. Orthotopic total artificial hearts have been used for implantation as bridging devices, and may represent an alternative circulatory support system in circumstances of established biventricular failure.

These devices are capable of maintaining end-organ perfusion and function for prolonged periods of time. The restoration of adequate blood flow can restore organ function, allowing the patient to become an appropriate candidate for transplantation.[23] Reliable pump filling and left heart decompression are best achieved by apical cannulation of the left ventricle. The distortion of the heart which accompanies apical cannulation is of little importance, since these devices are to be employed prior to transplantation. Outflow cannulation for these devices is end-to-side to the ascending aorta with Dacron tube grafts. Anticoagulation is accomplished in the early postoperative period with either heparin or dextran, and long-term anticoagulation is accomplished with warfarin.

Long-term VADs are under investigational device exemption (IDE) regulations of the FDA for Class III medical devices.[24] These devices are not commercially available and remain under investigation in anticipation of market approval. As a result, access to these devices is limited and the system costs are high.

Thoratec VAD System

The Thoratec VAD System (Thoratec Laboratories Corp., Berkeley, CA) components are a blood pump, inflow and outflow cannulas, and a pneumatic drive console. The blood pump is a single-chamber, seamless polyurethane pumping sac enclosed within a rigid polysulfone housing and is paracorporeal (Figure 27.2). Tilting disk prosthetic valves at the inflow and outflow ports provide unidirectional flow. The pumping mechanism uses pulses of air generated from the drive console transmitted via pneumatic hose to alternately compress and empty the pumping sac.

The Thoratec drive console consists of two completely independent drive modules and is capable of univentricular and biventricular support. The full 65-mL stroke volume is possible at heart rates of 20 to 100 bpm allowing pulsatile flow rates of 1.3 to 6.5 L/min. The drive module produces ejection of the blood pump by a pulse of air pressure and slight negative air pressure is used to assist blood pump filling. Volume loading and R-wave synchronous and asynchronous modes are available for pump-timing during circulatory support. The drive console is powered by alternating current, and contains an uninterruptible power supply battery that provides up to 40 minutes of backup power.

TABLE 27.3. Ventricular assistance for postcardiotomy cardiogenic shock.

	Number of patients	Percent weaned	Percent survival
Combined Registry[12]	965	45%	25%
Roller Pump[13]	72	42%	29%
Centrifugal Pump[14]	77	56%	35%
Abiomed BVS 5000[17]	31	55%	29%

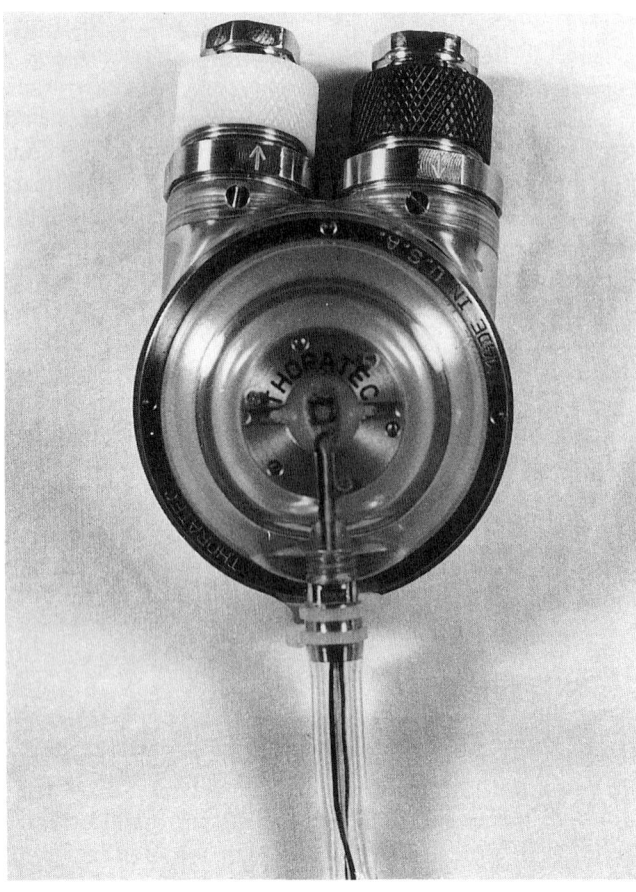

FIGURE 27.2. Thoratec blood pump (Courtesy Thoratec Laboratories, Berkeley, CA).

Paracorporeal placement of the Thoratec VAD represents a step between the freestanding short-term pumping devices and implantable pumps. The hybrid nature of the device is reflected in its clinical application for both PCCS and BTT. Thoratec Laboratories Corporation reports the results from ongoing application for PCCS support and bridge to transplantation.[25] As of August 1993, Thoratec VADs were implanted in 113 patients for PCCS, with 37% (42) weaned from the devices and 22% (25) long-term sursurvivors. Thoratec VAD was used as BTT in 249 patients with 64% (159) transplanted and 53% (133) survival. One-year actuarial survival posttransplant is 81%, similar to that achieved with primary cardiac transplantation.[26]

Novacor Left Ventricular Assist System (LVAS)

The Novacor LVAS (Novacor Division, Baxter Healthcare Corp., Oakland, CA) electrically powered left ventricular assist system employs a totally implantable pump with an external control console. The pump/drive unit is a dual pusher-plate sac-type pump coupled to a solenoid energy convertor encapsulated in a fiberglass-reinforced polymer shell (Figure 27.3). A cylindrical, seamless, polyurethane blood sac is bonded to the pusher plates and is symmetrically compressed during activation of the pusher plates, producing pulsatile flow. Inflow and outflow bioprosthetic valves provide unidirectional flow from the pump. Displacement transducers located on the pusher plates and solenoid signal pump information to the control console via a percutaneous vent tube. This vent tube, which also contains a power lead for transmission of electrical energy, is connected to the external console by a 20-foot extension cable. The pump is placed in the left upper abdominal quadrant anterior to the posterior rectus sheath.

Left ventricular apical cannulation is achieved with a semirigid plastic cannula connected to a woven Dacron conduit trasversing the diaphragm to the blood pump. Outflow cannulation requires an end-to-side Dacron tube graft anastomosis to the ascending aorta which also traverses the diaphragm (Figure 27.4). Proper timing of the blood pump allows decompression of the ventricle, which then serves as a low-pressure filling chamber or an atrium for the assist device.

The control console is modular in design with redundant circuits, and an uninterruptible power supply of 40 minutes, provided by battery backup. A signal monitor that provides transducer information, as well as electrocardiogram (ECG), arterial pressure, and left ventricular pressure, is located in the console. Volume loading and R-wave synchronous and asynchronous modes of operation can be used for circulatory support. The Novacor device is designed for long-term assistance in the counterpulsation mode using either R-wave synchronous timing or volume load timing. The blood pump volume is 70 mL, and average stroke volumes are 64 to 68 mL per beat.

The Novacor LVAD has been applied clinically for long-term circulatory support as a BTT.[27] In an international multicenter study on bridging to cardiac transplant, 129 patients received implants, with 60% receiving donor organ transplantation. There was a 51% survival rate (89% of the transplanted patients).[28] The mean implant duration was 42 days with the longest support time being 370 days, both suggesting long-term reliability. This system allows patient mobility, and even outpatient management at a residential apartment has been reported.[29] Long-term support patients have achieved nearly complete rehabilitation to NYHA Functional Class 1.

Thermo Cardiosystems HeartMate Left Ventricular Assist Device

The HeartMate LVAD (Thermo Cardiosystems Inc., Woburn, MA) consists of a pneumatically driven, implantable blood pump and an external console. The blood pump is a single pusher plate design with the pusher plate

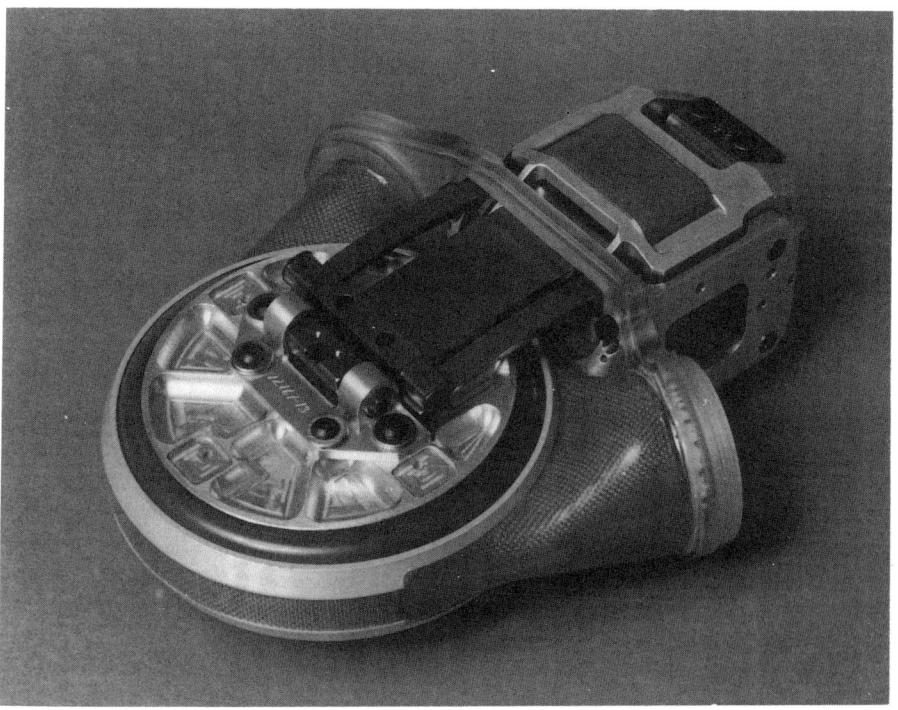

FIGURE 27.3. Novacor blood pump (Courtesy Novacor Division, Baxter Healthcare Corporation, Oakland, CA).

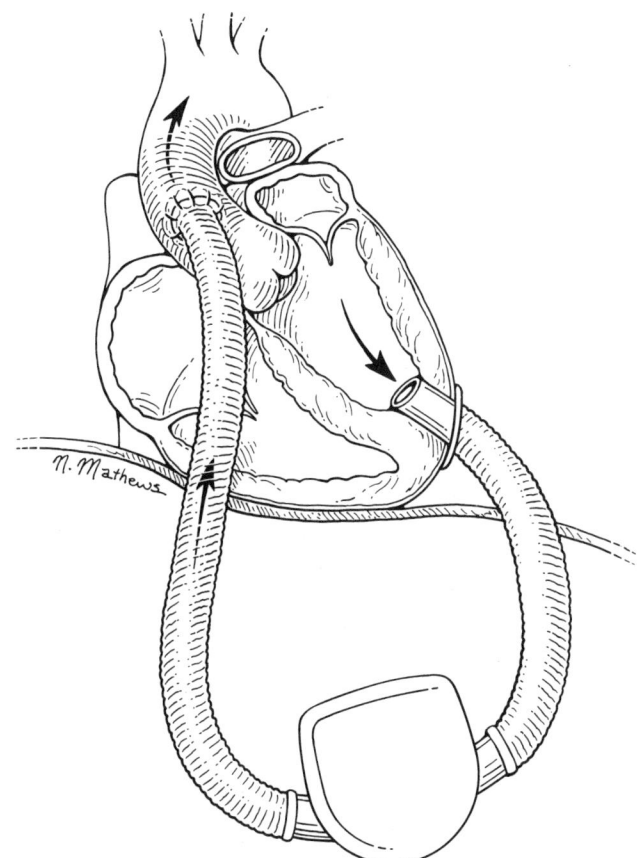

FIGURE 27.4. Inflow cannulation of left ventricular apex for LVAD with outflow cannulation of the ascending aorta.

bonded to a flexible diaphragm separating an air chamber and a blood chamber contained within a titanium housing (Figure 27.5). Pump ejection is created by pulsing compressed air through a transcutaneous hose to the air chamber of the blood pump which operates the blood pump diaphragm and forces blood through the outflow conduit. Inflow and outflow ports contain bioprosthetic valves to produce unidirectional flow. The inflow conduit of Dacron is connected to a left ventricular apical cannula, and outflow cannulation consists of an end-to-side Dacron tube graft to ascending aorta anastomosis. The blood-contacting surfaces of the HeartMate are textured, a unique feature that promotes the formation of a biological lining within the pump.[30] The internal surface of the titanium shell is lined with sintered titanium microspheres. The polyurethane diaphragm is integrally textured. These surfaces help reduce the risk of thromboembolic complications, and, because of this design, long-term anticoagulation with aspirin and dipyridamole is all that is recommended.[31]

The pump is implanted intraperitoneally in the left upper quadrant, with transdiaphragmatic inflow and outflow conduits. The pneumatic driveline passes percutaneously through the lower abdominal wall to the console. The console/driver is a self-contained unit that can be powered by alternating current and is supplied with rechargeable batteries that provide up to 40 minutes of support. The console has a continuous digital display of pump information, including pump flow, pump rate, and

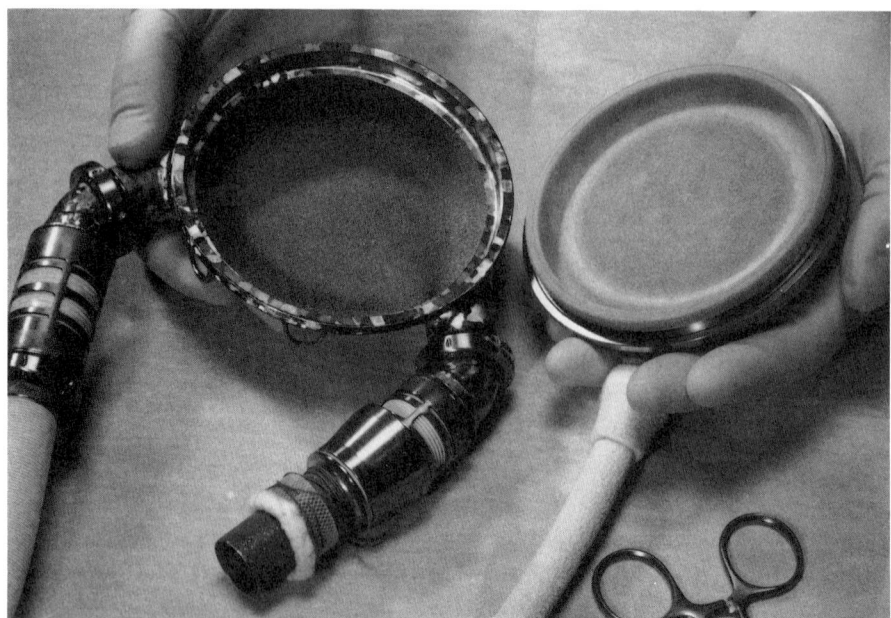

FIGURE 27.5. HeartMate blood pump demonstrating textured surfaces (Courtesy Thermo Cardiosystems Inc., Woburn, MA).

stroke volume. The console may be operated in volume loading, R-wave synchronous, or asynchronous modes for timing of the blood pump. The pump stroke volume of 83 mL allows outputs up to 10 L/min, depending on the beats per minute (range of 20 to 140 bpm).

The HeartMate has been used successfully as a BTT and is comparable to the Novacor LVAD as an interim support device. Thermo Cardiosystems Incorporated reported 123 devices implanted for BTT, with 67% of patients undergoing transplantation, and a survival rate of 58% (87% of those patients transplanted).[32] The texturing surface of the blood-contacting surfaces is a useful strategy with a low incidence of thromboembolism using minimal anticoagulation.

Symbion J-7 Total Artificial Heart

The Symbion J-7 Total Artificial Heart (TAH) (Symbion, Inc., Salt Lake City, UT) is a pneumatically driven device consisting of two pneumatic pumps designed for orthotopic implantation (Figure 27.6). The basic TAH pneumatic design consists of a flexible diaphragm contained within a semirigid housing of polyurethane molded with Dacron mesh. The diaphragm is composed of four polyurethane layers with graphite powder between the layers to prevent creasing of the diaphragms, which could lead to possible rupture. Air is pulsed to the ventricles through internal drivelines, producing diaphragm inflation and blood ejection. Diastolic filling collapses the diaphragm. Unidirectional flow is produced by tilting-disk Medtronic-Hall prosthetic valves at the inflow and outflow ports.

Orthotopic implantation of the device requires excision of the native ventricles along the atrioventricular groove. Atrial sewing cuffs are sutured to the remnant atria, and Dacron grafts are sutured end-to-end to the aorta and the pulmonary artery. The internal pneumatic drivelines are tunneled through subcutaneous tissue to exit on the anterior abdominal wall and then connect to external drivelines which are connected to the external drive console.

The external drive console uses compressed air supplied from an independent air source for pneumatic drive, and also contains two high-pressure air tanks for backup and patient transport. The console contains duplicated systems for TAH control, one of which serves as the primary controller, and the other as a backup. The console contains a personal computer that uses specialized software to monitor TAH function. The diastolic flow curve and the drive pressure waveform are constructed for each ventricular cycle by pneumotachometers and pressure transducers contained within the system. These hemodynamic measurements are used to optimize TAH function.

The Combined Registry for the Clinical Use of Mechanical Ventricular Assist Devices reported on 189 patients receiving pneumatic TAH as a BTT.[12] One-hundred thirty-five patients (71.4%) underwent transplantation and 67 (49.6%) achieved long-term survival. Although the rates of transplantation following TAH bridging were similar to those using heterotopic assist devices, the survival rates in this group of transplanted patients were significantly lower. This survival difference may be, in part, secondary to complications of TAH support.

Early application was complicated by thromboembolism as a result of pump design flaws and an incomplete understanding of long-term anticoagulation for patients with these systems. The pumps have been revised to eliminate thrombogenic elements, and long-term anticoagulation has subsequently improved, with more recent series

FIGURE 27.6. Symbion total artificial heart.

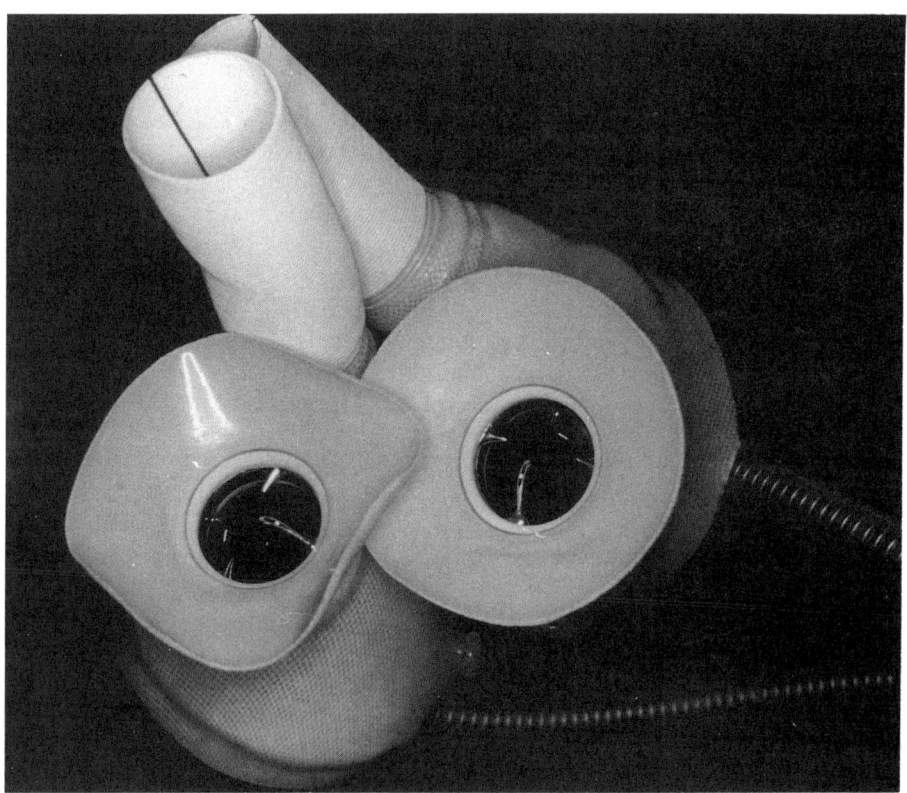

reporting fewer thromboembolic events. The mediastinal "dead space area" surrounding the TAH and the nonvascular TAH provide a focus for postoperative infection. Therefore, infection continues to be an important complication of this device.

Summary

Each of these systems has been used for long-term circulatory support and can be applied successfully in BTT procedures. Patient outcomes are similar with univentricular support devices, and results compare favorably with the experience of the Combined Registry for the Clinical Use of Mechanical Ventricular Assist Devices (Table 27.4). All of these VADs allow for patient mobility following implantation, and each provides pulsatile flow that appears to be important for long-term support. At present, these devices are not widely available and are still undergoing investigational trials for FDA approval. The growing demand for donor organs and the relatively stable pool of donor organs suggest that BTT procedures will be used increasingly for end-stage cardiac disease. Long-term support has demonstrated the ability of VADs to maintain end-organ function, and permit the recovery of reversible renal and hepatic insufficiency. The internally implanted devices are attractive because of less extrinsic hardware for potential contamination. They are the predecessors of totally implantable permanent circulatory support.

Assessment of Myocardial Recovery

Successful circulatory support for reversible myocardial injury following cardiac surgery requires appropriate patient selection, technically precise VAD implantation and perioperative care, and a means of assessing recovery of

TABLE 27.4 Ventricular assistance for bridge to transplantation.

	Number of patients	Percent transplanted	Percent survival
Combined Registry[12]	476	69%	46%
Thoratec VAD[26]	249	64%	53%
Novacor LVAS[28]	129	60%	51%
TCI HeartMate[32]	123	67%	58%

stunned myocardium. Appropriate patient selection begins with identifying those patients who have adequate myocardium for recovery from acute perioperative injury. Patients should have acceptable ventricular function preoperatively if myocardial recovery is to be expected. Patients with marginal ventricular function before the acute insult or with extensive infarction are not candidates for short-term VAD, and if transplantation is not an option, a VAD should not be considered. Following VAD implantation, the goal is to maintain adequate hemodynamics to support end-organ function. Pump flows are set to maintain cardiac index greater than 2.2 L/min/m^2, mean arterial blood pressure greater than 60 mm Hg, and left atrial filling pressure less than 20 mm Hg. Appropriate fluid and electrolyte therapy combined with rational pharmacologic support should be used to maintain these hemodynamic parameters. Correct early management includes assessment of intrinsic cardiac pump function.

The return of pulsatility in right or left ventricular ejection in patients who have atrial cannulation is often the earliest evidence of myocardial recovery. Objective evidence of myocardial recovery can be established by the ejection fraction and segmental ventricular function determined by radionuclide or echocardiographic studies.[33-35] Weaning is begun by decreasing pump flows in 1 L/min increments while monitoring hemodynamics and imaging ventricular function. IABP counterpulsation and judicious inotropic support are used for weaning from circulatory support. Patients maintaining adequate hemodynamics and left ventricular ejection fractions on decreasing pump flows are ready for removal of the VAD (Figure 27.7). Those patients whose ejection fraction deteriorates with decreasing pump flows are returned to circulatory support for 24 hours before weaning is again attempted.

Complications of VADs

Patients implanted with a VAD are critically ill so that the significant morbidity and mortality associated with these devices is expected. Bleeding, infection, and thromboembolic events are the most commonly occurring complications associated with both long- and short-term support. The Combined Registry for the Clinical Use of Mechanical Ventricular Assist Devices reported a bleeding complication rate of 40% to 50% in those patients with VAD implantation for treatment of PCCS, and bleeding was an independent predictor of ability to wean.[6] The bleeding complication rate is greatest following circulatory support for PCCS, since these patients have usually undergone prolonged CPB and have the coagulopathy that accompanies extended pump times that occur prior to device insertion. Bleeding is also a common complication following VAD insertion in BTT procedures. Extensive surgical dissection, multiple cannulation sites, anticoagulation, and CPB all contribute to the potential for bleeding in this setting. VAD patients should be quickly re-explored if bleeding occurs postoperatively. Central venous pressure, pulmonary artery pressures, and pump output must be carefully monitored, as any change in these variables may be an early sign of impending cardiac tamponade. In particular, if there is an unexplained decrease in pump output, the patient should be re-explored since cardiac tamponade is commonly the cause of this problem.

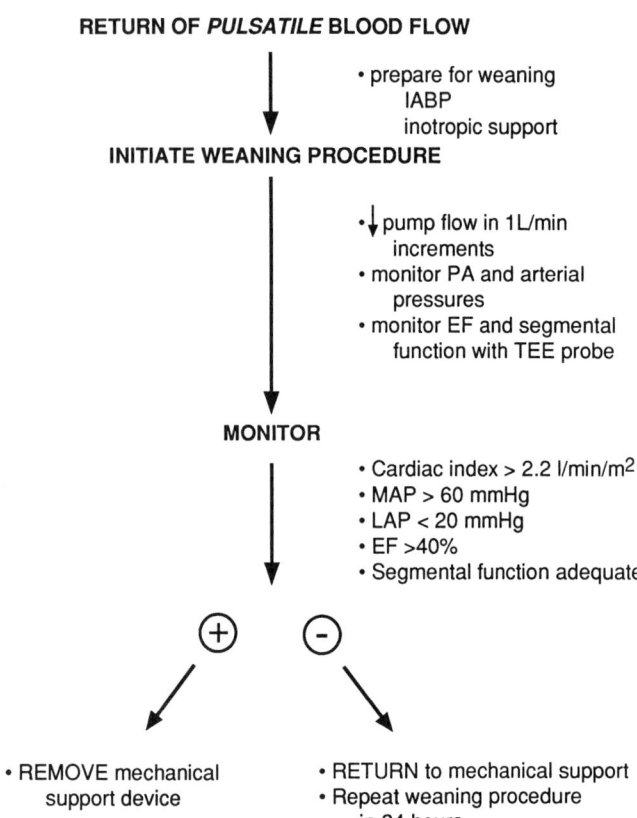

FIGURE 27.7. Management algorithm to wean circulatory support.

Infection represents a serious threat during mechanical circulatory support. Mortality as great as 76% has been reported for patients developing infection immediately before or during mechanical cardiac support.[36] Contamination of the device during implantation, postoperative wound infection, and remote site contamination can produce infection. Percutaneous drive lines and cannulas, which are continuously exposed to contamination from the patient's skin flora, can produce retrograde infection along the driveline tracts toward the device.[37] Dacron velour coating of percutaneous elements has been employed to encourage epithelial migration and the prevention of ascending infection. Bacteremia associated with the invasive monitoring required in these patients is another source of infection. Central venous catheters, arterial lines, bladder catheters, chest tubes, and endotracheal tubes must be removed as soon as possible to prevent ascending infections and resulting bacteremias. Enteral and parenteral nutrition should be administered to avoid the immunosuppressive effects of malnutrition. Importantly, broad-spectrum prophylactic antibiotics should be administered.

Thromboembolism is a continual threat following implantation of a foreign nonbiologic substance. Reported sites of thrombus formation include inlet and outlet cannulas, valves and valve mounts, pump housings and diaphragms, and other components of the assist device. Anticoagulation is required during VAD implantation to prevent the consequences of thromboembolic injury. Continuous intravenous heparin is used for short-term VAD support to maintain activated clotting times of 150 to 200 seconds. Anticoagulation for long-term VAD support includes continuous intravenous heparin or dextran therapy in the early postoperative period, followed by long-term maintenance with warfarin. The TCI Heart-Mate incorporates a unique design at the blood-biomaterial interface. The textured design of the blood-contacting surfaces of the blood pump promotes an intimal-like surface that deters thrombus formation.[30] As a result, anticoagulation regimens for this device consist of acetylsalicylic acid and dipyridamole. Further application of this methodology may limit thromboembolic complications while simplifying management of these devices.

Future Directions: The Totally Implantable Ventricular Assist Pump

The era of cardiac transplantation has allowed those patients suffering from untreatable cardiomyopathies to return to normal active lives. VADs presently serve an important temporary role as interim circulatory support prior to transplantation. Currently, research and development are under way toward the goal of totally implantable VADs. The aim of this next generation of devices is permanent circulatory support and full patient mobility, a possible alternative to cardiac transplantation.

Totally implantable devices require an implantable energy source and blood pump. Several groups are developing electrically powered devices. Efforts are being focused toward development of inductive coupling systems for power transmission, across intact skin, from a wearable battery pack to an implanted electronic controller (Figure 27.8). Numerous methods for converting electrical energy into blood-pumping capacity have been developed for the implantable pumps (Table 27.5). These devices will likely begin clinical application in this decade, illustrating the potential for VADs in the treatment of terminal heart failure.

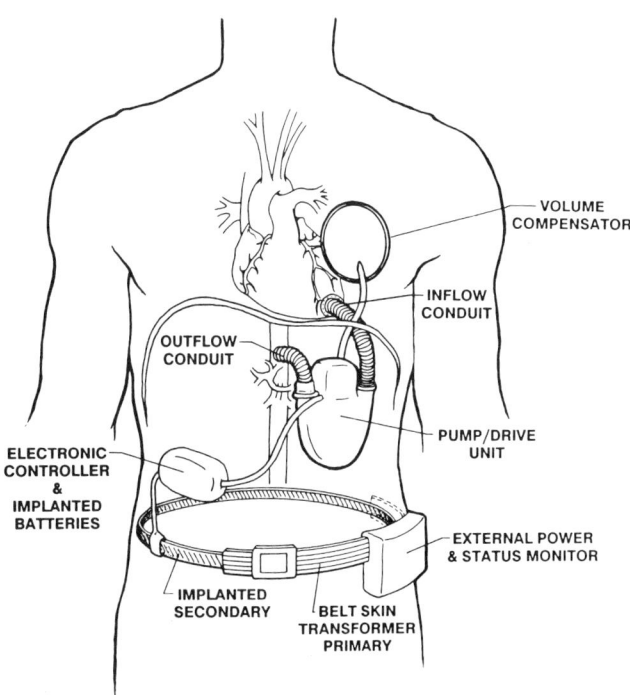

FIGURE 27.8. Totally implantable ventricular assist pump design of the Novacor LVAS (Courtesy Novacor Division, Baxter Healthcare Corporation, Oakland, CA).

Summary

Technological advancement in the field of VADs has paralleled the development of cardiac surgery with the recognition of PCCS and the advent of cardiac transplantation. PCCS is a potentially lethal complication of open-heart surgery, and circulatory support can be provided by short-term VADs until recovery of injured myocardium can resume pump function. The short-term VADs are designed for easy implantation and removal with minimal distortion of the heart and are suited to treatment of reversible processes. Long-term VADs have been designed for BTT procedures for patients awaiting cardiac transplantation. These systems allow patient mobility and are easily managed. Several devices are currently manufactured and have been successful for long-term support in clinical tri-

TABLE 27.5 Electromechanical energy convertors for totally implantable ventricular assist pump.

Development group	Convertor
Abiomed Cardiovascular Inc.	Electrohydraulic turbine
Nimbus Inc.	Thermal engine
Novacor Division, Baxter Healthcare Corp.	Solenoid
Pennsylvania State University	Reversing DC motor
Thermo Cardiosystems Inc.	Low-speed DC motor

als. All such long-term devices remain under IDE application and therefore are expensive and not widely available. Successful short- and long-term VAD use requires clinical expertise in the treatment of cardiogenic shock, experience in the care of circulation-assisted patients, and thorough knowledge of the complications of these devices. The future of ventricular assistance is a totally implantable system, eliminating percutaneous cannulas and drivelines, and completely freeing the patient from tethered support. Currently, these devices are in a pilot study, and it is likely that clinical trials will begin during this decade. A totally implantable system could be a viable alternative, providing long-term survival for patients ineligible for cardiac transplantation.

Pulsatile Versus Nonpulsatile Flow

A study on the subject of circulatory assistance requires contemplation of the flow pattern of the assist device. In broad terms, circulatory assist devices can be categorized as pulsatile or nonpulsatile. The native circulation produces pulsatile flow, and the pulsatility of flow is thought to provide hemodynamic and metabolic benefit. Theories for improved physiologic performance during pulsatile arterial flow focus on the effect of pulsatile flow on microcirculatory patency.[38,39] Capillary perfusion is facilitated by the increased energy contained in pulsatile flow and by the longer periods of microcirculatory patency occurring during peaks of pulsatile systolic pressure.[38,39] These effects reflect the findings of reduced tissue oxygen consumption, progressive acidosis, and lactate accumulation when pulsatility is omitted but total arterial flow and mean arterial pressure are maintained.[40,41]

Effect of Pulsatile Perfusion on End Organs

Organ structure and function studies emphasize the benefits of pulsatile flow. Cerebral cellular integrity, as measured by creatine kinase isoenzymes in cerebrospinal fluid, is better maintained with pulsatile perfusion than with nonpulsatile flow.[42] Murkin et al[43] assessed the effects of pulsatile and nonpulsatile perfusion on cerebral blood flow (CBF) during hypothermic CPB in man. They demonstrated that CBF is augmented with pulsatile perfusion and suggested that the observed reduction in CBF associated with nonpulsatile perfusion was consistent with the hypothesis of functional capillary closure during nonpulsatile flow. However, a larger study by this group[44] reported that neurologic and neuropsychologic outcomes after hypothermic CPB were similar in patients managed with pulsatile and nonpulsatile blood flow. Renal excretory functions are disturbed during nonpulsatile perfusion.[45] During pulsatile perfusion, outer cortical flow is preserved and renin release is reduced. This optimal intrarenal blood flow distribution preserves renal function.[45,46] Hepatic arterial flow and oxygen consumption are decreased by one-half during nonpulsatile perfusion when compared with native circulatory blood flow.[47] In contrast, extracorporeal pulsatile perfusion maintains hepatic arterial blood flow and metabolism comparable to that obtained with native circulation. Recently, one group of investigators demonstrated, in an acute ischemia canine model, that the inclusion of pulsatile perfusion with a percutaneous ventricle-bypass system improves myocardial blood flow.[48] Animals managed with pulsatile perfusion, compared to animals treated with nonpulsatile blood flow, had superior increases in aortic pressure and total cardiac output.

Hemodynamic Effects of Pulsatile Perfusion

Nonpulsatile blood flow is associated with several undesirable hemodynamic effects that should be considered during circulatory assistance. Nonpulsatile perfusion results in an increased systemic vascular resistance (SVR) when compared with pulsatile perfusion.[49,50] In part, this observed increase in SVR is secondary to increases in activation of the renin-angiotensin system.[51] Specific angiotensin II inhibitors have been shown to reduce SVR during nonpulsatile blood flow.[52] Increased SVR produces an increase in ventricular afterload, thereby increasing left ventricular work and impairing cardiac performance. Some studies suggest that pulsatile, compared to nonpulsatile, blood flow during cardiac surgery and CPB improves hemodynamics as reflected by the reduced requirements for inotropic drugs and IABP use in the pulsatile-CPB groups.[53-55]

Use of Pulsatile Perfusion in Short- and Long-Term Circulatory Support

Studies comparing the effects of pulsatile and nonpulsatile extracorporeal circulatory support largely have focused on their use during cardiac surgery and CPB. Short-term circulatory support usually combines nonpulsatile assistance with IABP counterpulsation, and therefore an element of pulsatility exists. The difference in patient outcomes between pulsatile and nonpulsatile flow in the setting of long-term circulatory support is probably significant, but remains unproven. Most devices in use for long-term support employ pumps that provide pulsatile flow. Although conclusive data are not available, there is near-uniform agreement that pulsatile flow is necessary for long-term assistance. Nonpulsatile devices have not been used for long-term applications but are quite successful in circumstances requiring short-term support. It is likely that the importance of pulsatility during circulatory assistance is proportional to the duration of assistance. This statement assumes that the physiologic benefits of pulsatility accrue over time.

Summary

Pulsatile flow seems to provide metabolic and hemodynamic advantage over nonpulsatile perfusion. The metabolic advantages are demonstrable in overall tissue perfusion and specific end-organ function. The hemodynamic effects of pulsatile perfusion improve overall metabolism and significantly reduce SVR, eliminating the increased afterload and increased ventricular work associated with nonpulsatile perfusion (a desirable goal during circulatory assistance when cardiac recovery is expected, ie, PCCS). An understanding of the pathophysiology of artificial circulatory assistance remains incomplete even for short-term assistance. The more complex situation of long-term assistance is even less well defined.

References

1. Pennington DG, Swartz M, Codd JE, et al. Intra-aortic balloon pumping in cardiac surgical patients: a nine-year experience. *Ann Thorac Surg* 1983;36:125–131.
2. Norman JC, Cooley DA, Igo SR, et al. Prognostic indices for survival during postcardiotomy intra-aortic balloon pumping. *J Thorac Cardiovasc Surg* 1977;74:709–720.
3. Downing TP, Miller DC, Stofer R, et al. Use of the intra-aortic balloon pump after valve replacement. *J Thorac Cardiovasc Surg* 1986;92:210–217.
4. Pennington DG, Merjavy JP, Swartz M, et al. The importance of biventricular failure in patients with postoperative cardiogenic shock. *Ann Thorac Surg* 1985;39:16–26.
5. Rose DM, Colvin SB, Culliford AT, et al. Long-term survival with partial left heart bypass following perioperative myocardial infarction and shock. *J Thorac Cardiovasc Surg* 1982;83:483–492.
6. Pae WE Jr, Miller CA, Matthews Y, et al. Ventricular assist devices for postcardiotomy cardiogenic shock. A combined registry experience. *J Thorac Cardiovasc Surg* 1992;104:541–552.
7. Pennington DG, Farrar DJ, Loisance D, et al. Panel discussion presented at the Circulatory Support Symposium of The Society of Thoracic Surgeons, San Francisco, November 16–17, 1991. *Ann Thorac Surg* 1993;55:206–212.
8. Pennington DG, Swartz MT. Temporary circulatory support in patients with postcardiotomy cariogenic shock. In: Spence PA, Chitwood WR, eds. *Cardiac Surgery: State of the Art Reviews.* Vol 5, no 3. Philadelphia: Hanley and Belfus; 1991:373–392.
9. Report to the Chairman, Subcommittee on Health, Committee on Ways and Means, House of Representatives. *Heart Transplants: Concerns About Cost, Access, and Availability of Donor Organs.* Washington: US General Accounting Office, 1989.
10. Copeland JG, Emery RW, Levinson MM, et al. The role of mechanical support and transplantation in treatment of patients with end-stage cardiomyopathy. *Circulation* 1985;72(suppl II):II-7,7–12.
11. Farrar DJ, Hill JD. Univentricular and biventricular Thoratec VAD support as a bridge to transplantation. *Ann Thorac Surg* 1993;55:276–282.
12. Pae WE Jr. Ventricular assist devices and total artificial hearts: a combined registry experience. *Ann Thorac Surg* 1993;55:295–298.
13. Rose DM, Corda M, Dunningham JR, et al. Roller pump ventricular assist device. Quaal SJ, Carter R, eds. *Cardiac Mechanical Assistance: Beyond Balloon Pumping.* St. Louis: Mosby; 1993:43–66.
14. Hoerr HR Jr, Kraemer MF, Williams JL, et al. In vitro comparison of blood handling by the constrained vortex and twin roller blood pumps. *J Extracorp Technol* 1987;19:316–321.
15. Oku T, Harasaki H, Smith W, et al. A comparative study of four nonpulsatile pumps. *Trans Am Soc Artif Intern Organs* 1988;34:500–504.
16. Magovern GJ Jr. The biopump and postoperative circulatory support. *Ann Thorac Surg* 1993;55:245–249.
17. Guyton RA, Schonberger JP, Everts PA, et al. Postcardiotomy shock: clinical evaluation of the BVS 5000 Biventricular Support System. *Ann Thorac Surg* 1993;56:346–356.
18. Taylor KM. Pulsatile perfusion. In: Taylor KM, ed. *Cardiopulmonary Bypass: Principles and Management.* Cambridge: Cambridge University Press; 1986:85–114.
19. Mavroudis C. To pulse or not to pulse. *Ann Thorac Surg* 1978;25:259–271.
20. Minami K, Korner MM, Vyska K, et al. Effects of pulsatile perfusion on plasma catecholamine levels and hemodynamics during and after cardiac operations with cardiopulmonary bypass. *J Thorac Cardiovasc Surg* 1990;99:82–91.
21. Farrar DG, Compton PG, Dajee H, et al. Right heart function during left heart assist and the effects of volume loading in a canine preparation. *Circulation* 1984;70:708–716.
22. Kormos RL, Gaisor T, Antaki J, et al. Evaluation of right ventricular function during clinical left ventricular assistance. *ASAIO Trans* 1989;35:547–550.
23. Burnett CM, Duncan JM, Frazier OH, et al. Improved multi-organ function after prolonged univentricular support. *Ann Thorac Surg* 1993;55:65–71.
24. US Department of Health and Human Services. *Regulatory Requirements for Medical Devices: A Workshop Manual.* FDA 89-4165. Rockville, MD: Center for Devices and Radiological Health.
25. Thoratec VAD Clinical Summary. In: Farrar DJ, ed. *Thoratec's Heartbeat 1993*; Vol 7.3:1–12.
26. Farrar DJ, Lawson JH, Litwak P, et al. Thoratec VAD system as a bridge to heart transplantation. *J Heart Transplant* 1990;9:415–422.
27. McCarthy PM, Portner PM, Tobler HG, et al. Clinical experience with the Novacor ventricular assist system. *J Thorac Cardiovasc Surg* 1991;102:578–587.
28. Portner PM. A totally implantable heart assist system: The Novacor Program. In: Akutsu T, Koyanagi H, eds. *Artificial Heart 4.* New York: Springer-Verlag; 1993:71–82.
29. Kormos RL, Murali S, Dew MA, et al. Chronic mechanical

circulatory support: rehabilitation, low morbidity and superior survival after heart transplant. *Ann Thorac Surg* 1994; 56:51-58.
30. Dasse KA, Chipman SD, Sherman CN, et al. Clinical experience with textured blood contacting surfaces in ventricular assist devices. *ASAIO Trans* 1987;33:418-425.
31. Burton NA, Lefrak EA, Macmanus Q, et al. A reliable bridge to cardiac transplantation: the TCI left ventricular assist device. *Ann Thorac Surg* 1993;55:1425-1431.
32. Thermo Cardiosystems HeartMate LVAD Experience Report. November 1993. Thermo Cardiosystems Inc.
33. Barzilai B, Davila-Roman VG, Eaton MH, et al. Transesophageal echocardiography predicts successful withdrawal of ventricular assist devices. *J Thorac Cardiovasc Surg* 1992;104:1410-1416.
34. Brack M, Olson JD, Pedersen WR, et al. Transesophageal echocardiography in patients with mechanical circulatory assistance. *Ann Thorac Surg* 1991;52:1306-1309.
35. Sekela ME, Verani MS, Noon GP. Comparison of hemodynamics and ejection fraction during left heart bypass. *Ann Thorac Surg* 1991;51:804-806.
36. Joyce LD, Johnson KE, Toninato CJ, et al. Results of the first 100 patients who received Symbion Total Artificial Hearts as a bridge to cardiac transplantation. *Circulation* 1989;80:(III)192-201.
37. von Recum AF, Park JB. Permanent percutaneous devices. *Crit Rev Bioeng* 1981;5:37-77.
38. Shepard RB, Simpson DC, Sharp JF. Energy equivalent pressure. *Arch Surg* 1966;93:730-740.
39. Takeda J. Experimental study of peripheral circulation during extracorporeal circulation with a special reference to a comparison of pulsatile flow with nonpulsatile flow. *Arch Jpn Chir* 1960;29:1407-1412.
40. Shepard RB, Kirklin JW. Relation of pulsatile flow to oxygen consumption and other variables during cardiopulmonary bypass. *J Thorac Cardiovasc Surg* 1969;58:694-702.
41. Jacobs LA, Klopp EH, Seamone W, et al. Improved organ function during cardiac bypass with a roller pump modified to deliver pulsatile flow. *J Thorac Cardiovasc Surg* 1969;58:703-712.
42. Taylor KM, Devlin BJ, Mittra SM, et al. Assessment of cerebral damage during open-heart surgery. A new experimental model. *Scand J Thorac Cardiovasc Surg* 1980;14:197-203.
43. Murkin JM, Farrar K. The influence of pulsatile vs nonpulsatile cardiopulmonary bypass on cerebral blood flow and cerebral metabolism. *Anesthesiology* 1989;71:A41.
44. Murkin JM, Martzke JA, Buchan AM, et al. Postoperative neurological and neuropsychological performance are not influenced by mode of pH-management or pulsatility during hypothermic cardiopulmonary bypass. *J Thorac Cardiovasc Surg*. In press.
45. Many M, Soroff HS, Birtwell WC, et al. The physiologic role of pulsatile and nonpulsatile blood flow: II Effects on renal function. *Arch Surg* 1967;95:762-766.
46. Many M, Soroff HS, Birtwell WC, et al. The physiologic role of pulsatile and non-pulsatile blood flow: III Effects of unilateral renal artery depulsation. *Arch Surg* 1968;97:917-923.
47. Mathie R, Desai J, Taylor KM. Hepatic blood flow and metabolism during pulsatile and non-pulsatile cardiopulmonary bypass. *Life Support Syst* 1984;2:303-305.
48. Hirofumi I, Yamaguchi A, Takashi I, et al. Evaluation of the pulsatility of a new pulsatile left ventricular assist device—the integrated cardioassist catheter—in dogs. *J Thorac Cardiovasc Surg* 1994;107:569-575.
49. Taylor KM. Vasopressor release and multiple organ failure in cardiac surgery. *Perfusion* 1988;3:1-16.
50. Minami K, Körner MM, Vyska K, et al. Effects of pulsatile perfusion on plasma catecholamine levels and hemodynamics during and after cardiac operation with cardiopulmonary bypass. *J Thorac Cardiovasc Surg* 1990;99:82-91.
51. Taylor KM, Bain WH, Morton JJ. The role of angiotensin II in the development of peripheral vasoconstriction during open-heart surgery. *Am Heart J* 1980;100:935-937.
52. Taylor KM, Casals J, Morton JJ, et al. The haemodynamic effects of angiotensin-converting enzyme inhibition after cardiopulmonary bypass in dogs. *Cardiovasc Res* 1980;14:199-205.
53. Bregman D, Bowman FO, Parodi EN, et al. An improved method of myocardial protection with pulsation during cardiopulmonary bypass. *Circulation* (suppl II) 1977;56:157-161.
54. Maddoux G, Pappas G, Jenkins M, et al. Effect of pulsatile and non-pulsatile flow during cardiopulmonary bypass on left ventricular ejection fraction early after aortocoronary bypass surgery. *Am J Cardiol* 1976;37:1000-1006.
55. Taylor KM, Bain WH, Davidson KG, et al. A comparative study of pulsatile and non-pulsatile cardiopulmonary bypass in 325 patients. *Proc Eur Soc Artif Org* 1979;6:238-242.

28
Intraaortic Balloon Pump Counterpulsation

John Parker Gott

Introduction

Intraaortic balloon pump (IABP) counterpulsation is most frequently used in patients undergoing cardiac operation to increase the likelihood of success in the face of marginal hemodynamics or frank circulatory failure. Balloon counterpulsation is a two-edged sword, however, with the potential for great therapeutic benefit as well as significant morbidity. While clearly efficacious, as evidenced by its low therapeutic index, the IABP must be clearly and compellingly indicated, and impeccable placement technique is crucial, particularly in those patients known to be at increased risk for IABP-related complications. Successful strategies to increase the margin of safety for balloon counterpulsation continue to evolve, and the balloon pump should retain, for the foreseeable future, a vital intermediary position in the therapeutic armamentarium for postcardiotomy pump failure. When pharmacologic measures are not sufficient, and total mechanical support is neither necessary nor feasible, the balloon pump may be lifesaving.

Historical Background

Twenty-five years have passed since the first successful implantation of an IABP in a human subject.[1] During those years, the efficacy of balloon counterpulsation in the treatment of cardiogenic shock has become firmly established. In the early 1950s experimental studies on the effects of a phase shift in the arterial pressure waveform suggested potential therapeutic use in patients with ischemic myocardial failure. Adrian and Arthur Kantrowitz, working in the laboratory of Carl Wiggers, designed an elegant, classic experiment which demonstrated the ability to increase coronary blood flow by over 50% by delaying arrival of the arterial pressure wave to the coronary circulation to coincide with diastole.[1] Early attempts to exploit the theoretical benefits of this concept of *phase shift diastolic augmentation* led to the construction of temporary ventricular support systems. These systems allowed rapid, timed removal and reinfusion of blood from major arterial sites, and provided myocardial support through diastolic pressure augmentation and afterload reduction.[2-4] But they also included many undesirable features, such as the need for major vascular access, risk of infection, and potential for damage to the formed elements of the blood, due to the high flow velocities.[3,5] The permanent implanted mechanical auxiliary ventricle of Kantrowitz et al demonstrated *clinically* that the concept of diastolic augmentation was valid and resulted in improved hemodynamic function. Long-term results, however, were disappointing.[3]

Many problems associated with these devices were solved by the development of a *temporary, internal, intravascular counterpulsator*, the forerunner of the current balloon pumps. Mouloupoulos et al[5] and Clauss and coworkers[6] demonstrated that the hemodynamic benefits attributable to the phase shift in the arterial wave form could be realized by coordinated inflation and deflation of a balloon passed into the aorta. Other systems followed, with significant improvements in balloon shape, size, composition, shuttle gas, and cardiac cycle timing. Placement of the balloon via the femoral artery was rapid, and obviated the need for a major operative procedure. Thus, in 1968 Kantrowitz and colleagues were able to report the first lifesaving application of the IABP for mechanical circulatory support of a patient in cardiogenic shock.[7] The clinical hemodynamic improvement was confirmed subsequently in a larger group of patients, and later by other investigators.[8-11] Widespread application and subsequent expansion of indications for the technique have resulted in over 70,000 IABP implantations annually.[12] Cooperation among basic scientists, clinicians, and industry has brought about rapid evolution of balloon and drive system design. Eloquent historical accounts by a principal participant in the development of the technology are available.[12,13]

Extraaortic Counterpulsation

The *intraaortic* balloon pump is not necessarily the ideal method for implementation of phase shift diastolic augmentation.[14] *Extraaortic* counterpulsation devices (EACPs) have been designed and employed experimentally[2] but have been used infrequently in patients.[4] Experimental EACPs are more effective at enhancing the myocardial oxygen supply/consumption ratio over a wider range of cardiac dysfunction, rhythm disturbance, and timing conditions when compared to the IABP. The various EACPs have in common the requirement that large cannulas be placed in the central arterial circulation for rapid withdrawal and reinfusion of blood. Moreover, the problem of obtaining safe, reliable, large-bore access to the arterial circulation, with the resultant risk of thromboembolism from an extraaortic counterpulsator situated proximal to the cerebral circulation, has not been adequately resolved.[14,15]

Since EACP technology is not readily available for clinical use, there will be no further discussion of these devices. The ease of insertion and widespread availability make the IABP the first-line therapy for mechanical circulatory support in a clinical setting.

IABP: Physiologic Considerations

General

The effects of IABP counterpulsation are variable and dependent upon the pre-existing physiologic state. Early experimental studies based on animal models of *cardiogenic shock* compared with *normal* control animals demonstrated that, in both situations, the myocardial oxygen demands are decreased by counterpulsation. The normal animal exhibits a decrease in left ventricular pressures, whereas the animal in cardiogenic shock shows a rise in mean arterial and left ventricular pressures.[16]

Intraortic balloon counterpulsation exerts its beneficial effects on the *failing circulation* mainly through two synergistic actions: *diastolic augmentation* of the arterial blood pressure, which improves coronary flow and thus oxygen delivery, and *afterload reduction*, which reduces left ventricular work and diminishes myocardial oxygen demand. The resultant reduction of ischemia and improvement in cardiac function is followed invariably by signs of improved systemic perfusion and renal function, clearing of the sensorium, resolution of pulmonary congestion, reversal of metabolic acidosis, and a decreased need for pharmacologic support.[9-11,17] The beneficial properties of diastolic augmentation and the reduced impedance to ejection offered by counterpulsation therapy are both affected in magnitude by patient and device variables. The balloon shape, diameter in relation to the aorta (occlusivity), volume, shuttle gas, timing, duration of inflation, and position all can be manipulated with a measurable change in efficacy.[18-21] Similarly, the patient's pre-existing cardiac mechanics, aortic compliance, volume status, and vascular tone affect the response to balloon counterpulsation.[20] The complex interaction among these mechanical and biological factors has been subjected to mathematical modeling that promises to facilitate balloon design improvements.[21]

Afterload Reduction

As the IABP is deflated just prior to systole, the aortic blood pool fills the volume that was occupied by the evacuated helium-filled balloon. Over and above this passive filling phenomenon, there is an active imparting of momentum to the aortic root blood column at the time of vacuum extraction of the balloon gas.[20] This results in a decreased impedance to left ventricular ejection. Left ventricular developed wall tension is lowered, effecting a decrease in myocardial oxygen demand and improved efficiency of cardiac energetics. The clinical significance of these effects is confirmed by the change in net myocardial lactate production to net myocardial utilization in 18 of 19 patients after IABP placement for cardiogenic shock.[11] This implies a dramatic reversal of myocardial oxygen supply-and-demand mismatch.

Diastolic Augmentation

Coronary blood flow is primarily controlled via autoregulatory mechanisms, with a minor role played by the autonomic nervous system.[22] Flow in the coronary circulation is phasic with roughly 70% of left ventricular coronary blood flow occurring during diastole. In the patient with impaired myocardial perfusion, the coronary vasculature is already maximally dilated through autoregulation, and significant increases in coronary flow come about only through increased perfusion pressure. This problem is obviously compounded in many patients by the presence of fixed atherosclerotic coronary stenoses. The IABP exerts its positive effect on the coronary flow through the addition of precisely timed, pulsatile external energy to the circulation in the form of diastolic pressure augmentation. The coronary blood flow in the failing heart may be increased as much as 100% after institution of balloon pumping. *Peak diastolic coronary blood flow velocity*, as determined by transesophageal echocardiography, is increased by a mean 117% ($p = 0.002$) during balloon counterpulsation.[23] The *coronary blood flow velocity in-*

terval is an analog of blood volume per unit of time through a sample segment of the coronary artery, and it is increased by a mean of 87% by the IABP ($p = 0.003$).[23]

In addition to increases in the volume of coronary blood flow, important changes in the *distribution* of flow help to explain the observed control of unstable angina, limitation of expected infarct size, and improved patient survival in subsets of acute coronary syndromes treated with the balloon pump. Initiation of IABP counterpulsation appears to improve flow through collateral pathways, supplementing circulation to the ischemic areas.

Collateral Coronary Flow

The anatomic existence of arterioarterial coronary collateral vessels is unquestioned—the physiologic significance in normal and disease states remains controversial. Nevertheless, the flow in these channels is responsive to metabolic and hemodynamic regulatory mechanisms. In the setting of occlusion of a major epicardial coronary artery, local metabolite formation favors vasodilation of these channels, which increases flow to the ischemic myocardium. After a critical closing pressure is exceeded, further changes in coronary flow occur based on the transcollateral *diastolic* blood pressure gradient. Little flow occurs in these collaterals during systole. Animal studies have demonstrated that aortic counterpulsation can significantly improve blood flow through coronary collaterals.[24] This increased flow can be demonstrated in large epicardial arteries distal to an acute occlusion and, thus, to the ischemic myocardium.[24-26] These animal studies explain the clinical benefit of balloon pumping in the treatment of unstable angina and in the patient with acute myocardial infarct, in whom improved diastolic pressure means myocardial salvage.

Prompt institution of balloon pumping would serve to minimize potential myocardial injury in the setting of acute myocardial ischemia. Different lines of research serve to support this thought. Results from a *canine* model of acute coronary occlusion, designed to assess collateral contribution to flow in acutely ischemic myocardium, suggest that the timing of IABP institution is important. The researchers demonstrated diminishing augmentation of coronary collateral flow with increasing delay before initiation of balloon counterpulsation after acute coronary occlusion.[27]

That temporal relationship also appears to hold true in the *clinical* setting. Patients with acute anterior myocardial infarction having IABP counterpulsation instituted early (4 hours after infarct) had significant reduction in electrocardiographic injury pattern (ST elevation) as compared with similar patients in whom IABP was started later (average 17 hours after infarct). The patients in whom the IABP was started late nevertheless benefitted *hemodynamically* and had elimination of persistent ischemic pain, despite failure to improve electrocardiographic evidence of injury.[17,27]

Circulatory Consequences of Intraaortic Counterpulsation

Initiation of IABP counterpulsation in patients in cardiogenic shock results in a variable but significant improvement in *cardiac index*. This improvement ranges from 10% to 43%.[9,11,28-31] In the representative series reported by Bardet et al[30] there was an increase in the mean cardiac index from the baseline 1.4 to 2.0 L/min/m^2 ($p = 0.001$). Ehrich et al[29] reported a reduction in filling pressures typified by the drop in *pulmonary capillary wedge pressure* from a mean of 20 mm Hg to 15 mm Hg after IABP placement (16 patients, $p = 0.04$). The effect on *heart rate* is usually negligible,[11,29,30] although Mueller and colleagues[28] found a significant decrease from a mean of 104 to 90 beats/min ($p = 0.05$). *Stroke index* increases significantly, as in the report from Ehrich et al,[29] from a mean of 15 to 20 mL/beat/m^2 ($p = 0.002$). The *systemic systolic blood pressure* drops. An example is taken from an early study by Buckley and associates[9] which showed a decrease from a mean of 87 mm Hg to 78 mm Hg ($p = 0.001$). The universal response of the *diastolic blood pressure* is elevation, and this is obviously consistent with intraaortic balloon inflation. The extensive, multicenter, cooperative trial reported by Scheidt and others[11] demonstrated a rise from a group mean of 53 mm Hg to 83 mm Hg ($p = 0.001$). There is no consistent response of the *mean systemic arterial pressure*. *Systemic vascular resistance* generally falls from a group mean of 2055 to 1471 dynes/s/cm^5 ($p = 0.01$)[29] but this is variable and dependent, to some degree, on concurrent drug therapy. The *time tension index*, an estimate of the myocardial oxygen demand, decreases by 10% to 19%,[16] while *blood flow* increases. This was elegantly documented in unstable angina patients by assessing great cardiac vein flows, which represent the myocardium supplied by the left anterior descending coronary artery. Flows increased from 52 to 67 mL/min ($p = 0.004$).[32] Table 28.1 summarizes the circulatory effects of IABP counterpulsation.

TABLE 28.1 Physiologic effects of IABP counterpulsation.

Cardiac index	↑
Pulmonary capillary wedge pressure	↓
Heart rate	↔
Stroke index	↑
Systemic systolic BP	↓
Systemic diastolic BP	↑
Mean systemic arterial pressure	Variable
Systemic vascular resistance	↓
Coronary blood flow	↑
Time tension index	↓

Indications for IABP Placement

General

Most indications for use of the IABP will be known to the readers of this text. The patient in whom left ventricular dysfunction leads to marginal performance will benefit hemodynamically from the mechanical assistance of the IABP. But the patient who cannot be weaned from cardiopulmonary bypass (CPB), despite maximal pharmacologic support, and after all significant, technically remediable cardiac defects have been treated, is the one with the most compelling indication for IABP therapy. Table 28.2 gives an overview of indications.

Prophylactic Use Prior to Elective Cardiac Operation

The vast majority of hemodynamically stable, nonischemic patients *do not* require or benefit from prophylactic IABP placement before cardiac surgery.[33] Although IABP is sometimes advocated prophylactically for those with left main stenosis or severe left ventricular dysfunction, current preoperative medical management, cardiac anesthesiology expertise, and myocardial protection techniques are associated with an IABP placement rate of only 1% to 2%.[34] These two studies, spanning almost a decade and a half of experience at Emory, would argue against prophylactic IABP placement in these subgroups.

TABLE 28.2. Indications for IABP support.

Postcardiotomy ventricular dysfunction
Unstable angina not responsive to medical management
Acute infarct
Postinfarct complications
    Pump failure
    Mechanical complications
        Ventricular septal defect
        Left ventricular aneurysm
        Mitral regurgitation/papillary muscle rupture
    Ventricular arrhythmias
    Postinfarct angina
Preoperative support of left main stenosis or other compelling coronary anatomy
Preoperative support of severe left ventricular dysfunction
High-risk cardiac catheterization or angioplasty (prophylactic)
Unsuccessful angioplasty
High-risk cardiac patient perioperatively for noncardiac surgery (prophylactic)
Selected, deteriorating cardiomyopathy patients awaiting transplantation
Right ventricular dysfunction
Myocarditis
Myocardial contusion
Septic shock (limited experience, controversial)

Prophylactic IABP Use in Noncardiac Operations

Georgeson et al[35] closely examined the risk/benefit ratio associated with the use of the IABP prophylactically placed for support of the cardiac patient undergoing noncardiac operations. It appears justifiable to use the IABP to minimize cardiac complications in high-risk heart patients for whom definitive cardiac operation is not feasible. Guidance in decision-making is aided by various risk-stratification schemes such as the Goldman classification.[35,36]

Right Ventricular Dysfunction

The IABP is an important therapeutic modality for the treatment of right ventricular dysfunction. The right ventricular myocardial perfusion gradient is approximated by the difference in systemic arterial pressure (which is low in this setting) and central venous pressure (typically high in this setting). The diastolic pressure augmentation of the IABP improves this net right ventricular perfusion gradient. The problem of right ventricular failure may occur after an acute myocardial infarct involving the right coronary artery or in the postcardiotomy surgical patient. The cardiac surgical patient may develop right ventricular failure postcardiotomy in the setting of an incompletely revascularized right ventricle, from suboptimal myocardial protection, or right ventriculotomy (intentional, as in tetralogy of Fallot repair, or inadvertent, as in injury at reentry for reoperation). The problem is also accentuated in the presence of right ventricular hypertrophy. The problem is compounded in the face of increased pulmonary vascular resistance or high pulmonary artery pressures. The IABP should be considered when volume loading and pharmacologic support have not been successful.

Viral Myocarditis

Recovery from severe, acute, nonischemic, nontraumatic cardiogenic shock with IABP assist (rather than more extensive mechanical circulatory support) has been recently documented. These patients were presumed to have had a viral myocarditis from which they recovered with excellent function over the ensuing days to weeks.[37]

IABP Before and After Cardiac Transplantation

The IABP is a valuable tool in the support of end-stage heart failure while the patient is awaiting cardiac transplantation.[38] The incidence of IABP use in this patient population varies from 9% to 29%.[39,40] In the Utah transplant experience, which included 401 patients from 1985 to 1990, the IABP was employed in 9% of the patients before transplantation.[39] The patients requiring IABP support did have significant morbidity; limb ischemia occurred in 15% of patients, necessitating IABP removal, thrombectomy, and/or limb amputation for resolution. The patients treated with an IABP *prior to* transplant had a 5-day average duration of therapy (range 1 to 28 days) and had the same rate of survival at 1 year after transplant as the group as a whole. The Texas Heart Institute results, with the IABP used *prior to* transplantation, correlated well with the Utah experience.[41] Patients requiring IABP support *after* transplantation (1.5%) showed very poor results, with only two of the five patients in the Utah Series[39] surviving for a significant period. Kanter et al,[42] reporting an earlier experience, had a uniformly poor outcome (0/5 long-term survivors) in *posttransplant* patients in whom the IABP was used alone or in combination with other forms of mechanical support after transplantation. The lesson from these two studies appears to be that those patients who require the IABP post-transplant should be considered for early retransplantation.

Myocardial Contusion

Myocardial contusion, most commonly associated with deceleration injury, has been successfully treated with the IABP. The association between the mechanism of injury for cardiac contusion and aortic transection must be borne in mind,[43] however, since placement of the balloon in an aorta with untreated transection could be catastrophic.

IABP Use in Ventricular Arrhythmias

In addition to its well-established hemodynamic benefits, the IABP may be helpful in suppressing ventricular arrhythmias in the setting of myocardial ischemia.[9,11,44]

Pediatric Use

An early experience with the IABP in the pediatric age group demonstrated greater effectiveness, better augmentation, and longer survival with older, larger children.[45] There are problems with balloon size and shape, as well as decreased efficacy due to the greater elasticity of the aorta in the young. The aorta may allow effective intraaortic balloon pumping by about 5 years of age, although the number of patients treated is too limited for definitive statements.[45] The iliac rather than the common femoral artery may be cannulated in the pediatric age group to minimize ischemic complications. Timing of the counterpulsation with the more rapid heart rates and low voltage remains a challenge for the trigger algorithms.[46]

Prophylactic IABP for High-Risk Angioplasty

Kreidick et al[47] electively and prophylactically placed IABPs in 21 patients deemed to be at high risk for angioplasty. Indications were anticipated multivessel angioplasty, severe left ventricular dysfunction, or fibrillation at diagnostic angiography. There were no major complications or deaths, and the authors felt that IABP was helpful in stabilizing patients and enhancing primary angioplasty success rates.

Contraindications

There are few absolute contraindications to intraaortic balloon pumping, although patients with hemodynamically significant aortic regurgitation are not considered good candidates.[7] Patients with a greatly limited life expectancy due to a noncardiac condition (eg, terminally ill cancer patients) would be poor candidates for support. Untreated aortic dissection or transection is a contraindication to balloon pump therapy.

Placement

General

The greatest source of morbidity and mortality attributable directly to the use of the IABP is the arterial access necessary for the placement and use of the balloon catheter. A thorough knowledge of the normal and the diseased vascular anatomy and physiology, as well as the effects of patient size, hemodynamic state, and pharmacologic support, will increase the margin of safety for use of the device. Prompt recognition and treatment of access complications, together with a thorough knowledge of alternative insertion sites, will maximize benefits and reduce risks associated with this valuable therapy.

Femoral Approach

The primary access route for the balloon pump is the retrograde approach to the common femoral artery. Placement should be successful by this route in well over 90% of patients.[35,44,48] With the currently available small-diameter catheters, the percutaneous approach is the method of choice for the initial attempt (Figure 28.1).

Preoperative preparation will facilitate IABP placement in the cardiac surgery patient who is a likely candidate for postoperative mechanical circulatory support.[49] This would include patients with pre-existing profound left ventricular dysfunction, those undergoing emergency operations for ischemia or mechanical complications of myocardial infarct (ventricular septal defect, papillary

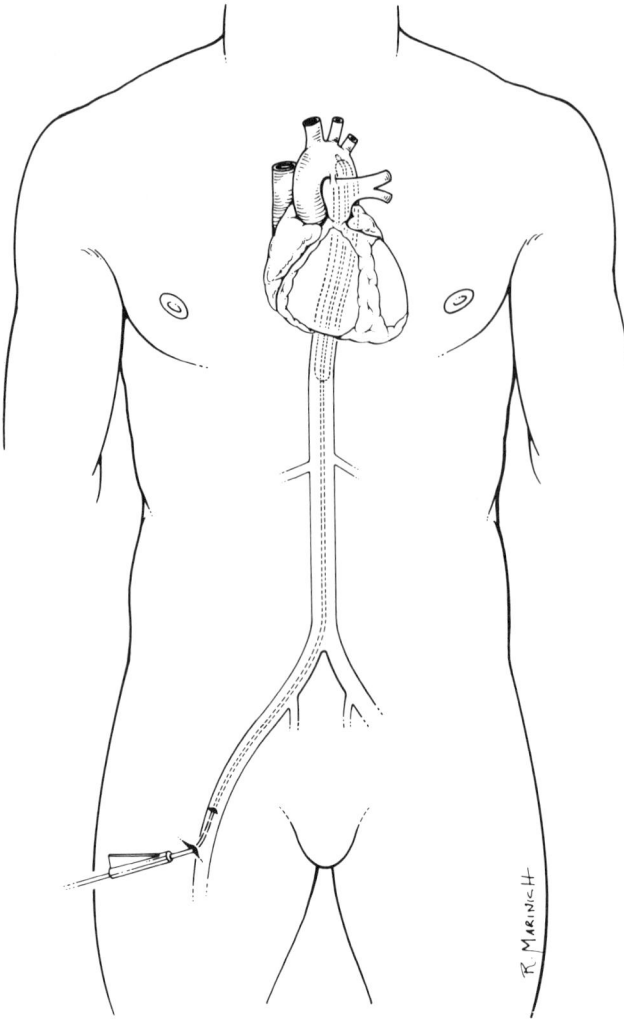

FIGURE 28.1. Percutaneous approach for IABP. Note proper positioning of IABP just past the left subclavian artery.

muscle rupture—although many of these patients would be expected to have balloon support under way preoperatively), and those who require lengthy, complex repair. The preparations are simple, but they greatly expedite subsequent balloon placement and function if balloon counterpulsation is required. Hospital personnel assigned to maintain and support the IABP should be alerted and the balloon pump should be brought into the operating room. An IABP console monitoring cable and electrodes should be attached in sites protected from skin preparation fluid, irrigation, and blood rundown. After the surgical drapes are in place, access to the common femoral artery may be assured by placement of a monitoring catheter through which a guide wire may subsequently be passed for placement of the balloon pump sheath, if needed. Preoperative attempts in this organized, nonhurried fashion, with pulsatile flow, improve the chance for a smooth and uneventful percutaneous balloon placement. Consider-

ation should be given to use of the femoral vessel not previously used for cardiac catheterization, due to the small but real chance for previous catheter-related bacterial colonization or frank infection. These contingencies can be deferred and dealt with when a decision is made to initiate balloon support, but at that point placement of an IABP is at the physiologic expense of additional cardiopulmonary bypass time.

When the decision is made to use the IABP, the sheath is placed percutaneously preferentially.[50] Establishment of pulsatile flow facilitates palpation of the femoral artery. If this is not successful, the common femoral vessel is exposed and the artery is cannulated under direct vision using the modified Seldinger technique. The IABP insertion length is estimated by using the sternomanubrial junction as the proximal extent of the device. The balloon is passed and secured. Balloon position may be checked by palpation of the descending aorta in the left pleural space, through the sternotomy incision.[51] Momentary reduction of the CPB flow facilitates palpation through the transiently decompressed aorta. Transesophageal echocardiography may be employed to assess balloon pump position.[23]

The tip of the IABP may move in or out as much as 4.5 cm with flexion and extension of the patient's hip.[52] This should be taken into account during intraoperative placement, using the typical frogleg position used for coronary bypass operations.

Balloon Placement in the Setting of Previous Peripheral Vascular Operation

The important clinical question regarding safety of placement of the IABP in patients with aortofemoral or aortoiliac vascular grafts for aneurysmal or occlusive disease has been thoughtfully addressed. This was studied retrospectively by LaMuraglia et al[53] in a group of 19 extremely ill patients. No infections, hemorrhagic events, or pseudoaneurysms were encountered, and thrombotic complications were low (2/19), comparing favorably with rates found with placement in native arteries. These patients all experienced hemodynamic improvement after successful placement and had a survival rate of 53% (again, comparable survival rates to those patients in whom balloon pumps were placed in native vessels). Recently placed grafts (<2 weeks postoperatively) should be approached with an open technique, since recent femoral operation makes exposure straightforward. These *nonmature* grafts may have the potential for anastomotic disruption at the time of placement, and in fact, this complication was thought to have caused the one death that occurred during emergency IABP placement in this series. Fluoroscopy, when available, should be employed, particularly with the Seldinger technique. This allows confirmation of correct intravascular wire placement. For a mature graft (≥ 2

years postoperatively), the percutaneous placement and removal technique is preferred, since it is expeditious and safe. The authors felt that optimal management of these patients included prophylactic antimicrobials directed against gram-positive organisms and heparin anticoagulation at 2½ times control activated partial thromboplastin time (PTT), unless the patients were in the postoperative period after cardiac operation. This group of patients was treated with low-molecular-weight dextran to minimize thrombotic complications.

IABP therapy can be offered to these patients with about the same risk as with others in need, provided management techniques as outlined are followed.

Techniques for IABP Use with Small, Stenotic, or Tortuous Femoral Vessels

Phillips et al[54] have described a modification of the percutaneous method for IABP placement that may decrease ischemic complications. The 9.5F balloon is passed over a guide wire which has been placed by the modified Seldinger technique in the common femoral artery. A pursestring suture is used at the small arterial puncture site for hemostasis. This eliminates the additional obstruction associated with the typical sheath. Its anticipated advantage awaits confirmation in comparative trials.

Modification of a 12F sheath to act as an internal stent, by placing multiple side holes, allowed maintenance of distal limb perfusion in a series of 11 patients with severe aortoiliac stenoses.[55]

Retroperitoneal exposure of the iliac artery is an option that may allow retrograde passage through a larger vessel.[48]

Alternative Access Routes

Multiple alternative IABP insertion sites exist, and the question to be answered is not whether the IABP can be placed, but rather what risk is acceptable for the expected benefit. Failure to achieve femoral access can be expected in approximately 5% of these patients, but the failure rate may be as high as 21% with some percutaneous techniques.[35,48,56-58]

Ascending Aortic Placement for IABP Support

If access via one femoral vessel cannot be achieved, attempts should be made to cannulate the opposite femoral vessel. If bilateral femoral attempts fail, then a re-evaluation of the risk-benefit ratio for the balloon is made. A decision is made whether or not to place the balloon into the descending aorta using an antegrade approach via the ascending aorta. This approach carries a higher risk than femoral access.[51] A direct 16-gauge needle puncture of the ascending aorta is made. This is followed by a guide wire, over which the balloon is passed into the descending aorta.[59] The balloon catheter is secured by an aortic purse string. Alternatively, a partial exclusion aortic clamp is used to place a long tube graft (polytetrafluoroethylene or Dacron) through which the balloon may be passed into the descending aorta. This technique carries a higher risk for aortic injury or atheroembolism due to the clamping of the aorta. Also, for the typical coronary bypass patient, space on the ascending aorta is at a premium, due to the proximal anastomoses.

Care must be taken not to advance the balloon below the diaphragm, as inadvertent cannulation of visceral vessels may occur with disastrous consequences. Palpation of the balloon in the descending aorta via the left pleural space confirms correct placement. The tube graft or IABP is brought out through the lower end of the sternal wound, which is closed in the standard fashion. Anticoagulation at some level during counterpulsation, and extreme care at removal *may* help to avoid a catastrophic cerebral,[58] coronary,[51] or renal[60] embolus. A fatal left main coronary embolus has been reported at ascending aortic balloon removal.[51] The balloon (with or without the graft) is removed ideally via sternal reentry, although some favor closed-chest removal.[51]

Subclavian Placement

When severe atherosclerosis or small caliber of the aortoiliofemoral system prevents safe retrograde intraaortic balloon pump passage, the subclavian artery may provide access. Resection of the middle third of the clavicle allows exposure of the third part of the right subclavian artery for IABP cannulation.[61] The balloon is placed through the innominate artery to the transverse arch, and then to the descending aorta (see Figure 28.2). Some form of anticoagulation is strongly recommended in this situation, as the foreign body lies in the path to the cerebral circulation.

The left subclavian approach is an alternative. Problems may be anticipated negotiating the guide wire or balloon into the descending aorta, due to the angle between the subclavian artery and aorta.

Axillary Artery Approach

Placement of the IABP into the descending aorta, antegrade from the axillary artery, was described in the early clinical series.[7] Occasional problems with ischemic complications in the upper extremity, despite extensive collaterals, should temper enthusiasm for this approach as a primary route (Figure 28.3).[7,11] McBride et al[62] have emphasized the advantage of patient ambulation with this route, and its suitability for the patient awaiting cardiac transplantation. The left approach is preferred, as placement from the right axillary artery to the descending aorta traverses the flow to the intracranial circulation. An open

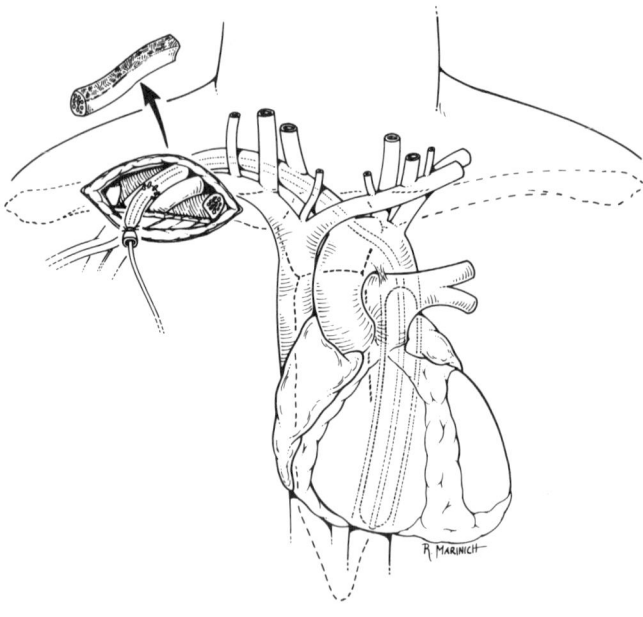

FIGURE 28.2. Alternative approach for IABP insertion. Antegrade approach to descending aorta via right subclavian artery. (Modified from Mayer,[61] by permission of *J Thorac Cardiovasc Surg*.)

technique, local anesthesia, and fluoroscopy are recommended for placement.[62]

Ascending Aortic Placement After Aortic Dissection

While generally considered relatively contraindicated, a novel approach to the use of the IABP after repair of a thoracic aortic dissection has been described.[63] The application of an IABP-containing tubular graft as a cul-de-sac on the ascending aorta allowed separation from CPB, and survival. The site of the aortic repair is spared from potential direct IABP trauma. The technical similarity to the vascular access for pulmonary artery balloon pumping is obvious (Figure 28.4).

IABP Management During CPB

The surgeon shares with the anesthesiologist, perfusionist, technicians, and nurses responsibility for actual surveillance of the device during CPB. While the patient is on

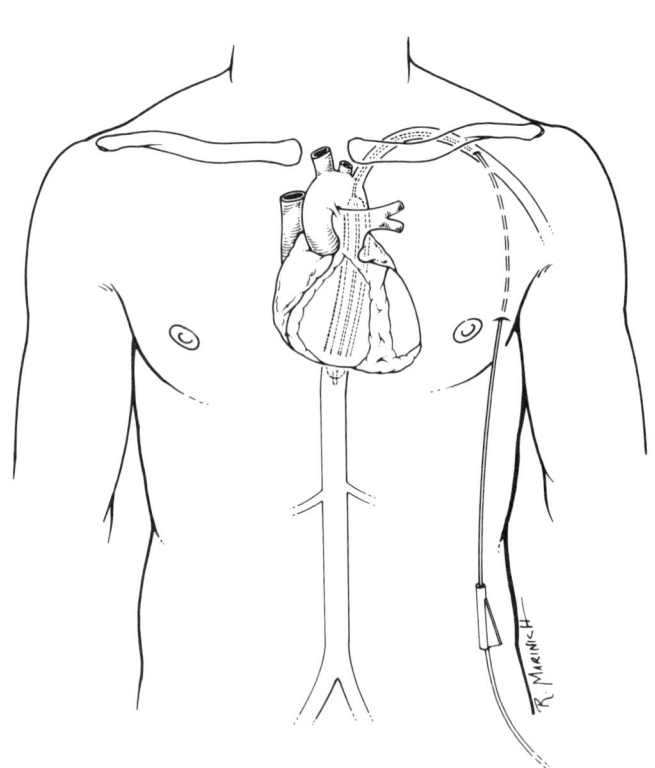

FIGURE 28.3. Alternative approach for IABP insertion. Antegrade approach to descending aorta via left axillary artery. (Modified with permission from the Society of Thoracic Surgeons [*Ann Thorac Surg* 1989;48:874–5].)

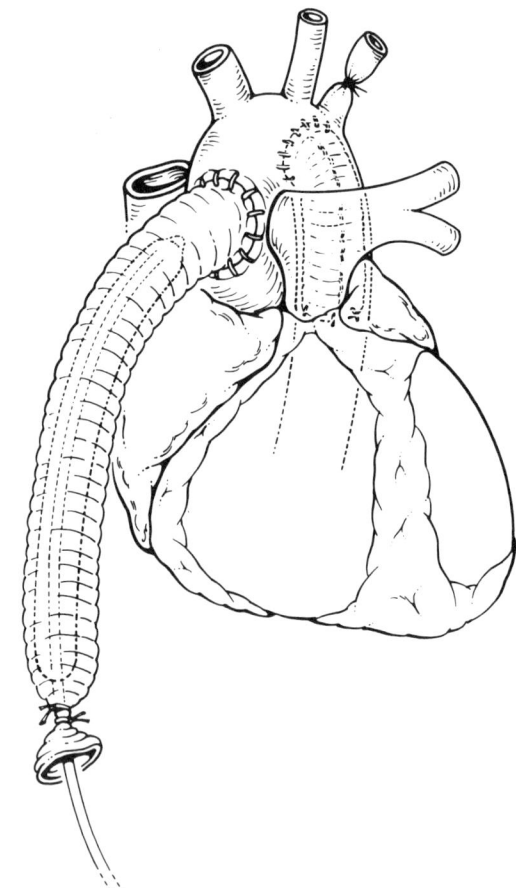

FIGURE 28.4. Alternative approach for IABP placement. IABP use in the setting of aortic dissection repair. Large vascular graft access cul-de-sac for IABP on ascending aorta. (Modified from S Hoka et al,[63] by permission of *J Cardiovasc Surg*.)

CPB, pumping is timed to the electrocardiogram (ECG), pacemaker, or, during periods of arrest, to an internal timing algorithm. Pumping is usually maintained at a low balloon volume or turned completely off while the patient is on CPB, and balloon volume is increased during weaning from the heart-lung machine. If the patient has been cannulated femorally for arterial return from the CPB circuit, it is prudent to keep balloon volumes low until the point of complete separation from bypass. This eliminates the potential for high pressures in the distal aorta and low flows in the proximal aorta (and, thus, in the cerebral and coronary circulation) due to the compartmentalizing effect of the aortic balloon at high volumes.

Conversely, when standard ascending aortic cannulation for CPB is used (as in the vast majority of patients), the same caveat regarding cyclic aortic compartmentalization may be used to advantage. While the patient is on CPB, the balloon volume may be judiciously increased, thereby using the intermittent descending aortic obstruction to increase cerebral and coronary perfusion pressure. The coronary circulation will obviously be excluded from this effect during the crossclamp period.

If the IABP has been placed preoperatively, and standard ascending aortic cannulation techniques have been employed, the balloon may be used to generate pulsatile flow during CPB. The benefits of pulsatile flow are apparent for prolonged periods of circulatory support, but more difficult to demonstrate for the duration of the typical short pump run. Internal IABP console timing may be employed to inflate and deflate at set balloon volumes during CPB.[64,65]

During hemostatic preparations for sternal wound closure, the electrocautery may interfere with balloon ECG timing. The arterial waveform is then employed for balloon triggering.

Pulmonary Artery Balloon Counterpulsation

Failure to separate from CPB, due to postcardiotomy right ventricular dysfunction unresponsive to pharmacologic and IABP therapy, poses a potentially lethal problem. Appropriate treatment would involve a total right ventricular assist device (RVAD). When the RVAD is not indicated or not available, pulmonary artery balloon counterpulsation (PABC) may salvage the patient with reversible right ventricular dysfunction.[66-68]

Animal studies have confirmed the hemodynamic benefit in models of right ventricular failure,[69-70] showing that right ventricular stroke work and cardiac output may be doubled. The important limitation to the efficacy of PABC is the necessity for some residual right ventricular function; total right ventricular support cannot be expected from pulmonary artery counterpulsation.

Symbas et al[67] have used PABC to wean three patients with severe postcardiotomy right ventricular failure from CPB, with one long-term survivor. The technique employs the same balloon catheter as used in the aorta placed into a cul-de-sac formed by a large vascular graft. The graft is sewn directly onto the main pulmonary artery. Balloon pump timing is by the pulmonary artery pressure waveform or the ECG (Figure 28.5).

General Management Principles During Intraaortic Counterpulsation

General

Balloon position is confirmed either fluoroscopically, by chest x-ray,[56] or by transesophageal echocardiography.[23] The tip should come to lie just past the origin of the left subclavian artery. Schematic representations of typical

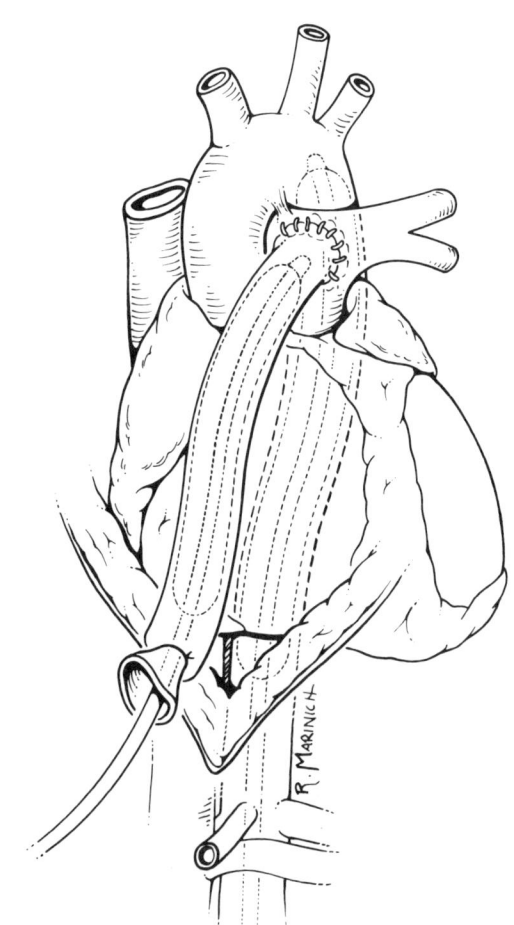

FIGURE 28.5. Pulmonary artery counterpulsation and IABP placement for postcardiotomy right ventricular failure. Large vascular graft forms cul-de-sac for balloon on main pulmonary artery. (Modified with permission from the Society of Thoracic Surgeons [*Ann Thorac Surg* 1984;37:167–168].)

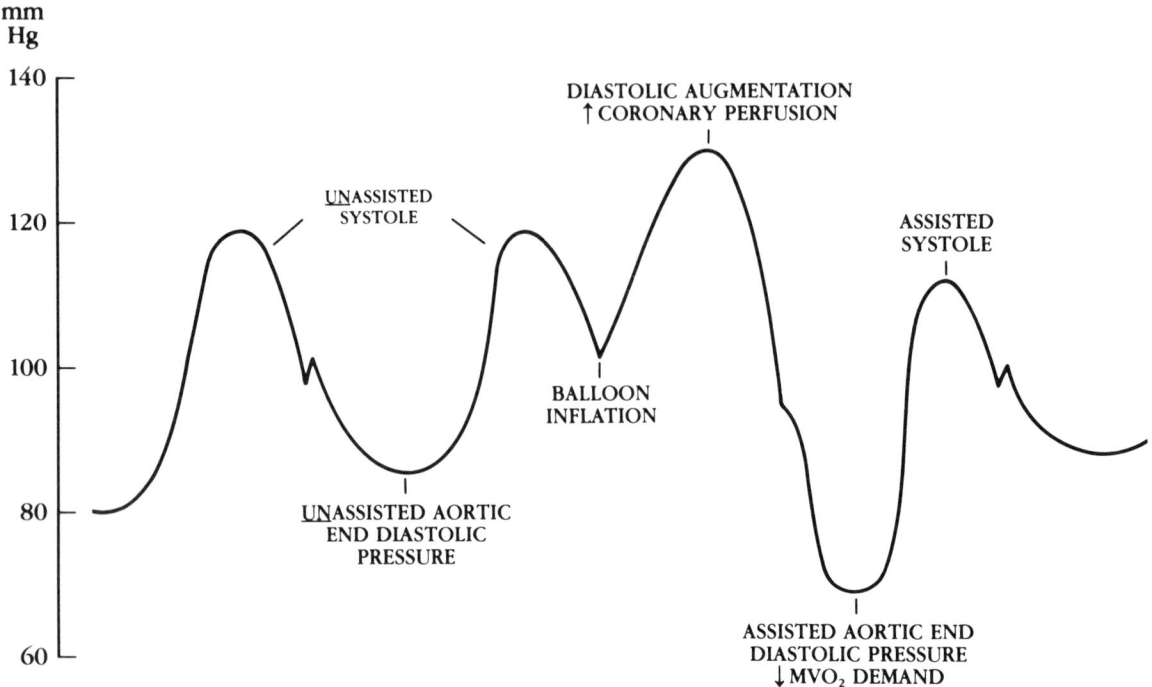

FIGURE 28.6. Schematic illustration of classic IABP waveforms. MVO_2 = myocardial oxygen consumption. (Illustration provided by Datascope Corporation.)

waveforms and timing considerations are given in Figures 28.6 to 28.10.

The length of treatment for IABP placed intraoperatively will be typically at least 24 hours and often a few days. The issue of *postoperative sedation* becomes an important management problem. In the intensive care unit, patients are often agitated and confused, and they have a propensity for removing access lines and support devices.

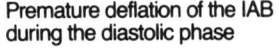

Timing Errors
Early Deflation

Premature deflation of the IAB during the diastolic phase

Waveform Characteristics:
- Deflation of IAB is seen as a sharp drop following diastolic augmentation
- Suboptimal diastolic augmentation
- Assisted aortic end diastolic pressure may be equal to or greater than the unassisted aortic end diastolic pressure
- Assisted systolic pressure may rise

Physiologic Effects:
- Sub-optimal coronary perfusion
- Potential for retrograde coronary and carotid blood flow
- Angina may occur as a result of retrograde coronary blood flow
- Sub-optimal afterload reduction
- Increased MVO_2 demand

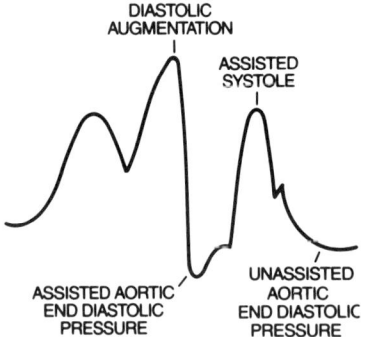

FIGURE 28.7–28.10. Timing errors and physiologic consequences. (Illustrations provided by Datascope Corporation.)

FIGURE 28.8. Timing errors and physiologic consequences. LVEDV = left ventricular end-diastolic volume; LVEDP = left ventricular end-diastolic pressure; MVO$_2$ = myocardial oxygen consumption. (Illustrations provided by Datascope Corporation.)

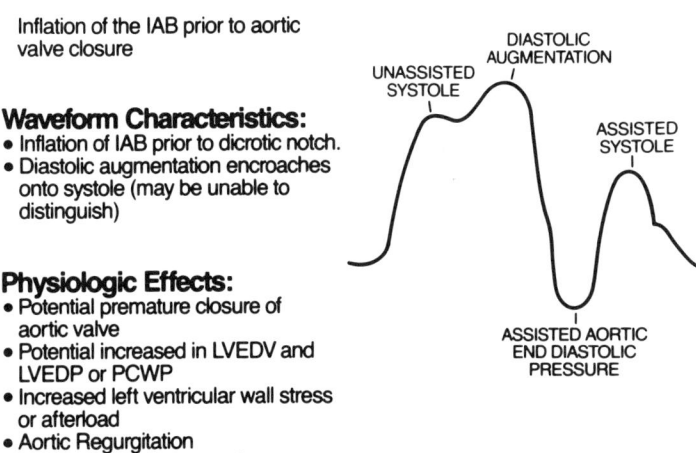

As patients with IABP have tenuous hemodynamics, sedative-hypnotic drugs chosen for postoperative sedation should have minimal cardiovascular depressant effects. Multiple therapies employing different drugs have been used successfully in the postoperative cardiac surgery patient. When compared to boluses of morphine sulfate and midazolam, sufentanil infusion with midazolam boluses, administered to postoperative coronary artery bypass surgery patients, has been shown to provide adequate sedation/analgesia and decrease significantly the incidence and severity of myocardial ischemia.[71] The short-acting sedative-hypnotic propofol compares favorably to midazolam and provides sedation without causing hemodynamic compromise.[72] A continuous, titrated intravenous infusion of chlorpromazine has been demonstrated to have satisfactory sedative properties and beneficial hemodynamic effects due to its α-blocking properties. This effect of chlorpromazine was associated with decreased systemic vascular resistance and improved cardiac index, as compared with the effects of sodium thiamylal on a concurrent nonrandomized group of IABP patients.[73]

Some authorities advocate *antimicrobial treatment* during IABP support.[57,74] If antimicrobials are administered prophylactically, a drug directed at typical skin organisms is a rational choice.

Should cardiopulmonary resuscitation (CPR) be necessary with the IABP in place, the balloon may be kept in the inflated position with a stopcock and large syringe. This may act as an internal aortic occluder and may improve cerebral and coronary perfusion during chest compressions.

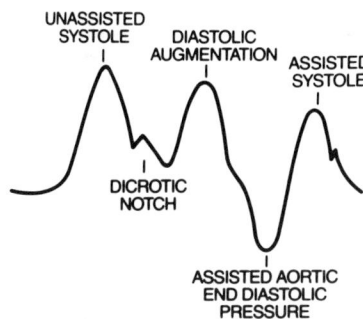

FIGURE 28.9. Timing errors and physiologic consequences. (Illustrations provided by Datascope Corporation.)

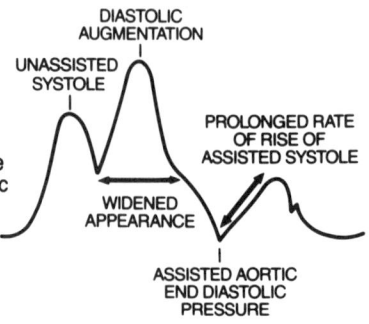

FIGURE 28.10. Timing errors and physiologic consequences. (Illustrations provided by Datascope Corporation.)

Anticoagulation

To minimize the chance for development of thrombus on the balloon surface, it is recommended that the balloon be kept in motion while in the intravascular position. For purposes of attempting to wean from mechanical assistance, the balloon may be kept in motion, but rendered nonsupportive, preferably by decreasing the balloon inflation volume, or by reduction of the inflation-to-cardiac cycle ratio.

Patients should be anticoagulated with heparin to a PTT 1.5 times normal.[7,74,75] Low-molecular-weight dextran is used in patients for whom heparin is not advisable (early postoperative period) or practical during balloon pump treatment. Low-molecular-weight dextran is administered 10 to 25 mL/h by continuous infusion.[9,29,48,75]

Hematologic Effects

Early clinical balloon pump experience demonstrated that development of thrombocytopenia was the prominent hematologic effect. Heparin, or low-molecular-weight dextran, does not appear to preserve platelet counts.[19] The platelet count will often drop as low as 20,000/mm^3 without bleeding problems, and few patients will require platelet transfusion. However, there may be synergistic or additive effects from concurrent drug therapy, notably amrinone. It appears prudent to ensure availability of platelets for transfusion if needed, in the face of low counts and anticipated percutaneous removal. Open removal, to ensure hemostasis and minimize the need for platelet transfusion, should be considered in these cases.

The effect on erythrocytes is inconsequential, with very little hemolysis evident. Human and animal studies show free hemoglobin levels in the range of 25–50 mg/dL, which should not pose a clinical problem.[9,58] Changes in red cell mass are more closely related to losses from operative procedures, balloon placement and removal, and laboratory sampling. There is as much as a fourfold increase in transfusion associated with an open, as opposed to a percutaneous, approach.[74] Finally, there is no significant effect on leukocyte cell types.[19]

Transesophageal Echocardiography and the IABP

The increasing use of transesophageal echocardiography (TEE) as an intraoperative monitoring and diagnostic adjunct offers the opportunity for observation of anatomic and physiologic changes associated with intraaortic balloon pumping. Katz et al[23] have demonstrated, in a small cohort, the ability to document and optimize placement and timing, to detect damage to the aortic wall (intimal injury), and to quantitate the augmentation of coronary blood flow during intraaortic balloon pumping. Intraoperative TEE guidance has been used to observe ascending aortic balloon passage, and is touted as improving the margin of safety for this route.[59]

Complications

Complications related to the use of the IABP range from trivial to fatal and re-emphasize the necessity of careful risk-benefit assessment in the decision to use the balloon.

From the initial large series, it was evident that *physician errors* in placement technique or management during support could prove disastrous and would negate the tremendous potential benefit of the device. Later series were able to document certain *patient attributes* that made IABP therapy a high-risk procedure. The *device characteristics* have led to an excellent safety record made possible through careful animal experimentation, good design and engineering, and industrial quality-improvement efforts. Predictably, most complications are mechanical in nature and relate to the placement and maintenance of a large foreign body in the arterial system. The overall IABP complication rate of approximately 20%,[35] major complication rate of around 10%,[48] and fatal complication rate of about 1%[48] should serve to focus decision-making and lower the threshold for use of counterpulsation therapy.

Risk Factors

General

Several factors may increase the risk of IABP treatment. Knowledge of these factors is crucial for estimation of the risk-benefit ratio for IABP placement in each patient. Table 28.3 lists patient and procedure characteristics that may be used for risk assessment for IABP therapy.

Peripheral Vascular Disease

There is a threefold increase in risk of IABP use in the presence of pre-existing peripheral vascular disease.[58] Limb ischemia associated with the IABP is secondary to IABP catheter size and resultant decreased effective residual arterial lumen at the insertion vessel. This explains the high incidence of complications with preexisting stenoses, the increased incidence of ischemic complications in women (because of their generally smaller vessels), and the lower incidence with smaller catheter sizes.[49,58]

Gender

Women, due to their smaller-caliber vessels, suffer up to a fourfold increase in incidence of vascular complications with IABP support compared with men.[58]

Route of Placement

Examination of the risk of percutaneous versus surgical placement of the IABP is confounded by differing patient populations and catheter sizes. Patients with pre-existing peripheral vascular disease have a two- to threefold increased incidence of vascular complications with the percutaneous route as opposed to the open technique.[49,58] A prospective randomized trial of percutaneous versus surgical placement with 12F catheters demonstrated a significantly increased risk for major vascular complications with the percutaneous approach.[74]

Catheter Size

New, small-diameter (10.5F) catheters appear to have a decreased incidence of complications (19%) versus the larger (12F) device (32%).[49] Iverson et al[49] concluded that an initial attempt at percutaneous placement is currently justified with the small device. Now that even smaller-diameter devices are available, the hope is that vascular complications will decrease further.

Diabetes

Diabetic patients have an increased risk of vascular and infectious complications; however, since the long-term outcome of IABP treatment in diabetic and nondiabetic patients is similar, indications for IABP placement are identical.[76]

Age

Age, at the upper extreme of life, does not appear to increase the risk for IABP-related complications. Sisto et al,[77] based on a decade of experience with no major complications in octogenarians, concluded that the IABP was safe and effective in this group, and advanced age should not exclude patients from the benefit of this mechanical support.

Duration of Balloon Pumping

The duration of IABP therapy has very little relevance in determining the risk of IABP support,[58] since most complications will be evident during the first day of such support.

TABLE 28.3. Conditions affecting risk for the IABP.

Obstruction to flow at insertion vessel resulting in ischemia or thrombosis
  ↑ risk
    Atherosclerosis
    Small stature (including pediatric population)
    Gender (women have smaller stature/smaller vessels)
  ↓ risk
    Smaller IABP catheter sizes
Anticoagulation during IABP treatment
  ↓ risk for thrombosis
Diabetes mellitus
  ↑ risk for infection/vascular complications; however, overall mortality same as nondiabetics
Open versus percutaneous placement
  Differences diminishing with new, smaller IABP catheters
Advanced age
  Negligible, if any, effect on risk
Duration
  After 24°–48° equivocal effect on significant morbidity

IABP Complications

General

The vast majority of IABP therapy complications are related to vascular problems. Some IABP complications and outcomes are shown in Figure 28.11 and Table 28.4 and discussed below.

Vascular

General

Vascular problems account for approximately 90% of the complications associated with IABP therapy. Thrombosis at the arterial insertion site is the most common vascular complication. There are also less common, yet potentially life- and limb-threatening, occurrences such as peripheral embolism, aortic dissection,[44] iliofemoral perforation,[44] laceration with retroperitoneal bleeding,[75] extremity ischemia due to the presence of the balloon catheter,[44] false aneurysm, and femoral stenosis after balloon removal.[49]

Ischemic Extremity

Half of the vascular complications will require an operative repair. Twenty-five percent of the vascular procedures for balloon-pump-related ischemia are done within 24 hours of balloon pump placement,[35] and approximately 95% of these operations will consist of thrombectomy. A small percentage of patients (5% of those requiring vascular operation or about ½% to 1% of all placements) have required limb amputation. Fortunately, about 90% of those with a vascular complication, whether

TABLE 28.4. IABP complications.

Vascular
  Ischemia
    Thrombosis
    Embolism
    Mechanical obstruction from catheter
    Dissection
    Stenosis after removal
  Bleeding
    Vascular perforation/retroperitoneal hematoma
  Dissection
  Pseudoaneurysm
Compartment syndrome
  Peroneal injury/foot drop
Infection
Renal dysfunction
Visceral injury
Paraplegia
Stroke
Balloon rupture
Lymph fistula

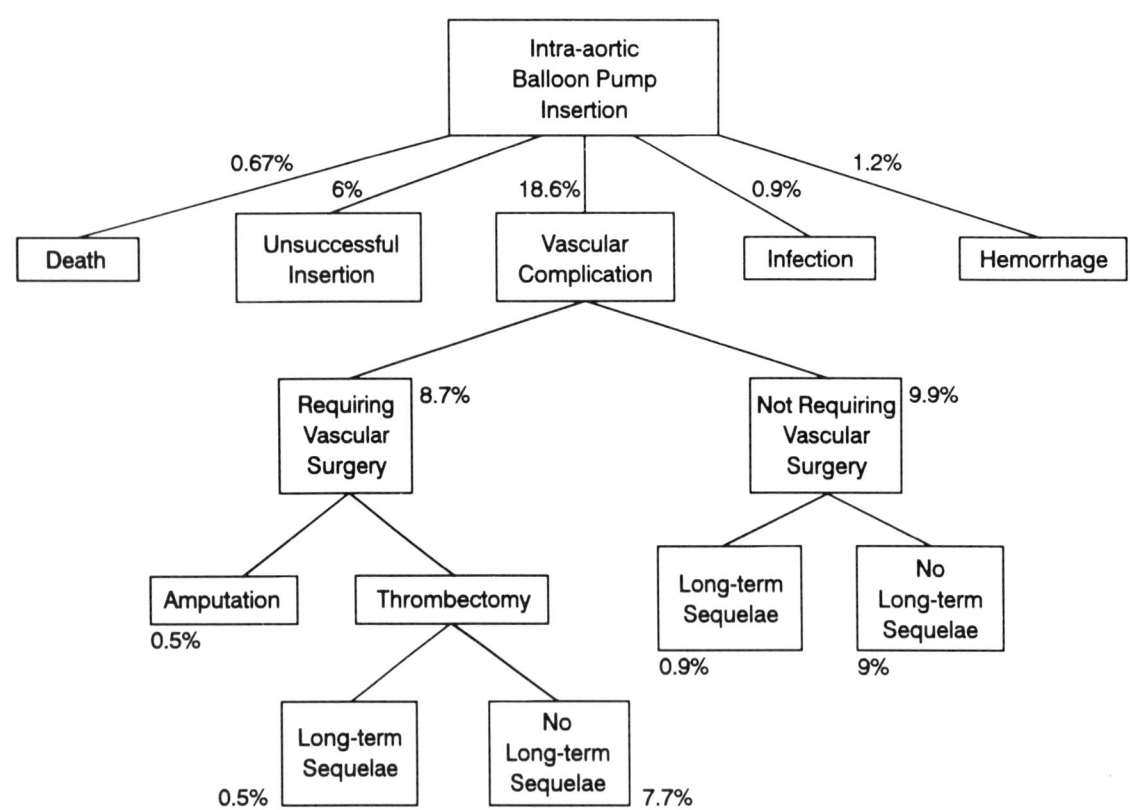

FIGURE 28.11. Complications associated with percutaneous intraaortic balloon pump use. (Modified from S Georgeson et al,[35] by permission of *Am J Medicine*.)

or not they required vascular procedure, will suffer no long-term sequelae.[35]

The recognition of an ischemic extremity after the initiation of IABP therapy necessitates a series of potentially difficult decisions and actions. A judgment as to the ongoing need for IABP support must be made. If the patient no longer requires support, or can be managed pharmacologically, the device is removed as outlined. If satisfactory perfusion of the extremity ensues, then careful observation is carried out until the patient's general condition allows further vascular testing. If removal of the device and attempted balloon catheter embolectomy/thrombectomy are not successful at restoring limb perfusion, then assessment of the level of arterial obstruction is made. If, at femoral exploration, the problem is found to be diminished inflow, treatment with a femorofemoral crossover graft should improve limb perfusion. If femoral arterial inflow is satisfactory, and the obstruction is distal, a femoropopliteal or distal bypass may be necessary to reestablish limb perfusion. A fasciotomy may be required for compartmental decompression, based on clinical judgment supplemented by compartment pressure measurement.

If the patient with an ischemic extremity remains dependent on balloon pump support for survival, the options include removal and replacement of the balloon at another site—the opposite common femoral artery or the iliac, subclavian, or axillary artery—or construction of a femorofemoral bypass below the IABP site. Ascending aorta IABP placement would be a major undertaking requiring sternal reentry.

Constant vigilance for the signs and symptoms of a developing compartment syndrome is crucial at this point.

Dissection

Arterial dissection that results from the advancement of the guide wire or balloon catheter occurs in 1.9% to 4% of IABP patients.[44-56] As these dissections or intimal flaps are not often appreciated as they develop, *any* resistance to advancement of the guide wire or IAB must be treated with extreme caution. Appropriate pressure waveforms and clinical improvement have been noted in patients who have subsequently been found to have had an intramural aortic placement. Fluoroscopic guidance at placement is desirable but is not always available in the operating room or intensive care unit. Specific treatment other than removal of the balloon pump is not always necessary.

Compartment Syndrome/Neuromuscular Injury

In addition to potential limb injury from frank impairment of arterial blood supply related to IABP placement, the soft tissues enclosed by the fascial compartments of the leg are at additional risk. *Formal, frequent neurovascular checks of the lower extremities are a mainstay of the care of the IABP patients.* However, due to incompletely understood pathophysiologic mechanisms, it is possible for the microcirculation of the musculature of the leg to be impaired to the point of tissue necrosis despite pedal blood flow by Doppler examination and pulses present at palpation. The insidious onset of the compartment syndrome is masked further by the frequently encountered patient obtundation related to sedation or transient central nervous system dysfunction. It appears that the syndrome may develop after some insult incites a change in membrane or capillary permeability, with a subsequent net increase in intracellular or extracellular fluid in the compartment. This in turn leads to an increase in compartment pressure, which may in turn exceed the capillary perfusion pressure and lead to tissue necrosis. Intracompartmental capillary perfusion may be impaired at a much lower compartmental pressure (less than 30 torr) than that which would lead to clinically appreciated changes in pedal arterial pulses. The end result may be the well-recognized clinical syndrome of peroneal nerve palsy and foot drop.[35] In a small group of patients, it has been demonstrated that continuous *experimental* monitoring of compartmental pressure in the balloon pump extremity represented an effective early warning system.[78] Early detection, based on a high index of suspicion, the neuromuscular examination, and compartmental pressure measurement, may prevent significant neuromuscular injury by early decompressive fasciotomy.

Infection

Infection related to IABP therapy occurs in about 4% of placements.[44] The majority of infections are related to an open technique and are confined to the wound. Most respond to local wound care, after removal of the IABP.[44,74]

An uncommon manifestation of infection related to IABP use is frank endarteritis. These endarteritides are more commonly associated with an open than with a percutaneous, placement technique; they may be due to either gram-positive or gram-negative bacteria; they may present late after removal; they may be associated with septic embolization distal to the insertion site; and they may require vascular resection and reconstruction with autologous tissue (typically saphenous vein patch or interposition).[44,79]

Infection of an ascending aortic conduit for antegrade IABP placement with subsequent fatal hemorrhage has been reported.[44]

Balloon Rupture

At least one documented episode of balloon rupture appears directly responsible for a patient death due to massive gas embolism.[11] This catastrophic event was probably due to improper balloon insertion technique.[11] Other episodes of balloon rupture with benign or serious sequelae have been documented.[58,80,81] Abrasive trauma from aortic atherosclerotic plaques at insertion, or during inflation cycles, appears to be a causative factor in some cases.[80] Helium in volumes approximating those used clinically in the IABP (20-40 mL), released into the descending aorta in the experimental model, is promptly distributed to cerebral and coronary vessels and is rapidly fatal.[20,82]

Renal Dysfunction

Renal dysfunction directly related to IABP may result from thrombus embolization from a motionless balloon left on standby for hours in a nonanticoagulated patient. There is no clear evidence that a balloon located at the diaphragmatic level, and otherwise functioning properly, plays any role in renal insufficiency. Renal dysfunction is usually attributable to the underlying circulatory state.[11]

Visceral Injury

Mesenteric infarction followed by sepsis and death has been attributed to IABP therapy.[11] In one report, cecal perforation during balloon pumping was recognized and treated by colon resection with survival.[44]

Paraplegia

The development of permanent spinal cord damage after intraaortic balloon counterpulsation is rare. Multiple mechanisms for the ischemic insult leading to spinal cord infarct and paraplegia have been documented.[83] Aortic dissection, related to IABP placement, may lead to spinal cord ischemia or infarction.[84] Occlusion of arterioles in the distribution of radicular spinal arteries, with cholesterol emboli, has been demonstrated in a case of postcardiotomy paraplegia. These emboli are presumed to have originated from aortic atheromatous plaque dislodged during intraoperative IABP placement or use.[85]

IABP Placement: Optimal Time of Therapy Initiation in Early Clinical Trials

IABP in patients with massively damaged ventricles improved hemodynamic variables but did not improve mortality rates. Thus, investigators hypothesized that IABP assistance would have its greatest clinical benefit in postinfarct cardiogenic shock patients with *reversible* ventricular dysfunction who had *early institution* of support prior to irretrievable loss of myocardium.[17,86,87] McEnany et al,[48] reporting a large institutional experience, were able to confirm these hypotheses and demonstrated the beneficial effect of early, definitive cardiac surgical treatment on outcome in these patients.

In the early IABP trials, the device often was not employed until all conventional treatment of that era proved ineffective. This resulted in a population of support patients in profound cardiogenic shock. The poor survival rates associated with the use of the device reflected the irreversible loss of left ventricular function. Most of these patients at postmortem examination were found to have lost greater than 40% of the left ventricular muscle mass. Although these early studies gave irrefutable evidence of immediate, important improvement in hemodynamics, it was most often too little and too late.

In the first large cooperative trial of IABP counterpulsation, there were only 15 hospital survivors out of 87 cardiogenic shock patients. This did not represent a change from the prevailing mortality rate of 85% for cardiogenic shock in that era.[11] There is a paucity of randomized studies directed at IABP efficacy questions. One study with a well-matched non-IABP-treated "control" group showed a survival advantage for the IABP-treated cohort in myocardial infarction.[88]

It was recognized that in order to improve patient survival rates, IABP intervention must occur prior to extensive left ventricular necrosis. Trials of early IABP support, with patients treated early in the course of myocardial failure, showed improvement in patient survival.

In the current era, the hospital patient survival is approximately 60% in patients treated with postcardiotomy IABP assistance. Those patients managed nonsurgically and receiving IABP assistance clearly represent a different pathophysiologic group, and have a hospital survival of about 30%.

Weaning from IABP Support

General

Although there are no hard and fast rules to ensure the readiness of a patient to be weaned from IABP, some guidelines are helpful.[89] Patients should have a mean arterial pressure $\geq$ 70 mm Hg, cardiac index $\geq$ 2.2 L/m^2/min, pulmonary capillary wedge pressure $\leq$ 18 mm Hg, and systolic or diastolic augmented pressures $\geq$ 90 mm Hg.

Improvement within 48 hours of IABP support to an index of 2.1 L/min/m^2 and systemic vascular resistance $\leq$ 2100 dynes/s/cm^{-5} is associated with ultimate successful weaning from IABP support.[90]

A reflex vasodilation[91] may occur in the alert patient with a good cardiac output and insignificant drug therapy requirements. These clinical observations suggest that the patient is ready for withdrawal of IABP support.

Few objective data are available about the effect of *balloon timing ratios* and balloon volumes during weaning from IABP support. Fuchs et al[32] have demonstrated no graded effect for inflation ratios less than 1:1. Ratios of 1:2 or 1:4 are the same as turning the balloon off in terms of augmentation of coronary blood flow. In contrast, the effect of *balloon volume reduction is* graded, and may be preferable if a gradual withdrawal from support is the goal.

Removal of a Balloon Catheter Placed Percutaneously

Meticulous technique should decrease the incidence of untoward sequelae after IABP removal. Potential complications of IABP removal include bleeding, hematoma formation, pseudoaneurysm, vascular thrombosis, and embolism.

The suture securing the device to the skin is removed and the entrance site prepared with a topical antimicrobial. The patient is draped with a towel, with the expectation of up to 100 mL of blood loss. The pump is turned off and a large syringe is used to evacuate the balloon gas. One hand should compress below the insertion site on the femoral vessel to minimize the chance for distal embolization of clot. The catheter is pulled back until the balloon meets the sheath, but not pulled through it, and the two are withdrawn simultaneously. The balloon entry tract is allowed to bleed freely for 2 or 3 pulses to expel thrombus and debris and compression is applied for 30 minutes[75] *by the clock*. The patient is kept supine for 24 hours after IABP removal, with a pressure dressing or a 5-pound weight over the arterial entry site. Close neuromuscular monitoring of the extremity allows prompt intervention if ischemia ensues. Vigilance must also be maintained for the development of retroperitoneal bleeding—an uncommon occurrence. If the patient has a low platelet count or is anticoagulated, the open technique for pump removal at the bedside can ensure hemostasis, with direct suture repair of the arterial defect.

Removal of Balloons Placed by Open Technique

Removal of the IABP by the open or surgical technique is considered for those patients with ischemic complications or significant potential for bleeding at the time of IABP removal. This may be done in the intensive care unit. Open removal allows balloon embolectomy and definitive repair of the vessel, and thus has been associated with a decrease in vascular complications. Patients with a prothrombin time greater than 16 seconds, PTT greater than 80 seconds, or platelet count less than 80,000 should be considered for open or surgical removal. Removal of percutaneously placed balloons requires an increased investment of the surgeon's time (holding pressure). However,

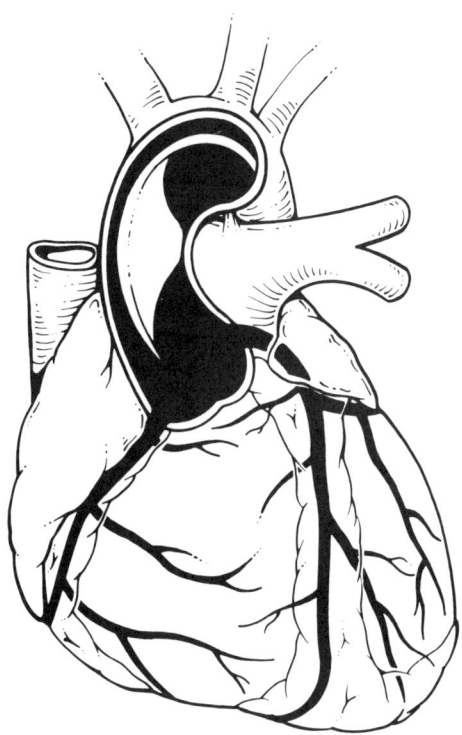

FIGURE 28.12. Investigative ascending aortic balloon counterpulsator. (Modified and used with permission ABIOMED Corp.)

when operating room personnel and equipment are factored into the equation, percutaneous removal is probably more cost effective than the open or surgical technical.[92] There is a low complication rate following removal of up to 11F devices percutaneously.[92]

Future Prospects

A new technology based on previously demonstrated principles is undergoing clinical trial. It has been shown that IABP effectiveness is enhanced with a more proximal IABP location and aortic occlusivity.[20,21,93,94] The Abiomed ICS 8000 device was designed to optimize balloon position and occlusivity with ascending aortic positioning of the balloon (Figure 28.12). Phase I human trials at the University of Louisville and the Massachusetts General Hospital have shown initial device safety.[95] A large-scale efficacy trial is planned to compare its circulatory support with conventional IABP treatment.

References

1. Kantrowitz A, Kantrowitz A. Experimental augmentation of coronary flow by retardation of the arterial pressure pulse. *Surgery* 1953;34:678–687.
2. Clauss RH, Birtwell WC, Albertal G, et al. Assisted circula-

tion. I. The arterial counterpulsator. *J Thorac Cardiovasc Surg* 1961;41:447-458.
3. Kantrowitz A, Akutsu T, Chaptal P-A, et al. A clinical experience with an implanted mechanical auxiliary ventricle. *JAMA* 1966;197:525-529.
4. Sugg WL, Rea, MJ, Webb WR, et al. Cardiac assistance (counter pulsation) in ten patients. *Ann Thorac Surg* 1970; 9:1-12.
5. Moulopoulos SD, Topaz S, Kolff WJ. Diastolic balloon pumping (with carbon dioxide) in the aorta – a mechanical assistance to the failing circulation. *Am Heart J* 1962;63: 669-675.
6. Clauss RH, Missier P, Reed GE, et al. Assisted circulation by counter-pulsation with an intraaortic balloon. Methods and effects. In: *Digest, 15th Annual Conference on Engineering in Medicine and Biology.* Chicago: Northwestern University; 1962;4:44.
7. Kantrowitz A, Tjonneland S, Freed PS, et al. Initial clinical experience with intraaortic balloon pumping in cardiogenic shock. *JAMA* 1968;203:135-140.
8. Kantrowitz A, Krakauer JS, Rosenbaum A, et al. Phase-shift balloon pumping in medically refractory cardiogenic shock: results in 27 patients. *Arch Surg* 1969;99:739-743.
9. Buckley MJ, Leinbach RC, Kastor JA, et al. Hemodynamic evaluation of intraaortic balloon pumping in man. *Circulation* 1970;46(suppl 2):130-134.
10. Bregman D, Kripke DC, Goetz RH. The effect of synchronous unidirectional intraaortic balloon pumping on hemodynamics and coronary blood flow in cardiogenic shock. *Trans Am Soc Artif Intern Organs* 1970;16:439-446.
11. Scheidt S, Wilner G, Mueller H, et al. Intra-aortic balloon counterpulsation in cardiogenic shock. Report of a cooperative clinical trial. *N Engl J Med* 1973;288:979-984.
12. Kantrowitz A. Origins of intraaortic balloon pumping. *Ann Thorac Surg* 1990;50:672-674.
13. Kantrowitz A. A moment in history: introduction of left ventricular assistance. *Trans Am Soc Artif Intern Organs* 1987;19:39-47.
14. Zelano JA, Ko W, Lazzaro R, et al. Comparison of an extraaortic counterpulsation device versus intraaortic balloon pumping in severe cardiac failure. *Trans Am Soc Artif Int Organs* 1991;37:M342-344.
15. Zelano JA, Ko W, Lazzaro R, et al. Evaluation of an extraaortic counterpulsation device in severe cardiac failure. *Ann Thorac Surg* 1992;53:30-37.
16. Schilt W, Freed PS, Khalil G, et al. Temporary nonsurgical intraarterial cardiac assistance. *Trans Am Soc Artif Int Organs* 1967;13:322-327.
17. Leinbach RC, Gold HK, Buckley MJ, et al. Reduction of myocardial injury during acute infarction by early application of intraaortic balloon pumping and propranolol. *Circulation* 1973(suppl 4);47-48:100.
18. Laird JD, Madras PN, Jones RT et al. Theoretical and experimental analysis of the intraaortic balloon pump. *Trans Am Soc Artif Int Organs* 1968;14:338-343.
19. Weber KT, Janicki JS, Walker AA. Intraaortic balloon pumping: an analysis of several variables affecting balloon performance. *Trans Am Soc Artif Intern Organs* 1972;18: 486-495.
20. Weber KT, Janicki JS. Intraaortic balloon counterpulsation. A review of physiologic principles, clinical results, and device safety. *Ann Thorac Surg* 1974;17:602-636.
21. Sun Y. Modeling the dynamic interaction between left ventricle and intraaortic balloon pump. *Am J Physiol* 1991;261: H1300-H1311.
22. Mountcastle VB, ed. *Medical Physiology.* St Louis: CV Mosby; 1974:999.
23. Katz ES, Tunick PA, Kronzon I. Observations of coronary flow augmentation and balloon function during intraaortic balloon counterpulsation using transesophageal echocardiography. *Am J Cardiol* 1992;69:1635-1639.
24. Evans JM, McGinnis GE, Brown BG, et al. Development of an intraaortic balloon assist device. *Artificial Heart Program Conference Proceedings* 1969;515-528.
25. Roy AJ, Lambert PB, Frank HA, et al. Immediate responses of collateral vessels to abrupt arterial occlusion. *Am J Physiol* 1964;206:1299-1303.
26. John HT, Warren R. The stimulus to collateral circulation. *Surgery* 1961;49:14-25.
27. Watson JT, Willerson JT, Fixler DE, et al. Temporal changes in collateral coronary blood flow in ischemic myocardium during intraaortic balloon pumping. *Circulation* 1973(suppl 4);47-48:100.
28. Mueller H, Ayres SM, Giannelli S, et al. Effect of isoproterenol, l-norepinephrine, and intraaortic counterpulsation on hemodynamics and myocardial metabolism in shock following acute myocardial infarction. *Circulation* 1972;45:335-351.
29. Ehrich DA, Biddle TL, Kronenberg MW, et al. The hemodynamic response to intraaortic balloon counterpulsation in patients with cardiogenic shock complicating acute myocardial infarction. *Am Heart J* 1977;93:274-279.
30. Bardet J, Masquet C, Kahn J-C, et al. Clinical and hemodynamic results of intraaortic balloon counterpulsation and surgery for cardiogenic shock. *Am Heart J* 1977;93:280-288.
31. Lazar JM, Ziady GM, Drummer SJ, et al. Outcome and complications of prolonged intraaortic balloon counterpulsation in cardiac patients. *Am J Cardiol* 1992;69:955-958.
32. Fuchs RM, Brin KP, Brinker JA, et al. Augmentation of regional coronary blood flow by intraaortic balloon counterpulsation in patients with unstable angina. *Circulation* 1983; 68:117-123.
33. Craver JM, Kaplan JA, Jones EL, et al. What role should the intraaortic balloon have in cardiac surgery? *Ann Surg* 1979;189:769-776.
34. Martin TD, Craver JM, Gott JP, et al. A prospective randomized trial of retrograde warm blood cardioplegia: myocardial benefit and neurologic threat. *Ann Thorac Surg* 1994;57:298-302; discussion 302-304.
35. Georgeson S, Coombs AT, Eckman MH. Prophylactic use of the intraaortic balloon pump in high-risk cardiac patients undergoing noncardiac surgery: a decision analytic view. *Am J Med* 1992;92:665-678.
36. Sin SC, Kowalchuk GJ, Welty FK, et al. Intraaortic balloon counterpulsation support in the high-risk cardiac patient undergoing urgent noncardiac surgery. *Chest* 1991;99:1342-1345.
37. Dembitsky WP, Moore CH, Holman WL, et al. Successful

mechanical circulatory support for non-coronary shock. *J Heart Lung Transplant* 1992;11:129-135.
38. Frazier OH, Nakatani T, Lammermeier DE, et al. Cardiac transplantation and mechanical circulatory assistance: the Texas Heart Institute experience. *J Jpn Assoc Thorac Surg* 1989;37:1873-1879.
39. Marks JD, Karwande SV, Richenbacher WE, et al. Perioperative mechanical circulatory support for transplantation. *J Heart Lung Transplant* 1992;11:117-128.
40. Oaks TE, Wisman CB, Pac WE, et al. Results of mechanical circulatory assistance before heart transplantation. *J Heart Transplant* 1989;8:113-115.
41. Lonquist JL, Duncan JM, Frazier OH, et al. Heart transplantation after mechanical circulatory support: four years' experience. *J Heart Lung Transplant* 1992;11:240-245.
42. Kanter KR, Pennington DG, McBride LR, et al. Mechanical circulatory assistance after heart transplantation. *J Heart Transplant* 1987;6:150-154.
43. Symbas P. *Cardiothoracic Trauma*. Philadelphia: WB Saunders Co; 1989:55.
44. Beckman CB, Geha AS, Hammond GL, et al. Results and complications of intraaortic balloon counterpulsation. *Ann Thorac Surg* 1977;24:550-559.
45. Pollock JC, Charlton MC, Williams WG, et al. Intraaortic balloon pumping in children. *Ann Thorac Surg* 1980;29:522-528.
46. Webster H, Veasy LG. Intraaortic balloon pumping in children. *Heart Lung* 1985;14:548-555.
47. Kreidich I, Davies DW, Lim R, et al. High-risk coronary angioplasty with elective intraaortic balloon pump support. *Int J Cardiol* 1992;35:147-152.
48. McEnany MI, Kay HR, Buckley MJ, et al. Clinical experience with intraaortic balloon pump support in 728 patients. *Circulation* 1978;58(suppl 1):124-132.
49. Iverson LIG, Herfindahl G, Ecker RR, et al. Vascular complications of intraaortic balloon counterpulsation. *Am J Surg* 1987;154:99-103.
50. Bregman D, Casaretta WJ. Percutaneous intraaortic balloon pumping: initial clinical experience. *Ann Thorac Surg* 1980;29:153-155.
51. Meldrum-Hanna WG, Deal CW, Ross DE. Complications of ascending aortic intraaortic balloon pump cannulation. *Ann Thorac Surg* 1985;40:241-244.
52. O'Rourke MF, Shepart KM. Protection of the aortic arch and subclavian artery during intraaortic balloon pumping. *J Thorac Cardiovasc Surg* 1973;65:543-546.
53. LaMuraglia, Vlahakes GJ, Moncure AC, et al. The safety of intraaortic balloon pump catheter insertion through suprainguinal prosthetic vascular bypass grafts. *J Vasc Surg* 1991;13:830-837.
54. Phillips SJ, Tannenbaum M, Zeff RH, et al. Sheathless insertion of the percutaneous intraaortic balloon pump: an alternate method. *Ann Thorac Surg* 1992;53:162.
55. Satoh H, Kobayashi T, Hiraishi T, et al. New side-holed sheath for intraaortic balloon pumping to maintain limb perfusion. *Ann Thorac Surg* 1992;54:794-796.
56. Grayzel J. Clinical evolution of the Percor percutaneous intraaortic balloon: cooperative study of 722 cases. *Circulation* 1982;66(suppl 1):223-226.
57. Martin RS, Moncure AC, Buckley MJ, et al. Complications of percutaneous intraaortic balloon insertion. *J Thorac Cardiovasc Surg* 1983;85:186-190.
58. Gottlieb SO, Brinker JA, Borkon AM, et al. Identification of patients at high risk for complications of intraaortic balloon counterpulsation: a multivariate risk factor analysis. *Am J Cardiol* 1984;53:1135-1139.
59. Kaplan LJ, Weiman DS, Langan N, et al. Safe intraaortic balloon pump placement through the ascending aorta using transesophageal ultrasound. *Ann Thorac Surg* 1992;54:374-375.
60. Baciewicz FA, Kaplan BM, Murphy TE, et al. Bilateral renal artery thrombotic occlusion: a unique complication following removal of a transthoracic intraaortic balloon. *Ann Thorac Surg* 1982;33:631-634.
61. Mayer JH. Subclavian artery approach for insertion of intraaortic balloon. *J Thorac Cardiovasc Surg* 1978;76:61-63.
62. McBride LR, Miller LW, Naunheim KS, et al. Axillary artery insertion of an intraaortic balloon pump. *Ann Thorac Surg* 1989;48:874-875.
63. Hoka S, Tashiro T, Haruta Y, et al. Modified application of intraaortic balloon pump after repair of thoracic dissecting aneurysm. *J Cardiovasc Surg* 1992;33:41-43.
64. Pappas G. Intrathoracic intraaortic balloon insertion for pulsatile cardiopulmonary bypass. *Arch Surg* 1974;109:842-843.
65. Mavroudis C. To pulse or not to pulse. *Ann Thorac Surg* 1978;25:259-271.
66. Miller DC, Moreno-Cabral RJ, Applebaum RE, et al. Pulmonary artery balloon counterpulsation for right ventricular failure. *Ann Thorac Surg* 1984;37:167-168.
67. Symbas PN, McKeown PP, Sanfora AH, et al. Pulmonary artery counterpulsation for treatment of intraoperative right ventricular failure. *Ann Thorac Surg* 1985;39:437-440.
68. Skillington PD, Couper GS, Peigh PS, et al. Pulmonary artery balloon counterpulsation for intraoperative right ventricular failure. *Ann Thorac Surg* 1991;51:658-660.
69. Jett GK, Siwek LG, Picone AL, et al. Pulmonary artery balloon counterpulsation for right ventricular failure. *J Thorac Cardiovasc Surg* 1983;86:364-372.
70. Spence PA, Weisel RD, Easdown J, et al. The hemodynamic effects and mechanism of action of pulmonary artery balloon counterpulsation in the treatment of right ventricular failure during left heart bypass. *Ann Thorac Surg* 1985;39:329-335.
71. Mangano DT, Siliciano D, Hollenbert M, et al. Postoperative myocardial ischemia: therapeutic trials using intensive analgesia following surgery. *Anesthesiology* 1992;76:342-353.
72. Grounds RM, Lalor JM, Lumley J, et al. Propofol infusion for sedation in the intensive care unit. Preliminary report. *Br Med J* 1987;294:397-400.
73. Mayumi H, Tokvnaga K. Constant intravenous infusion of chlorpromazine for both sedation and after load reduction in postcardiotomy patients under intraaortic balloon pumping. *Jpn Heart J* 1992;33:61-71.
74. Goldberg MJ, Rubenfire M, Kantrowitz A, et al. Intraaortic balloon pump insertion: a randomized study comparing percutaneous and surgical techniques. *J Am Coll Cardiol* 1987;9:515-523.
75. Shahian DM, Neptune WB, Ellis FH, et al. Intraaortic bal-

loon pump morbidity: a comparative analysis of risk factors between percutaneous and surgical techniques. *Ann Thorac Surg* 1983;36:644-653.
76. Wasfie T, Freed PS, Rubenfire M, et al. Risks associated with intraaortic balloon pumping in patients with and without diabetes mellitus. *Am J Cardiol* 1988;61:558-562.
77. Sisto DA, Hoffman DM, Fernandes S, et al. Is the balloon pump in octogenarians justified? *Ann Thorac Surg* 1992;54:507-511.
78. Glenville B, Crockett JR, Bennett JG. Compartment syndrome and intraaortic balloon. *Thorac Cardiovasc Surg* 1986;34:292-294.
79. Grantham RN, Munnell ER, Kanaly PJ. Femoral artery infection complicating intraaortic balloon pumping. *Am J Surg* 1983;146:811-814.
80. Rajani R, Keon WJ, Bedard P. Rupture of an intraaortic balloon. A case report. *J Thorac Cardiovasc Surg* 1980;79:301-302.
81. Haykal HA, Wang AM. Cardiothoracic diagnosis of delayed cerebral air embolism following intraaortic balloon catheter insertion. *Comput Radiol* 1986;10:307-309.
82. Furman S, Vijaynagar R, Rosenbaum R, et al. Lethal sequelae of intraaortic balloon rupture. *Surgery* 1971;69:121-129.
83. Scott IR, Goiti JJ. Late paraplegia as a consequence of intraaortic balloon pump support. *Ann Thorac Surg* 1985;40:300-301.
84. Seifert PE, Silverman NA. Late paraplegia resulting from intraaortic balloon pump. *Ann Thorac Surg* 1986;41:700 (letter).
85. Harris RE, Reimer KA, Crain BJ, et al. Spinal cord infarction following intraaortic balloon support. *Ann Thorac Surg* 1986;42:206-207.
86. Johnson SA, Scalon PJ, Loeb HS, et al. Treatment of cardiogenic shock in myocardial infarction by intraaortic balloon counterpulsation and surgery. *Am J Med* 1977;62:687-692.
87. Hagemeijer F, Laird J, Haalebos MMP, et al. Effectiveness of intraaortic balloon pumping without cardiac surgery for patients with severe heart failure secondary to a recent myocardial infarction. *Am J Caridol* 1977;40:951-956.
88. Lorente P, Gourgon R, Beaufils P, et al. Multivariate statistical evaluation of intraaortic counterpulsation in pump failure complicating acute myocardial infarction. *Am J Cardiol* 1980;46:124-134.
89. Bavin TK, Self MA. Weaning from intra-aortic balloon pump support. *Am J Nurs* 1991;10:54-59.
90. Quaal SJ. *Comprehensive Intra-aortic Balloon Pumping*. St Louis: The CV Mosby Company; 1984.
91. Brown BG, Goldfarb D, Gott VL. A vasomotor reflex contribution to systolic pressure reduction during diastolic augmentation. *Trans Am Soc Artif Int Organs* 1966;12:63-68.
92. Rohrer MJ, Sullivan CA, McLaughlin DJ, et al. A prospective randomized study comparing surgical and percutaneous removal of intraaortic balloon pump. *J Thorac Cardiovasc Surg* 1992;103:569-572.
93. Brown BG, Gundel WD, McGinnis GE, et al. Improved balloon diastolic augmentation with a double balloon catheter in the ascending and the descending thoracic aorta. *Ann Thorac Surg* 1968;6:127-135.
94. Chyong Y, Miura I, Ramez B, et al. Aortic root balloon pumping. *Jpn Heart J* 1971;12:263-274.
95. Ganzel BL, Gray LA Jr, Masden RR, et al. New percutaneous intra-arterial cardiac support system. *JACC* 1991;17:279A.

29
Extracorporeal Membrane Oxygenation for Severe Cardiorespiratory Failure

J. Devn Cornish

Throughout this volume, the efficacy of cardiopulmonary bypass (CPB) in providing short-term circulatory support is demonstrated. The need for such technology is undisputed, since 375,000 bypass operations are performed annually in the United States, where cardiovascular disease is the leading cause of death.[1] Respiratory diseases (not including respiratory complications of neoplastic conditions) are the third leading cause of death. Almost as soon as extracorporeal circulation was conceived as an adjunct to cardiac surgery, its developers recognized its potential application to the treatment of respiratory failure. In many ways, however, the latter is a much more convoluted enterprise. Since circulatory support cannot in any way "treat" underlying pulmonary conditions, at best it can be expected to provide a period of physiologically normal support of sufficient length to allow for intrinsic healing. The long-term use of extracorporeal circulation as a means of supporting patients with life-threatening respiratory (and/or cardiac) failure has come to be known as extracorporeal membrane oxygenation (ECMO) or extracorporeal life support (ECLS).

The purpose of this chapter is to provide the reader an overview of extracorporeal life support technology. This will be done by reviewing the mechanics of ECMO, the history of its development, the selection process used to identify candidate patients, and the reported effects of ECMO on patient survival and quality of life. For the sake of completeness, the application of ECMO to patients with primary circulatory failure, the financial implications of long-term perfusion support, and potential future developments in this field are also discussed.

What Is ECMO?

Extracorporeal membrane oxygenation (ECMO) is the use of a CPB system, similar to that used in the operating room, to supplement heart and lung function in patients at high risk of dying from cardiac and/or respiratory failure. It has been used with increasing frequency to treat neonates with severe respiratory distress since Barlett's[2] first successful case in 1975. Recently, it has been successfully applied to older pediatric and adult patients as well. ECMO differs from the heart-lung bypass used in the operating room in that it usually requires only cervical and/or femoral rather than intrathoracic cannulation, which can be performed under local rather than general anesthesia and is commonly done in the intensive care unit. It is continued not for 1 to 4 hours, as during cardiac surgery, but for periods generally ranging from 3 to 14 days. It is also significantly different in that the purpose of the procedure is not to provide support during the surgical repair of a cardiac lesion but rather to "buy time" in a state of physiologic normalcy during which intrinsic healing may occur. Since it often involves the cannulation and permanent ligation of the right common carotid artery and the right internal jugular vein, as well as long-term systemic heparinization, the decision to use ECMO should be made only after careful consideration of the alternatives.

The ECMO system consists essentially of a blood pump, an oxygenator, a countercurrent heat exchanger to rewarm the blood, and a control module that balances the rate of blood drainage from and return to the patient (Figure 29.1). The blood pump is usually a simple roller pump, although some centers employ a BioMedicus centrifugal pump. The oxygenator may be the original Avecor-Kolobow (Avecor Cardiovascular, Inc., Plymouth, MN) spiral coil sheet design or one of the newer hollow-fiber devices. Bubble oxygenators are not applicable to ECMO because of the high degree of associated trauma to blood components and because of the heightened risk of air embolization. The "oxygenator" is responsible for exchanging both oxygen and carbon dioxide with the blood. The heat exchanger rewarms the blood by exposing it, across metal tubing, to warm water, which circulates in a direction opposite to that of the blood. Those experienced with perfusion systems will immediately note that

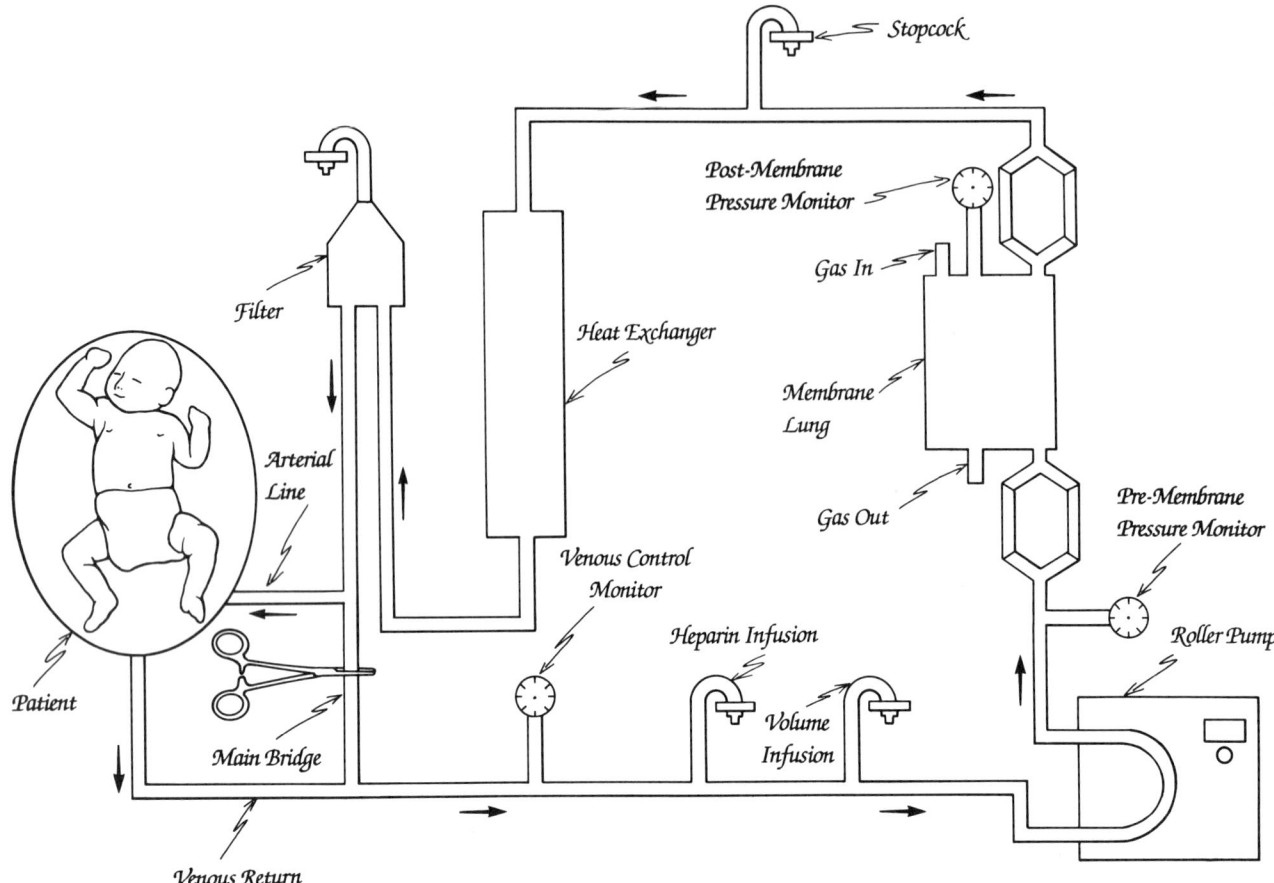

FIGURE 29.1. Typical circuit diagram for venoarterial ECMO in neonatal patients.

the heat exchanger, if separate from the oxygenator, is positioned in the circuit distal, not proximal, to the oxygenator. A broad variety of control modules are currently in use, but all function by servoregulating pump speed, so that the rate of drainage of blood from the patient is precisely and continuously equal to that of blood return to the patient. In other words, the ECMO circuit is a "closed" system as opposed to the open reservoir system commonly used in CPB.

Other devices may be added to the basic ECMO system. Some ECMO centers insert an arterial line filter in the circuit between the heat exchanger and the arterial cannula to trap any air, thrombi, or other emboli. Pressure monitors are often placed before and after the membrane to monitor the pressure of the circulating blood and to identify increasing resistance in the oxygenator (ie, increasing transmembrane pressure). Several different types of sensors have been applied to the blood path of ECMO circuits to measure the P_{O_2}, hemoglobin saturation, and other "blood gas" parameters in the circulating blood. In-line bubble detectors can identify microscopic air bubbles in the arterialized blood and automatically turn off the pump. Computerized modules are available from several manufacturers of perfusion equipment, which combine pressure monitoring, drainage and return coupling, and bubble detection in a single pump controller system. In addition, other "gadgets" are being introduced to make the system safer, simpler, easier to use, and even adaptable to patient transport.[3]

The ECMO procedure is conceptually simple. First, the ECMO system is primed with the freshest available banked blood (often leukodepleted and/or irradiated), and the acid-base balance and blood gases in the prime are adjusted to be similar to those of the patient (except for the P_{O_2}, of course). Next, the cannulation site(s) is (are) anesthetized, or the patient is given a general anesthetic, and the requisite vessels are cannulated. The drainage and return lines of the ECMO system are connected to the surgically inserted catheters, and pump flow is started. Blood flows by gravity from the patient to the control module which regulates pump speed, then on to the pump, the oxygenator, the heat exchanger, and finally back to the patient. In truth, ECMO follows the old adage, "out goes the bad blood, in goes the good blood." Although the "plumbing" of ECMO is quite straightforward, its clinical application is both complex and controversial. Before we consider the intricacies of modern ECMO, a brief review of the history of its development may be helpful.

History of the Development of Clinical ECMO

In the flow of time, disparate events may have overlapping effects of lasting importance. A simmering sense of frustration among American physicians at the seemingly endless tide of premature babies being born, developing respiratory distress (the dreaded "hyaline membrane disease"), and dying (at a rate of 25,000 per year) was brought to public attention by the death of President and Mrs. John F. Kennedy's premature baby at Boston Children's Hospital in August of 1963. More than a few investigators wondered whether CPB technology, as opposed to new and unproved infant respirators, could benefit these patients.

In 1965, Rashkind and coworkers,[4] using a femoral arteriovenous shunt and a bubble oxygenator, first attempted to employ extracorporeal circulation to support a neonate dying of respiratory failure. In 1969, Dorson and colleagues[5] reported the first use of a membrane oxygenator for the perfusion support of infants. Similar work was reported by White et al[6] and by Pyle and coworkers.[7] However, none of the infants so treated survived. Bartlett used ECMO to support a neonate in 1973, and treated the first neonatal ECMO survivor[2] in 1975. Subsequently, Drs. Bartlett,[8-11] Kolobow,[12-14] Salzberg and Krummel,[15,16] Hardesty,[17,18] and others did much to refine ECMO for the cardiopulmonary support of neonates with life-threatening lung disease.

The ECMO story reads quite differently with respect to the treatment of adults. The first adult patient to be offered long-term support with a membrane oxygenator for life-threatening pulmonary disease was a 24-year-old man treated by Dr. J. Donald Hill for "shock lung syndrome" following a motorcycle accident.[19] The perfusion lasted a total of 75 hours and had a favorable outcome. However, subsequent results were more variable. The early adult ECMO experience is best summarized in the 1979 report by Zapol et al[20] of a nine-hospital collaborative trial conducted under the auspices of the National Institutes of Health (NIH). Ninety patients were admitted to the study, of whom 48 were treated with mechanical ventilation alone and 42 were treated with mechanical ventilation plus partial venovenous, venoarterial, or mixed bypass support. Ultimately, only three of the control patients and four of the ECMO patients survived. Although there are many explanations for this disappointing outcome,[21] it had a chilling effect on the general level of enthusiasm for ECMO.

However, Bartlett and colleagues, encouraged by their local success, continued their development of neonatal ECMO. In 1984, they reported an overall survival rate of 80% in term infants supported on ECMO for persistent pulmonary hypertension.[22] Soon other centers began to report patient series with similar survival rates. Loe[23] from New Orleans reported 21/30 (70%) survivors; Short[24] from Washington, D.C., reported 18/23 (78%) survivors; and Bartlett[25] reported 72/100 (72%) survivors from his personal series in 1986. By 1987, Redmond[26] reported 36/40 survivors (90%) and Short[27,28] reported 84/100 survivors. A summary of the nationwide experience (18 centers) from the ECMO Registry as of June 1986 was published by Toomasian and others[29] in 1988. The survival rate in this group of 715 patients was 81%. The largest and most current summary of neonatal ECMO results is similarly derived from the ECMO Registry now maintained by the Extracorporeal Life Support Organization (ELSO).[30] This summary notes an overall survival rate of 83% among 3528 infants.

With the advent of improved equipment and methods, ECMO is again being used to treat older pediatric and adult patients. Gattinoni and colleagues[31-33] have shown dramatically improved results in the application of ECMO technology to adult patients, as have Snider and associates,[34] Wagner and colleagues,[35] Bindslev,[36] Bjertnaes et al,[37] Lennartz and Wagner,[38] and others.[39,40] In all, more than 500 adult patients have been treated with ECMO for life-threatening respiratory failure with an aggregate survival rate of around 45%. The substantial experience with adult ECMO in Europe has not been extensively published. The largest single-center experience reported to date is that from the University of Michigan[41] where 45% survival was reported for a group of 40 patients.

Long-term extracorporeal circulation has been applied, in adult patients, to the treatment of diseases as varied as chickenpox pneumonia,[42] peritonitis,[43] sickle chest syndrome,[44] refractory asthma,[45] and cardiogenic shock,[46] and has been used as a bridge to lung transplantation.[47-49] However, adult ECMO—or "$ECCO_2R$" (extracorporeal carbon dioxide removal), as its "low flow" version is sometimes called—must yet be viewed with caution because of the inherently poorer prognosis of patients with long-established cardiac, respiratory, or other diseases. It is also possible that the need for ECMO among adult patients may decrease as the success rate of "conventional" therapies improves[50] (and the same can be said, of course, with regard to neonates). Indeed, the recent report of a prospective randomized comparison of $ECCO_2R$ to pressure-controlled inverse ratio ventilation in adult patients with severe adult respiratory distress syndrome[51] showed no difference in survival between the two groups.

Simultaneously with the resurgence of adult ECMO (and generally in completely separate medical institutions) has come the cautious introduction of this technology into pediatric intensive care units. While the procedure is virtually the same as that used for neonatal patients, with the exception of some "upscaling" of size, the diseases for which its use is appropriate, the entry criteria by which patients should be selected, and the balance of its risks and benefits relative to "conventional" therapies are largely unknown. Growing comfort with neonatal ECMO in many centers, along with favorable results from pediatric ECMO in a few centers,[26,52-57] has inspired a multicenter study of pediatric respiratory failure and of the potential role of ECMO in its management. It is hoped that such a project will permit the promulgation of validated guidelines for pediatric ECMO.

To date, 629 pediatric ECMO cases have been reported to the ELSO registry, with an overall survival rate of 49%. O'Rourke and colleagues[58] have reviewed a more recent subset of these patients. In this group of 285 children, the survival rate was 47%. It is difficult to discern whether this represents an improvement in survival over that which would be expected without ECMO given the paucity of mortality predictors for respiratory failure in this age group.[59-61] Again, a prospective study is needed.

Selection Criteria for ECMO Patients

Although a detailed description of the clinical management of ECMO patients is beyond the scope of this chapter, several excellent summaries of technical methods and clinical management protocols have been prepared to which the interested reader is referred.[9,62-65] We shall consider more general issues, such as patient selection and patient outcomes.

The initial consideration must be patient selection. Neonates of less than 34 weeks' gestation have generally been excluded,[66] since their immature cerebral vascular structure is thought to render the risk of dying from an intracranial hemorrhage after systemic heparinization approximately the same as the risk of dying from the underlying heart or lung disease. Neonates with long-established fibrotic and scarring lung disease are also excluded, since it is unlikely that a period of 5 to 14 days on ECMO would produce sufficient healing to change the patient's ultimate prognosis. Using this kind of reasoning, a set of broadly accepted entry criteria has been developed for neonatal ECMO patients (Table 29.1).

Obviously, these criteria are not intended for older patients with respiratory failure. However, the general principles represented by them are broadly applicable. These can be summarized as follows: (1) "do no harm"; (2) reversibility of the underlying lung pathology; (3) absence of other pathologic conditions that might influence the prognosis independently of the degree of lung recovery; and (4) respiratory failure sufficiently severe as to be both life-threatening and unlikely to respond to less risky and invasive therapies. These principles are embodied in items 1, 2, 3-5, and 6 of Table 29.1, respectively.

It may be useful to review how these principles may be applied in general terms to nonneonates. First and fore-

TABLE 29.1. Patient selection criteria for neonatal ECMO.

1. Gestational age at least 34 weeks (birth weight < 2 kg a relative contraindication)
2. Not more than 10 days of mechanical ventilation (relative contraindication)
3. Absence of severe underlying nonpulmonary disease (eg, untreatable congenital heart disease, major malformation syndromes, major chromosomal anomalies, untreatable renal dysfunction)
4. Cranial ultrasound showing no evidence of intracranial hemorrhage (subependymal or "Grade I" hemorrhage a relative contraindication)
5. No uncontrolled bleeding or bleeding diathesis

AND

6. Evidence of severe, refractory respiratory failure as indicated by a) "Oxygenation Index" over 40 on 3 of 5 postductal blood gases at least 30 min apart but not more than 60 min apart (Oxygenation Index defined as Mean Airway Pressure × Fractional Inspired Oxygen Concentration × 100/postductal Pao$_2$). This is reported to correlate with an 80% mortality rate [25,70]

OR

b) AaDo$_2$ = P$_{atm}$ − 47 − Pao$_2$ − Pco$_2$ > 610 for 8 hours (80% mortality)[69] or > 600 for 12 hours (100% mortality)[77]

OR

c) Severe, refractory respiratory failure with sudden decompensation (defined loosely as Pao$_2$ less than 40 torr for 2 hours) unresponsive to maximal medical management in an unstable patient

most, one must ascertain that the use of ECMO for a given patient is not likely to impose more risk than benefit. It is imperative in making this decision that the most quantitative, authoritative, and objective information available be employed in assessing the balance of risks and benefits (ie, don't accept hearsay evidence). Rarely will this assessment be the basis for positively deciding to proceed with ECMO, but it often assists in identifying contraindications.

Second, there must be sound reason to believe that the lung injury, at the time the question is raised, is likely to be reversible within a reasonable period of ECMO support (usually taken to be 3-14 days, though much longer runs have been successful on occasion). At present, it is widely held that patients who have required mechanical ventilation for longer than 10 days are sufficiently unlikely to benefit from a course of ECMO as to make the associated risks unacceptable. It should be added that secondary lung injury, such as that caused by mechanical ventilation and by exposure to high oxygen concentrations, seems to occur more readily with advancing age. Thus, one might consider ECMO for a newborn who has had 12 days of ventilator support, but be anxious about ECMO for a teenager after 7 or 8 days at high ventilator settings.

Third, it is essential to consider the overall context in which respiratory failure has developed. Obviously, the presence of a lethal and untreatable nonpulmonary condition (such as inoperable congenital heart disease, an end-stage neoplasm, or a fatal chromosomal anomaly) renders the potential success of an ECMO run irrelevant. Other conditions may be equally important in defining the ultimate prognosis, but more difficult to quantify, such as brain injury or renal failure. Perhaps the most pressing circumstance in which this principle is raised is the patient with acute (or "adult") respiratory distress syndrome (ARDS) who develops multiorgan system failure. Since such secondary disease commonly contributes significantly to the patient's ultimate demise,[67,68] it has been suggested that the addition of one or two other organ system failures (besides respiratory failure) should disqualify a patient for ECMO.

Finally, before exposing a critical and unstable patient to the cannulation and ligation of major vessels, long-term systemic anticoagulation, potential secondary infection, potential mechanical malfunctions, and the other considerable risks of ECMO, there must be substantive evidence that the patient's respiratory failure is so unlikely to respond to less invasive and less risky measures as to justify the procedure. This is, at best, a very difficult task. No laboratory test for refractory and life-threatening respiratory failure exists. Predictive scales have been devised for neonatal,[25,29,30,69,70] pediatric,[59–61] and adult[20,71] patients; but none has been validated by a large-scale prospective trial, except for the criteria used in the NIH adult and pediatric ECMO study,[67] which may no longer be valid.[50] The predictive scales developed at one institution are not necessarily applicable to cases at the other centers where the patient population and standard treatment strategies are different.[72,73]

The Impact of ECMO on Survival

In order to determine the proper role of ECMO in the management of severe respiratory failure, one must ask whether this procedure in fact improves the survival rate among clearly moribund patients and, if so, how the improvement in survival is to be viewed in terms of the documented residual morbidity. There are two sources of data from which the question of survival may be addressed: anecdotal patient reports and published clinical trials.

Foremost among the anecdotal sources of ECMO patient data is the ECMO Registry. Although there may be hospitals routinely providing ECMO support to neonates, without either publishing their results or participating in national and international meetings on the subject, the paucity of even hearsay reports of such activity implies that virtually all infants treated with this modality have been reported to the Neonatal ECMO Registry which has been maintained since 1980 at the University of Michigan under the direction of Dr. Robert H. Bartlett. Recently expanded to include pediatric, adult, and cardiac cases, this Registry is now managed by ELSO, an international association of clinicians, researchers, inventors, and industry representatives formed to further the development and application of long-term perfusion support technology. Outcome data for 8419 neonates reported to the Registry[74] as of October 1993 demonstrate a survival rate of 81%. Similarly, survival rates have been reported for pediatric (309/629 or 49%), adult (33/95 or 35%), and cardiac (442/1001 or 44%) patients (with most of the adult cases to date having been managed in Europe and not yet submitted to the ELSO Registry). It is instructive to note the variations in survival rate by disease category (Tables 29.2, 29.3, 29.4, and 29.5). Also tabulated by the Registry are the patient and mechanical complication rates. Those for neonatal patients are shown in Tables 29.6 and 29.7, since they are roughly representative.

Data published from individual ECMO centers over the years,[22–28] as well as the two published summaries from the Registry,[29,30] provide greater clinical detail to lend credibility to the substantial survival rate demonstrated among neonatal ECMO patients. These and other investigations have provided data showing that the survival rate for similar patients (based on the use of a variety of predictive scales) without ECMO would be expected to be between 0% and 20%.[15,69,75–78] In contrast, others have reported substantially higher survival rates without ECMO among patients whom they believe to be similar to these ECMO patients.[72,73,79–82]

A controlled trial was conducted by Bartlett and colleagues[75] that included a statistical method designed to minimize the number of patients who would ultimately be assigned to whichever therapy proved to be less effective.

TABLE 29.2. Survival of neonatal ECMO patients by diagnosis.

Diagnosis	No.	Survived	Percent
Meconium aspiration syndrome	3127	2921	93
Respiratory distress syndrome	1008	842	84
Congenital diaphragmatic hernia	1625	952	59
Pneumonia/sepsis	1273	975	77
Air leak syndrome	33	22	67
Persistent pulmonary hypertension	1079	898	83
Other	274	213	78
Total	8419	6823	81

TABLE 29.3. Survival of pediatric ECMO patients by diagnosis.

Diagnosis	No.	Survived	Percent
Bacterial pneumonia	38	18	47
Viral pneumonia	156	78	50
Intrapulmonary hemorrhage	9	6	67
Aspiration	53	31	58
Pneumocystis	7	2	29
ARDS	164	73	45
Other	202	101	50
Total	629	309	49

Although this study demonstrated a significantly higher survival rate for the ECMO than for the conventionally treated group, the unfortunate consequence of their statistical strategy was that the control group consisted of a single patient, resulting in substantial criticism of the study.[83]

A more conventional controlled trial was then conducted by O'Rourke and colleagues.[84] In a two-phase approach, 39 infants were enrolled in the study comparing ECMO to conventional medical management for severe persistent pulmonary hypertension of the newborn (PPHN). In the first phase, infants were to be randomly assigned to one of the two treatments until 4 deaths occurred in either group. As it turned out, there were no deaths among 9 ECMO patients by the time that 4 of 10 conventionally treated infants had died. Thereafter, by design, patients were offered only the more successful of the two treatments (ie, ECMO) until the survival or mortality rate in that group reached statistical significance. This point was reached when 20 additional patients had been supported on ECMO, of whom 19 survived. Thus, the overall survival of the ECMO-treated infants was 97% (28/29), as compared to a survival rate of 60% (6/10) in the control group. Interpretation of this study has also been controversial.

Undoubtedly, discussions will continue over the propriety of employing an invasive and substantially risky therapy to treat neonatal patients with cardiac and/or respiratory failure. However, it is our belief that the considerable body of anecdotal and experimental evidence available justifies the conclusion that ECMO significantly improves survival in this group of patients.

ECMO Complications and Patient Follow-up Studies

If one accepts the argument that ECMO improves survival, the intuitive subsequent question is, "What are the survivors like?" Much concern and considerable controversy have centered on the question of ECMO-related complications,[85,86] and properly so. The risks of neurologic injury, including those potentially associated with ligation of the right common carotid artery and the right internal jugular vein, have been discussed in the literature at length.[87-102] The risk of bleeding is obviously increased during systemic heparinization,[103,104] and the potential for a sudden and catastrophic mishap exists, as noted by Zwischenberger and coworkers.[105] A wide variety of other adverse outcomes have been reported in ECMO patients, including leukopenia,[106] hemolysis,[107] myocardial "stun,"[108-110] arterial embolization,[111,112] cholestasis,[113] exposure to plasticizers,[114] persistent systemic hypertension,[115,116] vocal cord paralysis,[117] and potential sensorineural hearing loss.[118,119] However, taking all of the available data in combination, ECMO appears to add little to the risks attributable to the underlying diseases when

TABLE 29.4. Survival of adult ECMO patients by diagnosis.

Diagnosis	No.	Survived	Percent
Bacterial pneumonia	7	1	14
Viral pneumonia	10	7	70
Intrapulmonary hemorrhage	1	0	0
Aspiration	4	0	0
ARDS	25	14	56
Other respiratory	12	5	42
Cardiac transplant	11	3	27
Mitral valve replacement	2	0	0
Other cardiac	23	3	13
Total	95	33	35

TABLE 29.5. Survival of neonatal and pediatric cardiac ECMO patients by diagnosis.

Diagnosis	No.	Survived	Percent
Perioperative cardiac support	811	339	42
Cardiac transplant	49	20	41
Myocarditis	29	16	55
Myocardiopathy	38	25	66
Other diagnoses	74	42	57
Total	1001	442	44

TABLE 29.6. Patient complications associated with neonatal ECMO.

Complication	No. reported	% reported	% survived
Infarction/hemorrhage by ultrasound	1094	13	50
Infarction/hemorrhage by CT/MRI	290	3	84
Seizures	1127	13	66
Brain death	106	1	0
Other neurologic complications	359	4	71
Gastrointestinal hemorrhage	216	3	53
Bleeding at cannulation site	549	7	73
Bleeding at other surgical site	516	6	53
Hemolysis	822	10	72
Pulmonary hemorrhage	249	3	49
Other hemorrhagic complications	624	7	65
Serum creatinine > 1.5	863	10	58
Dialysis/hemofiltration	1104	13	59
Other renal complications	189	2	58
Cardiac arrhythmia	329	4	60
CPR required	199	2	49
Myocardial stun	517	6	64
Hypertension	925	11	76
Other cardiopulmonary complications	604	7	64
Pneumothorax	461	4	66
Other pulmonary complications	378	4	62
Culture proven infection	506	6	63
White blood cell count suspect	178	2	64
Other infectious complications	116	1	66
Hyperbilirubinemia	595	7	71

TABLE 29.7. Mechanical complications associated with neonatal ECMO.

Complication	No. reported	% reported	% survived
Oxygenator failure	390	5	62
Raceway tubing rupture	26	0	65
Other tubing rupture	94	1	78
Pump malfunction	146	2	80
Heat exchanger malfunction	100	1	73
Clots in blood path	1795	21	76
Air in circuit	467	6	74
Cannula problems	809	10	76
Hemofilter malfunction	64	1	50
Other mechanical complications	794	9	74

they are treated with "conventional" modalities. In newborns, it is difficult to know the true risks of the ECMO procedure, since only the very sickest of term and near-term neonates are supported with ECMO, many of whom suffer substantial morbidity before this intervention is ever instituted.

The growing clinical experience with neonatal ECMO has been accompanied by an increasing body of published data on the outcomes of these patients.[28,120-134] Although a detailed review of these data is beyond the scope of this chapter, a few salient points warrant emphasis. Obvious but often overlooked is the fact that ECMO survivors constitute a high-risk population. Although their clinical outcomes are surprisingly good, given the general severity of their conditions at the time they are considered for ECMO, handicaps and complications across the broad spectrum of the imaginable are observed. Overall, reported series demonstrate about 70% of survivors to have normal neurodevelopmental evaluations, with the remainder being variously divided between "suspect" and "delayed" groups. Similarly, about 70% of survivors are neurologically normal, with the others ranging between minimally and severely affected. However, 80% of survivors were free of any handicap at 1 to 7 years of age in the largest reported follow-up series[124] from an experienced ECMO center, and preliminary reports from another group of more than 100 5-year-old survivors show full-scale, verbal, and performance IQ scores to be normal for the group as a whole. Interestingly, the data do not demonstrate a predilection for lateralizing abnormalities on either side of the brain, whether the right common carotid artery is or is not reconstructed following venoarterial ECMO. Lower-birth-weight infants (2.0–2.5 kg) demonstrate a significantly higher mortality rate and greater incidence of major intracranial hemorrhages than do larger infants as well as a greater risk of developmental delay at 1 to 2 years.[129] Four to 12 percent of survivors exhibit sensorineural hearing loss.

These results compare favorably with those for infants with severe PPHN treated (generally in the "pre-ECMO" era) with conventional methods.[135-145] The most notable and consistent difference between the ECMO-treated and the conventionally treated groups is the higher incidence of sensorineural hearing loss reported from small series of the latter (around 25%). Of course, such comparisons must be made with caution, since they depend on outcomes derived from separate studies and are based on uncontrolled data.

ECMO for Primary Cardiac Failure

The discussion to this point has focused on the use of ECLS for patients with life-threatening respiratory failure, emphasizing the specific case of neonatal patients, since the bulk of our experience so far (and therefore the data) relates to that group. Experience with ECMO has now come full circle, and the technology that was initially developed to provide artificial support of the circulation is again being turned to that purpose. The differences between long-term perfusion support (ie, ECMO) and conventional intraoperative perfusion are several. The degree of support in ECMO is intended to be subtotal, with forward flow amounting to about 80% of the normal resting cardiac output. The cannulation route is intended to minimize the required surgery, and thus to limit the risk of bleeding during long-term anticoagulation; this in turn limits the achievable flow. Both because the flow is subtotal and because the cannulation need not be transthoracic, ECMO is generally not used for intraoperative support. Since the goal is to support intrinsic healing, the duration of the perfusion is typically days or weeks rather than hours; most commonly, "cardiac ECMO" cases run between 5 and 10 days. Given that a period of cardiac standstill is not anticipated, the level of anticoagulation need not be as aggressive as for conventional perfusion, with activated coagulation time (ACT) generally maintained between 180 and 220 seconds. Finally, if desired, the entire procedure can be performed with local anesthesia alone, although the patients in question are generally heavily sedated, and are often pharmacologically paralyzed, for reasons unrelated to the cannulation procedure.

As Table 29.5 indicates, 1001 patients have been supported with ECMO for primary cardiac failure, according to the data in the ELSO Registry. The bulk of these patients (811) were treated because of circulatory failure related to cardiac surgery. The complication rate for all cardiac support cases is substantial, with significant surgical bleeding occurring in 24%, arrhythmias in 15%, other cardiovascular complications in 15%, and mechanical malfunctions in about 25%. The reported survival rate of 42% for the perioperative subgroup is difficult to interpret, since no comparison group of patients with postoperative myocardial decompensation who were not given ECMO has been assembled. A controlled trial would obviously be most difficult to perform. Yet it is the general sense among physicians in the 70 or so centers offering this service that, without ECMO, the survival rate among these patients would be extremely low.

It is instructive to consider what has been published about the effects of venoarterial ECMO on the heart[109,146-152] and about the use of ECMO in cases of severe primary cardiac failure. As early as 1976, Bartlett and colleagues reported the successful use of "prolonged ECMO" for postoperative cardiac failure in an infant.[2] Subsequently, they employed ECMO as a means of preoperative stabilization and postoperative perfusion in 12 infants undergoing surgical repair of congenital heart lesions, all of whom survived.[153] In the same report, they noted five children treated with ECMO for postoperative cardiac failure, only one of whom survived. Morio and coworkers[154] in 1980 reported the use of prolonged ECMO for acute cardiac failure. In 1986, Cullen et al[155] utilized ECMO in a 9-month-old to manage fulminant and refractory pulmonary hypertension occurring after successful repair of a large ventricular septal defect, and suggested that this might be a very effective if uncommon application of ECMO technology. Following success at several centers with adults, Kanter and colleagues[156] reported using ECMO to treat refractory postoperative cardiac failure in 13 children, with 5 long-term survivors, all of whom had normal cardiac function. Similarly, Redmond and colleagues[26] treated 5 infants and 4 children with cardiac disease, of whom 3 and 1, respectively, survived, and Rogers et al[157] reported survival in 7 of their 10 patients. Weinhaus and colleagues[158] emphasized that outcomes were better if a period of postoperative stabilization could be achieved and if cervical rather than thoracic cannulation were used to minimize hemorrhagic complications.

In spite of growing experience with cardiac ECMO,[55] outcomes did not continue to improve, especially among patients placed on ECMO intraoperatively, until Klein and coworkers[159] suggested surgical decompression of the left as well as the right heart (using, for example, both left and right atrial drains). The reasoning, which was not new with this group,[160-163] is that venoarterial ECMO results in preload depletion of both ventricles and dramatically increased afterload of the left ventricle. This may in turn lead both to circulatory insufficiency and to sudden and massive pulmonary hemorrhage. It has been suggested that the effects of increased afterload on the failing heart may be further exacerbated by the preferential delivery of poorly saturated blood to the coronaries during ECMO.[164-168] It is thus not surprising that patients placed on venoarterial ECMO following a period of respiratory failure and severe hypoxia occasionally develop sudden cardiac failure.[108-110,169,170]

One of the more dramatic applications of ECMO has been its relatively recent use as a "bridge" to cardiac transplantation. Pennington and colleagues[171] reported in 1989 the use of a variety of circulatory support devices for this purpose. Seventeen patients were assisted, of whom two were placed on ECMO. Both died after transplantation, "in part as a result of ECMO complications." In 1990, Delius and coworkers[172] summarized the Ann Arbor experience using ECMO in this context. Three patients were placed on ECMO while awaiting cardiac transplantation, and three others were perfused for cardiac failure occurring after transplantation. None of the "bridge" patients survived, two of the post-transplant patients survived, and all of the patients awaiting transplantation developed contraindications while on ECMO, making them noncandidates for transplantation. The mean time of support in these two groups was 147.5 hours (range 70-370 hours).

In 1991, Galantowicz and Stolar[173] noted the use of ECMO as an adjunct to cardiac transplantation in 20 pediatric cases: as a bridge to transplantation in 4, in the immediate postoperative period in 10, and to treat late rejection in 6. Twelve were weaned from ECMO with 7 long-term survivors. Only one long-term survivor was in the "bridge-to-transplant" group. Pennington's group has used venoarterial ECMO quite extensively as a means of emergency stabilization for patients with cardiogenic shock,[174] including patients who either were awaiting transplantation or had suffered a transplant graft rejection. Over a 9-year period, they supported 38 patients, 9 of whom were long-term survivors. Although ECMO achieved hemodynamic stabilization in 35 of the 38 patients, it was concluded that ECMO should be exchanged for "more sophisticated devices" within 12 to 24 hours of cannulation. As a result of these and other similar experiences, enthusiasm for the use of ECMO in patients awaiting cardiac transplantation has waned substantially, especially for patients, such as neonates, for whom the delay is likely to be prolonged.

Financial Considerations

The initial cost of providing ECMO support is quite high, owing to the expense of the equipment, the extensive training required, the fact that the procedure is relatively "personnel-intense," and the extensive laboratory monitoring which must be performed. Some data, from both published and unpublished sources, are available relative to the costs of "respiratory" ECMO for neonatal patients. Based on discussions with a number of ECMO centers, the average cost of all goods and services utilized for a typical ECMO patient, excluding physician's fees, is generally between $5,000 and $6,500 per day during the run, whereas the average daily cost for a neonatal intensive care unit patient when not on ECMO is commonly $1,500 to $3,000 per day. Average cost data are not tabulated in the ELSO Registry; consequently, these figures represent only a rough approximation based on informal discussions among directors of ECMO centers. The average length of an ECMO run is 5.2 days, according to data from the Registry. If we take the average daily cost at $5,000, and the average run length at 5 days, the average cost of an ECMO run can be approximated at $25,000, excluding physician's fees. If the average daily cost of "routine" newborn ICU care is estimated at $2,000 per day, then the excess cost of the ECMO run is approximately $15,000. The actual amount billed against these costs may vary widely among hospitals and health care systems.

The average length of hospital stay for ECMO survivors at several centers is around 30 days, including time spent after return to the referring hospital prior to final discharge. This number is similar to the 25 days cited by

Pearson et al[175] for their group of ECMO survivors. However, we have not been able to reproduce the dramatic decrease in length of hospital stay for ECMO as compared to "pre-ECMO" survivors, as reported by Pearson (25.0 down from 75.8 days), since the duration of hospitalization among our comparable non-ECMO survivors (using either historical controls or prospectively followed "near-ECMO" patients) has been only slightly longer (34.7 days) than that of our ECMO survivors.

Taking these pieces of information together, we estimate that hospital costs for ECMO will run approximately $15,000 higher for the days on ECMO, but will be decreased by about $10,000 (5 days at $2,000 per day) due to the shortened total length of hospital stay. Obviously, these are approximations. Nonetheless, they highlight the fact that ECMO may not actually save money at its current stage of development. It is very likely, as the technology improves and the associated personnel and laboratory support requirements decrease, that neonatal ECMO will become less expensive, and may even save money over conventional therapy. In the meantime, it is hoped that administrators and other cost-conscious persons who make such decisions will find the improvement in survival to be sufficient justification for the small increase in cost.

Prospects for the Future

We are now entering a period of rapid technological development in ECMO. Ultra-thin-walled catheters are becoming available that might make alternate cannulation routes feasible for extracorporeal circulation, eliminating the necessity of carotid cannulation and ligation. A number of centers have reported their experience with carotid and jugular reconstruction following ECMO.[176-182] The technique for single-cannula venovenous bypass of neonates, long in development and well documented in the literature, has been refined by Kolobow,[14,183] Zwischenberger,[184,185] and others.[186,187] A multicenter clinical trial[188] and a retrospective comparison[189] have demonstrated the feasibility and desirability of this approach. It has even been shown to be effective in cases of marked circulatory insufficiency.[190] Today, most neonates requiring ECMO support do not need to have their carotid arteries instrumented at all. In France, the use of an older but clever pump system has made "tidal flow" venovenous bypass, using a conventional catheter, remarkably simple and very successful for both neonatal and pediatric patients.

A new, integrated, servo-regulated ECMO system that is small, easily transportable, computer-driven, simpler, and safer than existing devices is nearing the marketing stage. This device does not require a venous control module and will likely not require a heat exchanger in most applications. The pump draws directly from the patient, eliminating the need for "gravity feed" of blood to the pump, which in turn shortens the ECMO tubing circuit substantially. This and other tubing modifications have resulted in a circuit which has many fewer ports and connectors, making "anticoagulation" of the circuit much more feasible.

Several chemical treatments have now been licensed for sale which bind heparin to the plastics of the ECMO circuit. If the growing experience with these products is as positive as the initial reports would predict,[191-195] the consequences could be quite exciting. Not only may earlier and safer institution of bypass support in patients with respiratory failure be desirable, but ECMO might find relatively safe applications for premature babies with respiratory insufficiency.

New and less traumatic methods of pulmonary management during ECMO have been proposed, including concurrent high-frequency oscillatory ventilation[196,197] and higher levels of positive end-expiratory pressure (PEEP).[198,199] The goal in this approach is that ventilator-associated lung injury might be reduced along with the associated chronic pulmonary conditions, such as bronchopulmonary dysplasia in neonates.

The potential for providing complete respiratory support through a percutaneously placed double-lumen catheter, using a simplified computer-driven ECMO system and without the need for systemic anticoagulation, could revolutionize our approach to respiratory failure. It is thus likely, in the context of demonstrated clinical value and rapid technological improvements, that long-term perfusion support will play an important role in the future development of intensive care medicine.

Summary

Extracorporeal membrane oxygenation (ECMO) is a means for providing respiratory and/or circulatory support to critically ill patients for periods of days or weeks. It involves extracorporeal circulation just as intraoperative CPB does, but it does not require general anesthesia, a thoracotomy, or complete anticoagulation. Although the technology employed has its roots in the pioneering efforts of Gibbon, Dennis, and others, its acceptance as a "rescue" modality for medical intensive care patients is of much more recent date. It has been most frequently and successfully utilized to support term or near-term neonates with refractory respiratory failure associated with congenital diaphragmatic hernia, meconium aspiration, pneumonia, and similar conditions. In addition, favorable outcomes have been reported in older pediatric and adult patients with respiratory failure as well as in patients with isolated circulatory failure. The use of ECMO for non-neonates is still controversial, however, and patient selection criteria are not well defined.

As more experience is gained and the technology improves, it is conceivable that ECMO will come to be employed more extensively. It is likely that more premature infants will be supported as the risk of bleeding declines. Percutaneous cannulation and the availability of computer-controlled systems might make ECMO appealing for a larger subset of ventilated patients. The use of synchronized, pulsatile ECMO might make weeks of circulatory support feasible.

More novel applications might also be entertained. For example, extracorporeal circulation might find greater use for toxin removal or localized chemotherapy. Patients with chronic pulmonary insufficiency might receive nocturnal perfusion support for normalization of blood gases and acid-base balance much as periodic hemodialysis is employed today. Prototype devices already herald the day when artificial lungs will be implanted orthotopically for continuous respiratory supplementation. And the artificial uterus or artificial placenta may yet revolutionize our approach to extremely premature infants.

It is of paramount importance as such innovations are introduced that eagerness not be allowed to overrun careful experimentation. ECMO has been demonstrated to improve survival only in a small and carefully selected subset of critically ill newborns. The fact that we are able to adapt it to other applications does not necessarily mean that we should. More widespread use of this invasive, personnel-intense, and risky procedure must be based on carefully controlled trials.

References

1. Wegman ME. Annual summary of vital statistics-1990. *Pediatrics* 1991;88:1081-1092.
2. Bartlett RH, Gazzaniga AB, Jefferies MR, Huxtable RF, Haiduc NJ, Fong SW. Extracorporeal membrane oxygenation (ECMO) cardiopulmonary support in infancy. *Trans Am Soc Artif Intern Organs* 1976;22:80-93.
3. Cornish JD, Carter JM, Gerstmann DR, Null DM, Jr. Extracorporeal membrane oxygenation as a means of stabilizing and transporting high risk neonates. *ASAIO Trans* 1991;37:564-568.
4. Rashkind WJ, Freeman A, Klein D, Troft RW. Evaluation of a disposable plastic, low volume, pumpless oxygenator as a lung substitute. *J Pediatr* 1965;66:94-102.
5. Dorson WJ, Baker E, Cohen ML, et al. A perfusion system for infants. *Trans Am Soc Artif Intern Organs* 1969;15:155-160.
6. White JJ, Andrews HG, Risemberg H, Mazur D, Haller JA Jr. Prolonged respiratory support in newborn infants with a membrane oxygenator. *Surgery* 1971;70:288-296.
7. Pyle RB, Helton WC, Johnson FW, et al. Clinical use of the membrane oxygenator. *Arch Surg* 1975;110:966-970.
8. Bartlett RH, Gazzaniga AB, Huxtable RF, Schippers HC, O'Connor MJ, Jefferies MR. Extracorporeal circulation (ECMO) in neonatal respiratory failure. *J Thorac Cardiovasc Surg* 1977;74:826-833.
9. Bartlett RH, Gazzaniga AB. Extracorporeal circulation for cardiopulmonary failure. *Curr Probl Surg* 1978;15:1-96.
10. Bartlett RH, Gazzaniga AB, Huxtable RH, et al. Extracorporeal membrane oxygenation (ECMO) in newborn respiratory failure: technical consideration. *Trans Am Soc Artif Intern Organs* 1979;25:473-475.
11. Bartlett RH, Andrews AF, Toomasian JM, Haiduc NJ, Gazzaniga AB. Extracorporeal membrane oxygenation for newborn respiratory failure: forty-five cases. *Surgery* 1982;92:425-433.
12. Kolobow T, Bowman RL. Construction and evaluation of an alveolar membrane artificial heart-lung. *Trans Am Soc Artif Intern Organs* 1963;9:238-243.
13. Kolobow T, Gattinoni L, Tomlinson T, Pierce JE. An alternative to breathing. *J Thorac Cardiovasc Surg* 1978;75:261-266.
14. Kolobow T, Fumagalli R, Arosio P, Chen V, Buckhold DK, Pierce JE. The use of the extracorporeal membrane lung in the successful resuscitation of severely hypoxic and hypercapnic fetal lambs. *Trans Am Soc Artif Intern Organs* 1982;28:365-368.
15. Krummel TM, Greenfield LJ, Kirkpatrick BV, Mueller DG, Ormazabal M, Salzberg AM. Clinical use of an extracorporeal membrane oxygenator in neonatal pulmonary failure. *J Pediatr Surg* 1982;17:525-531.
16. Kirkpatrick BV, Krummel TM, Mueller DG, Ormazabal MA, Greenfield LJ, Salzberg AM. Use of extracorporeal membrane oxygenation for respiratory failure in term infants. *Pediatrics* 1983;72:872-876.
17. Griffith BP, Borovetz HS, Hardesty RL, Hung TK, Bahnson HT. Arteriovenous ECMO for neonatal respiratory support. A study in perigestational lambs. *J Thorac Cardiovasc Surg* 1979;77:595-601.
18. Hardesty RL, Griffith BP, Debski RF, Jeffries MR, Borovetz HS. Extracorporeal membrane oxygenation. Successful treatment of persistent fetal circulation following repair of congenital diaphragmatic hernia. *J Thorac Cardiovasc Surg* 1981;81:556-563.
19. Hill JD, O'Brien TG, Murray JJ, et al. Prolonged extracorporeal oxygenation for acute post-traumatic respiratory failure (shock-lung syndrome). Use of the Bramson Membrane Lung. *N Engl J Med* 1972;286:629-634.
20. Zapol WM, Snider MT, Hill JD, et al. Extracorporeal membrane oxygenation in severe acute respiratory failure. A randomized prospective study. *JAMA* 1979;242:2193-2196.
21. Pierce EC. Is extracorporeal membrane oxygenation a viable technique? *Ann Thorac Surg* 1981;31:102-104.
22. Andrews AF, Roloff DW, Bartlett RH. Use of extracorporeal membrane oxygenator in persistent pulmonary hypertension of the newborn. *Clin Perinatol* 1984;11:729-735.
23. Loe WA Jr, Graves ED III, Ochsner JL, Falterman KW, Arensman RM. Extracorporeal membrane oxygenation for newborn respiratory failure. *J Pediatr Surg* 1985;20:684-688.

24. Short BL, Pearson GD. Neonatal extracorporeal membrane oxygenation: a review. *J Intensive Care Med* 1986;1: 47-54.
25. Bartlett RH, Gazzaniga AB, Toomasian J, et al. Extracorporeal membrane oxygenation (ECMO) in neonatal respiratory failure. 100 cases. *Ann Surg* 1986;204:236-245.
26. Redmond CR, Graves ED, Falterman KW, Ochsner JL, Arensman RM. Extracorporeal membrane oxygenation for respiratory and cardiac failure in infants and children. *J Thorac Cardiovasc Surg* 1987;93:199-204.
27. Miller MK, Short BL, Glass P, Lotze A, Anderson KD. Outcome of 100 infants treated with extracorporeal membrane oxygenation (ECMO). *Pediatr Res* 1987;21:369A (Abstract).
28. Glass P, Miller M, Short B. Morbidity for survivors of extracorporeal membrane oxygenation: neurodevelopmental outcome at 1 year of age. *Pediatrics* 1989;83:72-78.
29. Toomasian JM, Snedecor SM, Cornell RG, Cilley RE, Bartlett RH. National experience with extracorporeal membrane oxygenation for newborn respiratory failure. Data from 715 cases. *ASAIO Trans* 1988;34:140-147.
30. Stolar CJ, Snedecor SM, Bartlett RH. Extracorporeal membrane oxygenation and neonatal respiratory failure: experience from the Extracorporeal Life Support Organization. *J Pediatr Surg* 1991;26:563-571.
31. Gattinoni L, Pesenti A, Kolobow T, Damia G. A new look at therapy of the adult respiratory distress syndrome: motionless lungs. *Int Anesthesiol Clin* 1983;21:97-117.
32. Gattinoni L, Pesenti A, Mascheroni D, et al. Low-frequency positive-pressure ventilation with extracorporeal CO_2 removal in severe acute respiratory failure. *JAMA* 1986;256:881-910.
33. Pesenti A, Gattinoni L, Kolobow T, Damia G. Extracorporeal circulation in adult respiratory failure. *ASAIO Trans* 1988;34:43-47.
34. Snider MT, Campbell DB, Kofke WA, et al. Venovenous perfusion of adults and children with severe acute respiratory distress syndrome. The Pennsylvania State University experience from 1982-1987. *Trans Am Soc Artif Intern Organs* 1988;34:1014-1020.
35. Wagner PK, Knoch M, Sangmeister C, Muller E, Lennartz H, Rothmund M. Adult respiratory distress syndrome. Associated morbidity and its surgical treatment. *Br J Surg* 1990;77:1395-1398.
36. Bindslev L, Bohm C, Jolin A, Hambraeus Jonzon K, Olsson P, Ryniak S. Extracorporeal carbon dioxide removal performed with surface-heparinized equipment in patients with ARDS. *Acta Anaesthesiol Scand Suppl* 1991;95:125-130.
37. Bjertnaes LJ, Olafsen K, Nilsen PA, et al. [Extracorporeal membrane oxygenation. A therapeutic alternative in acute heart and/or pulmonary failure?]. *Tidsskr Nor Laegeforen* 1991;111:1477-1480.
38. Lennartz H, Wagner P. [Extracorporeal membrane oxygenation and CO_2 elimination]. *Langenbecks Arch Chir Suppl Ii Verh Dtsch Ges Forsch Chir* 1990;P1113-9.:-9.
39. Pesenti A, Kolobow T, Gattinoni L. Extracorporeal respiratory support in the adult. *ASAIO Trans* 1988;34:1006-1008.
40. Sinard JM, Bartlett RH. Extracorporeal life support in critical care medicine. *J Crit Care* 1990;5:265-278.
41. Anderson H III, Steimle C, Shapiro M, et al. Extracorporeal life support for adult cardiorespiratory failure. *Surgery* 1993;114:161-172.
42. Clark GP, Dobson PM, Thickett A, Turner NM. Chickenpox pneumonia, its complications and management. A report of three cases, including the use of extracorporeal membrane oxygenation. *Anaesthesia* 1991;46:376-380.
43. Abdullaev EG, Babyshin VV. [Plasmapheresis with extracorporeal membrane oxygenation of the blood in the treatment of peritonitis]. *Klin Khir* 1989;4:47-48.
44. Gillett DS, Gunning KE, Sawicka EH, Bellingham AJ, Ware RJ. Life threatening sickle chest syndrome treated with extracorporeal membrane oxygenation. *Br Med J [Clin Res]* 1987;294:81-82.
45. King D, Smales C, Arnold AG, Jones OG. Extracorporeal membrane oxygenation as emergency treatment for life-threatening acute severe asthma. *Postgrad Med J* 1986;62: 855-857.
46. Pennington DG, Merjavy JP, Codd JE, Swartz MT, Miller LL, Williams GA. Extracorporeal membrane oxygenation for patients with cardiogenic shock. *Circulation* 1984;70: I130-I137.
47. Jurmann MJ, Haverich A, Demertzis S, Schaefers HJ, Wagner TO, Borst HG. Extracorporeal membrane oxygenation as a bridge to lung transplantation. *Eur J Cardiothorac Surg* 1991;5:94-97.
48. Jurmann MJ, Haverich A, Demertzis S, et al. Extracorporeal membrane oxygenation (ECMO): extended indications for artificial support of both heart and lungs. *Int J Artif Organs* 1991;14:771-774.
49. Demertzis S, Haverich A, Ziemer G, et al. Successful lung transplantation for posttraumatic adult respiratory distress syndrome after extracorporeal membrane oxygenation support. *J Heart Lung Transplant* 1992;11:1005-1007.
50. Suchyta MR, Clemmer TP, Orme JF Jr, Morris AH, Elliott CG. Increased survival of ARDS patients with severe hypoxemia (ECMO criteria). *Chest* 1991;99:951-955.
51. Morris AH, Wallace CJ, Menlove RL, et al. Randomized clinical trail of pressure-controlled inverse ratio ventilation and extracorporeal CO_2 removal for adult respiratory distress syndrome. *Am J Respir Crit Care Med* 1994;149:295-305.
52. Trento A, Thompson A, Siewers RD, et al. Extracorporeal membrane oxygenation in children. New trends. *J Thorac Cardiovasc Surg* 1988;96:542-547.
53. Klein MD, Arensman RM, Weber TR, Mottaghy K, Langer R, Nolte SH. Pediatric ECMO. Directions for new developments. *ASAIO Trans* 1988;34:978-985.
54. Frenckner B, Palmer K, Ehren H. [Preliminary experiences show good results. Extracorporeal membrane oxygenation in respiratory insufficiency in children.] *Lakartidningen* 1990;87:3505-6, 3511.
55. Anderson HL III, Attorri RJ, Custer JR, Chapman RA, Bartlett RH. Extracorporeal membrane oxygenation for pediatric cardiopulmonary failure. *J Thorac Cardiovasc Surg* 1990;99:1011-1019.

56. Adolph V, Heaton J, Steiner R, Bonis S, Falterman K, Arensman R. Extracorporeal membrane oxygenation for nonneonatal respiratory failure. *J Pediatr Surg* 1991;26:326–330.
57. Extracorporeal membrane oxygenation. Consensus development statement. Australian Association of Paediatric Teaching Centres, in conjunction with the National Health & Medical Research Council and Royal Children's Hospital, Melbourne. *Int J Technol Assess Health Care* 1991;7:100–105.
58. O'Rourke PP, Stolar CJ, Zwischenberger JB, Snedecor SM, Bartlett RH. Extracorporeal membrane oxygenation: support for overwhelming pulmonary failure in the pediatric population. Collective experience from the extracorporeal life support organization. *J Pediatr Surg* 1993;28:523–528.
59. Rivera RA, Butt W, Shann F. Predictors of mortality in children with respiratory failure: possible indications for ECMO. *Anaesth Intensive Care* 1990;18:385–389.
60. Timmons OD, Dean JM, Vernon DD. Mortality rates and prognostic variables in children with adult respiratory distress syndrome. *J Pediatr* 1991;119:896–899.
61. Tamburro RF, Bugnitz MC, Stidham GL. Alveolar-arterial oxygen gradient as a predictor of outcome in patients with nonneonatal pediatric respiratory failure. *J Pediatr* 1991;119:935–938.
62. Bartlett RH, Gazzaniga AB. Physiology and pathophysiology of extracorporeal circulation. In: Ionescu MI, Wooler GH, eds. *Current Techniques in Extracorporeal Circulation*. London: Butterworths; 1980:1–44.
63. Hirschl RB, Bartlett RH. Extracorporeal membrane oxygenation support in cardiorespiratory failure. *Adv Surg* 1988;21:189–211.
64. Zwischenberger JB, Bartlett RH. Extracorporeal circulation for respiratory or cardiac failure. In: Civetta JM, Taylor RW, Kirby RR, eds. *Critical Care*. 2nd ed. Philadelphia: Lippincott; 1992:1809–1820.
65. Bartlett RH. Extracorporeal life support for cardiopulmonary failure. *Curr Probl Surg* 1990;27:621–705.
66. Bui KC, LaClair P, Vanderkerhove J, Bartlett RH. ECMO in premature infants. Review of factors associated with mortality. *ASAIO Trans* 1991;37:54–59.
67. Bartlett RH, Morris AH, Fairley HB, Hirsch R, O'Connor N, Pantoppidan H. A prospective study of acute hypoxic respiratory failure. *Chest* 1986;89:684–689.
68. Montgomery AB, Stager MA, Carrico CJ, Hudson LD. Causes of mortality in patients with the adult respiratory distress syndrome. *Am Rev Respir Dis* 1985;132:485–489.
69. Beck R, Anderson KD, Pearson GD, Cronin J, Miller MK, Short BL. Criteria for extracorporeal membrane oxygenation in a population of infants with persistent pulmonary hypertension of the newborn. *J Pediatr Surg* 1986;21:297–302.
70. Hallman M, Merrit A, Jarvenpaa A, et al. Exogenous human surfactant for treatment of severe respiratory distress syndrome: a randomized prospective clinical trial. *J Pediatr* 1985;106:963–969.
71. Gattinoni L, Pesenti A, Caspani ML, et al. The role of total static lung compliance in the management of severe ARDS unresponsive to conventional treatment. *Intensive Care Med* 1984;10:121–126.
72. Cole CH, Jillson E, Kessler D. ECMO: regional evaluation of need and applicability of selection criteria. *Am J Dis Child* 1988;142:1320–1324.
73. Dworetz AR, Moya FR, Sabo B, Gladstone I, Gross I. Survival of infants with persistent pulmonary hypertension without extracorporeal membrane oxygenation. *Pediatrics* 1989;84:1–6.
74. Extracorporeal Life Support Organization. *ECMO Registry Report*. Ann Arbor, MI: University of Michigan; 1993.
75. Bartlett RH, Roloff DW, Cornell RG, Andrews AF, Dillon PW, Zwischenberger JB. Extracorporeal circulation in neonatal respiratory failure: a prospective randomized study. *Pediatrics* 1985;76:479–487.
76. Ormazabal MA, Kirkpatrick BV, Mueller DG. Alterations of A-a DO_2 in response to tolazoline as a predictor of outcome in neonates with persistent pulmonary hypertension. *Pediatr Res* 1980;14:607. Abstract.
77. Krummel TM, Greenfield LJ, Kirkpatrick BV, et al. Alveolar-arterial oxygen gradients versus the Neonatal Pulmonary Insufficiency Index for prediction of mortality in ECMO candidates. *J Pediatr Surg* 1984;19:380–384.
78. Marsh TD, Wilkerson SA, Cook LN. Extracorporeal membrane oxygenation selection criteria: partial pressure of arterial oxygen versus alveolar-arterial oxygen gradient. *Pediatrics* 1988;82:162–166.
79. Wung J, James LS, Kilchevsky E, James E. Management of infants with severe respiratory failure and persistence of the fetal circulation, without hyperventilation. *Pediatrics* 1985;76:488–494.
80. Hageman JR, Dusik J, Keuler H, Bregman J, Gardner TH. Outcome of persistent pulmonary hypertension in relation to severity of presentation. *Am J Dis Child* 1988;142:293–296.
81. Ortega M, Ramos AD, Platzker ACG, Atkinson JB, Bowman CM. Early prediction of ultimate outcome in newborn infants with severe respiratory failure. *J Pediatr* 1988;113:744–747.
82. Nading JH. Historical controls for extracorporeal membrane oxygenation in neonates. *Crit Care Med* 1989;17:423–425.
83. Ware JH, Epstein MF. Commentary: extracorporeal circulation in neonatal respiratory failure: a prospective randomized study. *Pediatrics* 1985;76:849–851.
84. ORourke PP, Crone RK, Vacanti JP, et al. Extracorporeal membrane oxygenation and conventional medical therapy in neonates with persistent pulmonary hypertension of the newborn: a prospective randomized study. *Pediatrics* 1989;84:957–963.
85. Watson JW, Brown DM, Lally KP, Null D, Clark R. Complications of extracorporeal membrane oxygenation in neonates. *South Med J* 1990;83:1262–1265.
86. Donn SM. ECMO indications and complications. *Hosp Pract [Off]* 1990;25:143–146, 149–150.
87. Bowerman RA, Zwischenberger JB, Andrews AF, Bartlett RH. Cranial sonography of the infant treated with extracorporeal membrane oxygenation. *AJR* 1985;145:161–166.
88. Cilley RE, Zwischenberger JB, Andrews AF, Bowerman

RA, Roloff DW, Bartlett RH. Intracranial hemorrhage during extracorporeal membrane oxygenation in neonates. *Pediatrics* 1986;78:699-704.
89. Taylor GA, Catena LM, Garin DB, Miller MK, Short BL. Intracranial flow patterns in infants undergoing extracorporeal membrane oxygenation: preliminary observations with Doppler US. *Radiology* 1987;165:671-674.
90. Taylor GA, Fitz CR, Miller MK, Garin DB, Catena LM, Short BL. Intracranial abnormalities in infants treated with extracorporeal membrane oxygenation: imaging with US and CT. *Radiology* 1987;165:675-678.
91. Taylor GA, Glass P, Fitz CR, Miller MK. Neurologic status in infants treated with extracorporeal membrane oxygenation: correlation of imaging findings with developmental outcome. *Radiology* 1987;165:679-682.
92. Pearlman JM, Altman DI, Powers WS, Volpe JJ. Cerebral injury and regional cerebral blood flow in newborn infants undergoing extracorporeal membrane oxygenation. *Ann Neurol* 1987;22:421. Abstract.
93. Schumacher RE, Barks JD, Johnston MV, et al. Right-sided brain lesions in infants following extracorporeal membrane oxygenation. *Pediatrics* 1988;82:155-161.
94. Campbell LR, Bunyapen C, Holmes GL, Howell CG Jr, Kanto WP Jr. Right common carotid artery ligation in extracorporeal membrane oxygenation. *J Pediatr* 1988;113:110-113.
95. Mitchell DG, Merton D, Desai H, et al. Neonatal brain: color Doppler imaging. Part II. Altered flow patterns from extracorporeal membrane oxygenation. *Radiology* 1988;167:307-310.
96. Taylor GA, Short BL, Glass P, Ichord R. Cerebral hemodynamics in infants undergoing extracorporeal membrane oxygenation: further observations. *Radiology* 1988;168:163-167.
97. Luisiri A, Graviss ER, Weber T, et al. Neurosonographic changes in newborns treated with extracorporeal membrane oxygenation. *J Ultrasound Med* 1988;7:429-438.
98. Slovis TL, Sell LL, Bedard MP, Klein MD. Ultrasonographic findings (CNS, thorax, abdomen) in infants undergoing extracorporeal membrane oxygenation therapy. *Pediatr Radiol* 1988;18:112-117.
99. Raju TN, Kim SY, Meller JL, Srinivasan G, Ghai V, Reyes H. Circle of Willis blood velocity and flow direction after common carotid artery ligation for neonatal extracorporeal membrane oxygenation. *Pediatrics* 1989;83:343-347.
100. Taylor GA, Fitz CR, Kapur S, Short BL. Cerebrovascular accidents in neonates treated with extracorporeal membrane oxygenation: sonographic-pathologic correlation. *AJR* 1989;153:355-361.
101. Lewin JS, Masaryk TJ, Modic MT, Ross JS, Stork EK, Wiznitzer M. Extracorporeal membrane oxygenation in infants: angiographic and parenchymal evaluation of the brain with MR imaging. *Radiology* 1989;173:361-365.
102. Short BL. Brain lesions and extracorporeal membrane oxygenation. *Pediatrics* 1989;83:634-635.
103. Sell LL, Cullen ML, Whittlesey GC, et al. Hemorrhagic complications during extracorporeal membrane oxygenation: prevention and treatment. *J Pediatr Surg* 1986;21:1087-1091.
104. Anderson HL III, Cilley RE, Zwischenberger JB, Bartlett RH. Thrombocytopenia in neonates after extracorporeal membrane oxygenation. *ASAIO Trans* 1986;32:534-537.
105. Zwischenberger JB, Cilley RE, Hirschl RB, Heiss KF, Conti VR, Bartlett RH. Life-threatening intrathoracic complications during treatment with extracorporeal membrane oxygenation. *J Pediatr Surg* 1988;23:599-604.
106. Zach TL, Steinhorn RH, Georgieff MK, Mills MM, Green TP. Leukopenia associated with extracorporeal membrane oxygenation in newborn infants. *J Pediatr* 1990;116:440-444.
107. Steinhorn RH, Isham Schopf B, Smith C, Green TP. Hemolysis during long-term extracorporeal membrane oxygenation. *J Pediatr* 1989;115:625-630.
108. Pyles LA, Einzig S, Stejskal EA, et al. Myocardial stunning during extracorporeal membrane oxygenation in newborn infants. *Crit Care Med* 1990;18:S244. Abstract.
109. Martin GR, Short BL, Abbott C, O'Brien AM. Cardiac stun in infants undergoing extracorporeal membrane oxygenation. *J Thorac Cardiovasc Surg* 1991;101:607-611.
110. Cater G, Lotze A, Miller M, Short B. Stunned myocardium in an infant treated with extracorporeal membrane oxygenation. *J Pediatr Surg* 1988;23:1011-1013.
111. Fink SM, Bockman DE, Howell CG, Falls DG, Kanto WP Jr. Bypass circuits as the source of thromboemboli during extracorporeal membrane oxygenation. *J Pediatr* 1989;115:621-624.
112. Vogler C, Sotelo Avila C, Lagunoff D, Braun P, Schreifels JA, Weber T. Aluminum-containing emboli in infants treated with extracorporeal membrane oxygenation. *N Engl J Med* 1988;319:75-79.
113. Shneider B, Maller E, VanMarter L, O'Rourke PP. Cholestasis in infants supported with extracorporeal membrane oxygenation. *J Pediatr* 1989;115:462-465.
114. Shneider B, Schena J, Truog R, Jacobson M, Kevy S. Exposure to di(2-ethylhexyl)phthalate in infants receiving extracorporeal membrane oxygenation. *N Engl J Med* 1989;320:1563.
115. Sell LL, Cullen ML, Lerner GR, Whittlesey GC, Shanley CJ, Klein MD. Hypertension during extracorporeal membrane oxygenation: cause, effect, and management. *Surgery* 1987;102:724-730.
116. Boedy RF, Goldberg AK, Howell CG Jr, Hulse E, Edwards EG, Kanto WP Jr. Incidence of hypertension in infants on extracorporeal membrane oxygenation. *J Pediatr Surg* 1990;25:258-261.
117. Schumacher RE, Weinfeld IJ, Bartlett RH. Neonatal vocal cord paralysis following extracorporeal membrane oxygenation. *Pediatrics* 1989;84:793-796.
118. Schumacher RE, Spak C, Kileny PR. Asymmetric brain stem auditory evoked responses in infants treated with extracorporeal membrane oxygenation. *Ear Hear* 1990;11:359-362.
119. Lott IT, McPherson D, Towne B, Johnson D, Starr A. Long-term neurophysiologic outcome after neonatal extracorporeal membrane oxygenation. *J Pediatr* 1990;116:343-349.
120. Krummel TM, Greenfield LJ, Kirkpatrick BV, et al. The early evaluation of survivors after extracorporeal membrane oxygenation for neonatal pulmonary failure. *J Pediatr Surg* 1984;19:585-590.

121. Towne BH, Lott IT, Hicks DA, Healey T. Long-term follow-up of infants and children treated with extracorporeal membrane oxygenation (ECMO): a preliminary report. *J Pediatr Surg* 1985;20:410–414.
122. Andrews AF, Nixon CA, Cilley RE, Roloff DW, Bartlett RH. One- to three-year outcome for 14 neonatal survivors of extracorporeal membrane oxygenation. *Pediatrics* 1986;78:692–698.
123. Adolph V, Ekelund C, Smith C, Starrett A, Falterman K, Arensman R. Developmental outcome of neonates treated with extracorporeal membrane oxygenation. *J Pediatr Surg* 1990;25:43–46.
124. Schumacher RE, Palmer TW, Roloff DW, LaClaire PA, Bartlett RH. Follow-up of infants treated with extracorporeal membrane oxygenation for newborn respiratory failure. *Pediatrics* 1991;87:451–457.
125. Garg M, Kurzner SI, Bautista DB, et al. Pulmonary sequelae at six months following extracorporeal membrane oxygenation. *Chest* 1992;101:1086–1090.
126. Griffin MP, Minifee PK, Landry SH, Allison PL, Swischuk LE, Zwischenberger JB. Neurodevelopmental outcome in neonates after extracorporeal membrane oxygenation: cranial magnetic resonance imaging and ultrasonography correlation. *J Pediatr Surg* 1992;27:33–35.
127. Paccioretti DC, Haluschak MM, Finer NN, Robertson CM, Pain KS, Hagler M. Auditory brain-stem responses in neonates receiving extracorporeal membrane oxygenation. *J Pediatr* 1992;120:464–467.
128. Park CH, Spitzer AR, Desai HJ, Zhang JJ, Graziani LJ. Brain SPECT in neonates following extracorporeal membrane oxygenation: evaluation of technique and preliminary results. *J Nucl Med* 1992;33:1943–1948.
129. Revenis ME, Glass P, Short BL. Mortality and morbidity rates among lower birth weight infants (2000 to 2500 grams) treated with extracorporeal membrane oxygenation. *J Pediatr* 1992;121:452–458.
130. Schwendeman CA, Clark RH, Yoder BA, Null DM Jr, Gerstmann DR, deLemos RA. Frequency of chronic lung disease in infants with severe respiratory failure treated with high-frequency ventilation and/or extracorporeal membrane oxygenation. *Crit Care Med* 1992;20:372–377.
131. Streletz LJ, Bej MD, Graziani LJ, et al. Utility of serial EEGs in neonates during extracorporeal membrane oxygenation. *Pediatr Neurol* 1992;8:190–196.
132. Flusser H, Dodge NN, Engle WE, Garg BP, West KW. Neurodevelopmental outcome and respiratory morbidity for extracorporeal membrane oxygenation survivors at 1 year of age. *J Perinatol* 1993;13:266–271.
133. Korinthenberg R, Kachel W, Koelfen W, Schultz C, Varnholt V. Neurological findings in newborn infants after extracorporeal membrane oxygenation, with special reference to the EEG. *Dev Med Child Neurol* 1993;35:249–257.
134. Weber TR, Westfall SH, Sotelo C, Vogler CA, Tracy T Jr. A clinical-pathological study of nonsurvivors of newborn ECMO. *J Pediatr Surg* 1993;28:135–137.
135. Brett C, Dekle M, Leonard CH, et al. Developmental follow-up of hyperventilated neonates: preliminary observations. *Pediatrics* 1981;68:588–591.
136. Bernbaum JC, Russell P, Sheridan PH, Gewitz MH, Fox WW, Peckham GJ. Long-term follow-up of newborns with persistent pulmonary hypertension. *Crit Care Med* 1984;12:579–583.
137. Ferrara B, Johnson DE, Chang PN, Thompson TR. Efficacy and neurologic outcome of profound hypocapneic alkalosis for the treatment of persistent pulmonary hypertension in infancy. *J Pediatr* 1984;105:457–461.
138. Sell EJ, Gaines JA, Gluckman C, Williams E. Persistent fetal circulation. Neurodevelopmental outcome. *Am J Dis Child* 1985;139:25–28.
139. Bifano EM, Pfannenstiel A. Duration of hyperventilation and outcome in infants with persistent pulmonary hypertension. *Pediatrics* 1988;81:657–661.
140. Ballard RA, Leonard CH. Developmental follow-up of infants with persistent pulmonary hypertension of the newborn. *Clin Perinatol* 1984;11:737–744.
141. Leavitt AM, Watchko JF, Bennett FC, Folsom RC. Neurodevelopmental outcome following persistent pulmonary hypertension of the neonate. *J Perinatol* 1987;7:288–291.
142. John E, Roberts V, Burnard ED. Persistent pulmonary hypertension of the newborn treated with hyperventilation: clinical features and outcome. *Aust Paediatr J* 1988;24:357–361.
143. Hendricks-Munoz KD, Walton JP. Hearing loss in infants with persistent fetal circulation. *Pediatrics* 1988;81:650–656.
144. Oelberg DG, Temple DM, Haskins KS, Bigelow RH, Adcock EW. Intracranial hemorrhage in term or near-term newborns with persistent pulmonary hypertension. *Clin Pediatr* 1988;27:14–17.
145. Klesh KW, Murphy TF, Scher MS, Buchanan DE, Maxwell EP, Guthrie RD. Cerebral infarction in persistent pulmonary hypertension of the newborn. *Am J Dis Child* 1987;141:852–587.
146. Martin GR, Short BL. Doppler echocardiographic evaluation of cardiac performance in infants on prolonged extracorporeal membrane oxygenation. *Am J Cardiol* 1988;62:929–934.
147. Walther FJ, van de Bor M, Gangitano ES, Snyder JR. Left and right ventricular output in newborn infants undergoing extracorporeal membrane oxygenation. *Crit Care Med* 1990;18:148–151.
148. Taylor GA, Martin GR, Short BL. Cardiac determinants of cerebral blood flow during extracorporeal membrane oxygenation. *Invest Radiol* 1989;24:511–516.
149. Martin GR, Chauvin L, Short BL. Effects of hydralazine on cardiac performance in infants receiving extracorporeal membrane oxygenation. *J Pediatr* 1991;118:944–948.
150. Karr SS, Martin GR, Short BL. Cardiac performance in infants referred for extracorporeal membrane oxygenation. *J Pediatr* 1991;118:437–442.
151. Kimball TR, Daniels SR, Weiss RG, et al. Changes in cardiac function during extracorporeal membrane oxygenation for persistent pulmonary hypertension in the newborn infant. *J Pediatr* 1991;118:431–436.
152. Kinsella JP, McCurnin DC, Clark RH, Lally KP, Null DM Jr. Cardiac performance in ECMO candidates: echocardiographic predictors for ECMO. *J Pediatr Surg* 1992;27:44–47.
153. Bartlett RH, Gazzaniga AB, Wetmore NE, Rucker R, Huxtable RF. Extracorporeal membrane oxygenation (ECMO)

154. Morio S, Yoshino Y, Yorozu H, et al. [Prolonged extracorporeal membrane oxygenation for acute cardiac failure (author's transl)]. *Kyobu Geka* 1980;33:296-300.
155. Cullen M, Splittgerber F, Sweezer W, Hakimi M, Arciniegas E, Klein M. Pulmonary hypertension postventricular septal defect repair treated by extracorporeal membrane oxygenation. *J Pediatr Surg* 1986;21:675-677.
156. Kanter KR, Pennington G, Weber TR, Zambie MA, Braun P, Martychenko V. Extracorporeal membrane oxygenation for postoperative cardiac support in children. *J Thorac Cardiovasc Surg* 1987;93:27-35.
157. Rogers AJ, Trento A, Siewers RD, et al. Extracorporeal membrane oxygenation for postcardiotomy cardiogenic shock in children. *Ann Thorac Surg* 1989;47:903-906.
158. Weinhaus L, Canter C, Noetzel M, McAlister W, Spray TL. Extracorporeal membrane oxygenation for circulatory support after repair of congenital heart defects. *Ann Thorac Surg* 1989;48:206-212.
159. Klein MD, Shaheen KW, Whittlesey GC, Pinsky WW, Arciniegas E. Extracorporeal membrane oxygenation for the circulatory support of chidlren after repair of congenital heart disease. *J Thorac Cardiovasc Surg* 1990;100:498-505.
160. Eugene J, McColgan SJ, Moore Jeffries EW, Ott RA, Haiduc NJ, Roohk HV. Cardiac assist by extracorporeal membrane oxygenation with in-line left ventricular venting. *Trans Am Soc Artif Intern Organs* 1984;30:99-102.
161. Eugene J, Ott RA, McColgan SJ, Roohk HV. Vented cardiac assistance: ECMO versus left heart bypass for acute left ventricular failure. *ASAIO Trans* 1986;32:538-541.
162. Kolobow T, Rossi F, Borelli M, Foti G. Long-term closed chest partial and total cardiopulmonary bypass by peripheral cannulation for severe right and/or left ventricular failure, including ventricular fibrillation. The use of a percutaneous spring in the pulmonary artery position to decompress the left heart. *ASAIO Trans* 1988;34:485-489.
163. Rossi F, Kolobow T, Foti G, Borelli M, Mandava S. Long-term cardiopulmonary bypass by peripheral cannulation in a model of total heart failure. The decompression of the left heart through a percutaneous helical spring positioned within the lumen of the tricuspid and pulmonary artery valves. *J Thorac Cardiovasc Surg* 1990;100:914-920.
164. Secker Walker JS, Edmonds JF, Spratt EH, Conn AW. The source of coronary perfusion during partial bypass for extracorporeal membrane oxygenation (ECMO). *Ann Thorac Surg* 1976;21:138-143.
165. Nowlen TT, Salley SO, Whittlesey GC, Kundu SK, Maniaci NA, Henry RL, Klein MD. Regional blood flow distribution during extracorporeal membrane oxygenation in rabbits. *J Thorac Cardiovasc Surg* 1989;98:1138-1143.
166. Smith HG, Whittlesey GC, Kundu SK, et al. Regional blood flow during extracorporeal membrane oxygenationin lambs. *ASAIO Trans* 1989;35:657-660.
167. Gerstmann DR, Nose K, Kinsella JP, Cornish JD. Left carotid artery (LCA) and coronary (CA) arterial flow partitioning during neonatal ECMO. *Pediatr Res* 1989;25:37A. Abstract.
168. Kinsella JP, Gerstmann DR, Rosenberg AA. The effect of extracorporeal membrane oxygenation on coronary perfusion and regional blood flow distribution. *Pediatr Res* 1992;31:80-84.
169. Dickson ME, Hirthler MA, Simoni J, Bradley CA, Goldthorn JF. Stunned myocardium during extracorporeal membrane oxygenation. *Am J Surg* 1990;160:644-646.
170. Rosenberg EM, Cook LN. Electromechanical dissociation in newborns treated with extracorporeal membrane oxygenation: an extreme form of cardiac stun syndrome. *Crit Care Med* 1991;19:780-784.
171. Pennington DG, McBride LR, Kanter KR, et al. Bridging to heart transplantation with circulatory support devices. *J Heart Transplant* 1989;8:116-123.
172. Delius RE, Zwischenberger JB, Cilley R, et al. Prolonged extracorporeal life support of pediatric and adolescent cardiac transplant patients. *Ann Thorac Surg* 1990;50:791-795.
173. Galantowicz ME, Stolar CJ. Extracorporeal membrane oxygenation for perioperative support in pediatric heart transplantation. *J Thorac Cardiovasc Surg* 1991;102:148-151.
174. Reedy JE, Swartz MT, Raithel SC, Szukalski EA, Pennington DG. Mechanical cardiopulmonary support for refractory cardiogenic shock. *Heart Lung* 1990;19:514-523.
175. Pearson GD, Short BL. An economic analysis of extracorporeal membrane oxygenation. *J Intensive Care Med* 1987;2:116-120.
176. Adolph V, Bonis S, Falterman K, Arensman R. Carotid artery repair after pediatric extracorporeal membrane oxygenation. *J Pediatr Surg* 1990;25:867-869.
177. Karl TR, Iyer KS, Sano S, Mee RB. Infant ECMO cannulation technique allowing preservation of carotid and jugular vessels. *Ann Thorac Surg* 1990;50:488-489.
178. Crombleholme TM, Adzick NS, deLorimier AA, Longaker MT, Harrison MR, Charlton VE. Carotid artery reconstruction following extracorporeal membrane oxygenation. *Am J Dis Child* 1990;144:872-874.
179. Spector ML, Wiznitzer M, Walsh Sukys MC, Stork EK. Carotid reconstruction in the neonate following ECMO. *J Pediatr Surg* 1991;26:357-359.
180. Moulton SL, Lynch FP, Cornish JD, Bejar RF, Simko AJ, Krous HF. Carotid artery reconstruction following neonatal extracorporeal membrane oxygenation. *J Pediatr Surg* 1991;26:794-799.
181. DeAngelis GA, Mitchell DG, Merton DA, et al. Right common carotid artery reconstruction in neonates after extracorporeal membrane oxygenation: color Doppler imaging. *Radiology* 1992;182:521-525.
182. Schaupp W, Brands W, Wirth H, Kachel W, Lasch P, Schmitt B. Reconstruction of the arteria carotis communis in newborn following extracorporeal membrane oxygenation (ECMO). *Eur J Pediatr Surg* 1992;2:78-80.
183. Solca M, Kolobow T, Huang HH, Chen V, Buckhold DK, Pierce JE. Respiratory distress syndrome in immature lambs. Prevention through antenatal accelerated conditioning of the lung. *Am Rev Respir Dis* 1984;129:979-984.
184. Andrews AF, Zwischenberger JB, Cilley RE, Drake KL. Venovenous extracorporeal membrane oxygenation (ECMO) using a double-lumen cannula. *Artif Organs* 1987;11:265-268.
185. Zwischenberger JB, Toomasian JM, Drake K, Andrews AF, Kolobow T, Bartlett RH. Total respiratory support

with single cannula venovenous ECMO: double lumen continuous flow vs. single lumen tidal flow. *Trans Am Soc Artif Intern Organs* 1985;31:610–615.
186. Otsu T, Merz SI, Hultquist KA. Laboratory evaluation of a double lumen catheter for venovenous neonatal ECMO. *ASAIO Trans* 1989;35:647–650.
187. Anderson HL III, Otsu T, Chapman RA, Bartlett RH. Venovenous extracorporeal life support in neonates using a double lumen catheter. *ASAIO Trans* 1989;35:650–653.
188. Anderson HL III, Snedecor SM, Otsu T, Bartlett RH. Multicenter comparison of conventional venoarterial access versus venovenous double-lumen catheter access in newborn infants undergoing extracorporeal membrane oxygenation. *J Pediatr Surg* 1993;28:530–534.
189. Delius R, Anderson H III, Schumacher R, et al. Venovenous compares favorably with venoarterial access for extracorporeal membrane oxygenation in neonatal respiratory failure. *J Thorac Cardiovasc Surg* 1993;106:329–338.
190. Cornish JD, Heiss KF, Clark RH, Strieper MJ, Boecler B, Kesser K. Efficacy of venovenous extracorporeal membrane oxygenation for neonates with respiratory and circulatory compromise. *J Pediatr* 1993;122:105–109.
191. Bindslev L, Eklund J, Norlander O, et al. Treatment of acute respiratory failure by extracorporeal carbon dioxide elimination performed with a surface heparinized artificial lung. *Anesthesiology* 1987;67:117–120.
192. Peters J, Radermacher P, Kuntz ME, et al. Extracorporeal CO_2-removal with a heparin coated artificial lung. *Intensive Care Med* 1988;14:578–584.
193. Marcolin R, Cugno M, Pesenti A, et al. Extracorporeal circulation in sheep with normal bleeding time using a surface heparinized circuit. *Trans Am Soc Artif Intern Organs* 1991;37:584–587.
194. van der Hulst VPM, Grundeman PF, Moulijn AC, Rutten PJJM, Klopper PJ. Long-term extracorporeal blood bypass in dogs at low flows without systemic heparinization. Heparin-coated versus uncoated circuits. *Trans Am Soc Artif Intern Organs* 1991;37:577–583.
195. Bindslev L. Adult ECMO performed with surface-heparinized equipment. *ASAIO Trans* 1988;34:1009–1013.
196. Cornish JD, Gerstmann DR, Clark RH, Carter JM, Null DM Jr, deLemos RA. Extracorporeal membrane oxygenation and high-frequency oscillatory ventilation: potential therapeutic relationships. *Crit Care Med* 1987;15:831–834.
197. Carter JM, Gerstmann DR, Clark RH, et al. High-frequency oscillatory ventilation and extracorporeal membrane oxygenation for the treatment of acute neonatal respiratory failure. *Pediatrics* 1990;85:159–164.
198. Keszler M, Subramanian KN, Smith YA, et al. Pulmonary management during extracorporeal membrane oxygenation. *Crit Care Med* 1989;17:495–500.
199. Keszler M, Ryckman FC, McDonald JV Jr, et al. A prospective, multicenter, randomized study of high versus low positive end-expiratory pressure during extracorporeal membrane oxygenation. *J Pediatr* 1992;120:107–113.

30
The Intravascular Oxygenator, IVOX®: Augmentation of Blood-Gas Transfer

Robert K. Wenger and JD Mortensen

Introduction: Physiologic Goals of Ventilation

The delivery of oxygen to the mitochondria, and the removal of carbon dioxide, is the ultimate goal of respiration. During physiologic respiration, the creation of negative intrathoracic pressure causes the flow of atmospheric air, containing 21% oxygen, to enter the lungs and transit the conducting airways, resulting in delivery to the bronchiole-alveolar complexes. Here, diffusion allows the oxygen to cross the alveolar membrane and enter into an oxyhemoglobin complex. The bound oxygen is then transported back to the left atrium, to the left ventricle, through the arterial tree, and, ultimately, to the mitochondria by simple diffusion. With normal respiratory function, and a normal metabolic state, oxygen delivery far exceeds tissue requirements. Interruption or impedance at any stage of this process, however, significantly affects oxygen delivery at the cellular level. As oxygen delivery lags behind the metabolic needs of the cells, the oxygen content of the circulating blood decreases, and hypoxemia ensues. Hypoxemia is, ultimately, the major threat to life.[1-3]

Augmentation of Oxygen Delivery

The simplest way to increase oxygen delivery is, of course, to increase the oxygen content of inspired air. This is usually initiated via nasal cannula or by oxygen face mask. However, the patient suffering acute respiratory failure (ARF) is tachypneic, with an increased minute ventilation and an increased right and left pulmonary blood-flow shunt, a state that makes difficult the delivery of high oxygen concentrations with these simple devices. Mechanical ventilation is more effective in increasing tissue oxygen delivery, and, when it is combined with positive-end-expiratory pressure (PEEP), adjustments in arterial pH (to shift the oxyhemoglobin dissociation curve), and optimization of hemoglobin as well as cardiac output, it can usually alleviate hypoxemia.[2-4]

Persistent hypoxemia in the face of maximal mechanical support may necessitate the use of an artificial membrane blood-gas exchanger. The system currently employed, extracorporeal membrane oxygenation (ECMO), uses extracorporeal perfusion of an external membrane blood-gas exchange, to augment oxygen delivery, and is described in Chapter 29 of this book. More recently, a new technology has been developed for adding oxygen to circulating venous blood without the need for extracorporeal perfusion. This is the intravenous oxygenator known as IVOX® (Cardiopulmonics, Inc., Salt Lake City, UT).[4-7]

Carbon Dioxide Elimination

Oxidation of carbon causes a continued production of carbon dioxide during the course of normal metabolism. By diffusion, carbon dioxide reaches the circulating blood, where it is transported to the lungs, crosses the alveolar-capillary membrane, again by diffusion, and is then expelled during the passive phase of respiration. Any increase in carbon dioxide production, or interference with the patient's ability to eliminate this metabolic end product, leads to hypercarbia, acidosis, and, ultimately, cellular dysfunction.[1-3]

Normal physiologic responses to hypercarbia include hyperventilation (if physically possible for the patient), increased cardiac output, and increased renal excretion. The physician is also able to aid in these physiologic responses, but, most frequently, mechanical ventilation is required to augment gas flow. Extracorporeal perfusion through a membrane blood-gas exchanger is an effective alternative to the problem of carbon dioxide removal. The intravenous oxygenator—IVOX—may also prove to be an effective, less invasive alternative.[7]

IVOX Design

Using the concept of gradient-drive gas exchange across a gas-permeable, liquid-impermeable membrane, the IVOX has been developed to assist patients in ARF by augmenting oxygen delivery and carbon dioxide removal.[4-6]

The IVOX device is an elongated, hollow-fiber membrane oxygenator fashioned from microporous polypropylene, which is placed within the venae cavae by venotomy. Proper insertion positions the proximal portion of the IVOX device near the caval bifurcation (Figure 30.1). The multiple hollow fibers of IVOX are joined together in a manifold that communicates with a double-lumen gas conduit, both proximally and distally (Figure 30.2).[4-6]

While the materials and the functional characteristics of the IVOX device are similar to those incorporated in the extracoporeal membrane oxygenator, there have been several specific design modifications. Most significantly, the intravenous placement of the device obviates the need for extracorporeal perfusion. The hollow fibers of the oxygenators are crimped, so that, once they are deployed, blood flows over the fibers in a disturbed, or nonlaminar fashion. This nonlaminar flow, combined with the low venous pressure and low velocity of blood flow in the caval system, maximizes blood-synthetic membrane contact, which, in turn, maximizes opportunity for gas exchange.

Two features were included in the design of the intravenous oxygenator to prevent the adverse consequences of free transfer of oxygen to the circulation. A vacuum pump pulls oxygen through the hollow fibers. Because the intraluminal gas pressure remains subatmospheric, any disruption of the fibers will result in blood entering the fibers, rather than gas entering the circulation. Moreover, all outer surfaces of the oxygenator are coated with an ultrathin, continuous siloxane film to prevent any open blood-gas interface or serum leakage into the hollow fibers. To prevent complications related to thrombosis, the surfaces of all components of the device are covalently bonded with heparin.[4-6]

Intravenous oxygenators are manufactured in sizes 7-, 8-, 9-, and 10-mm, as measured at the confluence of the

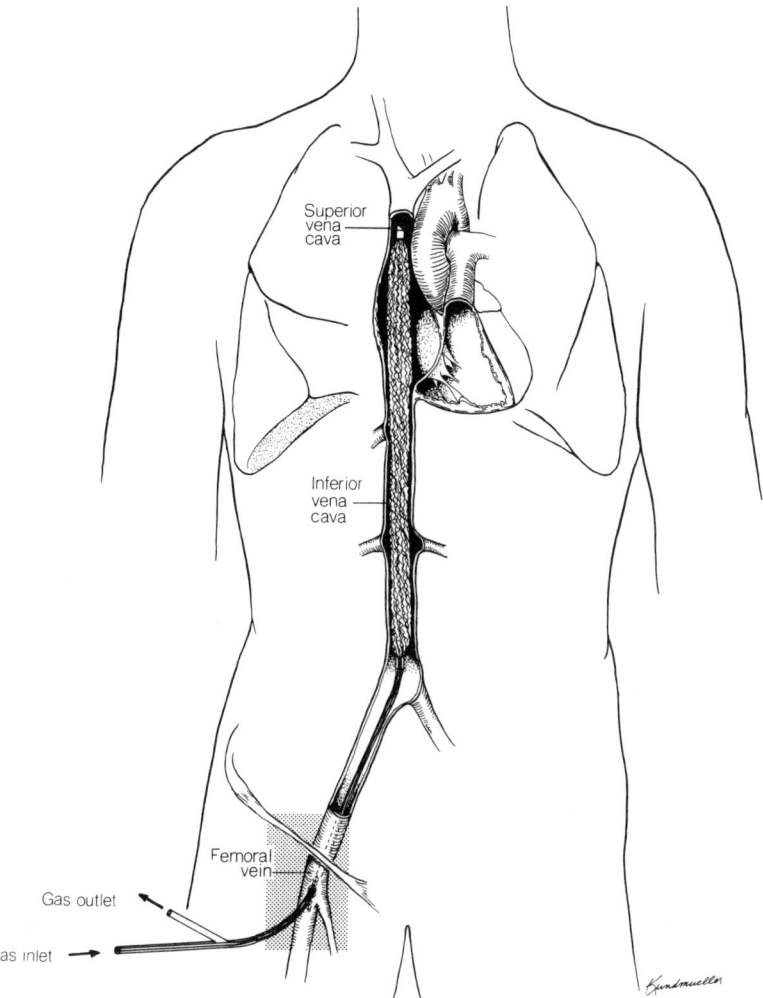

FIGURE 30.1. Diagram of IVOX in its intravenacaval position in a human patient. In this illustration, IVOX has been introduced into the body through a venotomy in the right common femoral vein, then advanced up the iliac vein and inferior vena cava, through the lateral aspect of the right atrium, and up the superior vena cava, with its tip lying in the superior vena cava. The crimped hollow fibers lie free in the venacaval bloodstream. The double-lumen gas conduit connects to the potted manifolds at the ends of the hollow fibers. The inner (inlet) gas conduit is connected to an oxygen source; the outer (outlet) gas conduit is connected to a vacuum pump which pulls the gas through the hollow fibers at controlled subatmospheric pressures. The IVOX device can safely remain functional in the venae cavae for up to 21 days; then (or whenever it is no longer needed), IVOX is removed and the access venotomy is repaired surgically.

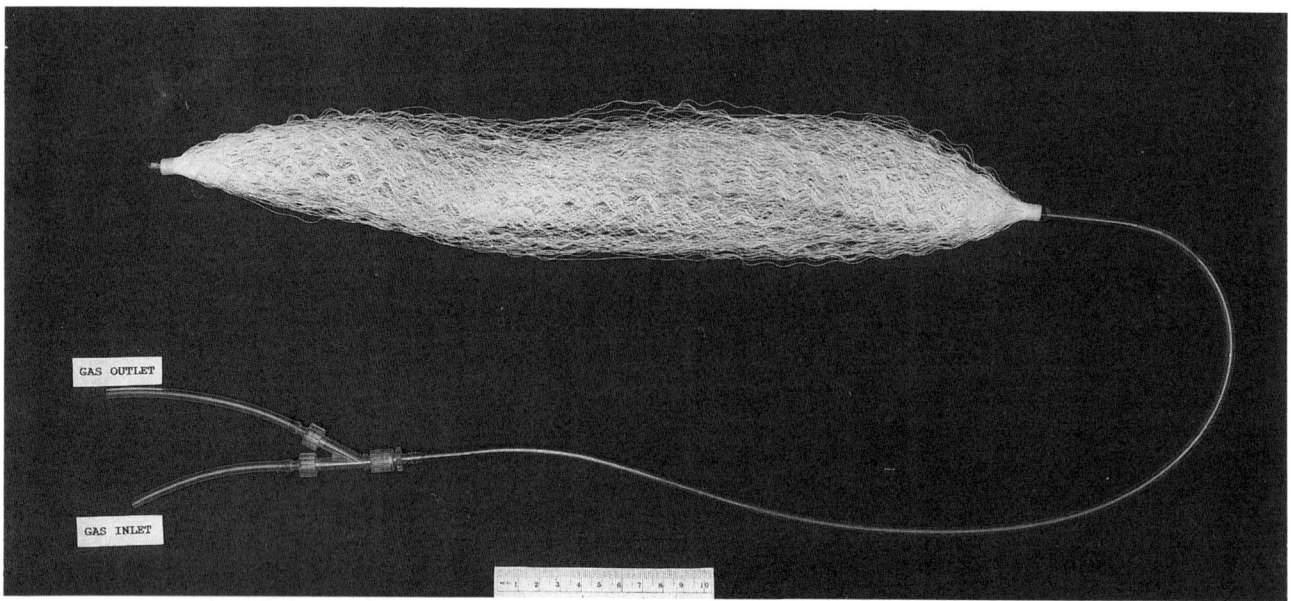

FIGURE 30.2. Photograph of the intravascular blood-gas exchanger (IVOX). The crimped hollow fibers (approximately 1000) lie free in the blood flowing in the superior vena cava, inferior vena cava, and right atrium en route to the right ventricle and lungs. Oxygen enters the inlet limb of the double-lumen gas conduit at atmospheric pressure. It is carried in the central gas conduit to the distal potting where it is distributed into the lumens of the hollow fibers. Gas exchange occurs with the blood outside each hollow fiber through the walls of the hollow fibers. Gas remaining in the hollow fiber lumens exits the body via the outer portion of the double-lumen gas conduit, being pulled through the device by suction applied to the gas outlet limb of the double-lumen gas conduit.

TABLE 30.1. IVOX mechanical/engineering specifications/characteristics.

Dimensional/mechanical specifications	IVOX size (mm)			
	7	8	9	10
Number of hollow fibers	589	703	894	1107
Length of each fiber	38 cm	41 cm	45 cm	50 cm
Length of crimped fiber bundle	30 cm	33 cm	37 cm	40 cm
Surface area of siloxane gas-transfer membrane	$0.21 \, m^2$	$0.32 \, m^2$	$0.41 \, m^2$	$0.52 \, m^2$
Outside diameter of furled fiber bundle	11.1 mm	12.0 mm	13.5 mm	14.6 mm
Outside diameter of insertional sheath	12.6 mm	13.5 mm	15.0 mm	15.8 mm
Nominal gas flow into and out of functioning IVOX device	2500 mL/min	2700 mL/min	3300 mL/min	3400 mL/min

Nominal gas pressure at various sites in a functioning IVOX device	All sizes of IVOX
O_2 inlet to gas conduit	+5 mm Hg
O_2 inlet to hollow fiber	−110 mm Hg
Gas outlet from hollow fibers	−210 mm Hg
Gas outlet at Y connector	−295 mm Hg
Vacuum delivered to gas outlet conduit	−355 mm Hg
I.D. of each hollow fiber	0.190 mm
O.D. of each hollow fiber	0.236 mm
Thickness of siloxane coating on each hollow fiber	0.001 mm

TABLE 30.2. Average quantitative gas transfer rates achieved by IVOX during the clinical trials.

IVOX size (mm)	Total experience (USA and international)	
	CO_2 transfer rate mL/min	O_2 transfer rate mL/min
7	40.3	43.8
8	45.6	60.2
9	54.2	60.1
10	72.5	71.0

fibers (Table 30.1). The largest oxygenator possible is utilized in order to maximize the surface area available for gas exchange, as well as to ensure complete filling of the venae cavae by the fibers. Failure of the fibers to fill the cavae will result in streaming of blood around the oxygenator, decreasing actual gas exchange.

The 10-mm IVOX is 400 mm in length, and consists of 1107 hollow fibers, each with an outer diameter of 236 μm, an inner diameter of 190 μm, and a wall thickness of 20 μm. The siloxane coating is 1-μm thick. Although the measured diameter of this size 10 device is 10 mm at its potted end, when furled for insertion, it reaches 13 to 15 mm at its widest point. The surface area of the gas transfer membrane is 0.52 m^2. In comparison, the 7-mm IVOX is 30 cm in length, consists of 589 fibers, and has a surface area of only 0.21 m^2 (Table 30.1).

Controlled ovine gas transfer experiments performed ex vivo established experimental gas-transfer indices for IVOX devices and demonstrated that, under ideal laboratory experimental conditions, up to 3.4 ml oxygen per minute per 100 cm^2 surface area could be transferred with current IVOX devices. The average gas transfer, achieved in human patients as a function of IVOX dimension, is summarized in Table 30.2. These data indicate that during clinical application in patients with ARF, an average of 40 to 72 mL/min of oxygen and carbon dioxide were transferred to and from circulatory blood. A variety of factors alter the rate of oxygen and carbon dioxide gas exchange; these are reviewed in Table 30.3.

Clinical Applications

As with any new support modality, a clear understanding of the objectives and limitations of the method is necessary, in order to define realistically the indications and contraindications for that modality.

Given the performance of the IVOX, both in the experimental model and in the current management of human respiratory failure, a primary objective of IVOX placement should be the temporary improvement of hypoxemia/hypercarbia in patients with moderate to severe, but potentially reversible, acute respiratory failure.

In cases of early, reversible acute respiratory failure, use of an IVOX device may adequately augment inadequate gas exchange, and avoid endotracheal intubation and positive pressure mechanical ventilatory support. In cases of moderately severe, reversible, acute respiratory failure, insertion of an IVOX device may decrease the time of ventilatory support by easing the weaning process and hastening extubation. This, in turn, decreases the risk of barotrauma and oxygen toxicity, and decreases length of stay in the intensive care unit. In cases of severe reversible acute respiratory failure, the use of an IVOX device is intended to reduce the intensity of mechanical ventilatory support (decrease F_iO_2, PEEP, minute volume, peak inspiratory pressure), thereby reducing the risk of barotrauma and oxygen toxicity. In the most severe cases of respiratory failure, when mechanical ventilatory support proves inadequate, an IVOX device may augment ventilatory support, thus giving the lungs additional time to recover. Finally, an IVOX may obviate the use of extracorporeal membrane oxygenation. These objectives are recapitulated in Table 30.4.[4,7]

Indications

While the clinical trials currently under way will more carefully define the indications for IVOX use, the currently perceived indications are as follows:

1. Unsatisfactory arterial blood gases despite oxygen administration by face mask or nasal cannula and when positive pressure mechanical ventilatory support is undesirable or hazardous.
2. Acute reversible airway obstruction not amenable to mechanical ventilatory support.

TABLE 30.3. Factors that influence gas transfer rate.

Size of the IVOX device (surface area of gas transfer membrane exposed to blood)
Flow rate of blood over IVOX hollow fibers (cardiac output/venous return of the subject with an indwelling IVOX)
Blood flow pattern around the IVOX hollow fibers (proper deployment of crimped hollow fibers, ratio of hollow-fiber volume to blood volume within the venae cavae, extent of mixing of blood flowing over the IVOX device)
P_{CO_2} and P_{O_2} in the blood exposed to IVOX (CO_2 and O_2 partial pressure gradients across the IVOX membrane)
Rate of gas flow through (into/out of) the IVOX device
Intraluminal pressure (vacuum) of gas within IVOX hollow fibers
Composition of gas delivered to IVOX
Hemoglobin content of circulating blood exposed to IVOX

TABLE 30.4. Objectives of IVOX Utilization.

In Severe, Reversible ARF
Augment inadequate mechanical ventilator support, thereby:
  —gain additional time for recovery of natural lungs.
  —possibly avoid extracorporeal perfusion
Reduce the intensity of mechanical ventilator support:
  —decrease the FiO_2
  —lower the PEEP, PIP, MAP
  —decrease the MV
  —decrease danger of barotrauma/oxygen toxicity
In Moderate Reversible ARF:
Decrease the time ventilator support is required:
  —hasten discontinuing ventilator
  —facilitate weaning from ventilator
  —shorten stay in ICU
  —decrease danger of barotrauma/oxygen toxicity
In Early, Reversible ARF:
Adequately augment the deficient blood gas exchange, while at the same time:
  —avoiding endotracheal intubation
  —avoiding utilization of closed system positive pressure mechanical ventilator support

3. Selected patients (postsurgical or post-trauma) whose tracheobronchial tree or pulmonary tissues cannot withstand increased airway pressures by means of positive pressure mechanical ventilation.
4. Failure of the patient to tolerate intubation, controlled ventilation, or the sedation/paralysis required for adequate mechanical ventilator support.
5. Mandatory mechanical ventilator support for patients with an active bronchopleural fistula or increasing mediastinal or subcutaneous emphysema.
6. Borderline gas exchange with mechanical ventilatory settings at maximum *safe* levels.
7. Unacceptable gas exchange despite maximal mechanical ventilatory support.[4]

Contraindications

Assessment of the performance of the IVOX device on the experimental animal model, as well as observations made during clinical trials, suggest a number of contraindications to its use:

1. Need for long-term support (>3 weeks)
2. Any contraindication to heparinization
3. Uncontrolled sepsis
4. Deep venous thrombosis
5. Unavailability of venous access
6. Advanced multiorgan failure
7. Depressed cardiac function despite inotropic support
8. Unavailability of trained personnel
9. Inability to monitor gas exchange and anticoagulation

These contraindications are related to the problems associated with device insertion, thromboembolism, and the possibility of hemorrhage. When assessing the risk of systemic heparinization, one must consider recent surgery and/or trauma, and the possibility of heparin resistance (antithrombin III deficiency, etc) or heparin-induced thrombocytopenia. The placement of a large intravascular device in the presence of an ongoing bacteremia or uncontrolled sepsis is obviously an undesirable intervention, since it has been shown that intravascular prosthetic devices may exacerbate the circulatory effects of sepsis. Moreover, the basic principle of the management of sepsis is removal of intravascular catheters. Assuming that IVOX placement was undertaken because of hypoxemia, resulting from adult respiratory distress syndrome (ARDS) accompanying sepsis, *and* that IVOX placement has improved the hypoxemia, it is reasonable to assume that device removal will lead to a worsening of the hypoxemic state. Maintaining the IVOX in a bacteremic patient, however, will lead to a worsening of the septis. The greatest "temptation" for inappropriate IVOX use, however, will be in patients unlikely to recover: those with advanced multiorgan system failure, those requiring support beyond the time limits currently imposed on IVOX, and those with irreversible respiratory failure.

Limitations of IVOX

It is clear from the design features, in vitro and in vivo experiments, and early clinical trials, that the IVOX should find a place in the management of ARF. The perceived indications and contraindications identify a large number of potential patients for this support modality. However, a number of limitations on its use are present, even when it may otherwise be indicated. These limitations include:

1. Current IVOX models are capable of providing only approximately ⅓–½ of the total metabolic gas transfer requirements of most adult ARF patients.
2. The safe duration of the device in the venae cavae is approximately 21 days.
3. Gas transfer membrane surface area is limited to 2100–5200 cm^2 by diameter of the device which can be inserted into the venae cavae.
4. Patient anatomy must allow adequate access to the vena cava by the right jugular or right femoral vein.
5. Patient must be able to tolerate anticoagulation.
6. Use of the device is limited to designated centers during clinical trials.[4]

Current Status of IVOX Clinical Trials

Between February 1990 and April 1991, 18 patients with ARDS received implantation of an IVOX device to augment blood-gas exchange, as Phase I of the US Food and

Drug Administration (FDA)-authorized IVOX clinical trials. The objective of these initial IVOX device implantations was to determine the risks and hazards of IVOX use. Data collected from these safety assessments demonstrated minimal adverse clinical, laboratory, or pathologic findings during or after use of the IVOX device.

As a result of the favorable safety record of the IVOX device during Phase I, the FDA approved entrance into Phase II of the clinical trials, commencing in May 1991. By mid 1993, 160 patients with advanced ARF, refractory to intensive mechanical ventilatory support, had received an IVOX device implantation in 35 international clinical trial centers. Although detailed data analysis is not complete, the following observations are apparent from review of the IVOX clinical trials database:

1. When used in accordance with the prescribed protocols, labels, and instructions, the IVOX device predictably transfers oxygen into, and carbon dioxide out of, circulating venous blood, in modest but measurable quantities, and without substantial decrease in gas transfer rate for up to 29 days after use.
2. During IVOX use, most hypoxemic patients in ARF experience a measurable increase in arterial Po_2, and most hypercarbic patients experience a measurable decrease in $Paco_2$.
3. These favorable changes in blood gases occur during IVOX use without increased intensity (usually with *decreased* intensity) of mechanical ventilator support.
4. Measures of lung function improve measurably in most ARF patients during IVOX use.
5. Most patients in severe ARF who have depressed hemodynamic function because of intensive mechanical ventilator support experience improvement in their hemodynamic state during IVOX use.
6. IVOX use as associated with significant IVOX-related complications or adverse events in 24.5% of the IVOX Clinical Trials patients.
7. IVOX use as currently implemented has certain inherent inadequacies and limitations. Most clinical trials investigators were pleased with the simplicity and convenience of IVOX use but would like:

   IVOX to transfer more gas
   IVOX to be easier to implant and remove
   IVOX use without systemic anticoagulation
   More information to adequately define the proper indications and contraindications for IVOX use.

Summary

Although clinical application of the current IVOX device in selected cases appears to be justified, further optimization of the device is appropriate to help satisfy the above list of desirable features developed by clinicians who have utilized IVOX. Objectives for future research and development pertaining to the IVOX device, include:

Increased gas transfer capability of the IVOX device
Simpler and more effective means for furling and unfurling the IVOX hollow-fiber bundle
Safer and simpler methods for implanting and explaining the IVOX device
Decreased fragility and susceptibility of the IVOX device to mechanical failure
Modification and clarification of the recommended indications and contraindications for IVOX use
Changes in training, accreditation, and supervision of IVOX users

Although research and development activities are currently being carried out to pursue these objectives, the findings from the IVOX clinical trials to date appear to be favorable enough to justify use of the IVOX device by properly qualified clinicians for augmentation of deficient blood-gas exchange of patients with moderate to severe, potentially reversible ARF. Applications for regulatory approval are currently being planned.

Selected Case Reports

The following case summaries are reported as illustrations of the effect of IVOX use in patients with acute respiratory failure:

Case 1

A 76-year-old Caucasian male underwent successful femoropopliteal bypass grafting for a severely ischemic left leg. On the third postoperative day, he became severely hypoxemic (Po_2 of 55 torr) and moderately hypercarbic (Pco_2 of 54 torr), despite closed-system mechanical ventilation at an F_iO_2 of 1.00 and PEEP of 10 cm H_2O. Chest x-ray supported the clinical diagnosis of ARDS. A 9-mm IVOX device was inserted through the right common femoral vein. Within 12 hours, the blood gases were markedly improved, with Pao_2 of 90 torr and $Paco_2$ of 32 torr, despite significant reduction in the ventilatory F_iO_2 (to 0.70) and PEEP (to 6 cm H_2O). After 6 days of IVOX augmentation of blood gas transfer, the lungs had regained sufficient function so that normal blood gases (Pao_2 = 80 torr; $Paco_2$ = 30 torr) were maintained with the ventilator delivering room air with no PEEP. Two days later, the endotracheal tube was removed. The patient thereafter left the ICU, completely recovered from his ARDS.

In this case, IVOX augmented blood-gas-transfer-facilitated recovery from ARDS, in a patient inadequately supported by intensive mechanical ventilation. The IVOX device permitted reduction in the magnitude of mechanical ventilator support, thereby possibly preventing mechanical ventilation-induced irreversible lung pathology. Approximately 30% of the advanced ARDS patients managed with IVOX during clinical trials followed a similar course to recovery.

Case 2

A 21-year-old Caucasian male developed a rapidly progressing viral pneumonitis that resulted in ARF. Despite mechanical ventilator support with an F_iO_2 of 0.55, PEEP of 12.5 cm H_2O, and minute ventilation of 17 L/min, his PaO_2 was 51 torr and his $PaCO_2$ was 38 torr. Rather than increase the magnitude of mechanical ventilatory assistance and risk adding the effects of barotrauma and oxygen toxicity to the lung dysfunction, insufficient blood-gas exchange was augmented with an IVOX device. Within 1 hour after IVOX insertion, the PaO_2 improved to 68 torr while the ventilatory F_iO_2 was reduced to 0.50, the MV to 11.0 L/min, and the PEEP to 8 cm H_2O (Figure 30.3). Thereafter, the F_iO_2 was decreased progressively to 0.30 on day 2, and to room air on day 6. The PaO_2 remained between 62 and 142 torr, and the $PaCO_2$ between 25 and 35 torr. Lung function (as indicated by compliance, intrapulmonary shunt, and oxygenation index) improved rapidly, and the chest x-ray cleared completely. On day 6 of IVOX use, the device was removed; 2 days later the patient was extubated. The patient fully recovered, returned to full activity, and had no clinical evidence of residual sequelae from his ARF or from the 6 days of IVOX use. The clinical course of this patient is summarized in Figure 30.3.

This case represents successful use of IVOX to augment deficient blood-gas exchange in patients with potentially reversible ARF, in whom lung function improved quickly without residual abnormalities. This favorable course occurred in approximately 30% of the ARF patients in whom IVOX was used in the Phase II clinical trials.

Case 3

A 33-year-old Hispanic, alcoholic, epileptic male aspirated vomitus during a seizure. Four days later, his aspiration pneumonitis progressed to full-blown ARDS, with hypoxemia refractory to intensive mechanical ventilatory assistance. With a PEEP of 12.5 cm H_2O, F_iO_2 of 1.00, and MV of 17.0 L/min, his PaO_2 was 38 torr (Figure 30.4). When he became hemodynamically unstable on the fifth day of ARDS, a 10-mm IVOX was inserted into his venae cavae via the right internal jugular vein. The device functioned well, transferring up to 95 mL O_2/min into the venous blood and removing up to 80 mL CO_2/min. During IVOX use, lung dysfunction improved to such a degree that mechanical ventilatory assistance could be reduced progressively. On the seventh day of IVOX support, ventilator F_iO_2 was 0.24, PEEP was 5 cm H_2O, and MV was 13.7 L/min, while PaO_2 was 64 torr and

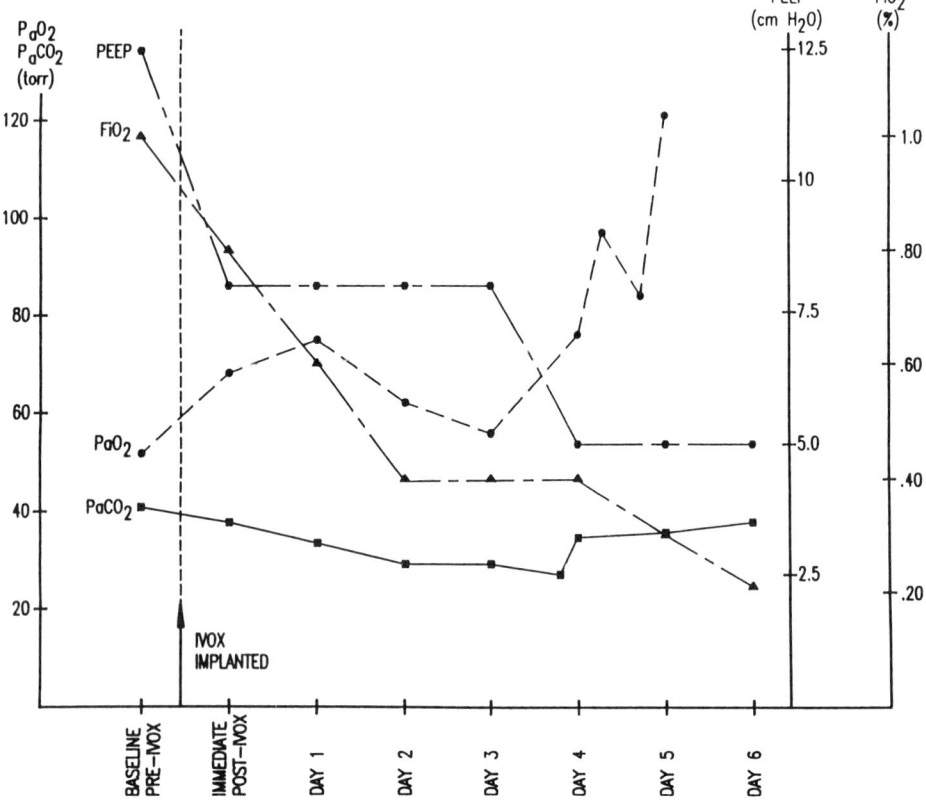

FIGURE 30.3. Respiratory variables in an ARF patient managed with an IVOX device. *Note the rapid decrease in the PEEP and F_iO_2 delivered by the mechanical* ventilator following insertion of an IVOX device. This was accompanied by recovery from the hypoxemia and hypercarbia associated with the patient's ARF. The patient made a complete recovery.

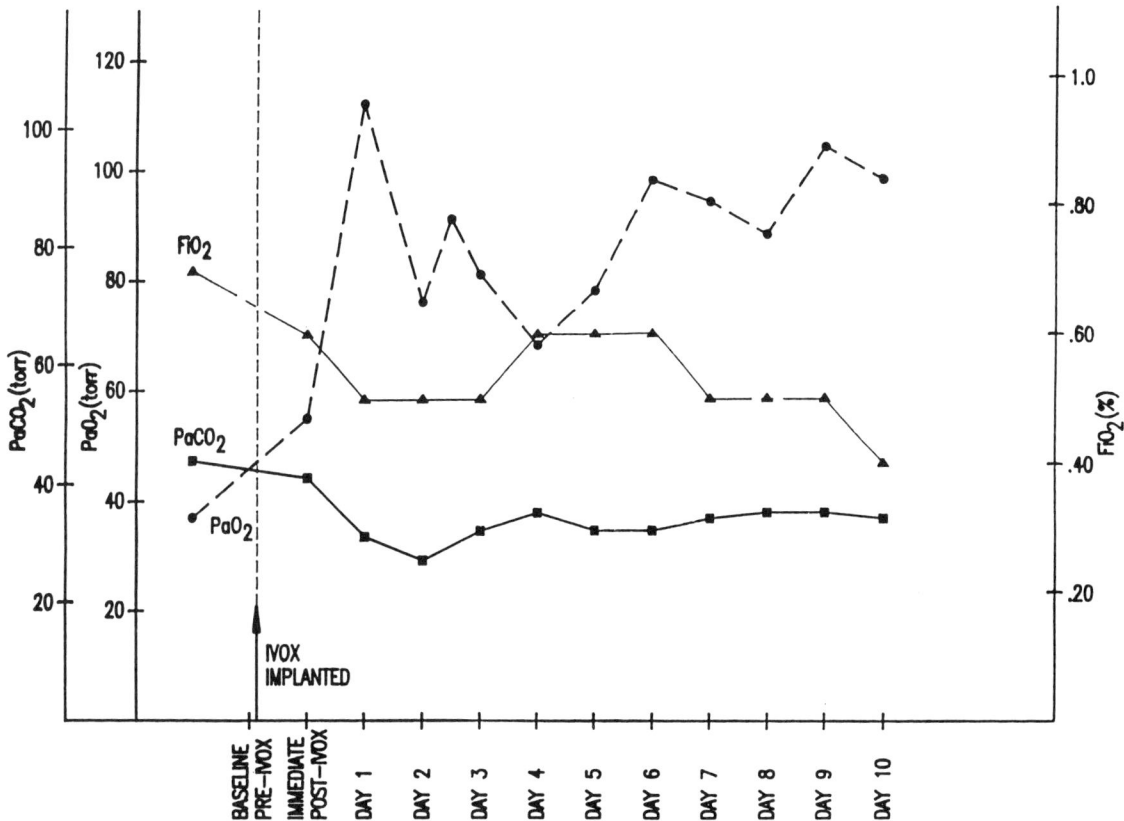

FIGURE 30.4. Respiratory variables in an ARDS patient managed with an IVOX device. *Note the improvement* in PaO_2 and $PaCO_2$ and the significant decrease in F_iO_2. This patient's native lung blood-gas transfer was augmented significantly by means of an IVOX device. However, death occurred a few days later from causes unrelated to his ARDS or to the IVOX device.

$PaCO_2$ was 32 torr. Chest x-ray evidence showed that interstitial edema and atelectasis had cleared considerably. Two days later, the IVOX device was removed and the patient's blood gases remained satisfactory with minimal support from the mechanical ventilator (Figure 30.4). However, 4 days after IVOX was removed, the patient developed the sepsis syndrome, requiring inotropic support and an increase in ventilator support, with an F_iO_2 of 0.40 and PEEP of 10 cm H_2O. Blood cultures were negative. The patient died suddenly the following day. Necropsy findings indicated the cause of death was acute hepatic failure with advanced liver degeneration and cirrhosis. There was no clinical or necropsy evidence of pathologic findings, injury, or harmful sequelae from the 9 days of IVOX implantation.

This case is representative of approximately 60% of the clinical trial patients. In these cases, considerable benefit was evident from IVOX use, in that blood gases improved and the magnitude of mechanical ventilation decreased, but the patient did not survive hospitalization, dying from causes other than inadequate respiration.

Several of the clinical trial investigators have reported their experience with the IVOX device,[8-21] but clinical trials are still under way, and data analysis is still in progress.

At this point, the most appropriate role for the IVOX device in the management of patients in ARF has not been determined. It appears evident that some patients in whom IVOX is used respond favorably, some receive no recognizable benefit, and some whose respiratory failure is reversed during IVOX use succumb to other (nonrespiratory) problems. Furthermore, the IVOX device cannot be distributed commercially or used widely until approval is granted by the appropriate regulatory agencies, both in the United States and internationally.

References

1. Guyton AC. *Textbook of Medical Physiology*. 8th ed. Philadelphia: WB Saunders; 1991:102–461.
2. Murray JF, Nodel JA. *Textbook of Respiratory Medicine*. Philadelphia: WB Saunders; 1988:2017–2034.
3. Levitsky MG. *Pulmonary Physiology*. 2nd ed. New York: McGraw Hill, 1986:136–156.
4. Mortensen JD. Augmentation of blood gas transfer by means of an intravascular blood gas exchanger (IVOX®). *Update in Intensive Care and Emergency Medicine* vol. 15, New York: Springer-Verlag; 1989:318–344.

5. Mortensen JD, Berry G, Winters S. IVOX: an intracorporeal device for temporary augmentation of blood gas transfer in subjects with acute respiratory insufficiency. *Cardiol Chronicle* 1990;4(4):1-60.
6. Mortensen JD, Berry G. Conceptual and design features of a practical, clinically effective intravenous mechanical blood oxygen carbon dioxide exchange device (IVOX). *Int J Artif Organs* 1989;12:384-389.
7. Mortensen JD. Intravascular oxygenator (IVOX): a new alternative method for augmenting blood gas transfer in patients with acute respiratory failure. *Artif Organs* 1992;16:75-82.
8. Kallis P, Al-Saady NM, Bennett D, et al. Clinical use of intravascular oxygenation. *Lancet* 1991;337:549.
9. Zwischenberger JB, Cox CS. A new intravascular membrane oxygenator to augment blood gas transfer in patients with acute respiratory failure. *Texas Medicine/The Journal* 1991;87:60-63.
10. Jurmann MJ, Demertzis S, Schaefers HJ, et al. Intravascular oxygenation for advanced respiratory failure. *ASAIO J* 1992;38:120-124.
11. von Segesser LK, Schaffner A, Stocker R, et al. Extended (29 days) use of intravascular gas exchanger. (Letter) *Lancet* 1992;339:1536.
12. Cox CS, Zwischenberger JB, Kurusz M. Development and current status of a new intracorporeal membrane oxygenator (IVOX). *Perfusion* 1991;6:291-296.
13. Kallis P, Al-Saady NM, Bennett ED, et al. Intravascular oxygenation with the IVOX. *Br J Hosp Med* 1992;47:824-828.
14. von Segesser LK, Weiss BM, Pasic M, et al. Temporary lung support using an intravascular gas exchanger. *Thorac Cardiovasc Surg* 1992;40:121-125.
15. High KM, Snider MT, Richard R, et al. Clinical trials of an intravenous oxygenator in patients with adult respiratory distress syndrome. *Anesthesiology* 1992;77:856-863.
16. Conrad S, Eggerstedt J, Romero M. Prolonged intracorporeal support of gas exchange with an intravascular oxygenator. *Chest* 1993;103:158-161.
17. Schmidt H, Bohrer H, Motsch J, et al. Intravenous oxygenator use in adult respiratory distress syndrome. *Anesthesiology* 1993;78:1193-1195.
18. Skolnick AA. Implantable lung-assist device being tested on patients with acute respiratory failure. *JAMA* 1991;266:1332-1333.
19. Gentilello LM, Jurkovich GJ, Gubler DK, et al. The intravascular oxygenator (IVOX®): preliminary results of a new means of performing extrapulmonary gas exchange. *J Trauma* 1993;35:399-404.
20. von Segesser LK, Pasic M, Tonz M, et al. Use of an intravascular gas exchanger: is low systemic heparinization safe? *Perfusion* 1993;8:449-458.
21. Tonz M, von Segesser LK, Leskosek B, et al. Quantitative gas transfer of an intravascular oxygenator. *Ann Thorac Surg* 1994;57:146-150.

Part VII
Special Considerations in Cardiopulmonary Bypass

31
Blood Conservation in Cardiac Surgery

James G. Cormack, Robert W. Bolen, and Dirk A. Maisel

Introduction

Cardiac operations are among the most commonly performed procedures in the United States, with some 300,000 performed annually. In most elective operations, if the patient starts with a normal hematocrit, there is no need for transfusion, providing the blood loss is less than 1 L, and is replaced with intravenous fluids. However, approximately two thirds of all blood transfusions are given in the perioperative period, and a significant portion of this blood is transfused during cardiac operations.[1] Blood loss during cardiac operations can be considerable, and it is important for physicians caring for these patients to do everything possible to minimize such loss. Consequent blood product transfusions may result in a life-threatening infection, transfusion reaction, or pathologic immunomodulation. Moreover, blood is a scarce resource and should not be wasted, since the cost of donation, storage, and processing of blood components is considerable and adds to the already high cost of heart disease therapy.

This chapter outlines the different risks associated with blood transfusion and discusses how to determine blood transfusion requirements based upon the physiologic response to anemia. The final section of this chapter describes the numerous blood conservation techniques available to reduce homologous blood product transfusion in cardiac surgery patients.

Risks Associated with Blood Transfusion

Infection

The most common transfusion-acquired infection is hepatitis, with a contagion risk of 7% to 12%.[2] Hepatitis B virus (HBV), hepatitis A virus (HAV), hepatitis C virus (HCV), non-A, non-B hepatitis virus (NANBV), cytomegalovirus (CMV), Epstein-Barr virus (EBV), human immunodeficiency virus types I and II (HIV), and human T-lymphocyte virus types I and II (HTLV) are the viruses that have been reported to cause infections in patients receiving blood transfusions.[2] Bacterial infections (most commonly *Salmonella* and *Staphylococcus*) occur in platelet concentrates, because platelets are stored at room temperature.[3] *Yersinia enterocolitica* and *Pseudomonas fluorescens* can replicate at 4°C and can infect even refrigerated blood products.[2] The spirochetes, *Treponema pallidum* (syphilis) and *Borrelia burgdorferi* (Lyme disease) can survive in blood products, although transfusion-associated Lyme disease has yet to be reported.[4] Blood transfusions may cause several types of parasitic infections, including malaria, toxoplasmosis, filariasis, kala-azar, Chagas' disease, and babesiasis.[2] Table 31.1 lists the types and frequency of infections that can occur following blood product transfusions.[2,5,6] The risk of infection is but one of the risks patients face when administered a blood transfusion; the problems of transfusion reactions and pathologic immunomodulation are discussed below.

Transfusion Reactions

Red blood cells, white blood cells, platelets, and proteins all can cause transfusion reactions. Table 31.2 lists the different types of transfusion reactions. Red blood cell reactions occur because the recipient forms antibodies against the donor red blood cell antigens. These reactions can be an immediate or delayed type of hemolytic response. Since 1975, 58% of transfusion-related deaths in the United States were secondary to hemolytic reactions.[7] Alloimmunization occurs by the same antibody mechanism as hemolytic reactions, but it is not commonly a problem following an initial transfusion, although it may make future cross-matching more difficult. Alloimmunization and febrile white blood cell reactions are common and oc-

TABLE 31.1. Types and frequency of infections following blood product transfusions.[1,5,6]

Type	Microorganism	Frequency
Viruses	Hepatitis A virus	Rare
	Hepatitis B Virus	1/200,000 units
	Hepatitis C virus	1/3300 units
	Non-A, non-B hepatitis virus	1/14 units (post-transfusion increase in serum transaminases)
	Epstein-Barr virus	Rare
	Cytomegalo virus	Rare
	Human immunodeficiency virus 1,2	1/225,000 units
	Human T-cell Lymphotrophic virus 1,2	1/50,000 units
Bacteria	Staphylococci	Rare
	Salmonella	Rare
	Yersinia enterocolitica	1/1,000,000 units
	Pseudomonas fluorescens	Rare
	Treponema pallidum	Rare
	Borrelia burgdorferi	Rare
Parasites	Babesia microtia	1/1,000,000 units
	Plasmodia (malaria)	1/1,000,000 units
	Trypanosoma (Chagas' disease)	1/1,000,000 units
	Toxoplasma	Rare
	Filaria	Rare
	Leishmania (kala azar)	Rare

cur when recipient antibody is formed against donor white blood cells. Other white cell-mediated phenomena include the potentially lethal graft-versus-host and acute lung injury reactions. Platelet reactions include post-transfusion purpura and alloimmunization. Protein transfusion reactions are a type of hypersensitivity reaction in which recipient antibody is formed against donor protein. IgA-deficient patients can have anaphylactoid reactions if transfused with IgA-containing blood products.

TABLE 31.2. Different types of transfusion reactions.

Red blood cell reactions
  Hemolytic—immediate
  Hemolytic—delayed
  Alloimmunization
White blood cell reactions
  Febrile
  Acute lung injury
  Graft versus host
  Alloimmunization
Platelet reactions
  Post-transfusion purpura
  Alloimmunization
Protein reactions
  Hypersensitivity
  Anaphylactoid
  Alloimmunization

Blood Products and Immunomodulation

The immunomodulatory effects of blood product transfusion result in an increased risk of cancer recurrence, altered transplant survival, and increased risk of postoperative infection. Perioperative transfusion may increase recurrence of colorectal, head and neck, soft tissue, lung, and breast cancer.[8] Whole blood transfusion seems to increase the risk of cancer recurrence more than transfusion of packed cells.[9,10] In the 1970s, preoperative blood transfusion was associated with increased survival of transplanted kidneys.[11] However, more effective immunosuppressive drug regimens have decreased the incidence of rejection of transplanted kidneys in nontransfused patients, so that blood transfusion prior to organ transplantation is no longer desirable.[12] An increased incidence of postoperative infections may occur in patients who have received blood transfusion during surgery for trauma,[13] colon resection,[14] hip replacement,[15] heart surgery,[16,17] and gastric cancer.[18] The mechanism for the immunomodulatory effects of blood transfusion is not well understood but may be due to decreased T-cell helper/suppressor ratios,[19] decreased natural killer cell activity,[20] or decreased lymphocyte responses to antigen.[21]

In addition to the problems of infection, transfusion reaction, and immunomodulation, blood product transfusion can result in untoward biochemical and embolic events. The biochemical effects of transfusion include acidosis, hyperkalemia, hypocalcemia, and decreased levels of 2,3-diphosphoglycerate. Hypervolemia, hypothermia, and air and clot embolization may also complicate blood transfusion. In addition to the risks of blood transfusion described above, some patients have strong religious beliefs that forbid transfusion of blood products. It is imperative that the medical team respect the wishes of such patients. This subject is discussed in detail in Chapter 32.

Determining Blood Product Transfusion Requirements and Physiologic Responses to Anemia

The first element of a comprehensive blood conservation program is to accept the lowest safe level of hemoglobin. The traditional lowest safe level of hemoglobin of 10 g/dL or a hematocrit of 30% for elective surgery has been challenged in recent years. Retrospective studies looking at perioperative complications,[22] or morbidity and mortality, suggest that a hemoglobin of 8 g/dL may be a more reasonable threshold for transfusion.[23] To determine a safe transfusion threshold, one must consider each patient individually, and have a thorough understanding of how the body compensates for anemia. The physiologic mechanisms that compensate for anemia depend on the patient's age, physical status, and oxygen requirements, and the rate and magnitude of hemoglobin loss. A patient compensates for anemia by increasing cardiac output, increasing oxygen extraction, and shifting the oxygen dissociation curve to the left (Table 31.3).

Cardiac output varies inversely with hematocrit; both blood viscosity and systemic vascular resistance decrease with a lower hematocrit, and thus cardiac output and blood flow is improved. As oxygen delivery is determined by blood flow (which is dependent on blood viscosity) and the oxygen content of arterial blood, there are data suggesting that oxygen delivery peaks at a hematocrit of 30%.[24] However, the tendency for the heart rate to increase and the blood pressure to decrease with decreasing hematocrit complicates the determination of safe lower limits of hematocrit in the clinical situation. Tachycardia decreases the time the heart is in diastole, predisposing the left ventricular endocardium to ischemia. In awake, hemodiluted dogs, the increase in cardiac output is predominantly due to an increase in heart rate, whereas in the anesthetized state, it is predominantly due to an increase in stroke volume.[25-27] In denervated or β-blocked, hemodiluted dogs, stroke volume increases, but cardiac output increases less than in control dogs, suggesting that patients on β-blockers may not be able to increase their cardiac output maximally in the face of hemodilution and decreased oxygen-carrying capacity.[25,26,28] Anesthetized healthy dogs tolerate a hematocrit of 15% without any endocardial-to-epicardial coronary blood flow redistribution (if heart rate and blood pressure remain normal[29]), and myocardial oxygen consumption and coronary sinus oxygen saturation remain constant until hematocrit falls below 20%.[30] Below a hematocrit of 20%, myocardial oxygen consumption decreases and coronary sinus oxygen saturation rises, implying an impairment in myocardial oxygen extraction.[30] In dogs with a 67% left anterior descending coronary artery stenosis, hemodilution to a hematocrit of 20% results in ischemic electrocardiographic (ECG) changes and a decrease in myocardial function.[31] Therefore, in healthy dogs, the lowest hematocrit that does not cause myocardial ischemia is likely between 15% and 20%, and in dogs with coronary artery disease, the "safe" hematocrit value is greater than 20%.

In healthy humans, the cardiac output increases significantly when hemoglobin is decreased below 7 g/dL.[1] However, older patients may be less able to increase cardiac output in response to hemodilution. In a study by Rosenberg and Wulff,[32] healthy anesthetized patients (average age of 68 years) who were hemodiluted from a hematocrit of 41% to a hematocrit of 28% showed no changes in heart rate, blood pressure, or cardiac output. However, in a study of awake patients undergoing major surgery who were hemodiluted to hematocrits of 27% to 29%, the group over 60 years of age and the group under 60 years of age had similar increases in cardiac output and adequate oxygen delivery.[33]

During hypothermic cardiopulmonary bypass (CPB), the increase in blood viscosity associated with low temperatures necessitates the implementation of hemodilution to preserve organ blood flow and oxygen delivery. Seventy-two hours after a 2-hour middle cerebral artery occlusion, rats with hematocrits of 44% had significantly greater neurologic injury than rats hemodiluted to hematocrits of 30% or 16% with diaspirin cross-linked hemoglobin.[34] In a study assessing cerebral oxygen delivery during hypothermia, patients with a hematocrit of 23% had better oxygen delivery than patients with a hematocrit of 28%.[35] However, at normal temperatures, hemodilution may predispose the brain and myocardium to ischemia. In a retrospective review of 99 patients who presented for autologous blood donation prior to coronary artery bypass surgery, one patient developed unstable angina 24 hours after donation.[36] In awake coronary artery bypass patients, 22% of the group with left ventricular dysfunction suffered ischemic ECG changes when hemodiluted from a hemoglobin of 14.1 to 9.6 g/dL.[37] In this study, patients with left ventricular dysfunction had a significant decrease in their cardiac index and mean arterial pressure and an increase in their pulmonary capillary wedge pressure and heart rate in comparison to the group with normal left ventricular function. In the normal group, heart rate and cardiac index increased significantly and no patient developed ischemic ECG changes.[37] In a study by Kim and colleagues,[38] postoperative cardiac surgery patients with normal ventricular function were found to similarly tolerate hematocrits of 23% and 34%; the 23% hematocrit group compensated for the decrease in oxygen carrying capacity by increasing their cardiac output. In a similar study, delayed recovery of myocardial function was found in those patients with a hematocrit of 21% to 24%, although this low-hematocrit group had significantly lower arterial blood pressure and did not have the compensatory increase in cardiac output present in the low-hematocrit group reported by Kim and colleagues.[38,39] Therefore, β-blockade, left ventricular dysfunction, coronary artery disease, and advanced age may limit the ability of the heart to compensate for anemia.

Increasing coronary artery blood flow is the primary mechanism for increasing oxygen delivery to the heart be-

TABLE 31.3. Physiologic compensation to anemia.

Increased cardiac output
    Decreased systemic vascular resistance
    Decreased viscosity
    Tachycardia
    Increased stroke volume
Increased oxygen extraction ratio
    Decreased mixed venous oxygen saturation
Oxygen dissociation curve shifts to right
    Increase in 2,3-diphosphoglycerate

Oxygen-Hemoglobin Dissociation Curve

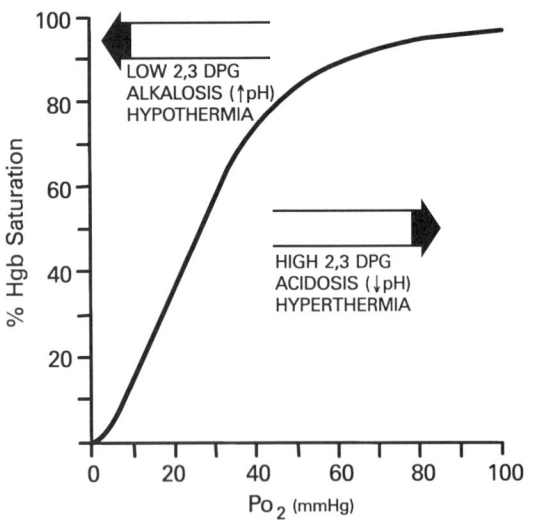

FIGURE 31.1. Factors affecting the dissociation of oxygen from hemoglobin. DPG = diphosphoglycerate.

cause the heart normally extracts the maximum possible amount of oxygen from the blood delivered to it (the heart normally extracts 60% to 70% of the oxygen delivered to it, whereas the whole body extraction ratio is only 25%). Increased peripheral oxygen extraction plays an important role when the hematocrit falls below 25%.[25,26] In a dog study, coronary artery blood flow increased 650% and cardiac output increased 220% during hemodilution from a hematocrit of 43% to 13%.[40] In a study of awake baboons, hemodilution to a hematocrit of 15% was well tolerated; however, the oxygen extraction ratio rose from 38% to 60%, and mixed venous oxygen saturation decreased from 70% to less than 50%, suggesting that, in baboons, extraction ratios greater than 50% and mixed venous saturations less than 50% are well tolerated.[41] In theory, one could measure oxygen delivery, consumption and extraction ratios, and mixed venous oxygen saturation, and red cells could be transfused when the extraction ratio is greater than 50% or the mixed venous saturation is less than 50%. But the determination of an extraction ratio is cumbersome and requires invasive monitoring.[42] In addition, the extraction ratio and mixed venous oxygen saturation only indicate global oxygen debt and may not uncover inadequate regional oxygen delivery.

Several factors affect the oxygen dissociation curve (Figure 31.1). Temperature, acid-base balance, and 2,3-diphosphoglycerate levels all affect the affinity of oxygen for the hemoglobin moiety. The oxygen dissociation curve shifts to the right with a decrease in hemoglobin because of an increase in 2,3-diphosphoglycerate. In dogs hemodiluted to a hematocrit of 20%, 2,3-diphosphoglycerate increased within 90 minutes.[43]

Thus, we can reduce blood transfusion in cardiac surgery by accepting lower hemoglobin values. There are several physiologic mechanisms to enhance oxygen delivery in the presence of a decreased hematocrit. However, one must identify which patients will be able to respond appropriately to a decrease in blood oxygen content, and which will not tolerate a lowered hematocrit. During hypothermic CPB in an uncomplicated operation on a patient less than 65 years of age, a hemoglobin value 6 g/dL is probably acceptable; postoperatively, in patients less than 65 years of age, a hemoglobin of 8 g/dL will not result in unacceptable oxygen delivery. Postoperative patients who are unable to increase their cardiac output or regional oxygen delivery to major end organs, those who have an increase in oxygen consumption or are critically ill, and those greater than 65 years of age should have a hemoglobin of at least 10 g/dL. In addition to accepting lower hemoglobin levels, we should practice as many practical and cost-effective blood conservation techniques as possible. This topic is discussed in the second part of this chapter.

Blood Conservation Techniques

The autotransfusion of blood is not a new idea. In the early 1800s, Blumdell reported autotransfusing vaginal blood to a young woman who was dying from postpartum hemorrhage.[44] In the nineteenth century, there were a few reports documenting the use of blood autotransfusion for various ailments (frostbite, carbon monoxide poisoning,[45] ectopic pregnancies[46]), but the lack of success associated with this technique precluded its widespread use. Today, blood autotransfusion is an important and commonly employed treatment modality and there are several effective blood conservation techniques used during cardiac surgery (Table 31.4). The indications, contraindications, and relative merit of each of these techniques are discussed in the second part of this chapter.

Autologous Donations

With autologous blood donation, the patient donates blood preoperatively for transfusion in the perioperative period. Iron is usually prescribed concomitantly, and

TABLE 31.4. Blood conservation techniques.

Autologous donation
Isovolemic hemodilution
Controlled hypotension
Pharmacologic interventions
Cell salvage
Ultrafiltration
Plasma sequestration

erythropoietin can be used to stimulate erythropoiesis in selected circumstances preoperatively.[47] Autologously donated blood preserved in a citrate-phosphate-dextrose-adenine (CPDA) preservative has a shelf life of 35 to 42 days. Autologous donation has been shown to significantly reduce homologous blood transfusion in patients undergoing elective cardiac surgery.[32,48] However, autologous donation before coronary artery bypass surgery has recently been shown not to be cost effective.[49] Contraindications to autologous donation are (1) a hematocrit less than 30%, (2) bacteremia, (3) emergency or urgent surgery, (4) severe respiratory, cerebrovascular, or cardiac disease (left main coronary artery disease, unstable angina, aortic stenosis, hypertrophic cardiomyopathy, ventricular arrhythmias, recent myocardial infarction, or congestive heart failure, and (5) signs or symptoms of ischemia on the day of donation. The side effects of autologous donation include volume overload, sepsis, transfusion reaction, and hypotension.[50]

Isovolemic Hemodilution

Isovolemic hemodilution is the isovolemic removal of whole blood during surgery for reinfusion later in the operative procedure. The guidelines for lowest acceptable hemoglobin are the same as those discussed previously. The usual technique is to remove a specified volume of whole blood into CPDA-preservative bags before CPB (Figure 31.2). The volume that can be removed in the prebypass period is determined by the following formula[51]:

$$\text{Volume removed} = \frac{\text{Estimated blood volume} \times (\text{HCT}_{initial} - \text{HCT}_{final})}{\text{HCT}_{mean}}$$

The removed blood should be labeled and can be stored in the operating room until transfused in the postbypass period. Gentle agitation during the storage period is important to prevent platelet clumping. The whole blood removed should be replaced with three times as much crystalloid or an equal amount of colloid solution. The return of the whole blood in the postbypass period after reversal of heparin provides autologous blood which contains coagulation factors and platelets that have not undergone the deleterious effects of CPB. Any patient who can safely tolerate a decrease in hemoglobin in the prebypass period is a candidate for isovolemic hemodilution. The contraindications to this technique include a hemoglobin level of less than 11 g/dL; renal insufficiency; severe respiratory, cardiovascular, or cerebrovascular disease; or age greater than 65 years.

Controlled Hypotension

Hypotension, induced by anesthetic or other vasoactive drugs, is effective in reducing blood loss in several different types of noncardiac surgical procedures.[52] The risk of hypotensive anesthesia including myocardial ischemia in the cardiac surgical patient would likely negate the benefits of reduced blood loss. However, it would be prudent in cardiac surgical procedures to prevent hypertension in order to minimize blood loss.

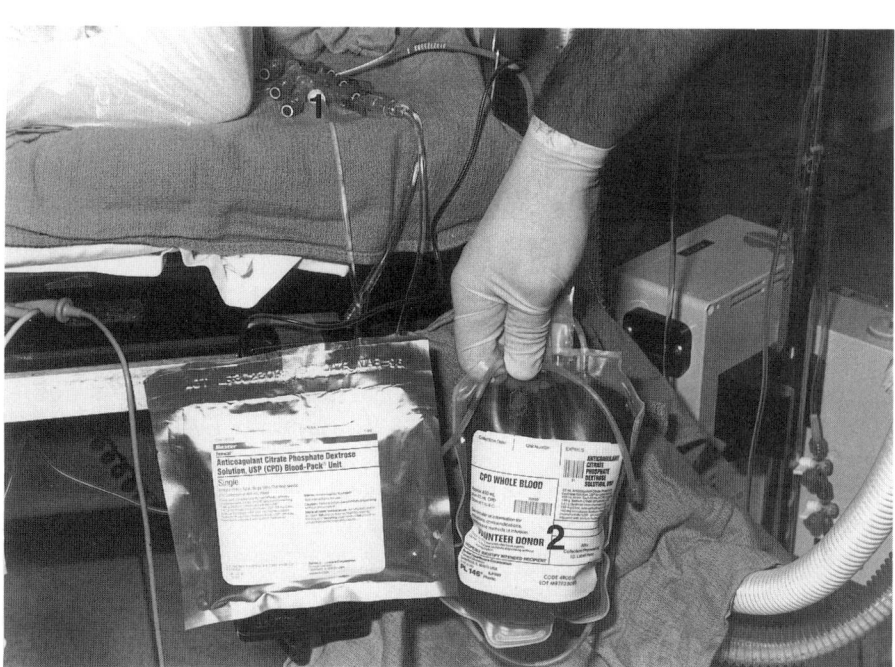

FIGURE 31.2. Removal of whole blood during cardiac surgery. Blood is easily drained from central venous lines (1) prior to heparinization and CPB for storage in CPDA-preservative bags (2).

Pharmacologic Interventions to Decrease Blood Loss

Antifibrinolytic therapy with ε-aminocaproic acid (EACA), tranexamic acid, or aprotinin has been shown to significantly reduce blood loss and homologous transfusion during cardiac surgery.[53-63] EACA and tranexamic acid are lysine analogs that bind to plasmin and plasminogen, thereby preventing clot lysis. Aprotinin inhibits not only plasmin but also trypsin and kallikrein. In some clinical settings, the cost of prophylactic antifibrinolytic therapy in elective primary cardiac operations may outweigh the benefits of reduced blood loss. Desmopressin (DDAVP) increases factor VIII:c and von Willebrand factor and may have a role in reducing bleeding during cardiac surgery.[64-66] DDAVP increases tissue plasminogen activator which can actually worsen the bleeding associated with CPB by increasing fibrinolysis. Large von Willebrand factor multimeters and prostacyclin (which can cause hypotension) are also released by DDAVP. These drug therapies are discussed further in Chapter 5.

Diuretics can be useful in blood conservation by increasing the rate at which the body excretes urine. As osmotic diuretic, such as mannitol, is often included in the heart-lung machine priming solution to facilitate the excretion of the priming and cardioplegic solutions infused during CPB. Loop diuretics can be used to increase urine output in those patients who are excessively hemodiluted or have renal insufficiency and require pharmacologic adjuncts to increase urine output.

Hemoconcentration and Ultrafiltration Devices

The crystalloid prime in the CPB circuit, cardioplegic solutions, and the administration of prebypass intravenous solutions put cardiac surgery patients at risk of fluid overload. Hemoconcentration, with either cell-salvage or ultrafiltration devices, is a technique that can be used to remove excess plasma water from patients supported on CPB. Ultrafiltration devices used with the heart-lung machine are similar to those originally created for dialysis patients. An ultrafiltrator is composed of a bundle of microporous fibers that permit removal of plasma water and dissolved solutes from the blood without the loss of proteins and clotting factors (Figure 31.3). The ultrafiltrate that crosses the fibers is similar to glomerular filtrate[67] and is collected in a waste bag and discarded. Ultrafiltration occurs when blood cells and proteins pass along the inside of a hollow fiber and back to the patient while water and permeable solutes pass through and to the outside of the fiber into a waste bag. Plasma volume is separated from blood at a rate dependent on the rate of blood flow through the device, the transmembrane pressure gradient (TMP), the red blood cell and protein concentrations,

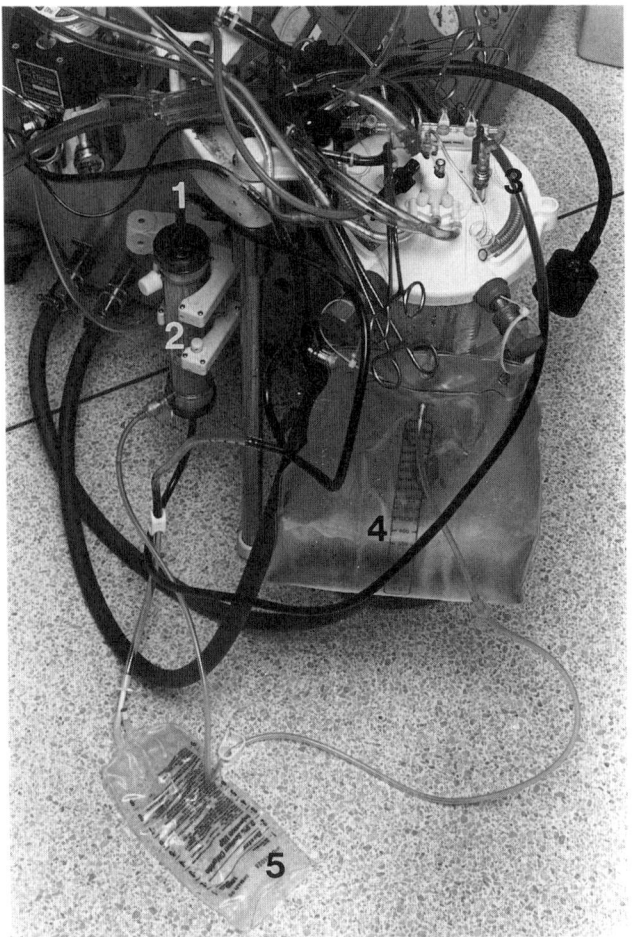

FIGURE 31.3. An ultrafiltration device. Blood (1) is circulated through the device (2) for the removal of excess fluid. Concentrated red cells (3) are returned to the venous reservoir and the ultrafiltrate is collected in a waste bag (4). A saline flush bag (5) completes the circuit.

the perfusate temperature, and the total surface area of the hemoconcentrator. The TMP is mathematically described as:

$$TMP = \frac{P_a + P_v}{2} + P_n - \frac{P_i + P_o}{2}$$

where P_a = arterial inlet pressure, P_v = venous outlet pressure, P_n = ultrafiltrate pressure of outlet, and P_i and P_o are the oncotic pressures at the inlet and outlet, respectively. The dimensions of ultrafiltrator fibers vary. Pore sizes range between 30 and 40 angstroms, fiber wall thickness is 40 μm, and the diameter is 200 μm.[68] With the elimination of excess plasma water and conservation of red blood cells, the hematocrit value increases because the same red cell mass is now in a smaller intravascular volume.

Most cardiac surgery patients tolerate the moderate

positive fluid balance associated with cardiac surgery and CPB without significant problems, so the benefits of ultrafiltration are limited to certain patient groups. In children, ultrafiltration of the extracorporeal circuit volume after CPB reduces homologous blood transfusion requirements, although additional protamine is required to counteract the heparin concentrated in the ultrafiltrate.[69] Ultrafiltration may decrease the incidence of pulmonary dysfunction after CPB[70] and is useful in maintaining fluid and electrolyte balance in patients with renal impairment.[71] Therefore, patients who will benefit from ultrafiltration include those with severe pulmonary dysfunction and those with renal insufficiency. Adverse effects associated with the use of ultrafiltration include leukopenia, complement activation, increased red blood cell trauma, and increased plasma hemoglobin.[72,73] Additionally, heparin retention in the ultrafiltrator is a potential problem.

Cell-Salvage Devices and Autotransfusion

Autotransfusion of blood from the cardiac surgical site is an effective way of reducing the need for homologous blood transfusion.[74-78] In the cardiac operating room, the cell-salvage machine is the most common method of performing autotransfusion. During CPB, a cell-salvage device can centrifuge blood removed from the venous line of the CPB circuit and then reinfuse the concentrated red cells into the venous reservoir (Figure 31.4). The use of cell salvage during CPB reduces the platelets, clotting proteins, and volume in the CPB circuit and is most helpful when there is excess volume but a low hematocrit in the patient-CPB circuit. This machine suctions blood from the surgical site through a double-lumen aspirator. The aspirated blood is mixed with the anticoagulant near the tip of the suction cannula and the anticoagulated aspirate is collected in a reservoir. When sufficient aspirate has collected in the reservoir, it is introduced to the spinning centrifuge bowl where it is centrifuged to concentrate the heavier red blood cells. The centrifuge bowl consists of an inner stationary subassembly and an outer rotating subassembly. Fluid enters and exits the centrifuge bowl via inlet and outlet ports. Blood is pumped into the spinning bowl through the inlet port and red blood cells are centrifuged toward the bowl's perimeter. The lower-density supernatant floats towards the bowl's inner core. As the bowl overflows, the lower-density supernatant — which includes the less dense plasma, platelets, cell stroma, activated clotting factors, extracellular potassium, free hemoglobin, anticoagulant, cardioplegic solution, hemolyzed cells and debris — is forced out the outlet port and into the waste bag. Once the bowl is nearly full of red cells, the bowl contents are washed with saline and the spinning action forces unwanted components into the waste bag. The saline wash removes any remaining platelets, plasma, he-

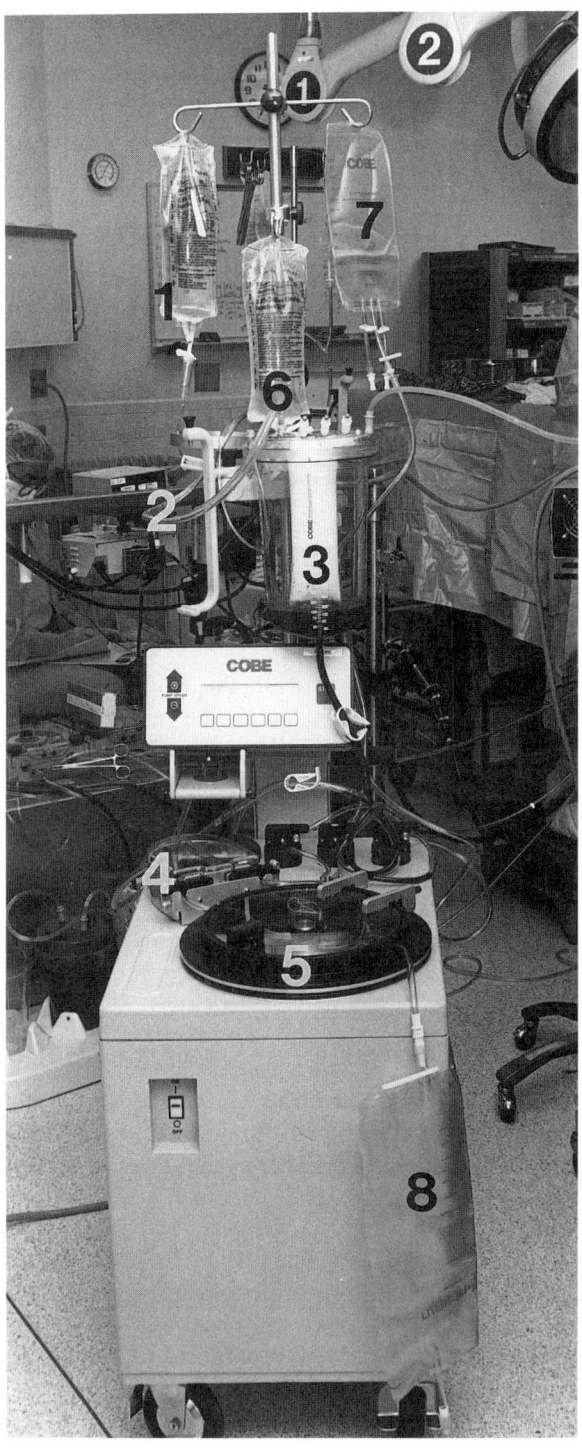

FIGURE 31.4. A cell salvage device. Blood is mixed with a heparinized saline (1) and suctioned through a double-lumen aspirator and tubing (2) to the cardiotomy reservoir (3). A roller-head pump (4) delivers the aspirate to the centrifuge and bowl (5). After the aspirate is centrifuged and washed with saline (6), it is pumped into a reinfusion bag (7) for storage and subsequent delivery to the patient. A waste bag (8) collects the supernatant.

molyzed cells, anticoagulant, or debris, as they are less dense than the red blood cells. After washing, the red blood cells are suspended in saline and pumped into the reinfusion bag.[79] The hematocrit in the bowl increases as more blood is pumped in and supernatant is forced out The hematocrit of the washed red blood cells is approximately 50% when the bowl is filled appropriately. A higher hematocrit can be obtained by filling the bowl until the red blood cell-supernatant interface is closer to the center of the bowl. Conversely, a lower hematocrit will be obtained if the filling is terminated by the operator before the standard interface level is reached.

If the patient is not systemically anticoagulated, an anticoagulant, such as heparin or sodium citrate, must be added to the aspirated blood as soon as possible to prevent clots from forming in the cell-salvage machine. Approximately 1 mL of anticoagulant solution (normal saline with 3 units heparin/mL) is mixed with 5 mL of aspirated blood.[79] Premixed citrate-phosphate-dextrose anticoagulant can be used in a 1:6–8 ratio of anticoagulant to aspirate.[79]

In another system that permits the collection of operating field blood for reinfusion to the patient, aspirated blood is collected in a suction canister with a plastic liner and filter that anticoagulates the blood as it is being aspirated. When the container is full, the unwashed aspirated solution is reinfused.[51]

Autotransfusion can also be utilized in the postoperative period, since blood shed into serosal cavities clots and then undergoes fibrinolysis.[51] Mediastinal blood has a hematocrit of 20% to 25%, free hemoglobin levels of 3–3.9 g/L, and small amounts of fibrinogen.[80-83] In routine cardiac surgical patients, autotransfusion of the shed mediastinal blood does not decrease homologous blood transfusion requirements and may cause coagulopathy by increasing the level of fibrin split products.[84,85] The platelets in shed mediastinal blood appear to have markedly decreased function[86] which may be due to a fibrinolytic mechanism.[87] However, in patients receiving aprotinin, autotransfusion of shed mediastinal blood may decrease homologous blood transfusion requirements[88] (Figure 31.5).

The complications of autotransfusion are air and/or fat emboli, pulmonary dysfunction, coagulopathy, renal dysfunction, sepsis, and dissemination of cancer. Contraindications to autotransfusion include any operation in which the operative field is contaminated by infection, malignant cells, gastric fluids, amniotic fluid, fibrin glue, topical thrombin, methylmethacrylate, topical antibiotics (not suitable for intravenous use), iodine antiseptic solutions, or the microfiber collagen Avitine.[79]

Plasma Sequestration Techniques

In plasma sequestration and plasmapheresis, whole blood is removed from the patient and separated into red cells,

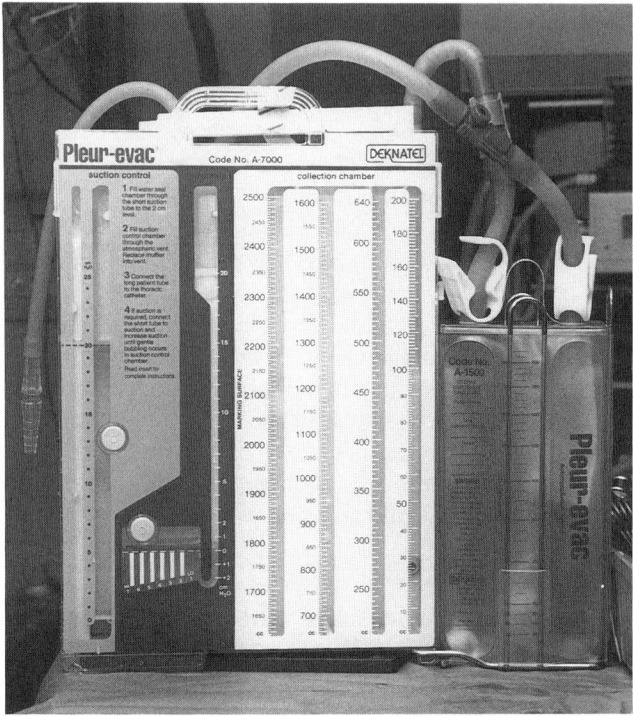

FIGURE 31.5. Mediastinal blood collection device with autotransfusion adapter. Shed mediastinal blood can be reinfused to the patient from the collection bag.

platelet-rich or platelet-poor plasma, and platelets. These procedures provide a method of preserving platelet function in a portion of the platelets prior to a platelet-damaging event such as CPB. Plasma sequestration provides autologous blood components that can be administered as needed, based on the patient's hematologic requirements. Plasmapheresis reduces serum albumin and protein levels, so that there is a risk of a decrease in colloid intravascular pressure, which may result in the accumulation of plasma water. Plasmapheresis should not be used in patients who are unable to tolerate a decreased hematocrit prior to CPB. Additionally, in patients treated with drugs that affect platelet function, platelet-rich plasma has no beneficial effect on postoperative bleeding.[89]

A "dedicated" plasmapheresis machine is manufactured by Plasma Collection System (Haemonetics Co., Braintree, MA), although several other manufacturers produce software products that permit an autotransfusion device to perform plasmapheresis. Plasmapheresis is similar to autotransfusion in that both processes have a microprocessor-controlled machine with centrifuges, collection reservoirs, pumps, and air detectors. However, a plasmapheresis machine is different from an autotransfusion machine in that plasmapheresis involves carefully controlled removal of whole blood from the patient's intravascular space rather than from the operative field. By altering the speed of the centrifuge, the operator can collect platelet-rich plasma by centrifuging at a slower speed; this allows the platelet fraction and plasma to be collected along with some red blood cells to form the platelet-rich plasma. At higher centrifuge speeds, the platelets separate into a buffy coat layer, allowing the collection of the platelet-poor plasma fraction. A cell-salvage machine performs plasma sequestration simply by spinning its centrifuge at a slower speed than that used for cell salvage, and inserting a Y-connector to allow the plasma to be collected into a sequestration reservoir separate from the waste bag (see Figure 32.4). The red blood cells can then be reinfused into the patient to conserve red cell mass.

Removal of whole blood for plasmapheresis can begin once central venous access has been established, and may be continued until 20% of the patient's intravascular volume is removed or the hematocrit falls to an unacceptable level. Volume replacement with 6% hetastarch,[90] crystalloid, or 5% albumin[91] solutions should begin prior to and during the plasmapheresis process. As the whole blood is removed from the patient, 1 mL of sodium citrate is added to every 12 mL of whole blood.[68] Twelve to 14 minutes is required to process 200 mL of whole blood,[90,92] and the average total processing time is between 30 and 57 minutes.[91,93] Generally, an adult patient will yield 1 to 2.5 × 10^{11} platelets per 600 mL of plasmapheresis product.[92,93] The collected blood products should be stored following accepted blood bank procedures. Platelets should receive gentle agitation to prevent platelet clumping. The blood products can be stored at operating room temperature for short periods of time, but if a prolonged time is expected prior to retransfusion, the blood bank should store the products until required. The blood products should be transfused after complete reversal of heparin with protamine.

Several studies have reported that patients treated with platelet-rich plasma have a decreased incidence of homologous blood transfusion during their hospitalization.[89-94] Patients receiving platelet-rich plasma have higher operative platelet counts,[90] improved platelet aggregability,[95] decreased postoperative bleeding,[96] and higher antithrombin III and fibrinogen levels.[97] Plasmapheresis has been shown to be more effective than autotransfusion alone, and platelet-rich plasma patients have a less positive fluid balance.[90] One study reported that the average number of transfusions was reduced from 13.67 to 6.32 homologous blood exposures per patient with the use of autotransfusion and platelet-rich plasma.[91] However, in primary cardiac surgery patients, plasmapheresis may not significantly decrease the need for homologous blood transfusion.[98,99]

Conclusion

Today, many patients undergoing cardiac surgery can leave the hospital without receiving any homologous blood product transfusions. By following a comprehensive blood conservation program and using the techniques outlined in this chapter, we can reduce the number of patients transfused to as little as 3.2% of elective coronary bypass surgeries.[100] Continued research and development of better blood conservation techniques will reduce this incidence of blood transfusion even further, resulting in safer and more cost-effective cardiac surgery in the future.

References

1. Consensus Conference: Perioperative red cell transfusion. *JAMA* 1988;260:2700-2703.
2. Faust RJ, Warner MA, Transfusion risks. *Int Anesthesiol Clinics* 1990;28:184-189.
3. Braine HG, Kickler TS, Charache P, et al. Bacterial sepsis secondary to platelet transfusion: an adverse effect on extended storage at room temperature. *Transfusion* 1986;26:391-393.
4. Aoki SK, Holland PV. Lyme disease: another transfusion risk? *Transfusion* 1989;29:646-650.
5. Dodd RY. The risk of transfusion-transmitted infection. *N Engl J Med* 1992;327:419-421.
6. Crosby ET. Perioperative haemotherapy: II. Risks and complications of blood transfusion. *Can J Anaesth* 1992;39:822-837.
7. Edinger SE. A closer look at fatal transfusion reactions. *Med Lab Observer* 1985;17:40-45.
8. Schriemer PA, Longnecker DE, Mintz PD. The possible immunosuppressive effects of perioperative blood transfusion in cancer patients. *Anesthesiology* 1988;68:422-428.
9. Blumberg N, Heal JM, Murphy P, et al. Association between transfusion of whole blood and recurrence of cancer. *Brit Med J* 1986;293:530-533.
10. Marsh J, Donnan PT, Hamer-Hodges DW. Association between transfusions with plasma and recurrence of colorectal carcinoma. *Br J Surg* 1990;77:623-626.
11. Opelz G, Sengar DPS, Mickey MR, et al. Effect of blood transfusions on subsequent kidney transplants. *Transplant Proc* 1973;5:253-259.
12. Opelz G. Improved kidney graft survival in non-transfused recipients. *Transplant Proc* 1987;19:149-152.
13. Nichols RL, Smith JW, Klein DB, et al. Risk of infection after penetrating abdominal trauma. *N Engl J Med* 1984;311:1065-1070.
14. Dawes LG, Aprahamian C, Condon RE, et al. The risk of infection after colon injury. *Surgery* 1986;100:796-803.
15. Murphy P, Heal JM, Blumberg N. Infection or suspected infection after hip replacement surgery with antologous or homologous blood transfusions. *Transfusion* 1991;31:212-217.
16. Miholic J, Hudec M, Domanig E, et al. Risk factors for severe bacterial infections after valve replacement and aortocoronary bypass operations: analysis of 246 cases by logistic regression. *Ann Thorac Surg* 1985;40:224-228.
17. Ottino G, DePaulis R, Pansini S, et al. Major sternal wound infection after open-heart surgery: a multivariate analysis of risk factors in 2,579 consecutive operative procedures. *Ann Thorac Surg* 1987;44:173-179.
18. Pinto V, Baldonedo R, Nicolas C, Barez A, Perez A, Aza

J. Relationship of transfusion and infectious complications after gastric carcinoma operations. *Transfusion* 1991;31:114-118.
19. Gascon P, Zoumbos NC, Young NS. Immunologic abnormalities in patients receiving multiple blood transfusions. *Ann Intern Med* 1984;100:173-177.
20. Ford CD, Warnick S, Sheets S, Quist R, Stevens LE. Blood transfusions lower natural killer cell activity. *Transplant Proc* 1987;19:1456-1457.
21. Fischer E, Lenhard V, Seifert P, Kluge A, Johannsen R. Blood transfusion-induced suppression of cellular immunity in man. *Hum Immunol* 1980;3:187-194.
22. Rawston RE, Preoperative hemoglobin levels. *Anaesth Intensive Care* 1976;4:175-185.
23. Carson JL, Spence RK, Poses RM, Bonavita G. Severity of anaemia and operative mortality and morbidity. *Lancet* 1988;1:727-729.
24. Messmer KFW. Acceptable hematocrit levels in surgical patients. *World J Surg* 1987;11:41-46.
25. Von Restorff W, Hofling B, Holtz J, Bassenge E. Effect of increased blood fluidity through hemodilution on general circulation at rest and during exercise in dogs. *Pflugers Arch* 1975;357;25-34.
26. Tarnow J, Eberlein HJ, Schneider E, et al. Hemodynamic interactions of hemodilution, anesthesia, propranolol pretreatment and hypovolemia. I. Systemic circulation. *Basic Res Cardiol* 1979;74:109-122.
27. Glick G, Plauth WH, Braunwald E, et al. Role of the autonomic nervous system in the circulatory response to acutely induced anemia in unanesthetized dogs. *J Clin Invest* 1964;43:2112-2124.
28. Escobar E, Jones NL, Rapaport E, et al. Ventricular performance in acute normovolemic anemia and effects of beta blockade. *Am J Physiol* 1966;211:877-884.
29. Crystal GJ. Coronary hemodynamic response during local hemodilution in canine hearts. *Am J Physiol* 1988;254:H525-H531.
30. Jan KM, Chien S. Effect of hematocrit variations on coronary hemodynamics and oxygen utilization. *Am J Physiol* 1977;233:H106-H113.
31. Geha AS, Baue AE. Graded coronary stenosis and coronary flow during acute normovolemic anemia. *World J Surg* 1978;2:645-652.
32. Rosenberg B, Wulff F. Hemodynamics following normovolemic hemodilution in elderly patients. *Acta Anaesthesiol Scand* 1981;25:402-406.
33. Vara-Thorbeck R, Guerrero-Fernandez Marcote JA. Hemodynamic responses of elderly patients undergoing major surgery under moderate normovolemic hemodilution. *Eur Surg Res* 1985;17:372-376.
34. Cole DJ, Drummond JC, Patel PM, et al. Hemodilution during cerebral ischemia in rats: effects of a molecular hemoglobin solution on neurologic outcome and brain injury. *Anesth Analg* 1994;78:S66. Abstract.
35. Roy RC, Prough DS, Rogers AT, et al. Higher hematocrit limits cerebral oxygenation during hypothermic nonpulsatile cardiopulmonary bypass. *Anesthesiology* 1989;71:A75.
36. Owings DV, Kruskall MS, Thurer RL, et al. Autologous blood donations prior to elective cardiac surgery. *JAMA* 1989;262:1963-1968.
37. Rao TLK, Montoya A. Cardiovascular, electrocardiographic and respiratory changes following acute anemia with volume replacement in patients with coronary artery disease. *Anesth Review* 1985;12:49-54.
38. Kim YD, Katz NM, Ng L, et al. Effects of hypothermia and hemodilution on oxygen metabolism and hemodynamics in patients recovering from coronary artery bypass operations. *J Thorac Cardiovasc Surg* 1989;97:36-42.
39. Weisel RD, Charlesworth DC, Mickleborough LL, et al. Limitations of blood conservation. *J Thorac Cardiovasc Surg* 1984;88:26-38.
40. Holtz J, Bassenge E, Von Restotff W, et al. Transmural differences in myocardial blood flow and in coronary dilatory capacity in hemodiluted conscious dogs. *Basic Res Cardiol* 1976;71:36-46.
41. Levine E, Rosen A, Sehgal L, et al. Physiologic effects of acute anemia: implications for a reduced transfusion trigger. *Transfusion* 1990;30:11-14.
42. Gould BA, Rosen AL, Sehgal LR, et al. O_2 extraction ratio: a physiologic indicator of transfusion need. *Transfusion* 1983;23:416.
43. Sunder-Plassmann L, Kessler M, Jesch F, et al. Acute normovolemic hemodilution: changes in tissue oxygen supply and hemoglobin-oxygen affinity. *Bibl Haematol* 1975;41:44-53.
44. Blumdell J. Experiments on the transfusion of blood. *Medico Chir Trans* 1818;9:56.
45. Halsted WS. Refusion in carbonic oxide poisoning. *New York Med J* 1883;38:625-629.
46. Tiber S. Ruptured ectopic pregnancy. *Calif West Med* 1934;41:16-20.
47. Goodnough LT, Rucnick S, Price TH, et al. Increased preoperative collection of autologous blood with recombinant human erythropoietin therapy. *N Engl J Med* 1989;321:1163-1168.
48. Love TR, Hendren WG, O'Keefe DD, et al. Transfusion of predonated autologous blood in elective cardiac surgery. *Ann Thorac Surg* 1987;43:508-512.
49. Birkmeyer JD, AuBuchon JP, Littenberg B, et al. Cost-effectiveness of preoperative autologous donation in coronary artery bypass grafting. *Ann Thorac Surg* 1994;57:161-169.
50. Miller AC, Scherba-Krugliak L, Toy PT, et al. Hypotension during transfusion of autologous blood. *Anesthesiology* 1991;74:624-628.
51. Stehling L. Autotransfusion and hemodilution. In: Miller RD, ed. *Anesthesia*. 3rd ed. New York: Churchill Livingstone; 1990:1501-1513.
52. Miller ED. Deliberate hypotension. In: Miller RD, ed. *Anesthesia*. 3rd ed. New York: Churchill Livingstone; 1990:1347-1367.
53. McClure PD, Izsak J. The use of epsilon-aminocaproic acid to reduce bleeding during cardiac bypass in children with congenital heart disease. *Anesthesiology* 1974;40:604-608.
54. Sterns LP, Lillehei CW. Effect of epsilon aminocaproic acid upon blood loss following open-heart surgery: an analysis of 340 patients. *Canad J Surg* 1967;10:304-307.
55. DelRossi AJ, Cernaianu AC, Botros S, et al. Prophylactic treatment of postperfusion bleeding using EACA. *Chest* 1989;96:27-30.

56. Midell AI, Hallman GL, Bloodwell RD, et al. Epsilon-aminocaproic acid for bleeding after cardiopulmonary bypass. *Ann Thorac Surg* 1971;11:577-582.
57. Vander Salm TJ, Ansell JE, Okike ON, et al. The role of epsilon-aminocaproic acid in reducing bleeding after cardiac operation: a double-blind randomized study. *J Thorac Cardiovasc Surg* 1988;95:538-540.
58. Horrow JC, Hlavacek J, Strong MD, et al. Prophylactic tranexamic acid decreases bleeding after cardiac operations. *J Thorac Cardiovasc Surg* 1990;99:70-74.
59. Horrow JC, Van Riper DF, Strong MD, et al. Hemostatic effects of tranexamic acid and desmopressin during cardiac surgery. *Circulation* 1991;84:2063-2070.
60. Royston D, Taylor KM, Birdstrup BP, et al. Effect of aprotinin on need for blood transfusion after repeat open-heart surgery. *Lancet* 1987;1289-1291.
61. Dietrich W, Barankay A, Dilthey G, et al. Reduction of homologous blood requirement in cardiac surgery by intraoperative aprotinin application: clinical experience in 152 cardiac surgical patients. *J Thorac Cardiovasc Surg* 1989;37:92-98.
62. Bidstrup BP, Royston D, Sapsford RN, et al. Reduction in blood loss and blood use after cardiopulmonary bypass with high dose aprotinin. *J Thorac Cardiovasc Surg* 1989;97:364-372.
63. Havel M, Teufelsbauer H, Knobl P, et al. Effect of intraoperative aprotinin administration on postoperative bleeding in patients undergoing cardiopulmonary bypass operation. *J Thorac Cardiovasc Surg* 1991;101:968-972.
64. Salzman EW, Weinstein MJ, Weintraub RM, et al. Treatment with desmopressin acetate to reduce blood loss after cardiac surgery. *N Engl J Med* 1986;314:1402-1406.
65. Ansell J, Klassen V, Lew R, et al. Does desmopressin acetate prophylaxis reduce blood loss after valvular heart operations? *J Thorac Cardiovasc Surg* 1992;104:117-123.
66. Mongan PD, Hosking MP. The role of desmopressin acetate in patients undergoing coronary artery bypass surgery. *Anesthesiology* 1992;77:38-46.
67. Silverstein ME, Ford CA, Lysaght MJ, et al. Treatment of severe fluid overload by ultrafiltration. *N Engl J Med* 1974;291:747-751.
68. Stammers AH. Extracorporeal devices and related technologies. In: Kaplan JA, ed. *Cardiac Anesthesia*. 3rd ed. Philadelphia: Saunders; 1993:995-1029.
69. Friesen RH, Tornabene MA, Coleman SP. Blood conservation during pediatric cardiac surgery: ultrafiltration of the extracorporeal circuit volume after cardiopulmonary bypass. *Anesth Analg* 1993;77:702-707.
70. Magilligan DJ, Oyama C. Ultrafiltration during cardiopulmonary bypass: laboratory evaluation and initial clinical experience. *Ann Thorac Surg* 1984;37:33-39.
71. Magilligan DJ. Indications for ultrafiltration in the cardiac surgical patient. *J Thorac Cardiovasc Surg* 1985;83:183-189.
72. Chenoweth DE, Cooper SW, Hugh TE, et al. Complement activation during cardiopulmonary bypass: evidence of generation of C3a and C5a anaphylatoxins. *N Engl J Med* 1981;304:497-506.
73. Craddick PR, Fehr J, Brigham KL. Complement and leucocyte-mediated pulmonary dysfunction in hemodialysis. *N Engl J Med* 1977;296:769-774.
74. Hiratzka LF, Richardson JV, Brandt B, et al. The effect of autologous blood salvage techniques upon bank blood usage and the cost of routine coronary revascularization. *Perfusion* 1986;1:239-244.
75. Breyer RH, Engelman RM, Rousou JA, et al. Blood conservation for myocardial revascularization. *J Thorac Cardiovasc Surg* 1987;93:512-522.
76. McCarthy PM, Popovsky MA, Schaff HV, et al. Effect of blood conservation efforts in cardiac operations at the Mayo Clinic. *Mayo Clinic Proc* 1988;63:225-229.
77. Laub GW, Dharan M, Riebman JB, et al. The impact of intraoperative autotransfusion on cardiac surgery. *Chest* 1993;104:686-689.
78. Khan RMA, Siddiqui AMA, Natrajan KM. Blood conservation and autotransfusion in cardiac surgery. *J Card Surg* 1993;8:25-31.
79. Cell Saver® Plus autologous blood recovery system owner's operating and maintenance manual. 1986 Haemonetics Corporation, Braintree, MA.
80. Hartz RS, Smith JA, Green D. Autotransfusion after cardiac operation. *J Thorac Cardiovasc Surg* 1988;96:178-182.
81. Solem J, Steen S, Tengborn L, et al. Mediastinal drainage blood: potentialities for autotransfusion after cardiac surgery. *Scand J Thorac Cardiovasc Surg* 1987;21:149-152.
82. Thurer RL, Lytle BW, Cosgrove DM, et al. Autotransfusion following cardiac operations: a randomized, prospective study. *Ann Thorac Surg* 1979;27:500-507.
83. Carter RF, McArdle B, Morrit GM. Autologous transfusion of mediastinal drainage blood: a report of its use following open heart surgery. *Anaesthesia* 1981;36:54-59.
84. Griffith LD, Billman GF, Daily PO, et al. Apparent coagulopathy caused by infusion of shed mediastinal blood and its prevention by washing of the infusate. *Ann Thorac Surg* 1989;47:400-406.
85. Ward HB, Smith RRA, Landis KP, et al. Prospective, randomized trial of autotransfusion after routine cardiac operations. *Ann Thorac Surg* 1993;56:137-141.
86. Kongsgaard UE, Hovig T, Brosstad F, et al. Platelets in shed mediastinal blood used for postoperation autotransfucion. *Acta Anaesthesiol Scand* 1993;37:265-268.
87. de Haan J, Schonberger J, Haan J, et al. Tissue-type plasminogen activator and fibrin monomers synergistically cause platelet dysfunction during retransfusion of shed blood after cardiopulmonary bypass. *J Thorac Cardiovasc Surg* 1993;106:1017-1023.
88. Schonberger J, Bredee J, Speekenbrink RG, et al. Autotransfusion of shed blood contributes additionally to blood saving in patients receiving aprotinin. *Eur J Cardiothorac Surg* 1993;7:474-477.
89. Giordano GF Sr, Giordano GF Jr, Rivers SL, et al. Determinants of homologous blood usage utilizing autologous platelet-rich plasma in cardiac operations. *Ann Thorac Surg* 1989;47:897-902.
90. Boldt J, Kling D, Zickmann B, et al. Acute preoperative plasmapheresis and established blood conservation techniques. *Ann Thorac Surg* 1990;50:62-68.
91. Giordano GF, Rivers SL, Chung GKT, et al. Autologous platelet-rich plasma in cardiac surgery: effect on intraoperative and postoperative transfusion requirements. *Ann Thorac Surg* 1988;46:416-419.

92. Tawes RL, Sydorak GR, Duvall TB, et al. The plasma collection system: a new concept in autotransfusion. *Ann Vasc Surg* 1988;64:304–306.
93. Jones JW, McCoy TA, Rawitscher RE, et al. Effects of intraoperative plasmapheresis on blood loss in cardiac surgery. *Ann Thorac Surg* 1990;49:585-590.
94. Smith JW. Haemonetics plasma collection system (PCS): automated collection of platelet-poor or platelet-rich plasma. *J Clin Apheresis* 1988;4:93-96.
95. Boldt J, Zickmann B, Ballesteros M, et al. Influence of acute preoperative plasmapheresis on platelet function n cardiac surgery. *J Cardiothorac Vasc Anesth* 1993;7:4-9.
96. Ferrari M, Zia S, Valbonesi M, et al. A new technique for hemodilution, preparation of autologous platelet-rich plasma and intraoperative blood salvage in cardiac surgery. *Int J Artif Organs* 1987;10:47-50.
97. Boldt J, von Borman NB, Kling D, et al. Preoperative plasmapheresis in patients undergoing cardiac surgery. *Anesthesiology* 1990;72:282-288.
98. Tobe CE, Vocelka C, Sepulvada R, et al. Infusion of autologous platelet rich plasma does not reduce blood loss and product use after coronary artery bypass. *J Thorac Cardiovasc Surg* 1993;105:1007-1014.
99. Wong CA, Franklin ML, Wade LD. Coagulation tests, blood loss, and transfusion requirements in platelet-rich plasmapheresed versus nonpheresed cardiac surgery patients. *Anesth Analg* 1994;78:29-36.
100. Ovrum E, Am Holen E, Abdelnoor M, et al. Conventional blood conservation techniques in 500 consecutive coronary artery bypass operations. *Ann Thorac Surg* 1991;52:500-505.

32
Religious Objections to Blood Transfusion

Robert B. Lee and Tomas D. Martin

Historical Aspect, Biblical Basis for Religious Beliefs

> Every moving animal that is alive may serve as food for you. As in the case of green vegetation, I do give it all to you. Only flesh with its soul—its blood—you must not eat. Genesis 9: 3,4[1]

God's admonition to Noah serves as the cornerstone scripture upon which Jehovah's Witnesses base their objection to transfusion of blood and blood products. The Jehovah's Witnesses are not a fanatic cult or religious eccentrics. They seek and comply with modern medical and surgical treatment, believing strongly in their religious duty to keep healthy the "bodily temple" God has given them. They do not partake of alcohol or recreational drugs and reject abortions, professing that they cherish and respect life too much to waste it.[2]

Numbering greater than 3.2 million worldwide, Witnesses are 750,000 strong in the United States.[3] Founded in the 1870s by Charles Taze Russell, a Pennsylvania lawyer, this nondenominational study group was joined by others forming the Watchtower Bible and Tract Society in 1881.[4,5] By 1909, they had become an international society with headquarters in Brooklyn, New York. They adopted their present name, Jehovah's Witnesses, in 1931 based on the Biblical scripture Isaiah 43:10 in which the Lord, Jehovah, said, "You are my witnesses."[6] Their doctrine of blood refusal was set forth in 1927 and again in 1944. Based on the Old Testament scriptures, they believe that the eating of blood was forbidden by God to Noah; since all mankind descended from Noah's family, the restriction applies to all who follow. God said, "I shall certainly set my face against the soul that is eating the blood, and I shall indeed cut him off from among his people"[7] thereby establishing the penalty for transgression as separation from God or loss of eternal life.

There is no mention in the Bible of blood transfusion as we know it today. The Witnesses believe that transfusion of blood and blood products was covered in principle, citing New Testament scripture commanding Christians to "keep abstaining from things sacrificed to idols and from blood and from things strangled [unbled meat] and from fornication. If you carefully keep yourselves from these things, you will prosper. Good health to you!"[8]

Witnesses firmly adhere to these tenets; yet, in keeping with their faith, they seek out the most modern medical and surgical therapies, having undergone major cardiovascular procedures[9] and even organ transplantation.[10] How, then, are we cardiovascular surgeons, anesthesiologists, and perfusionists to fulfill our Oath of Hippocrates while maintaining the bodily and spiritual integrity of the Jehovah's Witnesses? In this chapter, we will discuss the applicable legal precedents and outline perioperative management strategies for patients refusing blood product transfusion.

Legal Aspects: The Horns of a Dilemma

> Every person of adult years and sound mind has a right to determine what shall be done with his own body; and a surgeon who performs an operation without his patient's consent commits, . . . [a battery] for which he is liable in damages.
> Judge Benjamin Cardozo
> A.D. 1905[11]

There is a great volume of case law pertaining to the various philosophies, truths, and doctrines concerning consent to treatment and transfusion of blood products. Most of these precedents center around three aspects: (1) the patient's rights as guaranteed by the First Amendment,[4] (2) the case of minors, ie, parens patriae,[12,13] and (3) informed consent.[4]

A survey of a Witness congregation revealed that more than two thirds would file suit if transfused against their will.[5] Witnesses will readily sign the American Medical Association form relieving physicians and hospitals of liability (Figure 32.1). Most now wear a dated, witnessed

REFUSAL TO PERMIT BLOOD TRANSFUSION

DATE: _____ TIME: _____

I request that no blood or blood derivatives be administered to _____
Name of Patient

during this hospitalization. I hereby release Emory University, its personnel, and the attending physicians from any responsibility whatever for unfavorable reactions or any untoward results due to this refusal to permit the use of blood or its derivatives. I fully understand the possible consequences, including death, of such refusal and, if I am / the patient is pregnant, I understand such refusal may result in fetal death.

_____   _____
Witness   Patient Signature

                                  _____
                                  Signature of Person Authorized
                                  to Consent for Patient*

                                  Relationship to Patient:
                                  ❏ Parent   ❏ Guardian   ❏ Spouse

*When the patient is a minor (under 18 years of age), or an incompetent adult, the signature of a person authorized to consent for the patient is required. A parent or guardian is authorized to consent for a minor patient and a spouse or guardian may consent for an incompetent adult patient. The spouse, if available, should co-sign this form with the competent patient.

FIGURE 32.1. American Medical Association form relieving physicians and hospitals from liability for not transfusing blood products.

medical alert card prepared in consultation with medical and legal authorities (Figure 32.2).[2,14] These documents are considered binding on the patient and his estate, thereby protecting physicians and hospitals from negligence litigation. Justice Warren Burger has held that a malpractice proceeding "would appear unsupported" when the signed waiver is in effect. Furthermore, in the San Francisco Law Review, J. J. Paris wrote

> One commentator who surveyed the literature reported, 'I have not been able to find any authority for the statement that the physician would incur . . . criminal . . . liability by his *failure* to force a transfusion on an unwilling patient.' The risk seems more the product of a fertile legal mind than a realistic possibility.[14]

Thus, relative protection appears to exist for the physician who abides by the wishes of the Witnesses and does *not* transfuse, even when failure to transfuse results in ill effects or death of the patient. However, the physician must be aware of the legal precedents if he elects to authorize transfusion *without* consent of a Witness or his children.

Previous judiciary rulings can be grouped into three categories: (1) the legally competent adult, (2) the legally incompetent adult, and (3) the issue of minors. State courts rarely intervene when petitioned for the authority to transfuse a conscious, legally competent adult, ruling overwhelmingly in favor of the nonconsenting competent adult.[3] Article I of the Bill of Rights ("Congress shall make no law respecting an establishment of a religion, or prohibiting the free exercise thereof") is used as justification and foundation for the decision.

This legal precedent was set *In Regards to Brooks Estate* when the Illinois Supreme Court found in favor of Bernice Brooks, stating:

> Even though we may consider a patient's beliefs unwise, foolish or ridiculous, in the absence of overriding danger to society we may not permit interference therewith in the form of conservatorship established in the waning hours of her life for the sole purpose of compelling her to accept medical treatment forbidden by her religious principles and previously refused by her with full knowledge of the probable consequences.[4,15-17]

Although this would appear to be a clear mandate protecting competent adult Witnesses from transfusion, the courts have ordered transfusion of competent adults, such as pregnant females or adults with dependent children.[18] Cases in point are: *In the Matter of Melideo*,[19] the court

ADVANCE MEDICAL DIRECTIVE/RELEASE

I, _____, make this advance directive as a formal statement of my wishes. These instructions reflect my resolute decision.

I direct that **no blood transfusions** (whole blood, red cells, white cells, platelets, or blood plasma) be given to me under any circumstances, even if physicians deem such necessary to preserve my life or health. I will accept nonblood volume expanders (such as dextran, saline or Ringer's solution, or hetastarch) and other nonblood management.

This legal directive is an exercise of my right to accept or to refuse medical treatment in accord with my deeply held values and convictions. I am one of Jehovah's Witnesses, and I make this directive out of obedience to commands in the Bible, such as: "Keep abstaining . . . from blood." (Acts 15:28, 29) This is, and has been, my unwavering religious stand for _____ years. I am _____ years old.

I also know that there are various dangers associated with blood transfusions. So I have decided to avoid such dangers and, instead, to accept whatever risks may seem to be involved in my choice of alternative nonblood management.

I release physicians, anesthesiologists, and hospitals and their personnel from liability for any damages that might be caused by my refusal of blood, despite their otherwise competent care.

I authorize the person(s) named on the reverse to see that my instructions set forth in this directive are upheld and to answer any questions about my absolute refusal of blood.

Signature _____
Address _____ Date _____
                         Telephone _____
Witness _____
Witness _____

FIGURE 32.2. Release card carried by Jehovah's Witnesses documenting (1) their directive that they do not receive blood products; and (2) a form relieving physicians and/or hospitals from liability for not administering blood products.

ruled that promoting the welfare of children justified compulsory transfusion in pregnant women and mothers of young children.[18] *In Regards to Osborne*,[20] transfusion was allowed in a male Jehovah's Witness if loss of his income could leave his offspring to become wards of the state. Thus, based on the First Amendment, a conscious, competent adult who is not pregnant and has no dependents probably cannot be legally compelled to receive a blood transfusion against his or her religious beliefs if he or she makes these known to the physician.

Courts generally do *not* assume the right of self-determination for incompetent patients or minor children of nonconsenting adults. Two cases established conflicting precedents. The first, *Kennedy Memorial Hospital v Heston*, involved a 22-year-old unmarried Witness with a ruptured spleen following a motor vehicle accident.[21] The patient refused transfusion initially. While unconscious and thus "incompetent," she was transfused under court order. Several weeks later, after recovery, the patient and her mother sued to vacate the order under which transfusion had been authorized. The court held in part:

> . . . it seems correct to say that there is no constitutional right to die . . . we think it reasonable to resolve the problem by permitting the hospital and its staff to pursue their functions according to their professional standards. The solution sides with life, the conservation of which is, we think, a matter of state interest.[21]

By this ruling, the Supreme Court of New Jersey has supported and acknowledged the medical profession's ethical mandate as described by the Hippocratic Oath.

A conflicting view was expressed one year later by an Illinois Federal District Court when they found against the physician and hospital in the case *Holmes v Silver Cross Hospital*.[22] A 20-year-old male needed an emergency operation, to which he agreed on the condition of no transfusion. When he became unconscious from hemorrhagic shock, a guardian was appointed and a court-ordered transfusion authorized. The transfusion was instituted too late and the patient eventually died. The widow brought a civil rights action suit claiming violation of her husband's first amendment rights. The court dismissed the suit against the magistrate and the court-appointed guardian but required the physician and the hospital to stand trial and "show a grave and immediate danger" existed to an interest which the state might lawfully protect.[12]

When children are involved, courts intervene not to deny religious freedom, but because it is generally held that until children reach the age of majority they are *not* considered "capable" of accepting a given faith if the pursuit of its beliefs would be detrimental to their well-being. A Massachusetts court has held:

> . . . the right to practice religion does not include liberty to expose the child to . . . ill health or death . . . Parents may be free to become martyrs themselves. But it does not follow that they are free in identical circumstances to make martyrs of their children before they have reached the age of full and legal discretion when they can make the choice themselves.[23]

The courts are guided by the legal principle of parens patriae: the state has an overriding interest in the health and welfare of its citizens. The purpose of the court, to protect minors, has generally been accomplished by making the children temporary wards of the court, thereby giving the court clear jurisdiction in matters of welfare. In general, most states have statutes that define the neglected child as one whose parents cannot or will not provide proper care, including medical and surgical care. When the child is in jeopardy, the physician should present the plea and evidence to a judge, who in turn appoints a

TABLE 32.1. Perioperative pharmacologic interventions to minimize blood loss, facilitate (↑) hemoglobin (Hgb) synthesis, or increase (↑) O₂ delivery.

	↓ Blood loss	↑ Hgb synthesis	(↑) O₂ delivery
Preoperative	Discontinue anticoagulants and antiplatelet drugs Correct nutritional and hepatic abnormalities	Erythropoietin Folic acid Iron Vitamin K	
Intraoperative	Protamine reversal of heparin Desmopressin ε-Aminocaproic acid Minimize blood sample lab tests		Volume expansion Crystalloid Colloid-dextran, hetastarch
Postoperative	Same as intraoperative	Same as preoperative	Same as intraoperative Hyperbaric oxygen

guardian, usually the hospital administrator. The guardian can then authorize transfusion. The guardianship order, in most cases, stays in effect until the child is discharged from the hospital. Recently, there has been an increasing tendency by the courts not to accuse the parents of neglect and to respect the wishes of Witnesses concerning their children.[3]

Medical and Surgical Options

Witnesses are, in keeping with their religious philosophies, motivated to maintain their health and to seek the most modern medical and surgical options when good health fails. Complex abdominal surgery,[24] obstetric and gynecologic surgery,[25] spinal fusion,[26] and open-heart surgery[9,27] have been performed successfully in Witnesses without transfusion of blood products. Some Witnesses have even sought heart[10,28] and kidney[29] transplantation, with good success rates. More importantly, there has been no increase in morbidity or mortality under the conditions of "no transfusion."[24-27]

Preoperative assessment and planning are crucial. The exact wishes of the Witness patient must be elucidated, understood, and documented. Open communication must exist between the surgeon, the anesthesiologist, and the staff to provide care in accordance with the wishes of the patient. The patient should be interviewed apart from family members and congregation members to determine his exact wishes if death is imminent without transfusion. Some will accept transfusion under these circumstances. Parents of children needing transfusion are often relieved when the decision is taken from their hands and placed in the hands of the judicial system. Two issues in particular must be clarified prior to surgery. Most Witnesses accept blood scavenged intraoperatively by "cell-saver devices" as long as the "continuous circuit"[30] principle is maintained[2,27,30]; some will not accept it.[30-32] Blood shed into the mediastinal chest tubes and collected in autotransfusion devices is acceptable to some Witnesses, but not to all.[31,32] Predeposit of autologous blood or preoperative autologous donation with freeze drying is acceptable to a few, but not to many.[33]

Thus, the physician must have a clear understanding concerning what the particular patient's conscience will allow. The preoperative agreement should be clearly documented and considered binding by the surgeon. The surgeon and health care team should strictly adhere to the agreement regardless of events developing intraoperatively or postoperatively.[24] Once the physician-patient agreement is established, multiple methods for preventing

TABLE 32.2. Surgical techniques to minimize perioperative blood loss.

Meticulous technique
Electrocautery, laser surgery, argon beam coagulation, gamma knife radiosurgery
Increased numbers of surgical team to reduce operating time
Staged surgery
Endoscopy for identification and control of gastrointestinal bleeding
Arterial embolization
Tissue adhesives
Topical hemostatic agents: (Avitene[R], Gelfoam[R], Surgicel[R])

TABLE 32.3. Perioperative monitors to assess oxygen delivery and techniques to decrease blood loss.

Monitors
  Arterial catheters
  Oximetry pulmonary artery catheter
  Transcutaneous oxygen sensors
Techniques
  Hypotensive anesthesia
  Postoperative controlled hypotension
  Hypothermia
  Hemodilution
  Blood salvage
  Hemoconcentration

or controlling hemorrhage and managing the sequelae are at the surgeon's disposal. All the therapies and alternative treatments listed in Tables 32.1 to 32.3 are acceptable to the Jehovah's Witness.[34]

During the preoperative period, it is extremely important to correct all abnormalities of nutrition, liver function, and coagulation. In particular, all anticoagulants and antiplatelet drugs should be discontinued well in advance of surgery. It is also important in the preoperative period to determine total red cell mass and hemoglobin levels. There are no data to uphold the previously believed concept that 10 g/dL of hemoglobin is necessary for a safe anesthetic and favorable operative outcome. This commonly accepted level has never been firmly established by clinical or experimental endeavors. Data do exist, however, showing that patients with hemoglobin levels of 6 g/dL preoperatively can be operated upon safely when blood loss is kept at a minimum (<500 mL).[30,35,36] Additionally, chronically anemic patients can tolerate hemoglobin levels as low as 3 g/dL without significant difficulty.[37] However, few data exist evaluating the acceptable level of hemoglobin for patients with ischemic heart disease. Therefore, the surgeon should do everything possible to ensure as high a level of hemoglobin as possible. Ferrous sulfate and iron dextran have both been used preoperatively and postoperatively to increase hemoglobin levels.[37] Erythropoietin (Epogen, rh-EP), a drug that has been proven to stimulate red cell production, is now marketed in the United States and approved by the Food and Drug Administration. Several reports[30,38–40] have revealed successful use of rh-EP in Jehovah's Witnesses to stimulate bone marrow and improve hemoglobin levels.

Intraoperatively, multiple techniques can be utilized to limit blood loss,[27,35,41,42] and meticulous hemostasis is of the utmost importance (Table 32.2). Use of the electrocautery for hemostasis is well established, and newer modalities such as laser surgery and argon beam coagulation may prove useful. It has also been reported that limiting the size of the incision and obtaining a dry mediastinum before heparinization for cardiopulmonary bypass re-

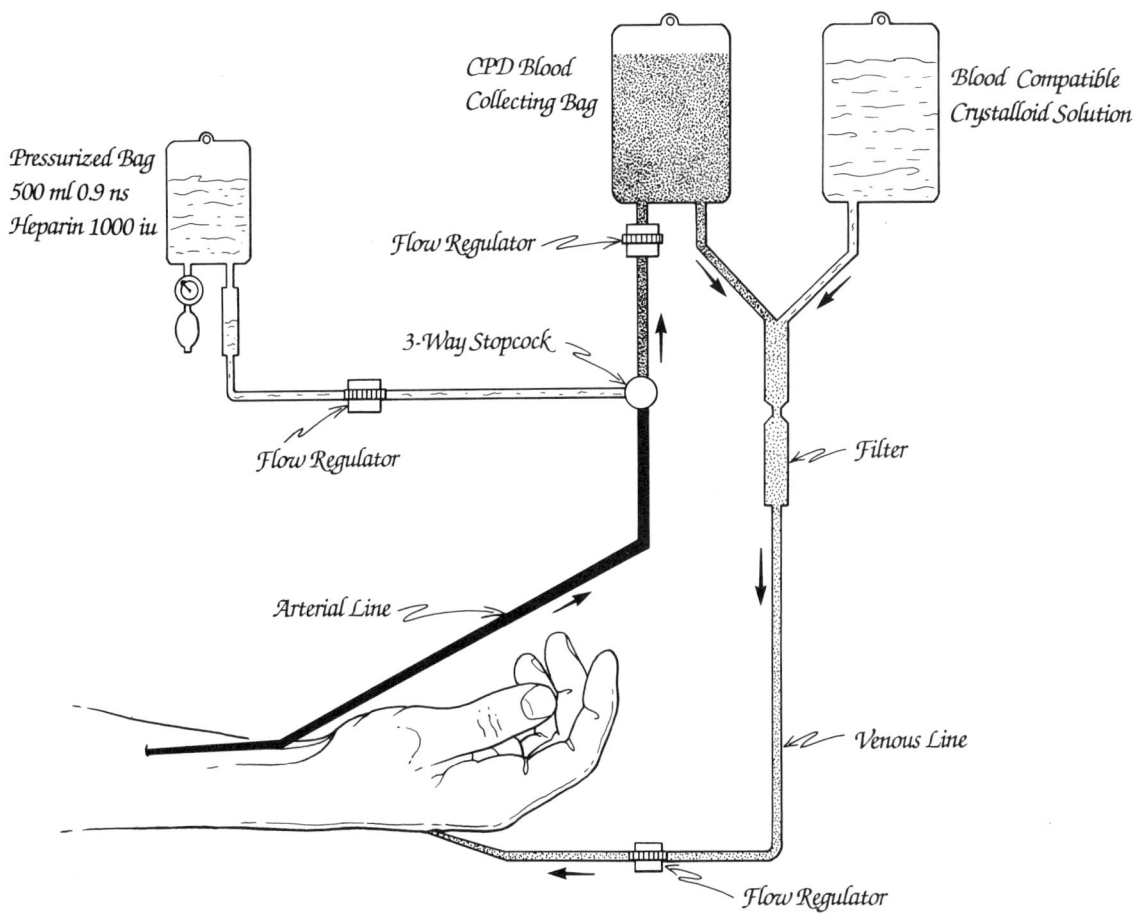

FIGURE 32.3. This system, accepted by Jehovah's Witnesses, permits simultaneous storage and circulation of blood. The arterial blood is collected at a faster rate than the venous reinfusion rate. The mandate that the blood does not lose contact with the body is fulfilled.

duces blood loss.[9,27] The surgeon may even want to consider using the saphenous vein only for coronary bypass rather than an internal mammary artery. At least one report has been published stating that use of the internal mammary artery may be associated with increased postoperative blood loss and increased mortality.[30] In our experience, bilateral mammaries have been associated with increased blood loss, with an increased rate of secondary operations for hemostasis. In the very complex case, staged procedures may also be considered when blood loss is expected to be high.

From an anesthetic standpoint, it is extremely important to use all available monitoring devices designed to assess oxygen delivery (Table 32.3). Beat-to-beat arterial pressure monitoring and pulmonary artery pressure monitoring as well as continuous mixed venous oxygen saturation measurement and pulse oximetry, allow on-line assessment of hemodynamics and oxygen delivery to assess the effects of relative anemia. Intraoperatively, and in the immediate postoperative period, volume expansion with crystalloid is acceptable. However, colloid in the form of dextran and hetastarch may be preferable for preventing postoperative edema. Artificial hemoglobin and fluorocarbon fluids (fluosol-DA 20%) may be the forerunners

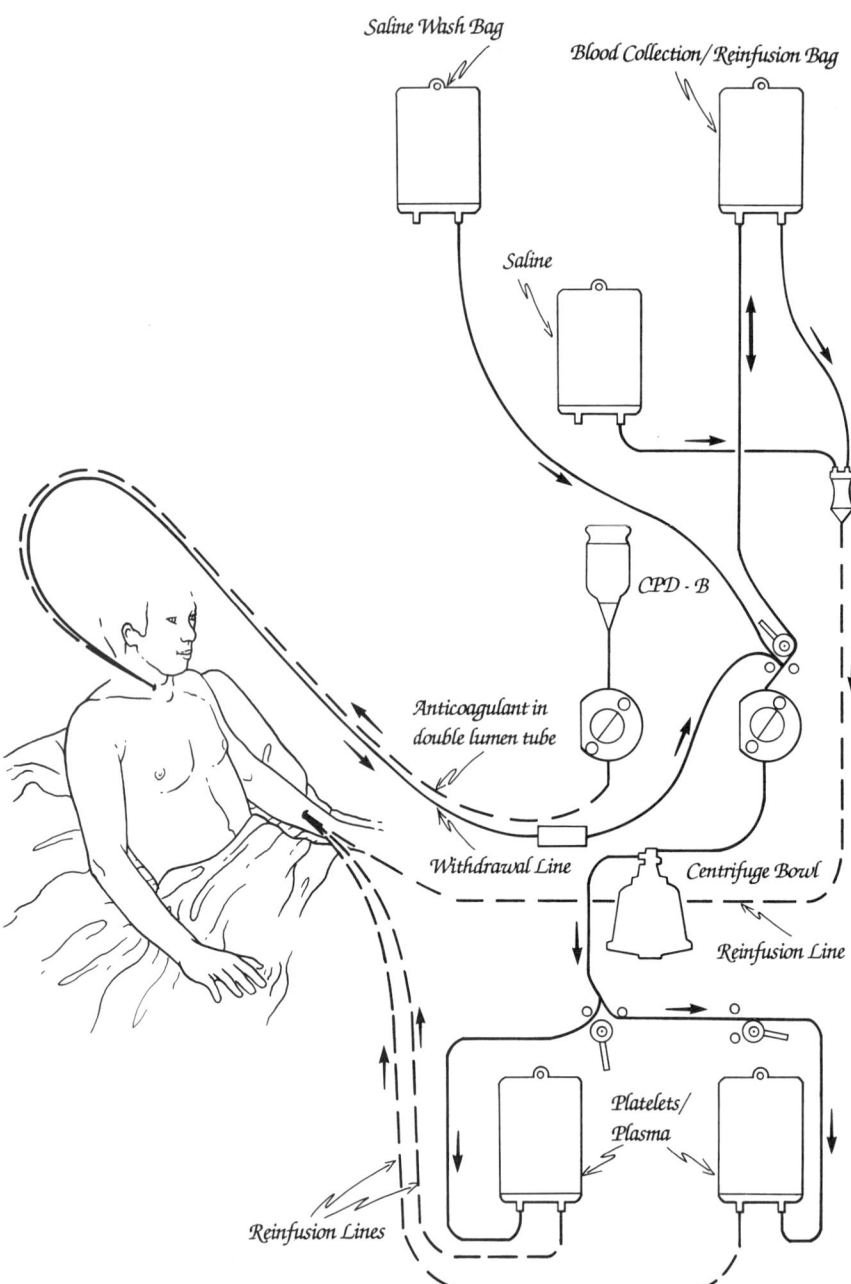

FIGURE 32.4. An alternative system to permit simultaneous storage and circulation of the blood. Additionally, blood centrifugation permits separation of individual blood components.

of artificial blood. These fluids carry large amounts of dissolved oxygen and have been used successfully in Jehovah's Witnesses in foreign countries.[43]

The greatest adjunct to intraoperative management of the Jehovah's Witnesses is blood conservation by use of cell-saver devices and autologous collection with reinfusion. Most Witnesses accept the use of cell-savers as long as the scavenged blood remains in contact with the body and the circulation.[2,30,45,46] Several methods have previously been described to accomplish this goal.[30,45,46] The system involves blood exiting the patient's body via an arterial cannula, and a coagulation and storage in collection bags with constant reinfusion at a slow rate (10–40 mL/min) through a venous cannula. As blood fills the reservoir, intravascular volume is kept stable by infusion of crystalloid plasma expanders. Volumes of 100 mL may be safely withdrawn prior to systemic heparinization for reinfusion after the patient is weaned from cardiopulmonary bypass and heparin reversed with protamine. It is feasible to withdraw a greater red cell volume as long as arterial oxygen saturation and mixed venous saturation are closely monitored to determine oxygen transport. Figures 32.3 and 32.4 illustrate previously used systems.

In the postoperative period, the amount of bleeding necessary to stimulate a return to the operating room for hemostasis should be markedly reduced in Witnesses, as opposed to those in whom transfusion of blood products might be considered. Any Witness who has mediastinal bleeding of 200 mL/h or greater for 2 hours or more should be returned to the operating room for hemostasis. The only postoperative laboratory studies that should be ordered are arterial blood gases and potassium levels. Even these must be limited to the minimal amount possible. Hemoglobin levels should not be checked in the postoperative period, as nothing can be done about low levels. Again, ferrous sulfate and iron dextran have been used in the postoperative period to increase hemoglobin levels. Erythropoietin has been used to stimulate bone marrow and improve hemoglobin levels.

Several drugs are also available to the surgeon and anesthesiologist that may help decrease blood loss. Certainly, protamine should be used in the appropriate concentrations and in the appropriate doses when heparin has been administered preoperatively or during cardiopulmonary bypass. Desmopressin (DDAVP) and Amikar (ϵ-aminocaproic acid) are now used fairly commonly and have been shown to be effective in decreasing postoperative bleeding and coagulopathies.[30,47] A new and exciting drug that is currently being tested in the United States is aprotinin. Aprotinin has been used in Europe for several years with great success in preventing postoperative bleeding and coagulopathies.[48] Aprotinin, similar to Amikar, is a fibrinolytic inhibitor and works by preventing the fibrinolysis that occurs when blood comes in contact with activation surfaces such as the pump tubing and oxygenator. The use of this drug and other antifibrinolytic drugs is discussed further in Chapter 31.

Conclusion

Jehovah's Witnesses are a religious group who seek the ultimate advances of modern medicine to maintain their health. However, they adamantly refuse transfusion of blood and blood products at the risk of death. No statutory law exists regarding transfusion of the patient who objects to transfusion on religious grounds. Legal precedents have been set such that competent adults are free from fear of legal interference. But incompetent adults, adults with dependent or unborn children, and minors may be made wards of the court or state when the court is petitioned to transfuse a person in jeopardy. There are many effective ways to minimize blood loss and avoid transfusion, not only in those who object to transfusion on a religious basis, but in the general population as well. Finally, the physician should attempt to understand and clarify the patient's wishes and beliefs and adhere to them.

References

1. Genesis 9:3,4. The Bible, New World Translation, Watchtower Bible and Tract Society of New York, Inc, 1984.
2. How can blood save your life? Watchtower Bible and Tract Society of New York, Inc., 1990.
3. Tierney WM, Weinberger M, Greene JY, et al. Jehovah's Witnesses and blood transfusion: physicians' attitudes and legal precedents. *South Med J* 1984;77:473–478.
4. Vercillo AP, Duprey SV. Jehovah's Witnesses and the transfusion of blood products. *NY State J Med*, 1988;88:493–494.
5. Findley FJ, Redstone PM. Blood transfusions in adult Jehovah's Witnesses: a case study of one congregation. *Arch Intern Med* 1982;142:606–607.
6. Isaiah 43:10: The Bible, New World Translation, Watchtower Bible and Tract Society of New York, Inc., 1984.
7. Leviticus 17:10.
8. Acts 15:22–29.
9. Ott DA, Cooley DA. Cardiovascular surgery in Johovah's Witnesses: report of 542 operations without blood transfusions. *JAMA* 1977;238:1256–1258.
10. Brunette CM, Duncan JM, Vega D, et al. Heart transplantation in Jehovah's Witnesses. *Arch Surg* 1990;125:1430–1433.
11. *Schoendorff v Society of New York Hospital*, 212 NY 125, 105 NE 92 (1914); see also *Marks v Williams*, 95 Minn. 261, 111 Am State Rpts 462, 104 NW 12 (1905).
12. Dornette WH. Jehovah's Witness and blood transfusion: the horns of a dilemma. *Anesth and Analg* 1973;52:272–278.
13. Studdard AP, Greene JY. Jehovah's Witnesses and blood transfusion: toward the resolution of a conflict of conscience. *Ala J Med Sci* 1986;23:454–459.
14. Dixon JL, Smalley MG. Jehovah's Witnesses: the surgical/ethical challenge. *JAMA* 1981;246:2471–2472.

15. *In re Brooks Estate*, 32 Ill. 2d 361, 205 NE 2d 435, 442 (1965).
16. Holman EJ. Adult Jehovah's Witnesses and blood transfusions. *JAMA* 1972;273,219(2):273-274.
17. Levin M. Religious objection to transfusion. *Mil Med* 1963;130:1024-1026.
18. Foley WJ, McGinn TJ. Jehovah's Witnesses and the question of blood transfusion. *Postgrad Med* 1973;53:109-113.
19. *In the Matter of Melideo*. 88 misc 2d974, 390 NY 52d, 523(1976).
20. *In Regards to Osborne*, 294 A2d, 372(GC Ct App 1972).
21. *Kennedy Memorial Hospital v Heston*, 58 NJ 576, 279 A 2d 670 (Superior Court 1971).
22. *Holmes v Silver Cross Hospital*, 340 F Supp 125 (DC Ill, 1972).
23. *Prince v Massachusetts*, 321 U S 158:88 1 ed. 645, 645 Ct 438; rehear den 32/US 804, 88 L ed 1090, 645 Ct 784 (1944).
24. Kambouris AA. Major abdominal operations on Jehovah's Witnesses. *Am Surg* 1987;53:350-356.
25. Bonakdar MI, Eckhous AW, Bacher BJ, Tabbilos RH, Peisner DB. Major gynecologic and obstetric surgery in Jehovah's Witnesses. *Obstet Gynecol* 1982;60:587-590.
26. Bowen JR, Angus PD, Huxster RR, MacEwen DG. Posterior spinal fusion without blood replacement in Jehovah's Witnesses. *Clin Orthop* 1985;198:284-288.
27. Folk FS, Bailey CP, Hirose T. Open heart surgery without blood transfusion. *J Natl Med Assoc* 1969;61:213-217.
28. Corno AF, Laks H, Stevenson LW, Clark S, Drinkwater DC. Heart transplantation in Jehovah's Witness. *J Heart Transplant* 1986;5:175-177.
29. Kaufman DB, Sutherland DE, Simmons RL, Ascher NA, Najarian JS. Transplantation in Jehovah's Witnesses. *Transplant Proc* 1987;19:3693.
30. Kaplan RF, Cuddeback J, Orsine L, Arkey I. Transfusions for Jehovah's Witnesses. *Anesth Analg* 1983;62:122-126.
31. Cooper JR. Perioperative considerations in Jehovah's Witnesses. *Int Anesthesiol Clin* 1990;28:210-215.
32. Shannon TA. Total exsanguination after refusal of blood transfusion. *N Engl J Med* 1982;306:544-545.
33. Popovsky MA, Moore SB. Autologous transfusion in Jehovah's Witnesses. *Transfusion* 1985;25:444-448.
34. Pioneering bloodless surgery with Jehovah's Witnesses. *Awake*, November 22, 1991:8-11.
35. Wong DH, Jenkins LC. Surgery in Jehovah's Witnesses. *Can J Anesth* 1989;36:578-585.
36. Spence RK, Carson JA, Poses R, McCoy S, Pello M, Alexander J. Elective surgery without transfusion: influence of preoperative hemoglobin level and blood loss on mortality. *Am J Surg* 1990;159:320-324.
37. Dudrick SJ, O'Donnell JJ, Raleigh DP, Matheny RG, Unkel SP. Rapid restoration of red blood cell mass in severely anemic surgical patients who refuse transfusion. *Arch Surg* 1985;120:721-727.
38. Boshkov LK, Tredget EE, Janowska-Wieczorek A. Recombinant human erythropoietin for a Jehovah's Witness with anemia of thermal injury. *Am J Hematol* 1991;37:53-54.
39. Koestner JA, Nelson LD, Morris JA Jr, Safcsak K. Use of recombinant human erythropoietin (r-HuEPO) in a Jehovah's Witness refusing transfusion of blood products: case report. *J Trauma* 1990;30:1406-1408.
40. Johnson PW, King R, Slevin ML, White H. The use of erythropoietin in a Jehovah's Witness undergoing major surgery and chemotherapy. *Brit J Cancer* 1991;63:476.
41. Grubbs PE Jr, Marini CP, Fleischer A. Acute hemodilution in an anemic Jehovah's Witness during extensive abdominal wall resection and reconstruction. *Ann Plast Surg* 1989;22:448-451.
42. Gollub S, Svigals R, Bailey CP, Hirose T, Schaefer C. Electrolyte solution in surgical patients refusing transfusion. *JAMA* 1971;215:2077-2083.
43. Ohyanagi H, Nakaya S, Okumura S, Saitoh Y. Surgical use of fluosol-DA in Jehovah's Witness patients. *Artif Organs* 1984(Feb);8(1):10-18.
44. Brown AS, Richman JH, Spence RK. Fluosol-DA, a perfluorochemical oxygen-transport fluid for the management of a trochanteric pressure sore in a Jehovah's Witness. *Ann Plast Surg* 1984;12:449-453.
45. Khine HH, Naidu R, Lowell H, MacEwen GD. A method of blood conservation in Jehovah's Witnesses: incirculation diversion and refusion. *Anesth Analg* 1978;57:279-280.
46. Lichtger B, Dupuis J, Siske J. Hemotherapy during surgery for Jehovah's Witnesses: a new method. *Anesth Analg* 1982;61:618-619.
47. Benk JB, Schwartz SI. From anesthesia to ethics. *Contemp Surg* 1977;11:39-41.
48. Royston D, Bidstrup D, Taylor KM, Sapsford RN. The effect of aprotinin on need for blood transfusion after repeat open heart surgery. *Lancet* 1987;2:1289-1291.

33
Medical-Legal Aspects of Cardiopulmonary Bypass

Tomas D. Martin and Charles R. Hatcher, Jr.

Introduction

It is imperative that a chapter on medical-legal issues be included in this book, since all members of the cardiopulmonary bypass (CPB) team (surgeons, anesthesiologists, perfusionists, and nurses) have significant potential medical liability in caring for patients undergoing CPB. The complexity of CPB, even with all of the current safeguards, makes it inevitable that problems will occur. It is not a question of *if*, but a question of *when*.

We will not attempt to cover all aspects of current medical-legal problems involving CPB, but will briefly discuss the basics of tort law, the group of statutes under which most medical malpractice cases are examined. We will discuss how tort law might be applied to CPB problems, a few of the more common problems that may lead to a lawsuit, and, finally, some suggestions on preventing problems and litigation.

Tort Liability

Tort law is a type of civil law that is concerned with civil wrongs, or wrongs of one individual against another, that do not violate a state or societal law. The primary basis for tort liability in medical malpractice suits is negligence. The standard definition of negligence in all situations of tort law is "the doing of what a reasonable person would *not* do under the circumstances."

Negligence

To prove negligence and recover damages in a medical malpractice case, four things must be proven:

1. Duty—that the physician owed the patient a duty to act given a particular situation and circumstances in conformity with patient care standards established by the profession.
2. Breach of Duty—that an act of commission or omission on the part of the physician violated the established patient care standards.
3. Proximate Cause—that the act of omission by the physician resulted in injury to the patient.
4. Damages—that the patient indeed suffered loss or damage as a result of the injury.

The "standard of care" can be defined as the knowledge, skill, and care ordinarily used by a well-qualified physician practicing under similar circumstances and in similar cases. In some cases "the standard of care" may be measured against the prevailing standards in the same or similar geographic locality. However, as communication, transportation, access to technological advances, and standards set by national medical organizations have improved, the so-called "strict locality rule" holds true in only a small number of jurisdictions.[1] This is especially true for specialists where geographical conditions typically have less of an impact, particularly in the specialized circumstances of extracorporeal circulation and cardiac surgery. All primary personnel involved in these cases (ie, surgeons, anesthesiologists, and perfusionists) have their own standards of care that are nationally based and not limited to an isolated geographic area. It is therefore the responsibility of each to keep abreast of the current "national standards" in their field of interest.

The issue of responsibility, however, is not always clear. Obviously, if there is a grave surgical technical misadventure, it is almost certainly the responsibility of the surgeon; or, if the anesthesiologist administers the wrong medication, he or she is usually responsible for his or her own actions. But who is responsible for the other personnel intimately involved with CPB (eg, the perfusionist)? Perfusionists carry their own malpractice insurance and, in many cases, are self-employed or are a part of a group of perfusionists who have no financial tie with the physician or hospital. In other circumstances, they are employees of the hospital, surgeon, or anesthesiologist. Under these circumstances, who is liable for their actions?

Vicarious Liability

According to the theory of vicarious liability, one party (A) may, under certain circumstances, be held liable for the actions of another (B) even though "A" is innocent of any personal fault. Two conditions are necessary in order to impose vicarious liability. First, the relationship between "A" and "B" must exist, with this relationship most commonly being an employer-employee relationship. Second, "B" must have been acting within the scope of the relationship when he or she committed the tort or injury.[2]

Several reasons have been used by the legal profession to justify vicarious liability. One is that it helps assure that the plaintiff will have a solvent defendant, or "deep pocket," from whom to obtain compensation. Another is that it helps assure that the loss will be borne by the party who can most afford the loss, and, finally, the threat of liability may serve to encourage "A" to exercise greater care in the management of those who work for him or her.

Several doctrines have been utilized by the courts to impart vicarious liability. Under the doctrine of *respondeat superior*, "let the master respond," the employer may be held liable whether or not the employer approved of the employee's actions or even knew or observed the negligent conduct. A surgeon, anesthesiologist, or hospital may thus be held vicariously liable for the actions of a perfusionist under their employ. The majority of these cases focus on the liability of hospitals and other health care institutions that arises out of the negligence of their employees.[3-5]

Another application of vicarious liability principles is to the doctrine of the *borrowed servant*. Under this doctrine, an employee or "servant" of one "master" is temporarily borrowed by another who exercises specific control over that person to accomplish a particular purpose. A surgeon or anesthesiologist who temporarily assumes control over a perfusionist, even though he or she is not his or her direct employer, may thus be held vicariously liable. An example of this is seen in an Ohio case in which a surgeon was sued for the actions of an assisting nurse anesthetist, not directly employed by the surgeon. Under the doctrine of the *borrowed servant*, the court found that a master-servant relationship did exist and that the surgeon did possess the right to control the actions of the anesthetist. The court therefore held the surgeon liable, stating "we seek only to ensure that where, in the operating room, a surgeon does control, or realistically possesses the right to control, events and procedures, he does so with a high degree of care."[6]

Similarly, some courts have referred to the chief surgeon in the operating room as the *captain of the ship*, and have held him or her responsible for negligence of other personnel in the operating room, *whether or not* the surgeon had the right to exercise control over their actions. In these cases, the surgeon has been considered the ad hoc employer of all personnel comprising the health care delivery team. This doctrine is applied in only a few states, including Georgia.

In *Swindle v St. Joseph's Hospital, Inc.*, the courts employed the captain of the ship doctrine to release the hospital from liability for alleged negligence in the performance of a surgical procedure, stating that "if a hospital employee committed any negligent act, such negligence would be imputed to the defendant surgeon."[7]

These doctrines are not uniformly upheld in all courts and vary among cases and particularly among states. Most courts have come to recognize that the operating theater today consists of multiple members, each with highly specialized and independent functions that may not come under the direct supervision of any one person. In most malpractice suits where negligence is alleged, all personnel (surgeons, perfusionists, anesthesiologists) and the hospital involved are named in the suit. It is then up to the courts to determine whether or not negligence has occurred and, if so, who is responsible. It seems usual, however, that in today's legal climate, and in most states, each person is legally responsible and liable for his or her own actions, with the doctrines of respondeat superior, the borrowed servant, and captain of the ship being upheld in only a few states and in specific cases.

Strict Liability

Equipment malfunction or failure is a different issue, and today most states apply the *strict liability doctrine* to most manufactured products. Under this doctrine, the plaintiff needs to prove that the product was unreasonably dangerous. That is, the product had a defect that existed at the time of marketing, and that defect led to harm of the user. The term "unreasonably dangerous" is also left up to the courts to define, and can have a very narrow or a very broad meaning.

Strict liability suits involving product failure or malfunction are usually directed against manufacturers. However, doctors and/or hospitals have been held liable on the basis of strict liability. The justification for this is that hospitals are thought to be able to absorb the cost of injuries; the hospitals and physicians are in the best position to discover defective products; and hospitals are felt to be in the optimal position to identify other parties who may also be held responsible. The number of cases where physicians have been held liable on a strict lability theory alone, however, is relatively few, and the odds that a member of the CPB team will be held liable for a product failure are very small.

Avoid Litigation

The best way for any member of the health care team, particularly the primary physician, to avoid litigation is to have a good rapport with the patient and his or her family. If a feeling of trust and confidence is instilled from the very beginning, then litigation problems should be few.

From a technical standpoint, the best way to avoid litigation, or defend, should litigation occur, is to keep abreast of the current trends in CPB and maintain an excellent safety record. Chapter 18 discusses safety during CPB.

References

1. Delaware Code of Annotated Statutes. 18 sec. 6801 (f) (supp 1984).
2. King JH. Vicarious liability. In: *The Law of Medical Malpractice in a Nutshell*. 2nd ed. St. Paul: West Publishing Co, 1986:231–250.
3. *Mazer v Lipshutz*, 327. F, 2d. 42 (3rd Cir 1963).
4. *Flagiello v Pennsylvania Hospital*, 417 Pa. 486, 308 A. 2d 193 (1965).
5. *Laznevick v General Hospital of Monroe County*, 499 F. supp, 146 (M.D. Pa 1980).
6. *Baird v Sickler*, 69 Ohio State 2D 652, 433 N.E. 2d 598 (1982).
7. *Swindle v St Joseph's Hospital, Inc.*, 161 Ga-App. 290, 291 S.E. 2d 1 (1982).

34
Warm-Blood Cardioplegia and Normothermic Cardiopulmonary Bypass

Robert A. Guyton

Introduction

Warm-blood cardioplegia represents an emerging and evolving technique in cardiac surgery, whose proponents claim it provides a remarkable improvement in myocardial protection.[1-6] These claims have been corroborated by researchers[7,8] and have led to an unusual interest in continuous warm-blood cardioplegia in recent years. For this reason, a special section of this text is devoted to warm-blood cardioplegia as a topic of particular current interest.

The technique of continuous blood cardioplegia, including retrograde infusion via the coronary sinus, has been suggested intermittently since 1957 in cardiac surgical literature.[9-12] These suggestions received little attention, however, until a Toronto group achieved extraordinary surgical success in high-risk patients with long crossclamp times,[6] in patients with acute postinfarction mitral insufficiency,[1] and in patients with recent myocardial infarction.[5] These studies led to an intense investigation of warm-blood cardioplegia by our institution, both in the laboratory setting and in clinical application.[13-18]

The basic concept of warm-blood cardioplegia is that myocardial oxygen demands are greatly reduced by asystole. Asystole at normothermia reduces myocardial oxygen demands to one tenth those of the beating working heart or one fifth those of the beating empty heart. If oxygen and nutrients are then supplied to the heart, even at a reduced rate, abundant substrate is available for maintenance of cellular metabolism. Indeed, since none of this substrate must be used to produce external work, all of it is available for maintenance of cellular homeostasis and, if necessary, reconstruction of damaged cellular elements and repletion of depleted cellular energy stores. Because the perfusion solution is blood-based, abundant buffering capacity is present, and free-radical scavengers are also continuously supplied.

The first large-scale clinical use of continuous warm cardioplegia was in Toronto, as an antegrade technique[3] — a cumbersome method requiring multiple cardioplegia infusion cannulas. Each coronary anastomosis was connected to the cardioplegia infusion system as the distal anastomosis was completed. The operative field tended to become cluttered, and the surgeon had to take care that each vein graft remained unkinked, so that flow could be delivered to the myocardium as homogeneously as possible.

The introduction of retrograde cardioplegic techniques[4,19] greatly simplified the cardioplegia delivery system. With this retrograde technique, a coronary sinus catheter is introduced via the right atrium into the coronary sinus. Induction of cardioplegic arrest is accomplished with antegrade infusion of cardioplegic solution into the aortic root. Cardioplegic arrest and nutrient flow are then maintained by retrograde infusion into the coronary sinus. The simplicity and other apparent advantages of this technique have made it very attractive and have led to widespread experimentation with warm-blood cardioplegic techniques. One survey suggested that 10% of cardiac surgeons had used these techniques by 1992, only two years after presentation of the extraordinary results from Toronto.[20]

Technique of Warm-Blood Cardioplegia

The method of warm-blood cardioplegia proposed by the Toronto investigators involved infusion, either antegrade or retrograde into the coronary sinus, of a mixture of one part of crystalloid solution to four parts of blood. The crystalloid solution originally used was Fremes solution, consisting of 5% dextrose in water (D_5W), 1 L; KCl, 100 mEq/L; magnesium, 18 mEq/L; THAM (trihydroxymethyl-aminomethane), 40 mL; and CPD (citrate-phosphate-dextrose), 20 mL. After induction of cardioplegia, the infusate was changed to a similar solution, with 40 mEq of potassium per liter in the crystalloid solution. The final concentration of potassium in the blood-crystalloid mixture infused into the heart was approximately 21 to 22 mEq/L in the high-potassium mixture and approximately 11 mEq/L in the low-potassium mixture. Antegrade infusion was accomplished with flows of approximately 200 mL/min, retrograde infusion with flows of at least 150 mL/min, and coronary sinus pressures maintained at less than 40 mm Hg.[1-5]

Problems with Clinical Application

The technique described above seemed simple enough, and it was advocated by some with almost evangelistic zeal. As the technique was applied in other institutions, however, problems were seen. The first and most difficult problem with continuous retrograde warm-blood cardioplegia (or, for that matter, continuous antegrade warm-blood cardioplegia) was found to be difficulty with visualization of the distal anastomosis for coronary bypass operations. Proponents of the antegrade technique have simply turned off the cardioplegic infusion for periods of 2 to 10 minutes to facilitate visualization of the anastomosis. Clinically, this interruption of cardioplegic infusion seems to be well tolerated. Experimental studies, however, have shown that there is at least some risk involved in interruption of warm-blood cardioplegia, particularly if one is attempting to resuscitate stunned or ischemically injured myocardium using the cardioplegic infusion.[21] Adequate visualization of the distal anastomosis can be accomplished without cessation of cardioplegia by local isolation of the coronary artery with small vascular clamps gently applied to the coronary artery and surrounding tissue, and/or by using a carbon dioxide gas blower to blow the blood away from the distal anastomosis.[22]

A second problem that occurred fairly frequently (in approximately 1 in 20 patients) with continuous warm-blood cardioplegia was that the heart began to beat during the cardioplegic infusion, and reinfusion of the high-potassium solution failed to restore complete cardioplegic arrest. This seemed to be the case particularly in patients with left main coronary obstruction, or in those patients whose noncoronary collateral flow might be expected to be high. When this occurred, cooling of the heart was used to increase the margin of safety for myocardial protection, and the administration of esmolol (50 or 100 mg, as a bolus) was used to achieve cardiac arrest. This continued beating of the heart is certainly troublesome and is incompletely explained. Continued cardiac contraction has been observed by this author despite sufficient cardioplegia to raise systemic potassium levels as high as 11 mEq/L.

Considerable concern has been expressed about the nonhomogeneous delivery of retrograde cardioplegic solutions, particularly with regard to nutrient flow to the right ventricle when a coronary sinus catheter is employed. The coronary sinus catheter often occludes the posterior interventricular vein, so that flow to the posterior part of the septum and to the right ventricle must occur by way of collaterals rather than by direct infusion into these venous systems. Studies of flow into the right ventricular myocardium, using colored microsphere and echocardiographic techniques,[23,24] have demonstrated that right ventricular nutrient flow is less than 10% of the nutrient flow in the free wall of the left ventricle. This observation conflicts with the observation that the right ventricle appears to be relatively well protected by retrograde warm-blood techniques.[25] It is possible that radioactive or colored microsphere techniques underestimate the potential substrate supply to the right ventricle, since these techniques reflect microspheres trapped in *capillary* beds. It may be that a large portion of the blood flow supplying substrate to the right ventricle, with retrograde techniques, is blood traveling through a venous plexus that entirely bypasses capillary beds. It is also possible that the atria and the right ventricle receive some of their nutrient supply from intracavitary blood. In any case, right ventricular protection has been less of a problem in clinical situations than one would expect it to be from experimental or theoretical considerations.

Another problem encountered in the initial application of warm-blood cardioplegia was systemic hyperglycemia and hyperkalemia, associated with the infusion of large quantities of glucose and potassium into the heart with the cardioplegic solution. Serum glucose levels as high as 400 to 500 mg% were frequently observed, and infusion of insulin was often necessary. A number of investigators have modified the crystalloid portion of their warm-blood solution to decrease the glucose content. Hyperkalemia was also a considerable problem. If a patient underwent an operation with a 2-hour crossclamp interval and infusion of cardioplegic solution at 200 mL/min (representing slightly more than 2 mEq/min of potassium), then the total amount of potassium infused would be well over 200 mEq. This systemic hyperkalemia can lead to a prolonged interval of asystole (or ineffective cardiac contraction) after the crossclamp is removed. It is advisable to treat this hyperkalemia prophylactically by diuretic administration (for example, administration of 20 mg of furosemide at the beginning of the crossclamp interval) to facilitate excretion of both crystalloid solution and potassium. An interval of asystole or ineffective cardiac contraction is ordinarily not a problem after crossclamp removal *unless* mild aortic insufficiency is present. If it is present, however, care must be taken to avoid ventricular distention in the interval between crossclamp removal and the beginning of effective left ventricular contraction. In an attempt to prevent systemic hyperkalemia, some investigators are using lower concentrations of potassium in the crystalloid component of the warm-blood cardioplegia solution after initial arrest.

The conduct of cardiopulmonary bypass (CPB) is also altered during warm heart surgery. Because the patient is warm, maintaining a reasonable perfusion pressure is a concern. α-Agonists often must be used during CPB to maintain systemic pressure above 50 mm Hg.[26] The mechanism of this vasodilation is incompletely understood, but it may be related to activation of cytokines or other vasodilators during warm CPB.[27]

Another important area of controversy is the appropriate flow rate for retrograde continuous warm-blood cardioplegia. The deceptively simple suggestion, made above, that flow rate should always exceed 150 mL/min with coronary sinus pressures less than 40 mm Hg is problematic. Often, particularly when the heart is elevated for a circumflex anastomosis, a coronary sinus infusion rate of 60 mL/min leads to a coronary sinus pressure of 60, 70, or even 80 mm Hg. One must accept either a lower flow rate or a higher pressure. When the heart is lowered back into the pericardial sac, the resistance of the coronary venous system ordinarily falls, and flow rates of 150 mL/min are usually achievable without excessive pressures. Some investigators have advocated the sampling of coronary arterial pH to assess the adequacy of retrograde flow, reasoning that if the blood leaving the heart via the coronary arteries closely approximates normal coronary sinus blood-gas values (a pH above 7.30), then nearly normal coronary metabolism will be maintained and myocardial functional recovery should be excellent. If, on the other hand, persistent acidosis exists in arterial efflux during retrograde coronary sinus infusion, then poor functional recovery of the ventricle is more likely.[28] Another group of investigators found that coronary sinus flows of 100 mL/min or less led to high lactate production and oxygen extraction during cardioplegic administration. Administration of retrograde warm-blood cardioplegia at 200 mL/min minimized lactate production and maintained pH within physiologic range. Further elevation of retrograde flow to 300 or even 500 mL/min led to no further improvement. Unfortunately, these investigators did not study flow rates between 100 and 200 mL/min. They therefore recommended a flow rate of at least 200 mL/min during retrograde warm-blood cardioplegia.[29]

Experimental Evaluation of Continuous Warm-Blood Cardioplegia

Hypothermic techniques of myocardial protection, using either oxygenated crystalloid solutions or intermittent cold-blood solutions, lead to excellent protection of normal hearts, with nearly 100% recovery of metabolism and function if the heart is metabolically and functionally intact prior to the cardioplegic arrest interval. Continuous warm-blood cardioplegia is most likely to be advantageous in the heart that is *not* metabolically and functionally intact prior to the cardioplegic interval. Because the heart is normothermic and because substrate is continuously being supplied, homeostatic mechanisms are intact and optimal conditions exist for continuous repair of damaged, stunned, or metabolically depleted myocardium during the crossclamp interval.[1,3,5] Two experimental studies demonstrate the ability of warm-blood cardioplegia to resuscitate stunned myocardium. The first of these is the evaluation of warm-blood cardioplegia in the presence of global ischemia,[13] and the second is a demonstration of its efficacy in the presence of regional myocardial ischemia.[14]

Brown and colleagues[13] developed a canine model of acute global myocardial ischemia followed by cardioplegic arrest. Fifteen minutes of global normothermic ischemia was followed by a 1-hour cardioplegic arrest interval. The warm-blood cardioplegic technique, delivered in a retrograde manner, was compared with the oxygenated crystalloid solution—developed and used successfully at Emory University—and with the intermittent antegrade cold-blood technique, with warm terminal reperfusion, advocated by Buckberg. After 60 minutes of cardioplegic arrest, the crossclamp was removed, the heart was reperfused, and hemodynamic end-points were determined 30, 60, and 90 minutes after crossclamp. A triaxial ultrasonic crystal system was used for determination of end-systolic pressure-volume relationships, diastolic function, and the preload-recruitable-stroke-work relationship. This experimental model showed no significant difference in systolic function among the three groups using the maximum elastance relationship. A linearized stress/strain regression analysis revealed that the left ventricle was stiffer in both the cold-blood and cold-crystalloid groups than in the warm-blood group (Figure 34.1). The preload-recruitable-stroke-work relationship revealed that the warm-blood group was significantly better than either the cold-blood group or the cold-crystalloid group (Figure 34.1). In addition, electrocardiographic analysis revealed that the ST segment elevation, which was almost uniformly present in the cold-blood and cold-crystalloid groups, was absent in the warm-blood group (Figure 34.2). This experimental study strongly suggests that warm-blood cardioplegia is at least as good as intermittent cold-blood cardioplegia, and is better than cold-crystalloid cardioplegia in the setting of global myocardial ischemia preceding cardioplegic arrest. The differences, however, were not prominent, and led to another study of the use of warm-blood cardioplegia in the setting of regional myocardial ischemia.

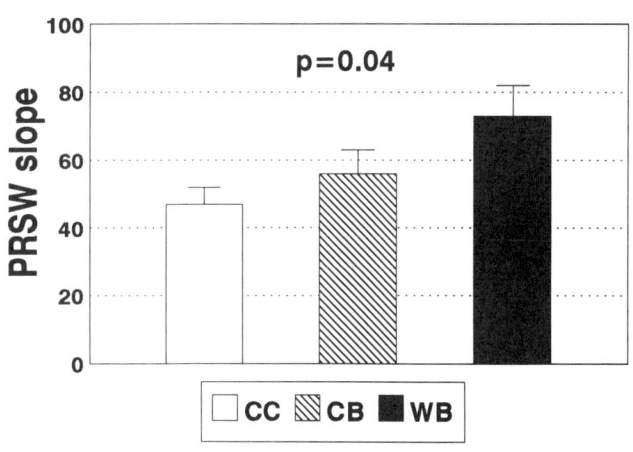

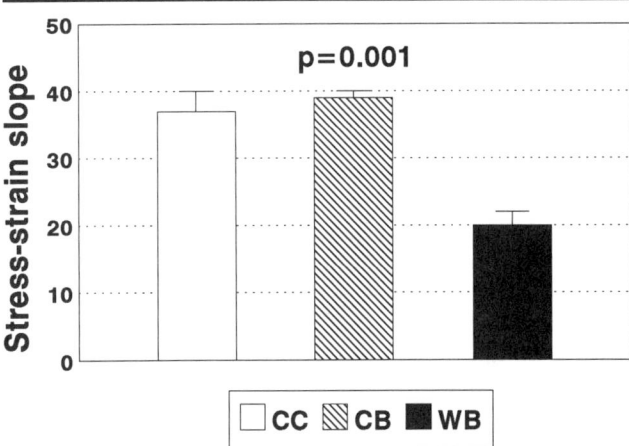

FIGURE 34.1. Left ventricular function after 60 minutes of cardioplegic arrest preceded by 15 minutes of global ischemia. *Top*: The preload-recruitable-stroke-work relationship revealed that warm-blood (WB) cardioplegia was superior to the cold-blood (CB) and cold-crystalloid (CC) groups. *Bottom*: A linearized stress-strain relationship revealed that the warm-blood group was also more compliant than the crystalloid group.

Horsley and colleagues,[14] using the same experimental preparation described by Brown et al, examined a canine model with a 45-minute occlusion of the left anterior descending artery (LAD), followed by a 1-hour cardioplegic arrest interval. Once again, cold oxygenated crystalloid cardioplegia, delivered intermittently, was compared with cold-blood cardioplegia delivered intermittently with warm terminal reperfusion and with continuous warm-blood cardioplegia, delivered antegrade for induction and then retrograde for maintenance. Hemodynamic function was evaluated at 30, 60, and 90 minutes. In this study, a clear separation existed between warm-blood, cold-blood, and cold-crystalloid cardioplegia, with warm-blood significantly superior to cold-blood, which in turn was significantly superior to cold-crystalloid cardioplegia. The superiority of warm-blood cardioplegia was demonstrated by the maximum elastance relationship and by the preload-recruitable-stroke-work relationship (Figure 34.3). Diastolic ventricular function, as assessed by the active stress/strain relationship, revealed that both of the blood groups were superior to the crystalloid group in this experimental preparation. Evaluation of regional myocardial adenosine triphosphate (ATP) levels revealed that ATP levels were restored to normal in the ischemic region (that is, the ATP levels in the LAD region were restored to the levels of the circumflex region) in the warm-blood group, but were not restored to normal in either the cold-crystalloid or the cold-blood groups (Figure 34.4). This experimental study strongly suggests that warm-blood cardioplegia is indeed effective in functional resuscitation of stunned myocardium, and also is effective in metabolic resuscitation, at least as measured by repletion of high-energy phosphate stores.

Yau and colleagues[30] in Toronto performed a randomized clinical trial to examine the effects of warm- versus cold-blood cardioplegia in humans. Pressure volume loops were constructed and ventricular function was assessed 3 hours after operation. End-systolic elastance and preload-recruitable-stroke-work were increased after warm-blood cardioplegia, compared to those variables in the

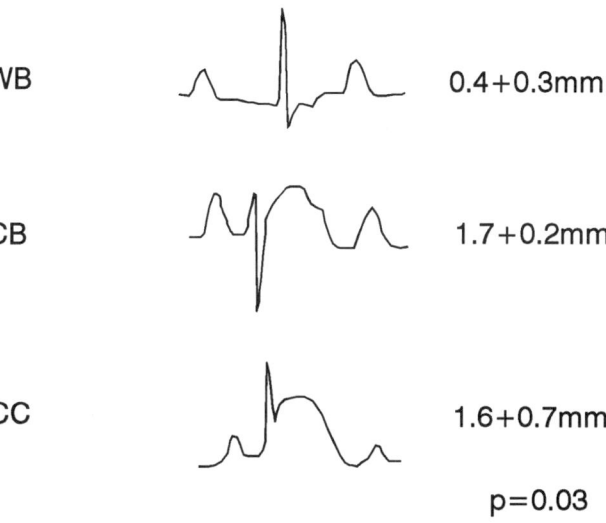

FIGURE 34.2. Typical electrocardiographic appearance after aerobic cardioplegia (WB, warm blood), cold-blood (CB), and cold-crystalloid cardioplegia (CC) from the study by Brown et al.[13] The average ST segment elevation was significantly lower with aerobic cardioplegia than it was with cold blood or cold crystalloid.

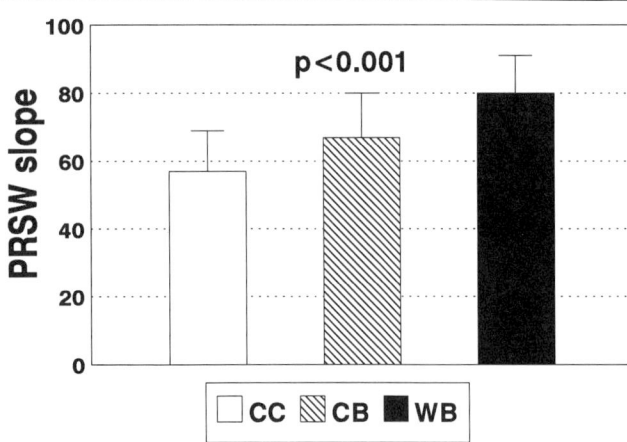

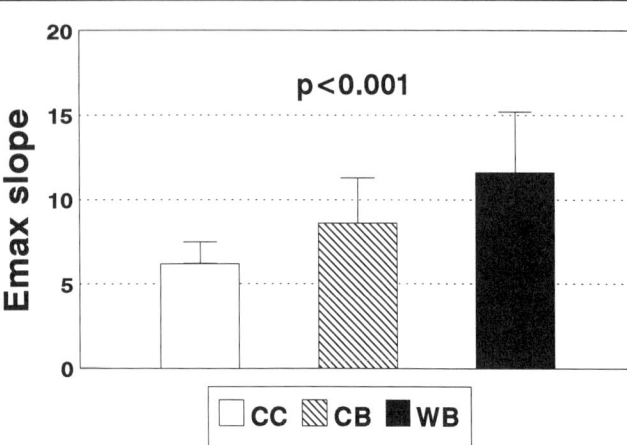

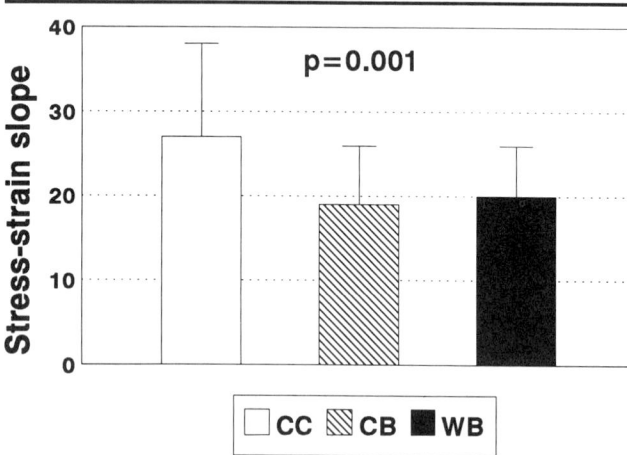

FIGURE 34.3. Functional recovery following 45 minutes of acute left anterior descending artery occusion, followed by 1 hour of cardioplegic arrest. Aerobic cardioplegia (WB, warm-blood) was superior to cold-blood cardioplegia (CB) and cold oxygenated crystalloid cardioplegia (CC) with regard to preload-recruitable-stroke-work (*top*), the maximum elastase (Emax) relationship (*middle*), and the stress-strain relationship (*bottom*) in this study.[14]

cold-blood group. Myocardial metabolism assessment in this investigation revealed greater myocardial lactate production in the warm-blood group but improved recovery of oxygen consumption during reperfusion. Total adenonucleotides were decreased in the warm-cardioplegia group, but the depletion of ATP was similar between groups. Myocardial CK-MB isoenzyme release was reduced in the warm group. This clinical study was conducted on patients without intentional ischemic compromise prior to the cardioplegic interval. The changes in metabolism were small and perhaps reflect some mild deterioration of metabolism in the warm group and protection in the cold group. Functional recovery, however, was definitely superior with warm-blood cardioplegia.

Clinical Trials

Two large prospective clinical trials of warm-blood cardioplegia have been reported. A prospectively randomized trial from Emory University conducted by Martin and colleagues[16] compared continuous retrograde warm-blood cardioplegia with oxygenated crystalloid cardioplegia delivered antegrade and retrograde. This study was initiated after the Emory surgeons had experience with continuous retrograde warm-blood cardioplegia in over 300 patients. The normothermic continuous retrograde technique described by Salerno and colleagues[4] was used. In patients randomized to the warm-blood group, systemic temperatures were maintained as close to 37°C as possible. This meant that active warming was often necessary and was done if the patient's systemic temperature fell below 36°C. In the cold-crystalloid group, oxygenated coldcrystalloid cardioplegia was delivered in an initial antegrade dose (1000 mL) at a temperature of 4° to 6°C. Additional cardioplegia solution was infused through the vein grafts as they were completed, and through the coronary sinus, aortic root, or a combination of these, to maintain myocardial hypothermia at the surgeon's discretion. In both groups, pump flows were maintained at 2.2 to 2.5 L/m^2, while the temperature was 32°C or greater and perfusion pressures were maintained at 50 to 70 mm Hg during normothermic perfusion. In the cold group, hypothermic perfusion was accomplished at 25° to 28°C.

One thousand and one patients were randomized, and as might be expected, the preoperative demographic char-

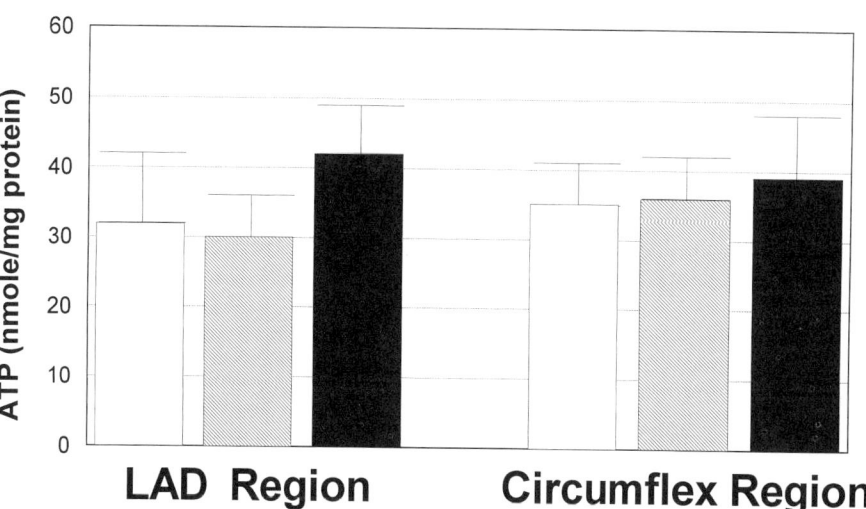

FIGURE 34.4. Myocardial ATP levels were restored to normal by warm-blood cardioplegia (WB) in the left anterior descending (LAD) artery region in a canine model of acute LAD artery occlusion (45 minutes) followed by 1 hour of cardioplegic arrest. Neither cold crystalloid (CC) nor cold-blood (CB) cardioplegia led to full restoration of myocadial ATP levels in the stunned region.[14]

acteristics of the two groups were nearly identical. Intraoperative variables were similar with regard to the number of bypass grafts (3.4 ± 1 in each group) and the use of the internal mammary artery (approximately 80% in each group). There was a significant difference in aortic cross-clamp times (40 minutes in the cold group and 46 minutes in the warm group), but CPB times were similar, at approximately 85 minutes in each group.

The analysis of outcome variables in this large randomized study revealed that the mortality rate for each group was very low (cold oxygenated crystalloid 1.6%, and warm-blood 1%). The Q-wave infarction rate was approximately 1% in each group, and the rate of intraaortic balloon bump (IABP) usage was approximately 1.5% to 2% in each group. The use of inotropic agents was 15% in each group. Therefore, as far as myocardial function recovery is concerned, there was a slight trend toward improved mortality in the warm group but this was not statistically significant.

A major difference was noted between the warm-blood group and the cold-crystalloid group with regard to neurologic events. In the warm group, 3.1% of patients, and, in the cold group, 1% suffered an acute perioperative (within 3 days of operation) cerebrovascular accident ($p < 0.02$). In addition, 5 patients in the warm group suffered a delayed cerebrovascular accident (more than 3 days after operation but during hospitalization) and 1 patient in the cold group suffered a delayed cerebrovascular accident. Two patients in the warm group and 1 patient in the cold group had postoperative encephalopathy. Therefore, the difference in total neurologic events between the two groups was 4.5% versus 1.4% ($p < 0.005$). This discovery of adverse neurologic sequelae resulting from the technique of warm-blood cardioplegia necessarily led to a re-evaluation of the technique. Myocardial protection was excellent, but a neurologic threat was also present.

While the study of retrograde warm-blood cardioplegia was being conducted at Emory, a large prospective study of antegrade normothermic blood cardioplegia was in progress in Toronto, comparing normothermic antegrade blood cardioplegia with hypothermic blood cardioplegia. No important differences were found in preoperative variables of the 1732 patients randomized. Mortality again showed a trend toward superior results with the warm technique (1.4% versus 2.6%, $p = 0.08$), and there was a significant difference in the two groups with regard to enzymatic detection of myocardial injury (12.6% versus 16.1%, $p < 0.05$). In addition, 6% of the patients in the warm-blood group suffered low-output syndrome versus 9.3% in the cold-blood group ($p = 0.02$). In contrast to the Emory study, there was no difference in stroke between the two groups (warm group 1.6%, and cold group 1.5%). The data from the large prospective evaluation of antegrade warm-blood cardioplegia in the Toronto group obviously encourage continuation of the warm-blood technique and a search for differences between the Emory application of the technique and the Toronto application.

Two major differences exist between the Toronto prospective randomized trial and the one conducted at Emory. First, the Toronto trial used an antegrade technique and the Emory trial a retrograde one. The suggestion has been made that the retrograde technique might flush atherosclerotic debris from the coronary arteries back into the aorta, debris that might then lodge in cerebral vessels after cardiac function is restored. Since retrograde techniques in cold-blood and cold-crystalloid cardioplegia have been extensively used without any detected neurologic sequelae, this possibility is considered unlikely. A second very important difference is that the CPB temperature in the Toronto series was allowed to drift down to 33°C or 34°C during the cardioplegia arrest interval. The patient was then rewarmed prior to termination of bypass. In the Emory series, patients were actively warmed to maintain normothermia. This means that the arterial blood temperature was 38°C or even 38.5°C at times during the bypass interval, and the brain may have been, in fact, mildly hyperthermic in some of these patients. As will be discussed below, this may be a very important consideration.

Current Techniques: Tepid Retrograde Continuous Blood Cardioplegia

Several studies of continuous aerobic cardioplegia agree with the Toronto randomized trial in the absence of adverse neurologic sequelae.[7,8] In general, these investigators have allowed the temperature during CPB to drift down slightly, and then rewarmed patients prior to discontinuation of CPB. This means that cerebral temperatures are slightly hypothermic when proximal anastomoses are being constructed and as the aortic crossclamp is manipulated. It is well known that micro- and macroembolism occur during CPB and that these events peak during manipulation of aortic clamps, inevitably leading to small areas of cerebral ischemia. Just a few degrees of hypothermia afford considerable cerebral protection from these transient ischemic insults.[31] For this reason, it appears that a slightly hypothermic CPB may be advantageous.

An experimental study has been undertaken to evaluate the myocardial protective and resuscitative effects of continuous aerobic cardioplegia at different temperatures. Bufkin and colleagues[17] developed a canine model of regional myocardial ischemia with a 75-minute occlusion of the left anterior descending artery, followed by a 60-minute cardioplegia arrest interval. Continuous blood cardioplegia was administered (antegrade induction and retrograde maintenance) at 18°, 28°, or 37°C. In animals receiving 18° or 28°C continuous blood cardioplegia, systemic temperatures of 28°C were used. The results of this study indicate that systolic ventricular function (maximum elastance) was not different among the three groups, although the maximum elastance was slightly higher in the 18° and the 28°C groups, compared to the 37°C group. Preload recruitable stroke-work, as a measure of global left ventricular performance, was significantly higher at 90 minutes after crossclamp removal in the 18°C group and the 28°C group, compared with the 37°C group. Diastolic function did not differ among the temperature groups at any time. There were small differences among the groups in myocardial ATP, myocardial blood flow, and myocardial oxygen consumption. This study indicated that 28°C appeared to be at least as good as, if not better than, 37°C in myocardial resuscitation after a 75-minute left anterior descending artery occlusion. This experimental study strongly supports the hypothesis that mildly hypothermic continuous blood cardioplegia may offer considerable advantage in myocardial protection and resuscitation. Hypothermic CPB offers a safety margin with regard to tissue perfusion, decreased complement activation, and whole-body systemic inflammatory response.[32,33] Hypothermic myocardial protection adds an additional margin of safety with regard to myocardial nutritive flow. The nutritive flow necessary to maintain myocardial metabolism at 28°C in the arrested state is approximately one half of the nutritive flow necessary to maintain metabolism at 37°C. Therefore, if for some reason a portion of the myocardium is receiving very low flows during continuous aerobic cardioplegia, it is likely to be better protected at 28° than at 37°C. One would have expected, however, the homeostatic mechanisms for cellular integrity and resuscitation to be more in balance at 37° than at 28°C. This remains an important topic of continued investigation.

Current Clinical Practice

Continuous aerobic cardioplegia is an evolving technique. Practitioners of this technique must watch the scientific literature for reports of adverse effects and for beneficial alterations in the technique.[18] The continuous aerobic technique currently (1994) being used at Emory University School of Medicine is antegrade induction of cardioplegic arrest with a high-potassium solution (1 part of crystalloid to 4 parts of blood, crystalloid solution containing 100 mEq of potassium chloride in 1 L of Plasmalyte with 20 mEq of sodium bicarbonate and 3 mL of $D_{50}W$ added). Cardioplegia is maintained by retrograde infusion of cardioplegic solution at a rate of at least 150 mL/min into a coronary sinus catheter. The crystalloid component of this solution (again a 4-to-1 mixture is used) contains 40 mEq of potassium chloride per liter. If systemic potassium levels rise above 6 or 7, or if a prolonged crossclamp interval is anticipated, a very low-potassium solution is used (15 mEq of potassium/L in the crystalloid component of the mixture). Temperatures of CPB are reduced to 30° to 32°C. The temperature of the cardioplegic infusion is identical to the systemic temperature. The continuous aerobic cardioplegia technique is favored for patients in whom there is evidence of preoperative myocardial ischemia or metabolic compromise. It is also generally used in valve patients who would be expected to have a slightly longer crossclamp interval than those undergoing routine coronary bypass. In routine coronary artery bypass cases, a cold oxygenated crystalloid cardioplegia technique is used because it allows superior visualization of distal anastomoses.

Summary

Continuous aerobic cardioplegic techniques appear to offer specific and important advantages in the resuscitation of metabolically compromised or depleted myocardium. An important adverse neurologic outcome was observed in the application of this technique when strict normothermia was maintained. The use of mildly hypothermic (or "tepid") continuous aerobic cardioplegia appears to offer all the advantages of normothermic continuous cardioplegic techniques without the disadvantages of systemic normothermia.

References

1. Panos A, Cristakis GT, Lichtenstein SV, et al. Operation for acute postinfarction mitral insufficiency using continuous oxygenated blood cardioplegia. *Ann Thorac Surg* 1989;48:816-819.
2. Lichtenstein SV, Salerno TA, Slutsky AS. Warm continuous cardioplegia versus intermittent hypothermic protection during cardiopulmonary bypass. Pro: warm continouous cardioplegia is preferable to intermittent hypothermic cardioplegia for myocardial protution during cardiopulmonary bypass. *J Cardiothorac Anesth* 1990;4:279-281.
3. Lichtenstein SV, Ashe KA, El-Daliti H, et al. Warm heart surgery. *J Thorac Cardiovasc Surg* 1991;101:269-274.
4. Salerno TA, Houck JP, Barrozo CAM, et al. Retrograde continuous warm blood cardioplegia: a new concept in myocardial protection. *Ann Thorac Surg* 1991;51:1023-1025.
5. Lichtenstein SV, Able JG, Salerno TA. Warm heart surgery and results of operation for recent myocardial infarction. *Ann Thorac Surg* 1991;52:455-460.
6. Lichtenstein SV, Abel JG, Panos A, et al. Warm heart surgery: experience with long cross-clamp times. *Ann Thorac Surg* 1991;52:1009-1013.
7. Kay GL, Aoki A, Zubiate P, et al. Superior myocardial protection by normothermic aerobic arrest over ischemic arrest for high-risk patients. Presented at the 28th Annual Meeting of The Society of Thoracic Surgeons, Orlando, Florida, February 3-5, 1992.
8. Vaughn CC, Opie JC, Florendo FT, et al. Warm blood cardioplegia. *Ann Thorac Surg* 1993;55:1227-1232.
9. Gott VL, Gonzalez JL, Zuhdi MN, et al. Retrograde perfusion of the coronary sinus for direct vision aortic surgery. *Surg Gynecol Obstet* 1957;104:319-328.
10. Gott VL, Gonzalez JL, Paneth M, et al. Cardiac retroperfusion with induced asystole for open-heart surgery upon the aortic valve or the coronary arteries. *Proc Soc Exp Biol Med* 1957;94:689-692.
11. Bomfim V, Kaijser L, Bendz R, et al. Myocardial protection during aortic valve replacement: cardiac metabolism and enzyme release following continuous blood cardioplegia. *Scan J Thor Cardiovasc Surg* 1981;15:141-147.
12. Khuri SF, Warner KG, Josa M, et al. The superiority of continuous cold blood cardioplegia in the metabolic protection of the hypertrophied human heart. *J Thorac Cardiovasc Surg* 1988;95:442-454.
13. Brown WM, Jay JL, Gott JP, et al. Warm blood cardioplegia: superior protection after acute myocardial ischemia. *Ann Thorac Surg* 1993;55:32-42.
14. Horsley WS, Whitlark JD, Hall JD, et al. Revascularization for acute regional infarct: superior protection with warm blood cardioplegia. *Ann Thorac Surg* 1993;56:1228-1238.
15. Martin TD, Craver JM, Weintraub WS, et al. Warm blood versus cold crystalloid cardioplegia: a case-matched comparison. Abstract. Presented at the 65th Scientific Session of the American Heart Association, New Orleans, Louisiana, November 16-19, 1992.
16. Martin TD, Craver JM, Gott JP, et al. Prospective, randomized trial of retrograde warm blood cardioplegia: myocardial benefit and neurologic threat. *Ann Thorac Surg* 1994;57:298-304.
17. Bufkin BL, Mellitt RJ, Gott JP, et al. Aerobic blood cardioplegia for revascularization of acute infarct: effects of delivery temperature on myocardial protection. Presented at the 13th Annual Meeting of The Society of Thoracic Surgeons, New Orleans, Louisiana, January 31, 1994.
18. Gutyon RA. Warm blood cardioplegia: benefits and risks. *Ann Thorac Surg* 1993;55:1071-1072.
19. Menasche P, Piwnica A. Cardioplegia by way of the coronary sinus for valvular and coronary surgery. *J Am Coll Cardiol* 1991;18:628-636.
20. Robinson LA. Cardioplegic solutions in the 90's: current perspective and national trends. Presented at Myocardial Preservation: Past Trends and Future Technology, Atlanta, Georgia, October 16-17, 1992.
21. Matsuura H, Lazar HL, Yang XM, et al. Detrimental effects of interrupting warm blood cardioplegia during coronary revascularization. *J Thorac Cardiovasc Surg* 1993;106:357-361.
22. Teoh KHT, Panos AI, Harmantas AA, et al. Optimal visualization of coronary artery anastomoses by gas jet. *Ann Thorac Surg* 1991;52:564.
23. Aronson S, Lee BK, Zaroff JG, et al. Myocardial distribution of cardioplegic solution after retrograde delivery in patients undergoing cardiac surgical procedures. *J Thorac Cardiovasc Surg* 1993;105:214-221.
24. Huang AH, Sofola IO, Bufkin BL, et al. Retrograde cardioplegia distribution is not affected by coronary arterial venting or by coronary sinus pressure. In preparation.
25. Lichtenstein SV, Abel JG, Slutsky A. Warm retrograde cardioplegia. Protection of the right ventricle in mitral valve operations. *J Thorac Cardiovasc Surg* 1992;104:374-379.
26. Christakis GT, Koch JP, Deemar KA, et al. A randomized study of the systemic effects of warm heart surgery. *Ann Thorac Surg* 1992;54:449-459.
27. Menasche P, Haydar S, Peynet J, et al. A potential mechanism of vasodilation after warm heart surgery. *J Thorac Cardiovasc Surg* 1994;107:293-299.
28. Gundry SR, Wang N, Bannon D, et al. Retrograde continuous warm blood cardioplegia: maintenance of myocardial homeostasis in humans. *Ann Thorac Surg* 1993;55:358-363.

29. Ikonomidis JS, Yau TM, Weisel RD, et al. Optimal flow rates for retrograde warm cardioplegia. *J Thorac Cardiovasc Surg* 1994;107:510–519.
30. Yau TM, Ikonomidis JS, Weisel RD, et al. Ventricular function after normothermic versus hypothermic cardioplegia. *J Thorac Cardiovasc Surg* 1993;105:833–844.
31. Hoff JT, Cerebral protection. *J Neurosurg* 1986;65:579–591.
32. Cavarocchi NC, Pluth JR, Schaff HV, et al. Complement activation during cardiopulmonary bypass. *J Thorac Cardiovasc Surg* 1986;91:252–258.
33. Moore FD Jr, Warner KG, Assousa S, et al. The effects of complement activation during cardiopulmonary bypass: attenuation by hypothermia, heparin, and hemodilution. *Ann Surg* 1988;208:95–103.

Index

Abortion, after surgery in pregnancy, 360
Absorption rate, for nonintravenously administered drug, and hypothermia, 59
Acetylcholine, effects of, and temperature, 63
Acid-base management
 acidosis
  and failure to wean from CPB, 292
  and intracellular enzyme function, 64
  lactic, as an indication of inadequate flow, 320
  during reperfusion, 50-51
  stomach wall, as an indicator of gut hypoperfusion, 158
 effect of, on cerebral vasodilation, 119-120
 during pediatric cardiopulmonary bypass, 322
 removal of acid, during cardiac arrest, 26
 status at the time of CPB weaning, 283
 See also Bicarbonate buffer; Buffer systems; pH
Acquired immune deficiency syndrome (AIDS), 176-177
Activated clotting time (ACT), 90
 before aortic cannulation, 272
 in ECMO, 440
 effect on
  of aprotinin, 105
  of protamine, 95
 for heparin reversal evaluation, 96
 for monitoring
  of heparin, during cardiac surgery, 91
  to prevent coagulopathy, 303
  to prevent DIC, 300
 predictive accuracy for postoperative bleeding, 102
 to verify effective anticoagulation, 275-276
 in pediatric patients, 317-318
Activation, of platelets, 97-98
Activity tests, for heparin, 90-91
Acute respiratory distress syndrome (ARDS), 152-153, 437
Acute respiratory failure (ARF), tachypnea in, 450
Adaptive immunity, 170
Adenine nucleotides, 43
Adenosine diphosphate (ADP), plasma levels of, in hemolysis, 97
Adrenal glands, responses to surgery, 185-189
Adrenal medulla, 187-189
Adrenergic agents, alpha, to maintain perfusion pressure, 28
Adrenergic agonists
 alpha, during warm heart surgery, 486
 beta, 64
 to maintain systemic blood pressure and perfusion pressure, 22
Adrenergic receptors
 beta blockade, 80
  in angina pectoris, 64
  stimulation or blockade of, effects on maternal-fetal physiology, 368t

Adrenocorticotropic hormone (ACTH), 182
 synthetic, administration during cardiopulmonary bypass, 185
Afterload
 of a centrifugal pump, 220
 reduction of, in intraaortic balloon pump counterpulsation, 414
Age
 effect of
  on drug levels, 61
  on drug metabolism, 58
 and risk
  in intraaortic balloon pump counterpulsation, 425
  of neuropsychologic dysfunction, 114, 127, 129
Air
 in the aorta, during surgery for mitral valve disease, 278
 in an aortic cannula, 273
 introduction of, to left heart chambers in venting, 32
Air embolism
 during aortic cannulation, 261-262
 due to balloon rupture, 427-428
 cerebral, 123, 125t
  reducing risk of, 48, 332
  risk in left ventricular decompression, 261
 coronary, myocardial dysfunction caused by, 290
 deairing the aorta, during surgery for mitral valve disease, 34
 frequency of accidents due to, 300-301
 management of, 304-305
 preventing, 302-303
 protection against, centrifugal pump use, 221
 in venovenous bypass, 392
 See also Emboli
Air lock, in a venous line, 262
Airways, injury to, 356-357
Albumin
 drugs bound to, 60-61, 65
 precoating for the ECC, 97, 230
  pediatric, 313
Alcuronium, 74-75
Aldosterone levels, in cardiopulmonary bypass, 60, 181, 185, 187
Alfentanil
 attenuation of stress response by, 190
 binding to equipment, 67
 clearance of, 66
 effect of hemodilution on plasma concentration of, 60, 65, 67
 elimination half-time, 62
 sensitivity to, and age, 61
Alkalosis, and neurologic injury after hypothermic arrest, 320
Alloimmunization, in blood transfusion, 461-462

Alpha-stat pH management, 52, 273-274, 322, 332
 and cerebral blood flow, 119, 135
ε-Aminocaproic acid (EACA; Amicar)
 inhibition of fibrinolysis by, 105-106
 to reduce blood loss, 466, 479
Aminophylline, for managing protamine reaction, 306
Amrinone, 293
 for afterload reduction, during separation from CPB, 324
 effect of
  on platelet count, 424
  during pregnancy, 368, 369f
 during weaning from CPB, 288
Anaerobiosis, duration of, and intracellular homeostasis, 43
Anaphylactic reactions, to protamine, 95, 105
Anaphylotoxins, complement fragments, 153
Anastomoses
 completion of, in a single crossclamp interval, 32
 distal coronary, visualizing during warm blood cardioplegia, 31
 visualizing during warm blood cardioplegia, 33
Ancrod (Arvin), 94
Anemia
 and level of uptake of drugs, 65
 physiologic responses to, 462-464
Anesthesia
 cardiac arrest during, 299
 damage during induction of, 22
 for intracranial surgery, 342
 neuropsychologic dysfunction following administration of, 116-117
 for pediatric cardiopulmonary bypass, 314-315
Anesthetic agents, 66-75
 and cerebral protection, 135-139, 332
 effect of
  on adrenocortical hormones, 185
  on antidiuretic hormone levels, 180-181
  on blood glucose levels, 184-185
  on catecholamine levels, 188-189
  on growth hormone release, 183
  on receptor-mediated events, 64
Aneurysms
 of the ascending aorta, 329-330
 cerebral, 340-341
  dissection of, 343
  outcomes of surgery for, 344-345
 profound hypothermia during surgery involving, 46
 traumatic, repair of, 353
Angina, produced by vasopressin, 180
Angiography
 diagnostic, for evaluating myocardial ischemia, 349
 fluorescein retinal, to follow retinal microvascular embolization, 132, 214

Angioplasty
   cardiopulmonary bypass-supported, 379–387
      alternatives to, 384–387
      high-risk, prophylactic IABP use in, 417
Angiotensin-converting enzyme (ACE) inhibitors, contraindication in the postoperative period, 163–164
Antegrade cerebral perfusion, in aortic arch surgery, 333–334, 334f
Anterior fontanel pressure (AFP), during DH-TCA, 120–121
Anti-arrhythmics, effect of, during pregnancy, 371–373
Antibiotics, 75–78. *See also* Prophylaxis
Anticoagulation, 88–90, 275–276
   heparin, reversal of, 94–97
   in intraaortic counterpulsation, 424
   with long-term ventricular assistance, 403
   for pediatric patients, 317–318
Antidiuretic hormone (ADH), 180–182
   levels of, in cardiopulmonary bypass, 60
Antifibrinolytic therapy, to decrease blood loss, 105–106, 466
Antigranulocyte antibody, and pulmonary edema, 151
Antihistamines, for managing protamine reaction, 306
Antiinflammatory drugs, postoperative use of, 175
Antimicrobials, timing and duration of prophylaxis, 176. *See also* Prophylaxis, antimicrobial
Anti-thrombin III (AT-III), 89, 90
Aorta, coarctation of, contraindication to pregnancy, 359
Aortic arch, 330–334
   cannulation modification for pediatric surgery, 318
   profound hypothermia in operations involving, 46
Aortic cannulation
   cerebral shower of emboli following, 123
   complications of, 261–263
Aortic disease
   and risk of neurologic dysfunction, 129
   stenosis, vulnerability resulting from, 21, 33–34
Aortic dissection, 272–273
   pressure change as a warning of, 304
Aortic regurgitation, myocardial protection in, 33–34
Aortic tract, atresia of, profound hypothermia during surgery involving, 46
Aortic wounds, 355
Aortoatriocaval cannulation, 257–263
Aprotinin, 104–105
   for anticoagulation, 94, 479
   to reduce blood loss, 466
   for immunodepression prevention, 175
Arachidonic acid, formation of, in cerebral ischemia, 125–126
Archimedean screw pumps, 226–227
Arginine vasopressin (AVP), and coagulant factor release, 100
Arrhythmias
   malignant, and failure to wean from CPB, 292
   postoperative, prevention of, 24
   ventricular
      intraaortic balloon pump counterpulsation use in, 417
      treating, 281
Arterial line filters, 233–235, 313
   flushing with carbon dioxide, 239
Arterial line pressure, monitoring, in pediatric cardiac surgery, 318–319
Arterial outlet port, in a bubble oxygenator, 201–202
Arteries
   cannulation of, to evaluate blood pressure, 267
   femoral, cannulation of, 329–330
   removal of cannula from, 284–285
Arteriovenous cannulation, femoral, 260
Arteriovenous malformations (AVM), intracranial surgery for, 344–345
Artifacts, distorting EEG readings, 271

Ascending aorta, 329–330
   atherosclerotic, management of, 130
   cannulation of, 258
   placement for IABP support, 419
      after aortic dissection, 420, 420f
Aspartate, for reperfusion after ischemic insult, 27
Aspirin, irreversible reaction with thromboxane A_2, 103
Asystole, myocardial oxygen demand in, 484–491
Atelectasis, left lung, 148
Atheroembolism, 262
Atracurium, metabolism of, 74–75
Atrial cannulas, double right, 259–260
Atrial natriuretic factor (ANF), and sodium excretion, 181
Atrial septal defects, hypothermia during repair of, 41
Atrial-ventricular (A-V) sequential pacing, in complete heart block, 281
Atriocaval cannulation, right, 258–259
Atrioventricular septal defects, repair of, 49
Atropine
   to avert bradycardia, with fentanyl or sufentanil, 315
   premedication with, pediatric patients, 315
Autologous blood recovery, during liver transplantation, 393
Automation of bypass monitoring, impediments to, 14–15
Autonomic function, changes in, during cardiopulmonary bypass, 60
Autoregulation, cerebral
   of blood flow, 119–122
   and carotid stenosis, 128
   with diabetes, 127
   loss of, during deep hypothermia, 322
   in pediatric cardiopulmonary bypass, 312
Autoregulatory plateau, 119
Autotransfusion of blood, 464–465, 467–468. *See also* Blood, conservation of
Axillary artery
   approach for IABP, 419–420, 420f
   catheterization of, in pediatric cardiac surgery, 316
Azathioprine, as a risk factor for pancreatitis, 159

Backup equipment, 303, 305
Bacteria, airborne, 173
Balloon rupture, IABP, 427–428
Ball valves, in perfusion circuit safety devices, 244–245
Barbiturates
   for cerebral protection, during cardiopulmonary bypass, 48, 67–68, 136–138, 341
   as induction agents, 67–68
   for intracranial surgery, 342
   in management of air embolism, 305
Benzodiazepines
   displacement from albumin, after heparin administration, 65
   sedative and amnestic properties, 68–70
Beta-blockade
   effect of, during pregnancy, 371
   effect on metabolic rate of the heart, 23
   in valve operations, 33
Bicarbonate buffer, 26
   in metabolic acidosis, 283
Binding, of drugs to equipment, 66, 68
Biochemical reactions, metabolic, 43
Biotransformation, of administered drugs, and hypothermia, 59
Bladder temperature, as a measure of core temperature, 51
Bleeding
   abnormal, after cardiopulmonary bypass, 101–104
   control of, in preparing to come off bypass, 282
   pharmacologic prophylaxis of, 104–106
Bleeding time, as a measure of platelet dysfunction, 99
Blender, monitoring oxygen to the oxygenator from, 244

Blood
   for cardioplegic solutions, 26–27
      cold, 29–30, 31, 32–33, 34
      warm, 30–31, 33, 34
   changes in, during cardiopulmonary bypass, 170–171
   conservation of, 238–239, 314, 461–469
   postoperative loss of, in oxygenation, 214
Blood-brain barrier, effect of hyperthermia on, 133
Blood film, thickness of, 10
Blood flow
   changes in, during cardiopulmonary bypass, 66, 415
   factors affecting requirements for, 45
   in pregnant patients, 364–365
   maximum, for a membrane oxygenator, 211–212
   monitoring of, 242–243
   renal, during cardiopulmonary bypass, 66, 160
   during venovenous bypass, in liver transplantation, 391
   See also Cerebral blood flow; Hepatic blood flow; Uterine blood flow
Blood gases
   augmentation of transfer, 450–457
   management of
      in a bubble oxygenator, 203–206
      and cerebral blood flow, 52, 135, 273–274
   measurement of, 244
Blood-gas exchange membranes, surface treatment of, 15
Blood groups, discovery of, 3
Blood pressure
   control of
      during intracranial surgery, 343
      during surgery on pregnant patients, 365
   diastolic, effect of IABP counterpulsation, 415
   monitoring of, 241–242, 267, 274–275
   systolic atrial, lowering for ascending aortic annulation, 258
   systolic systemic, effect of IABP counterpulsation, 415
   See also Hypertension; Hypotension
Blood products, immunomodulatory effects of, 462
Blood temperature, monitoring, 240–241
Blood urea nitrogen (BUN), after cardiopulmonary bypass, 160
Bradycardia, fetal, during maternal cardiopulmonary bypass, 363
Breakthrough ectopy, during lidocaine administration, 65
Breathing, effectiveness of effort, after cardiopulmonary bypass, 148
Bretylium, effect of, during pregnancy, 373
Bridge to transplantation (BTT)
   cardiac, ECMO for, 440
   ethical problems associated with, 400
   indication for ventricular assistance, 400
   with orthotopic total artificial hearts, 403
Bronchi, ruptured, repair of, 357
Bubble oxygenators, 4, 200–206
   bubble size, effect on gas transfer, 202–203
   complement fragments liberated in, 153
   versus membrane oxygenators, 212–214
   early models, 10
   microparticulate air produced by, 131–132
   platelet damage in, 98
   priming volume, 312
Buccal route, for drug administration, 58
Budd-Chiari syndrome, contraindication to venovenous bypass in, 392
Buffer systems
   blood, for maintaining pH of cardioplegic solutions, 26–27
   for crystalloid solutions, 28
   for maintaining pH of cardioplegic solutions, 26
   tham, 26, 283
   See also Acid-base management; Bicarbonate buffer; pH
Bundle branch block, right, 267

Index

Calcium
  effect on, of receptor-mediated events, 64
  hypocalcemia, for reperfusion after ischemic insult, 27
  as an inotrope, 293
  interaction with parathyroid hormone, 191
  levels of
    adjustment of, before separation from CPB, 323
    in cerebral ischemia, 124–125
    effect of hypothermia, 46, 64
    for reperfusion after ischemic insult, 27
  postoperative, after intracranial surgery, 343
  as a third messenger, 60
  for weaning from CPB, 286
Calcium channel blockers, effect of
  during pregnancy, 372
  on tolerance of ischemia, 24, 139
Calibration, of pump-side devices, 240
Cancer, risk of recurrence, after blood product transfusion, 462
Cannulas, 231–233
  placement of
    in portable cardiopulmonary bypass, 381, 383
    and venous return, 273
  in portable cardiopulmonary bypass units, 380
Cannulation
  aortic
    cerebral shower of emboli following, 123
    complications of, 261–263
  aortic arch, modification for pediatric surgery, 318
  aortoatriocaval, 257–263
  arterial, 329–330
    to evaluate blood pressure, 267
  of the ascending aorta, 258
  atriocaval, 258–259
  of femoral arteries, 329–330
  femoral arteriovenous, 260
  in hypoplastic left heart syndrome, 318
  in the pediatric patient, 318–319
  for reoperation, 261
  in surgery for acute aortic dissection, 330
  venous, 330
    complications of, 262–263
    in pediatric patients, 318–319
Capillary perfusion, improvement in, with hemodilution, 8
Capillary wedge pressure, pulmonary
  effect of IABP counterpulsation, 415
  indication for ventricular assistance, 399
Carbon dioxide
  elimination of, 450
    in an oxygenator, 200
  exchange of, 4, 10, 202–203, 204, 206, 210
  for flushing membrane oxygenators, 209–210
  modification of Pa_{CO_2} during surgery, 119
    and neuropsychologic dysfunction, 117
  solubility of, and temperature, 51
  See also Hypercarbia
Cardiac arrest, with potassium chloride, in intracranial surgery, 343
Cardiac disease, type of, and risk of neurologic dysfunction, 128
Cardiac failure, ECMO in, 440–441
Cardiac index
  improvement in, with IABP counterpulsation, 415
  indication for ventricular assistance, 399
Cardiac output, 269–270
Cardiac performance, postoperative, and renal failure, 163
Cardiac preload, 282
Cardiac tamponade, indication for reoperation, 101, 408
Cardiac transplantation, and intraaortic balloon pump counterpulsation, 416–417
Cardiac wounds, 353–355
Cardiogenic shock, 21
  intraaortic balloon pump counterpulsation in, 413
  postcardiotomy, ventricular assistance for, 225–226
Cardiomyopathy, end-stage, indication for ventricular assistance, 400

Cardioplegia
  early in reperfusion, 27
  and ECG monitoring, 266
  normothermic antegrade, versus hypothermic blood, 489–490
  to reduce oxygen consumption, 25
  in surgery after failed angioplasty, 350–351
  tepid retrograde continuous blood, 490
  warm-blood, 484–491
  warm-blood versus cold crystalloid, clinical trial, 488–489
  See also Crystalloid cardioplegia
Cardioplegic solutions
  cold blood, 34
    composition of, 30f
  filters for, 235
  potassium concentration in, 276
  pressure monitors for, 242
  requirements for, 25
  warm blood, composition of, 30f
Cardiopulmonary bypass
  discontinuation of, 281–294
    in pediatric patients, 322–324
  emergency, 347
  historical foundation, 3–16
  initiation of, 272–273
    pediatric patients, 319–321
  maintenance of, 263–278
    in pediatric patients, 321–322
  in pediatric patients, 311–325
Cardiotomy filters, 234
Cardiotomy suction system
  positive bacterial cultures from, 173–174
  stopping during protamine administration, 304
Cardioversion, for supraventricular tachycardia, 281–282
Carotid bruit, and postoperative neurologic deficit, 127–128
Carotid stenosis, and cerebral autoregulation, 128
Case reports, intravascular oxygenator use, 455–457
Catecholamines
  levels of, in cardiopulmonary bypass, 187–189
  response to
    and metabolic acidosis, 64
    in pregnant patients, 367, 367t
Catheterization, cardiac, 6
Catheters
  autoperfusion, 385
  balloon, removal of, 429
  for perfusion, in management of myocardial ischemia, 348–349
  pulmonary artery, in angioplasty, 350
  size of, and risk of intraaortic balloon pump counterpulsation, 425
Cefamandole, 76
  pharmacokinetics of, during cardiopulmonary bypass, 78
Cefazolin, comparison with cephalothin, 76
Ceftriaxone, pharmacokinetics of, during cardiopulmonary bypass, 78
Cells
  integrity of myocardial, effects of hypotension, 23
  integrity of phospholipid membranes, 43
Cell salvage, to conserve blood, 467
Central nervous system, 114–140
  nonintravenously administered drugs in, and hypothermia, 59
  recovery from ischemia, and hyperglycemia, 183
Central venous catheters, in pediatric cardiac surgery, 316
Central venous pressure, monitoring of, 267–268
Centrifugal pumps, 15, 220–222, 223f
  in portable cardiopulmonary bypass units, 380
  in venovenous bypass, potential complications of use, 392
  in ventricular assist devices, 401–402
Cephalexin, 75–76
Cephalosporins
  pharmacokinetics of, during cardiopulmonary bypass, 78
  prophylactic use of, 176

Cephalothin, comparison with cefazolin, in cardiopulmonary bypass, 76
Cerebral blood flow (CBF)
  autoregulation of, 52, 119, 274
    and extracorporeal perfusion flow rates, 48
  during cardiopulmonary bypass, 66
  effect of pulsatile perfusion on, 410
  failure to recover, after deep hypothermic total circulatory arrest, 120–121
  interrupting during aortic arch surgery, 331–334
  regulation of, and pH of blood, 51
Cerebral hypoperfusion, injury from, 122
Cerebral metabolic rate for oxygen ($CMRO_2$), 44, 341, f
Cerebral oxygen consumption, and flow rate, 322
Cerebral perfusion, and IABP during cardiopulmonary bypass, 421
Cerebral physiology, 118–122
Cerebroplegia, protective effects of, 140
Cerebrovascular disease, and risk of neuropsychologic dysfunction after cardiac surgery, 127–128
Chest drainage, usual levels of, 101
Children
  fentanyl levels in, 66–67
  thyroid function in cardiopulmonary bypass, 193
  See also Pediatric patients
Chlorpromazine, in postoperative intraaortic counterpulsation, 423
Choreoathetosis, and uneven cooling, 48
Chronic obstructive pulmonary disease (COPD)
  diastolic-to-occlusion pressure gradient in, 269
  and risk of pulmonary failure, 156
Cimetidine, effect of, on drug metabolism, 58
Circulation, of blood, sustaining mechanically, 3
Circulatory arrest
  in deep hypothermia, 120–121
  in pediatric cardiac surgery, 321
  with profound hypothermia, versus low-flow hypothermic perfusion, 49–50
  with surface cooling, 48
Circulatory shock, and ADH secretion stimulation, 180
Citrate toxicity, and hypothermia, 46
Clearance
  of alcuronium, 74
  of cefazolin, 78
  of cephalosporin, during cardiopulmonary bypass, 78
  of a drug from plasma, factors affecting, 66
  of a drug from the body, 57
    factors affecting, 63
  of fentanyl, in children, 67
  of fibrin degradation products, 101
  of heparin, 89–90
  of lidocaine, in cardiopulmonary bypass, 80
  of propofol, 70
  renal
    of administered drugs in hypothermia, 59
    of cefazolin, 78
  of thiopental, 68
  of tubocurarine, in cardiopulmonary bypass, 74
  See also Elimination half-time
Clinical systems, for myocardial protection, 27–31
Clinical trials, intravascular oxygenator, 454–455
Clonidine, attenuation of stress response by, 190
Coagulation, management of
  after intracranial surgery, 343
  predictive accuracy of tests in postoperative bleeding, 102
  See also Anticoagulation; Heparin
Coagulation cascade, 88–89
  activation of, and flow rate in venovenous bypass, 391
  effect on, of hypothermia with hemodilution, 46
  intrinsic, activation by factor XI, 99
Coagulopathy
  consumptive, 100–101
  dilutional, 97
  preventing, 303
Cognitive dysfunction, after CABG surgery, 115
Colchicine, effect of, on brain edema, 126

Collateral flow, noncoronary, effect on cardioplegic solutions, 25–26
Combined Registry for the Clinical Use of Mechanical Ventricular Assist Devices, 401–402, 403, 408
Compartment syndrome, 427
Complement
  activation of
    in cardiopulmonary bypass, 189
    in oxygenators, 213–214
      therapies for reducing, 157t
  levels of, in cardiopulmonary bypass, 60, 171–172
Complement cascade
  activation of, 171
  inflammation produced by, 170
  and innate immunity, 170
  role of, in lung injury, 153–154
Complement-split products, biologically significant, 153
Complexity, and vulnerability to accidents, 298
Compliance, of the respiratory system, 147–148, 156
Complications
  acute, in cardiopulmonary bypass, 272–273
  of aortoatrial cannulation, 261–262
  of autotransfusion of blood, 468
  of ECMO, 438–440
  of intraaortic balloon pump counterpulsation, 424–425, 426–428
  neurologic, after cardiac surgery, 115
  after percutaneous portable bypass, 384t
  during perfusion, management of, 304–306
  surveys of, 299–302
  of venous cannulation, 262–263
  of venovenous bypass, 392
  of ventricular assist device use, 408–409
Conduction, defined, 247
Conduits, for extracorporeal circulation, 229–233
Configurations, membrane, in a membrane oxygenator, 207
Congenital defects
  and maternal heart disease, 360
  repair of, 15–16, 199
  after surgery during pregnancy, 360
Congenital heart disease
  cardiopulmonary bypass during treatment of, 311
  metabolism of halothane in, 73
  myocardial protection in, 34
Congestive heart disease, and risk for pulmonary complications, 156
Conservation, blood, 314
Contact factors, changes in cardiopulmonary bypass, 99
Continuous-flow cardiopulmonary bypass versus deep hypothermic total cardiac arrest, 322
Contractility, myocardial, and strategy for weaning from CPB, 287f
Contraindications
  to autologous blood donation, 465
  to intraaortic balloon pump counterpulsation, 417
  to intravascular oxygenator use, 454
  to isovolemic hemodilution for blood conservation, 465
  to liver transplantation, 389
  to platelet transfusion, in heparin-induced thrombocytopenia, 93
  to transesophageal echocardiography, 342
  to venovenous bypass in liver transplantation, 392
Control groups, testing of, to assess neuropsychologic dysfunction, 116–117
Convection, defined, 247
Core hypothermia, 7
Core temperature, importance of, in warming after hypothermia, 253
Coronary artery, myocardial protection in reoperations on, 33
Coronary artery bypass graft (CABG), 114
  aprotinin for reduction of bleeding in, 104
  effects of pulsatile perfusion with, 122
  emergency, 103, 349–352
  postcardiotomy cardiogenic shock in, 400

prospective study of neurologic dysfunction after, 114–115
risk factors associated with postoperative pulmonary edema, 152
Coronary artery disease
  adaptation of myocardial protection techniques to, 31–33
  risks
    in induction of anesthesia, 22
    in thyroid hormone administration, 192–193
Coronary Artery Surgery Study (CASS), criteria from, for study of cardiopulmonary bypass, 238
Coronary blood flow, collateral, and intraaortic balloon pump counterpulsation, 415
Coronary occlusion, delayed, after angioplasty, 347
Coronary sinus pressure, for myocardial protection, 34
Coronary steal, in hemodilution, 22
Corticosteroids, effect of, in ischemic arrest, 24
Cortisol, levels of
  in cardiopulmonary bypass, 60, 186f
  in surgery, 185
Costs, of extracorporeal membrane oxygenation, 441–442
Coumadin therapy, effect of, on postoperative bleeding, 103, 106
Craniotomy, blood and perfusate management during, 343
Creatinine, levels of, after cardiopulmonary bypass, 160
Creatinine kinase BB, as a marker of cerebral ischemia, 322
Cross-circulation, 6
Crystalloid cardioplegia
  filters used in, 235
  oxygenated cold, 28–30
    in coronary artery disease, 31
    and poor left ventricular function, 32
Crystalloid solutions
  controlling composition of, 26, 28–29
  for perfusion hypothermia, 24
  for priming an extracorporeal circuit, 238
  in warm-blood cardioplegia, 484–485
Curare, effects of, and temperature, 63
Cytokines, interleukin family of, 172–173
Cytomegalovirus (CMV), transmission of, in blood transfusion, 461

1-Deamino-8-D-arginine vasopressin. See Desmopressin
DeBakey type I dissection, 330
Debubbling/defoaming, in bubble oxygenation, 200–201
Decompression, left ventricular, 261
Deep hypothermic-total circulatory arrest (DHTCA), 321–322, 340
  technique, 341–343
Defibrillation, during discontinuation of cardiopulmonary bypass, 281
Defibrination, overcoming, in oxygenators, 14
Defoaming compounds, silicone-based, 4
Depth filters, 234
Descending aorta
  approach to, for IABP insertion, 420f
  repair of, in trauma injury, 355
  thoracic, 334–336
Desferoxamine, reducing protease release with, 155
Desmopressin (DDAVP), 106
  reduction of bleeding by, 466, 479
Dexamethasone, in management of air embolism, 305
Dextran
  for anticoagulation, in long-term ventricular assistance, 403
  with long-term ventricular assistance, 409
Diabetes
  and pancreatic function in cardiopulmonary bypass, 185
  and risk of intraaortic balloon pump counterpulsation, 425
  and risk of neuropsychologic dysfunction after cardiac surgery, 127

Diaphragm pumps, 225
Diastolic augmentation, in intraaortic balloon pump counterpulsation, 414–415
Diazepam
  accumulation in blood, 69–70
  hepatic extraction ratio of, 58
  pharmacodynamics of, comparison with midazolam, 62
Digitalis, binding to tissue, 61
Digitalis glycosides, 78–79
Digoxin
  absorption by equipment, 78
  distribution of, 77f
  effect of, during pregnancy, 373
Diltiazem, effect of, on tolerance of ischemia, 24
Disease state, and drug distribution volumes, 66
Dissection
  acute aortic, 262
    cannulation in surgery for, 330
  arterial, from guide wire or balloon catheter, 427
Disseminated intravascular coagulation (DIC)
  cryoprecipitate transfusion in, 106
  frequency of, 300
Distal perfusion, in thoracoabdominal aortic procedures, 335–336
Distribution
  of a drug
    to a receptor area, 60–61
    after a single IV dose, 55–56
    effects of disease states, 66
  rate of, for nonintravenously administered drug, and hypothermia, 59
Diuretics
  and blood conservation, 466
  loop, 466
  to manage hyperkalemia in normothermic cardiopulmonary bypass, 485
Dobutamine, 292
  effect of, during pregnancy, 368, 369f
  for low pulse pressure, BP, 324
  for weaning from CPB, 286
Dopamine, 292
  effect of
    during pregnancy, 368, 369f
    on renal function, 163, 286
  for low pulse pressure, BP, 324
Dopexamine, 293
Down-regulation, in congestive heart failure, 64
Drugs
  antibiotics, 75–78
  antimicrobial, 176
  concentration of, changes due to hemodilution in CPB, 59–60
  dosage of, and free drug concentration, 64
  errors in administration of, 302, 306
    frequency, 300
    preventing, 304
  factors determining free concentration of, 64–66
  interactions with receptors, 60–64
  lungs as a reservoir for, 65
  metabolic products of, 55
  rate of administration, and free drug concentration, 65
  rectal route for administration of, 58
  routes for administration of, 58
  See also Anesthetic agents; Inotropic drugs; Opioids; particular drugs
Duration of cardiopulmonary bypass
  and infection prevention, 174
  and neurologic dysfunction, 135
  to pace rewarming, 50–51
  and renal dysfunction, 161
Duration of intraaortic balloon counterpulsation, and risks, 425
Dynamic priming volume, 210
Dysrhythmia, atrial, with excessive rewarming, 323

Echocardiography
  esophageal, for monitoring de-airing maneuvers, 278
  intraoperative, 324
    to identify risk for aortic emboli, 129
  See also Transesophageal echocardiography

Index

Edema
 cerebral
  from hypertension, 274
  from impaired drainage of the superior vena cava, 121
  from hemodilution, 149–151
  pulmonary, preexisting, and edema, 151
  after total cardiopulmonary bypass in infants, 49
Ejection from the left ventricle, 285–286
Elastance, in the respiratory system, 147
Elastase, release of, during cardiopulmonary bypass, 155
Electrical failure
 frequency of, 300, 301
 managing, 305
 preventing, 303
Electrocardiography (ECG), for monitoring, during cardiopulmonary bypass, 264–267
Electroencephalography (EEG)
 for central nervous system monitoring, 117–118, 331
 for detecting cortical ischemia, 270–271
 for monitoring cerebral effects of hypothermia, 48
Electrolytes
 changes in the excitotoxic cascade response, 124–126
 effect of, on receptor-mediated events, 64
 handling of, by the kidney during cardiopulmonary bypass, 66
 monitoring of, 244
 See also Calcium; Hyperkalemia; Hypokalemia; Potassium; Sodium-potassium pump
Elimination of drugs, 58–59
Elimination half-time
 for alcuronium, 74
 for alfentanil, 62
 for cefamandole, 76
 for cephalothin, during cardiac surgery, 77
 for a drug, defined, 57
 for esmolol, 371
 for fentanyl, 62
 for heparin, 89–90
 for isoflurane, 71
 for midazolam, 69
 for papaverine, 79
 for propofol, 70
 for sufentanil, 67
 for tubocurarine, during cardiopulmonary bypass, 74
 See also Clearance
Emboli
 aluminum, in infants in extracorporeal membrane oxygenation, 250
 and bubble oxygenator use, 131–132
 fat, 262
 gaseous, 233
 platelet, in myocardium and renal glomeruli, 233
 See also Air embolism; Microemboli; Thromboembolism
Enalapril, formation of active metabolites in liver, 58
Endarteritis, 427
Endocarditis
 infective, and risk of cerebral complications, 129
 prosthetic valvular, 169, 176
Endocrine system, 180–193
 changes in, during cardiopulmonary bypass, 60
β-Endorphin, levels of, in cardiopulmonary bypass, 60
Endotoxin, bacterial, release during cardiopulmonary bypass, 154–155, 158
Endotracheal intubation, introduction of, 21
Energy balance, maintaining in myocardial cells, 184. *See also* Metabolism; Oxygen/oxygenation
Enflurane, 70–71
 attenuation of stress response by, 190
 effect on, of hypothermia, 71
Enoximone, 293
Ephedrine
 effect of, during pregnancy, 368
 for weaning from CPB, 286

Epidural route, for drug administration, 58
Epinephrine, 292
 effect of, during pregnancy, 368
 levels of, in stress response, 97
 for low pulse pressure, BP, 324
 for managing protamine reaction, 306
 and stress response, 187
 for weaning from CPB, 286
Epstein-Barr virus (EBV), transmission of, in blood transfusion, 461
Equipment
 extracorporeal circuit, 379–381
 for pediatric cardiopulmonary bypass, 311–314
 reducing thrombogenicity of, 94, 131–132
 selection of, 238–239
Erythropoietin
 in autologous blood donation, 465
 to improve hemoglobin levels, 477
Esmolol
 effect of
  on maternal and fetal heart rates, 372
  during pregnancy, 371
 for ischemic arrest, 485
 preparing the heart for ischemic arrest, 23
Esophageal temperature, 270
Ethical considerations
 in bridge to transplantation (BTT), 400
 religious objections to blood transfusion, 473–483
Euthyroid sick syndrome, 192
Evaluation
 of heat exchanger performance, 250–251
 preoperative, for identification of risk factors, 174
Evoked potential (EP), cortical, monitoring, 120–121
Excitotoxic cascade response
 ischemic brain cells, 124–126, 133
 attenuation by anesthetics, 135
Extraaortic counterpulsation devices (EACPs), 414
Extracorporeal carbon dioxide removal ($ECCO_2R$), 435
Extracorporeal circuit
 assembling and monitoring, 238–246
 equipment, 379–381
 fatigue life of tubing, 229
 line separation in, managing, 306
Extracorporeal circulation
 ischemia as a complication of, 43
 oxygenators for, 199–215
 rewarming during, 50–51
Extracorporeal gas exchange, 3
Extracorporeal membrane oxygenation (ECMO), 250, 433–443
 pediatric, 312
Extraluminal flow (ELF) design, 13

Factor VIII, changes in, during cardiopulmonary bypass, 99
Femoral artery
 approach in intraaortic balloon pump counterpulsation, 417–418
 cannulation, alternative to aortoatrial cannulation, 261
 catheterization, in pediatric cardiac surgery, 316
 perfusion from, 262
Femorofemoral bypass, 336
Femorofemoral crossover graft, to improve limb perfusion, 427
Fenoldopam, effect of, on renal function, 163
Fentanyl
 attenuation of stress response by, 190
 binding of
  to equipment, 67
  to α-1-acid glycoprotein, 60
  to red cells, 65
  to tissue, 61
 clearance of, versus total plasma levels, in hypothermia, 66
 comparison with sufentanil, pharmacodynamic variables, 62
 dosages, for pediatric patients, 315

 effect of
  on blood glucose levels, 185
  on catecholamine levels, 188
 elimination half-time, 62
 hepatic extraction ratio of, 58
 for pediatric patients, 315
 sensitivity to, and age, 61
 sequestration in the lungs during CPB, 67
Fetal heart rate (FHR)
 after bypass discontinuation, 370f
 and maternal temperature, 367f
 monitoring, during maternal surgery, 363
Fibrinogen concentration, predictive accuracy for postoperative bleeding, 102
Fibrinolysis, 100–101
Fibrinolytic cascade, 88–89
Fick's law of diffusion, 210
Filling pressure, 267
Film coefficient, for convection, 249
Filters
 for extracorporeal circulation, 233–235, 313
 polyester, in a bubble oxygenator, 201
Flow obstruction, and failure to wean from CPB, 291
Flow rate, and degree of hypothermia, 321
Fluid dynamics, 248–249
Fluorometric assay, for heparin, 92
Food and Drug Administration (FDA), authorization of IVOX trials, 455
Forced expiratory volume (FEV_1), after cardiopulmonary bypass, 148
Free fatty acids, levels of, 60
Free radical scavenger
 mannitol as, 163
 thiopental as, 136
Fresh frozen plasma (FFP)
 for heparin-resistant patients, 92
 after intracranial surgery, 343
Functional residual capacity (FRC), after cardiopulmonary bypass, 148
Furosemide
 effect of
  on potassium levels, 276
  on renal blood flow, 163
 ototoxicity of, 163

Gas embolism, prevention of, with monitoring in the perfusion circuit, 244. *See also* Air embolism
Gas filters, 235
Gas-to-blood-flow ratio (GBFR), adjusting, to control arterial carbon dioxide pressure, 204–205
Gas transfer
 alveolar-to-arterial oxygen gradient, 149
 principles of, 202–203, 210
Gastrointestinal system, 157–159
Gender, and risk of intraaortic balloon pump counterpulsation, 425
Genetic predisposition, effect of, on drug metabolism, 58. *See also* Congenital defects
Glomerular filtration rate (GFR), during cardiopulmonary bypass, 160
Glomus jugulare tumors, intracranial surgery for, 344
Glucagon, levels of, in cardiopulmonary bypass, 60
Glucocorticoids, inhibition of neutrophil activation by, 155
Glucose, 277–278
 in cardioplegic solutions, 26
 levels of, during cardiopulmonary bypass, 183–185
 loading with, prior to surgery, 22
 management of, 134–135
 utilization of, and growth hormone secretion, 183
 See also Hyperglycemia
Glutamate
 neurotoxic effects of, in brain, 124–125
 for reperfusion after ischemic insult, 27
Glycoproteins
 α-1-acid, drugs bound to, 60, 65
 platelet, 98–99
Gonadotropic hormones, secretion during cardiopulmonary bypass, 182

Gott shunt, 336
G proteins, 60
Graft-versus-host reaction, in blood transfusion, 462
Growth hormone (GH), protective function after trauma, 182–183
Growth hormone-releasing factor (GHRF), 183

Hageman factor, activation of, in cardiopulmonary bypass, 171
Half-life. See Elimination half-time
Halothane
  and atropine premedication in pediatric patients, 315
  comparison with sufentanil, in pediatric cardiac surgery, 314
  effect of
    on blood glucose levels, 185
    on catecholamine levels, 188–189
    on the myocardium, 64
  effect on, of hypothermia, 71
  metabolism of, in congenital heart disease, 73
  studies of cerebroprotective effects of, 138
Heart
  preparation for induced arrest, 22–24
  repair of intracardiac defects, historic evolution of hypothermia for, 42
  See also Cardiac entries; Myocardial function entries
Heart block, risk of, during separation from CPB, 323–324
Heart-lung machine, 3–5
Heart rate, before discontinuing CPB support, 281–282, 291–292
Heat exchange, in extracorporeal systems, 247–253
Heat exchangers
  in bubble oxygenation, 200, 239
  comparisons of commercially available units, 252
  design of, 251–253
  in membrane oxygenators, 209
  monitoring temperature at, 240–241
  performance evaluation, 250–251
Heat transfer
  modes of, 247
  from water to blood, 249–250
Hemangioblastoma
  cerebellar, outcomes of surgery for, 344
  medullary, outcomes of surgery for, 344
Hematocrit
  adjusting before separation from CPB, 323
  calculating blood needed to meet, in pediatric CPB, 314
  and oxygen consumption, 463
Hematoma, presentation of dissection as, 262
Hemoconcentration
  to conserve blood, 466–467
  device for, 239
Hemodialysis, oxygenation during, 199
Hemodilution, 8, 97
  and coagulation factors, 88
  coronary steal in, 22
  effect on plasma opioid concentrations, 67
  isovolemic, to conserve blood, 465
  in pediatric cardiopulmonary bypass, 313–314
  and postoperative lung function, 149–151
  from priming volume, 210
  theoretical effects of cardiopulmonary bypass on, 59–60
Hemodynamics
  criteria for ventricular assistance, 399t
  during liver transplantation, 390
  during percutaneous portable bypass, 383–384
  and stress response, 189–190
  in ventricular assistance, 410
Hemoglobin
  lowest safe level of, criterion in transfusion, 462
  as a nephrotoxin, 161
  oxygen-binding capacity of, and temperature, 26–27
Hemolysis
  and choice of tubing, 230
  overcoming
    in oxygenators, 14
    in roller pump design, 224

Hemophilias
  desmopressin acetate to improve hemostasis in, 106
  replacement therapy planning in, 103
Hemopump, 385
Hemorrhage, and ADH secretion stimulation, 180
Hemostasis, 88–107
  to conserve blood, 477–478
  management of, after intracranial surgery, 343
  during orthotopic liver transplantation, 392–393
  postoperative, with heparin-bonded extracorporeal circulation circuits, 231
Hemostatic cascades, activation of, on ECC surfaces, 97–100
Heparin, 3–4, 14, 89
  administration of
    prior to cannulation, 257–258
    protocol, 92, 275–276
  effect of
    on free digitoxin concentrations, 78
    on platelet function, 97
    on thyroid hormones, 192
  in intraaortic balloon pump counterpulsation, 424
  with long-term ventricular assistance, 403, 409
  plasma levels of, 91–94
  rebound reaction, 96–97
  resistance to, 92, 300–301
  sensitivity to, 92
  with short-term ventricular assistance, 409
  source of, and thrombocytopenia, 94
Heparinase, activated clotting time assays and, 96
Heparin bonding
  to extracorporeal circuit components, 231
  reducing complement activation with, 155, 175
  to surfaces for arterial line filters, 234
  to surfaces for intravascular oxygenators, hollow-fiber design, 451
Heparinoid, synthetic, alternative to heparin, 94
Hepatic blood flow
  arterial, with pulsatile perfusion, 410
  after cardiopulmonary bypass, 158
Hepatic clearance (Cl_i), intrinsic, 58
Hepatic elimination of drugs, 58
Hepatic extraction ratio, 58
  for papaverine, 79
  for propofol, 70
Hepatic occlusion test, for determining need for venovenous bypass, 390
Hepatitis
  nosocomial, among cardiac surgery patients, 88
  transmission of, in blood transfusion, 461
Hexadrimethrine, alternative to protamine, for heparin reversal, 96
Hirudin, 94
Hoffman degradation, of atracurium, 75
Hollow fibers
  gas-permeable, 11
  in membrane oxygenators, 207, 208–209, 312
  IVOX, 451
  extraluminal flow (ELF) design, 13
Holmes v Silver Cross Hospital, 475
Homeostasis
  acid-base, effect of barbiturates on, 136
  disruption of, in hypothermia, 25
Hormonal changes in cardiopulmonary bypass
  correlation with outcome, pediatric procedures, 314
  summary, 193
Host tissues, attack on, by neutrophil response to immune system activation, 155
Human immunodeficiency virus (HIV), transmission of, in blood transfusion, 461
Human lymphocyte antigen (HLA), plateletapheresis compatible with, 106
Human-machine interactions, 14–15
Human T-lymphocyte virus (HLTV), transmission of, in blood transfusion, 461
Hydrophilic compounds, conversion of lipophilic drugs to, in liver, 58
Hydrostatic pressure, capillary, and pulmonary edema, 150
Hyperamylasemia, 158–159

Hyperbaric oxygen, in management of air embolism, 305
Hypercarbia
  normal physiologic responses to, 450
  tachycardia caused by, 281–282
  See also Carbon dioxide
Hyperemia
  cerebral, and pH-stat management, 332
  and reperfusion, 50
Hyperglycemia
  and neurologic dysfunction after cardiac surgery, 134–135, 277–278, 320
  in normothermic bypass with glucose administration, 183, 485
Hyperkalemia
  and failure to wean from CPB, 292
  to induce cardiac arrest, 25
  in normothermic cardiopulmonary bypass, 485
Hyperosmolar, hyperglycemic, nonketotic coma (HHNC), in noninsulin-dependent diabetics, 185
Hyperoxia, and cerebral blood flow, 122
Hyperreflexia, after cardiac surgery, 115
Hypertension
  during bypass, 274–275
  pulmonary
    contraindication to pregnancy, 359
    and hemodynamic instability, 324
    and weaning from cardiopulmonary bypass, 282, 289
  systemic, and risk of neuropsychologic dysfunction after cardiac surgery, 127
  and weaning from cardiopulmonary bypass, 291
  See also Blood pressure
Hyperthermia
  avoiding during rewarming, 50
  effect on tolerance for ischemia, 133
Hypocalcemia, in reperfusion after ischemic insult, 27
Hypokalemia, management of, 276–277
Hypoperfusion
  accidental, incidence of, 300–301, 302
  managing, 305–306
  monitoring of, and neuropsychologic dysfunction, 117
  preventing, 303–304
  See also Perfusion
Hypoplastic left heart syndrome
  cannulation in, 318
  profound hypothermia for surgery, 46
Hypotension
  controlled, for blood conservation, 465
  after initiation of cardiopulmonary bypass, 22, 23, 274–275, 319
  as a reaction to protamine, 95
  and risk of neurologic dysfunction, 130–131
  on weaning from cardiopulmonary bypass, 288, 291
  See also Blood pressure
Hypotension index (TM), 130
Hypothalamic temperature, 270
Hypothermia
  for air embolism management, 305
  in congenital heart disease, 34
  damage from, 22, 46
  deep, 6–7
    circulatory arrest in, 120–121
  defined, 40
  development of, during liver transplantation, 393
  effect of
    on activated clotting time, 317–318
    on enflurane, 71
    on intracellular pH, 45
    on pancreatic function, 183
    on pharmacodynamics, 59
    on pharmacokinetics, 59, 67
    on propofol levels, 70
  and elimination half-time, 66–67
  with fibrillatory arrest, 28
  hemodilution in, to preserve blood flow, 463
  history of clinical use, 40–43
  history of development of clinical uses, 40–43
  in intracranial surgery, rationale for, 341

Index

and low-flow cardiopulmonary bypass, 48–49
and low-flow hypothermic perfusion, for circulatory arrest, 49–50
in pediatric cardiac surgery, 319–320
in pediatric cardiopulmonary bypass, 313–314
profound, effect on cerebral autoregulation, 120, 331
rate of cooling, and postoperative cerebral dysfunction, 331
rationale for use of, in cardiac surgery, 44–45
to reduce metabolic rate during cardiac arrest, 24–25
in surgery after failed angioplasty, 351
systemic, 44
  effects on receptor function, 63–64
  for repair of defects in the heart, 41
techniques for inducing, 46–50
in transplantation, 35
ventricular fibrillation with, 281
Hypoxemia, ECMO for treating, 450

Iloprost, to prevent platelet activation, 98
Imidazole-buffering radicals, 45
Immune system, 169–177
  effect on, of cardiopulmonary bypass, 14
  normal, 169–170
Immunity, innate, 170
Immunoglobulins, 170, 173
  G (IgG), anti-heparin action of, 93
Indications
  for intraaortic balloon pump placement, 416–417
  for intravascular oxygenator use, 453–454
  for ventricular assistance, 399
Infants
  deep hypothermic total circulatory arrest (DHTCA) in, 120–121
  deep to profound hypothermia induced in, 46–47
  profound hypothermia induced in, 43
  See also Pediatric patients
Infarction
  mesenteric, in intraaortic balloon pump counterpulsation, 428
  myocardial, produced by vasopressin, 180
Infection
  in intraaortic balloon pump counterpulsation, 427
  rates of, and duration of procedure, 76
  risk factors
    in blood transfusion, 461
    and prevention, 173–176
    reactions at a blood-gas interface, 214
  in ventricular assistance, 408–409
  See also Prophylaxis
Inflammatory system
  activation by contact with tubing, 230
  normal, 170
Infusion pressure, for crystalloid cardioplegia, 28–29
Inotropic drugs
  common, for cardiac surgery, 292–293
  effects of, during pregnancy, 368–371
  support with, before weaning from CPB, 285–286
  and weaning
    from cardiopulmonary bypass, 286–287
    from ventricular assistance, 408
  See also Drugs
In Regards to Brooks Estate, 474
In Regards to Osborne, 475
Inspired oxygen concentration, level required in ARDS, 152–153
Insulin, plasma levels of, during cardiopulmonary bypass, 183
Intensive care, duration of stay in, and risk of infection, 175
Interleukins, 172–173
  IL-1, generation of, in membrane oxygenation, 14
Internal mammary artery (IMA)
  bilateral graft, and infection risk, 174–175
  as a bypass conduit, 351
  bypass graft, and lung preparation for weaning, 283
  dissection of, and A-a O_2 gradient, 149

In the Matter of Melideo, 474–475
Intraaortic balloon pump (IABP), 347
  in acute myocardial ischemia, after coronary angioplasty, 349
  in angioplasty, 385–386
  in cardiac trauma management, 355
  counterpulsation using, 413–429
  safety precautions in use of, 303
  with short-term circulatory support, 410
  use in PTCA, 384
  for weaning from ventricular assistance, 408
Intracellular environment
  alkalinization of, in hypothermia, 51
  calcium levels, in ischemia, 125
Intracranial surgery, 340–345
Intraoperative predictors, of neuropsychologic dysfunction after cardiac surgery, 128–135
Intravascular oxygenator (IVOX), 14, 450–457
  design of, 451–453
Intravenous injection
  bolus, and concentration in plasma, 55–56
  continuous, and concentration in plasma, 57–58
Intrinsic complexity, defined, 298
Intrinsic hepatic clearance (Cl_i), 58
Inulin, clearance of, indicator of GFR, 160
Iron
  to increase hemoglobin levels, 477, 479
  release of lactoferrin, during cardiopulmonary bypass, 155
Ischemia
  acute, myocardial protection in, 33
  central nervous system, neurochemistry of, 123–126
  cerebral
    monitoring for, 270
    protective anesthetics, 135
    from clamping the descending thoracic aorta, 334–335
  cortical, detection with EEG monitoring, 270
  defined, 43
  detection of, with ECG monitoring, 266–267
  effects of, on intracellular pH, 43–44
  focal temporary, effects of thiopental in, 137
  myocardial, 21
    intraaortic balloon pump counterpulsation in, 413, 415
    prior to cardioplegic arrest, 26–27
    produced by vasopressin, 180
    symptoms of, 347
  pathophysiology of, 43–44
  peripheral, in intraaortic balloon pump counterpulsation, 426–427
  sensitivity of organs to damage from, 45
  subendocardial, and blood pressure, 22
  and tachycardia, 281–282
Ischemic heart disease (IHD), 114
Isoflurane, 70–71
  attenuation of stress response by, 190
  effect on, of hypothermia, 71
  studies of cerebroprotective effects of, 138
Isoproterenol, 292–293
  effect of
    on myocardial recovery, 23, 288–289
    during pregnancy, 366–367, 369
    for low pulse pressure, BP, 324
    for managing protamine reaction, 306

Jehovah's Witnesses, objection to blood transfusion, 473–483

Kallikrein
  activation of coagulation-related systems by, 99, 170, 171
  inhibition of, with aprotinin, 104–105
Kennedy Memorial Hospital v Heston, 475
Ketamine, intramuscular injection of, for pediatric patients, 315
Kidneys. *See* Renal *entries*
Kinetics
  of drug elimination, first-order, 56
Kinin-bradykinin system, 171
Kinins, levels of, in cardiopulmonary bypass, 60

Labetolol, effect of, during pregnancy, 371
Lactic acidosis, as an indication of inadequate flow, 320. *See also* Acid-base management
Lactoferrin, release of, during cardiopulmonary bypass, 155
Law, and blood transfusion, 473–476
Left ventricular assist device (LVAD), 385
Left ventricular function
  and ischemia, with hemodilution, 463
  and myocardial protection, 31–33
Leukaphereis, complement activation during, 153
Leukocyte depletion, during reperfusion after ischemic insult, 27
Leukocytes, filtering, and reduced free radical formation, 155
Lidocaine, 80–81
  binding of, to α-1-acid glycoprotein, 60, 65
  effect of, during pregnancy, 373
  hepatic extraction ratio of, 58
  for membrane stabilization, 24
  pharmacokinetics of, postoperative, 80–81
  for reducing protease release, 155
Lidoflazine, effect of, on tolerance of ischemia, 24
Line filter, for reducing embolic load, 131–132
Lipid-soluble drugs, 62
Lipophilic compounds, metabolism of, in liver, 58
Lipoprotein lipase, interaction with heparin, 65
Liver function
  after cardiopulmonary bypass, 158
  after cardiopulmonary bypass in pediatric patients, 321
  and postoperative bleeding, 103, 106
  See also Hepati- *entries*
Liver transplantation, closed chest bypass for, 389–394
Loop diuretics, 466
Loose coupling, systemic, 298
Lorazepam, levels of, and administration schedule, 68–69
Low-birth-weight infants, mortality and morbidity of, in ECMO, 438–440
Low-flow hypothermic perfusion, 48
Lungs
  drug reservoir function, 65, 80–81
  preparing for cardiopulmonary bypass weaning, 283
  See also Pulmonary *entries*
Luteinizing hormone (LH), in cardiopulmonary bypass, 182
Luxury perfusion, 135
Lymphocytes
  B, 173
  T, 170, 173

Macroembolization, cerebral, and injury, 123
Macrophages, innate immunity and, 172
Malignant arrhythmias, and failure to wean from CPB, 292
Management
  of air embolism, 305
  of angioplasty patients with acute myocardial ischemia, 347–348
  of cardiopulmonary bypass
    for aortic arch surgery, 331–334
    for descending artery surgery, 335–336
    for thoracic aortic surgery, 330
  of IABP during cardiopulmonary bypass, 420–425
  of pH, during cardiopulmonary bypass, 51–52
  prevention of inflammatory response, during reperfusion after ischemic insult, 27
  surgical, in acute myocardial ischemia after angioplasty, 350–351
  See also Alpha-stat pH management; pH-stat management
Mannitol
  as a free radical scavenger, in reperfusion, 27
  during intracranial surgery, 343
  in management of air embolism, 305
  moderation of renal insult by, 162–163, ++163, 313
  in priming solution, 238
Marfan's syndrome, contraindication to pregnancy, 359

Markers, of acute lung injury, 152
Materials
　for heat-exchange devices, 250
　for membranes, 9-10
Mean arterial blood pressure (MAP)
　criteria for ventricular assistance, 399
　and uterine blood flow, 367
Measurement, of drug concentration in plasma, 55
Mechanical failure
　frequency of, 300, 301-302
　managing, 305
　preventing, 303
Mechanical pumps, for extracorporeal circulation, 220-227
Mechanical ventilation, prolonged, and diaphragmatic dysfunction, 148-149
Median sternotomy, and infection, 174
Mediastinitis, occurrence and mortality rates, 169
α-Melanocyte-stimulating hormone (α-MSH), 172-173
Membrane
　blood-gas exchanger, 450
　gas-permeable, 206
　microporous, 11
Membrane attack complex, 153
Membrane lungs
　blood gas management of, 210
　technology of, 10-11
Membrane oxygenation, 8-10
　activation of leukocytes, platelets and complement in, 175
　complement formation in, 153-154
　equipment for, 13-14, 206-211
　　sizing, 303
　　sizing for pediatric cardiopulmonary bypass, 311-312
Meperidine, premedication with, pediatric patients, 315
Mephentermine, effect of, during pregnancy, 369-370
Metabolism
　anaerobic, in cardiac arrest, 26
　balanced reactions in, and temperature, 25, 30
　demands of, and weaning from CPB, 292
　myocardial, methods for decreasing, 24t
　oxygen consumption, heart, 25f
　reducing requirements for
　　during ischemic arrest, 24
　　during reperfusion, 27
　See also Cerebral metabolic rate for oxygen (CMRO$_2$); Oxygen/oxygenation
Metaraminol, effect of, during pregnancy, 370
Methohexital
　effect of hemodilution on plasma level, 60
　levels and clearance of, during cardiopulmonary bypass, 68
Methoxamine, effect of, during pregnancy, 370
Methylprednisolone
　effect of, on cortisol levels, 185
　in management of air embolism, 305
　to reduce complement activation, 155
Metocurine, pharmacokinetics of, in cardiopulmonary bypass, 75
Metoprolol, effect of, during pregnancy, 371
Microemboli, 117-118
　cerebral injury from, 122-123
　gaseous
　　in oxygenators, 214
　　in venous reservoirs, 208
Midazolam
　pharmacodynamics of, 62, 69
　premedication with, pediatric patients, 315
Milrinone, 293
　effect of, during pregnancy, 370
　during weaning from CPB, 288
Mitral valve disease
　commissurotomy during pregnancy, outcomes, 360
　myocardial protection in, 34
Monitoring
　in cardiopulmonary bypass, 264-272
　of the central nervous system, 117-118

of evoked cortical potential, 120-121
of an extracorporeal circuit, 240-244
fetal, during maternal surgery, 363
of heparin levels, 90
during intracranial surgery, 342
invasive, of pediatric patients, 316-317
noninvasive, of pediatric patients, 315-316
of pregnant patients, and of fetuses, 361-363
of temperature, sites for, 51
Morbidity
　effect of religious objections to transfusions, 476
　in intraaortic balloon pump counterpulsation, before transplantation, 417
　in intracranial surgery, 344
　in supported percutaneous transluminal coronary angioplasty, 383-384
Morphine
　effect of, on antidiuretic hormone release, 180
　versus sufentanil, postoperative use in cardiopulmonary bypass, 423
Mortality rate
　effect of religious objections to transfusions, 476
　fetal, after surgery for heart disease in pregnant patients, 360
　in infection associated with mechanical cardiac support, 408-409
　in intracranial surgery, 340, 344
　in patients with gastrointestinal complications, 158
　in patients with jaundice, 158
　in pregnancy, association with heart disease, 359
　in use of mammary arteries for coronary bypass, 478
　in use of ventricular assistance, 401-402
Multiple-roller pump, 225
Multisystem organ failure (MSOF), after cardiopulmonary bypass, 152-153
Myeloperoxidase, release by neutrophils, 155
Myocardial functioning
　arrest, induced, 7
　contractility
　　effect on, of hypothermia, 46
　　evaluating, with intraoperative echocardiography, 285-286
　　optimization of, 282
　in contusion, intraaortic balloon pump counterpulsation in, 417
　defibrillation, 7-8
　depression of, in inhalation induction of anesthesia, 315
　dysfunctional, and failure to wean from CPB, 290
　preventing distention, with active venting, 28
　probability of infarction, and ischemia, 351
　protection in acute ischemia, 33
　recovery of, assessment of ventricular assistance, 407-408
Myocarditis, viral, intraaortic balloon pump counterpulsation in, 416
Myocardium, 21-35
Myocytes, reducing damage to, 27t

Namfamostat mesilate, reducing protease release with, 155
Narcotics, for intracranial surgery, 342
National Registry of Elective Cardiopulmonary-Bypass-Supported Coronary Angioplasty, 379
　initial report of, 383-384
Natural killer cells, 173
Nerve stimulator, for monitoring neuromuscular blocking agents, 271-272
Neurochemistry, of central nervous system ischemia, 123-126
Neurologic complications
　dysfunction
　　after cardiac surgery, 114-115
　　after hypothermia, with pH-stat management, 52
　　warm-blood versus cold crystalloid cardioplegia, 489
　　and temperature, 44
Neuromuscular blockade, 73-75, 271-272

Neuromuscular injury, in intraaortic balloon pump counterpulsation, 427
Neuromuscular transmission, changes in, with hypothermia, 63
Neuropsychologic dysfunction, after cardiac surgery, 115-116
Neutrophils
　activation of
　　in innate immunity, 172
　　therapies to reduce, 157t
　aggregation of, role of complement in, 153
　uptake in the lung
　　after cardiopulmonary bypass, 155, 171
　　and duration of cardiopulmonary bypass, 153
Nicotine, effect of, on antidiuretic hormone release, 180
Nifedipine
　effect of
　　during pregnancy, 372
　　on tolerance of ischemia, 24
　for reducing protease release, 155
Nitric oxide (endothelium-derived relaxing factor)
　stimulation by interleukin-1, 172-173
　for weaning from cardiopulmonary bypass, 289
Nitrogen exchange
　in a bubble oxygenator, 203
　in a membrane oxygenator, 210
Nitroglycerin, 79-80, 293-294
　adsorption of, on equipment, 79-80
　effect of, during pregnancy, 371
　interaction with heparin, 90
　for weaning from cardiopulmonary bypass, 289
Nitroprusside, 79, 293
　for afterload reduction, during separation from CPB, 324
　effect of, during pregnancy, 371
　for vasodilation during rewarming, 323
　for weaning from cardiopulmonary bypass, 289
Nitrous oxide
　comparison with fentanyl supplementation, 314
　effect of, on blood glucose levels, 185
　for pediatric cardiac surgery, 315
　studies of cerebroprotective effects of, 138
Norepinephrine, 187, 292
　β-adrenergic action of, 286-288
　effect of, during pregnancy, 370
　for managing protamine reaction, 306
Normal sinus rhythm (NSR), for coming off bypass, 281
Normothermic cardiopulmonary bypass, 484-491
Normothermic perfusion, 321

Obstruction, venous, 263
Open reservoir, in a membrane oxygenator, 208
Opioids, 66-67
　for blocking stress response in children, 190
　effects on, of hypothermia, 66-67
　for pediatric patients, 315
　See also Drugs
Opsonization, acute phase reactants in, 170
Oral route, for drug administration, 58
Orthotopic liver transplantation (OLT), 389
Orthotopic total artificial hearts, as bridging devices, 403
Osmotic diuresis, with mannitol administration, 163
Osmotic pressure, of extracellular fluid, regulation by ADH, 180
Ototoxicity, of furosemide, 163
Overheating, of blood, and ischemic brain injury, 253
Oxygen analyzer, in an oxygen-air blender line, 303
Oxygenators
　accidents associated with, 300, 302
　backup, 303
　clotting in, 96
　DeWall-Lillehie, 9f
　disposable, 4-5
　for extracorporeal circulation, 199-215
　frequency of failure, 300
　for pediatric cardiopulmonary bypass, 311-313
　platelet activation in, 98

Index

Oxygen demand, myocardial, effect of β-adrenergic receptor blockade on, 64
Oxygen dissociation curve, factors affecting, 464
Oxygen-hemoglobin dissociation curve, in hypothermia, 51
Oxygen/oxygenation
  adequacy of
    for fetuses in maternal heart surgery, 363
    and patient outcome, 300–301, 302
    protecting, 303
  arterial, during bypass, 274
  of cardioplegic solutions, 26, 28
  cerebral consumption of, and flow rate, 322
  delivery of, augmentation, 450
  ECMO for treating hypoxemia, 450
  effect of, on blood glucose levels, 185
  inspired, concentration required in ARDS, 152–153
  jugular venous
    for monitoring cerebral effects of hypothermia, 48
    saturation, monitoring, 118
  managing, in myocardial ischemia after angioplasty, 348
  metabolic requirement, 43
  mixed venous level of, monitoring in profound hypothermia, 49
  myocardial demand
    in asystole, 484–491
    in counterpulsation, 414, 415
  rate of consumption, as a function of temperature, 44
  during reperfusion, 27
  solubility of, and temperature, 51
Oxygen saturation
  monitoring, 243–244
  and weaning from bypass, 284

Pacemaker, 8
Pacing
  atrial, 281
  to correct heart block at separation from CPB, 323–324
Pancreas
  damage to, and mortality, 158–159
  function of, during cardiopulmonary bypass, 183–185
Pancuronium
  to avert bradycardia, with fentanyl or sufentanil, 315
  effects of, and temperature, 63, 74
Papaverine, 79
Paraaminohippurate (PAH) extraction, indicator of renal plasma flow, 160
Parallel plate, membrane configuration, 207
Paraplegia
  following descending aorta repair, 355
  following intraaortic balloon pump counterpulsation, 428
Parasitic infections, transmission by blood transfusion, 461
Parathyroid, 191
Partial thromboplastin time (PTT), 90
Partition coefficients
  during cardiac surgery, of isoflurane, enflurane, and halothane, 72–73
  in vitro, of isoflurane, enflurane, and halothane, 72
Partitioning, and timing of pharmacological effects of drugs, 62
Pathophysiology, of immune system responses during cardiopulmonary bypass, 169–173
Patients
  preparing for CPB weaning, 283
  selection of
    for ECMO, 436–437
    for liver transplantation, 389
    for ventricular assistance, 408
Peak diastolic coronary blood flow velocity, with intraaortic balloon pump counterpulsation, 414–415

Pediatric patients
  cardiopulmonary bypass in, 311–325
  intraaortic balloon pump counterpulsation for, 417
  liver transplantation in, with venovenous bypass, 393
  serum digoxin concentrations, during bypass, 79
  See also Children; Infants
Pentobarbital, premedication with, pediatric patients, 315
Pentothal, sodium
  in management of air embolism, 305
  and plasma epinephrine levels, 189
Penumbra region, of the ischemic brain, 123
Percutaneous transluminal coronary angioplasty (PTCA), 347, 379
  supported, 379–387
Performance factor, in heat exchange, 250
Perfusion
  accident prevention during, 302–304
  coronary, maintaining in hypothermia with fibrillatory arrest, 28
  regional, 321
    and delivery of drugs to receptor sites, 62
  renal, during liver transplantation, 391
  techniques, for managing pregnant patients, 363–364
  tissue, and nonpulsatile cardiopulmonary bypass, 60
  See also Hypoperfusion; Reperfusion
Perfusion circuits
  in portable cardiopulmonary bypass units, 380, 382f
  safety devices for, 244–245
Perfusion hypothermia, 24
Perfusion pressure
  cerebral (CPP), during alpha-stat acid-base management, 119–120
  maintaining
    in hypothermia with fibrillatory arrest, 28
    prior to cardiopulmonary bypass, 22
  modification of, during cardiopulmonary bypass, 117
Pericardial insulating pad, to reduce phrenic nerve damage, 148–149
Periodontal disease, preoperative evaluation of, 174
Peripheral tissues, uptake of administered drugs, and hypothermia, 59
Peripheral vascular disease, and risk of intraaortic balloon pump counterpulsation, 425
Permeability, capillary, after cardiopulmonary bypass, 150–151
Peroneal nerve palsy and foot drop, 427
Persistent pulmonary hypertension of the newborn (PPHN), ECMO for, 435, 438
Personnel, for extracorporeal circulatory support, 386–387
pH
  arterial, to assess retrograde flow, 486
  correction of, for temperature of samples, 51
  effect of, on receptor-mediated events, 64
  gastric, after cardiopulmonary bypass, 158
  intracellular
    effects of hypothermia, 45
    effects of ischemia on, 43–44
  management of, during cardiopulmonary bypass, 51–52, 332
  and renal excretion of drugs, 59
  of water, as a function of temperature, 45, 51
  See also Acid-base management; Alpha-stat pH management; Buffer systems
Pharmacodynamics
  defined, 55
  effects on, of hypothermia, 63, 75
  of heparin, 89–90
Pharmacokinetics
  defined, 55
  effects on
    of hypothermia, 67
    of systemic hypothermia, 63
  of heparin, 89–90

  of lidocaine, 80–81
  of protamine, 94
  single-compartment model, for isoflurane, 73
  theoretical effects of cardiopulmonary bypass on, 59–60
  of thiopental, changes with age, 61
  three-compartment model, 56
  two-compartment model, 56
Pharmacology
  and cognitive function after cardiopulmonary bypass, 139
  of interventions to decrease blood loss, 466
  of preparation for cardiopulmonary bypass, 23–24
  of preparation for weaning from cardiopulmonary bypass, 285–286
  strategies for cerebral protection, 135–140
  See also Anesthetic agents; Drugs
Phase shift diastolic augmentation, 413
Phenobarbital, effect of, on drug metabolism, 58
Phentolamine
  effect of, on growth hormone release in surgery, 183
  for vasodilation during rewarming, 323
Phenylephrine
  effect of, during pregnancy, 371
  for managing protamine reaction, 306
Phenytoin, binding of, to albumin, 60
Phospholipids, changes in, in cerebral ischemia, 125–126
Phrenic nerve, damage to, 148–149
pH-stat management
  effects on cerebral autoregulation, 66, 120, 135
  and gas analysis, 273–274
  of hypothermic cardiopulmonary bypass perfusion, 51, 332
Physiology
  in anemia, 462–464
  cerebral, 118–122
  considerations in intraaortic balloon pump counterpulsation, 414–415
Pipecuronium, pharmacokinetics of, in cardiopulmonary bypass, 75
Pituitary gland function, 180–183
Placement, and risk of intraaortic balloon pump counterpulsation, 425, 428
Plasma
  drug concentration in, 55–58
  uptake of drugs from, 61–62
Plasma membranes, drug equilibration across, 62–63
Plasmapheresis, perioperative, 104, 468–469
Plasma proteins
  binding of drugs to, 65
  concentration of, changes due to hemodilution in CPB, 59
Plasma sequestration, to conserve blood, 468–469
Plasmin
  circulating, effect on platelet function, 103
  generation of, and fibrinolysis, 100–101
Plasticizers, in polyvinyl chloride tubing, 229
Platelet-activating factor (PAF), formation of, in cerebral ischemia, 125–126
Platelet count, predictive accuracy for postoperative bleeding, 102
Platelets
  activation of, during cardiopulmonary bypass, 154
  activation sequence, in contract with ECC surfaces, 97–99, 171
  depletion of, and oxygenator design, 213
  dysfunction of, as a cause of postoperative bleeding, 102
  effect on function, in hypothermia, 46
  interactions with heparin, 90
  loss of
    in intraaortic counterpulsation, 424
    and oxygenator design, 207–208
  storage conditions, and transmission of bacterial infections, 461
  transfusion of, to control postoperative bleeding, 106, 343

Polar compounds, conversion of lipophilic drugs to, in liver, 58
Polycystic disease, liver, contraindication to venovenous bypass in, 392
Polyester, for screen filters, 234
Polyethylene membrane, 199
Polygeline, reducing complement activation with, 155
Polymorphonuclear neutrophil leukocyte (PMN) function, impairment in oxygenators, 214
Polypropylene, membrane for oxygenators, 206
Polytetrafluroethylene, microfibrillar, 11
Polyvinyl chloride, medical grade tubing of, 229, 239
Pores, membrane, for gas transfer, 206
Positioning, of pregnant patients, 361
Positive end expiratory pressure (PEEP), 450
   in ARDS, 152–153
Positive pressure ventilation, 3–4
   introduction of, 21
Positron emission tomography (PET), for cerebral blood flow observation, 119
Postcardiotomy cardiogenic shock (PCCS), indication for ventricular assistance, 400
Postperfusion lung syndrome (pump lung), 151
Potassium
   level of, in crystalloid cardioplegia solutions, 28, 30–31
   management of hypokalemia, 276–277
   monitoring during bypass, 276–277
   See also Hyperkalemia; Hypokalemia
Prebypass filters, 235
Pregnancy, and cardiopulmonary bypass, 359–373
Preload
   of a centrifugal pump, 220
   elevated, risk to the myocardium from, 22
   and failure to wean from CPB, 291
Premedication
   for pediatric cardiopulmonary bypass patients, 315
   for pregnant surgery patients, 361
Pressure, in the blood path of a membrane oxygenator, 211
Pressure gradient, across cannula, 233
Prime volume
   in a bubble oxygenator, 206
   in a membrane oxygenator, 210
   minimizing, 200
   for pediatric cardiopulmonary bypass, 312
Priming solution, 239
   addition of opioid to, 67
   for ECMO, 434
Procainamide, effect of, during pregnancy, 373
Procaine, for membrane stabilization, 24
Procoagulants, release of, during cardiopulmonary bypass, 99–100
Prolactin, levels of, in cardiopulmonary bypass, 182
Proliferation complexity, 298
Prophylaxis
   antimicrobial, 175–176
      during IABP placement, 419
      during IABP support, 423
   of bleeding, pharmacologic, 104–106
   use of intraaortic balloon pump placement, 416
      in angioplasty, 417
Propofol, 70
   attenuation of stress response by, 190
   effect on, of blood glucose levels, 185
   and neurological outcome in ischemia, 138–139
   for postoperative cardiac surgery management, 423
Propranolol
   effect of, during pregnancy, 371
   plasma levels of, during cardiopulmonary bypass, 80
   in preparing for ischemic arrest, 23
Prostacyclin (PGI_2)
   analog of, for preventing thrombocytopenia, 94
   effect of, on postoperative neuropsychologic dysfunction, 131
   platelet protection by, 94
   to prevent platelet activation, 98

Prostaglandins
   E_1, 294
   to prevent platelet activation, 98
   reducing protease release, 155
   for vasodilation, in separation from CPB, 324
   release of, in cardiopulmonary bypass, 189–190
Protamine, 4, 275
   accidental administration of, managing, 306
   and complement activation, 172
   dosage of, 96
   neutralization of heparin by, 91–92, 94–97
   reaction to, 300, 302
      preventing, 304
      and pulmonary edema, 151
      techniques for managing, 306
   to reduce blood loss after surgery, 479
   during weaning from CPB, 285
Protection, myocardial, basic concepts, 21–27
Protein binding, of drugs, 60
   effect of pH on, 64
Prothrombin time, predictive accuracy for postoperative bleeding, 102
Pseudoaneurysms, 354f
Pulmonary artery balloon counterpulsation (PABC), 421
Pulmonary artery catheters
   to determine intraventricular pressures, 269
   for monitoring intracardiac pressures, 267
   in pediatric cardiac surgery, 316–317
Pulmonary artery pressure, increase in, 269
Pulmonary hypertension
   contraindication to pregnancy, 359
   and hemodynamic instability, 324
Pulmonary vasoconstriction, in response to protamine, 95
Pulsatile blood flow
   and organ perfusion, 158, 410
   with ventricular assistance, 410–411
Pulsatile perfusion
   after air embolism, 305
   in aortic arch surgery, cerebral protection from, 333
   and catecholamine levels, 189
   after DHTCA, 121–122
   effect of
      on cortisol levels, 185
      on pancreatic function, 183
   equipment design, 212
   with reciprocating pumps, 225–226
Pulse oximetry, for monitoring pediatric patients, 316–317
Pump artifact, electrocardiographic, 264
Pump flow, and risk of neuropsychologic dysfunction, 130
Pump-oxygenators, 3
Pump pack, connecting to the oxygenator, 239
Pumps. See Centrifugal pumps; Reciprocating pump; Roller pumps; Rotary pumps

Radiation, for heat transfer
   defined, 247
Reaction time, in a membrane oxygenator, 212
Reception function, effect on administered drugs, in hypothermia, 59
Receptor-mediated events, factors affecting, 63–64
Receptors
   β-adrenergic blocking agents, 80
   affinity of, and systemic hypothermia, 63
   density of, and temperature, 64
   interactions with drugs, 60–64
   role in platelet dysfunction during cardiopulmonary bypass, 98–99
   subtype transformation, in systemic hypothermia, 63–64
Reciprocating pump, 225–226
Recirculation line, in a membrane oxygenator, 209
Red blood cells
   concentration of, changes due to hemodilution in CPB, 59
   packed, for managing hypoperfusion, 306

Redistribution
   of heparin, 89–90
   of opioid analgesics, 62–63
Religion, and blood transfusion, objections to, 473–483
Renal blood flow, during cardiopulmonary bypass, 66, 160
Renal elimination of drugs, 58–59. See also Clearance
Renal extraction ratio, 59
Renal failure
   after cardiopulmonary bypass, in pediatric patients, 321
   hemodynamically mediated, 162–163
   preexisting, and postbypass renal failure, 163
   preventing, 163–164
Renal function
   during bypass, 160–163
   defining, 159–160
   effect on, of pulsatile perfusion, 410
   after intraaortic balloon pump counterpulsation, 428
Renal functional reserve, change in after cardiac surgery, 162
Renin, levels of, in cardiopulmonary bypass, 60, 187
Reoperation
   advantage of central venous catheters in, 316
   cannulation for, 261
   coronary artery, myocardial protection in, 33
   rate of, 101–102
Reperfusion
   assuring metabolic quiescence initially, 28
   with cold blood cardioplegia, 33
   injury during, 45
      protective anesthetics, 135–136
   after ischemic insult, 27
   with oxygenated crystalloid cardioplegia, 32
   during surgery, 46
   surgical, effect on regional ejection fraction, 27
Resistance, chest wall, after coronary revascularization, 148
Respiratory distress, neonatal, and development of ECMO, 435
Respiratory system
   biochemistry of, 3
   changes expected after cardiac surgery, 147–149
   effects on, of cardiac surgery, 147–157
   failure of, postoperative, 155–157
Response time, of a monitoring device, 240
Resuscitation
   in acute ischemia, warm blood technique for, 33
   preoperative, and pulmonary edema, 150–151
Retina, abnormalities of, after cardiac surgery, 115
Retrograde cerebral perfusion (RCP)
   in air embolism accidents, 305
   during aortic arch surgery, 332–333
Retrograde infusion, in coronary artery reoperations, 33
Retrograde perfusion
   after air embolism, 305
Revascularization, papaverine administration during, 79
Right heart failure, and hemodynamic instability, 324
Right ventricular dysfunction
   IABP in, 416
   pulmonary artery balloon counterpulsation in, 421
Risk factors
   for aortic atherosclerotic diseases, 257
   in blood transfusion, 461–462
   in intraaortic balloon pump counterpulsation, 425
   for jaundice after cardiopulmonary bypass, 158
   for neurologic dysfunction after cardiac surgery, 126–135
   for postoperative bleeding, 102–104
Roller pumps, 4, 5, 222–225
   in ventricular assist devices, 401
Rotary pumps, 222–225
Runaway pumphead, 301

Index

Safety
  devices for, in extracorporeal circuit equipment, 240–244
  in IABP placement after peripheral vascular operations, 418–419
  margin of, in energy expenditure, 21–22, 25–27
  of an oxygenator, 200
  of perfusion circuits, devices for ensuring, 244–245
  procedures for ensuring, 298–307
St. Thomas solution, 29t, 30
Scavenging systems, gas, in a membrane oxygenator, 211
Screen filters, 234
Scrolled envelope, membrane configuration, 207
Secondary flows, membrane oxygenators, 11–13
Sedation
  postoperative, and intraaortic counterpulsation, 422–423
  with propofol, 70
Sepsis, after cardiopulmonary bypass, 152–153
Serine protease, factor XII, activation of, 99
Serotonin, levels of
  assays to detect heparin-induced thrombocytopenia, 93
  in cardiopulmonary bypass, 60
Sevoflurane, studies of cerebroprotective effects of, 138
Shunts, residual, and failure to wean from CPB, 292
Silicone compounds
  copolymer fibers, 11
  for defoaming, in bubble oxygenation, 199
  in membrane lungs, carbon dioxide transfer across, 10
  rubber, for membrane in oxygenators, 206
Single-roller pump, 224
Skin preparation, before surgery, 174
Small capillary and arteriolar dilatations (SCADs), and mortality, in cardiac surgery, 123
Sodium-potassium pump, 43
  response to hypothermia, 25
  response to ischemia, 124–125
Sonography, Doppler, transcranial, 118
Spallation, of tubing, during cardiopulmonary bypass, 229
Spinal cord, protecting, during repair of the descending aorta, 355
Spinal route, for drug administration, 58
Spirochetes, transmission by blood transfusion, 461
Stabilizers, in polyvinyl chloride tubing, 229
Staphylococcus aureus, 176
Staphylococcus epidermidis, 176
Starling equation, 149–150
Stationary film oxygenator, 4
Stenosis
  aortic, 21
    protection of the heart in, 33–34
  aortic valvular infundibular, correcting in a pregnant patient, 360
  carotid, and cerebral autoregulation, 128
Stents, intraluminal, evaluation of, 349
Sternotomy, repeat, risk of postoperative bleeding in, 104
Steroids
  in management of air embolism, 305
  for managing protamine reaction, 306
  and risk of pancreatitis, 159
Stone heart, 23
  prevention of, 33
Streptokinase therapy, and need for fresh frozen plasma and platelets, 103
Stress
  and α-1-acid glycoprotein levels, 65
  response to, 189–191
    and glucose concentrations, 277–278
    in pediatric cardiopulmonary bypass, 314
  of surgery, and neuropsychologic dysfunction, 116–117
Stroke
  neurochemistry of, 123
  and risk of neurodysfunction after cardiac surgery, 127–128
Stroke index, effect on, of intraaortic balloon pump counterpulsation, 415
Stroke volume, 324
Stunned myocardium
  indication for ventricular assistance in, 401, 403
  resuscitation in warm-blood cardioplegia, 486
Subclavian artery, for placement of IABP, 419
Subcutaneous drug administration, 58
Sufentanil
  attenuation of stress response by, 190
  clearance of, in children, 67
  comparison of
    with fentanyl, pharmacodynamic variables, 62
    with halothane/morphine, for pediatric cardiac surgery, 314
    with morphine, postoperative, in cardiopulmonary bypass, 423
  dosages for pediatric patients, 315
  stable plasma levels during surgery, 66
Superior vena cava syndrome, 320
Superoxide, release of, during cardiopulmonary bypass, 155
Superoxide dismutase, during reperfusion after ischemic insult, 27
Supported percutaneous transluminal coronary angioplasty (S-PTCA), 379–387
Surface contact, complement activation by, 172
Surface cooling, 46
  for infants, 46–48
Surface hypothermia, 6–7
Surfactant
  and pulmonary dysfunction, 149
  silicone, for defoaming in bubble oxygenation, 199
Surgery
  duration of, with low-flow hypothermic perfusion, 49
  intracranial, 340–345
  thoracic artery, 329–336
  valve
    coronary sinus retrograde infusion during, 29
    myocardial protection in, 33–34
  valve replacements in pregnant patients, fetal mortality, 360
  See also Reoperation
Survival, effect on, of ECMO, 437
Systemic cooling
  to enhance myocardial cooling, 24
  in hypothermia with fibrillatory arrest, 28
  in oxygenated cold crystalloid cardioplegia, 28
Systemic heparinization, 231
Systemic hypertension, and risk of neuropsychologic dysfunction after cardiac surgery, 127
Systemic hypothermia, 44
  effects of, on receptor function, 63–64
  for repair of defects in the heart, 41
Systemic vascular resistance (SVR), 190, 282
  in nonpulsatile perfusion, 410
Systems analysis, of safety in cardiopulmonary bypass, 298–299

Tachycardia
  fetal, during maternal cardiopulmonary bypass, 363
  and weaning from cardiopulmonary bypass, 281–282, 323
Teflon, in membrane oxygenators, 11
Temperature
  afterdrop in, 253
  of blood
    and ischemic brain injury, 253
    monitoring, 240–241
  and blood gas analysis, 273–274
  and blood glucose values, 183–184
  effect of, on receptor-mediated events, 63
  gradients in, and rate of heating or cooling, 247
  hypothalamic, 270
  maternal, and fetal heart rate, 367f
  monitoring, 240–241, 270
  myocardial probes for monitoring, 241
  optimum
    for cold blood cardioplegia
    for pregnant surgical patients, 365–366
  and pH of water, 45, 51
  studies of cerebroprotective effects of, 138
  and tolerance for cerebral ischemia, 132–134
  and toleration of low hematocrit, 463
  See also Hyperthermia; Hypothermia
Tetralogy of Fallot, correction of, in a pregnant patient, 360
Tham buffer (tris(hydroxymethyl)aminomethane), 26
  for metabolic acidosis, 283
Thermal conductance, unit, 248
Thermal conductivity
  of material for heat-exchange devices, 250
  and rate of heat flow, 248
Thermal potential, of a fluid, 250
Thermistor
  for monitoring temperature, 240–241
  placement in the pulmonary artery, 317
Thermocouple, for monitoring temperature, 240–241
Thermodilution, to determine cardiac output, 269–270, 317
Thiopental
  binding of, to albumin, 60
  effect of hemodilution on plasma concentration of, 60
  free and total levels of, during cardiopulmonary bypass, 67–68
  hepatic extraction ratio of, 58
  for intracranial surgery, 343
  reduction of oxygen demand by, 136–138
Thoracic aortic surgery, 329–336
Thoracoabdominal aorta, 334–336
Thoracotomy, compliance after, 147–148
Thrombin, heparin-resistant activity of, 97
Thrombin time (TT), 90–91
Thrombocytopenia
  heparin-induced, 90, 92–94
  in intraaortic counterpulsation, 424
Thromboelastogram (TEG), 102
Thromboembolism
  during aortic arch surgery, preventing, 332
  in ventricular assistance, 409
  See also Emboli; Microemboli
Thrombolytic therapy, and risk of postoperative bleeding, 103
Thromboplastin, use in heparin assay, 92
Thrombosis, in intraaortic balloon pump counterpulsation, 426
Thromboxane, levels of, in cardiopulmonary bypass, 60
Thrombus formation, 88
  intracardiac, and risk of stroke, 129
Thyroid, 191–193
Thyroid stimulating hormone (TSH), levels during cardiac surgery, 191–192
Thyroprotein (TP$_3$), 175
Thyrotropin-releasing hormone (TRH), in hypothermic cardiopulmonary bypass, 192
Tight coupling, systemic, 298
Timing, in intraaortic counterpulsation, 422–423, 423f, 428
Tissue binding, of drugs, 61
Tissue-type plasminogen activator (TPA), 100–101
  recombinant, 103–104
Tocodynamometer, for monitoring during surgery, 362
Topical hypothermic technique, 24
Total artificial heart, 406–407
Totally implantable ventricular assist pump, 409f
Trachea, ruptured, repair of, 357f
Tranexamic acid, to reduce blood loss, 466
Tranquilizers, effect of, on antidiuretic hormone release, 180
Transcranial Doppler (TCD) sonography, 118
  to study microemboli from oxygenation, 214
Transcutaneous drug administration, 58

Transesophageal echocardiography (TEE)
  for evaluating myocardial dysfunction, 290
  for evaluating pathology, in pregnant patients, 362
  for monitoring balloon pump position in IABP, 418
  for monitoring coronary blood flow in IABP, 414–415
  for monitoring during intracranial surgery, 342
  for monitoring during weaning from CPB, 282
  for monitoring IABP, 424
  for monitoring trapped air, 303
Transfusion filters, 235
Transfusions
  autologous, 104
  blood, risks of, 461–462
  of blood products
    and risk of ARDS, 152
    and risk of infection, 174
  effect of venovenous bypass on need for in liver transplantation, 391
  after percutaneous portable bypass, 383, 384
  platelet, for postoperative bleeding, 106
  prophylactic, 104
  rapid, in liver transplantation, 393
  reaction to, 461–462
Transient ischemia attack (TIA), and perioperative stroke risk, 127–128
Transmembrane pressure gradient (TMP), ultrafiltration, 466–467
Transplantation
  cardiac, and intraaortic balloon pump counterpulsation, 416–417
  liver, closed chest bypass for, 389–394
  myocardial protection in, 34–35
  pancreatitis associated with, 159
  See also Bridge to transplantation (BTT)
Transposition of the great arteries, 49
Trauma
  to blood, in oxygenators, 200
  chest, 353–357
Trends
  in anticoagulation, for cardiopulmonary bypass, 94
  in blood-gas exchange equipment, 15
  in extracorporeal membrane oxygenation (ECMO) development, 442
  in heat exchange equipment, 253
  in intraaortic balloon pump counterpulsation, 429
  in ventricular assist devices, 409–410
Tromethamine (THAM). See Tham buffer
Truncus arteriosus, 49
Tubing, for extracorporeal circulation, 229–231, 313
d-Tubocurarine
  effects of, and temperature, 63
  levels of, in cardiopulmonary bypass, 73–74
Tubular necrosis, 163
Twin-roller pump, 224–225
Tygon, super, 229

Ultrafiltration, to conserve blood, 466–467
Ultrasonography, algorithm for management of the atherosclerotic ascending aorta, 130
Ultrasound, for measuring blood flow, 242–243
Uncertainty complexity, defined, 298
Uremia, and hemostasis, 103

Uterine blood flow (UBF)
  decrease in
    conditions affecting, 368t
    during contractions, 362
  determinants of, 367
  effect on, of epinephrine, 368
Uterine contractions, association with cardiac surgery, 362–363
Uterine vascular resistance (UVR), 367
Uterine venous pressure (UVP), 367

Valve defects, surgical repair of, 15–16
Valve insufficiency, and failure to wean from CPB, 291
Valve operations
  coronary sinus retrograde infusion during, 29, f
  myocardial protection in, 33–34
  replacement in pregnant patients, fetal mortality in, 360
Vancomycin, for antibiotic prophylaxis, 176
van't Hoff's law, 45
Vascular resistance, systemic, 190, 282
  in nonpulsatile perfusion, 410
Vasoconstriction
  effects of drugs
    for managing protamine reaction, 306
    during pregnancy, 368–371
  in response to ADH, 180
Vasodilation
  cerebral, effect on the autoregulatory plateau, 119
  and reperfusion, 50
Vasodilators, 79–81, 293–294
  desmopressin, 106
  effect of, during pregnancy, 371
  promotion or uniform rewarming with, 323
  and weaning from cardiopulmonary bypass, 289
Vasopressin. See Antidiuretic hormone (ADH)
Vasopressors, effect of, on uterine blood flow, 370f
Vena cava, injury to, 263
Venous blood, oxygenation of, 199
Venous cannulation, in pediatric patients, 318–319
Venous oxygen saturation, to assess perfusion, 320
Venous reservoirs, design of, 208
Venous return
  decrease in
    evaluating in pediatric surgery, 320
    and venous cannulation, 262
  failure of, in cardiopulmonary bypass, 273
Venovenous bypass, rationale for, in orthotopic liver transplantation, 389
Ventilation
  maintaining, during initiation of cardiopulmonary bypass, 272
  physiologic goals of, 450
  reestablishing, 323
Venting
  active
    in hypothermia with fibrillatory arrest, 28
    techniques for, 23f, 32
  from an arterial line filter, 234
  of a bubble oxygenator, 202
  left ventricular, 261
    after initiation of cardiopulmonary bypass, 32
  to manage elevated pulmonary arterial pressure, 269
  to manage ventricular distention, 22–23
  passive, techniques for, 23f, 32
Ventricle pumps, 225–226

Ventricular arrhythmias
  intraaortic balloon pump counterpulsation use in, 417
  treating, 281
Ventricular assistance
  long-term, use of pulsatile devices for, 410–411
  for postcardiotomy cardiogenic shock, 225–226
  principles of, 399
Ventricular assist devices (VADs), 399–411
  long-term, 403–407
    for postcardiotomy cardiogenic shock, effectiveness of, 400
  short-term, 401–403
Ventricular distention, on initiation of cardiopulmonary bypass, 22–23
Ventricular dysfunction, management of, 286
Ventricular fibrillation, 7–8
  risk of subendocardial ischemia associated with, 22
Ventricular pacing, 281
Ventricular septal defects
  repair of, during pregnancy, 360
  repair of rupture, 356f
Verapamil, effect of
  during pregnancy, 372
  on tolerance of ischemia, 24
Visceral injury, in intraaortic balloon pump counterpulsation, 428
Viscoelastic monitoring, 102
Visual field defects, after cardiac surgery, 115
Vitamin K, and post-operative bleeding, 106
Volatile anesthetics, studies of cerebroprotective effects of, 138
Volume of distribution (V_d)
  and dilution, 65
  of a drug, 56–57
  effect on, of heart failure, 67
  of lidocaine, in cardiopulmonary bypass, 80–81
  of tubocurarine, in cardiopulmonary bypass, 74
Volume replacement, in plasmapheresis, 469
von Willebrand disease, desmopressin acetate to improve hemostasis in, 106
von Willebrand factor (vWF), 99–100, 106
von Willebrand receptors, 98–99

Warfarin
  displacement of, by phenylbutazone, 65
  in long-term ventricular assistance, 403, 409
Water, pH of, as a function of temperature, 51
Water vapor, transfer of, in a membrane oxygenator, 210
Waveforms, in intraaortic counterpulsation, 422, 422f
Weaning from cardiopulmonary bypass
  failure of, 289–292
    as an indication for IABP placement, 416
    due to postcardiotomy right ventricular dysfunction, 421
  inotropic drug support for, 351
  strategies with decreased myocardial contractility, 287f
Weaning from intraaortic balloon pump counterpulsation, 428–429
Whole blood clotting time (WBCT), 90
  effect on, of protamine, 95

Xanthine oxidase, in acidosis, 64
Xanthine oxidase inhibitors, for reperfusion after ischemic insult, 27

ISBN 0-387-94242-4